Damage-Associated Molecular Patterns in Human Diseases

Walter Gottlieb Land

Damage-Associated Molecular Patterns in Human Diseases

Volume 2: Danger Signals as Diagnostics, Prognostics, and Therapeutic Targets

Springer

Walter Gottlieb Land
Laboratoire d'ImmunoRhumatologie Moléculaire
LabEx TRANSPLANTEX
Université de Strasbourg
Strasbourg
France

German Academy for Transplantation Medicine
Munich
Germany

ISBN 978-3-030-53867-5 ISBN 978-3-030-53868-2 (eBook)
https://doi.org/10.1007/978-3-030-53868-2

This Springer imprint is published by the registered company Springer Nature Switzerland AG
The registered company address is: Gewerbestrasse 11, 6330 Cham, Switzerland

Foreword

The Munich SOD Trial: A Few Anecdotes

When searching for the scientific origin and foundation of this book on *Damage-Associated Molecular Patterns in Human Diseases*, one inevitably comes across a clinical study that we conducted in the late 1980s/early 1990s on kidney transplant patients and published in 1994: The Munich superoxide dismutase (SOD) trial [1]. I remember several anecdotal but remarkable stories around this trial that has led to the development of the *Injury Hypothesis* in Immunology [2–5]. Of interest, for example, is the launching phase of the clinical trial that started in 1986. The first step in initiating this trial came from me, who, at that time, was the Chairman of the Department of Experimental Surgery at the University of Heidelberg, Germany. In the late 1960s and early 1970s, I worked with Walter Land at the Institute of Surgical Research in Munich under Professor Walter Brendel, and we knew each other very well. In Heidelberg, one of the main topics of research was microcirculatory changes in ischemia/reperfusion injury in hamsters and hairless mice.

Together with Karl Arfors, Pharmacia International Experimental Medicine, of Uppsala, Sweden; Leopold Flohe and Hans Barth from Grünenthal, Aachen, Germany; and Gianfranco Rutili, Pharmacia, Uppsala, I visited Walter in his office at the Division of Transplantation Surgery, Klinikum Großhadern, University of Munich. The purpose of this visit was to discuss a clinical trial in kidney transplant patients, in which a new compound, the free radical scavenger recombinant (rh)-SOD, a powerful antioxidant, should be tested. The aim of the planned trial was to treat the renal allograft reperfusion injury with rh-SOD, intra-arterially administered to the donor organ during surgery shortly before the start of reperfusion (later on, we switched to the intravenous application via central venous catheter). The aim of the study (the primary endpoint) was improvement of early renal allograft function as a consequence of impairment/minimization of the oxidative ischemia/reperfusion injury to the allograft.

At a roundtable with experts in Walter Land's office in the Klinikum Grosshadern, after a relatively brief discussion, there was soon agreed on the initiation and performance of such a single-center, prospective, randomized, double-blind and placebo-controlled clinical trial in kidney transplant patients receiving ciclosporin-based immunosuppressive therapy. Notably, the background of the planned study had nothing to do with organ transplantation. Instead, the reperfusion of the renal allograft should be used as a model for successful resuscitation after cardiac arrest. A potentially significant improvement by rh-SOD of early renal allograft function via successful treatment of the reperfusion injury was planned as a surrogate marker for improved function of vital organs, such as the heart and lung, after successful resuscitation with an rh-SOD–containing resuscitation solution. In fact, the use of rh-SOD as a compound to be added to such solutions was the real marketing interest of the participating pharmaceutical companies.

After all the necessary preparatory steps were carefully done, the clinical trial was started by Land and his coworkers at the Transplant Division of the Klinikum Grosshadern (ward H5) in 1987. Unfortunately, the results of the clinical trial turned out to be not what we had hoped for. The primary endpoint of the study, early renal allograft function, proved not to be statistically significantly improved at the end of the trial. In fact, in view of this disappointing study outcome, there was a deep depression in all of the colleagues involved in the trial. The real bitter consequence, however, was that the participating pharmaceutical industry declined to continue such trials, for example, with the use of other dosages of rh-SOD.

Fortunately, however, this was not the end of the SOD trial, and its course finally converted to a happy end, and this is the story: At the 1990 Congress of The Transplantation Society held in San Francisco, Walter Land was invited to deliver a lecture on long-term results in kidney transplantation. For this reason, his coworkers looked at all the long-term data so far collected in the database, including the data obtained from those patients who were previously enrolled in the SOD trial. To our surprise, it was found that SOD-treated patients experienced fewer acute rejection episodes and better long-term survival. Over the next years, a careful and detailed retrospective analysis of the trial data confirmed these preliminary observations, which led to the first publication mentioned above. Today, we know that the reduction in incidences of reperfusion-induced rejection episodes was due to an inhibition/suppression by the free radical scavenger of reperfusion injury-induced DAMPs.

Of course, in those days, we wanted to restart similar clinical trials with rh-SOD in further patients, and, consequently, we planned a multicenter trial. However, to our great disappointment, the pharmaceutical industry that participated in the Munich SOD trial lost any marketing interest. Unfortunately, this kind of reluctance to produce and develop an antioxidative agent for clinical use in transplant patients has not changed inexplicably until today, although we had approached several other companies with this project. Obviously, the time-limited use of an antioxidant during surgery—in comparison with the long-term use of immunosuppressive drugs currently applied to transplant patients—did not evoke any marketing interests.

This policy is all the more a disaster because, today, it is now clear that not only ischemia/reperfusion injury but any injury, including bacteria/virus-induced injury, leads to the emission of DAMPs, which, in all these cases, induce a cytokine storm, which is associated with solid organ inflammation and/or a systemic hyperinflammatory syndrome. Indeed, a scientifically documented, in multicenter trials proven, inhibiting effect of SOD on a reperfusion injury-induced hyperinflammatory process–today known to be triggered by DAMPs-would have been a convincing stimulus to develop, in analogy to antioxidatively acting SOD, other compounds, this time aimed at suppressing bacterial/viral injury-induced DAMPs, which promote infection-caused hyperinflammation, clinically manifest as sepsis and multiple organ failure. At present, in the time of the Covid-19 pandemic, the availability of such novel drugs could have successfully contributed to a reduction of the case fatality rate. In fact, this is the reason that I am still not tired of demanding a public-private partnership model to foster the discovery and development of DAMP-inhibiting drugs.

Konrad Meßmer
Prof. em. Dr. med., Dr. h.c. mult.,
Former Chairman of Institute for
Surgical Research
Ludwig Maximilian University
Munich/Germany

References

1. Land W, Schneeberger H, Schleibner S, Illner WD, Abendroth D, Rutili G, et al. The beneficial effect of human recombinant superoxide dismutase on acute and chronic rejection events in recipients of cadaveric renal transplants. Transplantation. 1994;57:211–7. http://www.ncbi.nlm.nih.gov/pubmed/8310510.
2. Land W, Messmer K. The impact of ischemia/reperfusion injury on specific and non-specific, early and late chronic events after organ transplantation. Early events. Transplant Rev. 1996;10:108–27. http://linkinghub.elsevier.com/retrieve/pii/S0955470X96800164.
3. Land W, Messmer K. The impact of reperfusion injury on specific and non-specific, early and late chronic events after organ transplantation. Late chronic events. Transplant Rev. 1996;10:236–53. https://www.sciencedirect.com/science/article/abs/pii/S0955470X
4. Land W, Messmer K. The danger theory in view of the injury hypothesis: 20 years later. Front Immunol. 2012;3:349. http://www.ncbi.nlm.nih.gov/pubmed/23189080.
5. Land WG, Messmer K. The innate immune system: its rediscovery before toll was described. In: Hartmann G, Wagner H, editors. Innate immunity: resistance and disease-promoting principles. Else Kröner-Fresenius symposium, Basel, Karger, 2013, Vol. 4. pp. 24–8. https://doi.org/10.1159/000346531

Preface

This book is the continuation of the monograph on *DAMPs in Human Diseases*, whose Volume 1 has already been published in Springer International Publishing AG, part of Springer Nature, in 2018. Volume 2 of the book, which you now have in your hands, is again written for professionals from all medical and paramedical disciplines who are interested in the emerging and ambitious biomedical field of cell stress/tissue injury-induced inflammation and immunity in human diseases. Hence, again, it goes without saying that the book has not been written for experts in the field of innate immunity and related disciplines.

With reference to the title of the book, Volume 2 covers the practical and clinical aspects of DAMP-promoted human diseases. However, given the enormous increase in the number of incoming publications on DAMPs in human diseases that exceeded the allotted scope of the book, and contrary to the announcement made in Volume 1, the description of diseases had to be restricted to those disorders which are pathogenetically dominated by DAMPs, that is, polytrauma, solid organ injury, atherosclerosis, and cerebro-cardiovascular diseases; reserving other diseases such as metabolic, neurodegenerative, autoimmune, hematological, infectious, and malignant disorders for further publication.

The book is designed didactically and themes related in four parts, which cover 12 chapters altogether. Part I, Prologue, is devoted to some perspectives of the danger/injury model in Immunology as they have emerged today, for example, a modern holistic view of the universal defense system.

In Part II, some topics presented in Volume 1 of the book and of primary interest for clinicians are selectively updated, in particular, the SAMP-promoted resolution of inflammation and the DAMP-driven self-perpetuating process of fibrosis. Notably, these two topics are described with emphasis on epigenetic modifications because emerging evidence suggests DAMPs to drive these modifications. Indeed, science is moving fast, and so is the number of scientific publications! This also applies to research related to the danger/injury model in Immunology, including research on DAMPs and their cognate pattern recognition molecules. As a matter of fact, since submission of the manuscript to Vol. 1 of the book in January 2018, ~450 references on or related to DAMPs have been recorded in PubMed (deadline: October 2019). With the request of all authors' indulgence, they are not all reviewed here. Instead, only some of those topics described in Vol. 1 are briefly updated here that appear most relevant from the perspective of the book.

In Part III, the role of DAMPs and SAMPs in the selected human diseases is comprehensively outlined. Emphasis will be put on the role of DAMPs and SAMPs in the pathogenesis of human diseases, their use as biomarkers in diagnosis and prognosis, as well as their exploitation as targets for future therapeutic strategies. Since the publication of clinical data in these fields has just started, data from appropriate animal (rodent) studies are very often presented instead, to stress their future importance for the clinic. When it comes to clinical trials, they are usually specially marked.

Finally, Part IV, Epilogue, presents some insinuations on the future role of the "DAMPome" in the pathogenesis and treatment of human diseases.

Of note, all figures presented in this book are consciously oversimplified to spare the reader the burden of spending too much time with deciphering all the molecules and pathways involved.

My sources in writing this book mainly stem from the daily exploration of the MEDLINE database, especially PubMed (until October 2019). If not available online as a full-text article, I used the reprints requested by e-mail and sent by the corresponding authors in a thankful way. I want to use this opportunity to thank all these colleagues for their generosity.

Certainly, as already stressed in Volume 1, this book reflects just the beginning of a new era in medical/clinical practice that is rapidly growing. In particular, the phenomenon of regulated cell death has taken center stage as a crucial source of DAMPs emission. In fact, the intersection between cell death and the immune system is currently regarded as one of the hottest topics in modern biomedical research; it is this scenario that is central to homeostatic healing responses, critical human pathologies, and the development of novel therapeutics. Also, it can be noticed that researchers in the field of DAMPs are still trying to re-classify the DAMPs according to their personal viewpoints, knowledge, and area of interest, a policy that results in many different proposals of a proper DAMPs classification.

Accordingly, many topics here covered have to be re-written, modified, and amended in the near future. A veritable flood of new publications from this emerging research field awaits us.

Finally, having researched and written the book entirely on my own, I cannot blame others for its imperfections. Any errors or omissions have been made in good faith, and I plead for the reader's indulgence.

Prof. Conv. Univ. Strasbourg; Prof. em. Dr. med.
Walter Gottlieb Land

Acknowledgments

First and foremost, my dedication and heartfelt thanks go to my loving and supportive wife, Veronika, who provided me again with unending inspiration throughout the process of writing this book.

This publishing endeavor would certainly not have been possible without the moral and financial support of the German Academy for Transplantation Medicine, represented by the Council Members Prof. Dr. mult. Nikolaus Knoepffler (President), Prof. Dr. med. Bernhard Banas (Vice President), Priv.-Doz. Dr. med. Helmut Arbogast (Secretary-General and Treasurer), and Prof. Dr. med. Dietmar Abendrot (Historian). Furthermore, I am especially indebted to the distinguished members of the University of Strasbourg, Professor Seiamak Bahram, and Professor Jean Sibilia (Dean of the Medical Faculty) who supported my project and managed to hold my position as a Professeur Conventionné at the University of Strasbourg, France.

The completion of this project could not have been accomplished without the continuous support from some of my friends, to whom I am grateful for various reasons related to the project: Mr. Hildebrecht Braun, Dr. Peter Schmidt, Wolfgang Linss, and Hertha Jene.

Finally, I would also like to extend my thanks and appreciation to the whole Springer Nature staff, who edited my original prose and produced a high-quality product.

Contents

Abbreviations

4-HNE	4-hydroxynonenal
5-hmC	5-hydroxymethylcytosine
5mC	5-methylcytosine
8-OH-dG	8-hydroxy-2′-deoxyguanosine
A1AR	A1 adenosine receptors
A2AAR	A2A adenosine receptor
A3AR	A3 adenosine receptor
AA	Arachidonic acid
ABC	ATP-binding cassette
Abi-1	Abl interactor-1
Ac	Acetyl group
ACD	Accidental cell death
ACE	Angiotensin-converting enzyme
ACLF	Acute-on-chronic liver failure
ACS	Acute coronary syndrome
ADAMs	(short for: a disintegrin and metalloproteinase)
ADAMTS	ADAMs with a thrombospondin motif
aDMA	Asymmetric dimethylarginine
AGEs	Advanced glycation end products
AGO	Argonaute
AIDS	Acquired immune deficiency syndrome
AIM2	Absent in melanoma 2
AKI	Acute kidney injury
ALD	Alcoholic liver disease
ALF	Acute liver failure
ALI	Acute lung injury
ALRs	Absent in melanoma 2 (AIM2)-like receptors
alum	Aluminum hydroxide
ALX	Lipoxin A4
ALX/FPR2	Lipoxin receptor/*N*-formyl peptide receptor-2
AMPA	α-Amino-3-hydroxy-5-methyl-4-isoxazolepropionic acid
Ang I	Angiotensin I
Ang II	Angiotensin II

AnxA1	Annexin A1
AP-1	Activator protein-1
APAP	Acetaminophen
APCs	Antigen-presenting cells
ApoB	Apolipoprotein B
ApoE	Apolipoprotein E
ARDS	Acute respiratory distress syndrome
ARE	Antioxidant response element
ARF	Acute renal failure
ARs	Adrenergic receptors
ASC	Apoptosis-associated speck-like protein containing a caspase recruitment domain
ASH1	Absent, small, or homeotic disc 1
AT_1R	Angiotensin II AT1 receptor
ATF6α	Activating transcription factor 6 alpha
ATFs	Activating transcription factors
ATG	Autophagy-related
ATM	Ataxia telangiectasia mutated
ATR	Ataxia telangiectasia and Rad3 related
BBB	Blood–brain barrier
BCR	B cell receptor
BH4	Tetrahydrobiopterin
BIM	Bcl-2 interacting mediator of cell death
BiP	Binding immunoglobulin protein
BLT1	A leukotriene B4 receptor
BMPs	Bone morphogenic proteins
Bregs	Regulatory B cells
Bromo	Bromodomains
C3a, C5a	Complement fragments 3a and 5a
CAD	Coronary artery disease
CALR	Calreticulin
CaMKII	Ca^{2+}/calmodulin-dependent protein kinase II
cAMP	Cyclic adenosine monophosphate
CANTOS	Canakinumab Anti-inflammatory Thrombosis Outcomes Study
CARD	Caspase-activating and recruiting domain (also abbreviated as NLRC)
CARM1	Coactivator-associated arginine methyltransferase 1
CARS	Compensatory anti-inflammatory response syndrome
CAT	Category
CCAAT	Cytidine-cytidine-adenosine-adenosine-thymidine

CCLs	Chemokine (C-C motif) ligands
CCR4-NOT	Carbon catabolite repressor 4-negative on TATA
CCRs	CC-chemokine receptors
CD (e.g., CD40)	Cluster of differentiation (e.g., cluster of differentiation 40)
cDCs	Conventional dendritic cells
CE	Cerebral edema
CEP	Carboxyethyl pyrrole
CFH	Complement factor H
cGAMB	Cyclic GMP-AMP
cGAS	Cyclic GMP-AMP synthase
CHD	Coronary heart disease
ChemR23	Chemerin receptor 23 or chemoattractant receptor 23
ChOOHs	Hydroperoxide species
CHOP	Cytidine-cytidine-adenosine-adenosine-thymidine (CCAAT)—enhancer-binding homologous protein
Chpt	Chapter
Chromo	Chromodomains
CIITA	MHC class II transcription activator (transactivator)
cirRNA	Circular RNAs
CKD	Chronic kidney disease
CK-MB	Creatine kinase-muscle/brain
CL	Cardiolipin
CLRs	C-type lectin-like receptors
Clu	Clusterin
CMKLR1	Chemokine-like receptor 1
CMV	Cytomegalovirus
CNS	Central nervous system
COLIA2	Collagen, type I, α2
COLI–III	Collagen, type I–III
COPD	Chronic obstructive pulmonary disease
COX	Cyclooxygenases
CpG	Cytosine phospho-bound guanosine
CREB	cAMP response element-binding protein
CRP	C-reactive protein
CRS	Cytoreductive surgery
CSF	Cerebrospinal fluid
CT	Computed tomography
CTLA-4	Cytotoxic T lymphocyte-associated antigen-4
CTLD	C-type lectin-like domain
CTLs	$CD8^+$ cytotoxic T lymphocytes (= T cells)

CVD	Cardiovascular diseases
CXCLs	Chemokine (C-X-C motif) ligands
CYP2E1	Cytochrome P450 2E1
Cys2	Cystine
Cyt C	Cytochrome C
DAG	Diacylglycerol
DAI	DNA-dependent activator of IFN regulatory factors
DAMPs	Damage/danger-associated molecular patterns
DAPs	DNAX-activating proteins
DCP2	Decapping protein 2
DCs	Dendritic cells
DC-SIGN	Dendritic cell-specific intercellular adhesion molecule-3-grabbing non-integrin
DD	Death domain
DDR	DNA damage response
DED	Death effector domain
DGCR8	DiGeorge Syndrome Critical Region 8
DHA	Docosahexaenoic acid
DIC	Disseminated intravascular coagulation
DNA-PK	DNA-dependent protein kinase
DNGR-1	Dendritic cell natural killer lectin group receptor-1
DNMTs	DNA methylation is enhanced by DNA methyltransferases
DPA	*n*-3DPA, docosapentaenoic acid
DR5	Death receptor 5
Drosha	Ribonuclease III enzyme
DRV1/2	Resolving (RV) D1/D2 receptor 1/2
DSBs	Double-strand DNA breaks
dsRNA	Double-stranded ribonucleic acid
DUBs	Ubiquitin ligases/deubiquitinating enzymes
DUOX1	Dual oxidase 1
eATP	Extracellular ATP
ECM	Extracellular matrix
ECs	Endothelial cells
EDA	Extra domain A
eIF2α	Eukaryotic translation initiation factor 2 alpha
ELISA	Enzyme-linked immunosorbent assay
EMT	Epithelial-to-mesenchymal transition
eNOS	Endothelial nitric oxide synthase
EPA	Eicosapentaenoic acid
EpCs	Epithelial cells
Epi	Epinephrine
ER	Endoplasmic reticulum

ERK	Extracellular signal-regulated protein kinase
ERV/ChemR23	E-resolvin receptor (ERV)/chemoattractant receptor 23
ESCRT	Endosomal sorting complexes required for transport
ESG	Endothelial surface glycocalyx
ET-1,2,3	Endothelin-1,2,3
ET_A/ET_B	Endothelin receptors
ETC	Electron transport chain
EVs	Extracellular vesicles
EWAS	Epigenome-wide association studies
FACs	Focal adhesion complexes
FAD	Flavin adenine dinucleotide
FAK	Focal adhesion kinase
Fc	Fragment crystallizable (region)
FcRs	Fragment crystallizable receptors
fHA	Fragment of hyaluronan
FI–XIII	Factor I–XIII (coagulation, clotting factors)
fMet	*N*-formylmethionine
FNIII EDA	Extra domain A type III repeat of fibronectin
FNIII EDA/FNIII EDB	Alternatively spliced type III repeats extra domains A and B
Foxp3	Forkhead box protein 3
FP	Formyl peptides
FPRs	Formyl peptide receptors
FTL	Ferritin L
FZDs	Frizzled receptors
G proteins	Guanine nucleotide-binding proteins
GAGs	Glycosaminoglycans
GALs	Galectins
GAPs	GTPases-activating proteins
GARP	Glycoprotein-A repetitions predominant protein
GATA1/2/3	GATA-binding protein 1/2/3
GBD	Global burden of diseases, injuries, and risk factors study
GCL	Glutamate-cysteine ligase
GDP	Guanosine diphosphate
GEFs	Guanine nucleotide exchange factors
GLACIER	Goal of oxidized LDL and activated macrophage inhibition by exposure to a recombinant antibody
Glu	Glutamate
GPCRs (or GPRs)	G protein-coupled receptors
GPI	Glycosylphosphatidylinositol

GPXs	Glutathione peroxidases
GR	Glutathione reductase
GSDMD	Gasdermin D
GSH	Glutathione
GSKs	Glycogen synthase kinases
GSSG	Oxidized form of glutathione
GTP	Guanosine-5′-diphosphate
GWAS	Genome-wide association studies
H_2O_2	Hydrogen peroxide
HA	Hyaluronan
HATs	Histone acetylases
HCL	Hydrochloric acid
HCV	Hepatitis C virus
HDACs	Histone deacetylases
HDL	High-density lipoprotein
HDMBr	Hexadimethrine bromide
HDMs	Histone demethylases
HIF1α	Hypoxia-inducible factor 1-alpha
HIN	Hematopoietic interferon-inducible nuclear protein
HIPEC	Hyperthermic intraperitoneal chemotherapy
HIV	Human immunodeficiency virus
HLA	Human leukocyte antigen
HMGB1	High mobility group box 1 protein
HMTs	Histone methyltransferases
HMW	High-molecular-weight
hnRNPL	Heterogeneous nuclear ribonucleoprotein L
HO-1	Heme oxygenase-1
HOTTIP	HOXA distal transcript antisense RNA
HPA	Hypothalamic-pituitary-adrenocortical
HS/R	Hemorrhagic shock/resuscitation
HSCs	Hepatic stellate cells
HSFs	Heat shock transcription factors
HSPs	Heat shock proteins
HSR	Heat shock response
IAV	Influenza A virus
ICAM	Intercellular adhesion molecule
ICD	Immunogenic cell death
ICH	Intracerebral hemorrhage
ICU	Intensive care unit
iDCs	Immature dendritic cells
IFI16	Interferon-inducible protein 16
IFNs	Interferons
IFs	Intermediate filaments
Ig	Immunoglobulin

IHD	Ischemic heart disease
IKK	IκB kinase
IL(s)	Interleukin(s)
IL-1→x	Interleukin-1→x
IL1R1	IL-1 type I receptor
ILCs	Innate lymphoid cells
ILK	Integrin-linked kinase
iNOS	Inducible nitric oxide synthase
IRAK	Interleukin-1-receptor-associated kinase
IRE-1α	Inositol-requiring enzyme 1alpha
IRF	Interferon regulatory factor
IRI	Ischemia/reperfusion injury (also postischemic reperfusion injury)
ISS	Injury Severity Score
ITIM	Immunoreceptor tyrosine-based inhibition motif
iTregs	Inducible Foxp3^{+} regulatory T cells
JAK	Janus kinase
JHDM2A	jmjC domain-containing histone demethylation protein 2A
JmjC	Jumonji C
JMJD1A	Jumonji domain-containing protein 1A
JNK	c-Jun-N-terminal protein kinase
K	Histone lysine
KASH	Klarsicht, ANC-1, Syne homology
KDMs	Histone lysine demethylases
KEAP1	Kelch-like erythroid cell-derived protein with CNC homology (ECH)-associated protein 1
KIRs	Killer cell immunoglobulin-like receptors
KMTs	Histone lysine (K) methyltransferases
KO	Knockout (also denoted as "deficient" or −/−)
Ku	Ku70–Ku80
LAP	Latency-associated protein
LC-MS	Liquid chromatography-mass spectrometry
LDL	Low-density lipoprotein
LDL-C	Low-density lipoprotein cholesterol
LEF	Lymphoid enhancer factor
LGP2	Laboratory of genetics and physiology 2
LINC	Linker of the nucleoskeleton and cytoskeleton
lincRNA-EPS	LincRNA erythroid prosurvival
lincRNAs	Long intervening noncoding RNAs
LLC	Long latent complexes
LMW	Low molecular weight
lncRNAs	Long noncoding RNAs
LOX	Lipoxygenases

Lp(a)	Lipoprotein(a)
LPA	Lysophosphatidic acid
LPC	Lysophosphatidylcholine
LPE	Lysophosphatidylethanolamine
LPLs	Lysophospholipids
LPS	Lipopolysaccharide
LRPs	Low-density lipoprotein receptor-related proteins
LRRs	Leucine-rich repeats
LSDs	Lysine-specific demethylases
LSS	Laminar shear stress
LTB4	Leukotriene B4
LTBP	Latent TGF-β binding protein
LTs	Leukotrienes
LXA4	Lipoxin A4
LXRs	Liver X receptors
LXs	Lipoxins
LysoPS	Lysophosphatidylserine
M1 or M1-like	Macrophages with predominantly proinflammatory activities
M2 or M2-like	Macrophages with predominantly anti-inflammatory/proresolving/regenerative activities
mAbs	Monoclonal antibodies
MAC	Membrane attack complex
MALAT1	Metastasis-associated lung adenocarcinoma transcript 1
MAMPs	Microbe-associated molecular patterns
MAPKs	Mitogen-activated protein kinases
MARCO	Macrophage receptor with collagenous structure
MaRs	Maresins, for macrophage mediators in resolving inflammation
MARS	Mixed antagonist response syndrome
MAVS	Mitochondrial antiviral signaling proteins
MBL	Mannose-binding lectin
MBPs	Methyl-binding proteins
MCAO	Middle cerebral artery occlusion
MCP-1	Monocyte chemoattractant protein-1
MDA	Malondialdehyde
MDA5	Melanoma differentiation-associated gene 5
mDia2	Mammalian homolog of Diaphanous 2
Mdivi-1	Mitochondrial division inhibitor 1
MDSCs	Myeloid-derived suppressor cells
Me	Methyl group

MEG3	Maternally expressed gene 3
MELD	Model for end-stage liver disease
MHC-I	Major histocompatibility complex class I
MHC-II	Major histocompatibility complex class II
MI	Myocardial infarction
MICA	MHC class I polypeptide-related sequence A
MICB	MHC class I polypeptide-related sequence B
MICs	MHC class I chain-related proteins
miRISC	miRNA-induced silencing complex
miRNA	MicroRNA
MKL1	Megakaryoblastic leukemia 1
MLKL	Mixed lineage kinase domain-like protein
MLL	Mixed lineage leukemia
MMA	ω-NG-monomethylarginine
mmLDL	Minimally oxidized LDL
MMPs	Matrix metalloproteinases
MMR	Macrophage mannose receptor
mMRI	Molecular magnetic resonance imaging
MODS	Multiple organ dysfunction syndrome
MOF	Multiple organ failure
mPGES-1	Microsomal prostaglandin E2 synthase-1
MPT	Mitochondrial membrane permeability transition
MRFT-B	Myocardin-related transcription factor B (also known as MKL2, megakaryoblastic leukemia 2)
MRI	Magnetic resonance imaging
MRN	Mre11–RAD50–NBS1
MRS	Magnetic resonance spectroscopy
MRTF-A	Myocardin-related transcription factor A (also known as MKL1, megakaryoblastic leukemia 1)
MSCs	Mesenchymal stem cells
MSR1	Macrophage scavenger receptor 1
MSU	Monosodium urate
mtDNA	Mitochondrial DNA
mtFPs	Mitochondrial formyl peptides
mTOR	Mammalian target of rapamycin
MTs	Microtubules
MVBs	Multivesicular bodies
MyD88	Myeloid differentiation primary response gene 88
n-3DPA	Docosapentaenoic acid
NACHT domain	Neuronal apoptosis inhibitor protein (NAIP), MHC Class II transactivator/transcription activator (CIITA), plant het product (HET-E), and telomerase-associated protein 1 (TP1) protein

NADPH	Nicotinamide adenine dinucleotide phosphate
NAIP	Neuronal apoptosis inhibitor protein
NAPQI	*N*-acetyl-*p*-benzoquinone imine
NAs	Nucleic acids
NCCD	Nomenclature Committee on Cell Death
ncRNA	Noncoding RNAs
nDNA	Nuclear DNA
NE	Norepinephrine
NEAT1	The nuclear enriched abundant transcript 1
Nesprin proteins	Nuclear envelope spectrin repeat proteins
NETosis	Formation of NETs by neutrophils
NETs	Neutrophil extracellular traps
NF-κB	Nuclear factor-kappa B
NK cells	Natural killer cells
NKG2	Natural killer group 2
NKG2D	Natural killer group 2 D
NKT cells	Natural killer T cells
NLRP3	Nucleotide-binding and oligomerization domain (NOD, "NACHT")-like receptor family, pyrin domain-containing 3
NLRs	Nucleotide-binding oligomerization domain (NOD)-like receptors
NMDA	*N*-methyl-D-aspartate
NMHA-II	Nonmuscle myosin heavy chain IIA
NMII	Nonmuscle myosin II
NO	Nitric oxide
NOD	Nucleotide-binding oligomerization domain
NOX	Nicotinamide adenine dinucleotide phosphate-dependent oxidase
NOXO1	NADPH Oxidase Organizer 1
NPCs	Nuclear pore complexes
NPD1	Neuroprotectin D1
NPDS	American National Poison Data System
Nrf1/Nrf2	Nuclear factor-erythroid 2 p45-related factors 1/2
NSAIDs	Nonsteroidal anti-inflammatory drugs
NSTEMI	Non-ST-elevation myocardial infarction
$O_2^{\bullet-}$	Superoxide
OH	Hydroxyl radical
$ONOO^-$	Peroxynitrite
OSEs	Oxidation-specific epitopes
OSS	Oscillatory shear stress
OxCL	Oxidized cardiolipin
OxLDLs	Oxidized low-density lipoproteins
OxPE	Oxidized phosphatidylethanolamine

OXPHOS	Oxidative phosphorylation
OxPLs	Oxidized phospholipids
OxPS	Oxidized phosphatidylserines
P1Rs	P1 receptors, i.e., purin adenosine receptors
P2Rs	P2 receptors, i.e., purin ADP/ATP receptors
P2XRs	P2X purinoceptors
P2YRs	P2Y purinoceptors
PABPC	Poly(A)-binding protein C
PAN	Poly(A)-nuclease
PARP-1	Poly (ADP-ribose) synthetase-1
Parthanatos	Poly ADP-ribose polymer
PAX	Paxillin
PBMCs	Peripheral blood mononuclear cells
PC	Phosphatidylcholine
PCI	Percutaneous coronary intervention
PCR	Polymerase chain reaction
PCTR1	Protectin conjugate in tissue regeneration1
PD-1	Programmed cell death protein-1
PDCD4	Programmed cell death 4
pDCs	Plasmacytoid dendritic cells
PDGF	Platelet-derived growth factor
PD-L1/2	Programmed cell death protein ligand 1/2
Pds	Protectins
PE	Phosphatidylethanolamine
PECAM-1	Platelet endothelial cell adhesion molecule-1
PERK	Protein kinase RNA-like endoplasmic reticulum (ER) kinase
PET	Positron emission tomography
PGE2	Prostaglandin E2
PGF2α	Prostaglandin F2α
PGN	Peptidoglycan
PGs	Proteoglycans
PI3K	Phosphatidylinositol 3 kinase
PICS	Persistent inflammation, immunosuppression, and catabolism syndrome
PIKKs	Phosphatidylinositol 3 kinase-related kinases
PKA	Protein kinase A
PKC	Protein kinase C
PLOOH	Peroxyl radicals/phospholipid hydroperoxides
PM	Particulate matter
pMHC	Peptide/major histocompatibility complex
PMNs	Polymorphonuclear neutrophils
PMTs	Protein methyltransferases
Pol II	Polymerase II
poly (I:C)	Polyinosinic:polycytidylic acid

PPARγ/PPARδ	Peroxisome proliferator activating receptor gamma/delta
PPCI	Primary percutaneous coronary intervention
PPP	Pentose phosphate pathway
PRDXs	Peroxiredoxins
PRG4	Proteoglycan-4
PRMs	Pattern recognition molecules
PRMTs	Protein arginine (*R*) methyltransferases
PRP19	Pre-mRNA-processing factor 19
PRRs	Pattern recognition receptors
PRXs	Peroxiredoxins
PS	Phosphatidylserine (also abbreviated as PtdSer)
PtdSer	Phosphatidylserine
PTGR2	Prostaglandin reductase 2
PTMs	Posttranslational modifications
PUFAs	Polyunsaturated fatty acids
PUMA	p53 upregulated modulator of apoptosis
PYD	Pyrin domain (also abbreviated as NLRP)
R	Arginine
RAAS	Renin-angiotensin-aldosterone system
RAGE	Receptor for advanced glycation end products
RAS	Renin-angiotensin system
RCD	Regulated cell death
RGD	Sequence, arginylglycylaspartic acid (Arg-Gly-Asp) sequence
RhoA	Ras homolog gene family, member A
RIG-I	Retinoic acid-inducible gene (protein) I
RIP	Receptor-interacting protein
RIPK1–3	Receptor-interacting serine/threonine-protein kinase 1–3
RLH	Rig-I-like helicase
RLRs	Helicase retinoic acid-inducible gene I (RIG-I)-like receptors
RLRs	Rig I-like receptors
RN	Regulated necrosis
RNS	Reactive nitrogen species
ROCK	Rho-associated coiled-coil containing protein kinase
RORγt	Retinoic acid receptor-related orphan receptor-gamma t
ROS	Reactive oxygen species
RPA	Replication protein A
RT-PCR	Reverse transcription-polymerase chain reaction
RvD1/2	Resolving D1/2

RvE1	Resolving E1
Rvs	Resolvins, for: resolution phase interaction products
RXRα	Retinoid X receptor alpha
S1P	Sphingosine-1-phosphate
SAH	Subarachnoid hemorrhage
SAMPs	Suppressing/inhibiting DAMPs
sDMA	NG-asymmetric dimethylarginine
SET	Su(var)3-9, enhancer-of-zeste, trithorax
Setdb2	SET domain bifurcated 2
siRNA	Small interfering RNA
SIRS	Systemic inflammatory response syndrome
SIRTs	Sirtuins
SLRPs	Small leucine-rich proteoglycans
Smad	Similar to: mothers against decapentaplegic
SMCs	Smooth muscle cells
SMOCs	Supramolecular organizing centers
snoRNAs	Small nucleolar RNAs
SNPs	Single nucleotide polymorphisms
SNS	Sympathetic nervous system
SOCS	Suppressors of cytokine signaling
SOD	Superoxide dismutase
SPC	Sphingosylphosphorylcholine
SPECT	Photon emission computed tomography
SPMs	Specialized proresolving mediators
SPRY1	Protein-coding gene protein sprouty homolog 1
SRF	Serum response factor
SRs	Scavenger receptors
SSBs	Single-strand DNA breaks
ssDNA	Single-stranded DNA
ST2	Suppressor of tumorigenicity 2; originally: growth stimulation expressed gene 2
STAT 1/2/3/4	Signal transducer and activator of transcription 1/2/3/4
STEMI	ST-elevation myocardial infarction
STING	Stimulator of interferon genes
SUCNR1	Succinate receptor 1
SUN proteins	Sad1 Unc proteins
system xC-/xCT	Cystine/glutamate antiporter
T1DM	Type 1 diabetes mellitus
T2DM	Type 2 diabetes mellitus
TAAs	Tumor-associated antigens
TAB 1/2/3	Transforming growth factor-β-activated kinase1(TAK1)-binding protein 1/2/3

TAK1	Transforming growth factor-β-activated kinase 1
TAMs (**T**yro3, **A**xl, and **M**erTK)	MerTK receptor tyrosine kinases
TANK	Tumor necrosis factor (TNF)-receptor-associated factor (TRAF) family member-associated NF-κB activator
TAZ, WWTR1	WW domain-containing transcription regulator protein 1, also known as transcriptional co-activator with PDZ-binding motif
TBI	Traumatic brain injury
TBK1	TANK-binding kinase 1
TCA	Tricarboxylic acid
TCF	T cell factor
TCF/LEF	T cell factor/lymphoid enhancer factor
TCR	T cell receptor
TEA	Transcriptional enhancer factor
TEAD factors	Transcriptional enhancer factor (TEA) domain family members: a family of DNA-binding transcription factors
TET	Ten-eleven translocase
TF	Tissue factor
TF	Transcription factor
TGF-β	Transforming growth factor beta
TGIF	TGFβ-1 signaling pathway repressors 5′-TG-3c′-interacting factor
TGN	Trans Golgi network
Th1/Th2	T helper cell type 1/type 2
THP-1	A human monocyte cell line
THRIL	TNF and HNRNPL-related immunoregulatory long noncoding RNA
TIA	Transient ischemic attack
TIM 1–4	T cell immunoglobulin and mucin domain containing 1–4
TIMPs	Tissue inhibitors of metalloproteinases
TIR	Toll/IL-1
TLRs	Toll-like receptors
TNC	Tenascin-C
TNF	Tumor necrosis factor
TNFR	Tumor necrosis factor receptor
tolDCs	Tolerogenic dendritic cells
TRAF	Tumor necrosis factor (TNF) receptor-associated factor
TRAIL	TNF-related apoptosis-inducing ligand
TRALI	Transfusion-related acute lung injury
Tregs	T regulatory cells

TREMs	Triggering receptors expressed on myeloid cells
TREX1	Exonuclease 1
TRIF	Toll/IL-1(TIR)-domain containing adaptor inducing interferon-β
TRP	Transient receptor potential
TRPA1	Transient receptor potential cation channel subfamily A member 1
TRPC	Transient receptor potential cation channel subfamily
TRPM 2 or 8	Transient receptor potential melastatin member 2 or 8
TRPV1–4	Transient receptor potential vanilloid subtype 1–4
TRXs	Thioredoxins
TXNIP	Thioredoxin-interacting protein
TβRI/II	Transforming growth factor beta receptor I/II
TβRI–III	TGF-β type I–III receptor
ULBPs	UL16-binding proteins
UPR	Unfolded protein response
UTR	Untranslated region
UV	Ultraviolet
VCAM-1	Vascular cell adhesion molecule-1
VE-cadherin	Vascular endothelial cadherin
VEGFs	Vascular endothelial growth factors
VSMCs	Vascular smooth muscle cells
VWF	von Willebrand Factor
W	Tryptophan
WDR5	WD repeat-containing protein 5
WHO	World Health Organization
Wnt	Wingless-type
WPBs	Weibel-Palade bodies
XBP1	X-box binding protein 1
XOR	Xanthine oxidoreductase
XRN1	Exoribonuclease 1
YAP	Yes-associated protein
YB-1	Y-box binding protein-1
αARs/βARs	Alpha-adrenergic receptors and beta-adrenergic receptors
α-SMA	Alpha-smooth muscle actin

Part I

Prologue

Perspectives of the Danger/Injury Model in Immunology

1

1.1 Introduction

A quarter of century ago, in 1994, the danger/injury model in Immunology was formulated and published as the third major paradigm stating that the host immune system does not care about self and nonself but that it is any form of cell stress/tissue injury rather than the presence of foreign ("strange") nonself that elicits adaptive immunity. In other words, the danger/injury model held and still holds that the key triggers in instigating an innate/adaptive immune response are primarily not foreign antigenic stimulus and immune cells but endogenous molecules derived from cells and/or tissues in which distinct damage takes place. The model emerged from two sources: (1) its publication by Walter Land and the Munich transplant group on the basis of significant data from a clinical trial in transplant patients providing compelling evidence that tissue injury induces immunity [1] and (2) its description by Polly Matzinger in the form of an admirable, extremely plausible, self-coherent chain of argumentation on theoretical grounds resulting in the stringent conclusion that the self/nonself discrimination theory of immune responses is inappropriate [2].

However, scientific research always continues to advance, especially in the modern era of the Internet; thus, the danger/injury model in its original sense tends to become outdated. As a consequence, one has always to strive for attempts to integrate the model into new streams of scientific knowledge. Here, a few of those scientific streams should be briefly addressed.

1.2 A Modern Holistic View of the Universal Defense System

Since the beginning of the new millennium, emerging science and technology have stimulated a modern holistic view of the intrinsic nature of our universal defense system. It responds to any stress, including mental stress and any injury—may it be of infectious or sterile nature—the aim always being to maintaining and restoring cellular and organismal homeostasis, thereby guaranteeing our survival.

W. G. Land, *Damage-Associated Molecular Patterns in Human Diseases*,
https://doi.org/10.1007/978-3-030-53868-2_1

Cells of this universal defense system are specialized to recognize distinct cell stress/tissue injury-induced damage-associated molecular patterns (DAMPs) via pattern recognition molecules (PRMs)—traditionally called pattern recognition receptors (PRRs)—to initiate efferent defense responses. Accordingly, PRMs/PRRs may be defined as "innate homeostatic molecules/receptors," which sense DAMPs to trigger life-sustaining/life-saving defense responses.

These defensive responses are of different nature. Thus, compelling evidence has accumulated, indicating that the mammalian defense system mainly consists of four evolutionarily developed defense responses in terms of resistance modalities:

1. An innate immune response in terms of an inflammatory response
2. An adaptive immune response in terms of a specific T- and B-cell response (if cell stress/tissue injury is caused by or associated with nonself or altered-self antigens), that is, a response that is stimulated by nonself/altered-self-presenting cells (APCs) of the innate immune system such as dendritic cells (DCs)
3. A mechanically induced innate response in terms of an adaptive response to mechanical forces (e.g., regulation and control of blood pressure)
4. A fight-or-flight response in terms of a rapid physical response in the face of danger (Fig. 1.1)

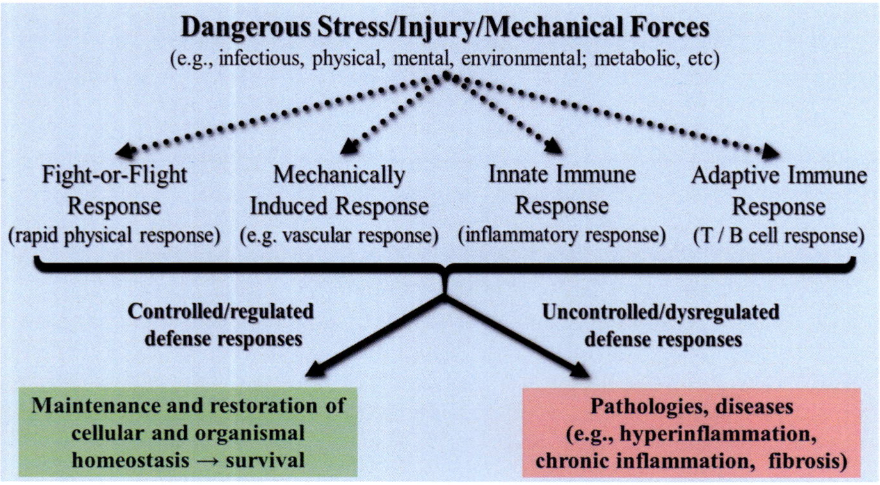

Fig. 1.1 Schematic presentation of a modern holistic view of the intrinsic nature of the universal defense system that responds to any stress including mental stress, any infectious or sterile injury, and mechanical forces. The aim of these various responses is always in maintaining and restoring organismal homeostasis. However, if uncontrolled, these defense responses can result in pathologies. Here, the system is exemplified by four evolutionarily developed defense responses: (1) the fight-or-flight response in terms of a rapid physical response; (2) the mechanically induced response (e.g., vascular response to increased blood pressure); (3) the innate immune response in terms of an inflammatory response; and (4)—if cell stress/tissue injury is caused by or associated with nonself or altered-self—the adaptive immune response in terms of a specific T- and B-cell response

From this modern holistic view of a universal defense system, a few aspects should be a bit closer addressed in the following.

An emerging topic in modern biomedicine refers to mechanosensation—mechanosignaling, that is, the conversion of mechanical forces into physiological responses. In fact, various types of cells in our body consistently respond to mechanical forces in daily life, a typical example being endothelial cells (ECs) lining the lumen of blood vessels. Equipped with stretch receptors located within the walls of the carotid sinus and aortic arch, they are vital for continuous blood pressure and heart rate regulation. Though mechanosensors are not considered to function as typical PRMs of the innate immune system, they refer to first-line host defense mechanisms that operate in the early stages of homeostatic disruption, may it be caused by infectious or sterile injury including mechanical forces. Like classical PRRs, mechanosensors play a crucial role in restoring and maintaining homeostasis, on the one hand, as well as, when dysregulated, may trigger pathologies and disorders, on the other hand. Hence, the functional properties to trigger homeostatic perturbation-induced defense responses qualify them as innate biomedical surveillance sensors that deserve to be included in the book (see Sect. 2.4).

1.2.1 The Fight-or-Flight Response

Also, the discussion about the fight-or-flight response (associated with the release of stress hormones) as a PRM-driven innate defense response has gained momentum in recent times. During the fight-or-flight response, the rise in circulating epinephrine and norepinephrine from the adrenal medulla and norepinephrine secreted from sympathetic nerve terminals cause increased blood pressure and cardiac output, relaxation of bronchial, intestinal and many other smooth muscles, mydriasis, and metabolic changes that increase levels of blood glucose and free fatty acids [3]. Thus, like an inflammatory response upon stress/injury, this defensive response is also aimed at protecting the life of an individual against acute stress/injury and serving to escape immediately from a dangerous situation. And this response appears to be a typical evolutionarily developed reaction. For example, in studies on *C. elegans* reported by Gupta and Singh [4], the immune response of the worm to a pathogen (*P. aeruginosa*) was shown to encompass a defensive flight response ("aversion response") of the worm against this bacterium. Notably, both the immune response and the flight (aversion) response were found to be controlled by a PRR, that is, a G protein-coupled receptor (GPCR). These studies nicely support the concept that psychological stress may well be able to trigger innate defensive responses such as a fight-or-flight response that have to be placed beyond the classical inflammatory/immune responses. Also, this example underlines the interweaving relationship between the innate immune system and the central nervous/psychoneural system (CNS): the topic of psychoneuroimmunology.

The four defense systems, together with the endocrine system and the microbiota, represent the major homeostatic control systems that take care of surveillance of homeostasis and initiate stress responses in case of a disruption of homeostasis (for additional information also compare Vol. 1 [5], Part II, Sect. 4.3, p. 36). The functional interactions of all these systems may determine the final orchestration of those PRM-triggered efferent responses, which, when controlled, result in the restoration of homeostasis or, when uncontrolled and dysregulated, constitute the pathogenesis of diseases such as inflammatory, degenerative, or autoimmune diseases.

1.3 The Continuously Evolving Story of DAMPs in Inflammation

The achievements of modern research in the field of inflammation are impressive and suggest a broad spectrum of innate defense responses that go far beyond that what was previously common knowledge (also compare Vol. 1 [5], Part I, Sect. 1.4, p. 9). For example, the injury-driven inflammatory defense response is now regarded to include a sequence of proinflammatory, antiinflammatory, proresolving, and tissue repairing/wound healing fibrogenic processes. When uncontrolled, these responses may lead to pathologies such as hyperinflammation, chronic nonresolving inflammation, or overshooting progressive fibrosis: the topic of this book.

Excitingly, there is first but accumulating evidence suggesting that DAMPs do not only activate innate immune cells such as M1-like macrophages and N1 neutrophils to promote inflammation but also modulate activated cells to change their phenotype from proinflammatory to proresolving traits. These transdifferentiated cells such as M2-like macrophages and N2 neutrophils possess inflammation-resolving properties including the capability to produce suppressing DAMPs (SAMPs), which in turn produce further SAMPs such as specialized proresolving mediators (SPMs) [6–11]. Interestingly, epigenetic modifications occurring during cell activation by various environmental stimuli have been described to drive this phenotype switch in inflammation [12]. On the other hand, there is emerging evidence for a role of DAMPs as critical inducers of epigenetic modifications [13–16]. Thus, it is tantalizing to think that DAMPs not only promote but also regulate homeostatic or pathological inflammatory responses via direct modification of gene expression: a new potential variant of the danger/injury model (Fig. 1.2). Further informative details of this burning issue in biomedicine will be presented in this book.

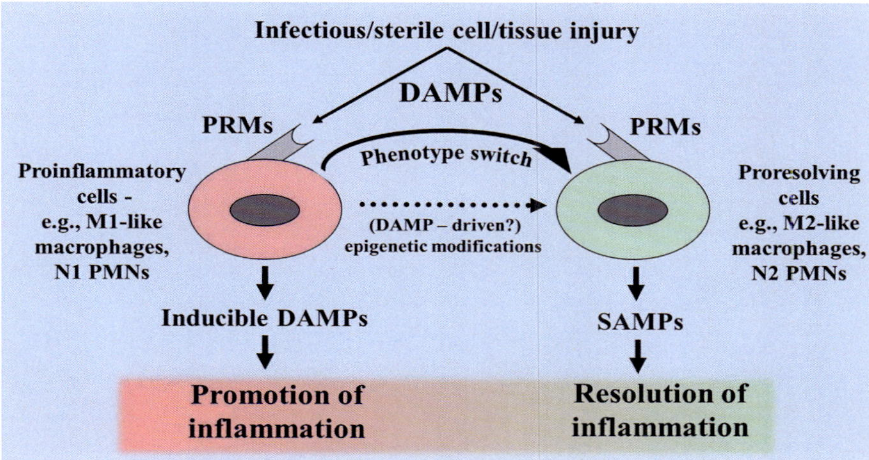

Fig. 1.2 Schematic conceptual model of injury-induced inflammation that is regulated by DAMP-triggered proinflammatory and SAMP-driven counterbalancing proresolving responses, aimed at returning to homeostasis. Increasing evidence suggests that DAMPs do not only activate PRM-bearing innate immune cells such as M1-like macrophages and N1 neutrophils to promote inflammation but also modulate activated innate immune cells to change their phenotype to inflammation-resolving traits. These transdifferentiated PRM-bearing cells, such as M2-like macrophages and N2 neutrophils, possess proresolving properties, including production of SAMPs, which in turn produce further SAMPs. Epigenetic modifications occurring during cell activation by various environmental stimuli (and triggered by DAMPs?) drive this phenotype switch. *DAMPs* damage-associated molecular patterns, *PMNs* polymorphonuclear leukocytes, *PRMs* pattern recognition molecules, *SAMPs* suppressing DAMPs. (Sources: [6–16])

1.4 DAMPs Across the Tree of Life

DAMPs do not only play a role in mammals, either in terms of homeostasis-preserving molecules or—when emitted in an uncontrolled and dysregulated way—in terms of disease-causing molecules. Indeed, modern evolutionary research tells us that all living creatures and organisms on our planet use these DAMPs to induce defense responses needed for their daily "struggle for life": from plants over invertebrates up to vertebrates including mammals and humans, "DAMPs across the tree of life" (Fig. 1.3) [17–19]. For example, DAMPs have been reported to trigger immunity and repair in plants [20], shrimps [21], and *Drosophila melanogaster* [22, 23]. Moreover, the discovery that DAMPs can modulate cellular functions via induction of epigenetic modifications implies a tremendous expansion of their role in host defense across the tree of life. Indeed, if this data could be confirmed and solidified in the future, they might have far-reaching consequences for social

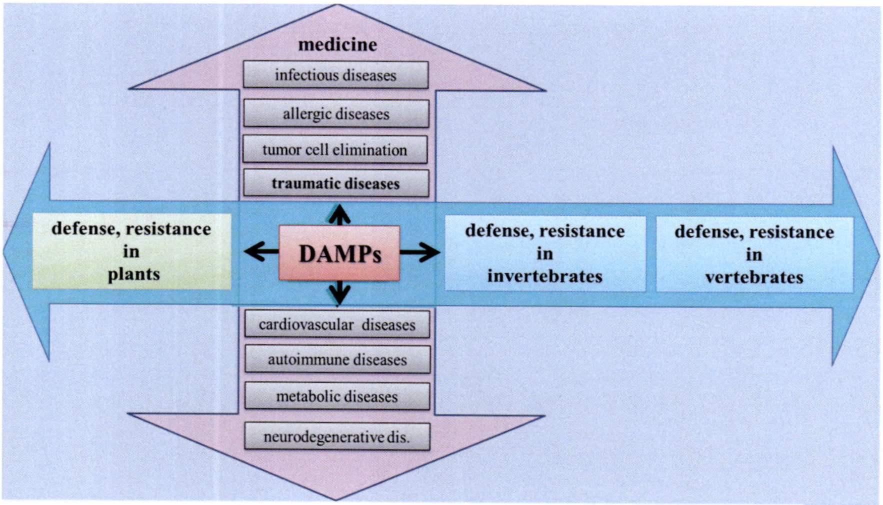

Fig. 1.3 The diagram should symbolize the world of DAMPs in health and diseases: The vertical level represents biomedicine, pointing to growing evidence for DAMPs to be pathogenetically involved in many human diseases. The horizontal level is related to modern research in evolution telling us that all living creatures and organisms on our planet use these DAMPs to induce defense responses needed for their daily "struggle for existence": from plants over invertebrates up to vertebrates, "DAMPs across the tree of life." (Sources: [17–19])

behavior via DAMP-induced epigenetic mechanisms that modify physiological processes, that is, DAMPs in terms of factors at the interface between species' biotic/abiotic environments and their genes. Unfortunately, however, the description of this emerging topic in evolutionary biology would go beyond the scope of this book.

References

1. Land W, Schneeberger H, Schleibner S, Illner WD, Abendroth D, Rutili G, et al. The beneficial effect of human recombinant superoxide dismutase on acute and chronic rejection events in recipients of cadaveric renal transplants. Transplantation. 1994;57:211–7. http://www.ncbi.nlm.nih.gov/pubmed/8310510.
2. Matzinger P. Tolerance, danger, and the extended family. Annu Rev Immunol. 1994;12:991–1045. http://www.ncbi.nlm.nih.gov/pubmed/8011301.
3. Tank AW, Lee WD. Peripheral and central effects of circulating catecholamines. Compr Physiol. 2015;5:1–15. https://doi.org/10.1002/cphy.c140007.
4. Gupta A, Singh V. GPCR signaling in C. elegans and its implications in immune response. Adv Immunol. 2017;136:203–26. https://linkinghub.elsevier.com/retrieve/pii/S0065277617300317.
5. Land WG. Damage-associated molecular patterns in human diseases. In: Injury-induced innate immune responses, vol. 1. Cham: Springer International Publishing AG; 2018. https://www.springer.com/de/book/9783319786544.

6. Fridlender ZG, Sun J, Kim S, Kapoor V, Cheng G, Ling L, et al. Polarization of tumor-associated neutrophil phenotype by TGF-β: "N1" versus "N2" TAN. Cancer Cell. 2009;16:183–94. https://linkinghub.elsevier.com/retrieve/pii/S1535610809002153.
7. Martinez FO, Helming L, Gordon S. Alternative activation of macrophages: an immunologic functional perspective. Annu Rev Immunol. 2009;27:451–83. http://www.ncbi.nlm.nih.gov/pubmed/19105661.
8. Martinez FO, Gordon S. The M1 and M2 paradigm of macrophage activation: time for reassessment. F1000Prime Rep. 2014;6:13.
9. Dalli J, Serhan C. Macrophage proresolving mediators—the when and where. Microbiol Spectr. 2016;4. http://www.ncbi.nlm.nih.gov/pubmed/27337457.
10. Prame Kumar K, Nicholls AJ, Wong CHY. Partners in crime: neutrophils and monocytes/macrophages in inflammation and disease. Cell Tissue Res. 2018;371:551–65. https://doi.org/10.1007/s00441-017-2753-2.
11. Halade GV, Norris PC, Kain V, Serhan CN, Ingle KA. Splenic leukocytes define the resolution of inflammation in heart failure. Sci Signal. 2018;11:eaao1818. http://www.ncbi.nlm.nih.gov/pubmed/29511119.
12. Kapellos TS, Iqbal AJ. Epigenetic control of macrophage polarisation and soluble mediator gene expression during inflammation. Mediators Inflamm. 2016;2016:1–15. http://www.ncbi.nlm.nih.gov/pubmed/27143818.
13. Crisan TO, Netea MG, Joosten LAB. Innate immune memory: implications for host responses to damage-associated molecular patterns. Eur J Immunol. 2016;46:817–8. https://doi.org/10.1002/eji.201545497.
14. Bekkering S, Quintin J, Joosten LAB, van der Meer JWM, Netea MG, Riksen NP. Oxidized low-density lipoprotein induces long-term proinflammatory cytokine production and foam cell formation via epigenetic reprogramming of monocytes. Arterioscler Thromb Vasc Biol. 2014;34:1731–8. https://doi.org/10.1161/ATVBAHA.114.303887.
15. Schnack L, Sohrabi Y, Lagache SMM, Kahles F, Bruemmer D, Waltenberger J, et al. Mechanisms of trained innate immunity in oxLDL primed human coronary smooth muscle cells. Front Immunol. 2019;10:13. http://www.ncbi.nlm.nih.gov/pubmed/30728822.
16. Neidhart M, Pajak A, Laskari K, Riksen NP, Joosten LAB, Netea MG, et al. Oligomeric S100A4 is associated with monocyte innate immune memory and bypass of tolerance to subsequent stimulation with lipopolysaccharides. Front Immunol. 2019;10:791. http://www.ncbi.nlm.nih.gov/pubmed/31037071.
17. Heil M, Land WG. Danger signals—damaged-self recognition across the tree of life. Front Plant Sci. 2014;5:578. http://www.ncbi.nlm.nih.gov/pubmed/25400647.
18. Heil M, Land WG, Tör M. Editorial: wound recognition across the tree of life. Front Plant Sci. 2016;7:1319. http://www.ncbi.nlm.nih.gov/pubmed/27635126.
19. Darwin C. On the origin of species by means of natural selection, or, The preservation of favoured races in the struggle for life. Mineola, NY: Dover; 2006. https://www.google.de/search?
20. De Lorenzo G, Ferrari S, Cervone F, Okun E. Extracellular DAMPs in plants and mammals: immunity, tissue damage and repair. Trends Immunol. 2018;39:937–50.
21. Soo TCC, Devadas S, Mohamed Din MS, Bhassu S. Differential transcriptome analysis of the disease tolerant Madagascar–Malaysia crossbred black tiger shrimp, Penaeus monodon hepatopancreas in response to acute hepatopancreatic necrosis disease (AHPND) infection: inference on immune gene response and in. Gut Pathog. 2019;11:39.
22. El Chamy L, Leclerc V, Caldelari I, Reichhart JM. Sensing of "danger signals" and pathogen-associated molecular patterns defines binary signaling pathways "upstream" of toll. Nat Immunol. 2008;9:1165–70.
23. Ming M, Obata F, Kuranaga E, Miura M. Persephone/Spätzle pathogen sensors mediate the activation of toll receptor signaling in response to endogenous danger signals in apoptosis-deficient Drosophila. J Biol Chem. 2014;289:7558–68.

Part II

A Select, Clinically Oriented Update of Topics Presented in "Damage-Associated Molecular Patterns in Human Diseases"; Volume 1: Injury-Induced Innate Immune Responses

Pattern Recognition Molecules

2

2.1 Introduction

Cells of the universal defense system, as briefly described in the prologue, are specialized to recognize cell stress/tissue injury-induced DAMPs via PRMs—traditionally called PRRs—to initiate efferent defense responses. Accordingly, PRMs/PRRs may be defined as "innate homeostatic molecules/receptors," which sense DAMPs to trigger life-sustaining/lifesaving defense responses (comprehensively described in Vol. 1 [1], Part II, Chpt. 5; also compare the recent review of Gong et al. [2]). In the following sections, the outstanding position of cellular PRRs in these scenarios is appreciated, and some of them are selectively and briefly updated. For information about the soluble humoral recognition molecules, the reader is referred to Vol. 1 [1], Part II, Sect. 5.4.

2.2 Cell-Associated "Classical" Pattern Recognition Receptors and Their Signaling

2.2.1 Introductory Remarks

The classical PRRs have been described in Vol. 1 [1], Part II, Sect. 5.2. As mentioned there, in the early research phase of innate immunity, signaling recognition molecules such as Toll-like receptors (TLRs) were termed "classical" PRRs and distinguished from "nonclassical" PRRs such as certain phagocytic receptors or receptors that can sense molecular perturbations. In the meantime, given recent discoveries of many other recognition molecules, these terms got blurred. Nowadays, the term "PRMs," covering all cellular and soluble humoral receptor groups, has gained acceptance and is increasingly used in international literature. In this book, just for didactic reasons, the term "classical" and "nonclassical" PRR is retained, though more or less arbitrarily chosen. In parallel, the term "PRMs" is also synonymously applied when referring to these molecules in a more general sense.

W. G. Land, *Damage-Associated Molecular Patterns in Human Diseases*,
https://doi.org/10.1007/978-3-030-53868-2_2

As outlined in Vol. 1 [1], Sect. 5.2, the "classical" cell-associated signaling PRRs—as here arbitrarily defined—include TLRs, *nucleotide-binding oligomerization domain* (NOD) *leucine-rich repeat* receptors (NLRs), *helicase retinoic acid-inducible gene I* (RIG-I)-*like receptors* (RLRs), *absent in melanoma 2* (AIM2)-*like receptors* (ALRs) along with other DNA receptors, *C-type lectin receptors* (CLRs), and the *receptor for advanced glycation end products* (RAGE) (compare [3–13]). These receptors or sensors collect information that is integrated and amplified by adapter or relay proteins to finally cumulate in a signaling pathway, which—via transcriptional processes—results in the activation of innate immune genes. The following effects may be cell-intrinsic or may be transferred to neighboring or distant cells. To meet the demands of various infectious or sterile insults timely and adequately, different modes of signal transduction have emerged. Thus, reversible signals transmitted through transient interactions or enzymatic activities, such as those in phosphorylation cascades, allow a rapid dose-dependent "tailor-made" homeostatic response.

2.2.2 Supramolecular Organizing Centers and Their Role as "Prion-Like" Proteins

2.2.2.1 General Remarks

Of note, newer studies on the nature of innate immune responses have provided stringent evidence indicating that intracellular signaling adaptor proteins may polymerize and assemble into structured, yet sometimes infinite, higher-order signaling machines for transmission of receptor activation information to cellular responses, called supramolecular organizing centers (SMOCs) [14]. These SMOCs (also denotes elsewhere as signalosomes) are now proposed to represent the principal subcellular sites of signal transduction in terms of signaling organelles of the innate immune system. Typically, these machines of the innate immune system allow for an all-or-none response that is only triggered once a threshold is exceeded. In other words, this molecular machinery allows efficient signal amplification, preceding enzyme activation that enables a response threshold to be reached. Indeed, this phenomenon of nucleated polymerization ensures that a small number of sensor proteins can activate many downstream signaling proteins (for key articles, see [15–17]). Up to date, three such SMOCs have been proposed: the TLR-induced myddosome [17, 18], the polymerization of inflammasome-associated *apoptosis-associated speck-like protein containing a caspase recruitment domain* (ASC), visible as so-called ASC specks, also denoted as "pyroptosomes" [16, 19], and the RLR-promoted polymerization of *mitochondrial antiviral signaling protein* (MAVS) [16].

2.2.2.2 Principle of Supramolecular Organizing Centers

The new concept of SMOCs includes the notion that nucleated polymerization may be a general principle in promoting the assembly of filamentous complexes upon stimulation to mediate innate immune signal transduction. As formulated by Kagan et al. [16]: "A sensor protein (receptor) in a pathway first becomes activated in the presence of ligands by overcoming auto-inhibition and subsequently oligomerizes. The oligomerized sensor then provides the platform to nucleate a downstream protein to polymerize into filaments."

Of note, as shown by Cai et al. [20, 21], MAVS and ASCs are mammalian proteins capable of switching into functional prions (= "prion-like" proteins), understanding prions as potentially adaptive mechanisms for phenotypic diversification and information storage [22]).

Indeed, as emphasized by Cai et al. [20]: "MAVS ^{CARD} and ASC ^{PYD} exhibit the cardinal hallmarks of prions, including irreversible conversion to stable filamentous structures, cytoplasmic multigenerational inheritance, and most importantly, an ability to template naïve molecules of the same protein into self-perpetuating conformations. For both MAVS and ASC, the tight regulation of nucleation followed by efficient polymerization produces a highly sensitive and robust 'digital' response to harmful insults."

2.2.2.3 Concluding Remarks

Also important to note here and reviewed by Franklin et al. [19] is the emerging evidence indicating that ASC specks are also released from inflammasome-activated cells and accumulate extracellularly in inflamed tissues, where they can continue to mature cytokines or be internalized by surrounding cells to further nucleate ASC specks in their cytosol. Regarding such function, and under adherence to the wide-ranging tenor of the book, the ASC specks may be considered inducible DAMPs [23] (see Sect. 3.5.4.2).

2.2.3 Toll-Like Receptors and Their Signaling

Toll-like receptors are type I membrane-associated innate immune receptors that, on the one hand, can sense microbe-associated molecular patterns (MAMPs) derived from useful commensal bacteria residing in our gastrointestinal tract to maintain homeostasis [24, 25] and, on the other hand, can recognize DAMPs (induced by infectious or sterile tissue injury) to promote inflammation and immunity. After activation, TLRs trigger signaling pathways leading—via activation of transcription factors—to the expression of innate immune genes that determine distinct functions of innate immune cells [3, 26–28]. Basically, TLRs mainly signal through two adaptor proteins, *myeloid differentiation primary response gene 88* (MyD88) and *Toll/IL-1(TIR)-domain-containing adaptor-inducing interferon-β* (TRIF). All TLRs, except TLR3, use MyD88 as their adaptor protein. This protein possesses a TIR domain that allows recruitment to TLRs following their activation but also contains an N-terminal death domain (DD), allowing members of the DD-containing *IL-1 receptor-associated kinase* (IRAK) family to be further recruited to the receptor complex [29]. This hetero-oligomeric structure comprising molecules of MyD88 and several IRAK members is termed the myddosome. As touched above, the myddosome is considered a SMOC [17] that plays a key role in MyD88-dependent signaling pathways to elicit vital inflammatory immune responses (reviewed by

Balka and De Nardo [18]). Interestingly, besides promoting inflammatory transcription factor activation, the myddosome reportedly drives the rapid induction of glycolysis, whereby the kinase *TANK-binding kinase 1* (TBK1) was identified as a myddosome component that promotes glycolysis [17].

Toll-like receptor 3 uses only TRIF as its adaptor [27, 28]. Although both MyD88 and TRIF pathways can activate *nuclear factor–kappa B* (NF-κB), interferon regulatory factor (IRF) family members, and *mitogen-activated protein kinase* (MAPK), they have preferences and distinct specificities and characteristics. The adaptor MyD88 activates mainly NF-κB family members and MAPK, and it tends to induce a proinflammatory response by producing proinflammatory cytokines such as interleukin (IL)-6 and IL-12. On the other hand, TRIF mainly activates IRF family members and tends to stimulate an antiviral response through the induction of interferon (IFN) [30] (for further details, see Vol. 1 [1], Part II, Sect. 5.2.2, and Part VI, Sect. 22.3.3, as well as Figs. 22.3 and 22.4; for a recent review, see [31]).

In sum, as outlined in Vol. 1, upon activation by MAMPs and DAMPs or DAMPs, the TLRs play a dominant role in triggering proinflammatory pathways that constitute the basis in the pathogenesis of many acute or chronic inflammatory diseases including autoimmune disorders.

2.2.4 Nucleotide-Binding and Oligomerization Domain-Like Receptors and Their Signaling

Nucleotide-binding and oligomerization domain-like receptors, the NLRs, are a group of evolutionarily conserved intracellular/cytosolic PRRs that are vitally essential to innate immunity and host physiology. In humans, there are 22 known NLRs, and the association of mutations and single nucleotide polymorphisms (SNPs) in their genes with human diseases reflects their key role in host defense [32]. The characteristic feature of mammalian NLRs is a central NOD domain, required for oligomerization, an N-terminal homotypic protein↔protein interaction domain, and a C-terminal series of *leucine-rich repeats* (LRRs) involved in agonist sensing or ligand binding. The NLRA subfamily includes only one member, the *major histocompatibility complex (MHC) Class II transactivator/transcription activator* (CIITA), and, similarly, the human NLRB subfamily also has just one member, the *neuronal apoptosis inhibitor protein* (NAIP). The NLRC subfamily consists of six members: NLRC1 (NOD1), NLRC2 (NOD2), NLRC3, NLRC4, NLRC5, and NLRX1. Finally, the NLR pyrin domain-containing subfamily (NLRP) consists of 14 members, NLRP1–14 (for further details, see Vol. 1 [1], Part II, Sect. 5.2.3, and [10, 33–37]).

The receptors NOD1 and NOD2 sense bacterial products in the host cytosol, thereby providing another level of microbial surveillance that is often associated with pathogen invasion. Like all PRMs, NODs contribute to homeostasis, here gut homeostasis, and have a fundamental role not only in the physiological development of the gastrointestinal system but also in inflammatory bowel disease. Furthermore, they have a proposed role in controlling the intestinal microbiota suggesting that this may have been a major selective pressure throughout evolution (for reviews, see [38–45]).

There are several potential mechanisms for intracellular bacterial recognition by NOD1 and NOD2 (reviewed in [46, 47]). In fact, host cells can internalize peptidoglycan (PGN)-derived MAMPs by multiple routes such as (1) phagocytosis of bacteria and subsequent bacterial degradation; (2) uptake of MAMP-containing Gram-negative bacterial outer membrane vesicles; (3) transport of MAMPs across host membranes via channels, pore-forming molecules, or bacterial secretion systems; (4) endocytosis; or (5) from neighboring cells. Upon sensing of their cognate MAMPs, NOD1 and NOD2 trigger signaling pathways resulting in the activation of NF-κB and MAPKs (reviewed in [33, 41, 46, 47]; for further details, see Vol. 1 [1], Part VI, Sect. 22.3.5). More recent data on the role of these PRRs in inflammation, immunity, and disease have been reviewed by Mukherjee et al. [48] and Platnich and Muruve [49].

2.2.5 NLRP3 Inflammasome-Dependent Inflammatory and Cell Death Pathways

2.2.5.1 General Remarks

Efferent inflammatory processes of the innate immune system are predominantly executed by inflammasomes, which are sizeable multi-molecular-weight protein complexes that can be regarded as key players in the regulation of cellular stress. As molecular platforms or molecular machines, they are formed in the cytosolic compartment in response to MAMPs and DAMPs or DAMPs alone. The most prominent member of those molecular machines is the NLRP3 inflammasome, whereby the NLRP3 sensor contains a central NOD ("NACHT") domain, an N-terminal pyrin (PYD) domain, and a C-terminal LRR domain (for additional information, see Vol. 1 [1], Part II, Sect. 5.2.3 and Fig. 5.3, p.50, as well as Part VI, Sect. 22.4.2, p.515, and Fig. 22.11, p.517 (for recent reviews, see [50–52]). Interestingly, a canonical type of NLRP3 activation and a noncanonical NLRP3 inflammasome activation have been described.

2.2.5.2 The Two Steps of Activation

The canonical activation of the NLRP3 inflammasome in macrophages is the results of two steps: a priming step (signal 1) and a subsequent real activating step (signal 2). Of note, however, since NLRP3 is not a receptor that directly/physically binds to a ligand but rather a sensor of molecular perturbations (reflected by dyshomeostatic Subclass IIC-4 DAMPs, partially emitted by preceding DAMP↔PRM interactions), the activation step is regarded as an indirect activation process. Of note, the action of MAMPs, originating from numerous pathogens, as well as DAMPs (= "NLRP3-priming DAMPs") was shown to stimulate the priming step, for example, via TLR4 that triggers NF-κB-mediated NLRP3 and pro-IL-1β expression. This priming step is obviously sufficient for human monocytes to mediate caspase-1 activation and IL-1β release [53]. It should be noted here that signal 1 is probably not restricted to the NF-κB-dependent transcriptional upregulation of NLRP3 and pro-IL-1β [54–57], as the NLRP3 inflammasome can be activated as early as 10 min when treated with signal 1 and signal 2 stimuli simultaneously [55]. The indirect activating step is triggered by MAMPs or DAMPs (= "NLRP3-activating DAMPs" = denoted throughout the book as Subclass IA-2 DAMPs). After full stimulation, NLRP3 recruits the adaptor protein ASC (containing a PYD domain and a *caspase activation and recruitment domain* [CARD]) that then undergoes prion-like polymerization, forming a single large spherical structure (denoted a "speck") in the perinuclear region (see also below). (Note: CARD belongs to the death domain superfamily, which is composed of the subfamilies of DDs, death effector domains (DEDs), and PYD along with CARDs [58], also compare Box 19.1 in Vol. 1 [1], Part V, Sect. 19.2.2.3.)

Then, ASC recruits and activates procaspase-1 (containing a CARD domain) into its cleaved form, caspase-1, to activate the downstream signaling cascade. This process is unequivocally required for the proteolytic processing of pro-IL-1β and pro-IL-18 into the mature IL-1β and IL-18 (= inflammatory path) in response to canonical inflammasome activators (i.e., NLRP3-priming MAMPs and DAMPs as well as NLRP3-activating DAMPs) (for further competent articles, see [59–65]). Caspase-1 activation also promotes the lytic cell death of pyroptosis (= cell death path), a subroutine of regulated necrosis (RN) that will be addressed in Sect. 4.3.5. There, it will also be mentioned that the gasdermin D (GSDMD) domain generates cell membrane pores, which are now believed to serve as a gate for extracellular release of mature IL-1β and IL-18 [66–70].

2.2.5.3 Mechanisms of NLRP3 Inflammasome Activation

As mentioned above, NLRP3 has a unique ability to sense a wide variety of MAMPs and DAMPs, indicating that these molecules likely elicit a common stress signal that is sensed by NLRP3. Nevertheless, despite more than 10 years of intensive research, the field has yet to reach a consensus opinion. Numerous studies have been performed dedicated to revealing NLRP3 activation mechanisms, in particular step 2 activation mechanisms. As described in Vol. 1 [1], Part VI, Sect. 22.4.2.2, and as reviewed by Yang et al. [51], these mechanisms so far reported include ion fluxes, reactive oxygen species (ROS) production, lysosomal destabilization ("frustrated phagocytosis," e.g., of air pollutants), and posttranslational modifications (PTMs; including phosphorylation and ubiquitination) of NLRP3. Of note, a study recently published by Zhong et al. [71] provided another new evidence suggesting that the generation of cytosolic oxidized mitochondrial DNA (mtDNA) may be the long-sought ligand for NLRP3 inflammasome activation by associating with the NLRP3 inflammasome complex. In fact, the authors even postulated that priming and activation of the NLRP3 inflammasome are coupled through the induction of new mtDNA synthesis and proposed further that NLRP3 is likely to recognize the presence of 8-hydroxy-2′-deoxyguanosine (8-OH-dG) on the oxidized DNA molecule (8-OHdG: an oxidized nucleoside and derivative of deoxyguanosine). Indeed, this is an interesting observation in that (1) cytosolic mtDNA is recognized as a critical DAMP (= IIC-2 DAMP sensed by *cyclic GMP-AMP (cGAMP) synthase* (cGAS), →

stimulator of interferon genes (STING); compare Sect. 3.4.4.2 and Table 3.1) and (2), when extracellularly released, has been found to act as a potent DAMP that, via TLR9-signaling, triggers robust inflammatory processes as, for example, observed in traumatic diseases (also compare Chap. 8). As also discussed by Yang et al. [51], the concept makes sense that NLRP3 perceives a common triggering pathway induced by intracellular processes, but does not directly interact with the various DAMPs so far described. Of interest in this context are very recent studies published by Chen and Chen [72] revealing a common triggering pathway for NRLP3 inflammasome activation (see also comment in [73]). Their exciting results showed that diverse NLRP3 stimuli result in the disassembly of the trans-Golgi network (TGN) (for TGN, also compare Vol. 1 [1], Part IV, Sect. 11.2.4.2 and Fig. 11.3). More specifically, the authors identified a common cellular signal triggered by diverse NLRP3 stimuli: the disassembly of TGN into (disassembled) dispersed TGN, to which NLRP3 is recruited through ionic bonding between its polybasic region and the phospholipid phosphatidylinositol-4-phosphate (PtdIns4P) on dispersed TGN. Dispersed TGN then serves as a scaffold for NLRP3 to aggregate and interact with ASC, which activates the downstream signaling cascade (for ASC as a SMOC, see below; also compare Fig. 2.1). Chen and Chen [72] then argue: "This mechanism of NLRP3 activation is reminiscent of the 'guard model' in plants, in which the disease resistant (R) proteins indirectly recognize virulent factors by monitoring the integrity of host targets, the 'pathogen-induced altered self … . By binding to dTGN as the 'altered self', NLRP3 indirectly senses a large variety of molecules associated with pathogens and other dangers."

In light of the danger/injury model, it is tempting to translate this conclusion into the following version cautiously: "This mechanism of NLRP3 activation is reminiscent of the robust host response to infection, in which PRMs recognize MAMPs derived from microbes to get an idea of the specificity and the nature of the pathogen involved. However, the PRMs, also, recognize pathogen-caused, injury-induced DAMPs in terms of constitutively expressed, injury-modified molecules to mount an efficient, robust defense response to infection. By binding to dispersed = modified TGN emerging as an IIC-6 DAMP (= cell-intrinsic modified DAMP, not yet included in Table 3.1), NLRP3 indirectly senses a large variety of molecules associated with pathogen-mediated infectious or nonpathogen-caused sterile injuries."

Nevertheless, to date, the final word has not yet been spoken, and there are still some open questions as articulated by Yang et al. [51]: "What factors ultimately determine the NLRP3 inflammasome activation? Is there a common signaling pathway targeted by NLRP3 inflammasome activation? Does the specific targeting of NLRP3 itself, and not other components (NEK7, ASC, caspase-1, or IL-1β) or up-/downstream factors of NLRP3 inflammasome produce therapeutic effects?"

2.2.5.4 Polymerization of ASC

Of note, as a result of the initial ASC oligomerization within the inflammasome, the ASC oligomers, in turn, nucleate large filamentous polymers of ASC^{PYD}, which are cross-linked by $ASC^{CARD} \leftrightarrow ASC^{CARD}$ interactions, forming the ASC specks. As touched above, sensor-nucleated polymerization of ASC is considered a

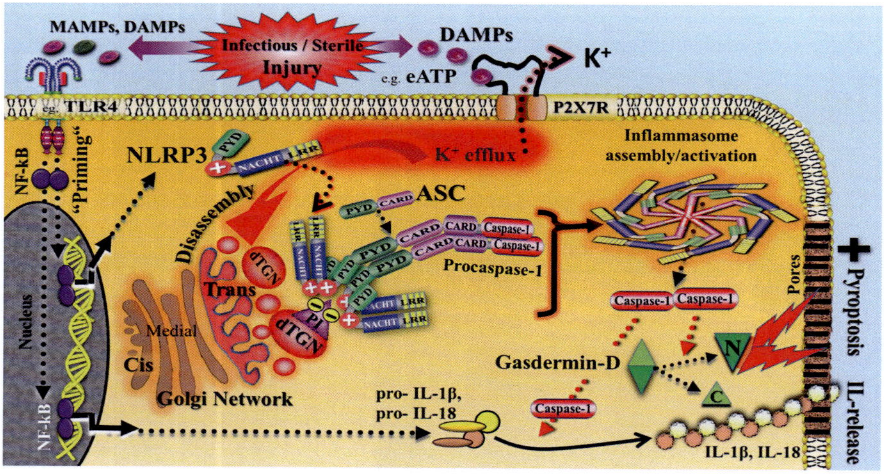

Fig. 2.1 Schematic diagram of a simplified narrative model illustrating infectious/sterile injury-induced activation of the NLRP3 inflammasome, whereby the new findings of Chen and Chen [72] are highlighted. The first priming step is regulated by MAMPs and a group of DAMPs that trigger PRR(TLR4)-mediated transcriptional pathways (NF-κB activation) to promote upregulation of NLRP3 and pro-IL-1β/pro-IL18 expression. Both "priming" MAMPs/DAMPs and "activating" DAMPs exemplified by eATP are required for NLRP3 inflammasome activation in macrophages. eATP-caused K+ efflux triggers disassembly of the trans-Golgi network (TGN) into multiple dispersed structures (dTGN), whereas cis- and medial-Golgi stacks remain intact. NLRP3 is recruited to and aggregates on the dispersed structures through ionic bonding between its conserved positively charged polybasic region and negatively charged phosphatidylinositol-4-phosphate (PI) that is exposed on the dTGN. The binding of NLRP3 to phosphatidylinositol-4-phosphate (a modified DAMP?) is essential for the inflammasome activation. Following aggregation on dTGN, NLRP3 promotes polymerization of the adaptor protein ASC via PYD–PYD interaction. In turn, the CARD domain of ASC recruits the CARD domain of procaspase-1 to form the NLRP3–ASC–procaspase-1 complex, denoted the activated NLRP3 inflammasome. Upon activation, the human inflammatory caspase-1 matures to its biologically active form and cleaves pro-IL-1β/pro-IL18 as well as Gasdermin D, releasing the N-terminal domain from the autoinhibitory Gasdermin D–C domain. Activated Gasdermin D-N then binds to lipids in the plasma membrane and forms large pores, leading to pyroptotic cell death and release of cellular contents such as matured (processed) IL-1β and IL-18 and DAMPs (not shown). (for additional information also compare Fig. 22.11, p. 517, in Vol. 1, Part VI, Sect. 22.4.2.2). *ASC* apoptosis-associated speck-like protein containing a caspase recruitment domain, *C* C-terminal domain, *CARD* caspase activating and recruiting domain, *dTGN* dispersed trans-Golgi network, *eATP* extracellular adenosine triphosphate, *K*$^+$ potassium, *NF-κB* nuclear factor–kappa B, *IL* interleukin, *LRRs* leucine-rich repeats, *N* N-terminal domain, *NACHT* (domain), neuronal apoptosis inhibitor protein (NAIP), MHC-Class II transactivator/ transcription activator (CIITA), plant het product (HET-E), and telomerase-associated protein 1 (TP1) protein, *NLRP3* NOD-like receptor family, pyrin domain containing 3, *PI,* phosphatidylinositol-4-phosphate, *PYD* pyrin domain, *P2X7R* P2X purinoceptor, *TGN* trans-Golgi network, *TLR4* Toll-like receptor 4. (Sources: [60–67, 72, 73]; and Vol.1 [1], Part VI, Sect. 22.4.2.2)

SMOC. This process has also been called "prion-like" polymerization [20, 21]. "Prionization" of the signal has been observed for all ASC-containing inflammasome tested so far, including the AIM2 inflammasome [74] (see below). As outlined and discussed by Franklin et al. [19], ASC specks are the sites of procaspase-1 recruitment and activation, thereby maximizing caspase-1 activation. They can be released from cells to disseminate inflammation in the extracellular space, or other cells after internalization and release from endosomes. Whether ASC specks are passively released from pyroptotic cells or whether they are secreted through more complex mechanisms remains to be investigated (for ASC specks operating as inducible DAMPs, see Sect. 3.5.4.2).

2.2.5.5 Concluding Remarks

Doubtlessly, NLRP3 inflammasome-dependent inflammatory and cell death pathways represent a powerful defense armamentarium serving as a crucial innate immune mechanism that protects the host from a wide variety of infectious and sterile injuries, notably viral infections. In particular, it is the emission of DAMPs from pyroptotic cells that constitutes this defense power. For example, inflammasome activation was demonstrated to prevent lethality upon influenza A virus infection [75]. However, if such DAMP-promoted pathways get uncontrolled and exaggerated, they may lead to fatal sepsis. In Sect. 4.3.5, the topic will be resumed.

2.2.6 Rig-I-Like Receptors and Their Signaling

2.2.6.1 General Remarks

The Rig-I-like receptor family encompasses three members, namely, RIG-I and *melanoma differentiation-associated gene 5* (MDA5) that trigger signaling pathways as well as the *laboratory of genetics and physiology 2* (LGP2) that functions as a regulator of RIG-I and MDA5 signaling. The receptors RIG-I and MDA5 can sense exogenous and endogenous cytosolic double-stranded RNA (dsRNA; such as endogenous non-coding RNAs) and, with their CARD domain, recruit and interact with the adaptor protein MAVS (also containing a CARD domain) to activate downstream signaling pathway via the transcription factors IRF3/IRF7 to induce production of type I IFNs (for MAVS, see also below). Here, it should be especially stressed that RNAs of nonviral and nonmicrobial origin operating as DAMPs have been shown to be recognized by RLRs (for competent articles, see [76–82]; for more details, see Vol. 1 [1], Sect. 5.2.4 and Fig. 5.4, and also Part VI, Sect. 22.3.6 and Fig. 22.7). For recent reviews on RLRs, the reader is directed to [83–85]. For example, Chow et al. [85] have comprehensively discussed recent insights into pathogen recognition by RLRs, related RNA helicases (RLHs), TLRs, and other RNA-sensing PRRs by focusing on emerging themes in innate immune signaling during virus infection.

2.2.6.2 Recognition by RIG-I-Like Receptors of Endogenous dsRNA Acting as Stress-Induced DAMPs

Finally, reports on the recognition by RLRs of endogenous dsRNA as stress-induced IIC-3 DAMPs are important from the perspective of the book [86, 87] (see Table 3.1). For example, as discussed by Khodarev et al. [86], certain stress stimuli such as oxidative stress and genotoxic stress associated with DNA damage can result in increased production of dsRNAs reflecting an "RNA stress." The cellular redistribution and accumulation of such aberrant dsRNA molecules to the compartments mimic a pathological state of viral invasion and, thus, provoke their recognition as DAMPs by RNA sensors (also compare [88, 89]). In this context, it should too be stressed that virus-induced activation of RIG-I, via receptor-interacting protein-1 (RIP-1) and NF-κB signaling, was found to lead to dramatic necroptosis indicating that viruses can trigger this subunit of regulated cell death (RCD), thereby providing a critical source of DAMPs needed for a robust antiviral defense response [90]. These findings were recently supported by studies on bone marrow-derived macrophages in mice demonstrating that sensing of intracellular RNA by RIG-I → MAVS pathway leads to activation of *receptor-interacting serine/threonine-protein kinase 3* (RIPK3) and necroptosis, requiring synergistic signaling through IFN and *tumor necrosis factor* (TNF) [91] (for necroptosis, see Sect. 4.3.3).

2.2.6.3 Polymerization of MAVs

Like ASC, aggregated MAVS has been proposed to act as a SMOC [16]. In fact, since its discovery, MAVS was reported to form detergent-insoluble aggregates on the surface of mitochondria upon activation of RIG-I/MDA5 (see [92]; also reviewed in [93]). Depending on its mitochondrial localization, aggregated MAVS is essential for its central function in mediating the signaling pathway upon activation of RIG-I. In other words, MAVS, like ASC, forms functional prion-like polymers to propagate immune signaling (reviewed by Cai et al. [21]). As emphasized by the authors, "following MAVS nucleation, irreversible and spontaneous polymerization ensues such that an all-or-none response is generated as long as the RIG-I stimulation threshold is reached." And further, "MAVS fibers are then able to recruit downstream signaling proteins to propagate a rapid and robust immune response."

2.2.6.4 Concluding Remarks

Of utmost importance from the tenor of the book is the new knowledge that RLRs can recognize various types of endogenous RNAs in their function as DAMPs to mediate an antiviral innate immune response. These host-derived "RNA-DAMPs" are sensed by RLRs upon virus-induced "unmasking" from the proteins that normally bind to these RNAs, or after their incorrect processing and/or subcellular mislocalization [87]. In this context, Lee et al. [87] argue: "In this case, recognition of 'self' represents an indirect mechanism of pathogen detection wherein the mammalian host senses viral manipulation of host RNA… metabolism, or virus-induced changes in the subcellular localization of host nucleic acids."

2.2.7 Cytosolic and Intranuclear DNA-Sensing Receptors

2.2.7.1 General Remarks

The repertoire of cytosolic DNA sensors encompasses a large list that includes ALRs such as AIM2 and *interferon-gamma-inducible protein 16* (IFI16), cGAS, the *DNA-dependent activator of IFN-regulatory factors* (DAI), and others (for more details, see Vol. 1 [1], Part II, Sects. 5.2.5 and 5.2.6 and Fig. 5.5; for key articles, see [94–100]).

These DNA sensors recognize exogenous bacterial and viral DNA or endogenous self-DNA (= IIC-2 DAMPs), present in the cytoplasm as a sign of infection or cell damage, and induce the production of type I and type III IFNs. Most of these DNA sensors utilize the adaptor proteins STING and TBK1 to induce type I IFN production (for more information, see Vol. 1 [1], Part VI, Sect. 22.3.7 and Fig. 22.8; for key articles, see [11, 26, 97, 101–104]). For recent reviews on cytosolic DNA sensors, the reader is referred to [105–108].

2.2.7.2 The Crucial Cytosolic cGAS→STING Signaling

From the perspective of the book, the cGAS→STING signaling is of considerable importance in that this pathway is involved in traumatic, autoinflammatory, and autoimmune disorders via recognition of endogenous nucleic acids (NAs). In their role as IIC-2 DAMPs, these NAs refer to mtDNA released from damaged mitochondria and/or nuclear DNA (nDNA) derived from (phagocytosed) dead cells or released from the damaged nucleus [104, 106] (also compare Fig. 2.2). The increasing importance of STING in human diseases culminates in emerging evidence suggesting that the activation of STING-dependent signaling is also implicated in the process of RCD, such as apoptosis, pyroptosis, necroptosis, and autophagy. Of note, the pro-death outcome is even predominant in certain cell types, like lymphocytes, myeloid cells, and hepatocytes (reviewed by Sun et al. [109]). For example, endogenous self-DNA from tumors is reportedly capable of activating the STING pathway, which contributes to augmenting an antitumor immune response [110, 111]. In addition, as also reviewed by Sun et al. [109], cGAS→STING-driven production of type I IFN and TNF was found to trigger RIPK3-dependent necroptosis [91], which again constitutes a source of DAMP emission. Moreover, a series of studies have revealed the interaction between pyroptosis and STING-dependent signaling [112], whereby mechanistically the transcription factor IRF1 is suggested to mediate this STING-driven subroutine of RN [113]: again another source of DAMP release.

Together, cGAS→STING signaling—regardless of whether it is activated by a viral infection or sterile injury—functions as a potent cell death pathway resulting in the emission of large amounts of DAMPs. In case of viral infection, this event elicits a strong antiviral defense response that may save the patient's life; in case of a severe polytrauma, this may result in a life-threatening systemic inflammatory response syndrome (SIRS). Additionally, it should be noted here that recent studies revealed a cGAS-independent noncanonical activation of STING by *ataxia telangiectasia mutated* (ATM) and IFI16 that mediates NF-κB signaling after nuclear DNA damage [114] (compare next section).

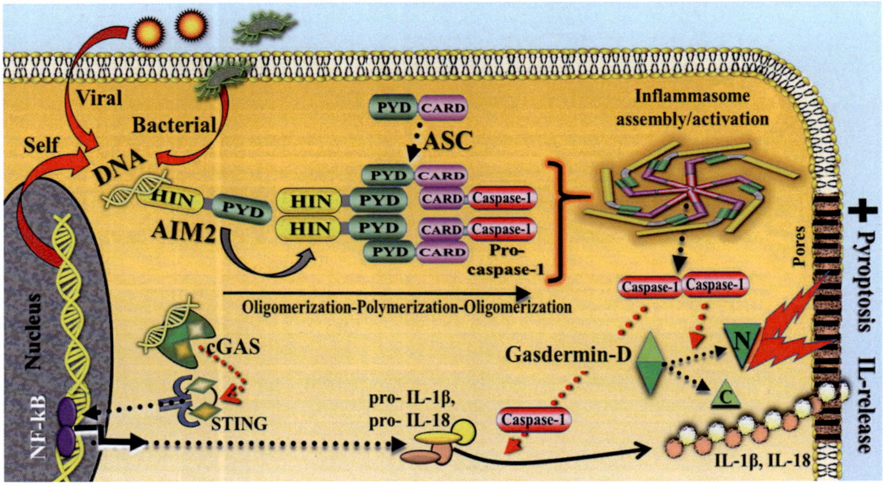

Fig. 2.2 Schematic diagram of a simplified narrative model illustrating viral, bacterial, and endogenous self-DNA activation of the AIM2 inflammasome. AIM2 is composed of an N-terminal pyrin domain (PYD) and a C-terminal HIN domain. Upon binding of dsDNA, AIM2 oligomerizes and recruits the adapter protein ASC via PYD–PYD interactions, associated with polymerization of the ASC protein. Then, pro-caspase-1 is recruited to the complex via CARD–CARD interaction to form the AIM2–ASC–pro-caspase-1 complex, denoted the activated AIM2 inflammasome. Upon activation, the human inflammatory caspase-1 matures and cleaves Gasdermin D, releasing the N-terminal domain from the autoinhibitory Gasdermin D–C domain. Activated Gasdermin D-N then binds to lipids in the plasma membrane and forms large pores, leading to pyroptotic cell death and release of cellular contents such as matured (processed) IL-1β and IL-18 and DAMPs (not shown). The model also illustrates the possibility that dsDNA activates the cGAS→STING pathway that, via transcriptional pathways (NF-κB activation), promotes upregulation of pro-IL-1β and pro-IL-18. (for cGAS→STING pathway, also compare Fig. 22.8 in Vol.1, Part VI, Sect. 22.3.7.3). *AIM2* absent in melanoma 2, *ASC* apoptosis-associated speck-like protein containing a caspase recruitment domain, *C* C-terminal domain, *CARD* caspase activating and recruiting domain, *cGAS* cyclic GMP-AMP synthase, *HIN* hematopoietic interferon-inducible nuclear protein, *NF-κB* nuclear factor–kappa B, *IL* interleukin, *LRR* leucine-rich repeats, *N* N-terminal domain, *PYD* pyrin domain, *STING* stimulator of interferon genes. (Sources: [11, 50, 52, 78, 94–96, 101, 131, 132], and Vol. 1 [1], Part VI, Sect. 22.4.2.2)

2.2.7.3 Intranuclear Receptors Sensing DNA Damage

This new group of receptors that can initiate the DNA damage response (DDR) has briefly been touched in Vol. 1 [1], Part II, Sect. 5.2.6.4. The receptors recognize *DNA double-strand breaks* (DSBs) or expression of the single-stranded DNA (ssDNA) and *replication protein A* (RPA)–ssDNA, respectively (denoted in the book as IIC-1 DAMPs). They include two highly conserved multiprotein complexes, *Mre11–RAD50–NBS1* (MRN) and *Ku70–Ku80* (Ku), which are considered the primary sensors of DSBs to subsequently activate the kinases ATM and DNA-dependent protein kinase (DNA-PK) [115–117]. Also, there is first evidence suggesting that the RPA [118] is a recognition molecule which is able to sense ssDNA as well as the protein *pre-mRNA-processing factor 19* (PRP19) that is thought to act as a sensor of RPA-ssDNA [119]; both sensors were shown to activate *ataxia telangiectasia and Rad3-related* (ATR) downstream (for more recent articles and reviews, see [120–123]). More recent studies published by Syed and Tainer [124] provided evidence for the DDR to be regulated in part from the MRN complex that forms a multifunctional DDR machine (for DDR, see Sect. 4.2.6). As pointed out by the authors, within its network assemblies, "MRN is the core conductor for the initial and sustained responses to DNA double-strand breaks, stalled replication forks, dysfunctional telomeres, and viral DNA infection."

2.2.7.4 Concluding Remarks

As with RLR-mediated signaling, cGAS→STING signaling can contribute to a robust antiviral innate immune response via recognition of endogenous mislocated cellular DNA. For example, mislocalization of mtDNA following virus-induced mitochondrial alterations, or apoptotic stimuli, is supposed to trigger cGAS→STING-mediated host immunity. In this context, Lee et al. [87] argue: "In this case, recognition of 'self' represents an indirect mechanism of pathogen detection wherein the mammalian host senses viral manipulation of host … DNA metabolism, or virus-induced changes in the subcellular localization of host nucleic acids."

Also, intranuclear receptors sensing damaged DNA in terms of IIC-1 DAMPs, thereby initiating the DDR, may contribute to efficient antiviral defense responses. In this context, Syed and Tainer [124] concluded: "The data reviewed here demonstrate how MRN interactions and resulting activities feed into cellular decision making in DNA stress responses, including viral defenses (typically considered to be only broadly related to the DDR)."

Together, the large list of cytosolic DNA sensors so far described is amazing and has raised the key issue on why so many DNA sensors exist and what is their relative role in DNA sensing in vivo and in different cell types. Also, this issue may be the reason why, despite the best efforts of researchers around the world, gene therapy has seen only limited success. Perhaps, the use of novel cGAS inhibitors [125, 126], together with previous administration of the DNA concerned under subimmunogenic conditions, that is, in the absence of injury, aimed at inducing tolerance [127–130], may be a future way of how the apply successful gene therapy.

2.2.8 The AIM2 Inflammasome-Dependent Inflammatory and Cell Death Pathways

The AIM2 inflammasome senses both endogenous mislocalized/altered-self DNA and nonself DNA generated during viral and intracellular bacterial infections (described in Vol. 1 [1], Part II, Sect. 5.2.5, and Part VI, Sect. 22.4.4). In contrast to the complexity of the NLRP3 inflammasome activation, inflammasome activation by AIM2 depends on the direct recognition of dsDNA only and thus does not need a second signal in terms of another subclass of DAMPs. But similar to the assembly of the NLRP3 inflammasome, the AIM2-triggered formation of an active inflammasome includes recruitment of the adaptor protein ASC and procaspase-1 (for ASC acting as a prion-like protein, see Sect. 2.2.5.4). Finally, the mature inflammatory caspase-1 processes proteolytically pro-IL-1β and pro-IL-18 into the mature IL-1β and IL-18, as well as promotes GSDMD-mediated pyroptotic cell death. The mature IL-1 and IL-18 are thought to be passively released through the GSDMD-induced cell membrane pores (Fig. 2.2) (for further reading, see [11, 50, 52, 78, 94–96, 101, 131, 132]).

Unexpectedly, as recently reported, AIM2 can also sense ionizing radiation-induced DNA damage in the nucleus [133]. In these studies, AIM2 was observed to act through the inflammasome pathway to promote caspase-1-mediated pyroptotic death in intestinal epithelial cells (EpCs) and bone marrow cells. Of high interest are also studies on a chemotherapy-induced intestinal mucositis mouse model showing that, besides sensing cell-intrinsic modified dsDNA (i.e., IIC-2 DAMPs), AIM2 in innate immune cells can recognize self-DNA delivered by exosomes that derived from intestinal EpCs exposed to chemotherapeutic agents [134]. Moreover, there is evidence (e.g., deduced from studies on mtDNA-triggered activation of the cGAS→STING pathway) suggesting that the AIM2 inflammasome may be activated by mtDNA, either in the form of cell-intrinsic IIC-2 DAMPs leaked by damaged mitochondria or in the form of circulating IA-1 DAMPs released from damaged cells (compare also [106, 135–138]).

Together, activation of the AIM2 inflammasome by both viral/bacterial infections and sterile cell stress/tissue injury are currently intensely discussed (Fig. 2.2). And the contribution of this inflammasome to efficient host defense against viral and bacterial infections may be explained by its property to promote a pyroptotic cell death that is associated with the release of large amounts of DAMPs (see also Sect. 4.3.5).

2.2.9 C-Type Lectin Receptors: A Remarkable Diverse Family of Proteins

The C-type lectin receptor superfamily is the largest and most diverse lectin family in animals and has been classified into 17 groups (I–XVII) based on phylogeny and structural and functional properties. The proteins consist predominantly of selectins, macrophage mannose receptor (MMR) family members, type II natural killer (NK)-cell receptors, and the *dendritic cell-specific intercellular adhesion molecule-3-grabbing non-integrin* (DC-SIGN) family. C-type lectin receptors are highly conserved soluble and transmembrane PRMs which recognize a diverse range of DAMPs and MAMPs and are defined by the presence of at least one *C-type lectin-like domain* (CTLD) (for details including signaling, see Vol. 1 [1], Part II, Sect. 5.2.7 and Fig. 5.6, and Part VI, Sect. 22.3.8 and Fig. 22.9). As other PRMs which sense tissue injury-induced DAMPs concomitant to infection to augment effector responses, *dendritic cell natural killer lectin group receptor-1* (DNGR-1) was demonstrated to perceive tissue injury concomitant with viral infections and facilitate antigen processing of viral antigens for cross-presentation to $CD8^+$ T cells [139–141] (for cross-presentation of exogenous antigens, see Vol. 1 [1], Part VIII, Sect. 31.3.5 and Fig. 31.5).

Here, the topic is not further pursued; instead, for further reading, the reader is referred to the review by del Fresno et al. [142]. Besides others, the authors concluded that research in this field had gained much attention "considering the diversity of members, ligands, expression pattern on clinically relevant cellular populations and their relevant function on the initiation, and regulation of immunity and inflammation."

2.2.10 Résumé

The story of classical PRMs is certainly not over yet. New aspects in sight include synergistic interaction between PRMs as, for example, documented between TLRs↔NLRs. As reported by Pashenkov et al. [143], potential practical implications of NOD-TLR synergy may be dual: "In sepsis, where synergistic effects probably contribute to excessive proinflammatory cytokine production, blockade of NOD1, and/or NOD2 in addition to TLR4 blockade may be required to achieve therapeutic benefit. On the other hand, synergistic combinations of relatively small doses of NOD and TLR agonists administered before infection could be used to boost innate resistance against bacterial pathogens." Such observations are of considerable importance for the future use of DAMPs as either therapeutic targets or therapeutics (see Sect. 7.4).

2.3 Cell-Associated "Nonclassical" Pattern Recognition Molecules and Their Signaling

2.3.1 Introductory Remarks

As already mentioned in Vol. 1 [1], Part II, Sect. 5.3.1 and above, the subdivision into "classical" and "nonclassical" recognition receptors used in this book has been chosen more or less arbitrarily. They encompass various groups of receptors including "dyshomeostasis"-sensing receptors, scavenger receptors (SRs), purinergic receptors, the natural killer group 2D (NKG2D) receptor, receptors able to sense metabolites, nociceptors, GPCRs, and fragment crystallizable (Fc) region receptors (FcRs). Typically, they play various roles within the broad field of MAMP/DAMP-driven innate immune functions. Here, the "nonclassical" PRMs are selectively and briefly resumed; relevant details concerning their role in initiating innate immune responses will be presented in the following chapters if and when appropriate.

2.3.2 Scavenger Receptors: With Focus on Their Ability to Recognize Apoptotic Cells

Scavenger receptors consist of a panoply of integral membrane proteins and soluble secreted extracellular domain isoforms that are structurally diverse and participate in a wide range of biological functions. These innate immune receptors are expressed predominantly by myeloid cells and recognize a variety of ligands, including DAMPs and MAMPs. As cell surface receptors, they typically bind multiple ligands and promote the removal of altered-self or nonself targets. As plasma membrane receptors, they mediate phagocytic recognition of microbes and/or apoptotic cells. Accordingly, they often function by mechanisms that include endocytosis and phagocytosis that ultimately lead to the elimination of degraded or harmful substances. By executing those functions, SRs play crucial roles in host homeostasis and operate as key regulators of inflammatory diseases, such as atherosclerosis. The receptors have been alluded to in Vol. 1[1], Part II, Sect. 5.3.3 and Fig. 5.8, and Part VI, Sect. 22.6. For more recent reviews, the reader is invited to refer to [144–147]. Here, however, the receptors recognizing apoptotic cells are resumed, because they play an increasing pathogenetic role in human diseases.

Recognition and engulfment of apoptotic cells, that is, the process termed "efferocytosis," involve a complex combination of signals (see Sect. 5.3.2.2; for additional information also compare Vol. 1 [1], Part V, Sect. 19.2.4, p. 435, and Part VI, Sect. 22.6.3.3, p. 562). The process is predominantly executed by phagocytes via the recognition of several molecules displayed on the surface of apoptotic cells, termed "eat-me" signals. The most characteristic molecule out of these "eat-me" signals is phosphatidylserine (PtdSer). Various PtdSer-specific receptors exist on phagocytes, including Tyro3, Axl, and the so-called MerTK receptor tyrosine kinases (the "TAMs," from the first letter of the three members Tyro3, Axl, and MerTK [148]); the *T-cell immunoglobulin and mucin domain-containing 1 and 4* ("TIM1 and 4") [149]; and the newly identified CD300 family (for reviews, see [150–152]) (for "eat me," also compare Vol. 1 [1], Part IV, Sect. 12.3.2). These numerous phagocytic receptors were found to bind apoptotic bodies directly or indirectly. For example, direct binding to PtdSer can be mediated by receptors of the TIM family. In other instances, soluble extracellular molecules bind to PtdSer and surface receptors, serving as bridging elements. One such molecule, MFG-E8 (also known as lactadherin), connects PtdSer to $\alpha V\beta 3$ integrins, which are efficient phagocytic receptors. Similarly, molecules such as Gas6 and protein S can bridge PtdSer to phagocytic receptors of the TAM family. Derivatives of PtdSer metabolism such lysophosphatidylserine (LysoPS) [153] also contribute to the recognition of apoptotic bodies. The function of most of the PtdSer and LysoPS recognition receptors consists in dampening inflammation by inducing the production of antiinflammatory mediators during the phagocytosis of apoptotic corpses (for LysoPS acting as a IIIC-5 DAMP (= SAMP), see Sect. 3.5.5.1, and also compare Vol. 1 [1], Part IV, Sect. 14.4.5). In addition, many PtdSer receptors are also capable of recognizing other ligands, with some receptors being categorized as scavenger receptors. Of interest are recent findings regarding members of the CD300 family that consists of both activating and inhibitory receptors. Inhibitory receptors, like CD300A, harbor *immunoreceptor tyrosine-based inhibition motifs* (ITIMs) within their intracellular tail to regulate signaling events [151] (for TAMs and ITIMs, also see Vol. 1 [1], Part II, Sect. 5.3.3.4).

2.3.3 Purinergic Receptors: Committed to Sense Extracellular Nucleotides

Purinergic receptors have been described in Vol. 1 [1], Part II, Sect. 5.3.4, and illustrated in Figs. 5.9 and 5.10. They include purine adenosine receptors (P1 receptors, P1Rs) and purine ADP/ATP receptors (P2 receptors, P2Rs) that are activated by the endogenous purines, adenosine, and ATP (plus ADP, UTP, UDP), respectively. On the basis of their signaling properties, P2Rs can be further subdivided into ionotropic P2X receptors (P2XRs) that are nucleotide-gated ion channels and metabotropic P2Y receptors (P2YRs) that are GPCRs. Extracellular purines, like pyrimidines, have significant and diverse effects on many biological processes, including smooth muscle contraction, neurotransmission, exocrine and endocrine secretion, the immune response, inflammation, platelet aggregation, pain, and modulation of cardiac function. There are 19 different receptor proteins for adenosine, adenine and uridine nucleotides, and nucleotide sugars. The majority are functionally expressed in blood vessels, as purinergic receptors in perivascular nerves, vascular smooth muscle cells (VSMCs), and ECs. They have been identified to play roles in the regulation of vascular contractility, immune function, and growth. The endogenous ligands for purine receptors acting as DAMPs, that is, ATP, ADP, UTP, UDP, and adenosine, can be released from different cell types within the vasculature as well as from circulating blood cells including erythrocytes and platelets. For example, in the central and peripheral nervous system, adenosine and ATP are recognized by these receptors as either neurotransmitters or neuromodulators. It is impressive to see the whole spectrum of purinergic receptors to trigger innate immune signaling pathways after recognition/binding to purines secreted by/released from damaged cells, including macrophages, DCs, leukocytes, nerves, platelets, and ECs, that is, pathways starting from instigation of acute inflammatory responses up to long-term (trophic) actions to stimulate cell proliferation. Accordingly, these receptors were shown to be involved in the pathogenesis of human diseases such as cardiovascular and neurological diseases (see also reviews by Burnstock [154–156]).

2.3.4 G Protein-Coupled Receptors: The Largest Family of Cell Surface Receptors

2.3.4.1 General Remarks

G protein-coupled receptors represent the largest family of cell surface receptors known, with an estimated total of more than 1000 members. They are—as the name indicates—able to couple to heterotrimeric G proteins composed of four main families: $G_{i/o}$, G_q, G_s, and G_{12}. The nature of GPCRs has briefly been overviewed in Vol. 1 [1], Part II, Sect. 5.3.5 and Fig. 5.11. As partially described there, GPCRs can be divided, on the basis of sequence homology, into six classes: Class A (rhodopsin-like), Class B (secretin receptor family), Class C (metabotropic glutamate), Class D (fungal mating pheromone receptors), Class E (cyclic AMP receptors), and Class F (frizzled/smoothened). Current notions hold that GPCRs are not static proteins, but rather dynamic structures capable of moving from one posture to the next and adopting unique functional characteristics at each transition. Further, a central feature of these receptors is their capability to interact with a large variety of ligands ranging from particles as small as protons to large proteins. These ligands include lipid-based inflammatory mediators such as prostaglandins, leukotrienes, and platelet-activating factor; vasoactive amines such as histamine and serotonin; nucleotides; signaling peptides and proteins such as vasoactive hormones (i.e., endothelin, catecholamines [norepinephrine], angiotensin II); the complement fragments C3b, C3a, and C5a; chemokines; proteases; bacterial or mitochondrial formylated peptides; and neurotransmitters. In other words, GPCRs, via sensing these various ligands, determine various functions in the body, including blood pressure regulation, contraction of the heart, immune responses, neurotransmission, hormone and enzyme release from exocrine and endocrine glands, and many others (for reviews, see [157, 158]). All these various ligands activate signaling by GPCRs linked to heterotrimeric G proteins composed of α, β, and γ subunits (for additional information, compare Vol. 1 [1], Part II, Sect. 5.3.5 and Fig. 5.11, p. 79). G protein-coupled receptors have also emerged as potential mechanosensors (reviewed in [157, 159, 160]). Indeed, this function has gained increasing attention and, thus, is addressed in more detail below (Sect. 2.4.3). Also, GPCRs have emerged as proton-sensing receptors [161–163].

Mechanistically, GPCR activation is induced by large conformational changes associated with the formation of the G protein-binding site, whereby most agonist-bound, activated-state GPCR structures show a modest contraction of the ligand binding. However, the molecular basis of this activation process is complex and complicated, and molecular understanding of the allosteric coupling between ligand binding and G protein interaction is emerging from structures of several GPCRs crystallized in inactive and active states, spectroscopic data, and computer simulations. Readers interested in detailed knowledge about this burning issue are referred to the competent reviews of Manglik and Kruse [164] and Weis and Kobilka [165].

2.3.4.2 G Protein-Coupled Receptor Signaling

G protein-coupled receptors can convert all these various stimuli into intracellular signals through different mechanisms [166, 167]. Signaling through GPCRs has been briefly touched in Vol. 1 [1], Part VI, Sect. 22.3.10 and is resumed here. In the classical model of receptor activation, GPCR signaling is mediated by guanine nucleotide-binding proteins (G proteins) upon ligand–receptor binding. In the basal state, Gα is anchored to the inner surface of cell membranes and bound to GPCR, guanosine diphosphate (GDP), Gβ, and Gγ. When a ligand such as an inducible DAMP activates GPCR, its signaling commences when the ligand-bound receptor binds to and catalyzes guanosine triphosphate (GTP) for GDP exchange within a Gα subunit (separated from Gβγ subunits whereby GTP binds to the G protein). Both GTP-bound Gα in the active form and the released Gβγ dimer can then go on with signaling to stimulate a number of downstream effectors [168] (for details compare Fig. 5.11, p. 79, in Vol. 1 [1], Part II). According to current concepts [169], initiation of signaling is promoted by a conformational selection at the level of the ligand/GPCR/G protein complex. In fact, crystallographic and other biophysical data have demonstrated how chemically diverse ligands stabilize highly conserved conformational changes on the intracellular side of the receptors, allowing many different extracellular stimuli to utilize shared downstream signaling molecules [164].

Although GPCRs primarily operate by coupling to G proteins, interaction with other scaffold proteins, such as β-arrestins, can influence signaling events [170]. In fact, by contrast to the classical concept, a modern concept, the so-called "biased activation" model, was proposed, upon uncovering the evidence of GPCR activation via the adaptor protein β-arrestin [171, 172]. By the way, β-arrestins are a highly conserved family of cytosolic adaptors that contribute to many immune functions by orchestrating the desensitization and internalization of cell surface GPCRs via well-studied canonical interactions. In cells of the innate and adaptive immune system, β-arrestins also subserve a parallel but less understood role in which they propagate, rather than terminate, intracellular signal transduction cascades (reviewed in [173]). To resume, in this biased activation mode, activated GPCRs recruit either the G protein-dependent pathways or the β-arrestin-dependent pathways (Fig. 2.3). Of note, certain ligands can preferentially trigger some of these signaling pathways, a phenomenon designated as biased agonism or functional selectivity [174]. In other words, this concept describes the ability of ligands to elicit different outcomes while

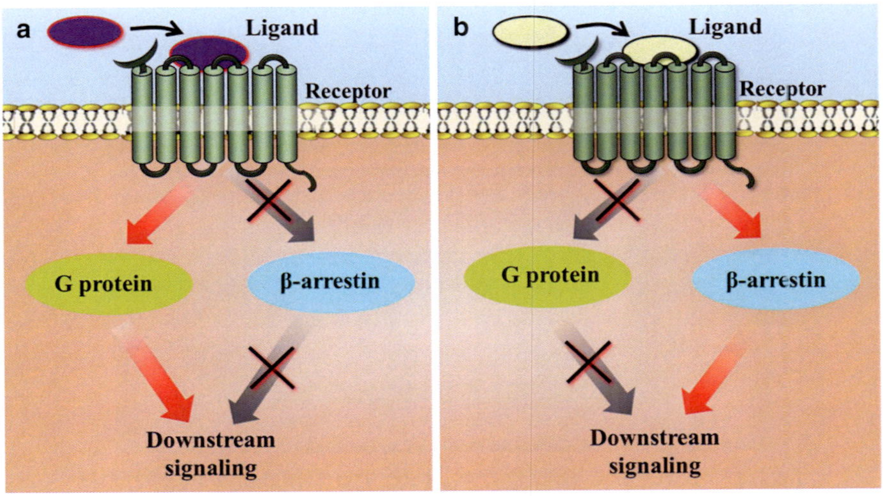

Fig. 2.3 Schematic diagram of a simplified model illustrating the biased activation of G protein-coupled receptors. Two major patterns of biased activation, (**a**) G protein-mediated biased signaling and (**b**) β-arrestin-mediated biased signaling, are shown. A given ligand that activates GPCRs can preferentially recruit either the G protein-dependent pathway or the β-arrestin-dependent pathway. (Sources: [176, 315])

acting on the same GPCR. Accordingly, biased ligands that can selectively influence beneficial signaling pathways may have a high therapeutic potential as drug candidates [170, 174]. Mechanistically, GPCR activation is again induced by large conformational change. After recruitment to activated GPCRs, ubiquitous arrestins mediate desensitization, uncoupling the receptor and G protein, and additionally act as those signaling scaffolds [175]. As discussed elsewhere [169], ligand-determined conformational changes within the bound arrestin influence both the avidity of GPCR-arrestin binding and arrestin engagement of downstream signaling. This scenario is in support of the notion that ligand binding-initiated conformational changes are transmitted through the receptor to impose functionally distinct conformations on intracellular effectors. However, the molecular mechanism of biased activation is still not fully understood. For the sake of completeness, it should be mentioned that, in addition to the two GPCR activation modes touched above, some novel modes of GPCR activation have been proposed including biased activation, intracellular activation, dimerization activation, transactivation, and biphasic activation. They are not further pursued here; for detailed information, the reader is referred to the comprehensive review of Wang et al. [176]). Depending on the effectors selected, downstream cascades are then initiated leading to activation of the *c-Jun-N-terminal protein kinase* (JNK), *signal transducer and activator of transcription* (STAT), phosphatidylinositol 3-kinase (PI3K), and MAPK/*extracellular signal-regulated protein kinase* (ERK) pathways (for reviews, see [169, 177–179]). Also, more recently performed studies reportedly demonstrate the existence, functionality, and architecture of internalized receptor complexes composed of a single GPCR, β-arrestin, and G protein, called "megaplexes" [179]. Another layer of complexity is added by emergent data showing that numerous GPCRs are also associated with various intracellular membranes where they may couple to different signaling systems, display unique desensitization patterns, and/or exhibit distinct patterns of subcellular distribution (for details, see [180]).

2.3.4.3 Endothelin Receptors

Endothelins (ETs) consist of three isoforms and are endothelium-derived vasoconstrictor peptides. All three isoforms of the ET family of peptides, ET-1, ET-2, and ET-3, are expressed in the human kidney, although ET-1 is the predominant isoform. Endothelin-1 is the most potent vasoconstrictor agent currently identified, and it was originally isolated and characterized from the culture media of aortic ECs. The two other isoforms ET-2 and ET-3 were subsequently identified (reviewed in [181]) (for ET-1 as an inducible DAMP, see Sect. 3.5.3.6).

Endothelin-1 and ET-2 bind to two GPCRs, ET_A and ET_B, whereas at physiological concentrations, ET-3 has little affinity for the ET_A receptor. The endothelin receptors are Class A (rhodopsin-like) GPCRs that constitute the largest transmembrane receptor family of the human genome (reviewed by Maguire and Davenport [182, 183]). Endothelin-1 signals via the subtypes ET_A and ET_B, which are Gαq-coupled and belong to GPCRs of the β-group of rhodopsin receptors, which are 21 amino acid long peptides derived from longer prepro-endothelin precursors (see [184]). Together, ET_A and ET_B are critical vasoactive receptors and together with the angiotensin II AT1 receptor (AT_1R, see below) play a crucial role in the pathogenesis of cardiovascular diseases (CVDs) like hypertension, heart failure, stroke, pulmonary hypertension, and cardiac hypertrophy—as will be outlined in Chaps. 10 and 11.

2.3.4.4 Adrenergic Receptors

Adrenergic receptors or adrenoreceptors (ARs) are also GPCRs that can sense epinephrine (Epi) (also called adrenaline) and norepinephrine (NE) (also called noradrenaline) that—besides dopamine—are catecholamines. Though not generally accepted and used, these molecules have been added to the list of inducible DAMPs as detailed in Sect. 3.5.3.4. The story of AR classification has been outlined by Tank and Lee Wong [185]. Originally, the ARs were divided into two broad classes, based upon their ability to either constrict or relax smooth muscle [186]. Their different function then resulted in the concept of two different subtypes, the alpha-ARs (αARs) and beta-ARs (βARs). Over time, however, it became clear that both αARs and βARs consist of at least two family members based on different responses to agonists and antagonists. Until today, nine different human ARs have been identified, classified first into the three classical families α-1 ARs and α-2 ARs and βARs, respectively (for more information, see again [185] and review in [187]). Alpha-1 ARs are further subdivided into the subtypes α-1a ARs and α-1b ARs (and a third subtype) and mediate many of the cardiovascular sympathetic responses to stress, particularly vasoconstriction and, during sustained stimulation, cardiac fibrogenic remodeling [188, 189]. All three receptors are coupled to G_q proteins, leading to activation of phospholipase C and the consequent increase in intracellular calcium and activation of protein kinase C. It is primarily the increase in intracellular calcium that evokes the contraction of smooth muscles rapidly after agonist occupation of αARs. Beta-ARs are subdivided into the subtypes β-1 ARs, β-2 ARs, and β-3 ARs and are particularly important in the regulation of the heart, smooth muscle contraction/relaxation, and metabolic activity [190, 191]. All three βARs couple to G_s proteins and activate adenylyl cyclase to promote intracellular cAMP generation. Depending on the tissue being studied, β-2 and β-3 ARs can also couple to G_i proteins and activate other pathways such as MAPK- and PI3K-mediated paths.

2.3.4.5 Formyl Peptide Receptor Family

The formyl peptide receptors (FPRs) are GPCRs that transduce chemotactic signals mainly in phagocytes, but also sessile innate immune cells such as ECs and mediate inflammatory responses, including cell adhesion, directed migration, granule release, and superoxide production. Also, they are implicated in tissue repair, angiogenesis, and protection against inflammation-associated tumorigenesis. In humans, members of the family include FPR1, FPR2, and FPR3 (reviewed in [192, 193]). In a prototype, FPRs have been shown to recognize MAMPs or DAMPs containing N-formylated methionine such as those produced in bacteria and mitochondria (mitochondrial DAMPs). The repertoire of FPR ligands, however, has expanded rapidly to include not only formyl peptides (FPs) from microbes but also endogenous non-formyl peptides of host origins, synthetic small molecules, and an eicosanoid.

Of note, first clues are suggesting that FPRs are also subject to agonistic activation via so-called functional selectivity or biased agonism, as mentioned above (compare Fig. 2.3). Clearly, this concept opens the way for developing novel FPR-based therapies [194]. In sum, there is no doubt that the FPR family of PRMs is of great importance in many clinically relevant scenarios, for example, in mtDNA-mediated hyperinflammation in trauma patients, as described in Sect. 8.3.3.3.

2.3.4.6 G Protein-Coupled Receptors to Sense Specialized Proresolving Mediators

There are peculiar inflammation-resolving members of the GPCR family that can sense the SPMs as ligands, which function as SAMPs (for SPMs, see Sect. 3.5.5.5). To date, SPMs were found to activate five separate GPCR receptors (reviewed in [195]): ALX/FPR2 or just ALX receptor; resolving *(RV) D1 receptor 1* (DRV1)/GPR32; resolving *(RV) D2 receptor* (DRV2/GPR18; a leukotriene B4 receptor BLT1; and the orphan GPCR ERV/chemerin receptor 23 (ChemR23). While named for the ligand used for identification (lipoxin A4 (LXA4), resolvin E1 (RvE1), resolvin D1 (RvD1), and resolvin D2 (RvD2), respectively), each receptor is capable of interacting with additional SPMs [195].

2.3.4.7 Frizzled Receptors

Frizzled receptors (FZDs) are a family of GPCRs (Class F) that serve as receptors for secreted Wingless-type (Wnt) ligands in the Wnt signaling pathway. The receptors are seven-transmembrane domain-spanning cell surface receptors, whereby ten members (FZD 1 to 10) have been identified within the FZD family in humans (reviewed in [196]). Frizzled proteins are the principal receptors for the Wnt family of ligands. They mediate canonical Wnt signaling together with *low-density lipoprotein receptor-related protein 5* (LRP5) and LRP6 co-receptors (for Wnt pathway, see also Box 2.1). Binding of canonical Wnt ligands (such asWnt1, Wnt3/3a, Wnt7a/b, Wnt8a/b, andWnt10a/b) to a complex of FZD receptors and LRP5/6 co-receptor leads to the accumulation of β-catenin. Following accumulation, β-catenin enters the nucleus and leads to the formation of complexes with T-cell factor (TCF)/*lymphoid enhancer factor proteins* (LEF proteins) and the activation of target genes (also compare Fig. 6.3 in Chap. 6). By contrast to this canonical pathway, the noncanonical pathways operate independently of β-catenin (planar cell polarity pathway and Wnt/Ca^{2+} pathway). Notably, the Wnt↔FZD signaling pathway is implicated in development and disease via maintenance of tissue homeostasis, regeneration, plasticity, and repair (reviewed in [197–200]). The pathway's role in fibrogenesis is briefly outlined in Sect. 6.5.3.4 in the context of myofibroblast activation (for Wnt as an inducible DAMP, see Sect. 3.5.4.5).

2.3.4.8 Proton-Sensing G Protein-Coupled Receptors

Proton-sensing GPCRs are Class A GPCRs that are expressed by various cells (by neutrophil macrophages, DCs, and ECs) and in various tissue and encompass four receptors, that is, GPR4, GPR65 (TDAG8), GPR68 (OGR1), and GPR132 (G2A). These GPCRs have been proposed to be activated by acidic extracellular pH through the protonation of several histidine residues of these receptors, once extracellular pH drops below the physiological range, that is, below the tightly controlled value of around pH 7.4 in blood and tissue (reviewed by Weiß et al. [163] and Justus et al. [201]).

A fundamental question in GPCR activation concerns the mechanism that couples agonist binding at the extracellular side with the conformational opening at the cytoplasmic face. As proposed by Zhang et al. [202, 203], it appears to be the dynamics of protonation, rather than protonation per se that affects the activation status of this Class A GPCR. In other words, it is a change in protonation status, together with proton transfer via conserved structural elements located in the transmembrane region that is the key element essential for signal transduction across the membrane. In this sense, this class of GPCRs may be regarded as mechanosensors able to sense proton-induced conformational changes. Indeed, the proton-sensing GPCRs trigger a plethora of signaling pathways that control critical processes in tumor growth and wound healing, such as neoangiogenesis, cell proliferation, and migration. Notably, these receptors have been shown to regulate inflammatory responses, qualifying them as typical receptors of the innate immune system (reported, e.g., in [204–206]). In fact, the demonstration of distinct GPCRs to sense protons such as generated in acidosis provides convincing evidence in support of the notion that receptors of the innate immune system have been evolutionarily developed to sense cell-extrinsic homeostatic danger signals/dyshomeostatic DAMPs that are comparable to cell-intrinsic dyshomeostatic DAMPs (for additional information also compare Vol. 1 [1], Part IV, Sect. 13.4.5, p. 289, and compare Sect. 2.4.5).

2.3.4.9 Adhesion G Protein-Coupled Receptors

The adhesion GPCRs represent the second-largest group of the human GPCR superfamily and are supposed to be evolutionarily ancient molecules conserved from *Tetrahymena* to mammals [146]. Thirty-three members have been discovered in mammals, and they have multiple features distinguishing them from the other classes of GPCRs. For example, unlike conventional GPCRs, adhesion GPCRs have extended ectodomains with various protein folds that facilitate protein↔protein interactions and, hence, putative cellular adhesive functions, in particular, in cell↔cell interactions. These PRMs are now termed ADGR (for adhesion G protein-coupled receptors) as a common dominator, followed by a letter and a number to denote each subfamily and subtype, respectively (for reviews, see [207–210]). Interestingly, the subtype ADGRB1 has been found to act as a macrophage receptor for the DAMP phosphatidylserine on apoptotic cells [211] and lipopolysaccharide (LPS) that may be regarded as an exogenous DAMP [212] (for lysophosphatidylserine acting as a putative inducible inflammation-resolving DAMP (= SAMP) and LPS, see Vol. 1 [1], Part IV, Sect. 11.2.6, and Sect. 14.4.5).

Together, adhesive GPCRs appear to be crucial receptors in innate and adaptive immunity and have gained increasing attention. Further studies will certainly provide us with some more information about their biological functions in health and disease.

2.3.4.10 Concluding Remarks

Impressively, it has become clear that GPCRs mediate the majority of cellular responses to external stimuli. However, their activation by ligands such as DAMPs is complex and still not fully understood. As outlined in this section, active states of GPCRs form small rearrangements of the ligand-binding or orthosteric site that are amplified into larger conformational changes. In this context, Weis and Kobilka [165] argue in the abstract of their article on "The Molecular Basis of G Protein-Coupled Receptor Activation": "Molecular understanding of the allosteric coupling between ligand binding and G protein or arrestin interaction is emerging from structures of several GPCRs crystallized in inactive and active states, spectroscopic data, and computer simulations. The coupling is loose, rather than concerted, and agonist binding does not fully stabilize the receptor in an active conformation. Distinct intermediates whose populations are shifted by ligands of different efficacies underlie the complex pharmacology of GPCRs."

2.3.5 Nociceptors: The Sensors of the Pain Pathway

Nociception is the process of transmission of painful signals by nociceptors (i.e., specialized primary sensory neurons essential for the perception of pain) in the primary afferent nerve fibers, which specifically respond to noxious stimuli (for additional information, see also Vol. 1 [1], Part II, Sect. 5.3.6, p.81). These noxious stimuli are detected by nociceptors and converted into electrical signals, which are then transmitted to the spinal cord, thalamus, and cerebral cortex via the discriminative pain pathway, leading to the final perception of pain [213, 214]. Several of the TLRs and RAGE have been implicated in playing critical roles in pain signaling [215]. In addition to these "familiar" PRRs, there appear to exist some special "non-classical" PRMs, including GPCRs [216, 217] and *transient receptor potential* (TRP) ion channels [218].

The TRP ion channels have emerged as a family of evolutionarily conserved ligand-gated ion channels that function as molecular detectors of damaging stimuli and, as mechanosensors, of mechanical forces. Several members of this family, at least six channels from three TRP family subtypes (*transient receptor potential vanilloid subtype 1–4* [TRPV1-4], *transient receptor potential cation channel subfamily M member 8* [TRPM8], and *transient receptor potential ankyrin 1* [TRPA1]), are expressed in nociceptors, where they act as transducers for danger signals from thermal, chemical, and mechanical stimuli, thereby playing crucial roles in the generation and development of pathological pain perception [218–220].

Importantly, as recently highlighted by Pinho-Ribeiro et al. [221], nociceptor sensory neurons do not only protect organisms from danger by eliciting pain and driving avoidance; but also an active crosstalk occurs operating between nociceptor neurons and the innate/adaptive immune system to regulate pain, host defense, and inflammatory diseases. The authors summarized: "Immune cells at peripheral nerve terminals and within the spinal cord release mediators that modulate mechanical and thermal sensitivity. In turn, nociceptor neurons release neuropeptides and neurotransmitters from nerve terminals that regulate vascular, innate, and adaptive immune cell responses. Therefore, the dialog between nociceptor neurons and the immune system is a fundamental aspect of inflammation, both acute and chronic. A better understanding of these interactions could produce approaches to treat chronic pain and inflammatory diseases." Nociceptors are sensitized by inflammatory mediators produced by the immune system, including cytokines, lipid mediators, and growth factors, and can also directly detect pathogens and their secreted products to produce pain during infection [222]. One may add that evidence accumulates supporting a role of both endogenous and exogenous DAMPs in activating those nociceptors (for additional information also compare Vol. 1 [1], Part IV, Sect. 15.3, p. 355).

2.3.6 The Superfamily of Immunoglobulin Receptors

2.3.6.1 General Remarks

The immunoglobulin superfamily is a heterogenic group of proteins built on a common fold, called the Ig fold, which is a sandwich of two beta sheets. Although members of the immunoglobulin superfamily share a similar immunoglobulin fold, they differ in their tissue distribution, amino acid composition, and biological role (reviewed in [223]). It is not the purpose of this section to examine these receptors in detail. Prominent members of this family are the human *killer cell immunoglobulin-like receptors* (KIRs) that have been addressed in Vol. 1 [1], Part II, Sect. 5.3.7.2, and are briefly touched again in the next section. Here, a few remarks are made to *the triggering receptors expressed on myeloid cells* (TREMs), which have recently gained increasing attention.

2.3.6.2 Recognition Receptors of Innate Lymphoid Cells

The family of innate lymphoid cells (ILCs) can be divided into three groups and has been addressed in more detail in Vol. 1 [1], Part III, Sect. 8.4. Numerous NK-cell receptors recognizing classic and nonclassic MHC-I molecules encoded by genes within the MHC locus have been identified, including the human KIRs and the conserved *CD94/natural killer group 2* (NKG2) receptor family. Typically, NK-cell function is regulated by a delicate balance between those germline-encoded activating and inhibitory receptors on their cell surface. Out of the NKG2 receptor family, the NKG2D receptor perceives any cell stress via recognition of an extensive repertoire of NKG2D ligands, denoted as Subclass IB-2 DAMPs that are upregulated on hyperproliferative, transformed, and damaged cells [224–226] (for these DAMPs, see Vol. 1 [1], Part IV, Section 12.3.3). For more details, the reader is referred to Vol. 1 [1], Part II, Sect. 5.3.7, as well as to recent review published by Rajalingam [227] emphasizing the diversity of KIRs and disease. Also, the reader is invited to read the article of Barrow and Colonna [228] that highlights the battery of specialized receptors of ILCs to sense not only DAMPs but also cytokines and other inflammatory mediators, metabolites, neuronal signals, hormones, and growth factors that are secreted by myeloid cells and specialized epithelial and stromal cells.

2.3.6.3 Triggering Receptors Expressed on Myeloid Cells

The TREM family comprises both activating and inhibitory receptors. Among these family members, TREM-1 represents the most studied activating receptor, whereas TREM-2 is known as an inhibitor of the inflammatory response (for reviews, see [229–231]). The receptor is expressed mostly on myeloid cells, including monocytes, macrophages, and neutrophils, and recognized as a potent amplifier of acute and chronic inflammation. TREM-1 plays a critical role in macrophage polarization and induces the M1-like macrophages. Following activation, TREM-1 results in downstream signaling through protein kinases that promote the secretion of proinflammatory cytokines. Because of the absence of signaling motifs, TREM-1 constitutively associates with DNAX-activating protein 12 (DAP12) for induction of intracellular signals (for DAP12, compare Vol. 1 [1], Part II, Sect. 5.3.7.3 and Fig. 5.12). Moreover, TREM-1 has also been shown to modulate signaling pathways induced by known classes of PRRs, such as TLRs and NLRs. However, the exact mechanisms through which TREM-1 influences TLR and NLR pathways are still largely elusive. Similar to DAMPs, TREM-1 is believed to play a crucial role in both acute and chronic forms of sterile inflammation. This may explain the similarities observed in the cascade of events occurring during sterile or infectious inflammation, including the activation of TREM-1 as an amplifier of TLRs [230]. Overall, TREM-1 was shown to be implicated in the pathogenesis of acute and chronic cardiovascular conditions, such as acute myocardial infarction, stroke, and atherosclerosis.

2.3.6.4 Concluding Remarks

Notably, both classes of receptors have gained increasing attention in research on CVDs for several reasons. For example, TREM-1 has an important role as an inflammatory orchestrator and player and functions by interacting with PRRs and their putative DAMPS and MAMPS. Hence, Kouassi et al. [230] have foreseen that "any intervention that will downplay the role of TREM-1 will be beneficial in the long run to prevent atherosclerosis and its detrimental consequences of acute myocardial infarction, stroke, or ischemia of the extremities."

2.3.7 Fragment Crystallizable Region Receptors: Tools of Cells to Bind to Antibodies

The Fc region (or just Fc) is the tail region of an antibody that interacts with cell surface receptors called FcRs and some proteins of the complement system. Members of the Fc receptor family are type I transmembrane proteins (except human *glycosylphosphatidylinositol* (GPI)-anchored FcγRIIIB) that produce activating (human FcγRI, FcγRIIA, FcγRIIC, FcγRIIIA, FcγRIIIB, and FcεRI) or inhibitory (human FcγRIIB) signals. The various types of FcRs are classified based on the type of antibody that they recognize. The Latin letter used to identify a type of antibody is converted into the corresponding Greek letter, which is placed after the "Fc" part of the name. For example, those that bind the most common class of antibody, immunoglobulin G (IgG), are called FcγRs, those that bind IgA are called FcαRs, and those that bind IgE are called FcεRs. Membrane FcRs trigger and regulate biological responses of cells on which they are expressed. Moreover, FcRs deliver signals when they are aggregated at the cell surface (for more information, see [232–238] and Vol. 1 [1], Part II, Sect. 5.3.8).

2.3.8 Résumé

As stated above, the distinction between "classical" and "nonclassical" recognition receptors as described here is rather arbitrary. Accordingly, "nonclassical" receptors are as important as their "classical" counterparts. This assessment is illustrated in addition to that alone that various classical/nonclassical PRMs are known to communicate in highly sophisticated crosstalks. Here, it is worth noting that a group of PRMs has recently gained special attention: the mechanosensors. They will, therefore, be discussed separately in the following section.

2.4 Cell-Associated "Nonclassical" Recognition Molecules: Mechanosensors

2.4.1 Introductory Remarks to Mechanosensitivity

All organisms from bacteria to humans are mechanosensitive. Numerous mechanical forces operate daily in our body and are consciously or unconsciously sensed by various types of cells. Among the five very well-known traditional human senses, sound and touch rely on mechanical forces, such as vibration and pressure that are perceived mainly by sensory neurons. Pulmonary cells experience inflation and deflation of the lungs to regulate their physiology. Muscle cell hypertrophy is primarily triggered by mechanical load/tensile forces during exercise and strength training. Endothelial cells lining the lumen of blood vessels are exposed to blood flow, causing a shear force on the cells (shear stress = the force per unit area exerted on a surface by a moving fluid). Tubular cells in the kidney sense osmotic pressure caused by ion transport across the cell membrane. Chondrocytes of the spine and joints of the lower extremities experience compressive forces. And last but not least, tensile forces occurring during cell–cell and cell–extracellular matrix (ECM) interactions determine the behavior and fate of cells (for further reading, see competent articles under [239–246]).

The capability of cells to sense, integrate, and respond to all these different stressful mechanical cues received from their microenvironment is vital for numerous biological processes, including maintenance of tissue homeostasis [247, 248]. Indeed, the field of mechanobiology has profoundly emerged in the past two decades, greatly increasing our knowledge of how mechanical stimuli orchestrate cell behavior. In particular, the seminal discoveries of special receptors that sense those stimuli—called mechanosensors—at the level of cell↔cell and cell↔ECM adhesion sites have enriched the knowledge of experts in this area of research tremendously. Though mechanosensors are not generally considered to function as typical PRMs of the innate immune system, they refer to first-line host defense mechanisms that operate in the early stages of homeostatic disruption, that is, a property that qualifies them as innate surveillance sensors (compare Fig. 1.1). Typically, however, when mechanical forces turn out to be too stressful and severe or persist over a long period of time, the elicited response may be inadequate leading to pathologies.

2.4.1.1 Mechanotransduction Pathways

The mechanosensors trigger mechanotransduction pathways, that is, a process by which cells convert mechanical stimuli from their extracellular microenvironment or cell-generated forces into biochemical signals to induce downstream cellular responses. Interestingly, some of those receptors, such as the GPCRs mentioned above and TRP ion channels, are known to trigger mechanically induced innate homeostatic surveillance responses as well (as will also be discussed in more detail below).

Accordingly, mechanoreceptors are responsible for the manifestation of many clinical phenomena. For example, as known by every physician, blood pressure is tightly regulated to guarantee that the body is prepared to meet the various activity demands. And indeed, within seconds and minutes, regulation of the blood pressure is initiated primarily by special mechanosensors, the baroreceptors, a class of stretch-sensitive neurons that are located primarily in the carotid artery sinuses and aortic arch [249].

However, as noted throughout the book, as with other innate homeostatic responses, when dysregulated or excessive, mechanosensor-triggered signaling pathways are reportedly involved in the pathogenesis of many human diseases, cardiovascular and fibrotic disorders being shining examples (see also Chaps. 6, 10, and 11).

To date, several mechanosensitive molecules have been described that trigger different signaling (mechanotransduction) pathways. They include stretch-activated ion channels, GPCRs, focal adhesion proteins (integrins), growth factor receptors, and phospholipid bilayer of the plasma membrane itself. Of note, mechanosensors do not get activated by physical binding to a cognate ligand. Thus, cells must use other mechanisms in sensing and responding to mechanical forces. However, these molecular mechanisms are still poorly understood. Generally, it is believed that mechanical forces induce changes in protein conformation.

2.4.1.2 Mechanical Force-Induced Conformational Changes

Conformational changes may be classified into six categories (reviewed by Chen et al. [250]):

1. Deformation of the global shape of mechanosensitive proteins, e.g., pore-forming membrane ion channels like TRP channels
2. Relative displacement of channels
3. Hinge movement (for proteins or their subunits that consist of two or more distinct globular domains connected by a hinge region, such as integrin)
4. Unfolding and unmasking a specific protein domain (to expose cryptic cleaving, binding, or enzymatic sites)
5. Translocation and rotation of a protein noncovalently complexed with a subunit or subunit of a polymeric filament (forming new bonds with the subunit from the other side)
6. Rearrangement of clustered proteins (which, through their mutual interactions, act on the adjacent structures and change their arrangement)

Here, some of those sensors are briefly and selectively described (for more information, the reader is referred to reviews and competent articles listed under [246, 251–253]).

2.4.2 Mechanosensitive Ion Channels

2.4.2.1 General Remarks

Mechanosensitive ion channels are evolutionarily conserved molecules that play a vital role in perceiving the mechanical signals experienced by various cell types [251]. The channels are pore-forming proteins that allow the flow of ions such as calcium, chloride, and/or potassium ions across plasma membranes. Mechanosensitive channels are currently regarded as major mechanosensors, transducing mechanical stimuli exerted on membranes of living cells into electrical or chemical intracellular signals [254, 255]. This category of channels can switch from "closed" to "open" state in response to stretch alone or to a direct mechanical force-induced membrane deformation (reviewed in [256]).

2.4.2.2 Transient Receptor Potential Channels

Mammalian TRP channels mediate the transmembrane flux of cations down their electrochemical gradients, thereby raising intracellular Ca^{2+} and Na^{+} concentrations and depolarizing the cell (reviewed in [257]). The channel proteins form six-transmembrane cation-permeable channels that may be grouped into six subfamilies on the basis of amino acid sequence homology (TRPV, TRPC, TRPM, TRPA, TRPP, and TRPML). Here, a few words are mentioned to TRPV and TRPC channels.

Transient Receptor Potential Vanilloid Family Channels

There is compelling evidence indicating that members of the TRPV family operate as critical mechanosensors through their membrane stretch-dependent properties, besides their role as nociceptors to perceive noxious stimuli (for additional information also compare Vol. 1 [1], Part II, Sect. 5.3.6, p. 81). One such receptor is TRPV2 that exerts several functions; among them, the mechanosensitive property has emerged. Earlier studies already suggested that TRPV2 channels in ECs may function as mechanosensors to transport Ca^{2+} in a stretch-dependent manner and showed further that the TRPV2 is critical for the maintenance of cardiac structure and function [258, 259].

More recent studies supported the idea by showing that TRPV2 channels play a key role in the function and structure of the heart, being involved in the cardiac compensatory mechanisms in response to pathologic or exercise-induced stress (reviewed in [260]). The authors discussed that "TRPV2 proteins form a part of cardiac stretch-activated channels and the major role of TRPV2 channels in the cardiac dystrophic Ca^{2+} signaling pathology is demonstrated. Nevertheless, mechanisms by which TPRV2 channels could play as mechanosensor for the mechano-electric coupling in healthy heart need to be understood."

Another crucial member of this family is TRPV4 that has also been demonstrated to act as a mechanosensitive ion channel. Activation of TRPV4 ion channels is associated with a massive influx of Ca^{2+} that licenses the cell to perform a vital role in regulating its functioning. As comprehensively reviewed by White et al. [261], "TRPV4 is now credited as being a major player in human physiology, crucially functioning not only in the maintenance of vascular tone and EC function, but also in the cardiac, respiratory, urinary, skeletal, and digestive systems, as well as in the central and peripheral nervous systems, while also being responsible for various channelopathy-induced hereditary diseases and pain of several different contexts of origin." This mechanosensor has been shown to respond to various stimuli on the endothelium, such as shear stress, pressure, acidic pH, and hypo-osmolarity [261–266]. Activation of endothelial TRPV4 was observed to result in vasodilatation. For example, in human coronary arterioles, blood flow-induced vasodilatation was shown to be mediated by TRPV4 that is accompanied by ROS generation [267].

Activation of TRPV4 is triggered by the application of force to the cell membrane, whether that mechanical force is generated by trauma, hypotonicity, or hypertonicity, to induce physiological effects. The mechanical pressure exerted on the cell membrane is thought to result in (some) deformation of the cell membrane, for example, in the form of cell stretch. However—as discussed by White et al. [261]—as to what constitutes the mechanism of action of such cell stretch or other deformation changes of the membrane, which induces the activation of TRPV4 is not entirely clear.

Transient Receptor Potential Canonical Family Channels

Transient receptor potential canonical channels are highly homologous, nonselective cation channels that form a family of voltage-sensitive calcium ion channels. These channels are highly abundant in the brain and kidney and have been implicated in numerous diseases, such as cancer, depression, addiction, and chronic kidney disease, among others. They are not further discussed here; instead, the reader is referred to informative articles under [268–271].

2.4.2.3 Piezo Family Proteins

Besides members of the TRPV family, the evolutionarily conserved Piezo family of proteins, including Piezo1 and Piezo2, has gained recent attention [272]. This family encodes the mammalian mechanosensitive cation channels that play critical roles in various mechanotransduction processes, such as mediated by touch, pain, and blood pressure. Mechanistically, the function of Piezo proteins is still not clear. It is suggested that the complex Piezo proteins can be deduced into discrete ion-conducting pore modules, which coordinate to fulfill their specialized function in mechanical sensing and transduction, ion permeation, and selection (compare Fig. 2.4; for reviews see Syeda et al. [273], Wang and Xiao [274], and Burke et al.

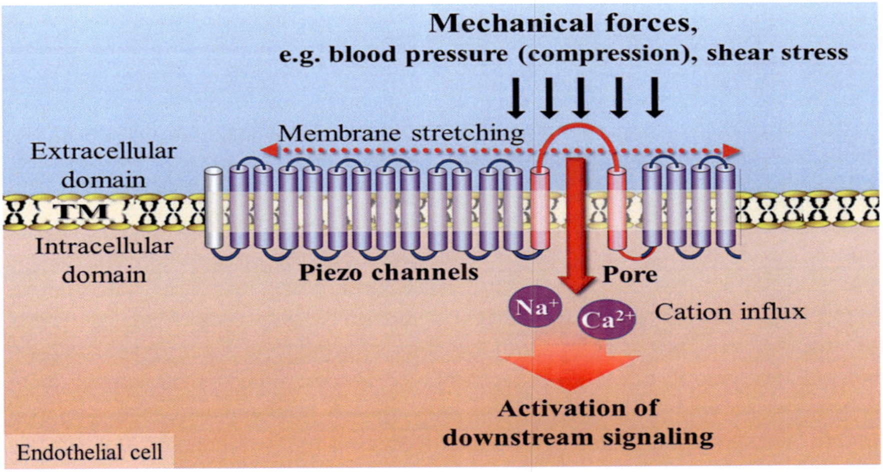

Fig. 2.4 Schematic diagram of a simplified model proposing activation of PIEZO ion channels by mechanical forces. The channels are supposed to be opened by force-induced motion associated with membrane tension resulting in altered conformational arrangement and gating of the channels. Mechanical forces promote cation influx via PIEZO channels. Shear stress or pressure-induced compression change surface tension in the cell membrane to activate the PIEZO channel that in turn leads to increased intracellular cations and activation of downstream signaling. *TM* transmembrane domain. (Sources: [273–275, 316])

[275]). Wang and Xiao state: "The identification and demonstration of Piezo proteins as the bona fide mechanosensitive cation channels has heralded a new era of research in the mechanotransduction field and tremendous progress has been made towards characterizing their physiological and pathophysiological significance, human diseases, biophysical properties, and molecular mechanisms." And Syeda et al. stress [273]: "… we show that mechanical perturbations of the lipid bilayer alone are sufficient to activate Piezo channels, illustrating their innate ability as molecular force transducers." Nota bene: this remark is reminiscent to the definition of danger signals in terms of dyshomeostasis-associated molecular patterns (IIC-4 DAMPs) sensed by various receptors such as *protein kinase RNA-like endoplasmic reticulum kinase* (PERK) (for additional information see Vol. 1 [1], Part IV, Sect. 13.4.5, p. 289, and Fig. 13.2, p. 290).

Of note, the mechanically activated ion channels Piezo1 and Piezo2 were recently discovered to function as the long-sought baroreceptor mechanosensors critical for acute blood pressure control (Zeng et al. [276] and Burke et al. [275]). Baroreceptors are a type of pressure sensors on specialized neurons that specifically perceive stretch within arterial walls, which happens when blood pressure elevates (also compare Fig. 2.4). When baroreceptors are stretched, they transmit afferent (sensory) signals to the autonomic nervous system. This information is then passed in rapid sequence to alter the total peripheral resistance and cardiac output maintaining blood pressure within a preset, normalized range. Two types of baroreceptors have been described, high-pressure arterial baroreceptors and low-pressure volume receptors, which are both stimulated by stretching of the vessel wall. Arterial baroreceptors are localized within the carotid sinuses and the aortic arch. Low-pressure volume receptors, or cardiopulmonary receptors, are located within the atria, ventricles, and pulmonary vasculature (for a comprehensive review, see Armstrong and Moore [277]).

A recent study revealed that both ion channels Piezo1 and Piezo2 are together required for arterial baroreceptor activity and function. This observation is an important finding in view of the fact that the baroreflex is critical in maintaining short-term blood pressure homeostasis in mammals. As commented elsewhere [278], this discovery has the potential to impact clinical practice if medications could be designed to target these receptors. Moreover, this new knowledge contributes to elucidating the phenomenon of "how a pure mechanical change or pressure change is translated to neuronal signaling in one of the most essential reflex mechanisms of the human body." Seen through "the glasses of the DAMPome," one might add that this discovery supports the concept of PRMs able to sense dyshomeostasis-associated molecular patterns, aimed at maintaining homeostasis.

2.4.2.4 Concluding Remarks

The experts' understanding of the biophysical principles of mechanosensitive channel gating mechanisms has significantly increased over the last decade. With regard to pathology of various diseases, there is accumulating evidence for mechanosensitive ion channels to play a critical role in many diseases such as CVD. For example, arterial baroreceptors have already been considered as a potential therapeutic target to improve the prognosis of patients with CVD and diabetes [279] (also compare Sect. 10.3.2.3).

2.4.3 Mechanosensitive G Protein-Coupled Receptors

2.4.3.1 General Remarks

Numerous GPCRs including angiotensin II AT1 receptors (AT_1R), the bradykinin B2, ET_A, the FPR1, the parathyroid hormone type 1, histamine H1, and muscarinic M5 have been proposed as mechanosensors [159]. Here, some of these receptors known to be involved in the pathogenesis of human diseases are briefly touched.

2.4.3.2 Gq/11 Protein-Coupled Angiotensin II Receptors

The octapeptide hormone angiotensin II (Ang II)—regarded in this book as an inducible DAMP as outlined in Sect. 3.5.3.5—acts through two pharmacologically distinct GPCRs, AT_1R and AT_2R [280, 281]. Human cells possess a single AT_1R, while two isoforms can be found in rats and mice. Expression of AT_1A (gene) was shown to be evident in vascular smooth muscle, kidney, liver, adrenal gland, brain, lung, heart, and some other tissues of adult mice [282].

The AT_1R is a prototypical GPCR that is expressed in many tissues and organs, including heart and vasculature, and is regarded as the main receptor that mediates the effects of the renin–angiotensin system (RAS) or renin–angiotensin–aldosterone system (RAAS). In fact, RAS constitutes a key hormonal system in the physiological regulation of blood pressure through peripheral and central mechanisms, whereby the receptor AT_1R plays a critical role. Then, the classic RAS encompasses the *angiotensin-converting enzyme (ACE)–Ang II–*AT_1R axis that promotes vasoconstriction, water intake, sodium retention, as well as increased oxidative stress, fibrosis, cellular growth, and inflammation (reviewed in [283, 284]). In addition, AT_1R was shown to be also involved in the regulation of salt–water homeostasis and, pathogenically, in disorders such as hypertension, heart failure, cardiovascular remodeling, renal fibrosis, inflammation, and metabolic disorders (reviewed in [285]). Notably, the AT_1R are activated not only by binding to Ang II (= ligand-dependent activation) but also by mechanical stress, qualifying them as mechanosensors (= ligand-independent activation). As such mechanosensors, the AT_1R was identified in VSMCs to mediate myogenic vasoconstriction, whereby mechanical receptor activation was supposed to be instigated by a conformational change of the receptor protein [286–289].

Stimulation of AT_1R results in pleiotropic signal transduction pathways that generate arrays of complex cellular responses. Upon binding with its ligand Ang II, AT_1R activates a series of downstream signaling molecules. The classical AT_1R path operates through recruiting heterotrimeric G proteins $G\alpha q/11$, $G\alpha 12/13$, and

Gβγ, which activate downstream effectors including phospholipase C, phospholipase A2, and phospholipase D. This classical pathway was demonstrated to promote vasoconstriction and hypertension. Moreover, AT_1R was found to signal G protein independently through β-arrestin-1 or β-arrestin-2, which stimulates cell growth and promotes cell survival via the ERK and Ca^{2+} pathways (reviewed in [290–292]; for recruitment of heterotrimeric G proteins, also compare Vol. 1 [1], Part II, Fig. 5.11 in Sect. 5.3.5, and for signaling pathways, see also Part VI, Sect. 22.3.10). Notably, in contrast to humans, rodents express two isoforms of the AT_1R, AT_1A, and AT_1B [293, 294]. Findings from more recent experimental studies in mice provided evidence suggesting that AT_1B receptors are not only essential for the extent of myogenic vasoconstriction but also determine the kinetics of the myogenic response [295].

Together, the AT_1R is a critical vasoactive receptor and, thus, as will be outlined in Chaps. 10 and 11 plays a crucial role in the pathogenesis of CVD.

2.4.3.3 Adhesion G Protein-Coupled Receptors

Adhesive GPCRs—briefly introduced above—have also been proposed to act as mechanosensors, though their mechanism of action is fully unknown (reviewed by Scholz et al. [296, 297]). For example, in a murine model of overload-induced muscle hypertrophy, GPR56 was found to be induced in humans by resistance exercise [298]. As a DAMP, the investigators identified collagen type III and argued that these findings imply that variations in GPR56 expression caused by disease or aging could affect the ability of a muscle to adapt to mechanical loading. And obviously, the capability of skeletal muscle to adapt to mechanical stimuli is vital for health and well-being. Other lines of studies in a *Drosophila melanogaster* model revealed that adhesive GPCR may generally process and modulate the perception of mechanical signals, linking these crucial stimuli to the sensory canon of the GPCR superfamily [299]. The authors concluded that the findings from their model provide an unprecedented opportunity to uncover features, which might prove of general relevance for the function and regulation of the entire adhesive GPCR class.

2.4.3.4 Wnt↔Frizzled Receptors

Frizzled receptors (class F GPCRs) sensing Wnt ligands (i.e., DAMPs) have also been observed to operate as mechanosensors (compare Box 2.1). Thus, experiments on murine models showed that endothelial noncanonical Wnt signaling regulates endothelial sensitivity to shear forces. Loss of Wnt5a/Wnt11 was found to render ECs more sensitive to shear, resulting in axial polarization and migration against the flow at lower shear levels [235]. Also, canonical Wnt-frizzled → β-catenin signaling has been shown to be activated by mechanical loading of osteocytes. In fact, β-catenin is considered a central molecule that is necessary to maintain bone homeostasis and mechanotransduction through maintenance of osteocyte viability [300, 301] (for Wnt-frizzled → β-catenin signaling, also compare Sect. 6.5.3.4 and Fig. 6.3).

Box 2.1 The Wnt Pathway

The Wnt pathway is a highly conserved innate immune signal transduction cascade that controls myriad biological phenomena throughout development and adult life of all animals. The name Wnt is resultant from a fusion of the name of the *Drosophila* segment polarity gene *wingless* and the name of the vertebrate homolog, integrated or int-1. Wnt proteins regulate a dizzying array of cellular processes, including cell fate determination, motility, polarity, primary axis formation, and organogenesis. Most recently, this pathway has also been implicated in stem cell renewal. The extracellular Wnt signal stimulates several intracellular signal transduction cascades, including the canonical or Wnt/β-catenin-dependent pathway and the noncanonical or β-catenin-independent pathway that can be divided into the *planar cell polarity* pathway and the Wnt/$Ca2^+$ pathway. All three pathways are activated by the binding of a Wnt-protein ligand to a so-called Frizzled family receptor (see also Sect. 2.3.4.7). The defective Wnt signaling is a causative factor for a number of pleiotropic human pathologies, including cancers of the breast, colon, and skin, skeletal defects, as well as human birth defect disorders. The role of Wnt in TGF-β signaling, that is, in fibrogenesis, is described in Chap. 6, Sect. 6.5.3.4 and Fig. 6.3.

For further reading, see [199, 317, 318]

2.4.3.5 Concluding Remarks

The unique action of several GPCRs as mechanosensors points out that these PRMs possess an enormous diversity of innate immune functions. Indeed, over the past years, these mechanosensitive receptors emerged as important players in recognizing DAMPs involved in chronic inflammatory processes. For example, in atherogenesis, prohypertensive DAMPs sensed by GPCRs in the form of mechanically induced dyshomeostatic DAMPs may be discussed to lead to the generation of *nicotinamide adenine dinucleotide phosphate* (NADPH) oxidases via GPCR signaling, thereby contributing to hypertension-mediated ROS production at the arterial wall (the topic will be resumed in Sect. 10.3.3).

2.4.4 Mechanosensitive Integrins (Focal Adhesion Proteins)

Integrins are transmembrane adhesion proteins that exist as heterodimers consisting of one α and one β subunit. The proteins interact with 156 known partners collectively referred to as the "integrin adhesome" [302]. Notably, integrins not only facilitate cell↔cell adhesion but also induce intracellular signaling and have recently been uncovered as mechanosensors providing additional complexity to the signaling pathways, termed mechanotransduction [303]. The adhesive proteins act as conduits of bidirectional signaling, directly connecting extracellular inputs to intracellular outputs. This connection allows transduction of mechanical forces generated by the nuclear actin retrograde flow and myosin II to the ECM through mechanosensitive focal adhesion proteins that are collectively termed the "molecular clutch." Upon ligand binding, integrins recruit numerous proteins to their cytoplasmic tails, leading to the assembly of diverse adhesion structures that differ in their morphology and subcellular localization as well as in their protein composition and mechanical properties (reviewed by Sun et al. [304]). As mechanosensors, these proteins can be regarded as bidirectional, that is, "inside-out and outside-in" transmembrane signaling machines that trigger mechanotransduction pathways through the ECM → integrin → focal adhesions → cytoskeleton → nucleus → mechanosensitive genes axis.

In view of a large number of interaction partners, a crosstalk of integrins with other membrane receptors and downstream signaling pathways takes place, including GPCRs and tyrosine kinase receptors affecting adrenergic and growth factor signaling (for further reading, see [305–309]).

Further details of the role of integrins in cellular mechanotransduction will be outlined when describing their function in progressive fibrosis (see Sect. 6.3, and also compare Figs. 6.1 and 6.2).

2.4.5 Résumé

As noted by the reader, the mechanisms of activating mechanosensors by various stimuli such as pressure, osmolarity, and shear stress are not fully understood. As a common denominator, conformational changes and dynamics are widely discussed and agreed upon to be critical to the mechanisms by which transmembrane receptors transmit signals across membranes [310]. Such deformative protein alterations may occur by changes in structure and dynamics, reorganization of protein↔protein interfaces, or changes in receptor oligomerization, whereby—as argued by Wang et al. about ligand binding [311]—protein dynamics appears to play a key and general role in receptor activation. Hence, concerning sensing mechanical forces without prove of ligand binding, the concept of perceiving homeostatic danger signals [312] by mechanosensors can still be continued to be maintained. Accordingly, and in the perspective of this book, stress/injury-caused molecular perturbances which induce those conformational changes of mechanosensors (or the whole cellular plasma membrane) are considered putative cell-extrinsic dyshomeostasis-associated molecular patterns, which—via activation of mechanosensors—convert extracellularly applied mechanical stimuli into intracellular (bio)chemical signaling pathways. Consequently, these dyshomeostatic DAMPs are newly added to the list of modified molecules as Subclass IIB-3 DAMPs (for details, see Sect. 3.4.3.3).

Nevertheless, the crucial question as to whether or not activation of mechanosensors upon the various mechanical stimuli is really due to perceiving homeostatic danger signals/IIB-3 DAMPs is still open. It may still be that as-yet-undiscovered (modified) molecules—generated in association with or without conformational changes—may act as physical ligands in terms of DAMPs. This possibility is supported by the recent discovery that NLRP3 (supposed to be activated by ion perturbation for a long time) is activated by binding to injury-induced *PtdIns4P* on dispersed TGN [72] (see Sect. 2.2.5.3).

2.5 Outlook and Future Perspectives

In this chapter, selected PRMs have been updated by focusing mainly on nonclassical receptors. Interestingly, some of the PRMs, subdivided here under nonclassical, have characteristic traits. For example, a central feature of GPCRs is their capability to interact with a large variety of ligands; nociceptors encompass classical, nonclassical, and a new type of receptors, the ion channels; recognition receptors of ILCs are confined to specific groups of lymphocytes, and Fc receptors amplify the action of antibodies. As a new family of receptors, mechanosensors have taken center stage operating as ion channels, GPCRs, or integrins. Together with soluble humoral recognition receptors (not revisited here), all these cellular PRMs impressively identify our innate immune system as a highly efficient and broadly defined organ of perception that intensely interacts with other homeostatic surveillance systems such as the CNS.

Perspectively, the therapeutic use of PRM antagonists as an effective treatment option remains an open question. To remember is the failure of TLR4 antagonists Eritoran and TAK-242 (resatorvid) to pass clinical trials as drugs against acute sepsis and septic shock. To date, the change of direction in TLR4-directed therapeutics is to use TLR4 antagonists for mitigation of acute and chronic inflammatory diseases due to TLR4 activation by endogenous factors such as ultraviolet radiation [313]. Nevertheless, as recently reviewed by Zaffaroni and Peri [314], ongoing clinical studies and a few licensed compounds demonstrate the potential of TLR4 modulators. The authors concluded: "Because of the very reduced number of chemicals in clinical phase of development as TLR4-based therapeutics, major efforts should be focused in the future to progress in the preclinical characterization of newly discovered hit compounds.... In parallel, it is still important to extend the chemical variety of TLR4 modulators by discovering new active molecules from natural sources (included fruits and vegetables) and from de novo designed synthetic molecules."

References

1. Land WG. Damage-associated molecular patterns in human diseases. In: Injury-induced innate immune responses, vol. 1. Cham: Springer International Publishing AG; 2018. https://www.springer.com/de/book/9783319786544.
2. Gong T, Liu L, Jiang W, Zhou R. DAMP-sensing receptors in sterile inflammation and inflammatory diseases. Nat Rev Immunol. 2020;20:95–112. https://doi.org/10.1038/s41577-019-0215-7.

3. Kawai T, Akira S. The role of pattern-recognition receptors in innate immunity: update on Toll-like receptors. Nat Immunol. 2010;11:373–84. http://www.ncbi.nlm.nih.gov/pubmed/20404851.
4. Hansen JD, Vojtech LN, Laing KJ. Sensing disease and danger: a survey of vertebrate PRRs and their origins. Dev Comp Immunol. 2011;35:886–97. http://www.ncbi.nlm.nih.gov/pubmed/21241729.
5. Jounai N, Kobiyama K, Takeshita F, Ishii KJ. Recognition of damage-associated molecular patterns related to nucleic acids during inflammation and vaccination. Front Cell Infect Microbiol. 2012;2:168. http://www.ncbi.nlm.nih.gov/pubmed/23316484.
6. Drummond RA, Brown GD. Signalling C-Type Lectins in Antimicrobial Immunity. PLoS Pathog. 2013;9:e1003417. http://www.ncbi.nlm.nih.gov/pubmed/23935480.
7. Lee EJ, Park JH. Receptor for advanced glycation endproducts (RAGE), its ligands, and soluble RAGE: potential biomarkers for diagnosis and therapeutic targets for human renal diseases. Genomics Inform. 2013;11:224–9. http://www.ncbi.nlm.nih.gov/pubmed/24465234.
8. Ratsimandresy RA, Dorfleutner A, Stehlik C. An update on PYRIN domain-containing pattern recognition receptors: from immunity to pathology. Front Immunol. 2013;4:440. http://www.ncbi.nlm.nih.gov/pubmed/24367371.
9. Unterholzner L. The interferon response to intracellular DNA: why so many receptors? Immunobiology. 2013;218:1312–21. http://www.ncbi.nlm.nih.gov/pubmed/23962476.
10. Zhong Y, Kinio A, Saleh M. Functions of NOD-like receptors in human diseases. Front Immunol. 2013;4:333. http://www.ncbi.nlm.nih.gov/pubmed/24137163.
11. Wu J, Chen ZJ. Innate immune sensing and signaling of cytosolic nucleic acids. Annu Rev Immunol. 2014;32:461–88. http://www.ncbi.nlm.nih.gov/pubmed/24655297.
12. Pontillo A, Crovella S. NOD-like receptors: a tail from plants to mammals through invertebrates. Curr Protein Pept Sci. 2017;18:311–22. http://www.eurekaselect.com/openurl/content.php?genre=article&issn=1389-2037&volume=18&issue=4&spage=311.
13. Sohn J, Hur S. Filament assemblies in foreign nucleic acid sensors. Curr Opin Struct Biol. 2016;37:134–44. http://www.ncbi.nlm.nih.gov/pubmed/26859869.
14. Qiao Q, Wu H. Supramolecular organizing centers (SMOCs) as signaling machines in innate immune activation. Sci China Life Sci. 2015;58:1067–72. http://www.ncbi.nlm.nih.gov/pubmed/26511517.
15. Wu H. Higher-order assemblies in a new paradigm of signal transduction. Cell. 2013;153:287–92. https://linkinghub.elsevier.com/retrieve/pii/S0092867413003358.
16. Kagan JC, Magupalli VG, Wu H. SMOCs: supramolecular organizing centres that control innate immunity. Nat Rev Immunol. 2014;14:821–6. http://www.nature.com/articles/nri3757.
17. Tan Y, Kagan JC. Innate immune signaling organelles display natural and programmable signaling flexibility. Cell. 2019;177:384–398.e11. http://www.ncbi.nlm.nih.gov/pubmed/30853218.
18. Balka KR, Nardo D. Understanding early TLR signaling through the Myddosome. J Leukoc Biol. 2019;105:339–51. https://onlinelibrary.wiley.com/doi/abs/10.1002/JLB.MR0318-096R.
19. Franklin BS, Latz E, Schmidt FI. The intra- and extracellular functions of ASC specks. Immunol Rev. 2018;281:74–87. http://www.ncbi.nlm.nih.gov/pubmed/29247990.
20. Cai X, Chen J, Xu H, Liu S, Jiang Q-X, Halfmann R, et al. Prion-like polymerization underlies signal transduction in antiviral immune defense and inflammasome activation. Cell. 2014;156:1207–22. https://linkinghub.elsevier.com/retrieve/pii/S0092867414001998.
21. Cai X, Xu H, Chen ZJ. Prion-like polymerization in immunity and inflammation. Cold Spring Harb Perspect Biol. 2017;9:a023580. http://www.ncbi.nlm.nih.gov/pubmed/27881448.
22. Holmes DL, Lancaster AK, Lindquist S, Halfmann R. Heritable remodeling of yeast multicellularity by an environmentally responsive prion. Cell. 2013;153:153–65. http://www.ncbi.nlm.nih.gov/pubmed/23540696.
23. Yatim N, Cullen S, Albert ML. Dying cells actively regulate adaptive immune responses. Nat Rev Immunol. 2017;17:262–75. https://doi.org/10.1038/nri.2017.9.

24. Chassaing B, Ley RE, Gewirtz AT. Intestinal epithelial cell toll-like receptor 5 regulates the intestinal microbiota to prevent low-grade inflammation and metabolic syndrome in mice. Gastroenterology. 2014;147:1363–1377.e17.
25. Yiu JHC, Dorweiler B, Woo CW. Interaction between gut microbiota and toll-like receptor: from immunity to metabolism. J Mol Med (Berl). 2017;95:13–20. http://www.ncbi.nlm.nih.gov/pubmed/27639584.
26. Pandey S, Kawai T, Akira S. Microbial sensing by Toll-like receptors and intracellular nucleic acid sensors. Cold Spring Harb Perspect Biol. 2014;7:a016246. https://doi.org/10.1101/cshperspect.a016246.
27. Leifer CA, Medvedev AE. Molecular mechanisms of regulation of Toll-like receptor signaling. J Leukoc Biol. 2016;100(5):927–41. http://www.ncbi.nlm.nih.gov/pubmed/27343013.
28. Liu Q, Ding JL. The molecular mechanisms of TLR-signaling cooperation in cytokine regulation. Immunol Cell Biol. 2016;94:538–42. http://www.ncbi.nlm.nih.gov/pubmed/26860369.
29. O'Neill LAJ, Bowie AG. The family of five: TIR-domain-containing adaptors in Toll-like receptor signalling. Nat Rev Immunol. 2007;7:353–64. http://www.ncbi.nlm.nih.gov/pubmed/17457343.
30. Takeuchi O, Akira S. Pattern recognition receptors and inflammation. Cell. 2010;140:805–20. http://www.ncbi.nlm.nih.gov/pubmed/20303872.
31. Vidya MK, Kumar VG, Sejian V, Bagath M, Krishnan G, Bhatta R. Toll-like receptors: significance, ligands, signaling pathways, and functions in mammals. Int Rev Immunol. 2018;37:20–36. http://www.ncbi.nlm.nih.gov/pubmed/29028369.
32. Ting JP-Y, Lovering RC, Alnemri ES, Bertin J, Boss JM, Davis BK, et al. The NLR gene family: a standard nomenclature. Immunity. 2008;28:285–7. http://www.ncbi.nlm.nih.gov/pubmed/18341998.
33. Caruso R, Warner N, Inohara N, Núñez G. NOD1 and NOD2: signaling, host defense, and inflammatory disease. Immunity. 2014;41:898–908. http://www.ncbi.nlm.nih.gov/pubmed/25526305.
34. Claes A-K, Zhou JY, Philpott DJ. NOD-like receptors: guardians of intestinal mucosal barriers. Physiology (Bethesda). 2015;30:241–50. http://www.ncbi.nlm.nih.gov/pubmed/25933824.
35. Motta V, Soares F, Sun T, Philpott DJ. NOD-like receptors: versatile cytosolic sentinels. Physiol Rev. 2015;95:149–78. http://www.ncbi.nlm.nih.gov/pubmed/25540141.
36. Kim YK, Shin JS, Nahm MH. NOD-like receptors in infection, immunity, and diseases. Yonsei Med J. 2016;57:5–14. http://www.ncbi.nlm.nih.gov/pubmed/26632377.
37. Wang X, Yi F. The nucleotide oligomerization domain-like receptors in kidney injury. Kidney Dis (Basel, Switzerland). 2016;2:28–36. http://www.ncbi.nlm.nih.gov/pubmed/27536689.
38. Chamaillard M, Hashimoto M, Horie Y, Masumoto J, Qiu S, Saab L, et al. An essential role for NOD1 in host recognition of bacterial peptidoglycan containing diaminopimelic acid. Nat Immunol. 2003;4:702–7. https://doi.org/10.1038/ni945.
39. Travassos LH, Carneiro LAM, Ramjeet M, Hussey S, Kim Y-G, Magalhães JG, et al. Nod1 and Nod2 direct autophagy by recruiting ATG16L1 to the plasma membrane at the site of bacterial entry. Nat Immunol. 2010;11:55–62. https://doi.org/10.1038/ni.1823.
40. Werts C, Rubino S, Ling A, Girardin SE, Philpott DJ. Nod-like receptors in intestinal homeostasis, inflammation, and cancer. J Leukoc Biol. 2011;90:471–82. http://www.jleukbio.org/cgi/doi/10.1189/jlb.0411183
41. Philpott DJ, Sorbara MT, Robertson SJ, Croitoru K, Girardin SE. NOD proteins: regulators of inflammation in health and disease. Nat Rev Immunol. 2014;14:9–23. https://doi.org/10.1038/nri3565.
42. Shibutani ST, Saitoh T, Nowag H, Münz C, Yoshimori T. Autophagy and autophagy-related proteins in the immune system. Nat Immunol. 2015;16:1014–24. http://www.ncbi.nlm.nih.gov/pubmed/26382870.
43. Rauch I, Tenthorey JL, Nichols RD, Al Moussawi K, Kang JJ, Kang C, et al. NAIP proteins are required for cytosolic detection of specific bacterial ligands in vivo. J Exp Med. 2016;213:657–65. https://doi.org/10.1084/jem.20151809.

44. Robertson SJ, Zhou JY, Geddes K, Rubino SJ, Cho JH, Girardin SE, et al. Nod1 and Nod2 signaling does not alter the composition of intestinal bacterial communities at homeostasis. Gut Microbes. 2013;4:222–31. http://www.ncbi.nlm.nih.gov/pubmed/23549220.
45. Robertson SJ, Geddes K, Maisonneuve C, Streutker CJ, Philpott DJ. Resilience of the intestinal microbiota following pathogenic bacterial infection is independent of innate immunity mediated by NOD1 or NOD2. Microbes Infect. 2016;18:460–71. http://www.ncbi.nlm.nih.gov/pubmed/27083475.
46. Caruso R, Núñez G. Innate immunity: ER stress recruits NOD1 and NOD2 for delivery of inflammation. Curr Biol. 2016;26:R508–11. http://linkinghub.elsevier.com/retrieve/pii/S0960982216304791.
47. Kaparakis-Liaskos M. The intracellular location, mechanisms and outcomes of NOD1 signaling. Cytokine. 2015;74:207–12. http://linkinghub.elsevier.com/retrieve/pii/S1043466615000770.
48. Mukherjee T, Hovingh ES, Foerster EG, Abdel-Nour M, Philpott DJ, Girardin SE. NOD1 and NOD2 in inflammation, immunity and disease. Arch Biochem Biophys. 2019;670:69–81. https://linkinghub.elsevier.com/retrieve/pii/S0003986118309378.
49. Platnich JM, Muruve DA. NOD-like receptors and inflammasomes: a review of their canonical and non-canonical signaling pathways. Arch Biochem Biophys. 2019;670:4–14. http://www.ncbi.nlm.nih.gov/pubmed/30772258.
50. Mathur A, Hayward JA, Man SM. Molecular mechanisms of inflammasome signaling. J Leukoc Biol. 2017;103:jlb.3MR0617-250R. http://www.ncbi.nlm.nih.gov/pubmed/28855232.
51. Yang Y, Wang H, Kouadir M, Song H, Shi F. Recent advances in the mechanisms of NLRP3 inflammasome activation and its inhibitors. Cell Death Dis. 2019;10:128. http://www.nature.com/articles/s41419-019-1413-8.
52. Place DE, Kanneganti T-D. Recent advances in inflammasome biology. Curr Opin Immunol. 2018;50:32–8. http://www.ncbi.nlm.nih.gov/pubmed/29128729.
53. Netea MG, Nold-Petry CA, Nold MF, Joosten LAB, Opitz B, van der Meer JHM, et al. Differential requirement for the activation of the inflammasome for processing and release of IL-1beta in monocytes and macrophages. Blood. 2009;113:2324–35. https://doi.org/10.1182/blood-2008-03-146720.
54. Gong Y-N, Wang X, Wang J, Yang Z, Li S, Yang J, et al. Chemical probing reveals insights into the signaling mechanism of inflammasome activation. Cell Res. 2010;20:1289–305. http://www.nature.com/articles/cr2010135.
55. Juliana C, Fernandes-Alnemri T, Kang S, Farias A, Qin F, Alnemri ES. Non-transcriptional priming and deubiquitination regulate NLRP3 inflammasome activation. J Biol Chem. 2012;287:36617–22. https://doi.org/10.1074/jbc.M112.407130.
56. Fernandes-Alnemri T, Kang S, Anderson C, Sagara J, Fitzgerald KA, Alnemri ES. Cutting edge: TLR signaling licenses IRAK1 for rapid activation of the NLRP3 inflammasome. J Immunol. 2013;191:3995–9. https://doi.org/10.4049/jimmunol.1301681.
57. Lin K-M, Hu W, Troutman TD, Jennings M, Brewer T, Li X, et al. IRAK-1 bypasses priming and directly links TLRs to rapid NLRP3 inflammasome activation. Proc Natl Acad Sci U S A. 2014;111:775–80. https://doi.org/10.1073/pnas.1320294111.
58. Ferrao R, Wu H. Helical assembly in the death domain (DD) superfamily. Curr Opin Struct Biol. 2012;22:241–7. http://www.ncbi.nlm.nih.gov/pubmed/22429337.
59. Bauernfeind FG, Horvath G, Stutz A, Alnemri ES, MacDonald K, Speert D, et al. Cutting edge: NF- B activating pattern recognition and cytokine receptors license NLRP3 inflammasome activation by regulating NLRP3 expression. J Immunol. 2009;183:787–91. https://doi.org/10.4049/jimmunol.0901363.
60. Man SM, Kanneganti T-D. Regulation of inflammasome activation. Immunol Rev. 2015;265:6–21. http://www.ncbi.nlm.nih.gov/pubmed/25879280.
61. Jo E-K, Kim JK, Shin D-M, Sasakawa C. Molecular mechanisms regulating NLRP3 inflammasome activation. Cell Mol Immunol. 2016;13:148–59. http://www.ncbi.nlm.nih.gov/pubmed/26549800.

62. Próchnicki T, Mangan MS, Latz E. Recent insights into the molecular mechanisms of the NLRP3 inflammasome activation. F1000Research. 2016;5:1–15. http://www.ncbi.nlm.nih.gov/pubmed/27508077.
63. Sharma D, Kanneganti T-D. The cell biology of inflammasomes: mechanisms of inflammasome activation and regulation. J Cell Biol. 2016;213:617–29. http://www.ncbi.nlm.nih.gov/pubmed/27325789.
64. Pellegrini C, Antonioli L, Lopez-Castejon G, Blandizzi C, Fornai M. Canonical and non-canonical activation of NLRP3 inflammasome at the crossroad between immune tolerance and intestinal inflammation. Front Immunol. 2017;8:36. https://doi.org/10.3389/fimmu.2017.00036/full.
65. Man SM, Karki R, Briard B, Burton A, Gingras S, Pelletier S, et al. Differential roles of caspase-1 and caspase-11 in infection and inflammation. Sci Rep. 2017;7:45126. http://www.nature.com/articles/srep45126.
66. He W, Wan H, Hu L, Chen P, Wang X, Huang Z, et al. Gasdermin D is an executor of pyroptosis and required for interleukin-1β secretion. Cell Res. 2015;25:1285–98. http://www.ncbi.nlm.nih.gov/pubmed/26611636.
67. Shi J, Zhao Y, Wang K, Shi X, Wang Y, Huang H, et al. Cleavage of GSDMD by inflammatory caspases determines pyroptotic cell death. Nature. 2015;526:660–5. http://www.ncbi.nlm.nih.gov/pubmed/26375003.
68. Vince JE, Silke J. The intersection of cell death and inflammasome activation. Cell Mol Life Sci. 2016;73:2349–67. http://www.ncbi.nlm.nih.gov/pubmed/27066895.
69. Man SM, Kanneganti T-D. Gasdermin D: the long-awaited executioner of pyroptosis. Cell Res. 2015;25:1183–4. http://www.ncbi.nlm.nih.gov/pubmed/26482951.
70. Shi J, Gao W, Shao F. Pyroptosis: Gasdermin-mediated programmed necrotic cell death. Trends Biochem Sci. 2017;42:245–54. https://linkinghub.elsevier.com/retrieve/pii/S0968000416301827.
71. Zhong Z, Liang S, Sanchez-Lopez E, He F, Shalapour S, Lin X-J, et al. New mitochondrial DNA synthesis enables NLRP3 inflammasome activation. Nature. 2018;560:198–203. http://www.nature.com/articles/s41586-018-0372-z.
72. Chen J, Chen ZJ. PtdIns4P on dispersed trans-Golgi network mediates NLRP3 inflammasome activation. Nature. 2018;564:71–6. http://www.nature.com/articles/s41586-018-0761-3.
73. Chen KW, Boucher D, Broz P. Divide to conquer: NLRP3 is activated on dispersed trans-Golgi network. Cell Res. 2019;29:181–2. http://www.nature.com/articles/s41422-018-0138-z.
74. Lu A, Magupalli VG, Ruan J, Yin Q, Atianand MK, Vos MR, et al. Unified polymerization mechanism for the assembly of ASC-dependent inflammasomes. Cell. 2014;156:1193–206. https://linkinghub.elsevier.com/retrieve/pii/S0092867414002001.
75. Thomas PG, Dash P, Aldridge JR, Ellebedy AH, Reynolds C, Funk AJ, et al. The intracellular sensor NLRP3 mediates key innate and healing responses to influenza A virus via the regulation of caspase-1. Immunity. 2009;30:566–75. https://linkinghub.elsevier.com/retrieve/pii/S107476130900140X.
76. Pichlmair A, Schulz O, Tan CP, Näslund TI, Liljeström P, Weber F, et al. RIG-I-mediated antiviral responses to single-stranded RNA bearing 5'-phosphates. Science. 2006;314:997–1001. https://doi.org/10.1126/science.1132998.
77. Kato H, Takeuchi O, Sato S, Yoneyama M, Yamamoto M, Matsui K, et al. Differential roles of MDA5 and RIG-I helicases in the recognition of RNA viruses. Nature. 2006;441:101–5. https://doi.org/10.1038/nature04734.
78. Schlee M, Hartmann G. Discriminating self from non-self in nucleic acid sensing. Nat Rev Immunol. 2016;16:566–80. http://www.ncbi.nlm.nih.gov/pubmed/27455396.
79. Loo Y-M, Gale M. Immune signaling by RIG-I-like receptors. Immunity. 2011;34:680–92. http://www.ncbi.nlm.nih.gov/pubmed/21616437.
80. Barik S. What really rigs up RIG-I? J Innate Immun. 2016;8:429–36. https://www.karger.com/Article/FullText/447947.

81. Ranoa DRE, Parekh AD, Pitroda SP, Huang X, Darga T, Wong AC, et al. Cancer therapies activate RIG-I-like receptor pathway through endogenous non-coding RNAs. Oncotarget. 2016;7:26496–515. http://www.ncbi.nlm.nih.gov/pubmed/27034163.
82. Hartmann G. Nucleic acid immunity. Adv Immunol. 2017;133:121–69. http://www.ncbi.nlm.nih.gov/pubmed/28215278.
83. Jiang Q-X. Structural variability in the RLR-MAVS pathway and sensitive detection of viral RNAs. Med Chem (Los Angeles). 2018;15:443–58. http://www.ncbi.nlm.nih.gov/pubmed/30569868.
84. Corby MJ, Raicu V, Frick DN. New techniques to study intracellular receptors in living cells: insights into RIG-I-like receptor signaling. Adv Exp Med Biol. 2019;1111:219–40. https://doi.org/10.1007/5584_2018_297.
85. Chow KT, Gale M, Loo Y-M. RIG-I and other RNA sensors in antiviral immunity. Annu Rev Immunol. 2018;36:667–94. http://www.ncbi.nlm.nih.gov/pubmed/29677479.
86. Khodarev NN, Intracellular RNA. Sensing in mammalian cells: role in stress response and cancer therapies. Int Rev Cell Mol Biol. 2019;344:31–89. http://www.ncbi.nlm.nih.gov/pubmed/30798990.
87. Lee J-H, Chiang C, Gack MU. Endogenous nucleic acid recognition by RIG-I-like receptors and cGAS. J Interferon Cytokine Res. 2019;39(8):450–8. http://www.ncbi.nlm.nih.gov/pubmed/31066607.
88. Roulois D, Loo Yau H, Singhania R, Wang Y, Danesh A, Shen SY, et al. DNA-demethylating agents target colorectal cancer cells by inducing viral mimicry by endogenous transcripts. Cell. 2015;162:961–73. https://linkinghub.elsevier.com/retrieve/pii/S0092867415009721.
89. Engel C, Brügmann G, Lambing S, Mühlenbeck LH, Marx S, Hagen C, et al. RIG-I resists hypoxia-induced immunosuppression and dedifferentiation. Cancer Immunol Res. 2017;5:455–67. http://cancerimmunolres.aacrjournals.org/lookup/doi/10.1158/2326-6066.CIR-16-0129-T.
90. Schock SN, Chandra NV, Sun Y, Irie T, Kitagawa Y, Gotoh B, et al. Induction of necroptotic cell death by viral activation of the RIG-I or STING pathway. Cell Death Differ. 2017;24:615–25. http://www.nature.com/articles/cdd2016153.
91. Brault M, Olsen TM, Martinez J, Stetson DB, Oberst A. Intracellular nucleic acid sensing triggers necroptosis through synergistic type I IFN and TNF signaling. J Immunol. 2018;200:2748–56. https://doi.org/10.4049/jimmunol.1701492.
92. Seth RB, Sun L, Ea C-K, Chen ZJ. Identification and characterization of MAVS, a mitochondrial antiviral signaling protein that activates NF-κB and IRF3. Cell. 2005;122:669–82. http://www.ncbi.nlm.nih.gov/pubmed/16125763.
93. Wu B, Hur S. How RIG-I like receptors activate MAVS. Curr Opin Virol. 2015;12:91–8. http://www.ncbi.nlm.nih.gov/pubmed/25942693.
94. Hornung V, Ablasser A, Charrel-Dennis M, Bauernfeind F, Horvath G, Caffrey DR, et al. AIM2 recognizes cytosolic dsDNA and forms a caspase-1-activating inflammasome with ASC. Nature. 2009;458:514–8. http://www.ncbi.nlm.nih.gov/pubmed/19158675.
95. Jakobs C, Perner S, Hornung V. AIM2 Drives Joint Inflammation in a Self-DNA Triggered Model of Chronic Polyarthritis. PLoS One. 2015;10:e0131702. http://www.ncbi.nlm.nih.gov/pubmed/26114879.
96. Dubois H, Wullaert A, Lamkanfi M. General strategies in inflammasome biology. Curr Top Microbiol Immunol. 2016;397:1–22. http://www.ncbi.nlm.nih.gov/pubmed/27460802.
97. Dempsey A, Bowie AG. Innate immune recognition of DNA: a recent history. Virology. 2015;479–480:146–52. http://www.ncbi.nlm.nih.gov/pubmed/25816762.
98. Cai X, Chiu Y-H, Chen ZJ. The cGAS-cGAMP-STING pathway of cytosolic DNA sensing and signaling. Mol Cell. 2014;54:289–96. http://www.ncbi.nlm.nih.gov/pubmed/24766893.
99. Civril F, Deimling T, de Oliveira Mann CC, Ablasser A, Moldt M, Witte G, et al. Structural mechanism of cytosolic DNA sensing by cGAS. Nature. 2013;498:332–7. http://www.ncbi.nlm.nih.gov/pubmed/23722159.
100. Kuriakose T, Man SM, Subbarao Malireddi RK, Karki R, Kesavardhana S, Place DE, et al. ZBP1/DAI is an innate sensor of influenza virus triggering the NLRP3 inflammasome and

programmed cell death pathways. Sci Immunol. 2016;1:aag2045. http://www.ncbi.nlm.nih.gov/pubmed/27917412.
101. Xiao TS. The nucleic acid-sensing inflammasomes. Immunol Rev. 2015;265:103–11. http://www.ncbi.nlm.nih.gov/pubmed/25879287.
102. Gao D, Li T, Li X-D, Chen X, Li Q-Z, Wight-Carter M, et al. Activation of cyclic GMP-AMP synthase by self-DNA causes autoimmune diseases. Proc Natl Acad Sci U S A. 2015;112:E5699–705. http://www.ncbi.nlm.nih.gov/pubmed/26371324.
103. Ma Z, Damania B. The cGAS-STING defense pathway and its counteraction by viruses. Cell Host Microbe. 2016;19:150–8. http://www.ncbi.nlm.nih.gov/pubmed/26867174.
104. Ablasser A, Gulen MF. The role of cGAS in innate immunity and beyond. J Mol Med (Berl). 2016;94:1085–93. https://doi.org/10.1007/s00109-016-1423-2.
105. Khan S, Godfrey V, Zaki MH. Cytosolic nucleic acid sensors in inflammatory and autoimmune disorders. Int Rev Cell Mol Biol. 2019;344:215–53. http://www.ncbi.nlm.nih.gov/pubmed/30798989.
106. Kumar V. A STING to inflammation and autoimmunity. J Leukoc Biol. 2019;106(1):171–85. https://doi.org/10.1002/JLB.4MIR1018-397RR.
107. Bordignon V, Cavallo I, D'Agosto G, Trento E, Pontone M, Abril E, et al. Nucleic acid sensing perturbation: how aberrant recognition of self-nucleic acids may contribute to autoimmune and autoinflammatory diseases. Int Rev Cell Mol Biol. 2019;344:117–37. https://linkinghub.elsevier.com/retrieve/pii/S1937644818301072.
108. Abe T, Shapira SD. Negative regulation of cytosolic sensing of DNA. Int Rev Cell Mol Biol. 2019;344:91–115. http://www.ncbi.nlm.nih.gov/pubmed/30798991.
109. Sun F, Liu Z, Yang Z, Liu S, Guan W. The emerging role of STING-dependent signaling on cell death. Immunol Res. 2019;67(2–3):290–6. https://doi.org/10.1007/s12026-019-09073-z.
110. Woo S-R, Fuertes MB, Corrales L, Spranger S, Furdyna MJ, Leung MYK, et al. STING-dependent cytosolic DNA sensing mediates innate immune recognition of immunogenic tumors. Immunity. 2014;41:830–42. https://linkinghub.elsevier.com/retrieve/pii/S1074761314003938.
111. Gao P, Zillinger T, Wang W, Ascano M, Dai P, Hartmann G, et al. Binding-pocket and lid-region substitutions render human STING sensitive to the species-specific drug DMXAA. Cell Rep. 2014;8:1668–76. https://linkinghub.elsevier.com/retrieve/pii/S2211124714006731
112. Webster SJ, Brode S, Ellis L, Fitzmaurice TJ, Elder MJ, Gekara NO, et al. Detection of a microbial metabolite by STING regulates inflammasome activation in response to Chlamydia trachomatis infection. PLoS Pathog. 2017;13:e1006383. https://doi.org/10.1371/journal.ppat.1006383.
113. Man SM, Karki R, Malireddi RKS, Neale G, Vogel P, Yamamoto M, et al. The transcription factor IRF1 and guanylate-binding proteins target activation of the AIM2 inflammasome by Francisella infection. Nat Immunol. 2015;16:467–75. http://www.nature.com/articles/ni.3118.
114. Dunphy G, Flannery SM, Almine JF, Connolly DJ, Paulus C, Jønsson KL, et al. Non-canonical activation of the DNA sensing adaptor STING by ATM and IFI16 mediates NF-κB signaling after nuclear DNA damage. Mol Cell. 2018;71:745–760.e5. http://www.ncbi.nlm.nih.gov/pubmed/30193098.
115. Ciccia A, Elledge SJ. The DNA damage response: making it safe to play with knives. Mol Cell. 2010;40:179–204. http://linkinghub.elsevier.com/retrieve/pii/S1097276510007471.
116. Symington LS, Gautier J. Double-strand break end resection and repair pathway choice. Annu Rev Genet. 2011;45:247–71. http://www.ncbi.nlm.nih.gov/pubmed/21910633.
117. Symington LS. Mechanism and regulation of DNA end resection in eukaryotes. Crit Rev Biochem Mol Biol. 2016;51:195–212. http://www.ncbi.nlm.nih.gov/pubmed/27098756.
118. Blackford AN. Personal Communication.
119. Maréchal A, Zou L. DNA damage sensing by the ATM and ATR kinases. Cold Spring Harb Perspect Biol. 2013;5:a012716. http://www.ncbi.nlm.nih.gov/pubmed/24003211.
120. Shibata A, Jeggo P, Löbrich M. The pendulum of the Ku-Ku clock. DNA Repair (Amst). 2018;71:164–71. http://www.ncbi.nlm.nih.gov/pubmed/30177438.

121. Xu R, Xu Y, Huo W, Lv Z, Yuan J, Ning S, et al. Mitosis-specific MRN complex promotes a mitotic signaling cascade to regulate spindle dynamics and chromosome segregation. Proc Natl Acad Sci. 2018;115:E10079–88. http://www.ncbi.nlm.nih.gov/pubmed/30297404.
122. Johnson TE, Lee J-H, Myler LR, Zhou Y, Mosley TJ, Yang S-H, et al. Homeodomain proteins directly regulate ATM kinase activity. Cell Rep. 2018;24:1471–83. http://www.ncbi.nlm.nih.gov/pubmed/30089259.
123. Wang Z, Gong Y, Peng B, Shi R, Fan D, Zhao H, et al. MRE11 UFMylation promotes ATM activation. Nucleic Acids Res. 2019;47:4124–35. http://www.ncbi.nlm.nih.gov/pubmed/30783677.
124. Syed A, Tainer JA. The MRE11–RAD50–NBS1 complex conducts the orchestration of damage signaling and outcomes to stress in DNA replication and repair. Annu Rev Biochem. 2018;87:263–94. http://www.ncbi.nlm.nih.gov/pubmed/29709199.
125. Hall J, Brault A, Vincent F, Weng S, Wang H, Dumlao D, et al. Discovery of PF-06928215 as a high affinity inhibitor of cGAS enabled by a novel fluorescence polarization assay. PLoS One. 2017;12:e0184843.
126. Vincent J, Adura C, Gao P, Luz A, Lama L, Asano Y, et al. Small molecule inhibition of cGAS reduces interferon expression in primary macrophages from autoimmune mice. Nat Commun. 2017;8:750. http://www.ncbi.nlm.nih.gov/pubmed/28963528.
127. Dresser DW. Specific inhibition of antibody production. II. Paralysis induced in adult mice by small quantities of protein antigen. Immunology. 1962;5:378–88. http://www.ncbi.nlm.nih.gov/pubmed/13887798.
128. Land W, Seifert J, Fateh-Moghadam A, Hopf U, Brendel W. Immunological tolerance induced in adult dogs by small amounts of horse IgG. Transplantation. 1969;8:748–50.
129. Brendel W, Land W, Hopf U, Seifert J. Induction of tolerance in man to horse-IgG. Lancet. 1969;2:1141–2. http://www.ncbi.nlm.nih.gov/pubmed/4188086.
130. Verginis P, McLaughlin KA, Wucherpfennig KW, von Boehmer H, Apostolou I. Induction of antigen-specific regulatory T cells in wild-type mice: visualization and targets of suppression. Proc Natl Acad Sci U S A. 2008;105:3479–84. https://doi.org/10.1073/pnas.0800149105.
131. Lugrin J, Martinon F. The AIM2 inflammasome: sensor of pathogens and cellular perturbations. Immunol Rev. 2018;281:99–114. http://www.ncbi.nlm.nih.gov/pubmed/29247998.
132. Man SM, Karki R, Kanneganti T-D. AIM2 inflammasome in infection, cancer, and autoimmunity: Role in DNA sensing, inflammation, and innate immunity. Eur J Immunol. 2016;46:269–80. http://www.ncbi.nlm.nih.gov/pubmed/26626159.
133. Hu B, Jin C, Li H-B, Tong J, Ouyang X, Cetinbas NM, et al. The DNA-sensing AIM2 inflammasome controls radiation-induced cell death and tissue injury. Science. 2016;354:765–8. https://doi.org/10.1126/science.aaf7532.
134. Lian Q, Xu J, Yan S, Huang M, Ding H, Sun X, et al. Chemotherapy-induced intestinal inflammatory responses are mediated by exosome secretion of double-strand DNA via AIM2 inflammasome activation. Cell Res. 2017;27:784–800. https://doi.org/10.1038/cr.2017.54.
135. Zhang Q, Itagaki K, Hauser CJ. Mitochondrial DNA is released by shock and activates neutrophils via p38 map kinase. Shock. 2010;34:55–9. http://content.wkhealth.com/linkback/openurl?sid=WKPTLP:landingpage&an=00024382-201007000-00010.
136. Boyapati RK, Tamborska A, Dorward DA, Ho G-T. Advances in the understanding of mitochondrial DNA as a pathogenic factor in inflammatory diseases. F1000Research. 2017;6:169. http://www.ncbi.nlm.nih.gov/pubmed/28299196.
137. Bai J, Cervantes C, Liu J, He S, Zhou H, Zhang B, et al. DsbA-L prevents obesity-induced inflammation and insulin resistance by suppressing the mtDNA release-activated cGAS-cGAMP-STING pathway. Proc Natl Acad Sci. 2017;114:12196–201. http://www.ncbi.nlm.nih.gov/pubmed/29087318.
138. Bae JH, Jo SI, Kim SJ, Lee JM, Jeong JH, Kang JS, et al. Circulating cell-free mtDNA contributes to AIM2 inflammasome-mediated chronic inflammation in patients with type 2 diabetes. Cell. 2019;8:328. https://www.mdpi.com/2073-4409/8/4/328.
139. Zelenay S, Keller AM, Whitney PG, Schraml BU, Deddouche S, Rogers NC, et al. The dendritic cell receptor DNGR-1 controls endocytic handling of necrotic cell antigens to favor

cross-priming of CTLs in virus-infected mice. J Clin Invest. 2012;122:1615–27. http://www.jci.org/articles/view/60644.
140. Iborra S, Izquierdo HM, Martínez-López M, Blanco-Menéndez N, Reis e Sousa C, Sancho D. The DC receptor DNGR-1 mediates cross-priming of CTLs during vaccinia virus infection in mice. J Clin Invest. 2012;122:1628–43. http://www.jci.org/articles/view/60660.
141. Iborra S, Martínez-López M, Khouili SC, Enamorado M, Cueto FJ, Conde-Garrosa R, et al. Optimal generation of tissue-resident but not circulating memory T cells during viral infection requires crosspriming by DNGR-1+ dendritic cells. Immunity. 2016;45:847–60. https://linkinghub.elsevier.com/retrieve/pii/S1074761316303430.
142. del Fresno C, Iborra S, Saz-Leal P, Martínez-López M, Sancho D. Flexible signaling of myeloid C-type lectin receptors in immunity and inflammation. Front Immunol. 2018;9:804. http://www.ncbi.nlm.nih.gov/pubmed/29755458.
143. Pashenkov MV, Murugina NE, Budikhina AS, Pinegin BV. Synergistic interactions between NOD receptors and TLRs: mechanisms and clinical implications. J Leukoc Biol. 2019;105:669–80. http://www.ncbi.nlm.nih.gov/pubmed/30517768.
144. Pombinho R, Sousa S, Cabanes D. Scavenger receptors: promiscuous players during microbial pathogenesis. Crit Rev Microbiol. 2018;44:685–700. http://www.ncbi.nlm.nih.gov/pubmed/30318962.
145. Patten DA, Shetty S. More than just a removal service: scavenger receptors in leukocyte trafficking. Front Immunol. 2018;9:2904. http://www.ncbi.nlm.nih.gov/pubmed/30631321.
146. Gulati A, Kaur D, Krishna Prasad GVR, Mukhopadhaya A. PRR function of innate immune receptors in recognition of bacteria or bacterial ligands. Adv Exp Med Biol. 2018;1112:255–80. http://www.ncbi.nlm.nih.gov/pubmed/30637703.
147. Nakayama M. Macrophage recognition of crystals and nanoparticles. Front Immunol. 2018;9:103. http://www.ncbi.nlm.nih.gov/pubmed/29434606.
148. Rothlin CV, Carrera-Silva EA, Bosurgi L, Ghosh S. TAM receptor signaling in immune homeostasis. Annu Rev Immunol. 2015;33:355–91. http://www.ncbi.nlm.nih.gov/pubmed/25594431.
149. Freeman GJ, Casasnovas JM, Umetsu DT, DeKruyff RH. TIM genes: a family of cell surface phosphatidylserine receptors that regulate innate and adaptive immunity. Immunol Rev. 2010;235:172–89. http://www.ncbi.nlm.nih.gov/pubmed/20536563.
150. Flannagan RS, Jaumouillé V, Grinstein S. The cell biology of phagocytosis. Annu Rev Pathol Mech Dis. 2012;7:61–98. http://www.ncbi.nlm.nih.gov/pubmed/21910624.
151. Voss OH, Tian L, Murakami Y, Coligan JE, Krzewski K. Emerging role of CD300 receptors in regulating myeloid cell efferocytosis. Mol Cell Oncol. 2015;2:e964625. https://doi.org/10.4161/23723548.2014.964625.
152. Penberthy KK, Ravichandran KS. Apoptotic cell recognition receptors and scavenger receptors. Immunol Rev. 2016;269:44–59. https://doi.org/10.1111/imr.12376.
153. Frasch SC, Bratton DL. Emerging roles for lysophosphatidylserine in resolution of inflammation. Prog Lipid Res. 2012;51:199–207. http://www.ncbi.nlm.nih.gov/pubmed/22465125.
154. Burnstock G, Ralevic V. Purinergic signaling and blood vessels in health and disease. Pharmacol Rev. 2014;66:102–92. http://www.ncbi.nlm.nih.gov/pubmed/24335194.
155. Burnstock G. Purinergic signaling in the cardiovascular system. Circ Res. 2017;120:207–28. http://www.ncbi.nlm.nih.gov/pubmed/28057794.
156. Burnstock G. Purinergic signalling and neurological diseases: an update. CNS Neurol Disord Drug Targets. 2017;16:257–65. http://www.ncbi.nlm.nih.gov/pubmed/27658510.
157. Audet M, Stevens RC. Emerging structural biology of lipid G-protein coupled receptors. Protein Sci. 2019;28(2):292–304. http://www.ncbi.nlm.nih.gov/pubmed/30239054.
158. Karageorgos V, Venihaki M, Sakellaris S, Pardalos M, Kontakis G, Matsoukas M-T, et al. Current understanding of the structure and function of family B GPCRs to design novel drugs. Hormones. 2018;17:45–59. http://www.ncbi.nlm.nih.gov/pubmed/29858864.
159. Storch U, Schnitzler MM, Gudermann T. G protein-mediated stretch reception. Am J Physiol Circ Physiol. 2012;302:H1241–9. http://www.ncbi.nlm.nih.gov/pubmed/22227128.

160. Zhou XE, Melcher K, Xu HE. Structural biology of G protein-coupled receptor signaling complexes. Protein Sci. 2018;28:487–501. http://www.ncbi.nlm.nih.gov/pubmed/30311978.
161. Okajima F. Regulation of inflammation by extracellular acidification and proton-sensing GPCRs. Cell Signal. 2013;25:2263–71. http://www.ncbi.nlm.nih.gov/pubmed/23917207.
162. Zhu H, Cheng X, Niu X, Zhang Y, Guan J, Liu X, et al. Proton-sensing GPCR-YAP signalling promotes cell proliferation and survival. Int J Biol Sci. 2015;11:1181–9. http://www.ncbi.nlm.nih.gov/pubmed/26327812.
163. Weiß KT, Fante M, Köhl G, Schreml J, Haubner F, Kreutz M, et al. Proton-sensing G protein-coupled receptors as regulators of cell proliferation and migration during tumor growth and wound healing. Exp Dermatol. 2017;26:127–32. https://doi.org/10.1111/exd.13209.
164. Manglik A, Kruse AC. Structural basis for G protein-coupled receptor activation. Biochemistry. 2017;56:5628–34. http://www.ncbi.nlm.nih.gov/pubmed/28967738.
165. Weis WI, Kobilka BK. The molecular basis of G protein–coupled receptor activation. Annu Rev Biochem. 2018;87:897–919. http://www.ncbi.nlm.nih.gov/pubmed/29925258. [cited 2019 Jul 11].
166. Kobilka BK. G protein coupled receptor structure and activation. Biochim Biophys Acta Biomembr. 1768;2007:794–807. http://www.ncbi.nlm.nih.gov/pubmed/17188232.
167. Luttrell LM, Maudsley S, Bohn LM. Fulfilling the promise of "Biased" G protein-coupled receptor agonism. Mol Pharmacol. 2015;88:579–88. https://doi.org/10.1124/mol.115.099630.
168. Vilardaga J-P, Bünemann M, Feinstein TN, Lambert N, Nikolaev VO, Engelhardt S, et al. GPCR and G proteins: drug efficacy and activation in live cells. Mol Endocrinol. 2009;23:590–9. https://doi.org/10.1210/me.2008-0204.
169. Luttrell LM. GPCR signaling rides a wave of conformational changes. Cell. 2016;167:602–3. http://linkinghub.elsevier.com/retrieve/pii/S0092867416313873.
170. Rajagopal S, Rajagopal K, Lefkowitz RJ. Teaching old receptors new tricks: biasing seven-transmembrane receptors. Nat Rev Drug Discov. 2010;9:373–86. http://www.nature.com/articles/nrd3024.
171. Wootten D, Christopoulos A, Marti-Solano M, Babu MM, Sexton PM. Mechanisms of signalling and biased agonism in G protein-coupled receptors. Nat Rev Mol Cell Biol. 2018;19:638–53. http://www.nature.com/articles/s41580-018-0049-3.
172. Bologna Z, Teoh J, Bayoumi AS, Tang Y, Kim I. Biased G protein-coupled receptor signaling: new player in modulating physiology and pathology. Biomol Ther (Seoul). 2017;25:12–25. http://www.ncbi.nlm.nih.gov/pubmed/28035079.
173. Ahmadzai MM, Broadbent D, Occhiuto C, Yang C, Das R, Subramanian H. Canonical and noncanonical signaling roles of β-Arrestins in inflammation and immunity. Adv Immunol. 2017;136:279–313. http://www.ncbi.nlm.nih.gov/pubmed/28950948.
174. Kenakin T. Collateral efficacy in drug discovery: taking advantage of the good (allosteric) nature of 7TM receptors. Trends Pharmacol Sci. 2007;28:407–15. http://linkinghub.elsevier.com/retrieve/pii/S0165614707001551.
175. Luttrell LM, Gesty-Palmer D, Sibley DR. Beyond desensitization: physiological relevance of arrestin-dependent signaling. Pharmacol Rev. 2010;62:305–30. https://doi.org/10.1124/pr.109.002436.
176. Wang W, Qiao Y, Li Z. New insights into modes of GPCR activation. Trends Pharmacol Sci. 2018;39:367–86. https://linkinghub.elsevier.com/retrieve/pii/S0165614718300245,
177. Pierce KL, Premont RT, Lefkowitz RJ. Seven-transmembrane receptors. Nat Rev Mol Cell Biol. 2002;3:639–50. https://doi.org/10.1038/nrm908.
178. Bachelerie F, Graham GJ, Locati M, Mantovani A, Murphy PM, Nibbs R, et al. An atypical addition to the chemokine receptor nomenclature: IUPHAR review 15. Br J Pharmacol. 2015;172:3945–9. http://www.ncbi.nlm.nih.gov/pubmed/25958743.
179. Thomsen ARB, Plouffe B, Cahill TJ, Shukla AK, Tarrasch JT, Dosey AM, et al. GPCR-G protein-β-Arrestin super-complex mediates sustained G protein signaling. Cell. 2016;166:907–19. http://linkinghub.elsevier.com/retrieve/pii/S0092867416309102.
180. Jong Y-JI, Harmon SK, O'Malley KL. GPCR signalling from within the cell. Br J Pharmacol. 2018;175:4026–35. http://www.ncbi.nlm.nih.gov/pubmed/28872669.

181. Levin ER. Endothelins. N Engl J Med. 1995;333:356–63. http://www.ncbi.nlm.nih.gov/pubmed/7609754.
182. Maguire JJ, Davenport AP. Endothelin receptors and their antagonists. Semin Nephrol. 2015;35:125–36. http://www.ncbi.nlm.nih.gov/pubmed/25966344.
183. Maguire JJ. Evidence for biased agonists and antagonists at the endothelin receptors. Life Sci. 2016;159:30–3. http://www.ncbi.nlm.nih.gov/pubmed/26898124.
184. Braasch I, Schartl M. Evolution of endothelin receptors in vertebrates. Gen Comp Endocrinol. 2014;209:21–34. http://www.ncbi.nlm.nih.gov/pubmed/25010382.
185. Tank AW, Lee WD. Peripheral and central effects of circulating catecholamines. Compr Physiol. 2015;5:1–15. https://doi.org/10.1002/cphy.c140007.
186. Ahlquist RP. A study of the adrenotropic receptors. Am J Physiol. 1948;153:586–600. https://doi.org/10.1152/ajplegacy.1948.153.3.586.
187. Scanzano A, Cosentino M. Adrenergic regulation of innate immunity: a review. Front Pharmacol. 2015;6:171. http://journal.frontiersin.org/Article/10.3389/fphar.2015.00171/abstract.
188. Graham RM, Perez DM, Hwa J, Piascik MT. alpha 1-adrenergic receptor subtypes. Molecular structure, function, and signaling. Circ Res. 1996;78:737–49. http://www.ncbi.nlm.nih.gov/pubmed/8620593.
189. Cotecchia S. The α1-adrenergic receptors: diversity of signaling networks and regulation. J Recept Signal Transduct Res. 2010;30:410–9. https://doi.org/10.3109/10799893.2010.518152.
190. Philipp M, Hein L. Adrenergic receptor knockout mice: distinct functions of 9 receptor subtypes. Pharmacol Ther. 2004;101:65–74. http://www.ncbi.nlm.nih.gov/pubmed/14729393.
191. Wachter SB, Gilbert EM. Beta-adrenergic receptors, from their discovery and characterization through their manipulation to beneficial clinical application. Cardiology. 2012;122:104–12. https://www.karger.com/Article/FullText/339271.
192. He H-Q, Ye R. The formyl peptide receptors: diversity of ligands and mechanism for recognition. Molecules. 2017;22:455. http://www.ncbi.nlm.nih.gov/pubmed/28335409.
193. Chen K, Bao Z, Gong W, Tang P, Yoshimura T, Wang JM. Regulation of inflammation by members of the formyl-peptide receptor family. J Autoimmun. 2017;85:64–77. https://linkinghub.elsevier.com/retrieve/pii/S0896841117304377.
194. Raabe CA, Gröper J, Rescher U. Biased perspectives on formyl peptide receptors. Biochim Biophys Acta Mol Cell Res. 1866;2019:305–16. http://www.ncbi.nlm.nih.gov/pubmed/30521870.
195. Chiang N, Serhan CN. Structural elucidation and physiologic functions of specialized pro-resolving mediators and their receptors. Mol Aspects Med. 2017;58:114–29. http://linkinghub.elsevier.com/retrieve/pii/S0098299717300195.
196. Dijksterhuis JP, Petersen J, Schulte G. WNT/Frizzled signalling: receptor-ligand selectivity with focus on FZD-G protein signalling and its physiological relevance: IUPHAR review 3. Br J Pharmacol. 2014;171:1195–209. https://doi.org/10.1111/bph.12364.
197. Chien AJ, Conrad WH, Moon RT. A Wnt survival guide: from flies to human disease. J Invest Dermatol. 2009;129:1614–27. http://www.ncbi.nlm.nih.gov/pubmed/19177135.
198. van Amerongen R, Nusse R. Towards an integrated view of Wnt signaling in development. Development. 2009;136:3205–14. https://doi.org/10.1242/dev.033910.
199. Najdi R, Proffitt K, Sprowl S, Kaur S, Yu J, Covey TM, et al. A uniform human Wnt expression library reveals a shared secretory pathway and unique signaling activities. Differentiation. 2012;84:203–13. https://linkinghub.elsevier.com/retrieve/pii/S0301468112000874.
200. Wang Y, Chang H, Rattner A, Nathans J. Frizzled receptors in development and disease. Curr Top Dev Biol. 2016;117:113–39. http://www.ncbi.nlm.nih.gov/pubmed/26969975.
201. Justus CR, Dong L, Yang LV. Acidic tumor microenvironment and pH-sensing G protein-coupled receptors. Front Physiol. 2013;4:354. https://doi.org/10.3389/fphys.2013.00354/abstract.
202. Zhang XC, Sun K, Zhang L, Li X, Cao C. GPCR activation: protonation and membrane potential. Protein Cell. 2013;4:747–60. http://www.ncbi.nlm.nih.gov/pubmed/24057762.

203. Zhang XC, Cao C, Zhou Y, Zhao Y. Proton transfer-mediated GPCR activation. Protein Cell. 2015;6:12–7. https://doi.org/10.1007/s13238-014-0106-4.
204. Chen A, Dong L, Leffler NR, Asch AS, Witte ON, Yang LV. Activation of GPR4 by acidosis increases endothelial cell adhesion through the cAMP/Epac pathway. PLoS One. 2011;6:e27586. https://doi.org/10.1371/journal.pone.0027586.
205. Onozawa Y, Fujita Y, Kuwabara H, Nagasaki M, Komai T, Oda T. Activation of T cell death-associated gene 8 regulates the cytokine production of T cells and macrophages in vitro. Eur J Pharmacol. 2012;683:325–31. https://linkinghub.elsevier.com/retrieve/pii/S0014299912002476.
206. Dong L, Li Z, Leffler NR, Asch AS, Chi J-T, Yang LV. Acidosis activation of the proton-sensing GPR4 receptor stimulates vascular endothelial cell inflammatory responses revealed by transcriptome analysis. PLoS One. 2013;8:e61991. https://doi.org/10.1371/journal.pone.0061991.
207. Yona S, Lin H-H, Siu WO, Gordon S, Stacey M. Adhesion-GPCRs: emerging roles for novel receptors. Trends Biochem Sci. 2008;33:491–500. http://linkinghub.elsevier.com/retrieve/pii/S0968000408001850.
208. Hamann J, Aust G, Araç D, Engel FB, Formstone C, Fredriksson R, et al. International Union of Basic and Clinical Pharmacology. XCIV. Adhesion G protein-coupled receptors. Pharmacol Rev. 2015;67:338–67. https://doi.org/10.1124/pr.114.009647.
209. Hamann J, Petrenko AG. Introduction: history of the adhesion GPCR field. Handb Exp Pharmacol. 2016;234:1–11. https://doi.org/10.1007/978-3-319-41523-9_1.
210. Lin H-H, Hsiao C-C, Pabst C, Hébert J, Schöneberg T, Hamann J. Adhesion GPCRs in regulating immune responses and inflammation. Adv Immunol. 2017;136:163–201. http://www.ncbi.nlm.nih.gov/pubmed/28950945.
211. Das S, Owen KA, Ly KT, Park D, Black SG, Wilson JM, et al. Brain angiogenesis inhibitor 1 (BAI1) is a pattern recognition receptor that mediates macrophage binding and engulfment of Gram-negative bacteria. Proc Natl Acad Sci U S A. 2011;108:2136–41. https://doi.org/10.1073/pnas.1014775108.
212. Park D, Tosello-Trampont A-C, Elliott MR, Lu M, Haney LB, Ma Z, et al. BAI1 is an engulfment receptor for apoptotic cells upstream of the ELMO/Dock180/Rac module. Nature. 2007;450:430–4. http://www.nature.com/articles/nature06329.
213. Fitzgerald M. The development of nociceptive circuits. Nat Rev Neurosci. 2005;6:507–20. https://doi.org/10.1038/nrn1701.
214. Dubin AE, Patapoutian A. Nociceptors: the sensors of the pain pathway. J Clin Invest. 2010;120:3760–72. http://www.ncbi.nlm.nih.gov/pubmed/21041958.
215. Kato J, Svensson CI. Role of extracellular damage-associated molecular pattern molecules (DAMPs) as mediators of persistent pain. Prog Mol Biol Transl Sci. 2015;131:251–79. http://www.ncbi.nlm.nih.gov/pubmed/25744676.
216. Palazzo E, Marabese I, Luongo L, Guida F, de Novellis V, Maione S. Nociception modulation by supraspinal group III metabotropic glutamate receptors. J Neurochem. 2016;141(4):507–19. http://www.ncbi.nlm.nih.gov/pubmed/27363363.
217. Geppetti P, Veldhuis NA, Lieu T, Bunnett NW. G protein-coupled receptors: dynamic machines for signaling pain and itch. Neuron. 2015;88:635–49. http://www.ncbi.nlm.nih.gov/pubmed/26590341.
218. Dai Y. TRPs and pain. Semin Immunopathol. 2016;38:277–91. http://www.ncbi.nlm.nih.gov/pubmed/26374740.
219. Mickle AD, Shepherd AJ, Mohapatra DP. Sensory TRP channels: the key transducers of nociception and pain. Prog Mol Biol Transl Sci. 2015;131:73–118. http://www.ncbi.nlm.nih.gov/pubmed/25744671.
220. Parenti A, De Logu F, Geppetti P, Benemei S. What is the evidence for the role of TRP channels in inflammatory and immune cells? Br J Pharmacol. 2016;173:953–69. http://www.ncbi.nlm.nih.gov/pubmed/26603538.

221. Pinho-Ribeiro FA, Verri WA, Chiu IM. Nociceptor Sensory neuron–immune interactions in pain and inflammation. Trends Immunol. 2017;38:5–19. http://www.ncbi.nlm.nih.gov/pubmed/27793571.
222. Baral P, Udit S, Chiu IM. Pain and immunity: implications for host defence. Nat Rev Immunol. 2019;19:433–47. http://www.nature.com/articles/s41577-019-0147-2.
223. Halaby DM, Mornon JPE. The immunoglobulin superfamily: an insight on its tissular, species, and functional diversity. J Mol Evol. 1998;46:389–400. https://doi.org/10.1007/PL00006318.
224. Vivier E, Raulet DH, Moretta A, Caligiuri MA, Zitvogel L, Lanier LL, et al. Innate or adaptive immunity? The example of natural killer cells. Science. 2011;331:44–9. http://www.ncbi.nlm.nih.gov/pubmed/21212348.
225. Raulet DH, Gasser S, Gowen BG, Deng W, Jung H. Regulation of ligands for the NKG2D activating receptor. Annu Rev Immunol. 2013;31:413–41. http://www.ncbi.nlm.nih.gov/pubmed/23298206.
226. Lanier LL. NKG2D receptor and its ligands in host defense. Cancer Immunol Res. 2015;3:575–82. http://www.ncbi.nlm.nih.gov/pubmed/26041808.
227. Rajalingam R. Diversity of killer cell immunoglobulin-like receptors and disease. Clin Lab Med. 2018;38:637–53. http://www.ncbi.nlm.nih.gov/pubmed/30420058.
228. Barrow AD, Colonna M. Innate lymphoid cell sensing of tissue vitality. Curr Opin Immunol. 2019;56:82–93. https://linkinghub.elsevier.com/retrieve/pii/S0952791518300542.
229. Arts RJW, Joosten LAB, van der Meer JWM, Netea MG. TREM-1: intracellular signaling pathways and interaction with pattern recognition receptors. J Leukoc Biol. 2013;93:209–15. https://doi.org/10.1189/jlb.0312145.
230. Kouassi K, Gunasekar P, Agrawal D, Jadhav G. TREM-1; Is it a pivotal target for cardiovascular diseases? J Cardiovasc Dev Dis. 2018;5:45. http://www.ncbi.nlm.nih.gov/pubmed/30205488.
231. Tammaro A, Derive M, Gibot S, Leemans JC, Florquin S, Dessing MC. TREM-1 and its potential ligands in non-infectious diseases: from biology to clinical perspectives. Pharmacol Ther. 2017;177:81–95. http://www.ncbi.nlm.nih.gov/pubmed/28245991.
232. Daëron M. Fc receptor biology. Annu Rev Immunol. 1997;15:203–34. http://www.ncbi.nlm.nih.gov/pubmed/9143687.
233. Kraft S, Kinet J-P. New developments in FcεRI regulation, function and inhibition. Nat Rev Immunol. 2007;7:365–78. http://www.ncbi.nlm.nih.gov/pubmed/17438574.
234. Gould HJ, Sutton BJ. IgE in allergy and asthma today. Nat Rev Immunol. 2008;8:205–17. https://doi.org/10.1038/nri2273.
235. Platzer B, Stout M, Fiebiger E. Functions of dendritic-cell-bound IgE in allergy. Mol Immunol. 2015;68:116–9. http://www.ncbi.nlm.nih.gov/pubmed/26052071.
236. Hayes J, Wormald M, Rudd P, Davey G. Fc gamma receptors: glycobiology and therapeutic prospects. J Inflamm Res. 2016;9:209–19. http://www.ncbi.nlm.nih.gov/pubmed/27895507.
237. Pincetic A, Bournazos S, DiLillo DJ, Maamary J, Wang TT, Dahan R, et al. Type I and type II Fc receptors regulate innate and adaptive immunity. Nat Immunol. 2014;15:707–16. http://www.ncbi.nlm.nih.gov/pubmed/25045879.
238. Bournazos S, Ravetch JV. Diversification of IgG effector functions. Int Immunol. 2017;29:303–10. https://academic.oup.com/intimm/article/29/7/303/3787477.
239. Dewey CF, Bussolari SR, Gimbrone MA, Davies PF. The dynamic response of vascular endothelial cells to fluid shear stress. J Biomech Eng. 1981;103:177–85. http://www.ncbi.nlm.nih.gov/pubmed/7278196.
240. Magid A, Law DJ. Myofibrils bear most of the resting tension in frog skeletal muscle. Science. 1985;230:1280–2. http://www.ncbi.nlm.nih.gov/pubmed/4071053.
241. Freeman PM, Natarajan RN, Kimura JH, Andriacchi TP. Chondrocyte cells respond mechanically to compressive loads. J Orthop Res. 1994;12:311–20. https://doi.org/10.1002/jor.1100120303.

242. Beck FX, Burger-Kentischer A, Müller E. Cellular response to osmotic stress in the renal medulla. Pflugers Arch. 1998;436:814–27. https://doi.org/10.1007/s004240050710.
243. Orr AW, Helmke BP, Blackman BR, Schwartz MA. Mechanisms of mechanotransduction. Dev Cell. 2006;10:11–20. https://linkinghub.elsevier.com/retrieve/pii/S153458070500482X.
244. Eftestøl E, Egner IM, Lunde IG, Ellefsen S, Andersen T, Sjåland C, et al. Increased hypertrophic response with increased mechanical load in skeletal muscles receiving identical activity patterns. Am J Physiol Physiol. 2016;311:C616–29. http://www.ncbi.nlm.nih.gov/pubmed/27488660.
245. Baratchi S, Khoshmanesh K, Woodman OL, Potocnik S, Peter K, McIntyre P. Molecular sensors of blood flow in endothelial cells. Trends Mol Med. 2017;23:850–68. https://linkinghub.elsevier.com/retrieve/pii/S1471491417301259.
246. Lim C-G, Jang J, Kim C. Cellular machinery for sensing mechanical force. BMB Rep. 2018;51(12):623–9. http://www.ncbi.nlm.nih.gov/pubmed/30293551.
247. Matthews BD, Overby DR, Mannix R, Ingber DE. Cellular adaptation to mechanical stress: role of integrins, Rho, cytoskeletal tension and mechanosensitive ion channels. J Cell Sci. 2006;119:508–18. https://doi.org/10.1242/jcs.02760.
248. Barnes JM, Przybyla L, Weaver VM. Tissue mechanics regulate brain development, homeostasis and disease. J Cell Sci. 2017;130:71–82. https://doi.org/10.1242/jcs.191742.
249. Wehrwein EA, Joyner MJ. Regulation of blood pressure by the arterial baroreflex and autonomic nervous system. Handb Clin Neurol. 2013;117:89–102. https://linkinghub.elsevier.com/retrieve/pii/B9780444534910000080.
250. Chen Y, Ju L, Rushdi M, Ge C, Zhu C. Receptor-mediated cell mechanosensing. Mol Biol Cell. 2017;28:3134–55. http://www.ncbi.nlm.nih.gov/pubmed/28954860.
251. Kocer A. Mechanisms of mechanosensing — mechanosensitive channels, function and re-engineering. Curr Opin Chem Biol. 2015;29:120–7. http://www.ncbi.nlm.nih.gov/pubmed/26610201.
252. Martinac B. The ion channels to cytoskeleton connection as potential mechanism of mechanosensitivity. Biochim Biophys Acta. 1838;2014:682–91. https://linkinghub.elsevier.com/retrieve/pii/S0005273613002551.
253. Luis Alonso J, Goldmann WH. Cellular mechanotransduction. AIMS Biophys. 2016;3:50–62. https://doi.org/10.3934/biophy.2016.1.50.
254. Gillespie PG, Walker RG. Molecular basis of mechanosensory transduction. Nature. 2001;413:194–202. http://www.nature.com/articles/35093011.
255. Hamill OP, Martinac B. Molecular basis of mechanotransduction in living cells. Physiol Rev. 2001;81:685–740. https://doi.org/10.1152/physrev.2001.81.2.685.
256. Reed A, Kohl P, Peyronnet R. Molecular candidates for cardiac stretch-activated ion channels. Glob Cardiol Sci Pract. 2014;2014:9–25. https://doi.org/10.5339/gcsp.2014.19.
257. Ramsey IS, Delling M, Clapham DE. An introduction to TRP channels. Annu Rev Physiol. 2006;68:619–47. http://www.ncbi.nlm.nih.gov/pubmed/16460286.
258. Katanosaka Y, Iwasaki K, Ujihara Y, Takatsu S, Nishitsuji K, Kanagawa M, et al. TRPV2 is critical for the maintenance of cardiac structure and function in mice. Nat Commun. 2014;5:3932. http://www.nature.com/articles/ncomms4932.
259. Naruse K. Mechanomedicine. Biophys Rev. 2018;10:1257–62. http://www.ncbi.nlm.nih.gov/pubmed/30269290.
260. Aguettaz E, Bois P, Cognard C, Sebille S. Stretch-activated TRPV2 channels: role in mediating cardiopathies. Prog Biophys Mol Biol. 2017;130:273–80. http://www.ncbi.nlm.nih.gov/pubmed/28546113.
261. White JPM, Cibelli M, Urban L, Nilius B, McGeown JG, Nagy I. TRPV4: molecular conductor of a diverse orchestra. Physiol Rev. 2016;96:911–73. https://doi.org/10.1152/physrev.00016.2015.
262. Liedtke W, Choe Y, Martí-Renom MA, Bell AM, Denis CS, Sali A, et al. Vanilloid receptor-related osmotically activated channel (VR-OAC), a candidate vertebrate osmoreceptor. Cell. 2000;103:525–35. http://www.ncbi.nlm.nih.gov/pubmed/11081638.

263. Hartmannsgruber V, Heyken W-T, Kacik M, Kaistha A, Grgic I, Harteneck C, et al. Arterial response to shear stress critically depends on endothelial TRPV4 expression. PLoS One. 2007;2:e827. https://doi.org/10.1371/journal.pone.0000827.
264. Mendoza SA, Fang J, Gutterman DD, Wilcox DA, Bubolz AH, Li R, et al. TRPV4-mediated endothelial Ca2+ influx and vasodilation in response to shear stress. Am J Physiol Heart Circ Physiol. 2010;298:H466–76. https://doi.org/10.1152/ajpheart.00854.2009.
265. Bagher P, Beleznai T, Kansui Y, Mitchell R, Garland CJ, Dora KA. Low intravascular pressure activates endothelial cell TRPV4 channels, local Ca2+ events, and IKCa channels, reducing arteriolar tone. Proc Natl Acad Sci U S A. 2012;109:18174–9. https://doi.org/10.1073/pnas.1211946109.
266. Darby WG, Potocnik S, Ramachandran R, Hollenberg MD, Woodman OL, McIntyre P. Shear stress sensitizes TRPV4 in endothelium-dependent vasodilatation. Pharmacol Res. 2018;133:152–9. https://linkinghub.elsevier.com/retrieve/pii/S1043661817311143
267. Bubolz AH, Mendoza SA, Zheng X, Zinkevich NS, Li R, Gutterman DD, et al. Activation of endothelial TRPV4 channels mediates flow-induced dilation in human coronary arterioles: role of Ca2+ entry and mitochondrial ROS signaling. Am J Physiol Heart Circ Physiol. 2012;302:H634–42. https://doi.org/10.1152/ajpheart.00717.2011.
268. Feng S. TRPC channel structure and properties. Adv Exp Med Biol. 2017;976:9–23. http://www.ncbi.nlm.nih.gov/pubmed/28508309.
269. He Z. TRPC channel downstream signaling cascades. Adv Exp Med Biol. 2017;976:25–33. http://www.ncbi.nlm.nih.gov/pubmed/28508310.
270. Tai Y, Yang S, Liu Y, Shao W. TRPC channels in health and disease. Adv Exp Med Biol. 2017;976:35–45. https://doi.org/10.1007/978-94-024-1088-4_4.
271. Dryer SE, Roshanravan H, Kim EY. TRPC channels: regulation, dysregulation and contributions to chronic kidney disease. Biochim Biophys Acta Mol Basis Dis. 1865;2019:1041–66. http://www.ncbi.nlm.nih.gov/pubmed/30953689.
272. Geng J, Zhao Q, Zhang T, Xiao B. In touch with the mechanosensitive piezo channels: structure, ion permeation, and mechanotransduction. Curr Top Membr. 2017;79:159–95. https://linkinghub.elsevier.com/retrieve/pii/S1063582316300485.
273. Syeda R, Florendo MN, Cox CD, Kefauver JM, Santos JS, Martinac B, et al. Piezo1 channels are inherently mechanosensitive. Cell Rep. 2016;17:1739–46. http://www.ncbi.nlm.nih.gov/pubmed/27829145.
274. Wang Y, Xiao B. The mechanosensitive Piezo1 channel: structural features and molecular bases underlying its ion permeation and mechanotransduction. J Physiol. 2018;596:969–78. http://www.ncbi.nlm.nih.gov/pubmed/29171028.
275. Burke SD, Jordan J, Harrison DG, Karumanchi SA. Solving baroreceptor mystery: role of PIEZO ion channels. J Am Soc Nephrol. 2019;30(6):911–3. https://doi.org/10.1681/ASN.2019020160.
276. Zeng W-Z, Marshall KL, Min S, Daou I, Chapleau MW, Abboud FM, et al. PIEZOs mediate neuronal sensing of blood pressure and the baroreceptor reflex. Science. 2018;362:464–7. https://doi.org/10.1126/science.aau6324.
277. Armstrong M, Moore RA. Physiology, Baroreceptors. StatPearls. 2019. http://www.ncbi.nlm.nih.gov/pubmed/30844199.
278. Miglis MG, Muppidi S. Ion channels PIEZOs identified as the long-sought baroreceptor mechanosensors for blood pressure control, and other updates on autonomic research. Clin Auton Res. 2019;29:9–11. http://www.ncbi.nlm.nih.gov/pubmed/30604163.
279. Tu H, Zhang D, Li Y-L. Cellular and molecular mechanisms underlying arterial baroreceptor remodeling in cardiovascular diseases and diabetes. Neurosci Bull. 2019;35:98–112. http://www.ncbi.nlm.nih.gov/pubmed/30146675.
280. Hunyady L, Catt KJ. Pleiotropic AT1 receptor signaling pathways mediating physiological and pathogenic actions of angiotensin II. Mol Endocrinol. 2006;20:953–70. https://doi.org/10.1210/me.2004-0536.

281. Porrello ER, Delbridge LMD, Thomas WG. The angiotensin II type 2 (AT2) receptor: an enigmatic seven transmembrane receptor. Front Biosci. 2009;14:958–72. http://www.ncbi.nlm.nih.gov/pubmed/19273111.
282. Burson JM, Aguilera G, Gross KW, Sigmund CD. Differential expression of angiotensin receptor 1A and 1B in mouse. Am J Physiol. 1994;267:E260–7. https://doi.org/10.1152/ajpendo.1994.267.2.E260.
283. Chappell MC. Biochemical evaluation of the renin-angiotensin system: the good, bad, and absolute? Am J Physiol Heart Circ Physiol. 2016;310:H137–52. https://doi.org/10.1152/ajpheart.00618.2015.
284. Morris DL, Kahwaji CI. Angiotensin II. In: StatPearls. Treasure Island, FL: StatPearls; 2019. http://www.ncbi.nlm.nih.gov/pubmed/29763087.
285. Tóth AD, Turu G, Hunyady L, Balla A. Novel mechanisms of G-protein-coupled receptors functions: AT1 angiotensin receptor acts as a signaling hub and focal point of receptor cross-talk. Best Pract Res Clin Endocrinol Metab. 2018;32:69–82. http://www.ncbi.nlm.nih.gov/pubmed/29678287.
286. Mederos y Schnitzler M, Storch U, Gudermann T. AT1 receptors as mechanosensors. Curr Opin Pharmacol. 2011;11:112–6. http://www.ncbi.nlm.nih.gov/pubmed/21147033.
287. Mederos y Schnitzler M, Storch U, Meibers S, Nurwakagari P, Breit A, Essin K, et al. Gq-coupled receptors as mechanosensors mediating myogenic vasoconstriction. EMBO J. 2008;27:3092–103. https://doi.org/10.1038/emboj.2008.233.
288. Schleifenbaum J, Kassmann M, Szijártó IA, Hercule HC, Tano J-Y, Weinert S, et al. Stretch-activation of angiotensin II type 1a receptors contributes to the myogenic response of mouse mesenteric and renal arteries. Circ Res. 2014;115:263–72. https://doi.org/10.1161/CIRCRESAHA.115.302882.
289. Takezako T, Unal H, Karnik SS, Node K. Current topics in angiotensin II type 1 receptor research: Focus on inverse agonism, receptor dimerization and biased agonism. Pharmacol Res. 2017;123:40–50. http://www.ncbi.nlm.nih.gov/pubmed/28648738.
290. Mehta PK, Griendling KK. Angiotensin II cell signaling: physiological and pathological effects in the cardiovascular system. Am J Physiol Cell Physiol. 2007;292:C82–97. https://doi.org/10.1152/ajpcell.00287.2006.
291. Lymperopoulos A, Aukszi B. Angiotensin receptor blocker drugs and inhibition of adrenal beta-arrestin-1-dependent aldosterone production: implications for heart failure therapy. World J Cardiol. 2017;9:200. http://www.ncbi.nlm.nih.gov/pubmed/28400916.
292. Grisanti LA, Schumacher SM, Tilley DG, Koch WJ. Designer approaches for G protein–coupled receptor modulation for cardiovascular disease. JACC Basic Transl Sci. 2018;3:550–62. http://www.ncbi.nlm.nih.gov/pubmed/30175279.
293. Zhou J, Ernsberger P, Douglas JG. A novel angiotensin receptor subtype in rat mesangium. Coupling to adenylyl cyclase. Hypertens (Dallas, Tex 1979). 1993;21:1035–8. http://www.ncbi.nlm.nih.gov/pubmed/8389324.
294. Tian Y, Baukal AJ, Sandberg K, Bernstein KE, Balla T, Catt KJ. Properties of AT1a and AT1b angiotensin receptors expressed in adrenocortical Y-1 cells. Am J Physiol Metab. 1996;270:E831–9. https://doi.org/10.1152/ajpendo.1996.270.5.E831.
295. Mederos y Schnitzler M, Storch U, Gudermann T. Mechanosensitive G q/11 protein-coupled receptors mediate myogenic vasoconstriction. Microcirculation. 2016;23:621–5. http://www.ncbi.nlm.nih.gov/pubmed/27344060.
296. Scholz N, Monk KR, Kittel RJ, Langenhan T. Adhesion GPCRs as a putative class of metabotropic mechanosensors. Handb Exp Pharmacol. 2016;234:221–47. https://doi.org/10.1007/978-3-319-41523-9_10.
297. Scholz N, Guan C, Nieberler M, Grotemeyer A, Maiellaro I, Gao S, et al. Mechano-dependent signaling by Latrophilin/CIRL quenches cAMP in proprioceptive neurons. Elife. 2017;6:e28360. http://www.ncbi.nlm.nih.gov/pubmed/28784204.
298. White JP, Wrann CD, Rao RR, Nair SK, Jedrychowski MP, You J-S, et al. G protein-coupled receptor 56 regulates mechanical overload-induced muscle hypertrophy. Proc Natl Acad Sci U S A. 2014;111:15756–61. https://doi.org/10.1073/pnas.1417898111.

299. Scholz N, Gehring J, Guan C, Ljaschenko D, Fischer R, Lakshmanan V, et al. The adhesion GPCR latrophilin/CIRL shapes mechanosensation. Cell Rep. 2015;11:866–74. https://linkinghub.elsevier.com/retrieve/pii/S2211124715003836.
300. Kramer I, Halleux C, Keller H, Pegurri M, Gooi JH, Weber PB, et al. Osteocyte Wnt/beta-catenin signaling is required for normal bone homeostasis. Mol Cell Biol. 2010;30:3071–85. https://doi.org/10.1128/MCB.01428-09.
301. Duan P, Bonewald LF. The role of the wnt/β-catenin signaling pathway in formation and maintenance of bone and teeth. Int J Biochem Cell Biol. 2016;77:23–9. http://www.ncbi.nlm.nih.gov/pubmed/27210503.
302. Zaidel-Bar R, Itzkovitz S, Ma'ayan A, Iyengar R, Geiger B. Functional atlas of the integrin adhesome. Nat Cell Biol. 2007;9:858–67. http://www.nature.com/articles/ncb0807-858.
303. Walling BL, Kim M. LFA-1 in T cell migration and differentiation. Front Immunol. 2018;9:952. http://www.ncbi.nlm.nih.gov/pubmed/29774029.
304. Sun Z, Guo SS, Fässler R. Integrin-mediated mechanotransduction. J Cell Biol. 2016;215:445–56. http://www.ncbi.nlm.nih.gov/pubmed/27872252.
305. Mori S, Wu C-Y, Yamaji S, Saegusa J, Shi B, Ma Z, et al. Direct binding of integrin alphavbeta3 to FGF1 plays a role in FGF1 signaling. J Biol Chem. 2008;283:18066–75. https://doi.org/10.1074/jbc.M801213200.
306. Margadant C, Sonnenberg A. Integrin-TGF-beta crosstalk in fibrosis, cancer and wound healing. EMBO Rep. 2010;11:97–105. https://doi.org/10.1038/embor.2009.276.
307. Kim S-H, Turnbull J, Guimond S. Extracellular matrix and cell signalling: the dynamic cooperation of integrin, proteoglycan and growth factor receptor. J Endocrinol. 2011;209:139–51. https://joe.bioscientifica.com/view/journals/joe/209/2/139.xml
308. Teoh CM, Tam JKC, Tran T. Integrin and GPCR crosstalk in the regulation of ASM contraction signaling in asthma. J Allergy. 2012;2012:341282. https://www.hindawi.com/archive/2012/341282/.
309. Agarwal SK. Integrins and cadherins as therapeutic targets in fibrosis. Front Pharmacol. 2014;5:131. https://doi.org/10.3389/fphar.2014.00131/abstract.
310. Cournia Z, Allen TW, Andricioaei I, Antonny B, Baum D, Brannigan G, et al. Membrane protein structure, function, and dynamics: a perspective from experiments and theory. J Membr Biol. 2015;248:611–40. https://doi.org/10.1007/s00232-015-9802-0.
311. Wang Y, Bugge K, Kragelund BB, Lindorff-Larsen K. Role of protein dynamics in transmembrane receptor signalling. Curr Opin Struct Biol. 2018;48:74–82. https://linkinghub.elsevier.com/retrieve/pii/S0959440X17301173.
312. Gallo PM, Gallucci S. The dendritic cell response to classic, emerging, and homeostatic danger signals. Implications for autoimmunity. Front Immunol. 2013;4:138. http://www.ncbi.nlm.nih.gov/pubmed/23772226.
313. Dickinson SE, Wondrak GT. TLR4-directed molecular strategies targeting skin photodamage and carcinogenesis. Curr Med Chem. 2018;25:5487–502. http://www.eurekaselect.com/155201/article.
314. Zaffaroni L, Peri F. Recent advances on Toll-like receptor 4 modulation: new therapeutic perspectives. Future Med Chem. 2018;10:461–76. http://www.ncbi.nlm.nih.gov/pubmed/29380635.
315. Gurevich V, Gurevich E. Molecular Mechanisms of GPCR Signaling: A Structural Perspective. Int J Mol Sci [Internet]. 2017;18:2519. http://www.ncbi.nlm.nih.gov/pubmed/29186792.
316. Saotome K, Murthy SE, Kefauver JM, Whitwam T, Patapoutian A, Ward AB. Structure of the mechanically activated ion channel Piezo1. Nature [Internet]. 2018;554:481–6. http://www.nature.com/articles/nature25453.
317. Sun G, Irvine KD. Control of growth during regeneration. Curr Top Dev Biol. 2014;108:95–120. http://www.ncbi.nlm.nih.gov/pubmed/24512707.
318. Foulquier S, Daskalopoulos EP, Lluri G, Hermans KCM, Deb A, Blankesteijn WM. WNT signaling in cardiac and vascular disease. Pharmacol Rev. 2018;70:68–141. http://www.ncbi.nlm.nih.gov/pubmed/29247129.

3 The Growing World of DAMPs

3.1 Introduction

The evolutionarily determined function of DAMPs is to promote injury-, stress-, or molecular perturbation-induced defense responses, the aim always being to repair damaged tissue (i.e., to achieve restitutio ad integrum). The unique molecules accomplish this goal by promoting context-dependently proinflammatory and—in their function as SAMPs—inflammation-resolving pathways, as well as by driving profibrotic tissue-repairing paths. Moreover, in the presence of altered-self or nonself antigens, the DAMPs shape adaptive immune responses that have the same homeostasis-restoring aim. Furthermore, in light of a modern holistic view of the intrinsic nature of our universal defense system, DAMPs induced by mechanical forces at cell membranes may trigger homeostatic responses such as vascular responses upon altered blood pressure. Also, first experimental evidence suggests that DAMPs may be involved in fight-or-flight stress (defense) responses that are generated under the influence of the sympathoadrenal system and hypothalamic–pituitary–adrenocortical (HPA) axis [1–3] (also compare Fleshner and Crane [4] and Fig. 1.1). Cells of our universal defense system can execute these various defense responses using the PRMs mentioned in Chap. 2, which are specialized to recognize cell stress/tissue injury-induced DAMPs (Fig. 3.1). In case the insults are caused by pathogens, these recognition receptors simultaneously sense MAMPs.

Together, this universal defense system perceives any disruption of extra- and intracellular homeostasis as a consequence of inciting insults as reflected by the presence of DAMPs—be it of infectious or sterile nature. In this sense, the innate defense apparatus is now considered to be a significant biological system that has broad homeostatic functions, extending far beyond defending the host against pathogens. The system guarantees—in cooperation, interrelationship, and interaction with the psychoneuroendocrine homeostatic system and the microbiota—maintenance and restoration of cellular integrity of an organism. However, although initially beneficial, these DAMP-triggered, protection-intended tissue repair processes become pathogenic and can lead to pathologies and a considerable spectrum of diseases when they are dysregulated, uncontrolled, and exaggerated (compare Figs. 1.1, 3.1, and 3.2). In fact, this detrimental side of the coin,

W. G. Land, *Damage-Associated Molecular Patterns in Human Diseases*,
https://doi.org/10.1007/978-3-030-53868-2_3

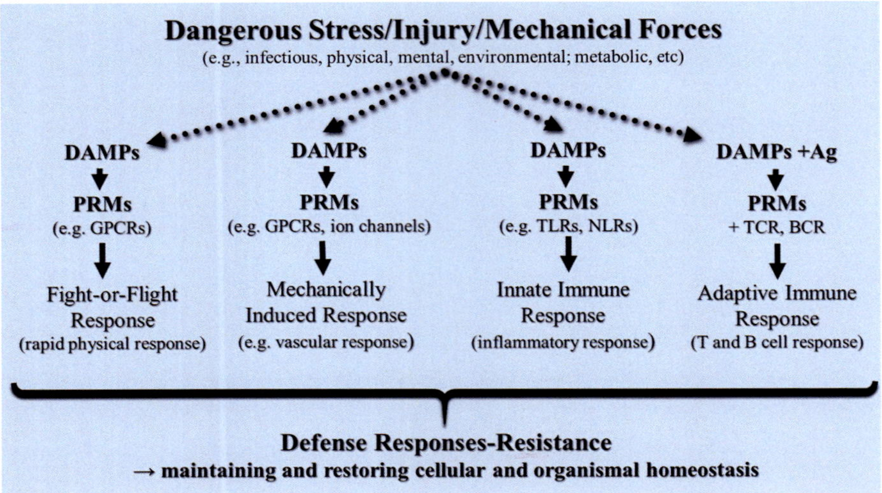

Fig. 3.1 Schematic illustration of the universal defense system that responds to any stress, including mental stress and any injury—may it be of infectious or sterile nature. Any stressful or injurious insult leads to the emission of DAMPs that are sensed by PRMs located on or in cells of the innate immune system. The aim of these defense responses is always for maintaining and restoring cellular and organismal homeostasis, thereby guaranteeing our survival (also compare Fig. 1.1). *BCR* B-cell receptor, *DAMPs* damage-associated molecular patterns, *GPCRs* G protein-coupled receptors, *NLRs* nucleotide-binding oligomerization domain (NOD) leucine-rich repeat receptors, *PRMs* pattern recognition molecules, *TCR* T-cell receptor, *TLRs* Toll-like receptors

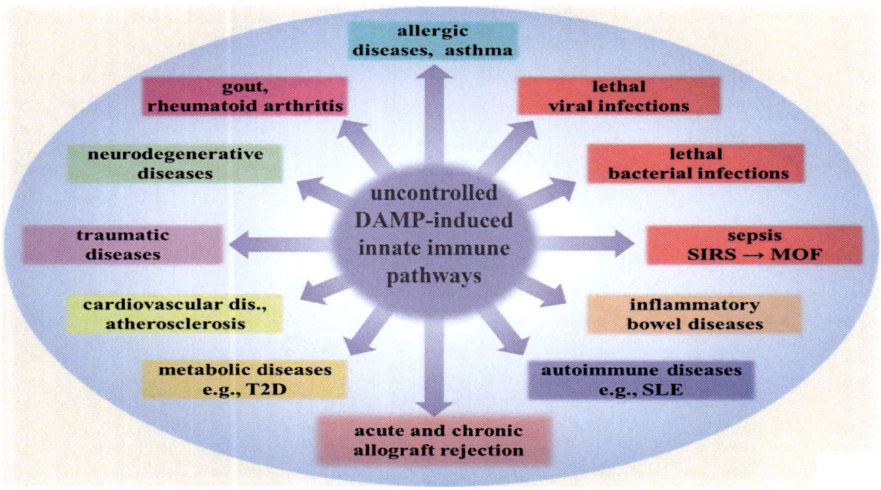

Fig. 3.2 Simplified diagram illustrating emerging evidence for a role of uncontrolled/dysregulated emission of DAMPs in the pathogenesis of many human diseases. *Dis.* Diseases, *MOF* multiple organ failure, *SIRS* systemic inflammatory response syndrome, *SLE* systemic lupus erythematosus, *T2D* type II diabetes mellitus

that is, the DAMP-promoted dysregulated and exaggerated innate defensive responses, will be the subject of the following chapters. As typical human disorders pathogenetically dominated by the work of DAMPs, systemic and organ-specific traumatic diseases, atherosclerosis, and CVD have been chosen to describe in this Vol. 2.

3.2 Classification of DAMPs

3.2.1 Introductory Remarks

At the time being, it can be noticed that researchers in the field of DAMPs are still trying to classify the DAMPs according to their personal viewpoints, knowledge, and field of interest. But this means automatically that many different proposals of a proper DAMPs classification are nowadays "on the market." Here, the classification of DAMPs as described in Vol. 1 [5], Part IV, Sect. 11.2, Table 11.1, is maintained and only slightly amended (addition of a few subclasses). Thus, constitutive and inducible DAMPs, as well as cell-extrinsic and cell-intrinsic dyshomeostatic DAMPs, were included (listed in Table 3.1). As the minimum criterion for inclusion of these molecules in this classification, the description of a cognate sensing/recognizing molecule was chosen. Of course, personally, the author does not agree with all of them, but the intention is to let the reader know what is going on in the world of DAMPs today. Interestingly, in this context, Gong et al. [6] stated correctly: "However, according to this broad definition of DAMPs, one could define every endogenous molecule linked to an inflammatory pathway as a DAMP, which seems unreasonable." Nevertheless, the world of DAMPs becomes "really colorful."

3.2.2 The Four Major Categories of DAMPs as Used in This Book

Thus, DAMPs are ordered in four major categories (CATs) by defining them roughly as endogenous and exogenous DAMPs, whereby the exogenous DAMPs (Cat. IV DAMPs) should refer to molecules invading a host from outside. Endogenous DAMPs are then further subdivided into constitutive and inducible DAMPs (compare Fig. 11.1 in Vol. 1 [5], Part IV).

Constitutive DAMPs are ad hoc, that is, immediately emitted DAMPs, either as native molecules (Cat. I DAMPs) or injury-modified molecules under various conditions (Cat. II DAMPs). Injury-induced alteration of these endogenous DAMPs can occur via conventional or unconventional types of PTMs of native molecules, for example, induced by oxidative or proteolytic processes (for more information about PTMs, see [7] and compare Vol. 1 [5], Part VI, Subchapter 25.3). Moreover, the alteration can be reflected not only by modification of a given molecule but also by changes of a molecular pattern, whereby the molecules per se are not biochemically modified. Such molecular perturbations reflect *homeostatic danger signals* [8] or *homeostasis-altering molecular processes* [9] or ***dyshomeostasis-associated molecular patterns*** [10]. Of note, these homeostatic danger signals are denoted

Table 3.1 Classification of DAMPs as used in this book

Category I: Endogenous DAMPs: Constitutively Expressed Native Molecules (Cat. I DAMPs)	
Class A: DAMPs passively released from necrotic cells	Subclass 1: DAMPs except for indirectly NLRP3-activating molecules Subclass 2: DAMPs indirectly activating the NLRP3 inflammasome
Class B: DAMPs exposed on the cell surface	Subclass 1: Phagocytosis-facilitating molecules ("chaperones") Subclass 2: MHC class I chain-related molecules
Category II: Endogenous DAMPs: Constitutively Expressed, Injury-Modified Molecules (Cat. II DAMPs)	
Class A: DAMPs released from the extracellular matrix	Subclass 1: Proteoglycans Subclass 2: Glycosaminoglycans Subclass 3: Glycoproteins
Class B: Cell-extrinsic modified DAMPs	Subclass 1: Oxidation-specific epitopes (membrane-bound) Subclass 2: Distinct structural sugar patterns (membrane-bound) Subclass 3: Cell-extrinsic dyshomeostasis-associated molecular patterns Subclass 4: Plasma-derived modified soluble molecules
Class C: Cell-intrinsic modified DAMPs	Subclass 1: Nuclear DNA breaks Subclass 2: Cytosolic DNA (nuclear and mitochondrial) Subclass 3: Cytosolic RNA (accumulated, processed) Subclass 4: Cell-intrinsic dyshomeostasis-associated molecular patterns Subclass 5: Abnormally accumulating metabolic molecules
Category III: Endogenous DAMPs: Inducible DAMPs (Cat. III DAMPs)	
Class A: Native molecules acting as inducible DAMPs	Subclass 1: Actively secreted molecules (also passively released) Subclass 2: Cytokines secreted by (DAMP-) activated cells Subclass 3: Full length interleukin-1 family members Subclass 4: Complement-related and vascular molecules Subclass 5: Galectins Subclass 6: NF-κB signaling in cross-priming Subclass 7: Eicosanoids Subclass 8: Vasoactive catecholamines, angiotensin II, endothelin-1
Class B: Modified Molecules Acting as Inducible DAMPs	Subclass 1: Processed interleukin-1 family members Subclass 2: Processed HMGB1 secreted by activated immune cells Subclass 3: Anaphylatoxins C3a and C5a Subclass 4: "Prion-like" polymers ("Specks") Subclass 5: Lysophospholipids Subclass 6: Peroxiredoxins Subclass 7: Wnt Proteins
Class C: Suppressing/inhibiting DAMPs ("SAMPs")	Subclass 1: Prostaglandin E2 Subclass 2: Adenosine (extracellular adenosine, cyclic AMP) Subclass 3: Annexin A1 Subclass 4: Specialized proresolving mediators Subclass 5: Lysophosphatidylserine, Lysophosphatidylethanolamine Subclass 6: Angiotensin (1-7)
Category IV: Exogenous DAMPs (Cat. IV DAMPs)	
Class A: Exogenous DAMPs indirectly sensed by NLRP3	Subclass 1: Aluminium salt Subclass 2: Asbestos fibres Subclass 3: Silica particles Subclass 4: Air pollution particles
Class B: Exogenous DAMPs sensed by nociceptors	Subclass 1: Noxious stimuli involved in thermosensation Subclass 2: Non-reactive compounds Subclass 3: Reactive electrophilic compounds Subclass 4: Vanilloids-capsaicin
Class C: Allergens	Subclass1: Metal Allergens

throughout the book as "dyshomeostatic DAMPs" (whereby DAMPs stand for ***d**ys-homeostasis-**a**ssociated **m**olecular **p**atterns*). Accordingly, such disruption of molecular homeostasis-reflecting DAMPs may be associated, for instance, with extracellular cell-extrinsic acidosis or disturbed osmolarity [11] (newly added in the classification as cell-extrinsic IIB-3 DAMPs). On the other hand, molecular perturbations indicating disruption of molecular homeostasis may be caused by cell-intrinsic intercompartmental dislocation of cellular molecules, unusual accumulation/aggregation of molecules, or intracellular perturbation of molecular patterns. These endogenous modified/native DAMPs—denoted as cell-intrinsic IIC-4 DAMPs—may directly or indirectly induce an inflammatory response.

Endogenous inducible DAMPs (Cat. III DAMPs) are molecules that are "newly made" by (DAMP)-activated cells upon cellular stress or tissue injury or even by cells undergoing (DAMP-promoted) RCD. Inducible DAMPs are generated via neo-transcription in terms of native proteins but also via neotranslation or PTMs in terms of modified proteins. This category of DAMPs is thought to amplify inflammatory responses mainly. Notably, they have recently been proposed to be critical for the generation of immunostimulatory DCs capable to cross-present exogenous antigens [12] (for DC cross-presentation, see Vol. 1 [5], Part VIII, Sect. 32.3.5).

As another category, exogenous DAMPs referring to molecules invading a host from outside have been included in this monograph. According to the perspective of the book, these Cat. IV DAMPs include various exogenous molecules, for example, aluminum salts, asbestos fibers, silica, and air pollution particles; noxious stimuli; some non-reactive compounds; reactive electrophilic compounds; vanilloids; and some allergens. Also, and at least as used in this book and discussed elsewhere [13, 14], MAMPs in terms of inherently injurious molecules derived from pathogens such as toxic LPS or in terms of intracellularly mislocated or pathologically accumulated microbial NAs - associated with endogenous molecular perturbations - may be regarded as exogenous danger signals in terms of DAMP. The interesting topic of exogenous DAMPs has been described in more detail in Vol. 1 [5], Part IV, Chpt. 15, and, thus, is only briefly touched at the end.

3.2.3 What About MAMPs, PAMPs, and DAMPs: A Personal View

In the context with exogenous DAMPs, a proposal is repeated that was already mentioned in Vol. 1. In relation to in vivo scenarios of infection-mediated inflammation and immunity, the following equation is proposed: exogenous MAMPs + endogenous DAMPs = operating as PAMPs in its original sense. For example, throughout this book, the term "MAMP/DAMP-induced inflammation" is used for "infection (= infectious injury)-mediated inflammation." Consequently, when referring to "any cell stress/any tissue injury," I use to articulate like: "any stress or injury is associated with the action of MAMPs and DAMPs or DAMPs (i.e., "MAMPs and DAMPs" in case of infective injury or "DAMPs" alone in case of sterile injury). Certainly, the reader should know that this interpretation of interrelationship between MAMPs and DAMPs is just a personal view and not generally accepted.

3.2.4 Résumé

Many attempts have been made to classify endogenous constitutive and inducible DAMPs into further classes and subclasses, whereby different aspects have been applied. For example, various classes of DAMPs can be identified based on (1) different families of their cognate recognition receptors; (2) their origin (e.g., cell-extrinsic/cell-intrinsic) or chemical nature; or (3) their different modes of emission, that is, (3a) passive release from a necrotic cell, (3b) intracellular active translocation to the plasma membrane and subsequent exposure on the surface of a stressed or dying cell, (3c) proteolytically mediated release from sequestered components of the ECM, (3d) intracellular mislocation from the nucleus into the cytosol (e.g., NAs), (3e) intranuclear DNA changes (e.g., manifested by DNA DSBs), and (3f) active secretion by a stressed or dying cell, either as activating or as inhibiting molecules (hereto, compare [15-24]). A few more details of these various emission forms are selectively added in the following subchapters.

3.3 Endogenous Constitutively Expressed DAMPs (Cat. I DAMPs)

3.3.1 Introductory Remarks

Endogenous DAMPs that are constitutively expressed in their native state are denoted as Cat. I DAMPs. Depending on their mode of emission, they comprise molecules passively released from necrotic cells (Cat. IA DAMPs) or actively exposed at the surface of stressed (or dying) cells (Cat. IB DAMPs). This category of danger signals includes molecules that are regarded as the "prototypical" or "historical" DAMPs, which marked the start of the era of DAMPs. High mobility group box 1 (HMGB1) and heat shock proteins (HSPs) can be found among these molecules but also proteins of entirely different nature, structure, and function such as MHC Class I chain-related proteins (MICs).

3.3.2 Constitutively Expressed Native DAMPs, Passively Released from Necrotic Cells (IA DAMPs)

DAMPs released from necrotic cells are described and illustrated in detail in Vol. 1 [5], Part IV, Sect. 12.2, and Figs. 11.2, 12.2, and 12.3. In principle, "everything from inside" a necrotic cell can theoretically be passively released into the extracellular/interstitial space to operate as a DAMP; examples are HMGB1, HSPs, S100 proteins, extracellular ATP (eATP), and NAs but also pro-forms of certain proteins such as cytokines, mitochondria, lysosomes, peroxisomes, and other organelles. In this book, the Cat. IA DAMPs are divided into (1) DAMPs except for indirectly NLRP3-activating molecules (Subclass IA-1 DAMPs) and (2) DAMPs indirectly activating the NLRP3 inflammasome (Subclass IA-2 DAMPs).

These Cat. IA DAMPs are of particular importance because they play a key role in the promotion of necroinflammatory responses as a common consequence of necrosis, in the form of either accidental cell death (ACD) or subroutines of RN such as necroptosis, ferroptosis, and pyroptosis (reviewed by Sarhan et al. [25]). The remarkable "clou" of these events is that bacterial/viral infection-caused RN of cells—via emission of large amounts of endogenous Cat. IA DAMPs—promotes robust host defense against the virus or the bacterium concerned (that is not mainly triggered by the pathogen per se!). Indeed, as stated by Tonnus and Linkermann [26, 27], growing evidence suggests a significant in vivo impact of RN on human diseases [26, 27]. The authors conclude "that targeting regulated necrosis in vivo represents a novel concept that requires the establishment of first-in-class compounds for clinical use."

3.3.3 Constitutive DAMPs, Exposed at the Cell Surface of Stressed or Dying Cells (IB DAMPs)

DAMPs exposed at the cell surface of stressed or dying cells denoted as Cat.1B DAMPs have been described in detail in Vol. 1 [5], Part IV, Sect. 12.3. They are divided into phagocytosis-facilitating molecules such as calreticulin (CALR) (Subclass IB-1 DAMPs) and MICs such as MHC Class I polypeptide-related sequence A and B (MICA/MICB) (Subclass IB-2 DAMPs), which have gained center stage as bona fide transplantation antigens [28].

The critical role of phagocytosis-facilitating IB-1 DAMPs lies in their function to facilitate antigen uptake. For example, CALR has a vital impact on the engulfment of tumor-associated antigens (TAAs) by phagocytosing DCs to increase the immunogenicity of cancer cells via the phenomenon of immunogenic cell death (ICD). However, it should be noted here that CALR does not only have an immunogenicity-increasing function acting as a DAMP but also exert an opposing immunosuppressive effect through its capability to promote phagocytosis of apoptotic cells by macrophages, a process called efferocytosis (compare Vol. 1 [5], Part IV, Sect. 12.3 and Fig. 12.5, and Part VI, Sect. 22.6.3.3). As will be pointed out in Sect. 5.3.2.2, efferocytosis is a carefully orchestrated process by which phagocytes are recruited to sites of cell death, recognize and engulf dying cells, and clear them in an "immunologically silent" manner. Importantly, this process is a vital prerequisite for the resolution of inflammation (reviewed in [29-31]; also see Sect. 5.3). One explanation for these two obviously contradictory effects may be that CALR exposed on dying tumor cells facilitates engulfment, processing, and presentation of nonself TAAs by DCs that initiates an adaptive anticancer immune response. On the other hand, CALR exposed on dying "self-cells" does not lead to the presentation of nonself antigens to instigate an adaptive immune response (see also similar discussion of this topic in [32]).

The MICs have recently been reviewed [33]. Expression of these DAMPs was shown to be regulated by a variety of stress pathways via different mechanisms (reviewed in [34]) (for stress responses, see Vol. 1 [5], Part V, Chpt. 18, and Sect.

4.2). For example, oxidative stress leads to accumulation of H_2O_2, which reportedly induces MICA and MICB and UL16-binding proteins (ULBPs) 1–4 via activation of the MAPK pathway. In contrast, heat shock can transcriptionally regulate MICA and MICB, as the promoter regions of the MIC genes have heat shock elements that can be recognized by heat shock factor 1 (HSF1). Also, the unfolded protein response (UPR) pathways during endoplasmic reticulum (ER) stress was demonstrated to result in upregulation of ULBP-related protein via the PERK → *activating transcription factor 4* (ATF4) → CHOP pathway (CHOP stands for cytidine–cytidine–adenosine–adenosine–thymidine (CCAAT)-enhancer-binding homologous protein) (reviewed in [34]) (for PERK–ATF4–CHOP pathway, also compare Vol. 1 [5], Part V, Fig. 18.6).

Importantly, compared to damage-modified molecules (Cat. II DAMPs), Cat. IB DAMPs have now taken over a similar crucial innate immune defending function in moderately stressful situations, which can be often observed in clinical situations.

3.3.4 Résumé

Certainly, the list of endogenous constitutively expressed native DAMPs as selectively resumed here refers to the more prominent DAMPs and thus is not complete. Of particular importance are the Class IA DAMPs because, as native molecules passively released from necrotic cells, they are now known to promote necroinflammatory responses. As mentioned, the phenomenon of necroinflammation as a common consequence of RN gains increasing attention, and growing evidence suggests a significant in vivo impact on human diseases. Compared to Class IA DAMPs, Class IB DAMPs have been neglected for a while. On the other hand, as also mentioned, they are now recognized as DAMPs, which are emitted by both stressed and succumbing cells in the early dying phase. As such, these DAMPs may take over an essential innate immune defending function together with damage-modified molecules (Cat. II DAMPs) in moderately stressful situations, in which no necrotic cell death occurs.

3.4 Endogenous Constitutively Expressed, Injury-Modified Molecules (Cat. II DAMPs)

3.4.1 Introductory Remarks

As described in Vol. 1 [5], Chap. 13, this category of DAMPs encompasses various endogenous molecules that undergo different modifications in their constitutional molecular structure upon cell stress and tissue injury, reflected by extra- or intracellular, biochemical, and/or spatially intercompartmental alterations. This category of DAMPs is characterized by different structures, localization, way of emission, and function and, consequently, is sensed by various PRMs. In the following, a brief selective look is taken at these DAMPs by sorting them into two cell-extrinsically modified classes and one cell-intrinsically modified class of molecules.

3.4.2 Damaged-Associated Molecular Patterns Derived from the Extracellular Matrix (IIA DAMPs)

Most but not all DAMPs derived from the ECM are proteolytically released and thus are modified DAMPs (Class IIA DAMPs). They have been described in Vol. 1 [5], Part IV, Sect. 13.2. Proteolysis is performed by certain proteases, which are either released from damaged/dying cells or actively secreted by DAMP-/cytokine-activated cells [35]. For example, specific metalloproteinases (MMPs) are known to act on ECM components to control processes in tissue repair, inflammation, and diseases [36]. These proteases can affect these and other events by proteolysis of ECM proteins. In fact, ECM proteolysis is a widely used mechanism for PTMs of proteins and refers to three principal processes: turnover, remodeling, and degradation. Turnover (or "accretion") is the normal, physiologic breakdown and replacement of a protein or protein complex; the term remodeling is used for describing the breakdown and clearance of ECM in tissues undergoing architectural changes; and the term degradation is being used to indicate the untimely, unregulated, or excessive matrix destruction due to inciting infectious or sterile insults. These MMP-cleaved components are released from the ECM following tissue injury to act in their soluble form as constitutively expressed modified DAMPs. They include proteins such as biglycan, decorin, and fibronectin – *extra domain A* (EDA) (reviewed in [15, 36]). Besides MMPs, other enzymes are involved in proteolysis of ECM components, including hyaluronidase [37] and heparanase [38]. However, there are some exceptions in that the proteoglycan versican is secreted and glycoprotein tenascin-C (TNC) is de novo synthesized (reviewed by Frewert et al. [39]). Such ECM-derived DAMPs reportedly trigger inflammatory processes, for example, via recruitment of leukocytes to sites of infectious and sterile injury. Their "dark side" refers to their ability to aggravate and prolong pathogen-induced inflammatory responses [40].

3.4.3 Cell-Extrinsic Modified DAMPs (IIB DAMPs)

3.4.3.1 General Remarks

The cellular plasma membrane is a privileged site of infectious and sterile tissue injury coming in from the intravasal space such as mechanical forces (damaging ECs) or the extravasal/extracellular environment (damaging, for instance, epithelial and parenchymal cells). Therefore, it is no wonder that many cell-extrinsic modified DAMPs can be found in these anatomic regions. In Vol. 1 [5], Part IV, Sect. 13.3, an attempt was made to define such DAMPs more precisely and denoted as Class IIB DAMPs by breaking them up in subdividing them into (1) membrane-bound oxidation-specific epitopes (OSEs), (2) distinct structural sugar patterns, and (3) plasma-derived modified molecules. Here, OSEs (Subclass IIB-1 DAMPs) and a newly introduced subclass of cell-extrinsic dyshomeostatic DAMPs are briefly addressed.

3.4.3.2 Oxidation-Specific Epitopes

As outlined in Vol. 1 [5], Part IV, Sect. 13.3.2.2, and Part V, Sect. 19.3.3.1, the OSEs are products of iron-dependent lipid peroxidation that is generally considered as a process under which oxidants such as ROS attack lipids containing carbon–carbon double bond(s), especially polyunsaturated fatty acids (PUFAs) that involve hydrogen abstraction from a carbon, with oxygen insertion resulting in lipid peroxyl radicals/phospholipid hydroperoxides (PLOOH). It is this process that leads to the generation of various highly reactive terminal degradation products with high stereospecificity, which include oxidized PtdSer, oxidized phospholipids (OxPLs) containing oxidized cardiolipin (OxCL), phosphatidylcholine (PC), or phosphatidylethanolamine (PE) headgroups, as well as fragments such as reactive aldehydes 4-hydroxynonenal (4-HNE), malondialdehyde (MDA), and 2-(ω carboxyethyl) pyrrole (CEP) (compare also Fig. 13.1 in Vol. 1 [5], Part IV, Sect. 13.3.2.2). Such OSEs including OxPLs and MDA-modified amino groups have been documented on the surface of damaged cells such as apoptotic cells and microvesicles (i.e., circular fragments of plasma membrane), as well as in form of damaged soluble circulating molecules such as oxidized low-density lipoproteins (OxLDLs) (note: oxidation of LDL refers to a complex process during which both the protein and the lipids undergo oxidative changes and form complex products = adducts). Notably, under homeostatic conditions, such lipid peroxidation products modulate and orchestrate a multitude of physiological processes; however, when present in too high concentration, they can cause cell death in the form of ferroptosis. Thus, obviously, there is a direct interconnection between the generation of OSEs and the event of ferroptotic cell death (for details of ferroptosis, see Sect. 4.3.4).

3.4.3.3 Cell-Extrinsic Dyshomeostasis-Associated Molecular Patterns

(Micro)environment-mediated mechanical stimuli to the cellular plasma membrane are sensed by mechanosensors. These cues include not only all components of force (strain, tensile and compressive forces, shear stress, and hydrostatic pressure) but also disturbed osmolarity (hypertonicity → cell shrinking with water egress; hypotonicity → cell swelling with water uptake), as well as substrate rigidity, topology, and adhesiveness (alluded to above in Sect. 2.4). This perception ability is vital for any cell to respond to the surrounding mechanical cues and adapt to the changing environment, the aim always being to maintain homeostasis (for review, see Chen et al. [41]). Mechanosensitive proteins contain a motif or motifs that can change the structure in response upon activation by such mechanical forces, termed mechanical or conformational changes (classified into six categories, see Sect. 2.4.1.2). If the molecular force to be sensed is exerted to a receptor, mechanopresentation would require a distinct conformational change-associated ligand (in terms of a modified DAMP) that is sensed by the mechanosensor concerned. Up to date, however, such mechanical force-induced molecules serving as ligands are not identified.

Thus, as already outlined in Sect. 2.4.5, instead of such putative ligands, cell stress/injury-induced molecular perturbances which induce those conformational changes of mechanosensors or the whole cellular plasma membrane are considered putative cell-extrinsic **d**yshomeostasis-**a**ssociated **m**olecular **p**atterns, which—via activation of mechanosensors—convert extracellularly applied mechanical stimuli into intracellular (bio)chemical signaling pathways.

An example of such dyshomeostatic DAMPs illustrating this scenario may refer to a mechanical sound wave that mediates a variation in pressure (compare Fig. 3.3; also [42]). A region of increased pressure on a sound wave is called compression of molecules (exemplifying, e.g., hypertension-induced molecular compression at the vessel lumen). A region of decreased pressure on a sound wave is called a rarefaction of molecules (exemplifying, e.g., ECM stiffness↔cell interaction-induced traction/tension force-induced molecular dilution; also compare Sect. 6.3 and Figs. 6.1 and 6.2). In other words, sound waves appear to be an appropriate model to illustrate perturbed displacement of molecules reflecting cell-extrinsic dyshomeostasis DAMPs. Hence, these putative DAMPs are tentatively added to the list of modified molecules as Subclass IIB-3 DAMPs (notably, the original Subclass IIB-3 DAMPs are renumerated to IIB-4 DAMPs; see also Table 3.1). Indeed, as a common denominator, such induced conformational changes and dynamics (conformational rearrangements) are widely discussed and agreed upon to be critical to the mechanisms by which transmembrane receptors transmit mechanical signals across membranes [43]. Of note, mechanistically, sensing of acidosis-associated protons (positively

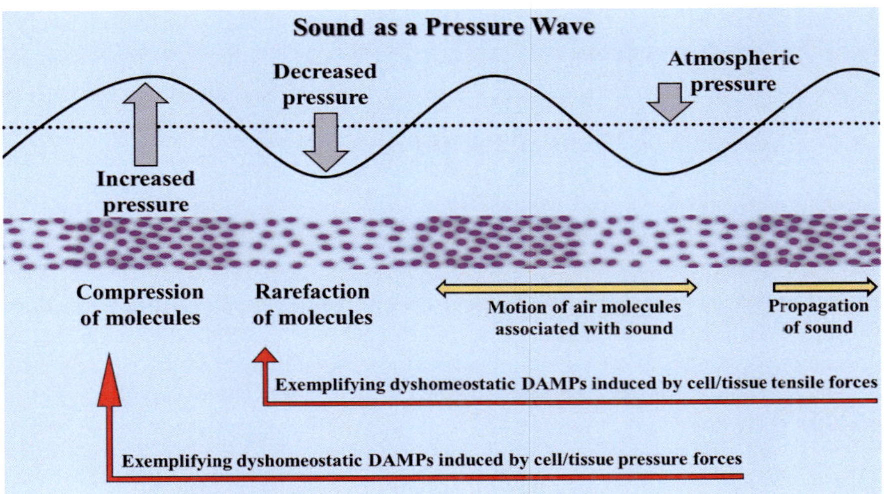

Fig. 3.3 Theoretical model of illustrating sound pressure wave-induced compression or rarefaction of molecules as an example of generation of putative cell-extrinsic dyshomeostatic DAMPs induced by pressure forces or tension/traction forces which can arise, for example, from high blood pressure exerted on vascular cells or ECM stiffness ↔ cell interaction (also compare Sect. 6.3 and Figs. 6.1 and 6.2). (Source: [42])

charged hydrogens ions) by class-A GPCR mechanosensors may also be due to the perception of such dyshomeostatic DAMPs. In fact, as suggested by Zhang et al. [44, 45], activation of GPCR by sensing of protons may be a consequence of the dynamics of protonation of these sensors in terms of conformational changes, rather than protonation process per se.

Together, these molecular perturbation-caused conformational changes of mechanosensors in terms of a change in the shape of a macromolecule (without chemically modifying it) lead to their activation to trigger intracellular downstream signaling pathways. Accordingly, damaging force-induced, perturbed, and displaced molecular patterns that promote conformational changes may be regarded—in analogy to cell-intrinsic dyshomeostatic DAMPs—as cell-extrinsic dyshomeostatic DAMPs that are sensed by distinct mechanosensors.

Here, however, it is appropriate for the reader to know that such cell-extrinsic dyshomeostatic DAMPs have neither been discussed elsewhere in the literature nor generally agreed upon (therefore, they may be called "putative"). Nevertheless, regarding the increasing importance of mechanobiology in maintaining and restoring homeostasis, they are tentatively included in this book on DAMPs.

3.4.3.4 Concluding Remarks

Oxidative PTMs of proteins and lipids result in the development of OSEs, which represent a powerful subclass of DAMPs capable of instigating and maintaining efficiently innate immune efferent and adaptive autoimmune responses. Together with cell-extrinsic dyshomeostatic DAMPs, they are taking care of restoring and maintaining homeostasis to guarantee health and, on the other hand, are involved in the pathogenesis of human diseases such as chronic inflammatory and autoimmune disorders (i.e., OSEs) and atherosclerosis (i.e., OSEs, dyshomeostatic DAMPs).

3.4.4 Cell-Intrinsic Modified DAMPs (IIC DAMPs)

3.4.4.1 General Remarks

Endogenous cell-intrinsic DAMPs refer to molecules that are not passively released from necrotic cells but emerge within cells upon cell stress or damage. As described in Vol. 1 [5], Part IV, Sect. 13.4, this class of DAMPs is denoted as IIC DAMPs that encompass all forms of nuclear or cytosolic, constitutive, or modified molecules, including cell organelles. Doubtlessly, apart from intracellularly located exogenous NAs derived from viruses or bacteria, self NAs can be regarded as the most critical cell-intrinsic endogenous DAMPs.

3.4.4.2 A Brief Summing Up of Cell-Intrinsic Modified DAMPs

In order to spare the reader the annoying task of returning to the pages on Section 11.2.5 in Part IV of Vol. 1 [5], the most important points of this class of DAMP are cursorily resumed here.

Unusual intracellular accumulation of NAs can induce an innate immune response, whereas physiological amounts of endogenous NAs can be tolerated by a sensing PRM and at least not induce a signaling pathway. Moreover, the sensing threshold of a PRM and its signaling cascade can also be subject to modulation [46]. Slight lesions, for example, in the form of discontinuation of intracellular molecules, can also lead to their recognition by PRMs. For example, in the nucleus, DSBs and ssDNA generated upon DNA damage may act as DAMPs (denoted as IIC-1 DAMPs) to be sensed by special receptors located in the nucleus [47] (see also Sect. 2.2.7.3 and for additional information Vol. 1 [5], Part IV, Sect. 13.4.2, p. 285, and Part V, Sect. 18.6.3, p. 410).

Besides the accumulation of NAs, intracellular molecules can dislocate/mislocate or translocate to be recognized as DAMPs. An example of dislocated molecules recognized as DAMPs refers to DNA (IIC-2 DAMPs), leaked from mitochondria (denoted mtDNA) or the nucleus (denoted nDNA) upon cellular damage, or RNA (IIC-3 DAMPs), pathologically accumulated or processed in the cytosol (described in Vol. 1 [5], Part IV, Sects. 13.4.3 and 13.4.4; also compare Sects. 2.2.6.2 and 2.2.7.2). Indeed, our innate immune system noticed every molecule that has left its "homeostatic location" ("breaching of compartmentalization"). Thus, the appearance of NAs in the cytosol signals danger because they should not be there under homeostatic conditions! A typical example of translocation refers to the preapoptotic trafficking of the chaperone CALR from the ER toward the plasma membrane to get exposed at the cell surface during ICD [48]. Another similar example may be reflected by the upregulation of MICs in the ER during stress that are translocated to the cell surface to be exposed at the cell membrane [34, 49, 50].

Another kind of signaling intracellular danger to the innate immune defense system refers to molecular perturbations without any modification of the molecules themselves which remain undamaged and intact, similar and in analogy to sound waves where molecules are compressed or are spread apart (compare Fig. 3.3; and for additional information Vol. 1 [5], Part IV, Sect. 13.4.5, p. 289, and Figs. 11.4, p. 199, and 13.2, p. 290). The interpretation of such molecular perturbations, when occurring extracellularly, has been denoted above as putative cell-extrinsic dyshomeostatic DAMPs. Here, such intracellular perturbations indicating a disturbance/loss of cellular/cytoplasmic homeostasis are denoted as cell-intrinsic dyshomeostatic DAMPs (also compare [8-10]). These DAMPs may intracellularly signal any dangerous pathological stress (e.g., ER stress) such as caused by hypoxia, acidosis, redox imbalance, and intracellular ion perturbations. Accordingly, this subclass of DAMPs (IIC-4 DAMPs) reflecting perturbed molecular homeostasis of a cell is intrinsically associated with any cellular stress be it of infectious or sterile nature.

Finally, accumulating metabolic molecules are included in the class of cell-intrinsic modified DAMPs. As outlined in Vol. 1 [5], Part IV, Sect. 13.4.6 and Fig. 13.3, new insights into intracellular metabolism in DCs and macrophages have stimulated modern notions about a contributing role of metabolism-derived DAMPs in the activation of these key cells of the innate immune system (denoted as metabolic IIC-5 DAMPs). Intriguingly, both cell types have been shown to undergo profound metabolic reprogramming not only in response to environmental cues, such as hypoxia or nutrient alterations, but importantly also in response to DAMP-triggered activation of PRMs. In fact, the activation process of DCs and macrophages is metabolically characterized by a switch toward glycolysis and away from oxidative phosphorylation (OXPHOS)—similar to the Warburg effect ("aerobic glycolysis") in tumors [51, 52] (for more details, see Vol. 1 [5], Part VI, Sect. 24.4). Such metabolic DAMPs include succinate and *thioredoxin-interacting protein* (TXNIP). Of note, succinate as a Krebs cycle intermediate has been shown to operate as an extracellular DAMP when recognized by the "nonclassical" PRR GPR91, also denoted as succinate receptor 1 (SUCNR1). In fact, according to the current paradigm, succinate triggers GPR91-signaling pathways to indicate local stress that may affect cellular metabolism. In this function, succinate is engaged in processes related to innate immunity and inflammation (for further reading, see [53-59]). Thioredoxin-interacting protein is supposed to be significantly generated during ER stress (mostly associated with oxidative stress, under which TXNIP dissociates from the thioredoxin-1 (TRX-1)/TXNIP complex [60]). This metabolic DAMP, as an intracellular amplifier of oxidative stress, has been identified to play a vital role in the canonical activation of the NLRP3 inflammasome leading to release of IL-1β and pyroptosis [61–64]. Clinically, TXNIP was shown to be involved in the pathogenesis of human diseases often associated with ER stress such as type I diabetes mellitus (T1DM) and type II diabetes mellitus (T2DM) [65], neurodegenerative diseases, CVD, stroke, inflammation, metabolic syndrome, myocardial ischemia/reperfusion injury (IRI), and infarction [66–68].

3.4.4.3 Concluding Remarks

In sum, the class of cell-intrinsically modified DAMPs encompasses—as defined for this book—several subclasses such as (1) nuclear DNA breaks, (i.e., DSBs and SSBs = processed DNA), (2) cytosolic DNA (accumulated and mislocated), (3) cytosolic RNA (accumulated and processed), and (4) perturbed intracellular molecular patterns without modifying the molecules per se. Also, another fifth subclass has been included by addressing accumulating metabolic molecules. As with all other DAMPs, this Class IIC of DAMPs can serve as potent tools for innate immune defense, however, when emitted in an uncontrolled way, may contribute to pathologies including chronic infective/sterile inflammatory and autoimmune diseases. Certainly, this list of modified DAMPs as selected here is not complete and will probably change shortly, in particular, by adding further newly discovered cell stress/tissue injury-altered molecules.

3.4.5 Résumé

The category of endogenous constitutively expressed but injury-modified molecules as selectively resumed in this section refers to the more prominent DAMPs, which are of different structure, localization, and function. Apparently, evolution, from the very beginning, has taken care to furnish damaged mammalian cells with clear-cut stigmatic markers, which enable the PRMs to recognize them as danger-signaling molecules correctly. Such markers act as DAMPs to signal any infectious or sterile intracellular perturbation, cell stress, and tissue injury, wheresoever they are located and whatsoever their distinct nature is. One of the greatest achievements in the evolutionary development of PRMs appears to be their ability to distinguish between the cytosolic presence of useful physiological and harmful pathophysiological NAs, that is, to respond only to the accumulation of pathological NAs operating as DAMPs. The result is a harmonic orchestration of innate immune effector responses, which are tailor-made in accordance with the underlying nature and strength of the injurious insult.

3.5 Endogenous Inducible DAMPs (Cat. III DAMPs)

3.5.1 Introductory Remarks

Endogenous inducible DAMPs, defined as a separate category for this book, have been outlined in Vol. 1 [5], Part IV, Chpt. 14. These DAMPs refer to molecules such as peculiar cytokines, which are generated, secreted, and emitted by stress/injury-activated innate immune cells in the course of the primary innate immune response. In most cases, cell activation (eventually resulting via stress responses in RCD) is induced by MAMPs plus DAMPs in case of infectious stress/injury or DAMPs alone in case of sterile stress/injury. Notably, included in the definition of inducible DAMPs is their ability to activate other innate immune cells on their own, thereby promoting another wave of proinflammatory or antiinflammatory/inflammation-resolving innate immune responses.

If one includes inducible DAMPs as a separate category of damage-associated molecules in a book, it is necessary to point out that there are some uncertainties and inconsistencies in their definition. On the one hand, scientific articles referring to inducible DAMPs emitted by activated cells do not expressively refer to a putative involvement of MAMP/DAMP-induced activation of these cells. In such a few cases, the term inducible DAMPs is nevertheless applied in the tenor of the book. Moreover, other cytokines known to be secreted by DAMP-activated cells and demonstrated to activate other types of PRM-bearing innate immune cells have not been addressed in the literature at all, though regarded by the author as putative inducible DAMPs. For example, throughout this book, the transforming growth factor-beta (TGF-β) has been chosen to call as an inducible DAMP, because this molecule is known to activate PRM-bearing myofibroblasts as the key cells in fibrogenesis. On the other hand, some of such inducible DAMPs have also been denoted elsewhere as stressorins [69] and—by referring to cytokines of the IL-1 family—even highlighted by Martin [17] as the real canonical DAMPs of the immune system. To add another level of complexity, a few such molecules mentioned below are proposed by the author himself for the first time. In sum, the definition of the category of inducible DAMPs is still not only blurred and nebulous but also not generally accepted in international literature.

Together, when reading this section, the reader should take these reservations into account and be aware that the molecules presented here as putative inducible DAMPs cannot be momentarily regarded as standard knowledge in the field of innate immunity. Accordingly, the reader may decide to her or his discretion either to use still the traditional terms such as cytokines, inflammatory mediators, and stress hormones or to accept the new term inducible DAMPs.

3.5.2 Generation and Active Secretion of Inducible DAMPs

Inducible DAMPs can be generated by neo-transcription to act as native inducible DAMPs (Class IIIA) or by neo-translation or PTMs to operate as modified inducible DAMPs (Class IIIB). In cells dying from RCD, the occurrence of such DAMPs directly depends on the type of cell death pathway engaged (also compare Yatim et al. [12]). Even of note, many cytokines that act as inducible DAMPs are released by active secretion via unconventional secretion pathways [70] (for secretion mechanisms of inducible DAMPs, including cytokines, see Vol. 1 [5], Part IV, Sect. 11.2.4 and Fig. 11.3 as well as Part VI, Sect. 22.5.2 and Figs. 14.1, 14.2, 14.4). Also worthwhile to mention is that exosomes in the form of extracellular vesicles (EV) play an increasing role in transferring biomolecules such as RNA, DNA, proteins, enzymes, and lipids, which may act as inducible DAMPs [4, 71].

All these secondarily produced DAMPs operate in synergy with constitutively expressed DAMPs and may act as critical danger signals, which promote and expand excessive sterile inflammatory processes such as observed in SIRS. The third class of this Category III refers to inducible SAMPs (Class IIIC DAMPs) that operate as suppressing/inhibiting DAMPs. These molecules emitted by DAMP-activated innate immune cells upon infectious or sterile stress/injury are determined to mitigate or resolve inflammation, to promote repair processes, and to suppress cytotoxic adaptive immune responses, in one word, to establish restoration and maintenance of homeostasis following the first proinflammatory phase.

3.5.3 Endogenous Native Molecules Operating as Inducible DAMPs (IIIA DAMPs)

3.5.3.1 General Remarks

The subclasses sorted into this class, so far published and described in Vol. 1 [5], Part IV, Sect. 14.2, refer to various inducible native DAMPs, which include (1) molecules that are also "classically" emitted, that is, passively released from necrotic cells such as HSPs, eATP, and S100 A proteins (IIIA-1 DAMPs), whereby secretion of these molecules via exosomes plays an increasing role (see below); (2) cytokines, which are neo-transcribed in MAMP+DAMP- or DAMP-activated PRM-bearing innate immune cells (e.g., neutrophils, M1-like macrophages [72–74]) such as TNF (compare Fig. 3.4) and type I IFNs (IIIA-2 DAMPs); (3) full-length IL-1 family member such as pro-IL-1α and pro-IL-33 (IIIA-3 DAMPs); (4) complement-related and vascular molecules such as properdin and molecules released from *Weibel–Palade bodies* (WPBs) such as the *von Willebrand factor* (VWF), P-selectin, and uromodulin (IIIA-4 DAMPs); (5) galectins (GALs) (IIIA-5 DAMPs); and

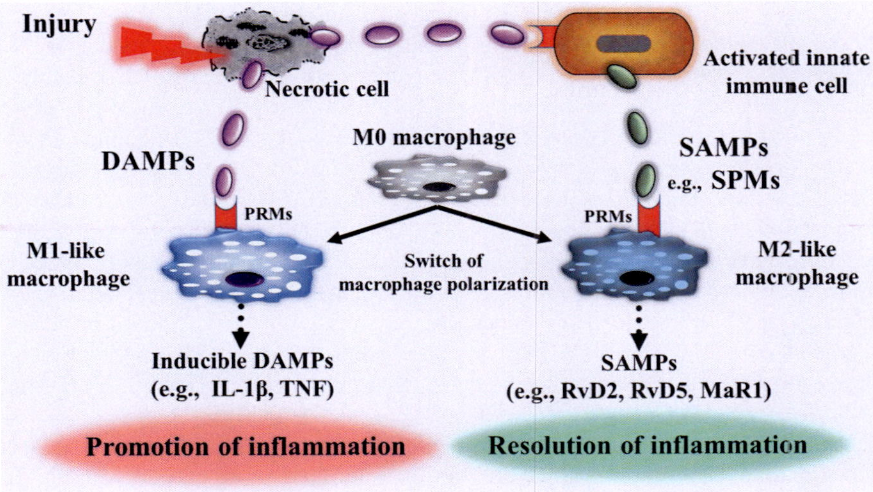

Fig. 3.4 Conceptual model of production of proinflammatory inducible DAMPs (exemplified by IL-1β, TNF) by DAMP-activated M1-like macrophages during promotion of inflammation and antiinflammatory/proresolving inducible SAMPs (exemplified by the SPMs RvD2, RvD5, MaR1) by SAMP-activated M2-like macrophages during resolution of inflammation. *IL-1β* interleukin-1beta, *MaR1* maresin1, *M0* resting macrophages, *PRMs* pattern recognition molecules, *RvD2/5* resolving D2/D5, *SPMs* specialized proresolving mediators, *TNF* tumor necrosis factor. (Sources: [72–74, 98, 208–213, 273])

finally (6) the transcription factor NF-κB (IIIA-6 DAMPs). Of note, three more molecules that may also be regarded as inducible DAMPs are added to this list: eicosanoids denoted as IIIA-7 DAMPs, as well as catecholamines and Ang II denoted as vasoactive IIIA-8 DAMPs (together with ET-1, see below).

Notably, native inducible DAMPs, secreted by DAMP-activated cells upon infectious injury, may be able to amplify an innate defense response against pathogens. Such an example has been reported by Niessner et al. [75] referring to atherosclerotic plaques, where IFN-α functions as an inflammatory amplifier. The authors observed that IFN-α sensitizes APCs toward pathogen-derived TLR4 ligands by upregulating TLR4 expression, thereby intensifying the production of proinflammatory mediator substances such as TNF, IL-12, and MMP-9.

3.5.3.2 Exosome-Transferred, Secreted Inducible DAMPs

An emerging source of non-cell death mechanism for cellular release of DAMPs is their inclusion in exosomes. Indeed, exosomes have gained increasing attention in different biological research fields (plants–microorganisms, animals) over the past decade and, thus, deserve a few more words in the context of secreted inducible DAMPs (for a recent review, see [76]). Studies have shown that different types of exosomes are produced under normal physiological or various pathological conditions and participate in various life activities. Exosomes are biovesicles of 30–100 nm in size that are actively secreted through an exocytosis pathway into surrounding body fluids upon fusion of multivesicular bodies (MVBs) (i.e., organelles of the endocytic pathway) and the plasma membrane (briefly touched in Vol. 1 [5], Part IV, Sect. 11.2.4.3). Exosomes, together with plasma membrane-budded microvesicles and apoptotic bodies (both considered to be larger than 100 nm), belong to the three main types of EVs. Functionally, exosomes are vehicles that carry a complex cargo of proteins, lipids, and NAs (e.g., messenger (m)RNA, micro (mi)RNA, DNA), that is, various subclasses of IIIA-1DAMPs (known to be released from necrotic cells) that are now secreted and delivered to (even distant) target cells including innate immune cells. Via this property, exosomes can horizontally transfer information via cell↔cell communication, for example, to reprogram recipient cells epigenetically. Of crucial importance, for example, is the secretion of DNA fragments-containing exosomes that has been proposed as a model in which exosome secretion maintains cellular homeostasis by removing harmful cytoplasmic DNA from cells [77].

Exosome biogenesis starts within the endosomal system. Initially, early endosomes mature into late endosomes or MVBs, and during this process, the endosomal membrane invaginates to generate vesicles in the lumen of the organelles. The *endosomal sorting complexes required for transport* (ESCRT) machinery is important in this process (for ESCRT machinery, see Box 3.1, and [78-80]; for further reading concerning exosome biogenesis, purification, etc., see [4, 71, 81-83]).

Box 3.1 The Endosomal Sorting Complexes Required for Transport (ESCRT) Pathway

The *endosomal sorting complexes required for transport* (ESCTR) pathway mediates cellular membrane remodeling that results in membranes bending/budding away from the cytoplasm and fission reactions. The machinery comprises five core cytosolic protein complexes, known as ALIX, ESCRT-I, ESCRT-II, ESCRT-III, and Vps4 (an AAA ATPase, i.e., ATPases associated with diverse cellular activities). The complexes are typically recruited to target membranes by site-specific adaptors that bind one or both of the early-acting ALIX and ESCRT-I/ESCRT-II. Following, these factors nucleate assembly of ESCRT-III subunits into membrane-bound filaments that recruit the Vps4. Together, ESCRT-III filaments and Vps4 remodel and dismantle cellular membranes. The ESCRT machinery plays a vital role in a number of cellular processes, including unconventional protein secretion, multivesicular body (MVB) biogenesis, autophagosome closure, plasma membrane repair, exovesicle shedding, nuclear pore complex quality control, nuclear envelope repair after rupture, endolysosomal repair, cytokinetic abscission during mitotic exit (the process by which the membrane connecting two daughter cells is cleaved), and viral budding (the process by which specific types of viruses exit cells).

For further reading, see [78-80].

Prominent in the perspective of the book is the phenomenon that exosomes can be released from both stressed living cells and dying apoptotic cells. For example, studies on several in vitro stress models (e.g., ionizing radiation- and cisplatin-induced cell stress, hypoxia-mediated stress, ER stress) have shown that cellular stress increases exosome secretion [84–89]. In studies on apoptotic cells, the release of exosomes (together with microvesicles and apoptotic bodies) from apoptotic cells has also been reported (reviewed in [71, 90]). Apoptosis may be activated deliberately by a variety of injurious stimuli, including certain types of severe cell stress and insults or in response to extracellular signals triggered by specific death-inducing ligands, for example, TNF. In particular, the extrinsic pathway is involved in injury-induced immune function (for intrinsic and extrinsic apoptotic pathways, see Vol. 1 [5], Part V, Sect. 19.2, and Fig. 19.3). Also of interest in this context are studies on an in vitro stress model showing that severe ER stress induced by two distinct mechanisms in *BeWo* choriocarcinoma cells (a cell line used to model trophoblast) can result in the release of EVs carrying proinflammatory DAMPs [91]. In another recently reported in vitro study on human and mouse cholangiocyte cell lines, EVs from both cell lines were found to contain the DAMP S100A11, a ligand for the receptor for RAGE [92].

Of note, however, exosomes/microvesicles released from apoptotic cells have been shown not only to activate proinflammatory pathways [93–96] but may also promote proresolving/immunosuppressive responses through release of soluble cytokine receptors and stimulation of SPMs in macrophages, respectively [96–98] (for SPMs, see below). That DAMPs such as HMGB1 and eATP packed in exosomes and other EVs are the real players in promoting these responses is well appreciated and has already been documented [4, 95, 99–101].

Collectively, these studies clearly show that stressed/apoptotic cell-associated exosome secretion contributes to the emission of inducible DAMPs, which can aggravate and amplify context-dependently proinflammatory or proresolving innate immune responses.

3.5.3.3 Eicosanoids

Eicosanoids have been briefly addressed in Vol. 1 [5], Part VI, Sect. 22.5.13, in the chapter on *Inflammatory Mediator Substances of the Innate Immune System*. Growing evidence, however, may allow these molecules to be included in the list of inducible DAMPs. Indeed, there is convincing evidence suggesting that innate immune cells, including macrophages, are activated by PRMs such as TLRs and purinergic receptors to produce eicosanoids. These molecules, classically divided into prostaglandins and leukotrienes (LTs), are bioactive lipid products primarily derived from the oxidation of arachidonic acid (AA) and related PUFAs, which regulate a diverse set of physiological and pathological processes ranging from inflammatory responses to tissue repair and chronic tissue remodeling [102, 103].

Leukotriene B4 (LTB4) is an endogenous lipid mediator of inflammation derived from AA by the sequential action of cytosolic phospholipase A2 and 5-lipoxygenase. Acting as a key chemoattractant, LTB4 is a proinflammatory lipid mediator that recruits inflammatory cells such as neutrophils by interacting with two major

GPCRs, the high-affinity receptor BLT1 and the low-affinity receptor BLT2 [104–106]. The molecule is mainly secreted by neutrophils and macrophages after MAMP/DAMP↔ PRR-triggered activation and, thus, may be regarded as an inducible DAMP. For example, harmful neutrophil degranulation was shown to induce the activation of macrophages, which produces LTB4 (besides TNF). The lipid mediator LTB4 is a potent neutrophil chemoattractant, and recently, its role as a dominant molecule that amplifies many arms of phagocyte antimicrobial effector function has been unveiled. However, excessive LTB4 production may contribute to disease severity in chronic inflammatory diseases such as diabetes and arthritis, which could potentially be involved in weak host defense in these groups of patients (for further reading, see [107-110]).

Of note, however, endogenous lipid mediators do not possess proinflammatory properties in general. By contrast, another group of lipid mediators functions as typical antiinflammatory/proresolving molecules: the SPMs, as will be further outlined in Sect. 3.5.5.5.

3.5.3.4 Catecholamines

Another subclass of native molecules may also be tentatively included in this class of inducible DAMP: the stress-induced, HPA axis-mediated catecholamines (note for the reader: these molecules are not generally accepted as inducible DAMPs). Catecholamines are endogenous neurosignaling mediators and hormones, which are integral in maintaining homeostasis by promptly responding to any stressor (for recent reviews including the following text, see Tank and Lee Wong [111] and Lymperopoulos et al. [112]). Although Epi and NE are structurally related, they have differing effects. Epinephrine has more wide-ranging effects, whereas NE has a more specific action working mainly on alpha receptors to increase and maintain blood pressure. Also, both catecholamines derive from two major sources in the whole organism. All of the circulating Epi in the body and a significant amount of circulating NE derive from the adrenal chromaffin cells located in the adrenal medulla, which are cells that synthesize, store, and release Epi (mainly) and NE. On the other hand, circulating NE is partially derived from the adrenal medulla, but the remainder stems from the overflow of NE secreted in synapses at target effector organs innervated by postganglionic sympathetic nerves (for a comprehensive review, see [113]). Notably, the secretion of catecholamines from adrenal chromaffin cells is controlled in a complex way via a variety of membrane receptors, the vast majority of which are GPCRs, including ARs, which act as "presynaptic autoreceptors" in this regard (see also Sect. 2.3.4.4).

Physical challenges, increased physical activity, and psychological/emotional, thermal, or environmental stress trigger stress responses, which require altered activity of visceral organs, glands, and smooth muscles. These changes in activity also encompass the "fight-or-flight" response and must occur promptly and immediately, or the organism may not survive. During such a stressful situation, the sympathetic nervous system is rapidly stimulated, resulting in large amounts of Epi and NE secreted by adrenal chromaffin cells and NE produced by sympathetic nerves. Both catecholamines then are sensed by innate immune GPCRs to initiate the necessary, appropriate defense responses. In fact, this evolutionarily developed function of Epi and NE may tentatively qualify them as inducible DAMPs (for a modern holistic view of the universal defense system, also compare Sect. 1.2).

In humans, plasma Epi and NE levels increase two- to tenfold after exposure to different types of stress [114–116]. Interestingly, in some situations, Epi levels are more elevated than NE concentrations. For example, a substantial increase in circulating Epi compared to NE can be observed after surgical stress [117]. As also reviewed by Tank and Wong [111], the main direct effects of Epi and NE on peripheral tissues as, for example, observed during a fight-or-flight response include (1) increased blood pressure, heart rate, and contractility; (2) smooth muscle contraction in blood vessels leading to vasoconstriction; (3) smooth muscle relaxation in blood vessels associated with vasodilation in the skeletal muscle, heart, and brain; (4) increased glycogenolysis and gluconeogenesis in the liver; (5) increased lipolysis in adipose tissue; and (6) prolonged mydriasis. Again, all these responses are mediated by the interaction of the catecholamines with a select subset of GPCRs, that is, as mentioned above, the ARs expressed on the target organs. These receptors mediate the sympathetic response to stress by triggering signaling pathways resulting in changes in organ and smooth muscle function. Also, as also reviewed by Tank and Lee Wong [111], circulating catecholamines can alter memory via effects on afferent sensory nerves impacting the central nervous system function. While these rapid responses may be necessary for survival, sustained elevation of circulating catecholamines for prolonged periods can also produce pathological conditions, such as atherosclerosis often associated with hypertension and cardiac hypertrophy (as outlined in Chap. 10).

3.5.3.5 Angiotensin-II

Angiotensin II—here included in the list of inducible DAMPs—has also been regarded as such as stress-induced molecule elsewhere [118, 119]. The generation of Ang II within this system is complex: First, the RAS (or (RAAS) is a regulatory cascade that plays major physiological roles in blood pressure regulation, fluid volume, and electrolyte homeostasis (sodium–potassium balance) (recently reviewed by Satou et al. [120] and Takimoto-Ohnishi and Murakami [121]). Second, the molecule is an enzymatically cleaved product of protein angiotensinogen, an alpha-globulin. Initially, the protease renin enzymatically cleaves off two amino acids of angiotensinogen to form angiotensin I (Ang I), a decapeptide. Renin is synthesized by juxtaglomerular apparatus and collecting duct cells as an inactive form and secreted into the circulation upon metabolic stress, sympathetic activation (via catecholamines → β-adrenergic receptors), dehydration, hypotension in the afferent arterioles of renal glomerulus, and low levels of intratubular sodium (reviewed in [122-125]). Then, the ACE changes Ang I—the first and rate-limiting step in the RAS—to the bioactive form Ang II, primarily in the pulmonary endothelium, though this enzyme is present in the endothelium of other organs including the heart.

The classic RAAS encompasses the *ACE-Ang II-AT$_1$R* axis that homeostatically controls hemodynamic stability by regulating blood pressure, fluid volume, and sodium–potassium balance. However, as typically for inappropriately controlled innate defense mechanisms, dysregulation of this system associated with high levels of the RAAS molecules has been observed to play a significant pivotal role in pathologies, in particular, arterial hypertension. And chronic high pressure exerts mechanical stress—often associated with hypertension-induced oxidative stress—along the vascular system, heart, and kidneys that is associated with emission of DAMPs, which promotes chronic inflammatory and fibrogenic responses resulting in end-organ failure, mainly due to fibrosis (compare Sect. 6.4, and for further reading, see reviews in [125-128]).

3.5.3.6 Endothelin-1

Another vasoactive molecule acting as an inducible DAMP and emitted by exocytosis of WPBs is ET-1, a member of the endothelin family of proteins (ET-1, ET-2, and ET-3). Endothelin-1 is a very potent profibrotic vasoconstrictor with remarkably long-lasting action known to play multiple, complex roles in cardiovascular, neural, pulmonary, reproductive, and renal physiology. Under homeostatic conditions, this bioactive peptide is continuously released from the small vesicles of the constitutive pathway to interact with ET receptors to contribute to vasomotor tone. However, upon external insults such as physical and chemical insults, including shear stress, hypoxia, thrombin, and vasoactive factors, the molecule is also released from WPBs [129]. As published elsewhere, most of these insults can induce DAMPs such as shear stress-induced HMGB1 [130], hypoxia-induced HMGB1, mtDNA [131], and kinins [132–134].

Once released abluminally from ECs, ET-1 can interact with two main ET-1 receptors, ET_A and ET_B, which have different tissue and functional distributions. The peptide interacts mainly with ET_A receptors expressed on the underlying VSMCs but with a small population of ET_B receptors also mediating constriction in some but not all vessels (for a comprehensive review, see Davenport et al. [135]).

Together, it is the ET-1→ET-1 receptor signaling pathway that exerts the extraordinary vasoconstriction that may become pathogenic—as observed—in the human cardiovascular system. Thus, it is not surprising that ET receptor antagonists have been clinically developed and applied as potential novel therapeutics in mitigating IRI-induced pathologies such as myocardial infarction (MI) [136] but also in preventing long-term pathological effects such as severe chronic heart failure [137], persistent pulmonary hypertension [138], and arterial hypertension [139]. However, a final evaluation of the therapeutic benefits is apparently still missing.

3.5.3.7 Concluding Remarks

It is to be expected that the inducible DAMPs described in this section will gain the least acceptance in the future. Nevertheless, they have been tentatively mentioned here in the vision of a modern holistic view of our universal defense system. Certainly, future targeted studies—particularly evolution-oriented studies—will show whether or not such a tentative approach to the function of stress-/injury-induced molecules can be integrated into a holistic view on innate defense mechanisms across the tree of life.

3.5.4 Endogenous Modified Molecules Acting as Inducible DAMPs (IIIB DAMPs)

3.5.4.1 General Remarks

The subclasses sorted into this class, so far published and described in Vol. 1 [5], Part IV, Sect. 14.3, refer to processed IL-1 family members IL1α and IL-1β (IIIB-1 DAMPs); secreted HMGB1 (IIIB-2 DAMP) (for additional information compare Fig. 14.4, in Vol. 1 [5], Part IV, p. 326); anaphylatoxins (= complement fragments 3a and 5a, = C3a and C5a = IIIB-3 DAMPs); and "prion-like" polymers (IIIB-4 DAMPs). They are not all resumed here. Instead, a few more words to prion-like polymers are added. In addition, new subclasses, the lysophospholipids (LPLs, IIIB-5 DAMPs), peroxiredoxin-1 (PRDX1, IIIB-6 DAMP), and Wnt (denoted as IIIB-7 DAMPs), are briefly introduced.

3.5.4.2 Prion-Like Polymers ("Specks")

Prion-like polymers such as the ASC specks and aggregated MAVS have already been addressed as new candidates of inducible DAMPs in Vol. 1 [5], Part IV, Sect. 14.3.5, and concisely mentioned in Sects. 2.2.5.4 and 2.2.6.3. They are defined as molecules to propagate immune signaling and also principally regarded as an evolutionarily conserved mechanism of signal transduction in innate immunity (as such also outlined and competently discussed by Cai et al. [140]). Given the growing impact of ASC specks on the progression of inflammatory disorders such as neuroinflammation associated with Alzheimer's disease [141], they are briefly resumed here. The structure of ASC specks provides a unique signaling platform or compartment to control the activity of caspase-1 and likely other effectors. As competently reviewed by Franklin et al. [142], there is emerging evidence indicating that ASC specks are extracellularly released from inflammasome-activated cells and accumulate in inflamed tissues, where they can continue to mature cytokines or be internalized by surrounding cells to further nucleate ASC specks in their cytosol. As also outlined by Franklin et al. [142], the mechanisms by which ASC specks are released (or secreted?) and subsequently engulfed by neighbored cells remain largely unexplored. The efferent functions of ASC specks have also been described by the authors [142]: "(1) They can largely amplify the initial inflammasome signals by sustaining IL-1 cytokine production in the extracellular space; (2) boost T-cell responses via enhanced IL-1 signaling, or via cross-presentation of cytosolic co-aggregated antigens; (3) cause, or exacerbate autoimmunity by inducing the production of autoreactive anti-ASC, which were shown to boost IL-1β inflammation in vitro and in vivo; and potentially (5) entrap microbes, together with other pyroptotic cell corpses for clearance by neutrophils." Franklin et al. [142] finally concluded: "We strive to explain how ASC-dependent signaling achieves a well-balanced response to diverse threats by acting as a signaling hub that coordinates the innate and adaptive immune responses."

Together, ASC specks released by inflammasome-activated cells contribute to instigation and/or amplification of inflammatory and immune responses, thereby qualifying them as inducible DAMPs from the perspective of the book. The underlying mechanism, however, is different from other inducible DAMPs: they do not signal through distinct cognate PRMs to aggravate inflammatory processes, but instead—when engulfed by surrounding cells—they recruit and activate procaspase-1 again that causes both maturation and release of IL-1β and IL-18 as well as GSDMD-dependent pyroptosis (for additional information compare also Vol. 1 [5], Part VI, Sect. 22.4.2.2, p. 516, and Fig. 22.11, p. 517). Finally, pyroptotic cell death then may result in another wave of passively releases DAMPs.

3.5.4.3 Lysophospholipids

Lysophospholipids such as lysophosphatidic acid (LPA), sphingosine 1-phosphate (S1P), sphingosylphosphorylcholine (SPC), and lysophosphatidylcholine (LPC) may also be included in the list of inducible DAMPs (newly denoted as IIIB-5 DAMPs). Interestingly, Shao et al. [143] have proposed to call this group of endogenous metabolites "conditional DAMPs" in reference to their property to mediate homeostatic cellular functions at physiological concentrations but, at elevated levels, initiate sterile inflammatory pathways during various pathologies. Furthermore, the authors coined the term "conditional DAMP receptors" for the receptors of such endogenous metabolites, as they would trigger inflammatory signals when the concentration of their ligands reaches pathophysiological levels. Notably, such aberrant levels of most LPLs sensed by GPCRs as their prototypical receptors promote proinflammatory pathways to trigger innate immune responses leading to tissue oxidative and inflammatory injury. For example, increased levels of LPC were found in atherosclerotic models indicating a critical role of this DAMP as a proinflammatory mediator during the progression of the disorder [144–146]. By contrast, lysophosphatidylethanolamine (LPE) and LysoPS are supposed to exert antiinflammatory/proresolving effects [147, 148] and, thus, are listed under SAMPs (see next section).

3.5.4.4 Peroxiredoxins

Peroxiredoxins (PRDXs or PRXs) are a family of antioxidant proteins that remove ROS and other oxidative stress products. Some family members (PRDX1, PRDX2, PRDX4, PRDX5, PRDX6) have been reported to act as inducible DAMPs (newly denoted as IIIB-6 DAMPs) by stimulating secretion of proinflammatory cytokines via binding to TLR4 and TLR2, as well as (at least shown for PRDX1) interacting with NLRP3 (reviewed in [149-152]). The PRDX1 molecule is supposed to be secreted from stressed/damaged cells under PTMs (e.g., oxidation) via a nonclassical secretory pathway [153] or by an exosomal pathway [154]. Peroxiredoxin-1 was shown to be produced upon stress conditions (e.g., oxidative stress), especially during the acute inflammatory responses. For example, a study on liver injury models provided evidence suggesting that circulating PRDX1 can aggravate acute liver injury and elicit hepatic inflammation at least in part via activating the NLRP3 inflammasome signaling pathway [152]. As a final remark, it should not remain unmentioned that some PRDXs were reported to be also released from necrotic cells (e.g., see [150, 151]).

3.5.4.5 Wnt Proteins

Wnt proteins are a highly conserved family of secreted glycoproteins that serve as ligands for a diverse set of receptors that reportedly trigger signaling pathways to regulate several vital networks during tissue homeostasis including promotion of developmental and regenerative processes (reviewed in [155-157]) (also compare Sect. 2.3.4.7 and Box 2.1). It has been proposed that Wnt proteins are secreted, probably by stressed cells, under extensive PTMs in vesicles to bind to the GPCR receptor, that is, an observation suggesting these proteins to add tentatively to the list of inducible DAMPs (denoted as IIIB-7 DAMPs). Secreted Wnt protein then interacts with frizzled that triggers β-catenin-mediated signaling pathway in distant cells (for Frizzled, see Sect. 2.3.4.7; for more details of the Wnt →β-catenin pathway, see Sect. 6.5.3.4 and Fig. 6.3). There is growing evidence for Wnt signaling to be implicated in many diseases, including osteoporosis, neurodegenerative diseases, and CVDs (reviewed in [155-157]). Also, Wnt-triggered signaling pathways in terms of an interplay with TGF-β exert synergistic effects on myofibroblast differentiation, thereby promoting progressive fibrosis, a topic that will be described in more detail in Sect. 6.5.3.

3.5.4.6 Concluding Remarks

Again, this class of endogenous stress/injury-modified inducible DAMPs is not generally agreed upon. Nevertheless, some molecules such as PRDXs and LPLs have already been included in this subclass of DAMPs, though denoting them with other terms such as "conditional DAMPs" for LPLs [143]. Certainly, this emerging field of research is currently in motion, and, for the future, we can expect more exciting data, may they support or contradict this concept.

3.5.5 Inducible Suppressing DAMPs: The SAMPs (IIIC DAMPs)

3.5.5.1 General Remarks

As outlined in Vol. 1 [5], Part IV, Sect. 14.4, the concept of homeostasis is one that not only requires a fine balance between both proinflammatory mediators and antiinflammatory→proresolving mediators but also premises that this fine-tuned balance occurs in a time- and space-specific manner. In fact, as outlined many times throughout the book, strength-/time-/space-dysregulated, excessive, or chronic inflammatory responses are linked to the initiation and/or exacerbation of a variety of human diseases (for inflammation and resolution of inflammation, also see Vol. 1 [5], Part VI, Sect. 22.2, and compare Sect. 5.3 and Fig. 5.1). Accordingly, accumulating evidence now indicates that, besides activating DAMPs, suppressing DAMPs, that is, SAMPs, are actively secreted by DAMP-activated innate immune cells (mainly leukocytes and macrophages) upon stress and injury, which—in parallel to proinflammatory responses—convey antiinflammatory → proresolving processes and shape immunosuppressive responses. When the stressful and injurious stimuli are passed, for example, when toxic agents or pathogenic microbes are neutralized and eliminated, DAMPs for neutrophil recruitment cease abruptly choking continued recruitment, both events occurring in a contemporary way. Clearance of recruited neutrophils is then the option of choice to convert tissues to their normal homeostatic function, and, importantly, clearance must be timely before these short-lived cells disintegrate and pour their toxic phlogistic contents out, in other words as appropriately pronounced by Bratton and Henson [158]: "when the party is over, clean-up begins." Indeed, both events, "turn off" of neutrophil recruitment and the "turn on" of neutrophil removal, co-occur (compare Fig. 5.1). It is the work of SAMPs which contribute to this mechanism of correct resolution of inflammation, thereby avoiding pathogenic autoinflammatory processes and preventing adaptive autoimmune responses. These SAMPs include, but are not limited to, prostaglandin E2 (PGE2, IIIC-1 DAMPs)—recently reported to promote an antiinflammatory neutrophil phenotype and determine the outcome of inflammation resolution in vivo [159]; adenosine in form of intracellular cyclic adenosine monophosphate (cAMP) and extracellular adenosine (IIIC-2 DAMPs) [160–165]; annexin A1 (AnxA1, IIIC-3 DAMP) [166–169]; SPMs (IIIC-4 DAMPs) [170–172]; and PtdSer/LysoPS (IIIC-5 DAMPs) [173–179]. Here, as another LPL besides LysoPS, LPE (IIIC-5 DAMPs) should be added that was found to lower the level of proinflammatory mediators, but in contrast, to augment the antiinflammatory cytokine IL-10 [148]. Also, as a new molecule, angiotensin-(1-7) (Ang-[1-7]) can be included in the SAMP list. Among the various protective actions of Ang-(1-7), inhibition of inflammatory responses and protection of endothelial cell function are two of the most prominent (for further reading, see [180–182]).

3.5.5.2 The "Resolving SAMPs Axis"

As discussed and illustrated in Vol. 1 [5], Part IV, Sects. 14.4.2 and 14.4.3, and Fig. 14.5, the "resolving SAMPs axis" is typically implicated in the resolution of inflammation and composed of the sequelae of molecules, including "PGE2 ↔ EP2/EP4 → cAMP → protein kinase A (PKA) → AnxA1 ↔ FPR2 → proresolving pathways." This topic is not resumed here; however, within this axis, cAMP is being given increasing attention and therefore deserves a few more words.

3.5.5.3 Cyclic Adenosine Monophosphate

As outlined in Vol. 1 [5], Part IV, Sect. 14.4.2.3 and Fig. 14.5, intracellular cAMP is appreciated as a molecule able to suppress innate immune responses by inhibiting proinflammatory cytokine production. In particular, sustained elevations in intracellular cAMP concentrations were shown to be immunosuppressive, and emerging evidence suggests that cAMP compartmentalization may account, at least in part, for this effect [183]. This effect and other emerging data support a role for cAMP in some steps of the resolution process [163, 184, 185]. In particular, Sousa's group has documented that cAMP mimetics induce resolution of an established neutrophilic or eosinophilic inflammation by inducing caspase-dependent apoptosis of polymorphonuclear leukocytes [184].

3.5.5.4 Extracellular Adenosine

Besides intracellular cAMP, extracellular adenosine has also been identified as a SAMP (like cAMP termed as IIIC-2 DAMP), though, in the international literature, adenosine, when released into the extracellular space, is also denoted as a DAMP or alarmin (e.g., see [186, 187]). As outlined in Vol. 1 [5], Part II, Section 5.3.4.2, purine nucleoside adenosine is recognized by P1 receptors that are typical GPCRs (also compare Sect. 2.3.3). Adenosine is known as a significant determinant of the immunosuppressive tumor milieu contributing to cancer growth [188]. Preclinical data had already shown that targeting the adenosinergic receptor A2A relieves immunosuppression and potently inhibits tumor growth [150].

The antiinflammatory and immunosuppressive action of adenosine receptors has been previously described [189, 190]. Most of the antiinflammatory effects of this molecule have been assigned to the A2A adenosine receptor (A2AAR) subtype, which is expressed in many immune and inflammatory cells. Mechanistically, it is suggested that the antiinflammatory effects of the A2AAR, as seen in different cell types, are potentially mediated by a generalized suppression of inflammatory gene expression through inhibition of the NF-κB and *Janus kinase* (JAK)/STAT proinflammatory signaling pathways [189]. Studies on the A3 adenosine receptor (A3AR) revealed that administration of an agonist of this receptor promotes an antiinflammatory effect as observed in several experimental animal models [190]. Mechanistically, the authors discussed deregulation of signaling proteins including PI3K, IκB kinase (IKK), JAK2, and STAT1, resulting in decreased levels of NF-κB, known to mediate inflammatory effects (for these transcription factors, see Vol. 1 [5], Part VI, Sects. 22.3.3.2, 22.3.4.2, and 22.3.4.3; as well as Figs. 22.3, 22.5, and 22.6).

In a more recent article published by Antonioli et al. [191], current knowledge about the proresolving/immunosuppressive properties of extracellularly released adenosine when signaling through A2AAR was more specifically reviewed. The authors highlighted that (1) the stimulation of A2AAR seems to play a critical role in switching macrophages from M1-like to M2-like phenotype; (2) mature immunostimulatory DCs mainly express A2AARs, which reduce the release of proinflammatory cytokines; (3) A2AAR engagement mediates the inhibition of neutrophil adhesion to ECs; (4) stimulation of A2AARs reduces the phagocytic activity of neutrophils; (5) the activation of A2AARs downregulates ROS generation; (6) A2AARs are the most critical receptors in regulating lymphocyte activation, where the overall effect is suppressive; (7) A2AARs—similar to SPMs—upregulate the expression of the negative costimulatory molecules *cytotoxic T lymphocyte-associated antigen-4* (CTLA-4) and *programmed cell death protein-1* (PD-1) and suppress the expression of the positive costimulatory molecule CD40L (for these molecules, compare Vol. 1 [5], Part VIII, Fig. 32.1); (8) there is a self-reinforcing loop in the immunosuppressive activity of T regulatory cells (Tregs) via adenosine generation, that is, A2AAR engagement on Tregs induces the expansion of these cells, thereby causing additional immunosuppression; (9) adenosine can regulate the function of regulatory B cells (Bregs), a subset of immunosuppressive cells that support immunological tolerance; and (10) Bregs were able to regulate both their own function and T-cell activity via an adenosine signaling originating from the enzymatic degradation of ATP, released in the extracellular space from activated immune cells (for Tregs, see Vol. 1 [5], Part VIII, Sect. 33.4).

These various functions of adenosine may license them as a bona fide SAMP, this all the more since adenosine is known to accumulate in the extracellular space at sites of injured tissue and to play a crucial role in the modulation of immune responses and in restraining inflammatory tissue damage [192]. This is also emphasized by Antonioli et al. [191]: "Indeed, over the years, a number of studies have identified extracellular adenosine as a 'retaliatory metabolite', which indicates that it is generated as a result of cellular injury or stress, and that through interacting with specific G protein-coupled receptors, it regulates the immune/inflammatory cell functions … to protect tissues from injury and stress…"

3.5.5.5 Specialized Proresolving Mediators

The SPMs have received widespread attention as to their role in inflammatory processes as, for example, documented in a recently published book that presents detail advances in understanding their role in inflammatory conditions of the eye, brain, and cardiovascular system [193].

Specialized proresolving mediators are lipid mediators that represent a larger family of antiinflammatory/proresolving molecules (for additional information also compare Vol. 1 [1], Part IV, Sect. 14.4.4, p. 335). The lipids are produced in a spatiotemporally controlled manner from essential PUFAs that are either released enzymatically by phospholipase A2 from cell membranes for secondary conversion by biosynthetic enzymes or delivered with edema fluid from plasma to exudates.

It was the admirable work of the Serhan group (articles of the group found in [98, 170-172, 194-207]) who contributed most to current knowledge about the SPMs and, in particular, identified the three new families of lipid mediators. The SPMs—named in Vol. 1 [1], as IIIC-3 DAMPs, now in Vol. 2 throughout the book denoted as IIIC-4 DAMPs—include AA, eicosapentaenoic acid (EPA), docosapentaenoic acid (n-3DPA), and docosahexaenoic acid (DHA). They are grouped into four structurally distinct chemical families, the lipoxins (LXs); resolvins (Rvs, for resolution phase interaction products); protectins (Pds), including neuroprotectin D1 (NPd1); and maresins (MaRs, for macrophage mediators in resolving inflammation). Each SPM is structurally distinct, biosynthesized from EPA, n-3DPA, or DHA.

Of note, SPMs are produced by activated innate immune cells (e.g., M2-like macrophages [98, 208] (compare Fig. 3.4) which were primarily activated upon infectious and sterile stress and injury (for SAMP-driven transdifferentiation of M1-like to M2-like macrophages, also see [209-213]).

In addition to such insults, SPMs are produced by human vagus. The name of the superfamily "SPMs" was coined given the unique feature of each family member to possess potent antiinflammatory and proresolving actions with peculiar functions in the resolution phase, that is, functions which qualify these molecules as typical SAMPs. The SPMs exert their bioactions as SAMPs via binding to their cognate PRMs, including the GPCRs (see Sect. 2.3.4.6) and the chemokine-like receptor 1 (CMKLR1). However, the molecular identity of all cognate receptors involved in sensing SPMs remains elusive and awaits further investigation (for the various SPM-triggered proresolving/immunosuppressive responses, see Sect. 5.3.3.2).

3.5.5.6 Concluding Remarks

Doubtlessly, SAMP-promoted resolution of inflammation following favorable DAMP-induced inflammatory defense responses can be considered a fundamental process of our innate immune system that occurs in all human tissues and appears to be the key prerequisite for restoring and maintaining homeostasis. As the leading cells in this maneuver, phagocytes and specifically macrophages play a vital role in orchestrating this response as well as subsequent tissue repair and regeneration (for more details, see Sect. 5.3.3).

3.5.6 Damage-Associated Molecules Operating Context-Dependently as SAMPs or DAMPs

3.5.6.1 General Remarks

In the course of an increasing interest in research on DAMPs, the puzzling finding was made that some injury-induced molecules can function context-dependently either as SAMPs or DAMPs. For example, as already discussed in Vol. 1 [5], Part IV, Sect. 12.2.3.4, extracellular HSPs—either as constitutive or inducible DAMPs—appear to have functions in that they can influence the inflammatory and immunological balance in tissues. Thus, on the one hand, HSPs, in particular, HSP70 through interaction with TLR4, were demonstrated to promote proinflammatory responses [214]; on the other side, they were shown to possess antiinflammatory properties, thereby qualifying them as so-called DAMPERS [215].

Although the underlying mechanisms of this phenomenon are not fully understood, some others of such molecules are briefly mentioned here.

3.5.6.2 Transforming Growth Factor-Beta

The cytokine TGF-β, including its signaling, has been briefly reviewed in Vol. 1 [5], Part VI, Sect. 22.5.9 and Fig. 22.13. In mammals, the TGF-β subfamily of cytokines consists of three isoforms, TGF-β1, TGF-β2, and TGF-β3, which are known to be pivotal in the development and homeostatic immune responses. Whereas TGF-β2 and TGF-β3 play important roles in embryonic development, TGF-β1 is the most abundantly secreted isoform by immune cells that is implicated in controlling immune responses after birth. The molecule functions through its two types of cognate receptors (TβRI/II) that are structurally similar, both containing a glycosylated and disulfide-rich ectodomain, a single transmembrane segment, and a cytoplasmic kinase domain.

Notably, there is compelling evidence indicating that this cytokine can be regarded as a particular form of a stress-/injury-induced molecule, namely, to act context-dependently/context-specifically as an inducible either SAMP or DAMP. As emphasized by Kelly et al. [216], "there is still great uncertainty in many areas of the literature as to the exact function of TGF-β in different immune cells, with data showing dampening of immune cell function in many circumstances, but promotion of inflammation in others. Such a multifunctional nature could reflect the importance of different TGF-β doses in mediating different functional outcomes, and also the context-specific action of TGF-β signaling, which can synergize with other anti-inflammatory or proinflammatory signals to drive different responses."

The molecule has been shown to activate virtually every innate and adaptive immune cell including DCs, neutrophils, macrophages, NK cells, (myo)fibroblasts, and T and B cells, thereby regulating innate and adaptive immune responses as well as fibrogenic processes (for reviews, see [216-219]). The bioavailability of TGF-β is complex but of high interest. A full description of this scenario lies beyond the scope of the present section, but the reader is directed toward several excellent reviews that describe this topic comprehensively in detail (published by Kelly et al. [216], Hinz [220], Hinck et al. [221], and Robertson and Rifkin [222]). Here, some mechanisms of the secretion and activation of TGF-β are briefly outlined in an oversimplified way.

Secretion of TGF-β (TGF-β1) as a Latent Tripartite Complex

Production of TGF-β1 is a tightly regulated process. The molecule is secreted by many activated innate immune cells such as macrophages, fibroblasts, ECs, and VSMCs upon stress/injury. Notably, DAMP-activated fibroblasts preferentially secrete TGF-β [223–228]. When TGF-β is secreted from cells, it does not immediately function as an inducible DAMP but is tightly bound in a latent complex consisting of its dimeric pro-peptide referred to as *latency-associated peptide* (LAP) and a *latent TGF-β-binding protein* (LTBP). This tripartite complex of TGF-β, LAP, and LTBP is called the *large latent complex* (LLC). Within this complex, LAP confers latency to the cytokine, and the LTBP—as part of the ECM—functions to bind the growth factor to the ECM by covalent interactions between the N-terminal domain of LTBP and ECM proteins such as fibrillin and fibronectin. Also, LAP can link to *glycoprotein-A repetitions predominant protein* (GARP) in the LLC. In addition, LAP interacts with cell-surface integrins through its integrin-binding RGD motif/sequence (RGD, abbreviation for arginylglycylaspartic acid [Arg-Gly-Asp]). Thus, LAP holding TGF-β can be localized between the ECM and cell-surface integrins (compare Fig. 6.2). Finally, LAP assists in the conversion of the latent TGF-β to its active form, a process known as activation (reviewed in [220, 222]).

The functional significance of TGF-β's ECM localization – "caged in the straitjacket of LAP"—is still unclear. As argued by Hinz [220], given the vital role of TGF-β in coordinating homeostatic innate immune pathways of tissue repair, special security measures may have evolved to protect us against the disastrous consequences of uncontrolled dysregulated TGF-β1 signaling, that is, overshooting fibrotic processes, which eventually may affect the whole organism.

Activation of TGF-β: Release from the Extracellular Matrix

To function context-dependently as an inducible SAMP or DAMP by interacting with its receptor, mature TGF-β must be released from LAP. This action can be achieved through several mechanisms, including dissociation by acidic pH, oxidative stress, or proteolysis of LAP by MMPs and, most important, interaction with cell-surface integrins.

In fact, as reviewed [216], extremes of pH and heat have been shown to activate TGF-β in vitro, presumably by denaturing LAP. Reactive oxygen species can also activate TGF-β both in vitro and ex vivo, probably via oxidative modifications to LAP, associated with a loss in its ability to bind TGF-β. In mice and humans, the serine proteases plasmin and plasma kallikrein were observed to activate TGF-β in vitro via proteolytic cleavage of LAP. Another potential activator of TGF-β is thrombospondin, a protein that is either found in the ECM or secreted by multiple cell types. Thrombospondin was found to bind directly to TGF-β-associated LAP via interactions, thereby facilitating the release of active TGF-β.

Intriguingly, cell-surface integrins are considered well-established major activators of latent TGF-β. Integrins $\alpha_v\beta_6$ and $\alpha_v\beta_8$ are the best-described activators, but other α_v integrins, such as $\alpha_v\beta_1$, $\alpha_v\beta_3$, and $\alpha_v\beta_5$, have also been implicated in interacting with LAP and activating latent TGF-β. Doubtlessly, the best-studied mechanism for cell-surface integrin-mediated activation of latent TGF-β is direct activation by traction between cells and the ECM (= mechanical activation of TGF-β) (compare Fig. 6.2) (reviewed in [217, 220, 222, 229, 230]). Mechanistically, two pathways of TGF-β activation have been proposed as mediated by integrins: (1) integrins bind LAP at the cell surface, and this may make LAP more accessible to proteases such as MMPs that cleave LAP and release the active TGF-β; (2) the integrin-binding RGD sequence in LAP—bound via LTBPs to ECM and the cytoplasmic sequences of integrin that anchor it to the cell's actin/myosin cytoskeleton—mediates cell contraction. This traction provokes cell-extrinsic dyshomeostatic DAMPs, which trigger conformational change of LAP that disrupts the LAP-TGF-β interaction and releases the growth factor. In this way, a mechanical force can initiate TGF-β-mediated signaling events, a crucial mechanism that plays a pivotal role in TGF-β-promoted fibrogenesis [220] (for conformational change-provoking cell-extrinsic dyshomeostatic DAMPs [IIB-3 DAMPs], see Sect. 3.4.3.3).

Notably, more recently, the protein GARP was shown to be involved in TGF-β1 activation by Tregs. GARP is a transmembrane protein that binds latent-TGF-β1 and tethers it on the Treg surface. The role of GARP was studied mostly in Tregs; however, GARP is also expressed in non-immune cells, such as ECs and fibroblasts (for review, see [231]).

Together, the bioavailability of TGF-β is regulated in complex and diverse ways, and it appears to be evident that its function must be considered in the broader structural context of the ECM. In this regard, TGF-β can be seen as an unusual stress-/injury-induced molecule because it operates context-specifically and context-dependently as an inducible SAMP or DAMP. Its main homeostatic function appears to be the regulation of innate and adaptive immune as well as fibrogenic responses, whereby its role in resolution of inflammation and promotion of fibrogenesis is of particular importance. However, when uncontrolled, TGF-β-mediated signaling pathways can result in severe pathologies, the development of organ fibrosis being the most deleterious outcome, a topic that will be resumed in detail in Sect. 6.5.

3.5.6.3 Interleukin-33 and Certain Extracellular Matrix Compounds

As touched above, adenosine, when released into the extracellular space, has also been described as a molecule that not only acts as a SAMP as described here but also as a DAMP or alarmin [186, 187].

Moreover, there is evidence suggesting that IL-33 operates context-dependently as a DAMP or SAMP. Thus, IL-33, along with its receptor *suppression of tumorigenicity 2* (ST2), has been shown to modulate both the innate and adaptive immune system (for reviews, see [232, 233]). For example, on the one hand, IL-33 was found to act as a DAMP that may trigger sterile type II inflammatory and adaptive immune Th1 responses [234, 235]; on the other hand, in vitro and in vivo studies have described that the IL-33 plays a critical role in regulating the expansion and function of Tregs [236, 237].

Another group of molecules shown to play a bimodal role as DAMPs or SAMPs refers to some ECM compounds. As described in Vol. 1 [5], Part IV, Sect 13.2, and briefly resumed in Sect. 3.4.2, ECM-derived DAMPs reportedly trigger sterile inflammation, for example, via recruitment of leukocytes to sites of infectious and sterile injury. Recent research, however, has been published suggesting that some ECM-derived DAMPs such as biglycan and versican obviously possess a double bimodal role in that they are additionally involved in antiinflammatory and inflammation-resolving responses (reviewed by Meissner et al. [238] and Frevert et al. [39]). Of interest is hyaluronan (HA) that, as low-molecular-weight hyaluronan (LMW-HA), promotes proinflammatory pathways and, as high-molecular-weight hyaluronan (HMW-HA), is implicated in suppressing the inflammatory response. By contrast to such "hybrid" ECM-derived DAMPs, proteoglycan-4 (PRG4) could be demonstrated to only promote an antiinflammatory response (also reviewed in [39]).

3.5.6.4 Concluding Remarks

The existence of molecules that may function context-dependently as both DAMPs and SAMPs is an unsolved problem. And the list of molecules mentioned here is certainly not complete. For example, studies on S100A proteins in lung injury models [239, 240] suggest a proinflammatory role of S100A8 and an antiinflammatory protective role of S100A8/A9 or S100A9. Future studies should be envisaged to reveal the mechanisms that enable these injury-induced molecules to trigger either proinflammatory or antiinflammatory/resolving immune responses, depending on given circumstances. One may think of involvement of different types of innate immune cells or interaction with different PRMs or distinctive effects on different cell types.

3.5.7 Résumé

The accumulating body of evidence qualifying inducible DAMPs as molecules involved in inflammation-promoting and inducible SAMPs as antiinflammatory/inflammation-resolving responses is intriguing in that these functions demonstrate effective activity of our defense system even in scenarios of mild or moderate injury associated with stressed cells only, and not with cell death.

However, in situations in which the injury is severe, secreted inducible DAMPs cooperate in a tailor-made fashion with DAMPs passively released from necrotic cells, the "gross" result being the orchestration of robust *life-saving* host defense against *life-threatening* injuries such as caused by viral infections. On the other hand, the paradigm of the favorable and unfavorable role of DAMPs or SAMPs becomes striking here again: the cooperation of inducible DAMPs with released DAMPs may result in excessive amounts of DAMPs that may become the tragic nucleus for the development of excessive hyperinflammation diagnosed by physicians and clinicians as sepsis and/or SIRS. Moreover, excessive production of SAMPs in terms of a counterbalancing antiinflammatory/inflammation-hyperresolving response to excessive production of DAMPs may lead to a long-lasting counterbalancing *compensatory antiinflammatory response syndrome* (CARS) resulting in a state of immunosuppression. In fact, the CARS can be regarded as a disorder caused by hyperresolution following hyperinflammation in terms of a mirror-imaged counterregulation of SIRS (details of these scenarios will be presented in Sects. 5.4, 8.3.3, and 8.3.4).

3.6 Exogenous DAMPs: The Emerging Role of Ambient Air Pollutants

As already mentioned above, exogenous IV DAMPs include various exogenous molecules such as aluminum salts, asbestos fibers, and silica particles (IVA DAMPs); noxious stimuli; some non-reactive compounds; reactive electrophilic compounds; vanilloids (IVB DAMPs); and some allergens (IVC DAMPs). They have been described in more detail in Vol. 1 [5], Part IV, Chap. 15, and thus are not resumed again. Here, however, a few remarks should be dedicated to air pollutants, which are increasingly implicated in a wide range of health effects.

In fact, ambient air pollution is considered to be the world's biggest challenges to human health, estimated to account for seven million deaths worldwide every year. As most deleterious compounds, nitrogen oxides, sulfur oxides, ozone, and particulate matter (PM)—especially particulate matter with aerodynamic diameter below 2.5 μm (PM2.5)—have been identified. As these tiny particles penetrate through the nasal passage deep into the lungs, affecting both the respiratory and vascular systems, they cause and exacerbate a number of diseases, ranging from acute/chronic airway inflammation, CVDs, asthma, and chronic obstructive pulmonary disease (COPD) up to cancer (for reviews, see [241-246]).

Whereas pollutants such as nitrogen oxides, sulfur oxides, and ozone are toxic substances supposed to induce oxidative injury-induced endogenous DAMPs [247, 248], particulates can be regarded as bona fide exogenous IVA-4 DAMPs (newly added to Table 3.1) able to trigger local and systemic proinflammatory (profibrotic) innate immune responses [249, 250]. Mechanistically, indirect activation of the NLRP3 inflammasome appears to be the key event by which the particulate matter—when operating as exogenous DAMPs—elicit those detrimental inflammatory processes (for NLRP3 inflammasome, see Sect. 2.2.5 and Fig. 2.1). In support of such a mechanism are experiments on mice demonstrating that PM2.5 induces acute lung inflammation (ALI) associated with a significant increase of IL-1β production in murine lung tissues and bronchoalveolar lavage fluid [251]. The interesting experiments provided evidence suggesting that PM2.5-induced ALI may be caused in part to the generation of IL-1β and activation of TLR4/MyD88 signaling pathway and NLRP3 inflammasome may be involved in this process. Also, in other lines of studies in mice [252], long-term PM2.5 exposure was found to induce lung inflammation and fibrosis, whereby resveratrol was shown to alleviate these adverse effects via inhibiting autophagy-related NLRP3 inflammasome activation.

Accordingly—as will be discussed in Sect. 7.4.3 in more detail—administration of SAMPs might be a therapeutic option to treat such pollution-related chronic (nonresolving) airway inflammatory diseases. Interestingly, such a therapeutic approach using SPMs has already been proposed elsewhere (see [253]).

3.7 Role of DAMPs in Trained Immunity

3.7.1 The Emerging Concept of Trained Immunity

The emerging concept of "trained immunity"—de facto an innate immune memory—has been briefly addressed in Vol. 1 [1], Part VI, Sect. 24.2.4. The concept has been developed by the *Radboud* University group around Netea [254–256]. The model holds that cells of the innate immune system such as monocytes, macrophages, DCs, and NK cells can establish a memory of past stimulation via a process of metabolic and epigenetic reprogramming that allows modifying their response (either hyperresponsive or hyporesponsive) upon secondary challenges with an infectious or sterile insult similar or unrelated to the first one. This process results in enhanced cytokine production and provides more effective protection against reinfection but—in case of sterile insults—may also promote chronic inflammation. The fundamental mechanism of this phenomenon is epigenetic reprogramming that supports the acquisition of trained immunity, with selective changes in histone methylation and acetylation associated with the acquisition of a trained phenotype [257].

Tremendous progress in this exciting research field, in particular, in atherosclerosis and CVD research has been noticed during the past 2 years as mirrored by many recent original publications (see [258-267]). Here, the topic of DAMP-induced trained immunity, as already introduced in Vol. 1 [5], Part VI, Sect. 24.2.4.4, is briefly resumed.

3.7.2 DAMP-Induced Trained Immunity

In earlier studies, DAMP-promoted trained immunity has already been shown for IIB-1 DAMPs (OSEs), namely, OxLDL [268] and lipoprotein A containing OxPLs [269]. Mechanistically, induction of trained immunity was supposed to be mediated through DAMP-induced epigenetic regulation of transcriptional programs. More recent in vitro studies on peripheral blood monocytes from healthy donors, published by Neidhart et al. [270], could confirm these early observations. In this study, the investigators succeeded in showing that certain rheumatoid arthritis-related DAMPs (such as oligomeric S100A4, HMBG1, HSP90, and TNC) can also induce trained immunity via epigenetic reprogramming involving histone methylase PRDM8. Indeed, this discovery indicates PRDM8 to play a pivotal role in DAMP-induced trained immunity. Interestingly, this trained immunity-inducing effect was particularly pronounced by oligomeric S100A4, less by HMBG1, HSP90, or TNC. Successful induction of trained immunity was demonstrated by increased production of cytokines (IL-1β, IL-6, and TNF) by monocytes exposed to these DAMPs upon restimulation with LPS. As a synopsis of their experiments (some of them demonstrating bypass of endotoxin tolerance by DAMPs, not quoted here), the authors [270] proposed that histone methylase PRDM8 plays a pivotal role in DAMP-induced trained immunity. They further suggested that DAMP-induced trained immunity may reflect a crucial mechanism in chronically persistent inflammation, as seen in many diseases such as rheumatoid arthritis and atherosclerosis.

3.7.3 Résumé

The discovery that DAMPs can modulate cellular functions via induction of epigenetic modifications implies a tremendous expansion of their role in host defense across the tree of life. Moreover, if this data could be confirmed and solidified in the future, they might have far-reaching consequences for social behavior via DAMP-induced epigenetic mechanisms that modify physiological processes, that is, DAMPs in terms of factors at the interface between our biotic/abiotic environments and our genes.

3.8 Outlook and Future Perspectives

As already discussed in Vol. 1, any actual approach (including updates at the time of writing) to define and classify DAMPs is just a momentary snapshot to show what is going on in this emerging biomedical area. Thus, the topic—particularly, as inducible DAMPs are concerned—is still debatable and will be revisited in the future as our knowledge of the world of DAMPs increases. For example, further research may well show that not all the molecules mentioned here do operate as bona fide DAMPs, that is, to promote or—as SAMPs—to resolve inflammation in homeostatic and/or pathological situations.

We have not reached the end of the narrative that evolution has created and left us. In particular, the emerging, growing evidence for the existence of a universal defense system that has evolutionarily evolved across the tree of life—from plants over invertebrates to vertebrates including humans [271, 272]—has opened our eyes for a wide-ranging role of DAMPs in nature. Generated during any stress, including mental stress and any injury, may it be of infectious or sterile nature, these "miracle molecules" work permanently as molecular defenders to guarantee our organismal homeostasis. The bitter pill is that those DAMPs do not only induce innate homeostatic responses but, when emitted in excess, cause pathologies. The intense clinical exploration of their pathogenetic role in human diseases is just at the beginning, but the first clinical data have already been reported. Indeed, practitioners and clinicians will soon learn from such targeted scientific publications how to use this new information to make a proper diagnosis and chose the most effective treatment for their patients suffering from those human diseases, where they play a dominant pathogenetic role. The following chapters on a first series of human diseases are written to assist in this endeavor.

References

1. Goldstein DS, Kopin I. Adrenomedullary, adrenocortical, and sympathoneural responses to stressors: a meta-analysis. Endocr Regul. 2008;42:111–9. https://www.ncbi.nlm.nih.gov/pubmed/18999898.
2. Goldstein DS. Adrenal responses to stress. Cell Mol Neurobiol. 2010;30:1433–40. http://www.ncbi.nlm.nih.gov/pubmed/21061156.
3. Carter JR, Goldstein DS. Sympathoneural and adrenomedullary responses to mental stress. Compr Physiol. 2014;5:119–46. http://www.ncbi.nlm.nih.gov/pubmed/25589266.
4. Fleshner M, Crane CR. Exosomes, DAMPs and miRNA: features of stress physiology and immune homeostasis. Trends Immunol. 2017;38:768–76. https://linkinghub.elsevier.com/retrieve/pii/S1471490617301539.
5. Land WG. Damage-associated molecular patterns in human diseases. In: Injury-induced innate immune responses, vol. 1. Cham: Springer International Publishing AG; 2018. https://www.springer.com/de/book/9783319786544.
6. Gong T, Liu L, Jiang W, Zhou R. DAMP-sensing receptors in sterile inflammation and inflammatory diseases. Nat Rev Immunol. 2020;20(2):95–112.
7. Cao X. Self-regulation and cross-regulation of pattern-recognition receptor signalling in health and disease. Nat Rev Immunol. 2016;16:35–50. https://doi.org/10.1038/nri.2015.8.
8. Gallo PM, Gallucci S. The dendritic cell response to classic, emerging, and homeostatic danger signals. Implications for autoimmunity. Front Immunol. 2013;4:138. http://www.ncbi.nlm.nih.gov/pubmed/23772226.

9. Liston A, Masters SL. Homeostasis-altering molecular processes as mechanisms of inflammasome activation. Nat Rev Immunol. 2017;17:208–14. https://doi.org/10.1038/nri.2016.151.
10. Land WG. Emerging role of innate immunity in organ transplantation part II: potential of damage-associated molecular patterns to generate immunostimulatory dendritic cells. Transplant Rev (Orlando). 2012;26:73–87. http://www.ncbi.nlm.nih.gov/pubmed/22074784.
11. Danziger J, Zeidel ML. Osmotic homeostasis. Clin J Am Soc Nephrol. 2015;10:852–62. https://doi.org/10.2215/CJN.10741013.
12. Yatim N, Cullen S, Albert ML. Dying cells actively regulate adaptive immune responses. Nat Rev Immunol. 2017;17:262–75. https://doi.org/10.1038/nri.2017.9.
13. Khodarev NN. Intracellular RNA sensing in mammalian cells: role in stress response and cancer therapies. Int Rev Cell Mol Biol. 2019;344:31–89. http://www.ncbi.nlm.nih.gov/pubmed/30798990.
14. Fischer S. Pattern recognition receptors and control of innate immunity: role of nucleic acids. Curr Pharm Biotechnol. 2019;19:1203–9. http://www.ncbi.nlm.nih.gov/pubmed/30636600.
15. Schaefer L. Complexity of danger: the diverse nature of damage-associated molecular patterns. J Biol Chem. 2014;289:35237–45. http://www.ncbi.nlm.nih.gov/pubmed/25391648.
16. Bianchi ME. DAMPs, PAMPs and alarmins: all we need to know about danger. J Leukoc Biol. 2007;81:1–5. http://www.ncbi.nlm.nih.gov/pubmed/17032697.
17. Martin SJ. Cell death and inflammation: the case for IL-1 family cytokines as the canonical DAMPs of the immune system. FEBS J. 2016;283:2599–615. http://www.ncbi.nlm.nih.gov/pubmed/27273805.
18. Kavita U, Mizel SB. Differential sensitivity of interleukin-1 alpha and -beta precursor proteins to cleavage by calpain, a calcium-dependent protease. J Biol Chem. 1995;270:27758–65. http://www.ncbi.nlm.nih.gov/pubmed/7499244.
19. Zheng Y, Humphry M, Maguire JJ, Bennett MR, Clarke MCH. Intracellular interleukin-1 receptor 2 binding prevents cleavage and activity of interleukin-1α, controlling necrosis-induced sterile inflammation. Immunity. 2013;38:285–95. http://linkinghub.elsevier.com/retrieve/pii/S1074761313000484.
20. Lu B, Wang H, Andersson U, Tracey KJ. Regulation of HMGB1 release by inflammasomes. Protein Cell. 2013;4:163–7. https://doi.org/10.1007/s13238-012-2118-2.
21. Rendon-Mitchell B, Ochani M, Li J, Han J, Wang H, Yang H, et al. IFN-gamma induces high mobility group box 1 protein release partly through a TNF-dependent mechanism. J Immunol. 2003;170:3890–7. http://www.ncbi.nlm.nih.gov/pubmed/12646658.
22. Rubartelli A, Lotze MT. Inside, outside, upside down: damage-associated molecular-pattern molecules (DAMPs) and redox. Trends Immunol. 2007;28:429–36. http://www.ncbi.nlm.nih.gov/pubmed/17845865.
23. Land WG, Agostinis P, Gasser S, Garg AD, Linkermann A. Transplantation and damage-associated molecular patterns (DAMPs). Am J Transplant. 2016;16:3338–61. http://www.ncbi.nlm.nih.gov/pubmed/27421829.
24. Liu X, Wang C. The emerging roles of the STING adaptor protein in immunity and diseases. Immunology. 2016;147:285–91. http://www.ncbi.nlm.nih.gov/pubmed/26643733.
25. Sarhan M, Land WG, Tonnus W, Hugo CP, Linkermann A. Origin and consequences of necroinflammation. Physiol Rev. 2018;98:727–80. https://doi.org/10.1152/physrev.00041.2016.
26. Tonnus W, Linkermann A. "Death is my Heir"—ferroptosis connects cancer pharmacogenomics and ischemia-reperfusion injury. Cell Chem Biol. 2016;23:202–3. http://www.ncbi.nlm.nih.gov/pubmed/26971867.
27. Tonnus W, Linkermann A. The in vivo evidence for regulated necrosis. Immunol Rev. 2017;277:128–49. http://www.ncbi.nlm.nih.gov/pubmed/28462528.
28. Carapito R, Jung N, Kwemou M, Untrau M, Michel S, Pichot A, et al. Matching for the nonconventional MHC-I MICA gene significantly reduces the incidence of acute and chronic GVHD. Blood. 2016;128:1979–86. http://www.ncbi.nlm.nih.gov/pubmed/27549307.
29. Green DR, Oguin TH, Martinez J. The clearance of dying cells: table for two. Cell Death Differ. 2016;23:915–26. http://www.nature.com/articles/cdd2015172.

30. Elliott MR, Koster KM, Murphy PS. Efferocytosis signaling in the regulation of macrophage inflammatory responses. J Immunol. 2017;198:1387–94. http://www.ncbi.nlm.nih.gov/pubmed/28167649.
31. Greenlee-Wacker MC. Clearance of apoptotic neutrophils and resolution of inflammation. Immunol Rev. 2016;273:357–70. http://www.ncbi.nlm.nih.gov/pubmed/27558346.
32. Schcolnik-Cabrera A, Oldak B, Juárez M, Cruz-Rivera M, Flisser A, Mendlovic F. Calreticulin in phagocytosis and cancer: opposite roles in immune response outcomes. Apoptosis. 2019;24:245–55. https://doi.org/10.1007/s10495-019-01532-0.
33. Zingoni A, Molfetta R, Fionda C, Soriani A, Paolini R, Cippitelli M, et al. NKG2D and its ligands: "One for All, All for One.". Front Immunol. 2018;9:476. http://www.ncbi.nlm.nih.gov/pubmed/29662484.
34. Hosomi S, Grootjans J, Huang Y-H, Kaser A, Blumberg RS. New insights into the regulation of natural-killer Group 2 Member D (NKG2D) and NKG2D-ligands: endoplasmic reticulum stress and CEA-related cell adhesion molecule 1. Front Immunol. 2018;9:1324. https://doi.org/10.3389/fimmu.2018.01324/full.
35. Schaefer L. Personal communication.
36. Apte SS, Parks WC. Metalloproteinases: a parade of functions in matrix biology and an outlook for the future. Matrix Biol. 2015;44–46:1–6. http://www.ncbi.nlm.nih.gov/pubmed/25916966.
37. Jiang D, Liang J, Noble PW. Hyaluronan as an immune regulator in human diseases. Physiol Rev. 2011;91:221–64. http://www.ncbi.nlm.nih.gov/pubmed/21248167.
38. Jin H, Zhou S. The functions of heparanase in human diseases. Mini Rev Med Chem. 2017;17:541–8. http://www.ncbi.nlm.nih.gov/pubmed/27804885.
39. Frevert CW, Felgenhauer J, Wygrecka M, Nastase MV, Schaefer L. Danger-associated molecular patterns derived from the extracellular matrix provide temporal control of innate immunity. J Histochem Cytochem. 2018;66:213–27. http://www.ncbi.nlm.nih.gov/pubmed/29290139.
40. Nastase M-V, Janicova A, Wygrecka M, Schaefer L. Signaling at the crossroads: matrix-derived proteoglycan and reactive oxygen species signaling. Antioxid Redox Signal. 2017;27:855–73. https://doi.org/10.1089/ars.2017.7165.
41. Chen Y, Ju L, Rushdi M, Ge C, Zhu C. Receptor-mediated cell mechanosensing. Mol Biol Cell. 2017;28:3134–55. http://www.ncbi.nlm.nih.gov/pubmed/28954860.
42. Zeng L, Smith C, Poelzer GH, Rodriguez J, Corpuz E, Yanev G. Illustrations and supporting texts for sound standing waves of air columns in pipes in introductory physics textbooks. Phys Rev Spec Top Phys Educ Res. 2014;10:020110. https://doi.org/10.1103/PhysRevSTPER.10.020110.
43. Cournia Z, Allen TW, Andricioaei I, Antonny B, Baum D, Brannigan G, et al. Membrane protein structure, function, and dynamics: a perspective from experiments and Theory. J Membr Biol. 2015;248:611–40. https://doi.org/10.1007/s00232-015-9802-0.
44. Zhang XC, Sun K, Zhang L, Li X, Cao C. GPCR activation: protonation and membrane potential. Protein Cell. 2013;4:747–60. http://www.ncbi.nlm.nih.gov/pubmed/24057762.
45. Zhang XC, Cao C, Zhou Y, Zhao Y. Proton transfer-mediated GPCR activation. Protein Cell. 2015;6:12–7. https://doi.org/10.1007/s13238-014-0106-4.
46. Roers A, Hiller B, Hornung V. Recognition of endogenous nucleic acids by the innate immune system. Immunity. 2016;44:739–54. http://www.ncbi.nlm.nih.gov/pubmed/27096317.
47. Mavragani I, Nikitaki Z, Souli M, Aziz A, Nowsheen S, Aziz K, et al. Complex DNA Damage: A Route to Radiation-Induced Genomic Instability and Carcinogenesis. Cancers (Basel). 2017;9:91. http://www.ncbi.nlm.nih.gov/pubmed/28718816.
48. van Vliet AR, Agostinis P. When under pressure, get closer: PERKing up membrane contact sites during ER stress. Biochem Soc Trans. 2016;44:499–504. http://www.ncbi.nlm.nih.gov/pubmed/27068961.
49. Carapito R, Bahram S. Genetics, genomics, and evolutionary biology of NKG2D ligands. Immunol Rev. 2015;267:88–116. http://www.ncbi.nlm.nih.gov/pubmed/26284473.
50. Carapito R. Personal Communication.

51. Kelly B, O'Neill LAJ. Metabolic reprogramming in macrophages and dendritic cells in innate immunity. Cell Res. 2015;25:771–84. http://www.ncbi.nlm.nih.gov/pubmed/26045163.
52. O'Neill LAJ, Pearce EJ. Immunometabolism governs dendritic cell and macrophage function. J Exp Med. 2016;213:15–23. http://www.ncbi.nlm.nih.gov/pubmed/26694970.
53. Ariza AC, Deen PMT, Robben JH. The succinate receptor as a novel therapeutic target for oxidative and metabolic stress-related conditions. Front Endocrinol (Lausanne). 2012;3:22. http://www.ncbi.nlm.nih.gov/pubmed/22649411.
54. de Castro FM, Aguiar CJ, da Rocha Franco JA, Gingold RN, Leite MF. GPR91: expanding the frontiers of Krebs cycle intermediates. Cell Commun Signal. 2016;14:3. http://www.ncbi.nlm.nih.gov/pubmed/26759054.
55. Gilissen J, Jouret F, Pirotte B, Hanson J. Insight into SUCNR1 (GPR91) structure and function. Pharmacol Ther. 2016;159:56–65. http://www.ncbi.nlm.nih.gov/pubmed/26808164.
56. Rubic T, Lametschwandtner G, Jost S, Hinteregger S, Kund J, Carballido-Perrig N, et al. Triggering the succinate receptor GPR91 on dendritic cells enhances immunity. Nat Immunol. 2008;9:1261–9. http://www.ncbi.nlm.nih.gov/pubmed/18820681.
57. Littlewood-Evans A, Sarret S, Apfel V, Loesle P, Dawson J, Zhang J, et al. GPR91 senses extracellular succinate released from inflammatory macrophages and exacerbates rheumatoid arthritis. J Exp Med. 2016;213:1655–62. http://www.ncbi.nlm.nih.gov/pubmed/27481132
58. Williams NC, O'Neill LAJ. A Role for the Krebs cycle intermediate citrate in metabolic reprogramming in innate immunity and inflammation. Front Immunol. 2018;9:141. http://www.ncbi.nlm.nih.gov/pubmed/29459863.
59. Mills EL, Kelly B, O'Neill LAJ. Mitochondria are the powerhouses of immunity. Nat Immunol. 2017;18:488–98. http://www.ncbi.nlm.nih.gov/pubmed/28418387.
60. Nakka VP, Prakash-babu P, Vemuganti R. Crosstalk between endoplasmic reticulum stress, oxidative stress, and autophagy: potential therapeutic targets for acute CNS injuries. Mol Neurobiol. 2016;53:532–44. http://www.ncbi.nlm.nih.gov/pubmed/25482050.
61. Zhou R, Tardivel A, Thorens B, Choi I, Tschopp J. Thioredoxin-interacting protein links oxidative stress to inflammasome activation. Nat Immunol. 2010;11:136–40. http://www.ncbi.nlm.nih.gov/pubmed/20023662.
62. Schroder K, Zhou R, Tschopp J. The NLRP3 inflammasome: a sensor for metabolic danger? Science. 2010;327:296–300. https://doi.org/10.1126/science.1184003.
63. Gu C, Liu S, Wang H, Dou H. Role of the thioredoxin interacting protein in diabetic nephropathy and the mechanism of regulating NOD-like receptor protein 3 inflammatory corpuscle. Int J Mol Med. 2019;43:2440–50. http://www.ncbi.nlm.nih.gov/pubmed/31017263.
64. Kim S-K, Choe J-Y, Park K-Y. TXNIP-mediated nuclear factor-κB signaling pathway and intracellular shifting of TXNIP in uric acid-induced NLRP3 inflammasome. Biochem Biophys Res Commun. 2019;511:725–31. http://www.ncbi.nlm.nih.gov/pubmed/30833078.
65. Omar DF, Kamal MM, El-Hefnawy MH, EL-Mesallamy HO. Serum vitamin D and its upregulated protein, thioredoxin interacting protein, are associated with beta-cell dysfunction in adult patients with Type 1 and Type 2 diabetes. Can J Diabetes. 2018;42:588–94. http://www.ncbi.nlm.nih.gov/pubmed/29980378.
66. Wang BF, Yoshioka J. The emerging role of thioredoxin-interacting protein in myocardial ischemia/reperfusion injury. J Cardiovasc Pharmacol Ther. 2017;22:219–29. http://www.ncbi.nlm.nih.gov/pubmed/27807222.
67. Mahmood DFD, Abderrazak A, El Hadri K, Simmet T, Rouis M. The thioredoxin system as a therapeutic target in human health and disease. Antioxid Redox Signal. 2013;19 1266–303. http://www.ncbi.nlm.nih.gov/pubmed/23244617.
68. Nasoohi S, Ismael S, Ishrat T. Thioredoxin-interacting protein (TXNIP) in cerebrovascular and neurodegenerative diseases: regulation and implication. Mol Neurobiol. 2018;55:7900–20. https://doi.org/10.1007/s12035-018-0917-z.
69. Rider P, Voronov E, Dinarello CA, Apte RN, Cohen I. Alarmins: feel the stress. J Immunol. 2017;198:1395–402.
70. Daniels M, Brough D. Unconventional pathways of secretion contribute to inflammation. Int J Mol Sci. 2017;18:102. http://www.ncbi.nlm.nih.gov/pubmed/28067797.

71. Gurunathan S, Kang M-H, Jeyaraj M, Qasim M, Kim J-H. Review of the isolation, characterization, biological function, and multifarious therapeutic approaches of exosomes. Cell. 2019;8:307. https://www.mdpi.com/2073-4409/8/4/307.
72. Tarique AA, Logan J, Thomas E, Holt PG, Sly PD, Fantino E. Phenotypic, functional, and plasticity features of classical and alternatively activated human macrophages. Am J Respir Cell Mol Biol. 2015;53:676–88. http://www.ncbi.nlm.nih.gov/pubmed/25870903.
73. Atri C, Guerfali F, Laouini D. Role of human macrophage polarization in inflammation during infectious diseases. Int J Mol Sci. 2018;19:1801. http://www.mdpi.com/1422-0067/19/6/1801.
74. Eisenman ST, Gibbons SJ, Verhulst P-J, Cipriani G, Saur D, Farrugia G. Tumor necrosis factor alpha derived from classically activated "M1" macrophages reduces interstitial cell of Cajal numbers. Neurogastroenterol Motil. 2017;29:e12984. http://www.ncbi.nlm.nih.gov/pubmed/27781339.
75. Niessner A, Shin MS, Pryshchep O, Goronzy JJ, Chaikof EL, Weyand CM. Synergistic proinflammatory effects of the antiviral cytokine interferon-alpha and Toll-like receptor 4 ligands in the atherosclerotic plaque. Circulation. 2007;116:2043–52. https://doi.org/10.1161/CIRCULATIONAHA.107.697789.
76. Jan A, Rahman S, Khan S, Tasduq S, Choi I. Biology, pathophysiological role, and clinical implications of exosomes: a critical appraisal. Cell. 2019;8:99. http://www.ncbi.nlm.nih.gov/pubmed/30699987.
77. Takahashi A, Okada R, Nagao K, Kawamata Y, Hanyu A, Yoshimoto S, et al. Exosomes maintain cellular homeostasis by excreting harmful DNA from cells. Nat Commun. 2017;8:15287. http://www.ncbi.nlm.nih.gov/pubmed/28508895.
78. McCullough J, Frost A, Sundquist WI. Structures, functions, and dynamics of ESCRT-III/Vps4 membrane remodeling and fission complexes. Annu Rev Cell Dev Biol. 2018;34:85–109. http://www.ncbi.nlm.nih.gov/pubmed/30095293.
79. Gatta AT, Carlton JG. The ESCRT-machinery: closing holes and expanding roles. Curr Opin Cell Biol. 2019;59:121–32. https://linkinghub.elsevier.com/retrieve/pii/S0955067419300237.
80. Han H, Hill CP. Structure and mechanism of the ESCRT pathway AAA+ ATPase Vps4. Biochem Soc Trans. 2019;47:37–45. http://www.ncbi.nlm.nih.gov/pubmed/30647138.
81. Sinha A, Alfaro J, Kislinger T. Characterization of protein content present in exosomes isolated from conditioned media and urine. Curr Protoc Protein Sci. 2017;87:24.9.1–24.9.12. http://www.ncbi.nlm.nih.gov/pubmed/28150884.
82. Hessvik NP, Llorente A. Current knowledge on exosome biogenesis and release. Cell Mol Life Sci. 2018;75:193–208. http://www.ncbi.nlm.nih.gov/pubmed/28733901.
83. Zhang Y, Liu Y, Liu H, Tang WH. Exosomes: biogenesis, biologic function and clinical potential. Cell Biosci. 2019;9:19. http://www.ncbi.nlm.nih.gov/pubmed/30815248.
84. Lehmann BD, Paine MS, Brooks AM, McCubrey JA, Renegar RH, Wang R, et al. Senescence-associated exosome release from human prostate cancer cells. Cancer Res. 2008;68:7864–71. https://doi.org/10.1158/0008-5472.CAN-07-6538.
85. King HW, Michael MZ, Gleadle JM. Hypoxic enhancement of exosome release by breast cancer cells. BMC Cancer. 2012;12:421. https://doi.org/10.1186/1471-2407-12-421.
86. Xiao X, Yu S, Li S, Wu J, Ma R, Cao H, et al. Exosomes: decreased sensitivity of lung cancer A549 cells to Cisplatin. PLoS One. 2014;9:e89534. http://www.ncbi.nlm.nih.gov/pubmed/24586853.
87. Beer L, Zimmermann M, Mitterbauer A, Ellinger A, Gruber F, Narzt M-S, et al. Analysis of the secretome of apoptotic peripheral blood mononuclear cells: impact of released proteins and exosomes for tissue regeneration. Sci Rep. 2015;5:16662. http://www.nature.com/articles/srep16662.
88. Kanemoto S, Nitani R, Murakami T, Kaneko M, Asada R, Matsuhisa K, et al. Multivesicular body formation enhancement and exosome release during endoplasmic reticulum stress. Biochem Biophys Res Commun. 2016;480:166–72. https://linkinghub.elsevier.com/retrieve/pii/S0006291X16316837.
89. Desdín-Micó G, Mittelbrunn M. Role of exosomes in the protection of cellular homeostasis. Cell Adh Migr. 2017;11:127–34. https://doi.org/10.1080/19336918.2016.1251000.

90. Caruso S, Poon IKH. Apoptotic cell-derived extracellular vesicles: more than just debris. Front Immunol. 2018;9:1486. http://www.ncbi.nlm.nih.gov/pubmed/30002658.
91. Collett GP, Redman CW, Sargent IL, Vatish M. Endoplasmic reticulum stress stimulates the release of extracellular vesicles carrying danger-associated molecular pattern (DAMP) molecules. Oncotarget. 2018;9:6707–17. http://www.oncotarget.com/fulltext/24158.
92. Katsumi T, Guicciardi ME, Azad A, Bronk SF, Krishnan A, Gores GJ. Activated cholangiocytes release macrophage-polarizing extracellular vesicles bearing the DAMP S100A11. Am J Physiol Physiol. 2019;317(4):C788–99. http://www.ncbi.nlm.nih.gov/pubmed/31365294.
93. Théry C, Ostrowski M, Segura E. Membrane vesicles as conveyors of immune responses. Nat Rev Immunol. 2009;9:581–93. http://www.nature.com/articles/nri2567.
94. Meckes DG, Raab-Traub N. Microvesicles and viral infection. J Virol. 2011;85:12844–54. [cited 2019 May 22]. https://doi.org/10.1128/JVI.05853-11.
95. Buzas EI, György B, Nagy G, Falus A, Gay S. Emerging role of extracellular vesicles in inflammatory diseases. Nat Rev Rheumatol. 2014;10:356–64. http://www.nature.com/articles/nrrheum.2014.19.
96. Bretz NP, Ridinger J, Rupp A-K, Rimbach K, Keller S, Rupp C, et al. Body fluid exosomes promote secretion of inflammatory cytokines in monocytic cells via Toll-like receptor signaling. J Biol Chem. 2013;288:36691–702. https://doi.org/10.1074/jbc.M113.512806.
97. Sagini K, Costanzi E, Emiliani C, Buratta S, Urbanelli L. Extracellular vesicles as conveyors of membrane-derived bioactive lipids in immune system. Int J Mol Sci. 2018;19:1227. http://www.ncbi.nlm.nih.gov/pubmed/29670015.
98. Dalli J, Serhan C. Macrophage proresolving mediators—the when and where. Microbiol Spectr. 2016;4. http://www.ncbi.nlm.nih.gov/pubmed/27337457.
99. Ayna G, Krysko DV, Kaczmarek A, Petrovski G, Vandenabeele P, Fésüs L. ATP release from dying autophagic cells and their phagocytosis are crucial for inflammasome activation in macrophages. PLoS One. 2012;7:e40069. https://doi.org/10.1371/journal.pone.0040069.
100. Schiller M, Heyder P, Ziegler S, Niessen A, Claßen L, Lauffer A, et al. During apoptosis HMGB1 is translocated into apoptotic cell-derived membranous vesicles. Autoimmunity. 2013;46:342–6. https://doi.org/10.3109/08916934.2012.750302.
101. Park SJ, Kim JM, Kim J, Hur J, Park S, Kim K, et al. Molecular mechanisms of biogenesis of apoptotic exosome-like vesicles and their roles as damage-associated molecular patterns. Proc Natl Acad Sci U S A. 2018;115:E11721–30. http://www.ncbi.nlm.nih.gov/pubmed/30463946.
102. Dennis EA, Norris PC. Eicosanoid storm in infection and inflammation. Nat Rev Immunol. 2015;15:511–23. http://www.ncbi.nlm.nih.gov/pubmed/26139350.
103. Esser-von BJ. Eicosanoids in tissue repair. Immunol Cell Biol. 2019;97:279–88. http://www.ncbi.nlm.nih.gov/pubmed/30680784.
104. Malawista SE, de Boisfleury CA, van Damme J, Serhan CN. Tonic inhibition of chemotaxis in human plasma. Proc Natl Acad Sci U S A. 2008;105:17949–54. https://doi.org/10.1073/pnas.0802572105.
105. Lämmermann T, Afonso PV, Angermann BR, Wang JM, Kastenmüller W, Parent CA, et al. Neutrophil swarms require LTB4 and integrins at sites of cell death in vivo. Nature. 2013;498:371–5. http://www.nature.com/articles/nature12175
106. Zinn S, Sisignano M, Kern K, Pierre S, Tunaru S, Jordan H, et al. The leukotriene B4 receptors BLT1 and BLT2 form an antagonistic sensitizing system in peripheral sensory neurons. J Biol Chem. 2017;292:6123–34. http://www.ncbi.nlm.nih.gov/pubmed/28242764.
107. Yokomizo T. Leukotriene B4 receptors: novel roles in immunological regulations. Adv Enzyme Regul. 2011;51:59–64. https://linkinghub.elsevier.com/retrieve/pii/S0065257110000579.
108. Brandt SL, Serezani CH. Too much of a good thing: how modulating LTB4 actions restore host defense in homeostasis or disease. Semin Immunol. 2017;33:37–43. https://linkinghub.elsevier.com/retrieve/pii/S1044532316300793.
109. Tavares N, Afonso L, Suarez M, Ampuero M, Prates DB, Araújo-Santos T, et al. Degranulating neutrophils promote leukotriene B 4 production by infected macrophages to kill Leishmania amazonensis parasites. J Immunol. 2016;196:1865–73. http://www.ncbi.nlm.nih.gov/pubmed/26800873.

110. Le Bel M, Brunet A, Gosselin J. Leukotriene B 4, an endogenous stimulator of the innate immune response against pathogens. J Innate Immun. 2014;6:159–68. https://www.karger.com/Article/FullText/353694.
111. Tank AW, Lee WD. Peripheral and central effects of circulating catecholamines. Compr Physiol. 2015;5:1–15. https://doi.org/10.1002/cphy.c140007.
112. Lymperopoulos A, Brill A, McCrink KA. GPCRs of adrenal chromaffin cells & catecholamines: the plot thickens. Int J Biochem Cell Biol. 2016;77:213–9. https://linkinghub.elsevier.com/retrieve/pii/S1357272516300218.
113. Goldstein DS, Eisenhofer G, Kopin IJ. Sources and significance of plasma levels of catechols and their metabolites in humans. J Pharmacol Exp Ther. 2003;305:800–11. https://doi.org/10.1124/jpet.103.049270.
114. Chamberlain KG, Pestell RG, Best JD. Platelet catecholamine contents are cumulative indexes of sympathoadrenal activity. Am J Physiol Metab. 1990;259:E141–7. https://doi.org/10.1152/ajpendo.1990.259.2.E141.
115. Tosti-Croce C, Lucarelli C, Betto P, Floridi A, Rinaldi R, Salvati A, et al. Plasma catecholamine responses during a personalized physical stress as a dynamic characterization of essential hypertension. Physiol Behav. 1991;49:685–90. http://www.ncbi.nlm.nih.gov/pubmed/1881970.
116. Brenner IK, Zamecnik J, Shek PN, Shephard RJ. The impact of heat exposure and repeated exercise on circulating stress hormones. Eur J Appl Physiol Occup Physiol. 1997;76:445–54. https://doi.org/10.1007/s004210050274.
117. Mannelli M, Gheri RG, Selli C, Turini D, Pampanini A, Giusti G, et al. A study on human adrenal secretion. Measurement of epinephrine, norepinephrine, dopamine and cortisol in peripheral and adrenal venous blood under surgical stress. J Endocrinol Invest. 1982;5:91–5. https://doi.org/10.1007/BF03350497.
118. Erridge C. Endogenous ligands of TLR2 and TLR4: agonists or assistants? J Leukoc Biol. 2010;87:989–99. http://www.ncbi.nlm.nih.gov/pubmed/20179153.
119. McCarthy CG, Goulopoulou S, Wenceslau CF, Spitler K, Matsumoto T, Webb RC. Toll-like receptors and damage-associated molecular patterns: novel links between inflammation and hypertension. Am J Physiol Heart Circ Physiol. 2014;306:H184–96. https://doi.org/10.1152/ajpheart.00328.2013.
120. Satou R, Penrose H, Navar LG. Inflammation as a regulator of the renin-angiotensin system and blood pressure. Curr Hypertens Rep. 2018;20:100. http://www.ncbi.nlm.nih.gov/pubmed/30291560.
121. Takimoto-Ohnishi E, Murakami K. Renin–angiotensin system research: from molecules to the whole body. J Physiol Sci. 2019;69:581–7. http://www.ncbi.nlm.nih.gov/pubmed/31028527.
122. Kurtz A. Renin release: sites, mechanisms, and control. Annu Rev Physiol. 2011;73:377–99. http://www.ncbi.nlm.nih.gov/pubmed/20936939.
123. Peti-Peterdi J, Gevorgyan H, Lam L, Riquier-Brison A. Metabolic control of renin secretion. Pflügers Arch Eur J Physiol. 2013;465:53–8. http://www.ncbi.nlm.nih.gov/pubmed/22729752.
124. Mendez M. Renin release: role of SNAREs. Am J Physiol Integr Comp Physiol. 2014;307:R484–6. http://www.ncbi.nlm.nih.gov/pubmed/24944251.
125. Muñoz-Durango N, Fuentes CA, Castillo AE, González-Gómez LM, Vecchiola A, Fardella CE, et al. Role of the renin-angiotensin-aldosterone system beyond blood pressure regulation: molecular and cellular mechanisms involved in end-organ damage during arterial hypertension. Int J Mol Sci. 2016;17:797. http://www.mdpi.com/1422-0067/17/7/797.
126. Chappell MC. Biochemical evaluation of the renin-angiotensin system: the good, bad, and absolute? Am J Physiol Heart Circ Physiol. 2016;310:H137–52. https://doi.org/10.1152/ajpheart.00618.2015.
127. Morris DL, Kahwaji CI. Angiotensin II. In: StatPearls. Treasure Island, FL: StatPearls; 2019. http://www.ncbi.nlm.nih.gov/pubmed/29763087.

128. Mirabito Colafella KM, Danser AHJ. Recent advances in angiotensin research. Hypertens (Dallas, Tex 1979). 2017;69:994–9. https://doi.org/10.1161/HYPERTENSIONAHA.117.08931.
129. Stow LR, Jacobs ME, Wingo CS, Cain BD. Endothelin-1 gene regulation. FASEB J. 2011;25:16–28. https://doi.org/10.1096/fj.10-161612.
130. Qin W, Mi S, Li C, Wang G, Zhang J, Wang H, et al. Low shear stress induced HMGB1 translocation and release via PECAM-1/PARP-1 pathway to induce inflammation response. PLoS One. 2015;10:e0120586. http://www.ncbi.nlm.nih.gov/pubmed/25793984.
131. Liu Y, Yan W, Tohme S, Chen M, Fu Y, Tian D, et al. Hypoxia induced HMGB1 and mitochondrial DNA interactions mediate tumor growth in hepatocellular carcinoma through Toll-like receptor 9. J Hepatol. 2015;63:114–21. http://www.ncbi.nlm.nih.gov/pubmed/25681553.
132. Scharfstein J, Schmitz V, Svensjö E, Granato A, Monteiro AC. Kininogens coordinate adaptive immunity through the proteolytic release of Bradykinin, an endogenous danger signal driving dendritic cell maturation. Scand J Immunol. 2007;66:128–36. http://www.ncbi.nlm.nih.gov/pubmed/17635790.
133. Monteiro AC, Scovino A, Raposo S, Gaze VM, Cruz C, Svensjo E, et al. Kinin danger signals proteolytically released by gingipain induce fimbriae-specific IFN- and IL-17-producing T cells in mice infected intramucosally with Porphyromonas gingivalis. J Immunol. 2009;183:3700–11. http://www.ncbi.nlm.nih.gov/pubmed/19687097.
134. Yoshino O, Yamada-Nomoto K, Kobayashi M, Andoh T, Hongo M, Ono Y, et al. Bradykinin system is involved in endometriosis-related pain through endothelin-1 production. Eur J Pain. 2018;22:501–10. http://www.ncbi.nlm.nih.gov/pubmed/29034546.
135. Davenport AP, Hyndman KA, Dhaun N, Southan C, Kohan DE, Pollock JS, et al. Endothelin. Pharmacol Rev. 2016;68:357–418. https://doi.org/10.1124/pr.115.011833.
136. Adlbrecht C, Wurm R, Humenberger M, Andreas M, Redwan B, Distelmaier K, et al. Peri-interventional endothelin-A receptor blockade improves long-term outcome in patients with ST-elevation acute myocardial infarction. Thromb Haemost. 2014;112:176–82. http://www.ncbi.nlm.nih.gov/pubmed/24695986.
137. Packer M, McMurray JJV, Krum H, Kiowski W, Massie BM, Caspi A, et al. Long-Term effect of endothelin receptor antagonism with bosentan on the morbidity and mortality of patients with severe chronic heart failure. JACC Heart Fail. 2017;5:317–26. http://www.ncbi.nlm.nih.gov/pubmed/28449795.
138. Kuntz M, Leiva-Juarez MM, Luthra S. Systematic review of randomized controlled trials of endothelin receptor antagonists for pulmonary arterial hypertension. Lung. 2016;194:723–32. http://www.ncbi.nlm.nih.gov/pubmed/27506903.
139. Yuan W, Cheng G, Li B, Li Y, Lu S, Liu D, et al. Endothelin-receptor antagonist can reduce blood pressure in patients with hypertension: a meta-analysis. Blood Press. 2017;26:139–49. http://www.ncbi.nlm.nih.gov/pubmed/27808564.
140. Cai X, Xu H, Chen ZJ. Prion-like polymerization in immunity and inflammation. Cold Spring Harb Perspect Biol. 2017;9:a023580. http://www.ncbi.nlm.nih.gov/pubmed/27881448.
141. Venegas C, Kumar S, Franklin BS, Dierkes T, Brinkschulte R, Tejera D, et al. Microglia-derived ASC specks cross-seed amyloid-β in Alzheimer's disease. Nature. 2017;552:355–61. http://www.nature.com/articles/nature25158.
142. Franklin BS, Latz E, Schmidt FI. The intra- and extracellular functions of ASC specks. Immunol Rev. 2018;281:74–87. http://www.ncbi.nlm.nih.gov/pubmed/29247990.
143. Shao Y, Nanayakkara G, Cheng J, Cueto R, Yang WY, Park J-Y, et al. Lysophospholipids and their receptors serve as conditional DAMPs and DAMP receptors in tissue oxidative and inflammatory injury. Antioxid Redox Signal. 2017;28:973–86. https://doi.org/10.1089/ars.2017.7069.
144. Li X, Fang P, Li Y, Kuo Y-M, Andrews AJ, Nanayakkara G, et al. Mitochondrial reactive oxygen species mediate lysophosphatidylcholine-induced endothelial cell activation. Arterioscler Thromb Vasc Biol. 2016;36:1090–100. https://doi.org/10.1161/ATVBAHA.115.306964.
145. Ojala PJ, Hirvonen TE, Hermansson M, Somerharju P, Parkkinen J. Acyl chain-dependent effect of lysophosphatidylcholine on human neutrophils. J Leukoc Biol. 2007;82:1501–9. https://doi.org/10.1189/jlb.0507292.

146. Wang X, Li Y-F, Nanayakkara G, Shao Y, Liang B, Cole L, et al. Lysophospholipid receptors, as novel conditional danger receptors and homeostatic receptors modulate inflammation-novel paradigm and therapeutic potential. J Cardiovasc Transl Res. 2016;9:343–59. https://doi.org/10.1007/s12265-016-9700-6.
147. Frasch SC, Bratton DL. Emerging roles for lysophosphatidylserine in resolution of inflammation. Prog Lipid Res. 2012;51:199–207. https://linkinghub.elsevier.com/retrieve/pii/S0163782712000197.
148. Hung ND, Kim MR, Sok D-E. 2-Polyunsaturated acyl lysophosphatidylethanolamine attenuates inflammatory response in zymosan A-induced peritonitis in mice. Lipids. 2011;46:893–906. http://doi.wiley.com/10.1007/s11745-011-3589-2
149. Cao Z, Lindsay JG. The peroxiredoxin family: an unfolding story. Subcell Biochem. 2017;83:127–47. http://www.ncbi.nlm.nih.gov/pubmed/28271475.
150. Gülke E, Gelderblom M, Magnus T. Danger signals in stroke and their role on microglia activation after ischemia. Ther Adv Neurol Disord. 2018;11:175628641877425. http://www.ncbi.nlm.nih.gov/pubmed/29854002.
151. Knoops B, Becker S, Poncin MA, Glibert J, Derclaye S, Clippe A, et al. Specific interactions measured by AFM on living cells between peroxiredoxin-5 and TLR4: relevance for mechanisms of innate immunity. Cell Chem Biol. 2018;25:550–559.e3. http://www.ncbi.nlm.nih.gov/pubmed/29551349.
152. He Y, Li S, Tang D, Peng Y, Meng J, Peng S, et al. Circulating Peroxiredoxin-1 is a novel damage-associated molecular pattern and aggravates acute liver injury via promoting inflammation. Free Radic Biol Med. 2019;137:24–36. https://linkinghub.elsevier.com/retrieve/pii/S089158491832416X.
153. Chang JW, Lee SH, Lu Y, Yoo YJ. Transforming growth factor-beta1 induces the non-classical secretion of peroxiredoxin-I in A549 cells. Biochem Biophys Res Commun. 2006;345:118–23. https://linkinghub.elsevier.com/retrieve/pii/S0006291X06009156.
154. Mullen L, Hanschmann E-M, Lillig CH, Herzenberg LA, Ghezzi P. Cysteine oxidation targets peroxiredoxins 1 and 2 for exosomal release through a novel mechanism of redox-dependent secretion. Mol Med. 2015;21:98–108. https://doi.org/10.2119/molmed.2015.00033.
155. Najdi R, Proffitt K, Sprowl S, Kaur S, Yu J, Covey TM, et al. A uniform human Wnt expression library reveals a shared secretory pathway and unique signaling activities. Differentiation. 2012;84:203–13. https://linkinghub.elsevier.com/retrieve/pii/S0301468112000874.
156. Sun G, Irvine KD. Control of growth during regeneration. Curr Top Dev Biol. 2014;108:95–120. http://www.ncbi.nlm.nih.gov/pubmed/24512707.
157. Foulquier S, Daskalopoulos EP, Lluri G, Hermans KCM, Deb A, Blankesteijn WM. WNT signaling in cardiac and vascular disease. Pharmacol Rev. 2018;70:68–141. http://www.ncbi.nlm.nih.gov/pubmed/29247129.
158. Bratton DL, Henson PM. Neutrophil clearance: when the party is over, clean-up begins. Trends Immunol. 2011;32:350–7. http://linkinghub.elsevier.com/retrieve/pii/S1471490611000779.
159. Loynes CA, Lee JA, Robertson AL, Steel MJ, Ellett F, Feng Y, et al. PGE 2 production at sites of tissue injury promotes an anti-inflammatory neutrophil phenotype and determines the outcome of inflammation resolution in vivo. Sci Adv. 2018;4:eaar8320. http://www.ncbi.nlm.nih.gov/pubmed/30191175.
160. O'Callaghan G, Houston A. Prostaglandin E2 and the EP receptors in malignancy: possible therapeutic targets? Br J Pharmacol. 2015;172:5239–50. http://www.ncbi.nlm.nih.gov/pubmed/26377664.
161. Kawahara K, Hohjoh H, Inazumi T, Tsuchiya S, Sugimoto Y. Prostaglandin E2-induced inflammation: relevance of prostaglandin E receptors. Biochim Biophys Acta Mol Cell Biol Lipids. 1851;2015:414–21. http://www.ncbi.nlm.nih.gov/pubmed/25038274.
162. Hangai S, Ao T, Kimura Y, Matsuki K, Kawamura T, Negishi H, et al. PGE2 induced in and released by dying cells functions as an inhibitory DAMP. Proc Natl Acad Sci U S A. 2016;113:3844–9. https://doi.org/10.1073/pnas.1602023113.
163. Koga K, Takaesu G, Yoshida R, Nakaya M, Kobayashi T, Kinjyo I, et al. Cyclic adenosine monophosphate suppresses the transcription of proinflammatory cytokines via the phosphorylated c-Fos protein. Immunity. 2009;30:372–83. http://www.ncbi.nlm.nih.gov/pubmed/19285436.

164. Sokolowska M, Chen L-Y, Liu Y, Martinez-Anton A, Qi H-Y, Logun C, et al. Prostaglandin E2 inhibits NLRP3 inflammasome activation through EP4 receptor and intracellular cyclic AMP in human macrophages. J Immunol. 2015;194:5472–87. https://doi.org/10.4049/jimmunol.1401343.
165. Lima KM, Vago JP, Caux TR, Negreiros-Lima GL, Sugimoto MA, Tavares LP, et al. The resolution of acute inflammation induced by cyclic AMP is dependent on annexin A1. J Biol Chem. 2017;292(33):13758–73. http://www.ncbi.nlm.nih.gov/pubmed/28655761.
166. Perretti M, D'Acquisto F. Annexin A1 and glucocorticoids as effectors of the resolution of inflammation. Nat Rev Immunol. 2009;9:62–70. https://doi.org/10.1038/nri2470.
167. Gavins FNE, Hickey MJ. Annexin A1 and the regulation of innate and adaptive immunity. Front Immunol. 2012;3:354. http://www.ncbi.nlm.nih.gov/pubmed/23230437.
168. Sousa LP, Alessandri AL, Pinho V, Teixeira MM. Pharmacological strategies to resolve acute inflammation. Curr Opin Pharmacol. 2013;13:625–31. http://linkinghub.elsevier.com/retrieve/pii/S1471489213000416.
169. Sugimoto MA, Vago JP, Teixeira MM, Sousa LP. Annexin A1 and the resolution of inflammation: modulation of neutrophil recruitment, apoptosis, and clearance. J Immunol Res. 2016;2016:1–13. http://www.ncbi.nlm.nih.gov/pubmed/26885535.
170. Serhan CN. Pro-resolving lipid mediators are leads for resolution physiology. Nature. 2014;510:92–101. https://doi.org/10.1038/nature13479.
171. Basil MC, Levy BD. Specialized pro-resolving mediators: endogenous regulators of infection and inflammation. Nat Rev Immunol. 2015;16:51–67. http://www.ncbi.nlm.nih.gov/pubmed/26688348.
172. Serhan CN, Chiang N, Dalli J, Levy BD. Lipid mediators in the resolution of inflammation. Cold Spring Harb Perspect Biol. 2014;7:a016311. https://doi.org/10.1101/cshperspect.a016311.
173. Anderson HA, Maylock CA, Williams JA, Paweletz CP, Shu H, Shacter E. Serum-derived protein S binds to phosphatidylserine and stimulates the phagocytosis of apoptotic cells. Nat Immunol. 2003;4:87–91. https://doi.org/10.1038/ni871.
174. Frasch SC, Bratton DL. Emerging roles for lysophosphatidylserine in resolution of inflammation. Prog Lipid Res. 2012;51:199–207. http://www.ncbi.nlm.nih.gov/pubmed/22465125.
175. Frasch SC, Fernandez-Boyanapalli RF, Berry KAZ, Murphy RC, Leslie CC, Nick JA, et al. Neutrophils regulate tissue neutrophilia in inflammation via the oxidant-modified lipid lysophosphatidylserine. J Biol Chem. 2013;288:4583–93. http://www.ncbi.nlm.nih.gov/pubmed/23293064.
176. Zagórska A, Través PG, Lew ED, Dransfield I, Lemke G. Diversification of TAM receptor tyrosine kinase function. Nat Immunol. 2014;15:920–8. http://www.ncbi.nlm.nih.gov/pubmed/25194421.
177. Franz S, Muñoz LE, Heyder P, Herrmann M, Schiller M. Unconventional apoptosis of polymorphonuclear neutrophils (PMN): staurosporine delays exposure of phosphatidylserine and prevents phagocytosis by MΦ-2 macrophages of PMN. Clin Exp Immunol. 2015;179:75–84. http://www.ncbi.nlm.nih.gov/pubmed/24995908.
178. Griffiths HR, Gao D, Pararasa C. Redox regulation in metabolic programming and inflammation. Redox Biol. 2017;12:50–7. http://www.ncbi.nlm.nih.gov/pubmed/28212523.
179. Lemke G. Phosphatidylserine is the signal for TAM receptors and their ligands. Trends Biochem Sci. 2017;42:738–48. http://www.ncbi.nlm.nih.gov/pubmed/28734578.
180. McKinney CA, Fattah C, Loughrey CM, Milligan G, Nicklin SA. Angiotensin-(1–7) and angiotensin-(1–9): function in cardiac and vascular remodelling. Clin Sci. 2014;126(12):815–27.
181. Yue-Hui Zhang, Yong-huan Zhang, Xue-Fei Dong, Qing-Qing Hao, Xiao-Ming Zhou, Qing-Tao Yu, Shu-Ying Li, Xu Chen, Abdulai Fallah Tengbeh, Bo Dong, Yun Zhang, ACE2 and Ang-(1–7) protect endothelial cell function and prevent early atherosclerosis by inhibiting inflammatory response. Inflamm Res. 2015;64(3–4):253–60.
182. Serfozo P, Wysocki J, Gulua G, Schulze A, Ye M, Liu P, et al. Ang II (Angiotensin II) Conversion to Angiotensin-(1-7) in the Circulation Is POP (Prolyloligopeptidase)-

Dependent and ACE2 (Angiotensin-Converting Enzyme 2)-Independent. Hypertension. 2020;75(1):173–82.
183. Arumugham VB, Baldari CT. cAMP: a multifaceted modulator of immune synapse assembly and T cell activation. J Leukoc Biol. 2017;101:1301–16. http://www.ncbi.nlm.nih.gov/pubmed/28356349.
184. Sousa LP, Lopes F, Silva DM, Tavares LP, Vieira AT, Rezende BM, et al. PDE4 inhibition drives resolution of neutrophilic inflammation by inducing apoptosis in a PKA-PI3K/Akt-dependent and NF-kappaB-independent manner. J Leukoc Biol. 2010;87:895–904. https://doi.org/10.1189/jlb.0809540.
185. Laflamme C, Mailhot GB, Pouliot M. Age-related decline of the acute local inflammation response: a mitigating role for the adenosine A_{2A} receptor. Aging (Albany NY). 2017;9:2083–97. http://www.ncbi.nlm.nih.gov/pubmed/29064819.
186. Leonard CA, Schoborg RV, Borel N. Damage/Danger Associated Molecular Patterns (DAMPs) modulate Chlamydia pecorum and C. trachomatis Serovar E inclusion development in vitro. PLoS One. 2015;10:e0134943. http://www.ncbi.nlm.nih.gov/pubmed/26248286.
187. Patel N, Wu W, Mishra PK, Chen F, Millman A, Csóka B, et al. A2B adenosine receptor induces protective antihelminth type 2 immune responses. Cell Host Microbe. 2014;15:339–50. http://linkinghub.elsevier.com/retrieve/pii/S1931312814000596.
188. Di Virgilio F, Adinolfi E. Extracellular purines, purinergic receptors and tumor growth. Oncogene. 2017;36:293–303. http://www.ncbi.nlm.nih.gov/pubmed/27321181.
189. Milne GR, Palmer TM. Anti-inflammatory and immunosuppressive effects of the A 2A adenosine receptor. Sci World J. 2011;11:320–39. http://www.ncbi.nlm.nih.gov/pubmed/21298223.
190. Cohen S, Barer F, Bar-Yehuda S, IJzerman AP, Jacobson KA, Fishman P. A 3 adenosine receptor allosteric modulator induces an anti-inflammatory effect: in vivo studies and molecular mechanism of action. Mediators Inflamm. 2014;2014:1–8. http://www.ncbi.nlm.nih.gov/pubmed/25374446.
191. Antonioli L, Fornai M, Blandizzi C, Pacher P, Haskó G. Adenosine signaling and the immune system: when a lot could be too much. Immunol Lett. 2019;205:9–15. http://www.ncbi.nlm.nih.gov/pubmed/29702147.
192. Haskó G, Cronstein BN. Adenosine: an endogenous regulator of innate immunity. Trends Immunol. 2004;25:33–9. http://www.ncbi.nlm.nih.gov/pubmed/14698282.
193. Honn KV, Zeldin DC, editors. The role of bioactive lipids in cancer, inflammation and related diseases. Cham: Springer Nature Switzerland AG; 2019. https://www.springer.com/gp/book/9783030216368.
194. Serhan CN, Clish CB, Brannon J, Colgan SP, Chiang N, Gronert K. Novel functional sets of lipid-derived mediators with antiinflammatory actions generated from omega-3 fatty acids via cyclooxygenase 2-nonsteroidal antiinflammatory drugs and transcellular processing. J Exp Med. 2000;192:1197–204. http://www.ncbi.nlm.nih.gov/pubmed/11034610.
195. Serhan CN, Hong S, Gronert K, Colgan SP, Devchand PR, Mirick G, et al. Resolvins: a family of bioactive products of omega-3 fatty acid transformation circuits initiated by aspirin treatment that counter proinflammation signals. J Exp Med. 2002;196:1025–37. http://www.ncbi.nlm.nih.gov/pubmed/12391014.
196. Hong S, Gronert K, Devchand PR, Moussignac R-L, Serhan CN. Novel docosatrienes and 17S-resolvins generated from docosahexaenoic acid in murine brain, human blood, and glial cells. Autacoids in anti-inflammation. J Biol Chem. 2003;278:14677–87. https://doi.org/10.1074/jbc.M300218200.
197. Bannenberg GL, Chiang N, Ariel A, Arita M, Tjonahen E, Gotlinger KH, et al. Molecular circuits of resolution: formation and actions of resolvins and protectins. J Immunol. 2005;174:4345–55. http://www.ncbi.nlm.nih.gov/pubmed/15778399.
198. Serhan CN. Treating inflammation and infection in the 21st century: new hints from decoding resolution mediators and mechanisms. FASEB J. 2017;31:1273–88. https://doi.org/10.1096/fj.201601222R.

199. Serhan CN, Yang R, Martinod K, Kasuga K, Pillai PS, Porter TF, et al. Maresins: novel macrophage mediators with potent antiinflammatory and proresolving actions. J Exp Med. 2009;206:15–23. http://www.ncbi.nlm.nih.gov/pubmed/19103881.
200. Dalli J, Colas RA, Serhan CN. Novel n-3 immunoresolvents: structures and actions. Sci Rep. 2013;3:1940. http://www.nature.com/articles/srep01940.
201. Serhan CN. Pro-resolving lipid mediators are leads for resolution physiology. Nature. 2014;510:92–101. http://www.ncbi.nlm.nih.gov/pubmed/24899309.
202. Dalli J, Chiang N, Serhan CN. Elucidation of novel 13-series resolvins that increase with atorvastatin and clear infections. Nat Med. 2015;21:1071–5. http://www.nature.com/articles/nm.3911.
203. Serhan CN, Levy BD. Resolvins in inflammation: emergence of the pro-resolving superfamily of mediators. J Clin Invest. 2018;128:2657–69. http://www.ncbi.nlm.nih.gov/pubmed/29757195.
204. Chiang N, Dalli J, Colas RA, Serhan CN. Identification of resolvin D2 receptor mediating resolution of infections and organ protection. J Exp Med. 2015;212:1203–17. https://doi.org/10.1084/jem.20150225.
205. Kasuga K, Yang R, Porter TF, Agrawal N, Petasis NA, Irimia D, et al. Rapid appearance of resolvin precursors in inflammatory exudates: novel mechanisms in resolution. J Immunol. 2008;181:8677–87. http://www.ncbi.nlm.nih.gov/pubmed/19050288.
206. Serhan CN, Dalli J, Colas RA, Winkler JW, Chiang N. Protectins and maresins: new pro-resolving families of mediators in acute inflammation and resolution bioactive metabolome. Biochim Biophys Acta. 1851;2015:397–413. http://linkinghub.elsevier.com/retrieve/pii/S1388198114001619.
207. Serhan CN. Discovery of specialized pro-resolving mediators marks the dawn of resolution physiology and pharmacology. Mol Aspects Med. 2017;58:1–11. https://linkinghub.elsevier.com/retrieve/pii/S0098299717300183.
208. Werz O, Gerstmeier J, Libreros S, De la Rosa X, Werner M, Norris PC, et al. Human macrophages differentially produce specific resolvin or leukotriene signals that depend on bacterial pathogenicity. Nat Commun. 2018;9:59. http://www.ncbi.nlm.nih.gov/pubmed/29302056.
209. Li Y, Cai L, Wang H, Wu P, Gu W, Chen Y, et al. Pleiotropic regulation of macrophage polarization and tumorigenesis by formyl peptide receptor-2. Oncogene. 2011;30:3887–99. http://www.nature.com/articles/onc2011112.
210. Titos E, Rius B, González-Périz A, López-Vicario C, Morán-Salvador E, Martínez-Clemente M, et al. Resolvin D1 and its precursor docosahexaenoic acid promote resolution of adipose tissue inflammation by eliciting macrophage polarization toward an M2-like phenotype. J Immunol. 2011;187:5408–18. https://doi.org/10.4049/jimmunol.1100225.
211. Dalli J, Zhu M, Vlasenko NA, Deng B, Haeggström JZ, Petasis NA, et al. The novel 13S,14S-epoxy-maresinis converted by human macrophages to maresin 1 (MaR1), inhibits leukotriene A4 hydrolase (LTA4H), and shifts macrophage phenotype. FASEB J. 2013;27:2573–83.
212. Rius B, Titos E, Morán-Salvador E, López-Vicario C, García-Alonso V, González-Périz A, et al. Resolvin D1 primes the resolution process initiated by calorie restriction in obesity-induced steatohepatitis. FASEB J. 2014;28:836–48. http://www.ncbi.nlm.nih.gov/pubmed/24249635.
213. Herová M, Schmid M, Gemperle C, Hersberger M. ChemR23, the receptor for chemerin and resolvin E1, is expressed and functional on M1 but not on M2 macrophages. J Immunol. 2015;194:2330–7. https://doi.org/10.4049/jimmunol.1402166.
214. Calderwood SK, Murshid A, Gong J. Heat shock proteins: conditional mediators of inflammation in tumor immunity. Front Immunol. 2012;3:75. https://doi.org/10.3389/fimmu.2012.00075/abstract.
215. van Eden W, Spiering R, Broere F, van der Zee R. A case of mistaken identity: HSPs are no DAMPs but DAMPERs. Cell Stress Chaperones. 2012;17:281–92. https://doi.org/10.1007/s12192-011-0311-5.
216. Kelly A, Houston SA, Sherwood E, Casulli J, Travis MA. Regulation of innate and adaptive immunity by TGFβ. Adv Immunol. 2017;134:137–233. http://www.ncbi.nlm.nih.gov/pubmed/28413021.

217. Travis MA, Sheppard D. TGF-β activation and function in immunity. Annu Rev Immunol. 2014;32:51–82. http://www.annualreviews.org/doi/10.1146/annurev-immunol-032713-120257.
218. Sanjabi S, Oh SA, Li MO. Regulation of the immune response by TGF-β: from conception to autoimmunity and infection. Cold Spring Harb Perspect Biol. 2017;9:a022236. https://doi.org/10.1101/cshperspect.a022236.
219. Carthy JM. TGFβ signaling and the control of myofibroblast differentiation: implications for chronic inflammatory disorders. J Cell Physiol. 2018;233:98–106. https://doi.org/10.1002/jcp.25879.
220. Hinz B. The extracellular matrix and transforming growth factor-β1: tale of a strained relationship. Matrix Biol. 2015;47:54–65. https://linkinghub.elsevier.com/retrieve/pii/S0945053X15001055.
221. Hinck AP, Mueller TD, Springer TA. Structural biology and evolution of the TGF-β family. Cold Spring Harb Perspect Biol. 2016;8:a022103. https://doi.org/10.1101/cshperspect.a022103.
222. Robertson IB, Rifkin DB. Regulation of the bioavailability of TGF-β and TGF-β-related proteins. Cold Spring Harb Perspect Biol. 2016;8:a021907. https://doi.org/10.1101/cshperspect.a021907.
223. Pintavorn P, Ballermann BJ. TGF-beta and the endothelium during immune injury. Kidney Int. 1997;51:1401–12. http://www.ncbi.nlm.nih.gov/pubmed/9150451.
224. Nacu N, Luzina IG, Highsmith K, Lockatell V, Pochetuhen K, Cooper ZA, et al. Macrophages produce TGF-beta-induced (beta-ig-h3) following ingestion of apoptotic cells and regulate MMP14 levels and collagen turnover in fibroblasts. J Immunol. 2008;180:5036–44. http://www.ncbi.nlm.nih.gov/pubmed/18354229.
225. El-Karef A, Yoshida T, Gabazza EC, Nishioka T, Inada H, Sakakura T, et al. Deficiency of tenascin-C attenuates liver fibrosis in immune-mediated chronic hepatitis in mice. J Pathol. 2007;211:86–94. https://doi.org/10.1002/path.2099.
226. Zhang W, Lavine KJ, Epelman S, Evans SA, Weinheimer CJ, Barger PM, et al. Necrotic myocardial cells release damage-associated molecular patterns that provoke fibroblast activation in vitro and trigger myocardial inflammation and fibrosis in vivo. J Am Heart Assoc. 2015;4:e001993. http://www.ncbi.nlm.nih.gov/pubmed/26037082.
227. Wang Q, Wang J, Wang J, Hong S, Han F, Chen J, et al. HMGB1 induces lung fibroblast to myofibroblast differentiation through NF-κB-mediated TGF-β1 release. Mol Med Rep. 2017;15:3062–8. http://www.ncbi.nlm.nih.gov/pubmed/28339089.
228. Lee WJ, Song SY, Roh H, Ahn HM, Na Y, Kim J, et al. Profibrogenic effect of high-mobility group box protein-1 in human dermal fibroblasts and its excess in keloid tissues. Sci Rep. 2018;8:8434. http://www.ncbi.nlm.nih.gov/pubmed/29849053.
229. Dong X, Zhao B, Iacob RE, Zhu J, Koksal AC, Lu C, et al. Force interacts with macromolecular structure in activation of TGF-β. Nature. 2017;542:55–9. http://www.nature.com/articles/nature21035.
230. Hinz B. It has to be the αv: myofibroblast integrins activate latent TGF-β1. Nat Med. 2013;19:1567–8. http://www.nature.com/articles/nm.3421.
231. Stockis J, Dedobbeleer O, Lucas S. Role of GARP in the activation of latent TGF-β1. Mol Biosyst. 2017;13:1925–35. http://www.ncbi.nlm.nih.gov/pubmed/28795730.
232. Hodzic Z, Schill EM, Bolock AM, Good M. IL-33 and the intestine: the good, the bad, and the inflammatory. Cytokine. 2017;100:1–10. http://www.ncbi.nlm.nih.gov/pubmed/28687373.
233. Cayrol C, Girard J-P. Interleukin-33 (IL-33): a nuclear cytokine from the IL-1 family. Immunol Rev. 2018;281:154–68. http://www.ncbi.nlm.nih.gov/pubmed/29247993.
234. de Kouchkovsky DA, Ghosh S, Rothlin CV. Induction of sterile type 2 inflammation. Nat Mater. 2019;18:193–4. http://www.ncbi.nlm.nih.gov/pubmed/30783225.
235. Mehraj V, Ponte R, Routy J-P. The dynamic role of the IL-33/ST2 axis in chronic viral-infections: alarming and adjuvanting the immune response. EBioMedicine. 2016;9:37–44. http://www.ncbi.nlm.nih.gov/pubmed/27397514.

236. Duan L, Chen J, Zhang H, Yang H, Zhu P, Xiong A, et al. Interleukin-33 ameliorates experimental colitis through promoting Th2/Foxp3+ regulatory T-cell responses in mice. Mol Med. 2012;18:753–61. http://www.ncbi.nlm.nih.gov/pubmed/22426954.
237. Cui G, Li Z, Ren J, Yuan A. IL-33 in the tumor microenvironment is associated with the accumulation of FoxP3-positive regulatory T cells in human esophageal carcinomas. Virchows Arch. 2019;475(5):579–86. http://www.ncbi.nlm.nih.gov/pubmed/31062086.
238. Meissner M, Viehmann SF, Kurts C. DAMPening sterile inflammation of the kidney. Kidney Int. 2019;95:489–91. https://linkinghub.elsevier.com/retrieve/pii/S0085253819300079.
239. Chakraborty D, Zenker S, Rossaint J, Hölscher A, Pohlen M, Zarbock A, et al. Alarmin S100A8 activates alveolar epithelial cells in the context of acute lung injury in a TLR4-dependent manner. Front Immunol. 2017;8:1493. https://doi.org/10.3389/fimmu.2017.01493/full.
240. Hiroshima Y, Hsu K, Tedla N, Wong SW, Chow S, Kawaguchi N, et al. S100A8/A9 and S100A9 reduce acute lung injury. Immunol Cell Biol. 2017;95:461–72. http://www.ncbi.nlm.nih.gov/pubmed/28074060.
241. 7 million deaths annually linked to air pollution. Cent Eur J Public Health. 2014;22:53–59. http://www.ncbi.nlm.nih.gov/pubmed/24844108. [cited 2019 Jul 16].
242. WHO. Ambient and household air pollution and health. Geneva: WHO. World Health Organization; 2019. https://www.who.int/airpollution/data/en/.
243. Mannucci P, Franchini M. Health effects of ambient air pollution in developing countries. Int J Environ Res Public Health. 2017;14:1048. http://www.ncbi.nlm.nih.gov/pubmed/28895888.
244. Chen R, Yin P, Meng X, Liu C, Wang L, Xu X, et al. Fine particulate air pollution and daily mortality. a nationwide analysis in 272 Chinese cities. Am J Respir Crit Care Med. 2017;196:73–81. http://www.ncbi.nlm.nih.gov/pubmed/28248546.
245. Turner MC, Krewski D, Diver WR, Pope CA, Burnett RT, Jerrett M, et al. Ambient air pollution and cancer mortality in the cancer prevention study II. Environ Health Perspect. 2017;125:087013. http://www.ncbi.nlm.nih.gov/pubmed/28886601.
246. De Grove KC, Provoost S, Brusselle GG, Joos GF, Maes T. Insights in particulate matter-induced allergic airway inflammation: focus on the epithelium. Clin Exp Allergy. 2018;48:773–86. https://doi.org/10.1111/cea.13178.
247. Zielinska B, Samy S, McDonald JD, Seagrave J. HEI Health Review Committee. atmospheric transformation of diesel emissions. Res Rep Health Eff Inst. 2010:5–60. http://www.ncbi.nlm.nih.gov/pubmed/20572366.
248. Müller L, Jaspers I. Epithelial cells, the "switchboard" of respiratory immune defense responses: effects of air pollutants. Swiss Med Wkly. 2012;142:w13653. http://doi.emh.ch/smw.2012.13653. [cited 2019 Jul 16].
249. Kuroda E, Coban C, Ishii KJ. Particulate adjuvant and innate immunity: past achievements, present findings, and future prospects. Int Rev Immunol. 2013;32:209–20. https://doi.org/10.3109/08830185.2013.773326.
250. Tsai D-H, Riediker M, Berchet A, Paccaud F, Waeber G, Vollenweider P, et al. Effects of short- and long-term exposures to particulate matter on inflammatory marker levels in the general population. Environ Sci Pollut Res Int. 2019;26:19697–704. https://doi.org/10.1007/s11356-019-05194-y.
251. Wang H, Song L, Ju W, Wang X, Dong L, Zhang Y, et al. The acute airway inflammation induced by PM2.5 exposure and the treatment of essential oils in Balb/c mice. Sci Rep. 2017;7:44256. http://www.nature.com/articles/srep44256.
252. Ding S, Wang H, Wang M, Bai L, Yu P, Wu W. Resveratrol alleviates chronic "real-world" ambient particulate matter-induced lung inflammation and fibrosis by inhibiting NLRP3 inflammasome activation in mice. Ecotoxicol Environ Saf. 2019;182:109425. https://linkinghub.elsevier.com/retrieve/pii/S0147651319307559.
253. Thatcher TH, Woeller CF, McCarthy CE, Sime PJ. Quenching the fires: pro-resolving mediators, air pollution, and smoking. Pharmacol Ther. 2019;197:212–24. https://linkinghub.elsevier.com/retrieve/pii/S0163725819300142.
254. Netea MG, Quintin J, van der Meer JWM. Trained immunity: a memory for innate host defense. Cell Host Microbe. 2011;9:355–61. http://linkinghub.elsevier.com/retrieve/pii/S1931312811001284.

255. Netea MG, Latz E, Mills KHG, O'Neill LAJ. Innate immune memory: a paradigm shift in understanding host defense. Nat Immunol. 2015;16:675–9. https://doi.org/10.1038/ni.3178.
256. Netea MG, Joosten LAB, Latz E, Mills KHG, Natoli G, Stunnenberg HG, et al. Trained immunity: a program of innate immune memory in health and disease. Science. 2016;352:aaf1098. http://www.ncbi.nlm.nih.gov/pubmed/27102489.
257. Saeed S, Quintin J, Kerstens HHD, Rao NA, Aghajanirefah A, Matarese F, et al. Epigenetic programming of monocyte-to-macrophage differentiation and trained innate immunity. Science (80-). 2014;345:1251086. https://doi.org/10.1126/science.1251086.
258. Riksen NP, Netea MG. Be aware, innate immune cells remember. Aging (Albany NY). 2018;10:2218–9. http://www.ncbi.nlm.nih.gov/pubmed/30215600.
259. Lacy M, Atzler D, Liu R, de Winther M, Weber C, Lutgens E. Interactions between dyslipidemia and the immune system and their relevance as putative therapeutic targets in atherosclerosis. Pharmacol Ther. 2019;193:50–62. http://www.ncbi.nlm.nih.gov/pubmed/30149100.
260. Riksen NP, Stienstra R. Metabolism of innate immune cells. Curr Opin Lipidol. 2018;29:1. http://www.ncbi.nlm.nih.gov/pubmed/30020200.
261. Dominguez-Andres J, Netea MG. Long-term reprogramming of the innate immune system. J Leukoc Biol. 2019;105:329–38. http://www.ncbi.nlm.nih.gov/pubmed/29999546.
262. Norata GD. Trained immunity and cardiovascular disease: is it time for translation to humans? Cardiovasc Res. 2018;114:e41–2. http://www.ncbi.nlm.nih.gov/pubmed/29897493.
263. Pirillo A, Bonacina F, Norata GD, Catapano AL. The interplay of lipids, lipoproteins, and immunity in atherosclerosis. Curr Atheroscler Rep. 2018;20:12. http://www.ncbi.nlm.nih.gov/pubmed/29445885.
264. Leentjens J, Bekkering S, Joosten LAB, Netea MG, Burgner DP, Riksen NP. Trained innate immunity as a novel mechanism linking infection and the development of atherosclerosis. Circ Res. 2018;122:664–9. http://www.ncbi.nlm.nih.gov/pubmed/29367213.
265. Christ A, Günther P, Lauterbach MAR, Duewell P, Biswas D, Pelka K, et al. Western diet triggers NLRP3-dependent innate immune reprogramming. Cell. 2018;172:162–175.e14. http://www.ncbi.nlm.nih.gov/pubmed/29328911.
266. van der Heijden CDCC, Noz MP, Joosten LAB, Netea MG, Riksen NP, Keating ST. Epigenetics and trained immunity. Antioxid Redox Signal. 2018;29:1023–40. http://www.ncbi.nlm.nih.gov/pubmed/28978221.
267. Groh L, Keating ST, Joosten LAB, Netea MG, Riksen NP. Monocyte and macrophage immunometabolism in atherosclerosis. Semin Immunopathol. 2018;40:203–14. http://www.ncbi.nlm.nih.gov/pubmed/28971272.
268. Bekkering S, Quintin J, Joosten LAB, van der Meer JWM, Netea MG, Riksen NP. Oxidized low-density lipoprotein induces long-term proinflammatory cytokine production and foam cell formation via epigenetic reprogramming of monocytes. Arterioscler Thromb Vasc Biol. 2014;34:1731–8. https://doi.org/10.1161/ATVBAHA.114.303887.
269. van der Valk FM, Bekkering S, Kroon J, Yeang C, Van den Bossche J, van Buul JD, et al. Oxidized phospholipids on lipoprotein(a) elicit arterial wall inflammation and an inflammatory monocyte response in humans. Circulation. 2016;134:611–24. https://doi.org/10.1161/CIRCULATIONAHA.116.020838.
270. Neidhart M, Pajak A, Laskari K, Riksen NP, Joosten LAB, Netea MG, et al. Oligomeric S100A4 is associated with monocyte innate immune memory and bypass of tolerance to subsequent stimulation with lipopolysaccharides. Front Immunol. 2019;10:791. http://www.ncbi.nlm.nih.gov/pubmed/31037071.
271. Heil M, Land WG. Danger signals—damaged-self recognition across the tree of life. Front Plant Sci. 2014;5:578. http://www.ncbi.nlm.nih.gov/pubmed/25400647.
272. Heil M, Land WG, Tör M. Editorial: wound recognition across the tree of life. Front Plant Sci. 2016;7:1319. http://www.ncbi.nlm.nih.gov/pubmed/27635126.
273. Chen S, Yang J, Wei Y, Wei X. Epigenetic regulation of macrophages: from homeostasis maintenance to host defense. Cell Mol Immunol. 2019;17(1):36–49. http://www.ncbi.nlm.nih.gov/pubmed/31664225.

The Growing Clinical Relevance of Cellular Stress Responses and Regulated Cell Death

4

4.1 Introduction

As outlined in Vol. 1 [1], Part V, the two topics of cell-intrinsic adaptive stress responses and RCD are cardinal features of the innate immune defense system and have to be seen in close interconnectedness. The common aim of both cellular events is to guarantee the survival of an individual in case of incoming dangerous, possibly life-threatening insults. To cope with such inciting insults and restore cellular homeostasis, the cell at first reacts with a defensive adaptive stress response. However, when such perturbations of the intracellular or extracellular microenvironment are too intense or prolonged, a form of RCD is initialized aimed at exposing or releasing an army of DAMPs used for intensified and extended defense of the whole organism. In other words, when defense at the cellular level fails, proliferative inactivation (cell cycle arrest/cellular senescence) or RCD of the stressed/injured cell and the associated emission of DAMPs directly operates at the level of the whole organism to restore organismal homeostasis (here, also compare [2]).

In the following, a brief update of both adaptive strategies to preserve and restore homeostasis is presented by focusing on recent publications in the field of RCD.

4.2 Cell-Autonomous Adaptive Stress Responses: From Cell Survival to Cell Death

4.2.1 Introductory Remarks

Beyond the well-characterized MAMP/DAMP engagement of PRMs leading to a variety of downstream efferent cellular and humoral responses, the innate immune defense program also depends on cell-autonomous, that is, cell-intrinsic responses which counteract any stressful insult [3]. Typically, constitutive cell-autonomous immunity mobilizes pre-existing molecules and processes to primarily and quickly

W. G. Land, *Damage-Associated Molecular Patterns in Human Diseases*,
https://doi.org/10.1007/978-3-030-53868-2_4

defend the cell and the host against infectious and sterile injury. Hence it can be considered as the very first line of innate immune defense. Cell-intrinsic stress responses include autophagic processes, the oxidative stress response, the heat shock response (HSR), the UPR, and the DDR (described and illustrated in Vol. 1 [1], Part V, Chpt.18 and Figs. 18.1 up to 18.7). Here, a few selected aspects of this important topic are briefly touched.

4.2.2 Autophagy: A Process Induced by DAMPs and a Source of DAMPs Emission

Autophagy is an evolutionarily highly conserved cytoprotective, self-digestive process in response to environmental stress to eukaryotic cells, by which cytoplasmic components such as defective/damaged or redundant organelles or protein aggregates are delivered to the lysosome for recycling and degradation. Autophagy is a lysosome-mediated degradation and recycling pathway that involves the formation of multiple membrane structures ranging from phagophores to autophagosomes and autophagolysosomes. The nature of the autophagic process and the various forms of autophagy are described in Vol. 1 [1], Part V, Subchapter 18.2, and Fig. 18.1, where the subsequent remarks are also outlined in more detail.

There is convincing evidence indicating that activation of the autophagic process is promoted by MAMPs and DAMPs or DAMPs [4, 5]. In more simple words, autophagy is a classical cell-protective and cell-autonomous process of the innate immune system aimed at maintaining and restoring homeostasis at both the cellular (cell-intrinsic) and organismal (cell-extrinsic) level [6]. Mechanistically, the biogenesis of autophagosomes needs the ordered intervention of autophagy-related (ATG) proteins that act on different modules. Thus, more than 30 ATG genes have been identified in humans that orchestrate the complex membrane dynamics involved in autophagic sequestration (reviewed in [7]). Notably, the autophagic process provides tremendous flexibility and capacity with regard to cargo, allowing entire organelles to be deleted via autophagy; however, this flexibility also means that autophagy must be tightly controlled in order to prevent inappropriate degradation, which—under pathological conditions—could lead to autophagy-dependent cell death (a form of RCD that mechanistically depends on the autophagic machinery) (for relevant papers, see [8–14]). It should be particularly noted that ROS and reactive nitrogen species (RNS) are reportedly considered the main early intracellular signal transducers sustaining autophagy, likely acting at multiple levels in the process [15]. However, it is still not entirely clear how these species exactly drive the process, but one may think of ROS-promoted emission of DAMPs, which are known to regulating autophagy (for additional information, see Vol. 1 [1], Part V, Sect. 18.2.5.3, p. 386). Intriguingly, growing evidence indicates that, in turn, autophagy regulates release and degradation of DAMPs in terms of inducible DAMPs (see Sect. 3.5). Interestingly, in more recent studies on a murine necroptotic tumor cell model, autophagy induced by the ICD inducer *shikonin* was found to contribute directly to DAMP upregulation [16]. The authors could show that the upregulated DAMPs exposed at the cell surface were able to activate the cocultured DCs. Given their findings, they concluded that the expression of autophagy-related exposed DAMPs appears to be critical for immunogenicity in cells undergoing necroptosis. Indeed, these observations are just one of many new insights into the interrelationship between autophagic processes and emission of DAMPs.

4.2.2.1 Role of Autophagy in Diseases

Autophagic processes are pathogenetically involved in many human diseases. As reviewed by Khandia et al. [17], autophagy is implicated in infectious and noninfectious diseases, either providing protection or worsening the disorder. Of note, autophagy has been observed to have dual roles in an antibacterial, antiviral, and cancer-suppressing capacity and by favoring bacterial and viral infections and tumor progression. Moreover, autophagic processes were shown to contribute to CVDs and autoimmune and neurodegenerative diseases. Given the critical role of autophagy in many diseases, a variety of drugs, biomolecules, chemicals, and epigenetic strategies have been developed to either promote or inhibit autophagy (reviewed in [17], and not further alluded to here).

For further recent articles on autophagocytic pathways, the reader is referred to [18–22]. The contribution of autophagy to the pathogenesis of atherosclerosis will be briefly mentioned in Chap. 10.

4.2.3 The Oxidative Stress Response

4.2.3.1 General Remarks

The oxidative stress response in terms of a potent antioxidative defense system has been described in Vol. 1 [1], Part V, Sect. 18.3. The antioxidative defense molecules comprise the following [23]: (1) agents that catalytically remove free oxygen radicals and other reactive species, for example, superoxide dismutase (SOD), catalase, peroxidase, and thiol-specific antioxidants; (2) proteins that minimize the availability of prooxidants such as iron ions, copper ions, and heme, for example, transferrins, haptoglobins, hemopexin, and metallothionein; (3) proteins that protect biomolecules against damage (including oxidative damage) by other mechanisms; and (4) low-molecular-mass agents that scavenge ROS and RNS, for example, glutathione (GSH), α-tocopherol, and (possibly) bilirubin and uric acid. In the past, it was fashionable to divide the antioxidative defense response into three main tiers: (1) antioxidant enzymes including SOD, catalase, glutathione peroxidase (GPX), and GSH; (2) detoxifying enzymes such as GPX (in particular GPX4), glutathione S-transferase, aldo-keto reductase, and aldehyde dehydrogenase; and (3) energy-dependent efflux pumps. As a fourth defense system, the antioxidant nutrients such as vitamins E and C as well as carotenoids were appreciated [24].

4.2.3.2 The Keap1↔Nrf2→ARE Pathway

Modern concepts now hold that the evolutionarily highly conserved, oxidant-promoted, *Kelch-like erythroid cell-derived protein with CNC homology*

(ECH)-associated protein 1 (Keap1) ↔ *nuclear factor-erythroid 2 p45-related factors 2* (Nrf2)-triggered *antioxidant response element* (ARE) pathway is the central command for a multifaceted cellular defense that serves to protect cells from ROS damage (for the Keap1↔Nrf2→ARE pathway, also compare Vol. 1 [1], Part V, Sect. 18.3.3.3; for more recent reviews, see [25–28]). In particular, oxidative cell damage can be caused by the accumulation of lipid peroxides (lipid ROS) that has an essential role in driving the pathogenesis of multiple disease states and, at worst, can end up with ferroptotic cell death (see Sect. 4.3.4).

For this book only (and generally not accepted), Keap1 is regarded as a cell-intrinsic redox-sensitive protein that senses—via highly reactive cysteine residues—cell-intrinsic dyshomeostasis-associated molecular patterns (IIC-4 DAMPs), reflected by intracellular redox changes (compare Vol. 1 [1], Part II, Sect. 5.3.2, and Part IV, Sect. 13.4.5 and Sect. 3.4.4.2). The protein is a negative regulator of the transcription factor Nrf2 and the central hub for sensing endogenous and environmental oxidative and electrophilic stress. Mechanistically, it is proposed that oxidative stress modifies the ROS-sensing cysteine residues of Keap1, leading to loss of its polyubiquitination and degradation activity resulting in Nrf2 dissociation from Keap1, whereby Nrf2 becomes stabilized and accumulates to initiate a robust antioxidant response (for additional information compare Fig. 18.4 in Vol. 1 [1], Part V Sect. 18.3.3.3, p. 396). Indeed, the master transcription factor Nrf2 is a key regulator of the cellular antioxidant response, controlling the expression of genes that counteract oxidative and electrophilic stresses. For example, established Nrf2-regulated genes reportedly include Cu/Zn SOD, catalase, TRX, TRX reductase, glutathione reductase (GR), GPX, and ferritin L (FTL). Initiated is this Nrf2—triggered antioxidant response by activation of Keap1 that functions as a substrate adaptor protein for the degradation of Nrf2 (for additional information compare in Vol.1 [1]: Part II, Sect. 5.3.2, p. 68, and Part IV, Sect. 13.4.5, p. 289; for further reading, see [29–42]).

Of note, the Keap1↔Nrf2 pathway is now regarded as an evolutionarily highly conserved defense mechanism against oxidative and xenobiotic stress across the tree of life. As reviewed by Chen and Maltagliati [43], the powerful antioxidant action of Nrf2 manifests mainly through increased synthesis of GSH, activation of GSTs, or the peroxiredoxin system and increased expression of the antioxidative molecule heme oxygenase-1 (HO-1), in addition to the activity of classic antioxidant enzymes mentioned above (for peroxiredoxin, compare Sect. 3.5.4.4). Induction of other Nrf2-regulated genes such as the glutamate–cysteine ligase catalytic and regulatory subunit (i.e., *Gclc, Gclm*) contributes to an increased synthesis of GSH that is essential for detoxification of xenobiotics and oxidative products via the catalytic activity of GSTs. It is then the GSH that allows the GPX to remove hydrogen peroxides, in particular, PLOOH that is known to promote iron-dependent lipid peroxidation (see Sect. 3.4.3.2 and reviews in [43, 44]). In fact, GSH is one of the most important components of the cell-intrinsic antioxidant defenses. The molecule is a simple tripeptide consisting of glutamate, cysteine, and glycine, with the reactive thiol group on cysteine playing a critical functional role in the reduction of oxidized intracellular components. The cell obtains its cysteine via import of cystine (the oxidized dimer form of cysteine) from the extracellular environment via a cystine/glutamate antiporter, dubbed "system xC-/xCT". Imported cystine is then reduced via cystine reductase and used by two enzymes, glutamate-cysteine ligase (GCL) (previously known as *gamma glutamyl-cysteine synthetase*) and glutathione synthetase to generate GSH (also compare Fig. 4.2a, b).

4.2.3.3 Concluding Remarks

Under normal conditions, the oxidative stress response as executed by the potent cell-intrinsic Keap1↔Nrf2 pathway represents a powerful innate defense response that regulates the intracellular redox milieu and guarantees redox balance. However, in case of excessive production of ROS (including lipid ROS) and/or persistence of ROS production, this antioxidative defense pathway can be overridden and thus may fail in terms of a "sabotage," thereby paving the way for the development of ferroptosis [45–48] (see also Sect. 4.3.4).

4.2.4 The Heat Shock Response

The heat shock response has been addressed in Vol. 1 [1]: Part V, Sect. 18.4, and is only briefly resumed here. This defense response is one of the most ancient and evolutionarily conserved cytoprotective mechanisms found in nature and is induced

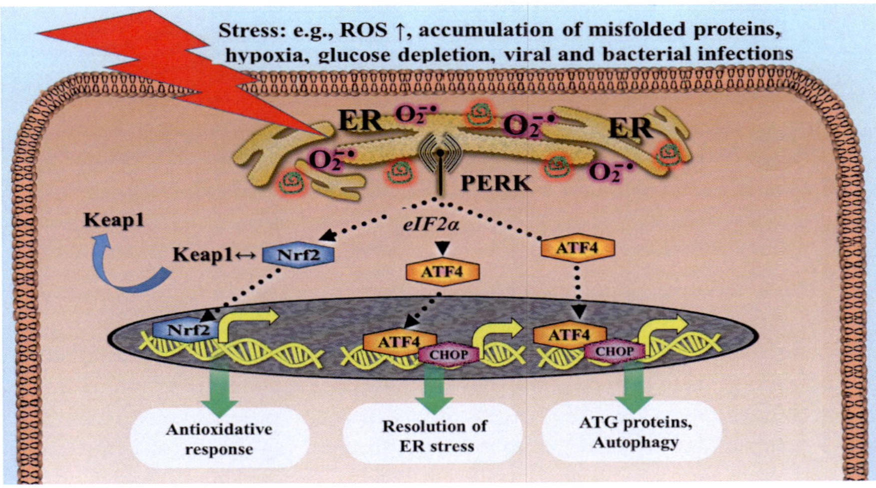

Fig. 4.1 Schematic scenario model of the PERK→Nrf2 and PERK→ATF4-mediated interconnectedness of the ER stress-promoted UPR with two other protective adaptive stress responses, autophagy and the antioxidative response (hereto compare in Vol 1, Part V, Fig. 18.4 in Sect. 18.3.3.3, and Fig. 18.6 in Sect. 18.5.2). *ARE* antioxidant response element, *ATG* autophagy-related, *ATF4* activating transcription factor 4, *ChOP* cytidine-cytidine-adenosine-adenosine-thymidine (CCAAT)-enhancer-binding homologous protein, *eIF2α* eukaryotic translation initiation factor 2 alpha, *ER* endoplasmic reticulum, *Keap1* Kelch-like erythroid cell-derived protein with CNC homology (ECH)-associated protein 1, *Nrf2* nuclear factor-erythroid 2 p45-related factors 2, *PERK* protein kinase RNA-like endoplasmic reticulum (ER) kinase. (Sources: [88–90, 103–105])

upon exposure of living cells to acute, subacute, or chronic stress conditions. This response is characterized by the expression of a group of phylogenetically conserved intracellular HSPs, which possess the capacity to recognize structures commonly found in the interior of proteins and to bind such structures. Thanks to this property, they form a chaperone network involved in correct protein folding, trafficking, and complex assembly (for reviews, see [49–55]). To be released from engagement with proteins after folding and take part in further rounds of activity, HSP70 and other chaperones utilize an intrinsic ATPase domain to hydrolyze ATP and assume a free conformation [56]. Once released, HSPs mediate protective cellular defense mechanisms, including regulation of apoptosis, the aim being to maintain and restore cellular protein homeostasis (proteostasis).

The HSR is recognized and accepted as a classical stress response in nearly all species across the tree of life. It reflects the desperate efforts of a cell to restore homeostasis and survive upon both infectious and sterile insults. Its products, the HSPs, operate as DAMPs in commission of the innate immune system to reach this goal. Notably, via this mechanism, an HSR, induced by infectious damage to a cell, can promote sterile inflammation. Whereas a successful HSR upon stress leads to restoration of cellular homeostasis and cell survival, an unsuccessful HSR may result in RCD, such as apoptosis [55].

4.2.5 Endoplasmic Reticulum Stress and the Unfolded Protein Response

4.2.5.1 General Remarks

The ER stress and the UPR have been addressed in Vol. 1 [1]: Part V, Sect. 18.5. Here, a few amendments are added that may be of interest to the reader from the perspective of the book (for more recent reviews, see [57–60]). The ER is the largest organelle in the cell spanning from the nuclear envelope to the cell membrane. It is mainly responsible for the correct folding and PTM-driven maturation of proteins destined to other organelles. As a subcellular organelle in the control of proteostasis, it is also accountable for calcium storage, detoxification of chemical compounds, and lipid biosynthesis as well as for the orchestration of the protein transport along the classical/conventional secretory pathway. Indeed, the ER delivers the modified protein components to their destination compartments, which include the ER itself, the Golgi apparatus, the plasma membrane, and the extracellular milieu or the endocytic and autophagic pathways. Plausibly, the multifunctional nature of this organelle requires a myriad of proteins, unique physical structures, and coordination with and response to perturbations in the intracellular environment. A series of chaperones such as CALR, folding enzymes, glucosidases, and carbohydrate transferases support and execute these processes.

Of note, oxidative protein folding characterized by intermolecular or intramolecular disulfide bond formation is considered the most common PTM that performs in the ER and has been identified as a significant source of H_2O_2 of the ER [61, 62]. To maintain the redox homeostasis of the ER, H_2O_2 is consumed by some oxidoreductases, GPX7/8, and ascorbate peroxidase to ensure the oxidative protein folding in order. Additionally, GSH also contributes to the removal of excessive ROS (reviewed in [63]). This kind of maintaining the homeostasis of ROS in the ER is considered vital for a cell. In case of too excessive accumulation of ROS, the redox homeostasis of the ER can be smashed, leading to accumulation of the misfolded proteins that cause ER stress [61, 64]. Thus, it is understandable that ER stress and oxidative stress usually interact and crosstalk with each other (also reviewed by Zhang et al. [63]).

Perturbation of ER-associated functions such as this excessive ROS production but also accumulation of unfolded/misfolded proteins, hypoxia, calcium and glucose depletion, or viral and bacterial infections reflects stress of the organelle and results in activation of an ER stress-coping response, the evolutionary conserved UPR [65–68]. For example, the processes of both IRI-mediated cell damage/cell death [69–71] and induction of the ICD of cancer cells [72–74] are characterized by demonstration of ER stress that is almost always associated with oxidative stress and vice versa [75].

4.2.5.2 Remediable Endoplasmic Reticulum Stress

To cope with ER stress, cells have the unique possibility to activate the UPR, a dynamic signaling network that orchestrates the recovery of homeostasis or triggers RCD modalities, depending on the level of damage. Perception of any perturbation of the ER is provided by three transmembrane sensor molecules of the UPR embedded in the ER membrane.

The Endoplasmic Reticulum Stress Sensors

The ER stress sensors are the PERK, *inositol-requiring protein 1α* (IRE-1α), and *activating transcription factor 6 alpha* (ATF6α) (described and illustrated in Vol. 1 [1]: Part V, Sect. 18.5.2 and Fig. 18.6). To remember: throughout this book, PERK is denoted as a sensor able to perceive cell-intrinsic dyshomeostatic DAMPs (IIC-4 DAMPs), here reflected by ER stress-associated molecular perturbations (see also Vol. 1 [1], Part IV, Sect 13.4.5). Under remediable ER stress conditions, the three sensors trigger signaling pathways to resolve ER stress aimed at maintaining cellular integrity. They are briefly described and illustrated in Vol. 1 [1], Part V, Sect. 18.5.2.2, and Fig. 18.6 (for reviews and original articles, see [67, 76–85]). Here, some aspects of the interconnectedness of the ER stress-promoted UPR with two other protective innate immune processes are resumed only: the antioxidant response and autophagy (Fig. 4.1).

Unfolded Protein Response and the Antioxidant Response

Strikingly, there is a considerable interconnectedness of the ER stress-promoted UPR with other innate immune processes. For example, as mentioned above, an increasing number of studies support the view that oxidative stress has a strong connection with ER stress. However, excessive accumulation of ROS may destroy this redox homeostasis that is vital for the proper function of the ER. Therefore, an efficient counterbalancing antioxidative defense response is mandatory for a cell to survive. Given this background, the role of UPR in maintaining redox homeostasis has gained increasing attraction in the field of targeted research [86]. For instance, findings from studies in rodents provided evidence showing that, upon oxidative stress associated with ER stress, activated PERK does not only lead to the activation (= phosphorylation) of the *eukaryotic translation initiation factor 2 alpha* (eIF2α, promoting activation of the transcription factor ATF4) but also—as a direct upstream molecule—the transcription factor Nrf2 that has been alluded to above in the context of the Keap1↔Nrf2→ARE antioxidant pathway [60, 87–90] (Fig. 4.1). Mechanistically, as also mentioned above, phosphorylation of Nrf2 results in Nrf2 dissociation from Keap1 associated with subsequent translocation to the nucleus [91]. Notably, Nrf2 can not only induce a panel of genes encoding antioxidant factors but also repress the transcription of genes encoding prooxidant proteins, such as TXNIP [92]. As briefly touched in Vol. 1 [1], Part IV, Sect. 13.4.6.3, and Part VI, Sect. 22.4.2.2, TXNIP—denoted as a metabolic DAMP (IIC-5 DAMP), besides the ASC—is another adaptor molecule which reportedly associates with NLRP3 [93–99] (for NLRP3 activation, compare also Sect. 2.2.5.3). Also, as known from earlier studies, the heterodimer consisting of both transcription factors Nrf2 and ATF4 translocates to the nucleus to bind to the stress-response element to induce *HO-1* gene expression [100]. As argued by Zhang et al. [63], "these studies indicate that PERK-NRF2 flux of UPR is a pivotal signaling pathway to restore the redox homeostasis in the ER, unrevealing a UPR-regulated antioxidant mechanism to keep ER redox homeostasis."

Together, these observations again demonstrate the close crosstalk between various cell-intrinsic defensive stress responses in terms of protective means, here, upon oxidative stress. Moreover, these observations lend further support to the suggestion that PERK operates as a molecule that senses dyshomeostatic perturbation of intracellular molecular patterns, this time caused by redox changes.

Unfolded Protein Response and Autophagy

Also, several signaling cascades triggered by the three sensors and Ca^{2+} are apparently potent inducers of autophagy at a cell-wide level that normally has an adaptive/protective function and consists of the three major types chaperone-mediated, macro-, and microautophagy, which are connected by crosstalk to receptor-mediated selective ER-phagy [101–103]. As reviewed by Song et al. [103], the ER stress-mediated autophagy is characterized by the generation of autophagosomes that include worn-out proteins, protein aggregates, and damaged organelles, whereby the autophagosomes of ER-phagy selectively include ER membranes. The three canonical branches of the UPR regulate autophagy at different stages in the process, induction, vesicle nucleation, and elongation. For example, PERK→ATF4 transcriptionally induces/regulates ATG12; and ATF4-mediated CHOP activation also transcriptionally induces/regulates ATG5 (compare Fig. 4.1). Following, ATG5, ATG12, and ATG16L create an ATG5/ATG12/ATG16L complex that involves the elongation process (for further reading, see [7, 103–105]; for ATG proteins, see Sect. 3.2.2 and Vol. 1 [1], Part V, Subchapter 18.2, and Fig. 18.1). Interestingly, recent evidence has indicated that UPR-induced autophagic processes are capable of alleviating the UPR, pointing to a crosstalk between these two innate immune defense mechanisms [106, 107].

Strikingly, as touched above and worthwhile to mention here again, a complex relationship reportedly exists between autophagy and DAMPs in cellular adaption to stress and injury and—when the stress response fails—cell death, a scenario that is characterized by a crosstalk between autophagy induction and secretion or release of DAMPs by dying cells. Indeed, growing evidence indicates that autophagic mechanisms are involved in regulating release and degradation of DAMPs including CALR, HMGB1, ATP, and DNA in several cell types [73, 108, 109]. This scenario may contribute to the observation that autophagy is also able to shape a supportive cellular immune response [110, 111]. Indeed, this kind of innate immune interrelationships is, for example, involved in mechanisms of both reperfusion-mediated cell injury and ICD of cancer cells (see [112–125]).

4.2.5.3 Irremediable Endoplasmic Reticulum Stress

In cases of prolonged or acutely severe irremediable ER stress, the balance is tipped in favor of pro-death signaling; that is, the UPR, now mediated by different biochemical pathways, may lead to proinflammatory and proapoptotic or proferroptotic responses resulting in RCD.

Unfolded Protein Response-Mediated Apoptosis

While the precise pathways of apoptosis induced by ER stress are not known, the upregulated PERK-triggered signaling cascade was shown to play an essential role [63, 126–129] (for additional information compare here also Fig. 18.6 in Vol. 1 [1], Part V, Sect. 18.5.2, p. 402). The transcription factor CHOP can induce apoptosis by both downregulating the anti-apoptotic protein Bcl-2 and transcriptionally upregulating proapoptotic proteins such as death receptor 5 (DR5), *p53 upregulated modulator of apoptosis* (PUMA), and *Bcl-2 interacting mediator of cell death* (BIM) (reviewed in [63, 128, 129]). Together, these proapoptotic proteins induce the release of cytochrome c from mitochondria, lead to loss of membrane potential, and initiate the caspase cascade.

Besides this strong PERK-governed proapoptotic pathway, the IRE1α-triggered cascade is also being discussed to contribute to apoptotic cell death (reviewed in [63, 129]) (for further details of apoptosis, see Vol. 1 [1], Part V, Sect. 19.2). Of note, because apoptosis may proceed to secondary necrosis in terms of a finely regulated process associated with the release of DAMPs [130], ER stress-induced UPR may not only result in a DAMP-promoted systemic defense response but—as the other side of the coin—contribute to DAMP-promoted inflammatory disorders.

Moreover, in case of excessive and/or prolonged ER stress, IRE-1α activation, through RNase-mediated decay of the microRNA *miR-17-5p*, was shown to elevate TXNIP expression to activate the NLRP3 inflammasome that may result in the release of IL-1β and pyroptosis (also compare [129, 131]). To remember: TXNIP (= IIC-5 DAMP) is an endogenous inhibitor of TRX, a major cellular thiol-reducing and antioxidant protein (compare also Sect. 3.2.3.2, and for additional information Vol. 1 [1], Part IV, Sect. 13.4.6.3, p. 292).

Unfolded Protein Response-Mediated Ferroptosis

In addition to those mentioned UPR-regulated autophagy and apoptosis, another subroutine of RCD has recently become the focus of scientific interest, namely, ferroptosis. This subroutine of RN apparently shares a piece of partially overlapping machinery with ER stress and oxidative stress, suggesting molecular interconnectivity between these three events [132]. Several reports suggest that loss of Ca^{2+} homeostasis in the ER that is associated with ER stress plays a fundamental role in ferroptosis induction [133, 134]. Interestingly, as reported by Lee et al. [135], recent studies showed that the ferroptotic agent-induced ER stress response plays a crucial role in the crosstalk between ferroptosis and other types of RCD. In fact, ferroptotic agents were found to induce the UPR and, subsequently, ER stress-mediated activation of the PERK→eIF2α→ATF4→CHOP pathway (for ferroptosis, see Vol. 1 [1], Part V, Sect. 19.3.3 and Sect. 4.3.4).

4.2.5.4 Concluding Remarks

Together, ER stress-induced UPR is not only a robust intracellular homeostatic stress response controlling proteostasis. The recently accumulated wealth of information on stress/injury-induced innate immune responses has also revealed that, in severe and/or prolonged ER stress, this stress response can also promote a systemic defense response via emission of large amounts of DAMPs, which may be released from subroutines of RN such as apoptosis → secondary necrosis, ferroptosis, and pyroptosis. Hence, these sequelae of innate immune events can also plausibly explain why ER stress has been observed to contribute to the pathogenesis of many diseases, including bacterial and viral infections, CVDs, neurodegenerative diseases, and autoimmune disorders (compare [136]). Thus, a thorough understanding of the ER stress response and its role in health and diseases has now opened the door to develop novel ER stress → DAMP-targeted therapies and stratifying patients into cohorts suitable for ER-targeted treatments. This new policy may be particularly crucial in virus- or bacteria-induced stress of the ER. The concept here is that it is the DAMP-activated innate defense responses that represent the real defense mechanisms against infection.

4.2.6 The DNA Damage Response

The DDR has been addressed in Vol. 1 [1], Part V, Sect. 18.6, and Fig 18.7 and is not resumed here. In sum, this stress response is controlled by three PI3K-related kinases (PIKKs): the ATM, the DNA-PK, and the ATR kinases. Various exogenous and endogenous factors, including ionizing radiation, chemical reactions, viral infections, oxidative stress, and replication stress, are known to induce diverse lesions in the DNA such as bulky adducts, collapsed DNA replication forks, DSBs, and single-strand DNA breaks (SSBs). As already mentioned in Sect. 2.2.7.3 and briefly touched in Vol. 1 [1], Part II, Sect. 5.2.6.4, two highly intranuclear multiprotein complexes, MRN and Ku, are considered the primary sensors of DSBs to activate ATM and DNA-PK subsequently. Also, there is first evidence suggesting that the RPA is a recognition molecule that can sense ssDNA as well as PRP19, which is thought to act as a sensor of RPA-ssDNA; both sensors were shown to activate ATR downstream. These recognition receptors enable cells in response to those DNA damages to initiate and activate a complex network of cellular signaling cascades that cooperate to sense and repair lesions in DNA. Indeed, the DDR orchestrates many processes, including execution of DNA repair, regulation of cell-cycle checkpoints, and commencement of protective transcriptional programs. However, when the damage is too severe, the stress response can drive initiation of cellular senescence and RCD.

4.2.7 Résumé

The brief description of adaptive stress responses should make clear that every cell of mammalian organisms intrinsically possesses powerful tools to react to potentially dangerous and harmful perturbations and injuries impacting from the microenvironment. The first line of the cell's defense refers to the instigation of distinct adaptive stress responses aimed at restoring cellular homeostasis. If these responses fail, the cell switches the lever by now envisaging RCD associated with the emission of DAMPs, intended to restore systemic organismal homeostasis. However, in case the dangerous and harmful perturbations and injuries are too severe or prolonged, all these defense responses get uncontrolled and overreact and, thus, may result in pathologies and diseases.

4.3 Regulated Cell Death: A Pivotal Source of DAMPs

4.3.1 Introductory Remarks

The various subroutines of RCD have been described in Vol. 1 [1], Part V, Chap. 19, by focusing on apoptosis (instigated by the intrinsic or extrinsic apoptotic pathway), necroptosis, pyroptosis, and NETosis (i.e., formation of neutrophil extracellular traps [NETs] by neutrophils). The event of RCD is of utmost importance as a productive source of DAMPs emission in human diseases, so its unique nature is selectively and briefly sketched here again.

As every living entity on our planet eventually dies, cells in a complex organism die as well. Under stressful and injurious conditions, cells in living tissue have only two options: to survive when the stress responses are successful or to die when they are unsuccessful. The character and the intensity of a cell's death can vary. In principle, cells may die either individually or in groups in an accidental manner, that is, in the form of an ACD or may succumb to an RCD. Accidental cell death is caused by extreme insults such as overwhelming thermal, chemical, or mechanical/

physical injuries, a typical example being freezing and thawing procedures. Notably, this kind of cell death is entirely uncontrolled and virtually immediate. Due to the typically accompanied rupture of the cellular plasma membrane, the process of ACD is associated with passive release of large amounts of intracellular compounds, organelles, and cell debris which can operate in the extracellular milieu as constitutive DAMPs (see Sect. 3.3.2). By contrast, RCD is caused by low or moderate stressful insults as can be observed, for example, during various kinds of infections or pathological tissue reperfusion; nevertheless, it finally also results in rupture of the cellular plasma membrane.

As already adumbrated above and in Vol. 1 [1], Part V, Chap. 17, in the situation of such incoming insults, the first reaction of our innate immune system is to mount a cell-intrinsic stress response associated with the emission of the first line of cell-intrinsic DAMPs. When these stress responses are successful and favorable, cellular homeostasis will be restored, and the cell will survive. However, when unsuccessful, stress responses may result in controlled destruction of the stressed cell, generally called RCD. Of utmost importance with respect to the emission of DAMPs is the event of RN: during this RN-associated dying process, a cell can initially continue with transcriptional activities, which include the capability to generate further DAMPs in terms of inducible DAMPs (see Sect. 3.5). At the end of the process, when the plasma membrane has definitely ruptured, constitutive DAMPs are passively released in large amounts. In this situation, both constitutive and inducible DAMPs, via activation of innate immune cells, evoke cell-extrinsic efferent responses in terms of inflammation and inflammation-related events such as phagocytosis. Accordingly, RCD in the context of injury ↔ host interactions can be seen as a continuation of the desperate efforts of a cell to save the life of the individual that harbors it. Of note, this controlled dying maneuver aimed at restoring organismal homeostasis highlights the intrinsic capacity of virtually every cell in metazoans to "altruistically" commit "suicide." Indeed, this pathway can be observed to occur in apoptosis, necroptosis, and pyroptosis and can be regarded as a form of cell suicide, where specific pro-death proteins are newly expressed and upregulated by various stimuli to promote death. In contrast to this pathway, the death path observed in ferroptosis is regarded as a kind of "sabotage" in terms of involving processes that preserve cell integrity such that, when disrupted, death occurs as a consequence of the cell's active, physiological state (compare also [137, 138]).

The increasing attention of the medical community to the different forms of RCD and their consequences is owed to the fact that they were found to contribute to human diseases such as cerebral or myocardial infarction (induced by accompanying reperfusion), cancer, infectious, autoimmune, and neurodegenerative diseases [139–141]. For example, RCD of infected cells functions as perhaps the most ancient firewall against lethal injury caused by pathogens by limiting replication and dissemination while concomitantly alerting neighboring cells to an impending threat. In fact, of considerable importance are recent reports showing that subroutines of RN such as necroptosis and pyroptosis can be induced by viruses. These observations are in strong support of the notion that it is the DAMPs released in large quantities from dying infected cells that elicit and amplify a robust antiviral defense response and not, as formerly proposed, the invading foreign virus per se and alone.

All in all, it has not come as a surprise that newly updated guidelines for the definition and classification of cell death subroutines have recently been published by the *Nomenclature Committee on Cell Death* (NCCD) by focusing on mechanistic and essential aspects of the process (see Galluzzi et al. [142] and Box 4.1). Here, only some selected updated topics of this immensely emerging research field in modern biomedicine are briefly presented.

Box 4.1 Regulated Cell Death: Operational Definitions (Published by Galluzzi et al. [142])

Accidental cell death (ACD) Virtually instantaneous and uncontrollable form of cell death corresponding to the physical disassembly of the plasma membrane caused by extreme physical, chemical, or mechanical cues.

Anoikis Specific variant of intrinsic apoptosis initiated by the loss of integrin-dependent anchorage.

Autophagy-dependent cell death A form of regulated cell death (RCD) that mechanistically depends on the autophagic machinery (or components thereof).

Autosis A specific instance of autophagy-dependent cell death that critically relies on the plasma membrane Na^+/K^+-ATPase.

Cell death Irreversible degeneration of vital cellular functions (notably ATP production and preservation of redox homeostasis) culminating in the loss of cellular integrity (permanent plasma membrane permeabilization or cellular fragmentation).

Cellular senescence Irreversible loss of proliferative potential associated with specific morphological and biochemical features, including the senescence-associated secretory phenotype (SASP). Cellular senescence does not constitute a form of RCD.

Efferocytosis Mechanism whereby dead cells and fragments thereof are taken up by phagocytes and disposed.

Entotic cell death A type of RCD that originates from actomyosin-dependent cell-in-cell internalization (entosis) and is executed by lysosomes.

Extrinsic apoptosis Specific variant of RCD initiated by perturbations of the extracellular microenvironment detected by plasma membrane receptors, propagated by caspase-8 and precipitated by executioner caspases, mainly caspase-3.

Ferroptosis A form of RCD initiated by oxidative perturbations of the intracellular microenvironment that is under constitutive control by glutathione peroxidase 4 and can be inhibited by iron chelators and lipophilic antioxidants.

Immunogenic cell death A form of RCD that is sufficient to activate an adaptive immune response in immunocompetent hosts.

Intrinsic apoptosis Type of RCD initiated by perturbations of the extracellular or intracellular microenvironment, demarcated by mitochondrial outer membrane permeabilization, and precipitated by executioner caspases, mainly caspase-3.

Lysosome-dependent cell death A type of RCD demarcated by primary LMP and precipitated by cathepsins, with optional involvement of mitochondrial outer membrane permeabilization and caspases.

Mitochondrial permeability transition (MPT)-driven necrosis Specific form of RCD triggered by perturbations of the intracellular microenvironment and relying on cyclophilin D.

Mitotic catastrophe Oncosuppressive mechanism for the control of mitosis-incompetent cells by RCD or cellular senescence. Per se, mitotic catastrophe does not constitute a form or RCD.

Mitotic death Specific variant of RCD (most often, intrinsic apoptosis) driven by mitotic catastrophe.

Necroptosis A modality of RCD triggered by perturbations of extracellular or intracellular homeostasis that critically depends on mixed lineage kinase domain-like protein (MLKL), receptor-interacting serine/threonine-protein kinase 3 (RIPK3), and (at least in some settings) on the kinase activity of RIPK1.

NETotic cell death A reactive oxygen species (ROS)-dependent modality of RCD restricted to cells of hematopoietic derivation and associated with neutrophil extracellular trap (NET) extrusion.

Parthanatos A modality of RCD initiated by poly(ADP-ribose) polymerase 1 (PARP1) hyperactivation and precipitated by the consequent bioenergetic catastrophe coupled to apoptosis inducing factor (AIF)-dependent and migration inhibitory factor (MIF)-dependent DNA degradation.

Programmed cell death (PCD) Particular form of RCD that occurs in strictly physiological scenarios, i.e., it does not relate to perturbations of homeostasis and hence does not occur in the context of failing adaptation to stress.

Pyroptosis A type of RCD that critically depends on the formation of plasma membrane pores by members of the gasdermin protein family, often (but not always) as a consequence of inflammatory caspase activation.

Regulated cell death Form of cell death that results from the activation of one or more signal transduction modules and hence can be pharmacologically or genetically modulated (at least kinetically and to some extent).

Source: Galluzzi et al. [142]

4.3.2 Apoptosis

The two major cellular signaling pathways, an intrinsic pathway that is initiated inside cells by mitochondrial release of proapoptotic factors and an extrinsic pathway that is initiated at the cell surface by death receptors, have been depicted and illustrated in Vol. 1 [1], Part V, Sect. 19.2, and Fig. 19.3.

Here, only a few remarks are added regarding possible immunogenicity of apoptotic cell death. Notably, apoptotic cells retain plasma membrane integrity and metabolic activity (to some degree) as the process progresses to completion. In vivo, such dying cells are rapidly cleared by macrophages or other cells with phagocytic activity, a process described in the literature as efferocytosis (see [143] and also compare Vol. 1 [1], Part VI, Sect. 22.6.3.3).

Importantly, apoptosis, due to consequent rapid efferocytosis, is usually immunologically silent [144]. The reason is apparent: there is no rupture of the plasma membrane allowing DAMPs to leave the cell. However, apoptosis is not always immunologically silent, as previously thought [145], but may well exert immunogenicity when progressing to secondary necrosis associated with the release of DAMPs [146]. Also, in response to certain stimuli, including anthracyclines, oxaliplatin, and hypofractionated irradiation, apoptosis was observed to mediate robust immunostimulatory effects [147, 148]. Moreover, autophagically or apoptotically dying cells were shown to contribute to DAMPs emission via secretion of inducible DAMPs such as ATP and type 1 IFNs [124, 149, 150]. Thus, when the incidence of apoptotic cell death is known to be pathogenetically involved in certain diseases, one has to take these findings into account.

4.3.3 Necroptosis

4.3.3.1 General Remarks

Necroptosis can be regarded as the by far best-studied RN subroutine leading—like all forms of RN—to plasma membrane perforation. The biochemical processes in necroptosis are distinct from those found in apoptosis; in particular, there is no caspase activation. As described and illustrated by us in Fig. 2 shown in [151], and Vol. 1 [1], Part V, Sect. 19.3.2, and Fig. 19.4, necroptosis is a kinase-mediated cell death that relies on RIPK3-mediated phosphorylation of the pseudokinase *mixed lineage kinase domain-like protein* (MLKL). This form of RN can be instigated by a variety of triggers, including TNF↔tumor necrosis factor receptor I (TNFRI), Fas, TNF-related apoptosis-inducing ligand (TRAIL), LPS, DNA, dsRNA, IFNs, ER stress, bacterial and viral infection, and anticancer drugs. Together, most of these triggers may be summarized as endogenous constitutive and inducible DAMPs (e.g., full-length biologically active IL-33 [152], TNF, and type 1 IFNs secreted by virus-activated cells). These stimuli mediate their efferent functions via signaling pathways and direct and indirect formation of necrosomes and execute necroptosis by MLKL activation via complex pathways under cooperation with the ESCRT-III machinery [153] (also compare Fig. 2 in [151]; additional information is illustrated in Fig. 19.4, p. 437, in Vol. 1 [1], Part V, Sect. 19.3.2).

4.3.3.2 The Release of DAMPs in Necroptosis

It has been proposed that MLKL forms pores in the plasma membrane to mediate plasma membrane rupture allowing release of DAMPs (discussed in [151]). Notably, however, the precise mechanism by which MLKL permeabilizes membranes to regulate the emission of DAMPs is by far not clear and still debated in the literature and will rely on future structural studies for resolution [154]. In this context, a recent report of Nakano et al. [155] on monitoring necroptosis and the release of DAMPs at the single cell resolution is of interest. First observations from this study revealed unexpectedly that the duration of the release of HMGB1 is divided into two modes: a burst-mode and a sustained-mode. The authors described and discussed [155]: "In a sustained mode cell, the release of HMGB1 continued more than 100 min, whereas the release of HMBG1 terminated within 10 min in a burst-mode cell. At this moment, the biological significance of two different modes of the release of HMGB1is unclear, one might surmise that a burst-mode cell might elicit strong immune responses to the surrounding micro-environment. Alternatively, sustained release of HMGB1 might induce another cellular response, such as recruitment of immune cells." Indeed, such studies will become most important in attempts to elucidate the dynamics of DAMPs release from various forms of RN, in particular, when induced by bacterial and viral infections.

4.3.3.3 Contribution of Necroptosis to Antiviral and Antibacterial Defense Programs

Among the various consequences of necroptotic cell death, its role in antiviral immune defense via DAMPs emission is of outstanding importance. In Fig. 19.5 in Vol. 1 [1], Part V, Sect. 19.3.2, such a scenario has been addressed as exemplified by influenza A virus (IAV) infection, whereby the DNA receptor DAI was identified as a link between viral replication and RIPK3 activation (also see [156]). Recent reports have confirmed and extended this finding (reviewed and discussed in [157, 158]). For example, DAI was reported to mediate IFN-induced necroptosis [159]; moreover, in this study, DAI-mediated necroptosis was found to be involved in acute SIRS, induced by TNF + IFN-γ in vivo. In another line of in vitro studies on macrophages and EpCs aimed at elucidating the mechanism of the IAV-mediated necroptosis process [160], the NS1 protein of IAV was shown to interact with MLKL. The interaction of NS1 with MLKL increases MLKL oligomerization and membrane translocation. Also, the MLKL-NS1 interaction was found to enhance MLKL-mediated NLRP3 inflammasome activation, leading to increased (IL-1β) processing and secretion. The authors [160] concluded that "these data provide insights into the critical role of NS1 in regulating pathogenesis and immunopathology during IAV infection by regulation of cell death and inflammatory responses."

Interestingly, a recent study provided first evidence suggesting that necroptosis may also drive antibacterial defense programs (see Meng et al. in [161]). In this study, bacterial lipids (lipid IVa or lipid A; i.e., microbial lipids in Gram-negative bacteria) were found to form a complex with HMGB1, released by activated immune cells or damaged tissue during bacterial infection. This complex was shown to trigger RIPK3- and TRIF-dependent immune responses. The authors argued that these findings "uncover a previously unrecognized mechanism by which host factors and bacterial components work in concert to orchestrate immune responses." In other words, this study supports the concept that both MAMPs and DAMPs work in concert to orchestrate host immune responses, a model that has been and still is being used throughout this book.

4.3.3.4 Concluding Remarks

Necroptosis has attracted considerable attention because it is apparently the solution for necrosis in general, probably the most widespread unmet clinical need in modern biomedicine. Indeed, necrosis associated with emission of large amounts of constitutive and inducible DAMPs occurs during trauma and SIRS, MI, cerebral stroke, cancer, pancreatitis, macular degeneration, and numerous other pathologies (reviewed in [151]). Unfortunately, however, reports on prevention of necroptosis by appropriate inhibitors are disappointing so far. Nevertheless, new hope shimmers on the horizon with the discovery of the small-molecule PK6 and its derivatives, a novel class of necroptosis inhibitors that can highly selectively suppress RIPK1 kinase activity and potently block necroptotic cell death, both in vitro and in vivo (see [162]). In view of their data, the authors conclude that further "understanding of the precise role of RIPK1 kinase activity in relevant diseases models will be critical for the development of valuable therapies using RIPK1 inhibitors."

4.3.4 Ferroptosis

4.3.4.1 General Remarks

The ferroptotic cascade has been described and illustrated by us in [151], Fig. 3, and Vol. 1 [1], Part V, Sect. 19.3.3, and Fig. 19.6 (for recent reviews, see Proneth and Conrad [163] and Lei et al. [164]). In these publications, besides others, GPX4 has been introduced and illustrated as the key ferroptosis regulator. This subroutine of RN in terms of a "sabotage" is an iron-dependent, oxidative form of RN that does not share morphological, biochemical, or genetic similarities with other forms of non-apoptotic cell death. Instead, morphological features of ferroptosis include a normal-sized nucleus free of chromatin condensation and dense miniature mitochondria with vestigial cristae.

As mentioned above in the context of the oxidative stress response, in case the potent cell-intrinsic, Keap1↔ Nrf2 pathway-driven antioxidative defense response to excessive production of ROS fails or is (e.g., pharmacologically) inhibited, ferroptosis will develop.

4.3.4.2 From Lipid Peroxidation to Ferroptosis

Before the development of this form of RN, accumulation of ROS production in excess affects macromolecules such as NAs, carbohydrates, lipids, and proteins leading to cellular dysfunction. One key example of this phenomenon is lipid peroxidation, which relies on ROS generation and iron availability. Indeed, lipid peroxidation is considered generally as a process under which oxidants such as ROS attack lipids containing carbon–carbon double bond(s), especially PUFAs that involve hydrogen abstraction from a carbon, with oxygen insertion resulting in lipid peroxyl radicals and hydroperoxides. This oxidative process of lipids can occur via three distinct mechanisms: (1) enzymatic oxidation by enzymes such as lipoxygenases (LOX), cyclooxygenases (COX), and cytochrome P450; (2) non-enzymatic, ROS-mediated oxidation that requires catalysis by transition metals or hemin; and (3) non-enzymatic, non-ROS-mediated oxidation. Each lipid oxidation mechanism finally leads to the generation of various highly reactive terminal degradation products with high stereospecificity, which include PS, OxPLs containing OxCL, PC, or PE headgroups, as well as fragments such as reactive aldehydes 4-HNE, MDA, and CEP (compare Sect. 3.4.3.2, and for reviews, see [165–174]; for more details of lipid peroxidation and its reactive products including the IIB-1 DAMPs OSEs, also compare Vol. 1 [1], Part IV, Sect. 13.3.2.2, and Part V, Sect. 19.3.3.1). Together, this scenario let suggest that lipid peroxidation with the generation of a first line of DAMPs (OSEs) mirrors a defense response against oxidative stress at the cellular level aimed at restoring cellular homeostasis. However, when this stress response fails as a consequence of excessive oxidative stress such as associated with IRI, the cell proceeds to RCD in the form of ferroptosis associated with release of large amounts of DAMPs, which operate at the level of the organism to restore organismal homeostasis (compare Fig. 4.2a).

4.3.4.3 The Release of DAMPs in Ferroptosis

The ferroptotic cell death is supposed to serve as a critical source for the release of DAMPs to trigger necroinflammation. However, the molecular mechanism that mediates the execution of ferroptosis as indicated by final plasma membrane rupture is unclear. Also, as in necroptosis, the regulation of DAMPs emission in ferroptosis is far from being understood. Nevertheless, such mechanisms are on the way to be uncovered. For example, the activation of autophagic processes (ferritinophagy, chaperone-mediated autophagy) has been reported to be involved in the execution of ferroptosis [175, 176]. Of interest in this context is the observation of Wen et al. [177], demonstrating that the DAMP HMGB1 is released by ferroptotic cells in an autophagy-dependent manner, mechanistically regulated through controlling HMGB1 acetylation as a form of PTM. This amazing finding gives rise to the consideration that release of DAMPs from necrotic cells is not always a passive process but can be actively regulated by PTMs (for HMGB1 acetylation, see Vol. 1 [1], Part IV, Sect. 14.3.3). Future targeted studies will certainly contribute to a solution to this puzzle.

4.3.4.4 The Role of NRF2 in the Ferroptotic Pathway

Some aspects of the cell-intrinsic Keap1↔ Nrf2 pathway in driving the antioxidative defense response are briefly touched in Sect. 4.2.3.2. Here, a few more remarks to the transcription factor Nrf2 are made that has emerged as another key regulator

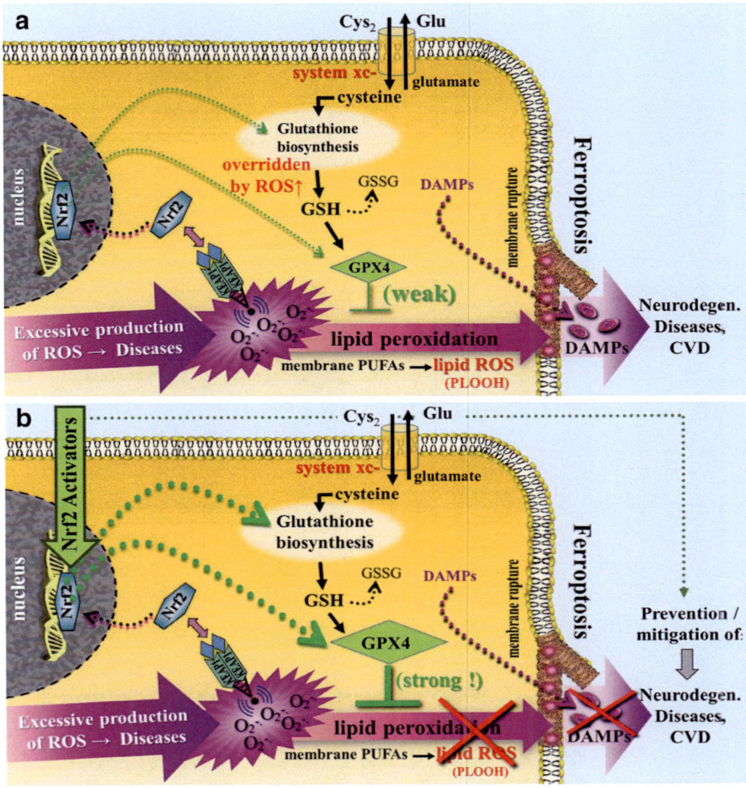

Fig. 4.2 (**a**) Schematic diagram of a simplified narrative model illustrating the unproven proposal that ferroptosis is involved in the pathogenesis of human disorders, e.g., neurodegenerative and cardiovascular diseases. Under homeostatic conditions, oxidative stress sensed by Keap1 leads to dissociation and subsequent translocation of the transcription factor Nrf2 to the nucleus where it binds to ARE and induces transcription of numerous cytoprotective antioxidant genes, including genes which contribute to increased biosynthesis of GSH associated with increased GPX4 production. GPX4 reduces PLOOH, thereby preventing lipid peroxidation. However, as illustrated in this figure, in case of prolonged and/or excessive production of ROS as observed in certain human diseases, this Nrf2→GPX4-mediated antioxidative response is overridden leading to iron-dependent lipid peroxidation that proceeds to ferroptosis associated with the release of DAMPs. Note: for the Keap1-Nrf2-mediated antioxidative stress response, also compare Sect. 4.2.3.2 and Fig. 18.4 in Vol. 1 [1], Part V, Sect. 18.3.3.3; for ferroptosis, also compare Fig. 19.6 in Vol. 1 [1], Part V, Sect. 19.3.3). *Cys2* cystine, *Glu* glutamate, *GPX4* glutathione-peroxidase 4, *GSH* glutathione, *GSSG* oxidized form of glutathione, *Keap1* Kelch-like erythroid cell-derived protein with CNC homology (ECH)-associated protein 1, *Nrf2* nuclear factor-erythroid 2 p45-related factors 2, *PLOOH* phospholipid hydroperoxides, *PUFAs* polyunsaturated fatty acids, *ROS* reactive oxygen species. (Sources: [1, 27, 42, 44, 182–184]) (**b**) This figure is a continuation of Fig. 4.2a (i.e., a model of involvement of ferroptosis in human diseases) schematically illustrating that administration of Nrf2 activators may be a therapeutic option in human diseases such as neurodegenerative diseases and CVD, in which oxidative stress is thought to be pathogenetically involved. Administration of Nrf2 activators is supposed to increase biosynthesis of GSH, thereby facilitating the GPX4-mediated prevention of lipid peroxidation resulting in prevention/mitigation of those diseases. *Cys2* cystine, *Glu* glutamate, *GPX4* glutathione-peroxidase 4, *GSH* glutathione, *GSSG* oxidized form of glutathione, *Keap1* Kelch-like erythroid cell-derived protein with CNC homology (ECH)-associated protein 1, *Nrf2* nuclear factor-erythroid 2 p45-related factors 2, *PLOOH* phospholipid hydroperoxides, *PUFAs* polyunsaturated fatty acids, *ROS* reactive oxygen species. (Sources: [27, 178–181])

of both lipid peroxidation and ferroptosis (for review, see Dodson et al. [46]). As mentioned above, Nrf2 is a master regulator of the antioxidant response and has been shown to regulate the activity of several ferroptosis and lipid peroxidation-related proteins. These targets can be divided into three broad classes: iron/metal metabolism, intermediate metabolism, and GSH synthesis/metabolism. If these Nrf2-promoted regulatory processes fail, are pharmacologically inhibited, or are overridden by ROS production in excess, ferroptosis occurs. Conversely, therapeutic targeting of Nrf2 using natural or synthetic activators of Nrf2 should be an option to mitigate the ferroptotic death pathway involved in human diseases (compare Fig. 4.2b). Interestingly, arguments in support of such a concept regarding protective effect of Nrf2 have already been presented and discussed elsewhere (compare [178–181]).

4.3.4.5 The Defense Response to Oxidative Stress Depending on Increasing Stress Intensity

Also, at this point, it seems worthwhile to note that our innate defense system operates against oxidative stress/injury on three levels, in each case adapted to the increasing intensity of oxidative insults (Fig. 4.3). All three levels have been addressed in this book: (1) the Keap1→Nrf2-initiated antioxidative response as the first attempt to restore and maintain homeostasis upon oxidative stress (see Sect. 4.2.3.2); (2) as an adjunct to the antioxidative response, the emission of OSEs (see Sect. 3.4.3.2), which represent a powerful subclass of DAMPs (IIB-1 DAMPs) capable of triggering robust innate defense pathways but also potentially pathogenic adaptive autoimmune responses; and (3)—as a culmination of defense against heavy and/or persistent oxidative stress—induction of ferroptosis associated with release of large amounts of DAMPs aimed at rescuing at least the organism that may be exposed to a severe oxidative injury-mediated threat (as described here and in Vol. 1 [1], Part V, Sect. 19.3.3). Again, this scenario shows the highly sophisticated, evolutionarily developed action of our defense system that always responds in a tailor-made fashion.

4.3.4.6 Role of Ferroptosis in Human Diseases

Given the knowledge that innate defense responses can lead to pathologies when uncontrolled and dysregulated, it is not a surprise that ferroptosis has been observed to play a role in human diseases (though a direct link between ferroptosis and human disease is still lacking). Thus, the activation of ferroptosis has been proposed to accelerate diseases whose pathogenesis is associated with oxidative stress, that is, disorders such as atherosclerosis, CVD, and neurodegenerative diseases (including Parkinson's and Alzheimer's disease) [182, 183]. Intriguingly, first experimental evidence for this concept derives from several studies, for example, from experiments on a mouse model with conditional deletion of GPX4 [184] showing that ablation of ferroptosis regulator GPX4 in forebrain neurons promotes cognitive impairment and neurodegeneration. Given these findings, the authors suggested that ferroptosis may be an important neurodegenerative mechanism in diseases such as Alzheimer's disease. Accordingly, future therapeutic

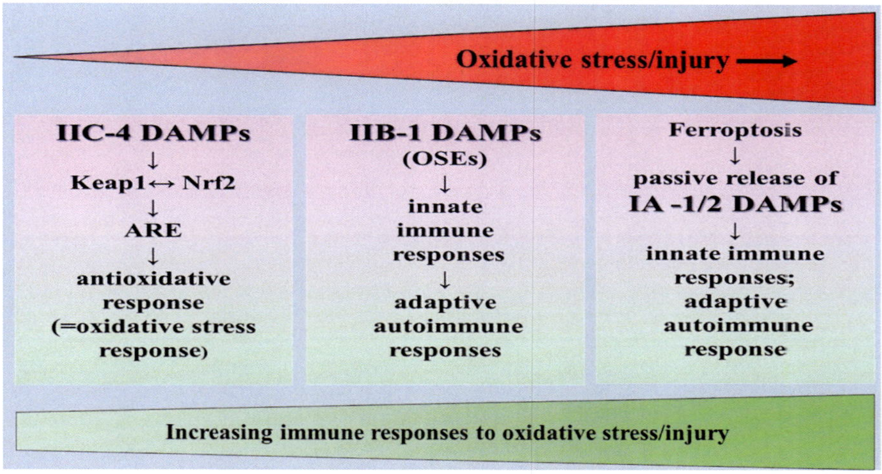

Fig. 4.3 DAMP-induced innate/adaptive responses of the innate immune system to oxidative stress/injury. Depending on the intensity of the oxidative insults, the tailored responses occur on three levels: (1) the Keap1-Nrf2-initiated antioxidative response aimed at restoring cellular homeostasis; (2) as an adjunct to the antioxidative response, the emission of OSEs representing a powerful subclass of DAMPs; and (3)—as a culmination of defense—induction of ferroptosis associated with release of large amounts of DAMPs aimed at restoring organismal homeostasis. *ARE* antioxidant response element, *Keap1* Kelch-like erythroid cell-derived protein with CNC homology (ECH)-associated protein 1, *Nrf2* nuclear factor-erythroid 2 p45-related factors 2, *OSE* oxidation-specific epitopes

options to treat human diseases found to be implicated by ferroptosis may include attempts to mitigate the ferroptotic death cascade. For example, therapeutic targeting of Nrf2 using natural or synthetic activators of Nrf2 could be such a strategy (Fig. 4.2b).

Conversely, in oncology, ferroptosis appears to play an essential role in inhibiting some types of cancers, such as hepatocellular carcinoma, pancreatic carcinoma, prostate, and breast cancer. In fact, cancer cells reportedly have often defects in cell death executioner mechanisms, which is one of the main reasons for therapy resistance. This new knowledge has encouraged emerging strategies of cancer therapy that are based on ferroptosis induction (for further reading, see [185–187]).

4.3.4.7 Concluding Remarks

Together, growing evidence suggests that cells succumbing from ferroptosis secrete DAMPs that activate the innate immune system to promote necroinflammatory responses, which may contribute to the development of human diseases such as CVD and neurodegenerative diseases. Nevertheless, there are many open questions such as regarding the nature of DAMPs released, as well as the exact ferroptotic death pathways implicated in those pathologies. Future studies will undoubtedly lead to a more precise molecular understanding of ferroptosis-promoted emission of necroinflammation-inducing DAMPs, allowing to develop sophisticated therapeutic concepts such as the use of Nrf2 activators and inhibitors in tackling disorders such as CVD and Alzheimer's disease, on the one hand, and resistant tumors, on the other hand.

4.3.5 Pyroptosis

4.3.5.1 General Remarks

The pyroptotic cell death, relevant for the demise of monocytes or macrophages but also other cell types such as EpCs, has been described and illustrated by us in [151], Fig. 4, and Vol. 1 [1], Part V, Sect. 19.3.4, and Fig. 19.7. Different from necroptosis and ferroptosis, but like apoptosis, pyroptosis is executed by caspases, here denoted as inflammatory caspases. The activation of the NLRP3 and AIM2 inflammasome as important DAMP-driven machines to mount inflammation is addressed in Sects. 2.2.5.3 and 2.2.8 and not resumed here again. Here, the mode of DAMPs release from this form of RN is again of interest and thus deserves a few more words.

4.3.5.2 The Release of DAMPs in Pyroptosis

In the initial phase of the pyroptotic pathway, caspases are activated within the inflammasomes, whose activation is the consequence of the interaction of their sensors/receptors with MAMPs and DAMPs or DAMPs. Although the molecular mechanisms of pyroptosis have not been fully elucidated, it is thought that cleavage of the pyroptotic executioner GSDMD by these inflammatory caspases is critical for this type of RN to occur, that is, caspase-1 and caspase-11 in murine macrophages and their human orthologs caspase-1, caspase-4, and caspase-5. However, other findings indicate that pyroptosis can also be driven by several other caspases, including caspase-3 [188]. Gasdermin D is cleaved by the caspases to release its N-terminal domain from inhibition by its C-terminal domain. The N-terminal fragment then rapidly moves to and targets the cell membrane fraction, where it induces the formation of a plasma membrane pore (see [189, 190] and compare Fig. 19.7 in Vol. 1 [1], Part V, Sect. 19.3.4). Of note, the GSDMD pore—thought to allow release of DAMPs —has been characterized at the ultrastructural level, consisting of 16 symmetric protomers with an inner diameter of ~10–14 nm [191]. By applying high-resolution (≤2 nm) atomic force microscopy, the N-terminal domain of GSDMD was observed to be inserted into a variety of lipid compositions, among which phosphatidylinositol 4,5-bisphosphate increases and cholesterol reduces insertion [192]. The investigation also revealed that the N-terminal domain of GSDMD, once inserted, assembles arc-, slit-, and ring-shaped oligomers, each of which being able to form transmembrane pores. It is this generated pore that is responsible for rapid plasma membrane permeabilization. Interestingly, however, the morphology of this pore is different from MLKL channel-mediated necroptosis [193].

4.3.5.3 Concluding Remarks

As expected, the pyroptotic pathway leading to release of large quantities of DAMPs has been recognized as a promising therapeutic target for inflammatory diseases, ranging from CVD, inflammatory bowel disease, T2DM, rheumatoid arthritis, cancer, to Alzheimer's disease (compare [194–198]). In particular, infectious disorders and hyperinflammation-associated sepsis are of high interest, whereby GDSMD is plausibly the focus of interest. In fact, researchers have already begun to search for small molecule inhibitors that block the function of GSDMD (recently reviewed by Pandeya et al. [199]). Thus, first clinical trials using GSDMD inhibitors to prevent DAMP-promoted inflammation in this way can be probably expected soon.

4.3.6 NETosis

The NETotic cell death has been described in Vol. 1 [1], Part V, Sect. 19.3.6. This subroutine of RCD is ROS-dependent and restricted to cells of hematopoietic derivation, that is, mainly neutrophils but also mast cells, eosinophils, and basophils. This cell death is associated with NET extrusion characterized by the release into the extracellular space of a meshwork of chromatin-containing and histone-containing fibers bound to granular and cytoplasmic proteins (= weblike structures). As outlined in Sect. 19.3.6 [1], three models for NETosis are being discussed to date: besides conventional suicidal NETosis, which occurs after several hours of stimulation, two types of nonsuicidal vital NETosis have been reported. In vital NETosis, neutrophils release NETs without showing disruption of the membrane.

Concomitant with the formation of NETs, many DAMPs are thought to be released, whereby NAs and histones appear to play a dominant role (for NAs and histones operating as IA-1 DAMPs, see Vol. 1 [1], Part IV, Sects. 12.2.4.3 and 12.2.4.4). This concept may be supported by recent studies showing that formation of NETs is dependent on pore-forming GSDMD (see [200, 201]).

Together, as with the other forms of RCD, NETosis is pathogenetically involved in many human inflammatory diseases, for example, sepsis, traumatic and autoimmune diseases, cancer, and coagulation-related disorders (also see [202–204]).

4.3.7 Résumé

As already stressed in Vol. 1 [1], Part IV, Sect. 19.3.8, the intersection between RCD and the immune system is currently appreciated as one of the hottest topics in biomedical and cell death research. It is critically central to homeostatic healing responses on the one hand and contributes to many human pathologies on the contrary. The "medium" of this scenario can be seen in the emission of various degrees of constitutive and inducible DAMPs, which—via induction of necroinflammation—can promote both innate and adaptive immune processes. As ideal diagnostic and therapeutic targets, they are supposed to play a dominant role in future medicine. At first, however, the molecular nature of the various necrosis pathways that mediate the pathological features of RN has to be more precisely specified. As concluded by Tonnus et al. in this context [205], "the extension of the arsenal of necrosis markers will allow pathological detection of specific molecular pathways rather than isolated morphological descriptions. These novel pieces of information will be extraordinarily helpful for clinicians as inhibitors of necroptosis (necrostatins), ferroptosis (ferrostatins), and inflammasomes have emerged in clinical trials."

4.4 Outlook and Future Perspectives

In this chapter, it has been attempted to collect recent experimental and clinical findings pointing to the growing relevance of stress responses and subroutines of RCD for clinical practice. This pleasing development is obviously due to the fact that three research disciplines have come together: research on adaptive stress responses, RCD, and DAMPs. It is this integration and interconnectedness of the three homeostasis-restoring molecular events that have enabled mammals to survive and reproduce until today—the secret of success being linking intrinsic cellular stress responses via DAMPs to organismal homeostasis. The other side of the coin of this phenomenon has already been particularized in Vol. 1 [1], Part V, Chpt. 20, and Fig. 20.1: the horror of a severe injury-induced "avalanche" of DAMPs in the form of SIRS often associated with multiple organ failure (MOF).

It is obvious, this scenario opens a novel perspective for clinicians and physicians on how to treat their patients in the future, considering three approaches: (1) early but cautious interference with stress responses (e.g., inhibition of oxidative stress/ER stress); (2) pharmacological inhibition of forms of RCD; and (3) the development of agents that interfere with DAMPs emission or promote activation of SAMPs (see Sect. 7.4). Indeed, much work awaits the researchers working in this emerging field of biomedicine.

References

1. Land WG. Damage-associated molecular patterns in human diseases. In: Injury-induced innate immune responses, vol. 1. Cham: Springer International Publishing AG; 2018. https://www.springer.com/de/book/9783319786544.
2. Galluzzi L, Yamazaki T, Kroemer G. Linking cellular stress responses to systemic homeostasis. Nat Rev Mol Cell Biol. 2018;19:731–45. http://www.ncbi.nlm.nih.gov/pubmed/30305710.
3. Moretti J, Blander JM. Cell-autonomous stress responses in innate immunity. J Leukoc Biol. 2017;101:77–86. http://www.ncbi.nlm.nih.gov/pubmed/27733577.
4. Deretic V, Saitoh T, Akira S. Autophagy in infection, inflammation and immunity. Nat Rev Immunol. 2013;13:722–37. https://doi.org/10.1038/nri3532.
5. Liu X, Cao H, Li J, Wang B, Zhang P, Dong Zhang X, et al. Autophagy induced by DAMPs facilitates the inflammation response in lungs undergoing ischemia-reperfusion injury through promoting TRAF6 ubiquitination. Cell Death Differ. 2017;24:683–93. http://www.ncbi.nlm.nih.gov/pubmed/28157209.
6. Choi AMK, Ryter SW, Levine B. Autophagy in human health and disease. N Engl J Med. 2013;368:651–62. http://www.ncbi.nlm.nih.gov/pubmed/23406030.
7. Shibutani ST, Saitoh T, Nowag H, Münz C, Yoshimori T. Autophagy and autophagy-related proteins in the immune system. Nat Immunol. 2015;16:1014–24. http://www.ncbi.nlm.nih.gov/pubmed/26382870.
8. Mizushima N. Autophagy: process and function. Genes Dev. 2007;21:2861–73. http://www.ncbi.nlm.nih.gov/pubmed/18006683.

9. He C, Klionsky DJ. Regulation mechanisms and signaling pathways of autophagy. Annu Rev Genet. 2009;43:67–93. https://doi.org/10.1146/annurev-genet-102808-114910.
10. Yang Z, Klionsky DJ. Eaten alive: a history of macroautophagy. Nat Cell Biol. 2010;12:814–22. https://doi.org/10.1038/ncb0910-814.
11. Yang Z, Klionsky DJ. Mammalian autophagy: core molecular machinery and signaling regulation. Curr Opin Cell Biol. 2010;22:124–31. http://linkinghub.elsevier.com/retrieve/pii/S0955067409002282.
12. Xu Z, Klionsky DJ. The AMPK-SKP2-CARM1 axis links nutrient sensing to transcriptional and epigenetic regulation of autophagy. Ann Transl Med. 2016;4:S7. http://atm.amegroups.com/article/view/11566/12702.
13. Glick D, Barth S, Macleod KF. Autophagy: cellular and molecular mechanisms. J Pathol. 2010;221:3–12. https://doi.org/10.1002/path.2697.
14. Mizushima N, Levine B, Cuervo AM, Klionsky DJ. Autophagy fights disease through cellular self-digestion. Nature. 2008;451:1069–75. https://doi.org/10.1038/nature06639.
15. Filomeni G, De Zio D, Cecconi F. Oxidative stress and autophagy: the clash between damage and metabolic needs. Cell Death Differ. 2015;22:377–88. http://www.nature.com/articles/cdd2014150.
16. Lin S-Y, Hsieh S-Y, Fan Y-T, Wei W-C, Hsiao P-W, Tsai D-H, et al. Necroptosis promotes autophagy-dependent upregulation of DAMP and results in immunosurveillance. Autophagy. 2018;14:778–95. http://www.ncbi.nlm.nih.gov/pubmed/29171784.
17. Khandia R, Dadar M, Munjal A, Dhama K, Karthik K, Tiwari R, et al. A comprehensive review of autophagy and its various roles in infectious, non-infectious, and lifestyle diseases: current knowledge and prospects for disease prevention, novel drug design, and therapy. Cell. 2019;8:674. https://www.mdpi.com/2073-4409/8/7/674.
18. Bhattacharjee A, Szabó Á, Csizmadia T, Laczkó-Dobos H, Juhász G. Understanding the importance of autophagy in human diseases using Drosophila. J Genet Genomics. 2019;46:157–69. http://www.ncbi.nlm.nih.gov/pubmed/31080044.
19. Kirkin V. History of the selective autophagy research: how did it begin and where does it stand today? J Mol Biol. 2020;432(1):3–27. http://www.ncbi.nlm.nih.gov/pubmed/31082435.
20. Pfister AS. Emerging role of the nucleolar stress response in autophagy. Front Cell Neurosci. 2019;13:156. http://www.ncbi.nlm.nih.gov/pubmed/31114481.
21. Wilkinson S. Emerging principles of selective ER autophagy. J Mol Biol. 2020;432(1): 185–205. http://www.ncbi.nlm.nih.gov/pubmed/31100386.
22. Yang M, Linn BS, Zhang Y, Ren J. Mitophagy and mitochondrial integrity in cardiac ischemia-reperfusion injury. Biochim Biophys Acta Mol Basis Dis. 2019;1865(9):2293–302. http://www.ncbi.nlm.nih.gov/pubmed/31100337.
23. Halliwell B, Gutteridge JMC. Free radicals in biology and medicine. 5th ed. Oxford: OUP; 2015. https://doi.org/10.1093/acprof:oso/9780198717478.001.0001.
24. Hayes JD, McLellan LI. Glutathione and glutathione-dependent enzymes represent a co-ordinately regulated defence against oxidative stress. Free Radic Res. 1999;31:273–300. http://www.ncbi.nlm.nih.gov/pubmed/10517533.
25. Panieri E, Saso L. Potential applications of NRF2 inhibitors in cancer therapy. Oxid Med Cell Longev. 2019;2019:1–34. http://www.ncbi.nlm.nih.gov/pubmed/31097977.
26. Wu S, Lu H, Bai Y. Nrf2 in cancers: a double-edged sword. Cancer Med. 2019;8:2252–67. http://www.ncbi.nlm.nih.gov/pubmed/30929309.
27. Liu Q, Gao Y, Ci X. Role of Nrf2 and its activators in respiratory diseases. Oxid Med Cell Longev. 2019;2019:1–17. http://www.ncbi.nlm.nih.gov/pubmed/30728889.
28. Doonan LB, Hartigan A, Okamura B, Long PF. Stress-free evolution: the Nrf-coordinated oxidative stress response in early diverging metazoans. Integr Comp Biol. 2019;59:799–810. http://www.ncbi.nlm.nih.gov/pubmed/31120488.
29. Hayes JD, Dinkova-Kostova AT. The Nrf2 regulatory network provides an interface between redox and intermediary metabolism. Trends Biochem Sci. 2014;39:199–218. http://www.ncbi.nlm.nih.gov/pubmed/24647116.

30. Itoh K, Wakabayashi N, Katoh Y, Ishii T, Igarashi K, Engel JD, et al. Keap1 represses nuclear activation of antioxidant responsive elements by Nrf2 through binding to the amino-terminal Neh2 domain. Genes Dev. 1999;13:76–86. http://www.ncbi.nlm.nih.gov/pubmed/9887101.
31. Kaspar JW, Niture SK, Jaiswal AK. Nrf2:INrf2 (Keap1) signaling in oxidative stress. Free Radic Biol Med. 2009;47:1304–9. http://www.ncbi.nlm.nih.gov/pubmed/19666107.
32. Niture SK, Khatri R, Jaiswal AK. Regulation of Nrf2—an update. Free Radic Biol Med. 2014;66:36–44. http://www.ncbi.nlm.nih.gov/pubmed/23434765.
33. Zhang Y, Xiang Y. Molecular and cellular basis for the unique functioning of Nrf1, an indispensable transcription factor for maintaining cell homoeostasis and organ integrity. Biochem J. 2016;473:961–1000. http://www.ncbi.nlm.nih.gov/pubmed/27060105.
34. Taguchi K, Yamamoto M. The KEAP1-NRF2 system in cancer. Front Oncol. 2017;7:85. http://www.ncbi.nlm.nih.gov/pubmed/28523248.
35. Deshmukh P, Unni S, Krishnappa G, Padmanabhan B. The Keap1–Nrf2 pathway: promising therapeutic target to counteract ROS-mediated damage in cancers and neurodegenerative diseases. Biophys Rev. 2017;9:41–56. http://www.ncbi.nlm.nih.gov/pubmed/28510041.
36. Saito R, Suzuki T, Hiramoto K, Asami S, Naganuma E, Suda H, et al. Characterizations of three major cysteine sensors of Keap1 in stress response. Mol Cell Biol. 2015;36:271–84. http://www.ncbi.nlm.nih.gov/pubmed/26527616.
37. Dinkova-Kostova AT, Kostov RV, Canning P. Keap1, the cysteine-based mammalian intracellular sensor for electrophiles and oxidants. Arch Biochem Biophys. 2017;617:84–93. http://www.ncbi.nlm.nih.gov/pubmed/27497696.
38. Sihvola V, Levonen A-L. Keap1 as the redox sensor of the antioxidant response. Arch Biochem Biophys. 2017;617:94–100. http://www.ncbi.nlm.nih.gov/pubmed/27769838.
39. Katoh Y, Itoh K, Yoshida E, Miyagishi M, Fukamizu A, Yamamoto M. Two domains of Nrf2 cooperatively bind CBP, a CREB binding protein, and synergistically activate transcription. Genes Cells. 2001;6:857–68. http://www.ncbi.nlm.nih.gov/pubmed/11683914.
40. Chen X-L, Kunsch C. Induction of cytoprotective genes through Nrf2/antioxidant response element pathway: a new therapeutic approach for the treatment of inflammatory diseases. Curr Pharm Des. 2004;10:879–91. http://www.ncbi.nlm.nih.gov/pubmed/15032691.
41. Cleasby A, Yon J, Day PJ, Richardson C, Tickle IJ, Williams PA, et al. Structure of the BTB domain of Keap1 and its interaction with the triterpenoid antagonist CDDO. PLoS One. 2014;9:e98896. https://doi.org/10.1371/journal.pone.0098896.
42. Lee J-M, Johnson JA. An important role of Nrf2-ARE pathway in the cellular defense mechanism. J Biochem Mol Biol. 2004;37:139–43. http://www.ncbi.nlm.nih.gov/pubmed/15469687.
43. Chen QM, Maltagliati AJ. Nrf2 at the heart of oxidative stress and cardiac protection. Physiol Genomics. 2018;50:77–97. http://www.ncbi.nlm.nih.gov/pubmed/29187515.
44. Maiorino M, Conrad M, Ursini F. GPx4, lipid peroxidation, and cell death: discoveries, rediscoveries, and open issues. Antioxid Redox Signal. 2018;29:61–74. http://www.ncbi.nlm.nih.gov/pubmed/28462584.
45. Cao JY, Poddar A, Magtanong L, Lumb JH, Mileur TR, Reid MA, et al. A genome-wide haploid genetic screen identifies regulators of glutathione abundance and ferroptosis sensitivity. Cell Rep. 2019;26:1544–1556.e8. http://www.ncbi.nlm.nih.gov/pubmed/30726737.
46. Dodson M, Castro-Portuguez R, Zhang DD. NRF2 plays a critical role in mitigating lipid peroxidation and ferroptosis. Redox Biol. 2019;23:101107. https://linkinghub.elsevier.com/retrieve/pii/S2213231718310267.
47. Liu Q, Wang K. The induction of ferroptosis by impairing STAT3/Nrf2/GPx4 signaling enhances the sensitivity of osteosarcoma cells to cisplatin. Cell Biol Int. 2019;43(11):1245–56. http://www.ncbi.nlm.nih.gov/pubmed/30811078.
48. Shin D, Kim EH, Lee J, Roh J-L. Nrf2 inhibition reverses resistance to GPX4 inhibitor-induced ferroptosis in head and neck cancer. Free Radic Biol Med. 2018;129:454–62. http://www.ncbi.nlm.nih.gov/pubmed/30339884.
49. Hightower LE. Heat shock, stress proteins, chaperones, and proteotoxicity. Cell. 1991;66:191–7. http://www.ncbi.nlm.nih.gov/pubmed/1855252.

50. Schlesinger MJ. Heat shock in vertebrate cells. Cell Stress Chaperones. 1996;1:213–4. http://www.ncbi.nlm.nih.gov/pubmed/9222606.
51. Land W. Allograft injury mediated by reactive oxygen species: from conserved proteins of Drosophila to acute and chronic rejection of human transplants. Part II: Role of reactive oxygen species in the induction of the heat shock response as a regulator of innate. Transplant Rev. 2003;17:31–44. http://linkinghub.elsevier.com/retrieve/pii/S0955470X0380006X.
52. Beere HM. "The stress of dying": the role of heat shock proteins in the regulation of apoptosis. J Cell Sci. 2004;117:2641–51. http://www.ncbi.nlm.nih.gov/pubmed/15169835.
53. Westerheide SD, Morimoto RI. Heat shock response modulators as therapeutic tools for diseases of protein conformation. J Biol Chem. 2005;280:33097–100. http://www.ncbi.nlm.nih.gov/pubmed/16076838.
54. Land WG. Innate alloimmunity. Part 2. Innate immunity and allograft rejection. Ankara, Lengerich: Baskent University, Pabst Science; 2011. ISBN 9783899677386.
55. Kennedy D, Jäger R, Mosser DD, Samali A. Regulation of apoptosis by heat shock proteins. IUBMB Life. 2014;66:327–38. http://www.ncbi.nlm.nih.gov/pubmed/24861574.
56. Kityk R, Vogel M, Schlecht R, Bukau B, Mayer MP. Pathways of allosteric regulation in Hsp70 chaperones. Nat Commun. 2015;6:8308. https://doi.org/10.1038/ncomms9308.
57. So J-S. Roles of endoplasmic reticulum stress in immune responses. Mol Cells. 2018;41:705–16. http://www.ncbi.nlm.nih.gov/pubmed/30078231.
58. Almanza A, Carlesso A, Chintha C, Creedican S, Doultsinos D, Leuzzi B, et al. Endoplasmic reticulum stress signalling—from basic mechanisms to clinical applications. FEBS J. 2019;286:241–78. https://doi.org/10.1111/febs.14608.
59. Adams CJ, Kopp MC, Larburu N, Nowak PR, Ali MMU. Structure and molecular mechanism of er stress signaling by the unfolded protein response signal activator IRE1. Front Mol Biosci. 2019;6:11. https://doi.org/10.3389/fmolb.2019.00011/full.
60. Limia C, Sauzay C, Urra H, Hetz C, Chevet E, Avril T. Emerging roles of the endoplasmic reticulum associated unfolded protein response in cancer cell migration and invasion. Cancers (Basel). 2019;11:631. http://www.ncbi.nlm.nih.gov/pubmed/31064137.
61. Malhotra JD, Kaufman RJ. Endoplasmic reticulum stress and oxidative stress: a vicious cycle or a double-edged sword? Antioxid Redox Signal. 2007;9:2277–94. http://www.ncbi.nlm.nih.gov/pubmed/17979528.
62. Qin M, Wang W, Thirumalai D. Protein folding guides disulfide bond formation. Proc Natl Acad Sci U S A. 2015;112:11241–6. https://doi.org/10.1073/pnas.1503909112.
63. Zhang Z, Zhang L, Zhou L, Lei Y, Zhang Y, Huang C. Redox signaling and unfolded protein response coordinate cell fate decisions under ER stress. Redox Biol. 2018;25:101047. https://linkinghub.elsevier.com/retrieve/pii/S2213231718308954.
64. Tu BP, Weissman JS. Oxidative protein folding in eukaryotes: mechanisms and consequences. J Cell Biol. 2004;164:341–6. https://doi.org/10.1083/jcb.200311055.
65. Schröder M, Kaufman RJ. The mammalian unfolded protein response. Annu Rev Biochem. 2005;74:739–89. http://www.ncbi.nlm.nih.gov/pubmed/15952902.
66. Ron D, Walter P. Signal integration in the endoplasmic reticulum unfolded protein response. Nat Rev Mol Cell Biol. 2007;8:519–29. http://www.ncbi.nlm.nih.gov/pubmed/17565364.
67. Wang Q, Groenendyk J, Michalak M. Glycoprotein quality control and endoplasmic reticulum stress. Molecules. 2015;20:13689–704. http://www.ncbi.nlm.nih.gov/pubmed/26225950.
68. Díaz-Villanueva JF, Díaz-Molina R, García-González V. Protein folding and mechanisms of proteostasis. Int J Mol Sci. 2015;16:17193–230. http://www.ncbi.nlm.nih.gov/pubmed/26225966.
69. Xie Y, Hou W, Song X, Yu Y, Huang J, Sun X, et al. Ferroptosis: process and function. Cell Death Differ. 2016;23:369–79. https://doi.org/10.1038/cdd.2015.158.
70. Hofmans S, Vanden Berghe T, Devisscher L, Hassannia B, Lyssens S, Joossens J, et al. Novel ferroptosis inhibitors with improved potency and ADME properties. J Med Chem. 2016;59:2041–53. http://www.ncbi.nlm.nih.gov/pubmed/26696014.
71. Kuznetsov G, Bush KT, Zhang PL, Nigam SK. Perturbations in maturation of secretory proteins and their association with endoplasmic reticulum chaperones in a cell culture model for

epithelial ischemia. Proc Natl Acad Sci U S A. 1996;93:8584–9. http://www.ncbi.nlm.nih.gov/pubmed/8710914.
72. Garg AD, Agostinis P. ER stress, autophagy and immunogenic cell death in photodynamic therapy-induced anti-cancer immune responses. Photochem Photobiol Sci. 2014;13:474–87. http://www.ncbi.nlm.nih.gov/pubmed/24493131.
73. van Vliet AR, Martin S, Garg AD, Agostinis P. The PERKs of damage-associated molecular patterns mediating cancer immunogenicity: from sensor to the plasma membrane and beyond. Semin Cancer Biol. 2015;33:74–85. http://linkinghub.elsevier.com/retrieve/pii/S1044579X15000255.
74. Rodvold JJ, Mahadevan NR, Zanetti M. Immune modulation by ER stress and inflammation in the tumor microenvironment. Cancer Lett. 2016;380:227–36. http://www.ncbi.nlm.nih.gov/pubmed/26525580.
75. Dandekar A, Mendez R, Zhang K. Cross talk between ER stress, oxidative stress, and inflammation in health and disease. Methods Mol Biol. 2015;1292:205–14. http://www.ncbi.nlm.nih.gov/pubmed/25804758.
76. Martinon F, Glimcher LH. Regulation of innate immunity by signaling pathways emerging from the endoplasmic reticulum. Curr Opin Immunol. 2011;23:35–40. http://www.ncbi.nlm.nih.gov/pubmed/21094031.
77. Tabas I, Ron D. Integrating the mechanisms of apoptosis induced by endoplasmic reticulum stress. Nat Cell Biol. 2011;13:184–90. http://www.ncbi.nlm.nih.gov/pubmed/21364565.
78. Wang S, Kaufman RJ. The impact of the unfolded protein response on human disease. J Cell Biol. 2012;197:857–67. http://www.ncbi.lm.nih.gov/pubmed/22733998.
79. Cao SS, Kaufman RJ. Endoplasmic reticulum stress and oxidative stress in cell fate decision and human disease. Antioxid Redox Signal. 2014;21:396–413. http://www.ncbi.nlm.nih.gov/pubmed/24702237.
80. Hetz C, Chevet E, Oakes SA. Proteostasis control by the unfolded protein response. Nat Cell Biol. 2015;17:829–38. http://www.ncbi.nlm.nih.gov/pubmed/26123108.
81. Zhu X, Yao F, Yao Y, Dong N, Yu Y, Sheng Z. Endoplasmic reticulum stress and its regulator XBP-1 contributes to dendritic cell maturation and activation induced by high mobility group box-1 protein. Int J Biochem Cell Biol. 2012;44:1097–105. http://www.ncbi.nlm.nih.gov/pubmed/22504285.
82. Finka A, Sharma SK, Goloubinoff P. Multi-layered molecular mechanisms of polypeptide holding, unfolding and disaggregation by HSP70/HSP110 chaperones. Front Mol Biosci. 2015;2:29. http://www.ncbi.nlm.nih.gov/pubmed/26097841.
83. Spiro RG, Zhu Q, Bhoyroo V, Söling HD. Definition of the lectin-like properties of the molecular chaperone, calreticulin, and demonstration of its copurification with endomannosidase from rat liver Golgi. J Biol Chem. 1996;271:11588–94. http://www.ncbi.nlm.nih.gov/pubmed/8626722.
84. Trevelin SC, Lopes LR. Protein disulfide isomerase and Nox: new partners in redox signaling. Curr Pharm Des. 2015;21:5951–63. http://www.ncbi.nlm.nih.gov/pubmed/26510433.
85. Carreras-Sureda A, Pihán P, Hetz C. The unfolded protein response: at the intersection between endoplasmic reticulum function and mitochondrial bioenergetics. Front Oncol. 2017;7:55. http://www.ncbi.nlm.nih.gov/pubmed/28421160.
86. Eletto D, Chevet E, Argon Y, Appenzeller-Herzog C. Redox controls UPR to control redox. J Cell Sci. 2014;127:3649–58. https://doi.org/10.1242/jcs.153643.
87. Cullinan SB, Zhang D, Hannink M, Arvisais E, Kaufman RJ, Diehl JA. Nrf2 is a direct PERK substrate and effector of PERK-dependent cell survival. Mol Cell Biol. 2003;23:7198–209. https://doi.org/10.1128/MCB.23.20.7198-7209.2003.
88. Zhang G, Yang W, Jiang F, Zou P, Zeng Y, Ling X, et al. PERK regulates Nrf2/ARE antioxidant pathway against dibutyl phthalate-induced mitochondrial damage and apoptosis dependent of reactive oxygen species in mouse spermatocyte-derived cells. Toxicol Lett. 2019;308:24–33. https://linkinghub.elsevier.com/retrieve/pii/S0378427418317752.
89. Chen ZJ, Chen JX, Wu LK, Li BY, Tian YF, Xian M, et al. Induction of endoplasmic reticulum stress by cadmium and its regulation on Nrf2 signaling pathway in kidneys of rats. Biomed Environ Sci. 2019;32:1–10. http://www.ncbi.nlm.nih.gov/pubmed/30696534.

90. Sun J, Yu X, Huangpu H, Yao F. Ginsenoside Rb3 protects cardiomyocytes against hypoxia/reoxygenation injury via activating the antioxidation signaling pathway of PERK/Nrf2/HMOX1. Biomed Pharmacother. 2019;109:254–61. http://www.ncbi.nlm.nih.gov/pubmed/30396083.
91. Cullinan SB, Diehl JA. PERK-dependent activation of Nrf2 contributes to redox homeostasis and cell survival following endoplasmic reticulum stress. J Biol Chem. 2004;279:20108–17. https://doi.org/10.1074/jbc.M314219200.
92. Ma Q. Role of nrf2 in oxidative stress and toxicity. Annu Rev Pharmacol Toxicol. 2013;53:401–26. https://doi.org/10.1146/annurev-pharmtox-011112-140320.
93. Jo E-K, Kim JK, Shin D-M, Sasakawa C. Molecular mechanisms regulating NLRP3 inflammasome activation. Cell Mol Immunol. 2016;13:148–59. http://www.ncbi.nlm.nih.gov/pubmed/26549800.
94. Elliott EI, Sutterwala FS. Initiation and perpetuation of NLRP3 inflammasome activation and assembly. Immunol Rev. 2015;265:35–52. http://www.ncbi.nlm.nih.gov/pubmed/25879282.
95. Harijith A, Ebenezer DL, Natarajan V. Reactive oxygen species at the crossroads of inflammasome and inflammation. Front Physiol. 2014;5:352. http://www.ncbi.nlm.nih.gov/pubmed/25324778.
96. Santos CXC, Tanaka LY, Wosniak J, Laurindo FRM. Mechanisms and implications of reactive oxygen species generation during the unfolded protein response: roles of endoplasmic reticulum oxidoreductases, mitochondrial electron transport, and NADPH oxidase. Antioxid Redox Signal. 2009;11:2409–27. http://www.ncbi.nlm.nih.gov/pubmed/19388824.
97. Zhou R, Tardivel A, Thorens B, Choi I, Tschopp J. Thioredoxin-interacting protein links oxidative stress to inflammasome activation. Nat Immunol. 2010;11:136–40. http://www.ncbi.nlm.nih.gov/pubmed/20023662.
98. Kim S, Joe Y, Jeong SO, Zheng M, Back SH, Park SW, et al. Endoplasmic reticulum stress is sufficient for the induction of IL-1β production via activation of the NF-κB and inflammasome pathways. Innate Immun. 2014;20:799–815. http://www.ncbi.nlm.nih.gov/pubmed/24217221.
99. Bronner DN, Abuaita BH, Chen X, Fitzgerald KA, Nuñez G, He Y, et al. Endoplasmic reticulum stress activates the inflammasome via NLRP3- and Caspase-2-driven mitochondrial damage. Immunity. 2015;43:451–62. http://www.ncbi.nlm.nih.gov/pubmed/26341399.
100. He CH, Gong P, Hu B, Stewart D, Choi ME, Choi AM, et al. Identification of activating transcription factor 4 (ATF4) as an Nrf2-interacting protein. Implication for heme oxygenase-1 gene regulation. J Biol Chem. 2001;276:20858–65. https://doi.org/10.1074/jbc.M101198200.
101. Luhr M, Torgersen ML, Szalai P, Hashim A, Brech A, Staerk J, et al. The kinase PERK and the transcription factor ATF4 play distinct and essential roles in autophagy resulting from tunicamycin-induced ER stress. J Biol Chem. 2019;294:8197–217. http://www.ncbi.nlm.nih.gov/pubmed/30926605.
102. Zhang Y, Qu X, Jiang L. An oasis in the desert of cancer chemotherapeutic resistance: the enlightenment from reciprocal crosstalk between signaling pathways of UPR and autophagy in cancers. Biomed Pharmacother. 2017;92:972–81. https://linkinghub.elsevier.com/retrieve/pii/S0753332217312350.
103. Song S, Tan J, Miao Y, Zhang Q. Crosstalk of ER stress-mediated autophagy and ER-phagy: involvement of UPR and the core autophagy machinery. J Cell Physiol. 2018;233:3867–74. http://www.ncbi.nlm.nih.gov/pubmed/28777470.
104. Kang X, Yang W, Feng D, Jin X, Ma Z, Qian Z, et al. Cartilage-specific autophagy deficiency promotes ER stress and impairs chondrogenesis in PERK-ATF4-CHOP-dependent manner. J Bone Miner Res. 2017;32:2128–41. http://www.ncbi.nlm.nih.gov/pubmed/28304100.
105. Zheng W, Xie W, Yin D, Luo R, Liu M, Guo F. ATG5 and ATG7 induced autophagy interplays with UPR via PERK signaling. Cell Commun Signal. 2019;17:42. http://www.ncbi.nlm.nih.gov/pubmed/31060556.
106. Khan MM, Yang W-L, Wang P. Endoplasmic reticulum stress in sepsis. Shock. 2015;44:294–304. http://www.ncbi.nlm.nih.gov/pubmed/26125088.

107. Cominacini L, Mozzini C, Garbin U, Pasini A, Stranieri C, Solani E, et al. Endoplasmic reticulum stress and Nrf2 signaling in cardiovascular diseases. Free Radic Biol Med. 2015;88:233–42. http://www.ncbi.nlm.nih.gov/pubmed/26051167.
108. Zhang Q, Kang R, Zeh HJ, Lotze MT, Tang D. DAMPs and autophagy: cellular adaptation to injury and unscheduled cell death. Autophagy. 2013;9:451–8. https://doi.org/10.4161/auto.23691.
109. Garg AD, Dudek AM, Ferreira GB, Verfaillie T, Vandenabeele P, Krysko DV, et al. ROS-induced autophagy in cancer cells assists in evasion from determinants of immunogenic cell death. Autophagy. 2013;9:1292–307. http://www.ncbi.nlm.nih.gov/pubmed/23800749.
110. Ma Y, Galluzzi L, Zitvogel L, Kroemer G. Autophagy and cellular immune responses. Immunity. 2013;39:211–27. http://www.ncbi.nlm.nih.gov/pubmed/23973220.
111. Bhattacharya A, Eissa NT. Autophagy as a stress response pathway in the immune system. Int Rev Immunol. 2015;34:382–402. http://www.ncbi.nlm.nih.gov/pubmed/25699578.
112. Martins I, Wang Y, Michaud M, Ma Y, Sukkurwala AQ, Shen S, et al. Molecular mechanisms of ATP secretion during immunogenic cell death. Cell Death Differ. 2014;21:79–91. http://www.ncbi.nlm.nih.gov/pubmed/23852373.
113. Kalogeris T, Baines CP, Krenz M, Korthuis RJ. Cell biology of ischemia/reperfusion injury. Int Rev Cell Mol Biol. 2012;298:229–317. http://www.ncbi.nlm.nih.gov/pubmed/22878108.
114. Whelan RS, Kaplinskiy V, Kitsis RN. Cell death in the pathogenesis of heart disease: mechanisms and significance. Annu Rev Physiol. 2010;72:19–44. http://www.ncbi.nlm.nih.gov/pubmed/20148665.
115. Lee W-S, Yoo W-H, Chae H-J. ER stress and autophagy. Curr Mol Med. 2015;15:735–45. http://www.ncbi.nlm.nih.gov/pubmed/26391548.
116. Pyo JO, Nah J, Jung YK. Molecules and their functions in autophagy. Exp Mol Med. 2012;44:73–80. http://www.ncbi.nlm.nih.gov/pubmed/22257882.
117. Thapalia BA, Zhou Z, Lin X. Autophagy, a process within reperfusion injury: an update. Int J Clin Exp Pathol. 2014;7:8322–41. http://www.ncbi.nlm.nih.gov/pubmed/25674198.
118. Li L, Tan J, Miao Y, Lei P, Zhang Q. ROS and autophagy: interactions and molecular regulatory mechanisms. Cell Mol Neurobiol. 2015;35:615–21. http://www.ncbi.nlm.nih.gov/pubmed/25722131.
119. Kroemer G, Galluzzi L, Brenner C. Mitochondrial membrane permeabilization in cell death. Physiol Rev. 2007;87:99–163. http://www.ncbi.nlm.nih.gov/pubmed/17237344.
120. Galluzzi L, Morselli E, Kepp O, Kroemer G. Targeting post-mitochondrial effectors of apoptosis for neuroprotection. Biochim Biophys Acta. 1787;2009:402–13. http://www.ncbi.nlm.nih.gov/pubmed/18848916.
121. Broughton BRS, Reutens DC, Sobey CG. Apoptotic mechanisms after cerebral ischemia. Stroke. 2009;40:e331–9. http://www.ncbi.nlm.nih.gov/pubmed/19182083.
122. Galluzzi L, Vitale I, Abrams JM, Alnemri ES, Baehrecke EH, Blagosklonny MV, et al. Molecular definitions of cell death subroutines: recommendations of the Nomenclature Committee on Cell Death 2012. Cell Death Differ. 2012;19:107–20. http://www.ncbi.nlm.nih.gov/pubmed/21760595.
123. Halestrap AP, Richardson AP. The mitochondrial permeability transition: a current perspective on its identity and role in ischaemia/reperfusion injury. J Mol Cell Cardiol. 2015;78:129–41. http://www.ncbi.nlm.nih.gov/pubmed/25179911.
124. Ayna G, Krysko DV, Kaczmarek A, Petrovski G, Vandenabeele P, Fésüs L. ATP release from dying autophagic cells and their phagocytosis are crucial for inflammasome activation in macrophages. PLoS One. 2012;7:e40069. http://www.ncbi.nlm.nih.gov/pubmed/22768222.
125. Garg AD, Dudek AM, Agostinis P. Calreticulin surface exposure is abrogated in cells lacking, chaperone-mediated autophagy-essential gene, LAMP2A. Cell Death Dis. 2013;4:e826. http://www.ncbi.nlm.nih.gov/pubmed/24091669.
126. Urra H, Dufey E, Lisbona F, Rojas-Rivera D, Hetz C. When ER stress reaches a dead end. Biochim Biophys Acta. 1833;2013:3507–17. http://linkinghub.elsevier.com/retrieve/pii/S016748891300311X.

127. Han J, Back SH, Hur J, Lin Y-H, Gildersleeve R, Shan J, et al. ER-stress-induced transcriptional regulation increases protein synthesis leading to cell death. Nat Cell Biol. 2013;15:481–90. http://www.nature.com/articles/ncb2738.
128. Chang T-K, Lawrence DA, Lu M, Tan J, Harnoss JM, Marsters SA, et al. Coordination between two branches of the unfolded protein response determines apoptotic cell fate. Mol Cell. 2018;71:629–636.e5. https://linkinghub.elsevier.com/retrieve/pii/S1097276518305136.
129. Hetz C, Papa FR. The unfolded protein response and cell fate control. Mol Cell. 2018;69:169–81. https://linkinghub.elsevier.com/retrieve/pii/S1097276517304446.
130. Galluzzi L, Kroemer G. Secondary necrosis: accidental no more. Trends Cancer. 2017;3:1–2. https://linkinghub.elsevier.com/retrieve/pii/S2405803316301893.
131. Chen D, Dixon BJ, Doycheva DM, Li B, Zhang Y, Hu Q, et al. IRE1α inhibition decreased TXNIP/NLRP3 inflammasome activation through miR-17-5p after neonatal hypoxic–ischemic brain injury in rats. J Neuroinflammation. 2018;15:32. http://www.ncbi.nlm.nih.gov/pubmed/29394934.
132. Dixon SJ, Patel DN, Welsch M, Skouta R, Lee ED, Hayano M, et al. Pharmacological inhibition of cystine-glutamate exchange induces endoplasmic reticulum stress and ferroptosis. Elife. 2014;3:e02523. http://www.ncbi.nlm.nih.gov/pubmed/24844246.
133. Maher P, van Leyen K, Dey PN, Honrath B, Dolga A, Methner A. The role of Ca2+ in cell death caused by oxidative glutamate toxicity and ferroptosis. Cell Calcium. 2018;70:47–55. https://linkinghub.elsevier.com/retrieve/pii/S014341601730074X.
134. Periyasamy P, Shinohara T. Age-related cataracts: Role of unfolded protein response, Ca2+ mobilization, epigenetic DNA modifications, and loss of Nrf2/Keap1 dependent cytoprotection. Prog Retin Eye Res. 2017;60:1–19. https://linkinghub.elsevier.com/retrieve/pii/S1350946217300575.
135. Lee Y-S, Lee D-H, Choudry HA, Bartlett DL, Lee YJ. Ferroptosis-induced endoplasmic reticulum stress: cross-talk between ferroptosis and apoptosis. Mol Cancer Res. 2018;16:1073–6. https://doi.org/10.1158/1541-7786.MCR-18-0055.
136. Land WG. The role of damage-associated molecular patterns (DAMPs) in human diseases: part II: DAMPs as diagnostics, prognostics and therapeutics in clinical medicine. Sultan Qaboos Univ Med J. 2015;15:e157–70. http://www.ncbi.nlm.nih.gov/pubmed/26052447.
137. Dixon SJ. Ferroptosis: bug or feature? Immunol Rev. 2017;277:150–7. http://www.ncbi.nlm.nih.gov/pubmed/28462529.
138. Green DR. The coming decade of cell death research: five riddles. Cell. 2019;177:1094–107. https://linkinghub.elsevier.com/retrieve/pii/S009286741930443X.
139. Zhe-Wei S, Li-Sha G, Yue-Chun L. The role of necroptosis in cardiovascular disease. Front Pharmacol. 2018;9:721. http://www.ncbi.nlm.nih.gov/pubmed/30034339.
140. Linkermann A, Stockwell BR, Krautwald S, Anders H-J. Regulated cell death and inflammation: an auto-amplification loop causes organ failure. Nat Rev Immunol. 2014;14:759–67. http://www.nature.com/articles/nri3743.
141. Vanden Berghe T, Linkermann A, Jouan-Lanhouet S, Walczak H, Vandenabeele P. Regulated necrosis: the expanding network of non-apoptotic cell death pathways. Nat Rev Mol Cell Biol. 2014;15:135–47. http://www.ncbi.nlm.nih.gov/pubmed/24452471.
142. Galluzzi L, Vitale I, Aaronson SA, Abrams JM, Adam D, Agostinis P, et al. Molecular mechanisms of cell death: recommendations of the Nomenclature Committee on Cell Death 2018. Cell Death Differ. 2018;25:486–541. http://www.nature.com/articles/s41418-017-0012-4.
143. Green DR, Oguin TH, Martinez J. The clearance of dying cells: table for two. Cell Death Differ. 2016;23:915–26. http://www.nature.com/articles/cdd2015172.
144. Fuchs Y, Steller H. Live to die another way: modes of programmed cell death and the signals emanating from dying cells. Nat Rev Mol Cell Biol. 2015;16:329–44. http://www.nature.com/articles/nrm3999.
145. Green DR, Ferguson T, Zitvogel L, Kroemer G. Immunogenic and tolerogenic cell death. Nat Rev Immunol. 2009;9:353–63. http://www.ncbi.nlm.nih.gov/pubmed/19365408.
146. Sachet M, Liang YY, Oehler R. The immune response to secondary necrotic cells. Apoptosis. 2017;22:1189–204. http://www.ncbi.nlm.nih.gov/pubmed/28861714

147. Kepp O, Senovilla L, Vitale I, Vacchelli E, Adjemian S, Agostinis P, et al. Consensus guidelines for the detection of immunogenic cell death. Oncoimmunology. 2014;3:e955691.
148. Galluzzi L, Buqué A, Kepp O, Zitvogel L, Kroemer G. Immunogenic cell death in cancer and infectious disease. Nat Rev Immunol. 2017;17:97–111. http://www.ncbi.nlm.nih.gov/pubmed/27748397.
149. Sistigu A, Yamazaki T, Vacchelli E, Chaba K, Enot DP, Adam J, et al. Cancer cell-autonomous contribution of type I interferon signaling to the efficacy of chemotherapy. Nat Med. 2014;20:1301–9. http://www.nature.com/articles/nm.3708.
150. Catelas I, Petit A, Zukor DJ, Antoniou J, Huk OL. TNF-alpha secretion and macrophage mortality induced by cobalt and chromium ions in vitro-qualitative analysis of apoptosis. Biomaterials. 2003;24:383–91. http://www.ncbi.nlm.nih.gov/pubmed/12423593.
151. Sarhan M, Land WG, Tonnus W, Hugo CP, Linkermann A. Origin and consequences of necroinflammation. Physiol Rev. 2018;98:727–80. https://doi.org/10.1152/physrev.00041.2016.
152. Shlomovitz I, Erlich Z, Speir M, Zargarian S, Baram N, Engler M, et al. Necroptosis directly induces the release of full-length biologically active IL-33 in vitro and in an inflammatory disease model. FEBS J. 2019;286:507–22. https://doi.org/10.1111/febs.14738.
153. Gatta AT, Carlton JG. The ESCRT-machinery: closing holes and expanding roles. Curr Opin Cell Biol. 2019;59:121–32. https://linkinghub.elsevier.com/retrieve/pii/S0955067419300237
154. Petrie EJ, Czabotar PE, Murphy JM. The structural basis of necroptotic cell death signaling. Trends Biochem Sci. 2019;44:53–63. https://linkinghub.elsevier.com/retrieve/pii/S0968000418302299.
155. Nakano H, Murai S, Yamaguchi Y, Shirasaki Y, Nakabayashi O, Yamazaki S. Development of novel methods that monitor necroptosis and the release of DAMPs at the single cell resolution. Cell Stress. 2019;3:66–9. http://www.ncbi.nlm.nih.gov/pubmed/31225501.
156. Upton JW, Shubina M, Balachandran S. RIPK3-driven cell death during virus infections. Immunol Rev. 2017;277:90–101. https://doi.org/10.1111/imr.12539.
157. Nailwal H, Chan FK-M. Necroptosis in anti-viral inflammation. Cell Death Differ. 2019;26:4–13. http://www.nature.com/articles/s41418-018-0172-x.
158. Frank D, Vince JE. Pyroptosis versus necroptosis: similarities, differences, and crosstalk. Cell Death Differ. 2019;26:99–114. http://www.nature.com/articles/s41418-018-0212-6.
159. Yang D, Liang Y, Zhao S, Ding Y, Zhuang Q, Shi Q, et al. ZBP1 mediates interferon-induced necroptosis. Cell Mol Immunol. 2020;17(4):356–68. http://www.nature.com/articles/s41423-019-0237-x.
160. Gaba A, Xu F, Lu Y, Park H-S, Liu G, Zhou Y. The NS1 protein of Influenza A virus participates in necroptosis by interacting with MLKL and increasing its oligomerization and membrane translocation. J Virol. 2019;93:e01835–18. https://doi.org/10.1128/JVI.01835-18.
161. Meng R, Gu L, Lu Y, Zhao K, Wu J, Wang H, et al. High mobility group box 1 enables bacterial lipids to trigger receptor-interacting protein kinase 3 (RIPK3)-mediated necroptosis and apoptosis in mice. J Biol Chem. 2019;294:8872–84. https://doi.org/10.1074/jbc.RA118.007040.
162. Hou J, Ju J, Zhang Z, Zhao C, Li Z, Zheng J, et al. Discovery of potent necroptosis inhibitors targeting RIPK1 kinase activity for the treatment of inflammatory disorder and cancer metastasis. Cell Death Dis. 2019;10:493. http://www.ncbi.nlm.nih.gov/pubmed/31235688.
163. Proneth B, Conrad M. Ferroptosis and necroinflammation, a yet poorly explored link. Cell Death Differ. 2019;26:14–24. http://www.ncbi.nlm.nih.gov/pubmed/30082768.
164. Lei P, Bai T, Sun Y. Mechanisms of ferroptosis and relations with regulated cell death: a review. Front Physiol. 2019;10:139. http://www.ncbi.nlm.nih.gov/pubmed/30863316.
165. Esterbauer H, Schaur RJ, Zollner H. Chemistry and biochemistry of 4-hydroxynonenal, malonaldehyde and related aldehydes. Free Radic Biol Med. 1991;11:81–128. http://www.ncbi.nlm.nih.gov/pubmed/1937131.
166. Niki E, Yoshida Y, Saito Y, Noguchi N. Lipid peroxidation: mechanisms, inhibition, and biological effects. Biochem Biophys Res Commun. 2005;338:668–76. http://linkinghub.elsevier.com/retrieve/pii/S0006291X05017766.
167. Bochkov VN, Oskolkova OV, Birukov KG, Levonen A-L, Binder CJ, Stöckl J. Generation and biological activities of oxidized phospholipids. Antioxid Redox Signal. 2010;12:1009–59. http://www.ncbi.nlm.nih.gov/pubmed/19686040.

168. Lee S, Birukov KG, Romanoski CE, Springstead JR, Lusis AJ, Berliner JA. Role of phospholipid oxidation products in atherosclerosis. Circ Res. 2012;111:778–99. http://www.ncbi.nlm.nih.gov/pubmed/22935534.
169. Yin H, Xu L, Porter NA. Free radical lipid peroxidation: mechanisms and analysis. Chem Rev. 2011;111:5944–72. https://doi.org/10.1021/cr200084z.
170. Ayala A, Muñoz MF, Argüelles S. Lipid peroxidation: production, metabolism, and signaling mechanisms of malondialdehyde and 4-hydroxy-2-nonenal. Oxid Med Cell Longev. 2014;2014:360438. http://www.hindawi.com/journals/omcl/2014/360438/.
171. Salomon RG. Structural identification and cardiovascular activities of oxidized phospholipids. Circ Res. 2012;111:930–46. http://www.ncbi.nlm.nih.gov/pubmed/22982874.
172. Bochkov V, Gesslbauer B, Mauerhofer C, Philippova M, Erne P, Oskolkova OV. Pleiotropic effects of oxidized phospholipids. Free Radic Biol Med. 2017;111:6–24. http://www.ncbi.nlm.nih.gov/pubmed/28027924.
173. Thomas CP, O'Donnell VB. Oxidized phospholipid signaling in immune cells. Curr Opin Pharmacol. 2012;12:471–7. http://linkinghub.elsevier.com/retrieve/pii/S1471489212000367.
174. O'Donnell VB, Murphy RC. New families of bioactive oxidized phospholipids generated by immune cells: identification and signaling actions. Blood. 2012;120:1985–92. https://doi.org/10.1182/blood-2012-04-402826.
175. Kang R, Tang D. Autophagy and ferroptosis—what's the connection? Curr Pathobiol Rep. 2017;5:153–9. https://doi.org/10.1007/s40139-017-0139-5.
176. Wu Z, Geng Y, Lu X, Shi Y, Wu G, Zhang M, et al. Chaperone-mediated autophagy is involved in the execution of ferroptosis. Proc Natl Acad Sci U S A. 2019;116:2996–3005. https://doi.org/10.1073/pnas.1819728116.
177. Wen Q, Liu J, Kang R, Zhou B, Tang D. The release and activity of HMGB1 in ferroptosis. Biochem Biophys Res Commun. 2019;510:278–83. http://www.ncbi.nlm.nih.gov/pubmed/30686534.
178. Yamazaki H, Tanji K, Wakabayashi K, Matsuura S, Itoh K. Role of the Keap1/Nrf2 pathway in neurodegenerative diseases. Pathol Int. 2015;65:210–9. http://www.ncbi.nlm.nih.gov/pubmed/25707882.
179. Sun Y, Yang T, Leak RK, Chen J, Zhang F. Preventive and protective roles of dietary Nrf2 activators against central nervous system diseases. CNS Neurol Disord Drug Targets. 2017;16:326–38. http://www.ncbi.nlm.nih.gov/pubmed/28042770.
180. Abdalkader M, Lampinen R, Kanninen KM, Malm TM, Liddell JR. Targeting Nrf2 to suppress ferroptosis and mitochondrial dysfunction in neurodegeneration. Front Neurosci. 2018;12:466. https://doi.org/10.3389/fnins.2018.00466/full.
181. Ge Z-D, Lian Q, Mao X, Xia Z. Current status and challenges of NRF2 as a potential therapeutic target for diabetic cardiomyopathy. Int Heart J. 2019;60:512–20. http://www.ncbi.nlm.nih.gov/pubmed/30971629.
182. Tang M, Chen Z, Wu D, Chen L. Ferritinophagy/ferroptosis: iron-related newcomers in human diseases. J Cell Physiol. 2018;233:9179–90. http://www.ncbi.nlm.nih.gov/pubmed/30076709.
183. Liguori I, Russo G, Curcio F, Bulli G, Aran L, Della-Morte D, et al. Oxidative stress, aging, and diseases. Clin Interv Aging. 2018;13:757–72. http://www.ncbi.nlm.nih.gov/pubmed/29731617.
184. Hambright WS, Fonseca RS, Chen L, Na R, Ran Q. Ablation of ferroptosis regulator glutathione peroxidase 4 in forebrain neurons promotes cognitive impairment and neurodegeneration. Redox Biol. 2017;12:8–17. https://linkinghub.elsevier.com/retrieve/pii/S2213231717300277.
185. Lu B, Chen XB, Ying MD, He QJ, Cao J, Yang B. The role of ferroptosis in cancer development and treatment response. Front Pharmacol. 2018;8:992. http://www.ncbi.nlm.nih.gov/pubmed/29375387.
186. Hassannia B, Vandenabeele P, Vanden Berghe T. Targeting ferroptosis to iron out cancer. Cancer Cell. 2019;35(6):830–49. http://www.ncbi.nlm.nih.gov/pubmed/31105042.

187. Friedmann Angeli JP, Krysko DV, Conrad M. Ferroptosis at the crossroads of cancer-acquired drug resistance and immune evasion. Nat Rev Cancer. 2019;19(7):405–14. http://www.ncbi.nlm.nih.gov/pubmed/31101865.
188. Shi J, Gao W, Shao F. Pyroptosis: Gasdermin-mediated programmed necrotic cell death. Trends Biochem Sci. 2017;42:245–54. https://linkinghub.elsevier.com/retrieve/pii/S0968000416301827.
189. Sborgi L, Rühl S, Mulvihill E, Pipercevic J, Heilig R, Stahlberg H, et al. GSDMD membrane pore formation constitutes the mechanism of pyroptotic cell death. EMBO J. 2016;35:1766–78. https://doi.org/10.15252/embj.201694696.
190. Qiu S, Liu J, Xing F. 'Hints' in the killer protein gasdermin D: unveiling the secrets of gasdermins driving cell death. Cell Death Differ. 2017;24:588–96. http://www.ncbi.nlm.nih.gov/pubmed/28362726.
191. Ding J, Wang K, Liu W, She Y, Sun Q, Shi J, et al. Pore-forming activity and structural autoinhibition of the gasdermin family. Nature. 2016;535:111–6. http://www.ncbi.nlm.nih.gov/pubmed/27281216.
192. Mulvihill E, Sborgi L, Mari SA, Pfreundschuh M, Hiller S, Müller DJ. Mechanism of membrane pore formation by human gasdermin-D. EMBO J. 2018;37:e98321. http://www.ncbi.nlm.nih.gov/pubmed/29898893.
193. Chen X, He W-T, Hu L, Li J, Fang Y, Wang X, et al. Pyroptosis is driven by non-selective gasdermin-D pore and its morphology is different from MLKL channel-mediated necroptosis. Cell Res. 2016;26:1007–20. http://www.nature.com/articles/cr2016100.
194. Rojas J, Bermudez V, Palmar J, Martínez MS, Olivar LC, Nava M, et al. Pancreatic beta cell death: novel potential mechanisms in diabetes therapy. J Diabetes Res. 2018;2018:1–19. http://www.ncbi.nlm.nih.gov/pubmed/29670917.
195. Yuan Y-Y, Xie K-X, Wang S-L, Yuan L-W. Inflammatory caspase-related pyroptosis: mechanism, regulation and therapeutic potential for inflammatory bowel disease. Gastroenterol Rep. 2018;6:167–76. http://www.ncbi.nlm.nih.gov/pubmed/30151200.
196. Jia C, Chen H, Zhang J, Zhou K, Zhuge Y, Niu C, et al. Role of pyroptosis in cardiovascular diseases. Int Immunopharmacol. 2019;67:311–8. http://www.ncbi.nlm.nih.gov/pubmed/30572256.
197. Lee C, Do HTT, Her J, Kim Y, Seo D, Rhee I. Inflammasome as a promising therapeutic target for cancer. Life Sci. 2019;231:116593. http://www.ncbi.nlm.nih.gov/pubmed/31228512.
198. Dempsey C, Rubio Araiz A, Bryson KJ, Finucane O, Larkin C, Mills EL, et al. Inhibiting the NLRP3 inflammasome with MCC950 promotes non-phlogistic clearance of amyloid-β and cognitive function in APP/PS1 mice. Brain Behav Immun. 2017;61:306–16. http://www.ncbi.nlm.nih.gov/pubmed/28003153.
199. Pandeya A, Li L, Li Z, Wei Y. Gasdermin D (GSDMD) as a new target for the treatment of infection. MedChemComm. 2019;10:660–7. http://xlink.rsc.org/?DOI=C9MD00059C.
200. Sollberger G, Choidas A, Burn GL, Habenberger P, Di Lucrezia R, Kordes S, et al. Gasdermin D plays a vital role in the generation of neutrophil extracellular traps. Sci Immunol. 2018;3:eaar6689. http://www.ncbi.nlm.nih.gov/pubmed/30143555.
201. Chen KW, Monteleone M, Boucher D, Sollberger G, Ramnath D, Condon ND, et al. Noncanonical inflammasome signaling elicits gasdermin D–dependent neutrophil extracellular traps. Sci Immunol. 2018;3:eaar6676. http://www.ncbi.nlm.nih.gov/pubmed/30143554.
202. Berthelot J-M, Le Goff B, Neel A, Maugars Y, Hamidou M. NETosis: at the crossroads of rheumatoid arthritis, lupus, and vasculitis. Jt Bone Spine. 2017;84:255–62. http://www.ncbi.nlm.nih.gov/pubmed/27426444.
203. Jorch SK, Kubes P. An emerging role for neutrophil extracellular traps in noninfectious disease. Nat Med. 2017;23:279–87. http://www.ncbi.nlm.nih.gov/pubmed/28267716.
204. Kumar S, Gupta E, Kaushik S, Jyoti A. Neutrophil extracellular traps: formation and involvement in disease progression. Iran J Allergy Asthma Immunol. 2018;17:208–20. http://www.ncbi.nlm.nih.gov/pubmed/29908538.
205. Tonnus W, Meyer C, Paliege A, Belavgeni A, von Mässenhausen A, Bornstein SR, et al. The pathological features of regulated necrosis. J Pathol. 2019;247:697–707. https://doi.org/10.1002/path.5248.

DAMP-Promoted Efferent Innate Immune Responses in Human Diseases: Inflammation

5

5.1 Introduction

Across the tree of life, DAMP-promoted efferent innate immune responses serve as defense responses aimed at maintaining and restoring homeostasis. However, as repeatedly emphasized, although initially beneficial, when dysregulated, uncontrolled, and exaggerated, these protection-intended inflammatory and tissue repairing processes become pathogenic and can lead to pathologies and diseases (Vol.1 [1], Part II, Sect. 4.4 and Fig. 4.1; and [2]). Histopathologically, these disorders mostly manifest as aberrant inflammatory and fibrotic processes. Thus, most DAMP-promoted human disorders of entirely different etiology such as sepsis, CVD, neurodegenerative diseases, diabetes, obesity, and asthma, as well as classic inflammatory diseases, are associated with acute, hyperacute, or chronic inflammation with or without a fibrotic component. And to remind: typically, chronic inflammatory and fibrotic disorders are a consequence of disturbed "frustrated" resolution of inflammation.

In Vol.1 [1], first introductory remarks to these scenarios were already made. Here, the topic of dysregulated inflammatory processes is briefly resumed by focusing on updates of modern insights into SAMP-promoted resolution of inflammation and its failure resulting in chronic inflammation. Additionally, a model of hyperinflammation induced by excessive production of DAMPs followed by hyperresolution caused by counterbalancing production of SAMPs in excess is introduced.

Another aspect deserves a short update as well: whereas the mechanisms of initial activation and subsequent nuclear translocation of associated transcription factors for proinflammatory/antiinflammatory and profibrotic signaling pathways are rather well-characterized, how the transcription of genes concerned is finely controlled in the nucleus remains elusive. Therefore, an update of this emerging field of epigenetics is given additionally at the end of the chapter.

W. G. Land, *Damage-Associated Molecular Patterns in Human Diseases*,
https://doi.org/10.1007/978-3-030-53868-2_5

5.2 Inflammation: A Change in Viewpoints

The scenario of promotion and resolution of inflammation and their regulation has already been described in Vol. 1 [1], Part VI. In modern medicine, inflammatory disorders are formulated as a response of the innate/adaptive immune system to infectious or sterile injury, induced by MAMPs and DAMPs or DAMPs. As stressed in Part VI, many DAMP-promoted, PRM-triggered signaling pathways and transcription factors are involved in the inflammatory response, including NF-κB, MAPK, IRFs, PI3K → Akt → mTOR, and JAK/ STAT pathways (mTOR, mammalian target of rapamycin).

In Vol. 1 [1], Part VI, Sect. 22.2.2 and Figs. 22.1 and 22.2, the scenario of the promotion phase of acute inflammation has been sketched, but must be corrected here in a certain way. Indeed, recent data from inflammatory research has led to a change in viewpoints on the dynamic process of inflammation: DAMP-induced promotion of inflammation and SAMP-induced resolution of inflammation occur nearly in parallel, and not—as was suggested earlier on—in terms of two subsequent biphasic events (Fig. 5.1).

In the following, instead of resuming the essential proinflammatory pathways encountered in the acute phase of inflammation promotion, a special note is addressed to mechanisms involved in inflammation resolution, a topic that has been recently catapulted into the limelight of clinical inflammation research.

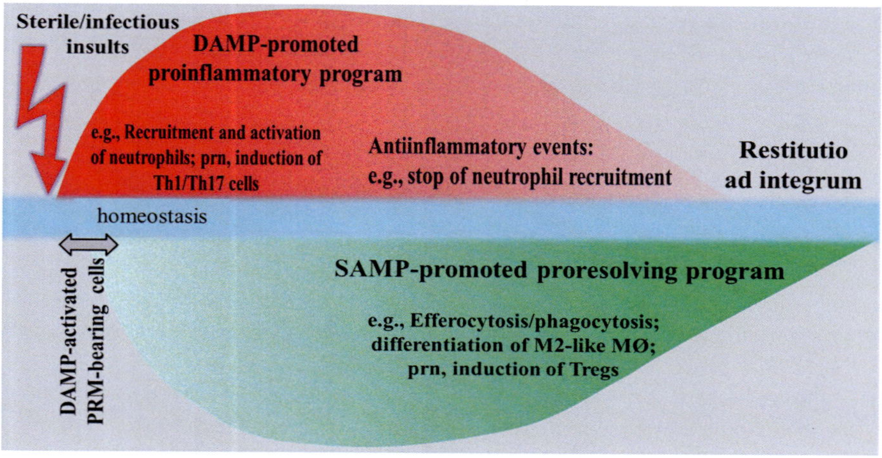

Fig. 5.1 Schematic diagram of a conceptual model illustrating an injury-induced controlled homeostatic inflammatory response leading to restitutio ad integrum. The initiating DAMP-promoted proinflammatory crescendo → decrescendo proceeds—slightly shifted but nearly in parallel—to a SAMP-promoted proresolving "reversed" crescendo → decrescendo. The short delay of the begin of the proresolving response (estimated about 3–6 h post-trauma) may be explained by the fact that SAMPs in terms of inducible suppressing DAMPs are secreted by DAMP-activated innate immune cells. *DAMPs* damage-associated molecular patterns, *MØ* macrophages, nrp pro re nata, *PRM* pattern recognition molecule, *Tregs* T regulatory cells, *Th1/17 cells* T helper cells type 1/17

5.3 Resolution of Inflammation

5.3.1 Introductory Remarks

As already pointed out in Vol. 1[1], Part VI, Sect. 22.2.3, resolution of inflammation is a tightly regulated multifactorial event that is characterized by the involvement of phenotypic, functional, regulatory, and epigenetic mechanisms. Of note, proresolution processes are not identical to antiinflammatory events. Antiinflammation, for example, refers to cessation of neutrophils recruitment and tissue infiltration, whereas resolution is elimination of these innate immune key cells by efferocytosis/phagocytosis (besides repairing tissue damage and replenishing blood and lymphatic vessels). As mentioned above, a typical feature of the antiinflammatory/proresolving phase is that it occurs nearly in parallel with acute proinflammatory processes, however, initially less predominantly and slightly delayed. A special role in these scenarios has to be ascribed to the SAMPs in terms of suppressing/inhibiting inducible DAMPs (see later for details) (Fig. 5.1). The SAMPs may be made accountable for such a model of slightly delayed begin of resolution mechanisms (estimated about 3–6 h post-trauma) since most of them are inducible suppressing molecules produced by DAMP-activated innate immune cells.

At the time being, research on these suppressing DAMPs is remarkably flourishing, and this is not a surprise. One has to realize: every minute during each day, MAMP/DAMP or DAMP-triggered acute inflammatory responses protect us from infectious injury mediated by invading microbes, or sterile injuries, for example, caused by minor accidents, but also from stressful insults occurring within, for example, metabolic damage caused by a dietary failure in diabetes. Most of these harmful challenges remain unnoticed because they are self-limited and naturally resolve without progressing to chronic inflammation. This "resolving scenario" is the work of SAMPs that operate "noiselessly."

5.3.2 Elimination and Transdifferentiation of Innate Immune Cells Involved in Resolution of Inflammation

5.3.2.1 General Remarks

As mentioned, resolution of inflammation is a tightly regulated multifactorial event that is characterized by several mechanisms. Certainly, and first of all, for resolution to occur effectively, the initiating infectious or sterile injurious agents must be eliminated that prompts the discontinuation of emission of DAMPs and subsequent shutdown of their triggered proinflammatory signaling pathways. Plausibly, if not occurring spontaneously under the assistance of negatively regulating innate immune pathways, this process has to be vigorously tackled therapeutically. In fact, this action, that is, the cessation of DAMPs production, allows the SAMPs to do their successful proresolving work. Furthermore, and addressed here, the effective resolution requires the death of inflammatory cells such as neutrophils and macrophages and, additionally, their differentiation into cells with preferentially antiinflammatory/proresolving capabilities.

5.3.2.2 Death of Inflammatory Cells and the Process of Efferocytosis

After recruitment of inflammatory innate immune cell into injured tissue, a peak of influx will be reached that is followed by the clearance of these cells: the start of resolution resulting in final restoration of functional homeostasis. Under normal physiological, that is, homeostatic conditions, inflammatory cell clearance is initiated by apoptosis as a form of "noninflammatory" RCD that avoids release of DAMPs (reviewed in [3, 4]; also see Vol. 1[1], Part V, Sect. 19.2). Apoptotic cells then are finally cleared by phagocytosing cells in a process known as efferocytosis (for additional information also compare Vol.1 [1], Part VI, Sect. 22.6.3.3, p. 562). As described there, efferocytosis is a carefully orchestrated process by which phagocytes are recruited to sites of cell death, recognize and engulf dying cells, and clear them in an "immunologically silent" manner. Doubtlessly, this process is essential for the maintenance of normal tissue homeostasis and a prerequisite for the resolution of inflammation (reviewed in [5-7]). Importantly, efferocytosis is not merely a passive event but a carefully orchestrated process aimed at efficiently clearing cells in early stages of cell death, while the plasma membrane is still intact. This maneuver hampers secondary necrosis, thereby preventing release of DAMPs. Indeed, this is an effective mechanism to prevent or at least minimize immunogenicity of a dying cell and, as a consequence, to maintain an immunologically tolerant state of tissues.

Efferocytosis can be generally categorized into four steps: (1) the release of "find-me" signals by dying cells to recruit phagocytes, (2) phagocyte recognition and engagement of "eat-me" signals on dying cells, (3) the engulfment of the cellular corpse, and (4) the processing, degradation, and immune response to the engulfed corpse. The "find-me" stage of efferocytosis is mediated by the secretion or release of numerous soluble factors that attract macrophages to the site of cell death, including the DAMP eATP and the chemokine (C-X3-C motif) ligand (CX3CL). There are also many "eat-me" signals on the surface of dying cells, which are recognized by specific "efferocytic receptors" on the phagocyte. They include the exposed DAMP CALR recognized by the scavenger receptor CD91 and a number of PtdSer molecules binding to several receptors such as GPCR, integrins, and TIM and TAM family PtdSer receptors (also compare [8, 9]; for "find-me" and "eat-me" signals, see Vol. 1 [1], Part IV, Sects. 12.2.5.2, p. 238 and 12.3.2.2, p. 246 and Fig. 12.5, p. 247; for efferocytosis receptors, see Sect. 2.3.2).

Following engulfment of apoptotic cells, multiple metabolic sensing pathways are reportedly engaged in macrophages that play essential roles in controlling phagocytosis and innate immune signaling. Among these metabolite-sensing mechanisms, the nuclear receptor family of transcriptional regulators represents a link between sensing of ingested apoptotic cells and the macrophage efferocytosis machinery. As reviewed elsewhere [10], studies using genetic and pharmacologic manipulation have identified multiple nuclear receptor family members as crucial regulators of efferocytosis, including the *liver X receptors* (LXRs) LXRα, LXRβ, *peroxisome proliferator activating receptor-gamma* [PPARγ], PPARδ, and *retinoid X receptor-alpha* (RXRα). Notably, as a master transcription factor, PPARγ can shift production from pro- to antiinflammatory mediators, alters macrophage trafficking, increases efferocytosis and phagocytosis, and promotes alternative M2-like macrophage activation [4, 11].

At this point, it should already be noted again—as outlined in Vol. 1 [1], Part V, Sect. 19.3 and above in Sect. 4.3—that, besides apoptosis, other forms of RCD have been described that can occur following inflammation, including necroptosis, ferroptosis, pyroptosis, and NETosis. All these subroutines of RN are known to be associated with the release of large amounts of DAMPs and, thus, may represent causal sources of nonresolving chronic inflammatory responses (see below).

5.3.2.3 Participation of Neutrophils and Macrophages in Inflammation Resolution

Neutrophils and macrophages are not only PRM-bearing innate immune cells to promote inflammation but are also involved in its resolution. For example, participation of neutrophils (also called alternative N2 neutrophils; see below) in the resolution phase of inflammation is documented by a report showing that oxidative burst-dependent NETosis is implicated in the resolution of necroinflammation [12]. These events are accompanied by further resolving processes, including clearance of proinflammatory dead cells and cytokines, as well as recruitment or phenotype switching of macrophages to antiinflammatory phenotype. In particular, the appearance of "antiinflammatory proresolving M2-like macrophages" is a characteristic sign of resolution. This transition from proinflammatory (classically activated) M1-like macrophages to antiinflammatory (alternatively activated) M2-like macrophages is a unique feature of macrophage plasticity that is transcriptionally [13], immunometabolically [14], and epigenetically [15, 16] regulated. Indeed, a striking example is the epigenetic control of M1-like or M2-like polarization that has been shown to rely on PTMs of histone proteins adjacent to inflammatory-related genes. Changes in methylation and acetylation of histones by methyltransferases, demethylases, acetyltransferases, and deacetylases can all impact how macrophage phenotypes are generated (reviewed in [17, 18]; see also Sect. 5.6, and compare Vol. 1 [1], Part III, Sect. 8.2.2.2 and Fig. 8.2 and Part VI, Sect. 22.2.3.2). M2-like macrophages—under epigenetic control, e.g., by histone methyltransferases (HMTs)—respond to IL-4/IL-13 and IL-10 and are mainly characterized by secretion of a variety of antiinflammatory mediators such as IL-10 and TGF-β1 [19] as well as chemokines such as *chemokine C-X-C motif ligand 10* (CXCL10), CXCL16, and *chemokine (C-C motif) ligand 5* (CCL5) [20] (for chemokines and their receptors, see Vol.1 [1], Part VI, Sect. 22.5.11 and Table 22.1). Also, they express cell surface receptors like *programmed death-ligand 1* (PD-L1) and PD-L2 that play significant roles in suppressing the immune system and quieting the inflammation (for additional information see also Vol. 1 [1], Part VIII, Sect. 33.3.5.4, p. 807).

Similar to the scenario of M1-like to M2-like polarization, transition of proinflammatory N1 neutrophils into inflammation-resolving N2 neutrophils has gained increasing attention in the research field of inflammation resolution. N2 neutrophils have been classified by Fridlender et al. [21] in the context of studies on tumor-associated neutrophils. The authors proposed that tumor-associated neutrophils—like tumor-associated macrophages—have differential states of activation/differentiation in that they can take an anti-tumorigenic phenotype (called an "N1-phenotype") versus a pro-tumorigenic phenotype (called an "N2 phenotype"). Given the observations that neutrophils can take on different phenotypes and functions during physiological conditions as well as in various diseases, the terms N1 and N2 neutrophils were adopted by researchers in the field of inflammation, whereby N1 neutrophils—in analogy to M1-like macrophages—were assumed to exert proinflammatory and N2 neutrophils, in analogy to M2-like macrophages, inflammation-resolving capabilities (also compare [22]).

5.3.2.4 Concluding Remarks

The scenario of elimination and transdifferentiation of innate immune cells in the resolving phase of inflammation is an impressive example of how evolution has solved the problem of achieving restitutio ad integrum following any tissue injury. Given the growing evidence for a role of DAMPs in the induction of epigenetic modifications (compare Sect. 3.7.2), one may discuss the unproven possibility that this mechanism is also involved in the epigenetically controlled polarization of macrophages into M2-like cells (also compare Fig. 5.1).

5.3.3 The Model of SAMP-Promoted Resolution of Inflammation

5.3.3.1 General Remarks

As outlined in Vol. 1 [1], Part IV, Sect. 14.4, every biological reaction in life is characterized by the action of both initially activating (agonists) and subsequently suppressing/inhibiting molecules (antagonists); the aim is not to cause dyshomeostasis. This life-protecting rule in biological systems includes regulation of the complex inflammatory processes: promotion of inflammation upon infectious and noninfectious/sterile cell stress and tissue injury and, subsequently, strictly regulated resolution of inflammation to ensure maintenance of homeostasis. Indeed, a fine-tuning of the inflammatory responses is the prerequisite to guarantee the outcome of inflammatory processes that strive for promotion of wound healing and tissue repair. As introduced in Sect. 3.5.5, it is the work of SAMPs—produced by DAMP-activated cells—that, in parallel to DAMP-triggered proinflammatory responses, convey antiinflammatory/proresolving processes and shape immunosuppressive responses. These unique regulating molecules have already been cursorily presented in separate sections in Vol. 1 [1], Part IV, Sect. 14.4, and Part VI, Sect. 22.2.3. They include, but are not limited to, PGE2 [23–25], cAMP [26–28], extracellular adenosine [29, 30], AnxA1 [31–34], SPMs [35–37], and PtdSer—lysoPS [38–44]. Some of these molecules will be re-addressed in the context of trauma in Sect. 8.3.4. Here, given the enormous progress made in recent research work, the topic of SPMs and their triggered responses are resumed and complemented.

5.3.3.2 Specialized Proresolving Mediator-Triggered Proresolving/Immunosuppressive Responses

The function of SPMs—produced, for example, by activated M2-like macrophages—reflects the intention of evolution to take care of providing counterregulation/counterbalance of biological defense responses for maintaining homeostasis. Thus, similar to AnxA1, SPMs were shown to contribute to resolution mechanisms by restricting neutrophil tissue recruitment and accumulation, neutralizing the activity of proinflammatory cytokines, and promoting macrophage phagocytosis. Intriguingly, during efferocytosis, phagocytic cells generate SPMs such as resolvins that serve as "autacoids" (i.e., biological factors acting like local hormones) to inhibit neutrophil activation, increase apoptotic cell expression of CC-chemokine receptor 5 (CCR5) for chemokine clearance, and provoke bacterial killing and efferocytosis by macrophages [36, 45].

Innate Immune Receptor-Mediated Functions of Specialized Proresolving Mediators

Notably, to mediate cell-type-specific actions, SPMs principally serve as ligands for select surface receptors, that is, proresolving GPCRs (for GPCRs and GPCR signaling, see Sect. 2.3.4, and compare Vol. 1 [1], Part II, Sect. 5.3.5.3, Fig. 5.11, and Part VI, Sect. 22.3.10). So far, four GPCR have been identified as the receptors for LXA4 and the D- and E-series of resolvins, namely, ALX/FPR2, DRV1/GPR32, DRV2/GPR18, and ERV1/ChemR23 [46] (see Sect. 2.3.4.6).

The distinct functions of SPMs are multifactorial and include the ability to terminate infiltration of inflammatory leukocytes into injured tissue and mediating stop signals to limit further leukocyte recruitment. Further, SPMs were shown to enhance macrophage phagocytosis of apoptotic leukocytes (efferocytosis) and cellular debris; in turn, efferocytosis promotes SPM production by macrophages, including LXA4, RvE1, and PD. Moreover, SPMs were demonstrated to decrease excessive oxidative stress [47], to augment bacteria-killing by phagocytes, to act at both the transcriptional and translational level, and to shorten the time to resolution by activation of endogenous resolution programs (see [48]). For example, RvE1 and RvE2 were found to stimulate the antiinflammatory cytokine IL-10 and phagocytosis potently; and LXA4, RvD1, and RvE1, as well as the maresin intermediate eMaR, were observed to stimulate transdifferentiation of M1-like to M2-like macrophages [49–53] (also compare, Fig. 3.4). Also, SPMs, in particular, the lipoxins, were observed to operate as chemoattractants that recruit monocytes, which, after differentiating into macrophages, enhance the overall efferocytic capacity of resolving lesions.

As already touched, specific SPMs are temporally and differentially regulated during both infections and sterile tissue responses to injury. Thus, as reported [54], in both *E. coli* and *Staphylococcus aureus* infections, RvD2 was shown to limit neutrophil infiltration and enhance phagocyte clearance of bacteria; after sterile injury from ischemia/reperfusion, the same SPM reportedly provides organ protection with decreased neutrophil infiltration to lungs. Interestingly, in this model,

RvD2 administration was demonstrated to increase tissue levels of other SPMs in a receptor-mediated manner to propel a positive-feedback loop for resolution. Of note, as reviewed by Duffney et al. [55], there is growing evidence suggesting that SPMs such as RvD, RvE1, can regulate DC activation markers, including suppression of signal 1 (expression of MHC), signal 2 (expression of costimulatory markers), and signal 3 (secretion of cytokines). Also, as recently reported elsewhere [56], SPMs (RvD2) can inhibit the priming and activation of the macrophage NLRP3 inflammasome. Moreover, in these experiments in mice, RvD2 was observed to increase the polarization of M2-like macrophages involved in the resolution of inflammation. Importantly, this study provides evidence for the ability of SPMs to limit inflammation and promote resolution by deactivating the NLRP3 inflammasome.

Interestingly, apart from their effect on DCs, neutrophils, and macrophages, SPMs were shown to augment a resolution mechanism mediated by the cytotoxic properties of NK cells that can promote granulocyte apoptosis for their clearance [57].

SPM-Modulated Adaptive Immune Responses

The important breakthroughs concerning the effects of SPMs on the key cell types involved in the development of adaptive immunity, namely, besides DCs, T cells, and B cells, were recently reviewed by Duffney et al. [55]. In a series of in vitro experiments performed by Chiurchiu et al. [58], the SPMs RvD1, RvD2, and MaR1 were shown to modulate adaptive immune responses in human peripheral blood lymphocytes. These lipid mediators were found to strongly reduce lineage-specific cytokine production by activated $CD4^+$ Th1 (i.e., IFN-γ) and $CD4^+$ Th17 cells (i.e., IL-17) as well as $CD8^+$ T cells (i.e., TNF, IFN-γ), but not to modulate T-cell inhibitory receptors (e.g., PD-1 and CTLA-4) or abrogate their capacity to proliferate (for PD-1 and CTLA-4, compare Vol. 1 [1], Part VIII, Sect. 33.3.5 and Fig. 33.3). Further targeted in vitro experiments revealed that the tested SPMs can prevent naïve $CD4^+$ T-cell differentiation into Th1 and Th17 by downregulating their signature transcription factors, T-bet and *retinoic acid receptor-related orphan receptor-gamma t* (RORγt) [58] (for Th cell subsets, see Vol. 1 [1], Part VIII, Sect. 32.4; and for these transcription factors, compare Vol. 1 [1], Part VIII, Sect. 32.4 and Fig. 32.4). Moreover, it could be demonstrated that SPMs can either up- or downregulate antibody production depending on the B-cell subset and specific SPM involved. Specialized proresolving mediators were also found to decrease cytokine production frequently. But—as too stressed by the investigators—some SPMs can also stimulate cytokine release in other cell types (reviewed in [55]).

This mechanism was found to be mediated by members of the GPCR family, that is, GPR32 and ALX/FPR2 (for GPCRs and GPCR signaling, see Sect. 2.3.4; and compare also Vol. 1 [1], Part II, Sect. 5.3.5.3, Fig. 5.11, and Part VI, Sect. 22.3.10). In these studies, the authors could also show that SPMs—concomitantly with Th1 and Th17 downregulation—enhance de novo generation and function of *inducible forkhead box protein 3 ($Foxp3^+$) regulatory T cells* (iTregs) via the GPR32 receptor (compare Fig. 5.1) (for additional information about iTregs, see Vol. 1 [1], Part VIII, Sect. 33.4.3.3, p. 813 and Fig. 33.4, p. 801). These findings are supported by another study on the property of the SPM MaR1 [59]. In these in vitro experiments, MaR1—together with TGF-β—was found to promote generation of iTregs.

Regulation of Lipid Mediators by Vagus Nerve and Vagotomy

Evidence obtained from studies in humans and experimental animal models support the notion that the vagus nerve can control the magnitude and duration of inflammation. Of note, there is now growing evidence for a role of the vagus nerve in regulating the resolution of infectious inflammation via control of SPMs. As reviewed by Serhan and Levy [48] and Serhan et al. [60], in experiments on mice, vagotomy was shown to reduce proresolving mediators, including the Lxs, Rvs, Pds, and MaRs, thereby delaying resolution in peritonitis. Also, vagotomy was found to delay resolution of *E. coli* infection in mice. Specifically, the right vagus could be demonstrated to regulate peritoneal ILC-3 number and peritoneal macrophage responses with lipid mediator profile signatures with elevated proinflammatory eicosanoids and reduced resolvins (for ILC-3, see Vol. 1 [1], Part III, Sect. 8.4.2 and Fig. 8.3). On the other hand, findings observed in other studies indicate that vagus stimulation increases proresolving mediators that can directly stimulate resolution of inflammation and infections by virtue of their ability to act on phagocytes to reduce and counterregulate proinflammatory mediator substances [35].

Moreover, results obtained with human vagus ex vivo provided evidence indicating that vagus can produce both proinflammatory eicosanoids, such as prostaglandins and leukotrienes, and the SPMs. Electrical stimulation of human vagus in vitro reduces both prostaglandins and leukotrienes and enhances resolvins and the other SPMs. Together, these interesting observations reveal a host protective mechanism mediated by vagus stimulation of SPMs that includes resolvins and the novel protective immunoresolvent agonist *protectin conjugate in tissue regeneration 1* (PCTR1) to regulate myeloid antimicrobial functions and resolution of infection. Hence—as stressed by Serhan and Levy [48]—"plasticity of neural networks and their innate immune system interactions are regulated by specific SPMs."

Role of SPMs in Resolution of Pain

Earlier studies in murine pain models had already revealed that RvE1 and RvD1 are effective in resolving inflammatory and postoperative pain [61, 62]. In these studies, the analgesic effects of resolvins was shown to be mediated by specific GPCRs that are widely expressed by neurons and can regulate TRP ion channels and spinal cord synaptic transmission (for TRP ion channels and GPCRs acting as exogenous DAMPs-sensing nociceptors, see Sect. 2.3.5, and Vol. 1 [1], Part IV, Sect. 15.3 and Fig. 15.1). Further studies then showed that SPMs convey their pain-relieving effect via inhibition of TRP ion channels. Thus, RvE1 was shown to block TRPV1 selectively, RvD1 to act via TRPA1, and RvD2 to operate via TRPV1 and TRPA1 [63].

5.3.3.3 Concluding Remarks

The role of SPMs as typical SAMPs in mechanisms of resolution is impressive and explains many puzzling inflammation-associated phenomena discovered in earlier times of research. Certainly, there is a great future of SPMs in using them as therapeutic targets or therapeutics. In this context, Serhan and Levy [48] conclude:

"SPMs have proven potent proresolving actions in a range of disease models...; given their potency, many drug development opportunities are possible. Human PMN swarming activates a temporal biosynthetic code that produces stop signals, e.g., LXA4 and resolvins, at critical PMN densities.... Temporal biosynthesis with lipid mediator class switching is documented in human blisters... and with specific drugs... (e.g., dexmedetomidine) that can prevent cognitive decline by activating SPMs...."

In the following chapters on traumatic diseases and atherosclerosis, the involvement of SPMs in their function as key SAMPs will be resumed when and if appropriate.

5.3.4 Résumé

The discovery of the phenomenon of resolution of inflammation as an active capacity of the innate immune system can be seen as a new dimension in clinical inflammation research and practice. Among medical circles, the topic gains increasing attention in the fields of the post-trauma hyperresolution phase and chronic inflammatory disorders. Further increase of our knowledge regarding the vital molecular and cellular mechanisms underlying this unique process will enable researchers and clinicians to explore and apply sophisticated therapeutic options to interfere—if necessary—with pathogenic proresolving pathways without compromising the proinflammatory healing processes (compare Chap. 7).

5.4 Hyperinflammation and Counterbalancing "Hyperresolution"

5.4.1 Introductory Remarks

For a long time, acute hyperinflammatory conditions are known to physicians as typical signs of patients suffering from sepsis in the course of bacterial, viral, or fungal infection. Indeed, patients with sepsis often present with high levels of fever, septic shock, respiratory failure, and, occasionally, MOF, a symptomology that led to the prevailing concept that sepsis represents an uncontrolled dysregulated acute inflammatory response. The discovery that various cellular and humoral proinflammatory mediators, including complement, are markedly elevated in septic patients (and when administered to animals reproducing some clinical features of sepsis) resulted in the concept of sepsis as a cytokine storm, today known as SIRS.

Soon, the recognition of an overshooting inflammatory nature of sepsis provided plausibly attractive targets for new antiinflammatory molecules designed to treat the life-threatening disease and prevent further propagation. New agents were designed to inhibit, bind, or neutralize the inflammatory mediators that were felt to be responsible for the network of events that culminated in the clinical manifestations.

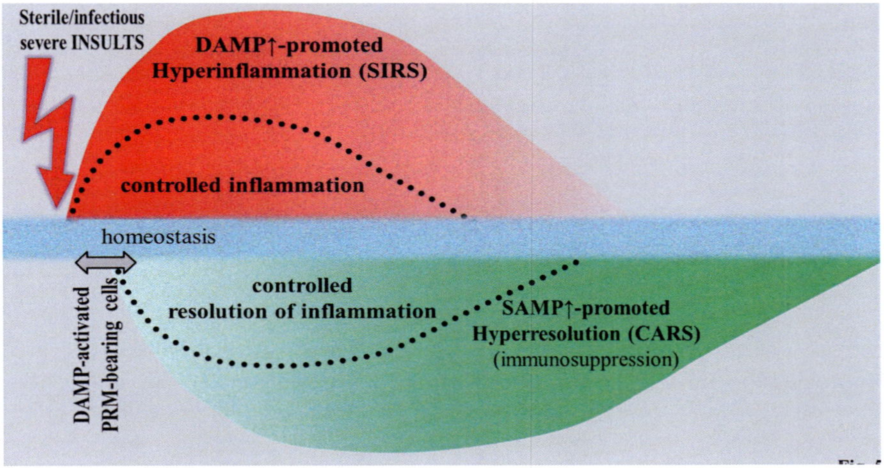

Fig. 5.2 Schematic diagram of a conceptual model illustrating the hyperinflammatory response in SIRS induced by excessive production of DAMPs that proceeds in parallel to a long-lasting hyperresolution response in CARS caused by counterregulating production of SAMPs in excess (the controlled homeostatic proinflammatory and resolving responses are faded in, separated by dotted lines). Clinically, the long-lasting hyperresolution phase is characterized by a state of immunosuppression. *CARS* compensatory anti-inflammatory response syndrome, *PRM* pattern recognition molecule, *SIRS* systemic inflammatory response syndrome

Disappointingly, however, targeted clinical trial then showed that most of these agents failed to cure the septic disease.

Intriguingly, it was this observation that paved the way to another previously undiscovered typical symptomatic feature of the disorder: the post-sepsis immunosuppression, today called CARS. Both syndromes, SIRS in terms of hyperinflammation and CARS in terms of post sepsis immunosuppression, have found their way into daily routine diagnostics in intensive care units (Fig. 5.2). Hence, a few more words should be added in the following.

5.4.2 Systemic Inflammatory Response Syndrome: An Example of Hyperinflammation

5.4.2.1 General Remarks

Already nearly three decades ago, continuous elucidation of knowledge about the complex pathophysiologic response involved in sepsis had culminated in the creation of the term SIRS (reviewed in [64-67]). Indeed, the SIRS concept derives from a 1991 consensus conference charged with the task of developing an easy-to-apply set of clinical parameters to aid in the early identification of potential candidates for entrance into clinical trials aimed at evaluating new treatments for sepsis. In this conference, broad definitions of sepsis and SIRS were proposed, along with detailed physiologic parameters by which a patient may be categorized [68, 69].

Of note, after 1991, when the concept of SIRS was created, several publications emerged heralding the efficacy of SIRS in predicting post-traumatic outcomes (reviewed in [70]). In 2005, Keel and Trentz wrote [71]: "In accordance with these pathophysiological mechanisms and definition of SIRS, the term polytrauma can be defined as a syndrome of combined injuries with an injury severity score (ISS) > 17 and consequent SIRS for at least 1 day, leading to dysfunction, or failure, of remote organs and vital systems, which themselves had not directly been injured." In 2006, Keel et al. stated [72] that "the severity of injury, estimated by the ISS... , and the gender determine the incidence of posttraumatic complications such as SIRS, sepsis, MODS, or mortality." In the following time, examples of such septic conditions were extended to include severe burns, IRI, and hemorrhagic shock.

5.4.2.2 Pathophysiology of SIRS

The pathophysiology of SIRs—often associated with a multiple organ dysfunction syndrome (MODS) or even MOF—is overwhelmingly dominated by hyperinflammatory processes as classically characterized by demonstration of elevated plasma levels of multiple powerful cellular and humoral proinflammatory mediators, which are comprehensively outlined and explained in Vol.1. [1], Part VI, Chaps. 22 and 23. As documented in many experimental and clinical studies, these sepsis-associated mediators include cytokines (e.g., TNF, IL-1α, IL-1β, and IL-6), chemokines, adhesion molecules, gaseous substances, vasoactive peptides, and cell stress markers (reviewed in [73-76]). Apart from these dysregulated inflammatory responses, other pathogenetic mechanisms have been described, which to mention, however, are beyond the scope of this section (for comprehensive reviews, see [66, 77, 78]). Instead, a few remarks are made to the issue of the imbalance in the redox system. In fact, during sepsis, biochemical changes lead to an imbalance in the redox system resulting in formation of an oxidant state, which appears to intensify SIRS and the downstream events. This is not a surprise since oxidative stress is known to promote emission of DAMPs. Indeed, the involvement of ROS and RNS such as nitric oxide (NO), peroxynitrite ($ONOO^-$), superoxide (O_2), hydrogen peroxide (H_2O_2), and hydroxyl radical (OH) has been reported to be involved in septic processes [66, 79]. In parallel, the antioxidative defense system is obviously disturbed (for this stress response, see Sect. 4.2.3, and compare Vol. 1 [1], Part V, Sect. 18.3). This kind of involvement of oxidative stress is a strong argument for the use of antioxidative therapy that has reportedly already been shown to be a beneficial adjuvant therapy of severe sepsis and septic shock (e.g., [80]).

5.4.2.3 Role of DAMPs in Sepsis and "Sepsis-Like" Hyperinflammation (SIRS)

In accordance with this new recognition of "sterile SIRS" as a severe "sepsis-like" complication in polytrauma patients, first clues to a critical role of DAMPs in the promotion of those hyperinflammatory responses were reported soon [81, 82]. In 2012, Ward wrote [82]: "Collectively, sufficient amounts of DAMPs can trigger a sepsis-like response resulting in a 'cytokine storm' [defined as presence of proinflammatory cytokines/chemokines in plasma and also referred to as the systemic inflammatory response syndrome (SIRS)]." Today, it is widely accepted by intensive care physicians that DAMPs systemically released in excess are the vital predominant molecules which induce PRM-triggered innate immune signaling pathways leading to SIRS [29, 83–88] (also compare Fig. 5.2). Basically, every DAMP proven to promote efferent proinflammatory pathways can be considered to be involved in the development of SIRS. As abundant sources of DAMPs emission, the various subroutines of RCD may be considered. Among those molecules, DAMPs of various classes have already been reported to activate innate immune responses in sepsis and sepsis-induced organ dysfunction, including HMGB1, HSPs, S100A8/9 proteins, histones, nDNA/mtDNA, and members of the IL-1 cytokine family (for corresponding articles, see [85, 89–93]; compare also Table. 3.1 in Chap. 3). Not to forget should be the anaphylatoxin C5a that was denoted as an inducible IIIB-3 DAMP in Vol. 1 [1], Part IV, Sect. 14.3.4. Indeed, in septic human beings, there is abundant evidence for complement activation and C5a production. In an experimental model of sepsis (cecal ligation and puncture model), interception of C5a or its receptors was shown to improve significantly survival in septic rodents, associated with mitigation of the consumptive septic coagulopathy as well as reduction of the hyperinflammatory response, reduced intensity of MOF, and septic shock (reviewed in [94, 95]).

Together, the pathogenetic role of DAMPs in pathogen-caused "infectious" sepsis is currently widely accepted (compare [96]). In Sect. 8.3.3, other DAMPs most critically involved in sterile "sepsis-like" disorders will be mentioned when and if appropriate.

5.4.2.4 Concluding Remarks

The emission of DAMPs upon severe sterile insults or MAMPs/DAMPs upon infectious injuries has impressively enriched modern insights into pathogenetic processes implicated in hyperinflammation—SIRS. More precisely stressed, given the parallelly running phases of promotion of inflammation and resolution of inflammation, the DAMPs:SAMPs ratio is high in that excessively emitted DAMPs outweigh (for DAMPs:SAMPs ratio, also see Sect. 7.3.3).

Nevertheless, the exact patho-innate immune mechanisms and direct involvement of DAMPs in the pathophysiology of sepsis is still not fully elucidated. In particular, it has to be explored whether there is a distinct pattern of DAMPs emission that may help differentiate between various forms of sepsis, for example, between sterile and infectious (bacterial or viral) sepsis. Exploration and final assessment of such DAMPs pattern may allow to define the exact roles of DAMPs in hyperinflammation further and develop specific inhibitors targeting DAMPs. Therapeutics targeting to DAMPs then may provide an innovative interventional approach for the clinical treatment of sepsis (see Chap. 7).

5.4.3 Compensatory Antiinflammatory Response Syndrome: An Example of Hyperresolution

5.4.3.1 General Remarks

For a long time, intensive care physicians had observed that patients with sepsis are prone to severe, sometimes lethal infectious diseases. In search of the causes during the 1970s and 1980s, researchers found out that many of these infected patients had acquired an impaired immune state characterized by various markers of immunosuppression. These observations were supported by other lines of clinical studies on sepsis patients treated—according to the prevailing concept of sepsis as a hyperinflammatory disease—with antiinflammatory agents. These studies failed to show a convincing beneficial effect and even suggested that harm could be done in some cases [97]. It was then Bone [98] who, by referring to this dilemma, coined the term CARS to help to describe the phenomenon of impaired immunity that was frequently observed in septic conditions. It became soon apparent that the CARS response essentially reverses many of the typical events encountered in SIRS. Guided by this new recognition, subsequent research over the last several decades then uncovered stepwise the antiinflammatory and immunosuppressive mechanisms that govern this disorder.

Today, CARS can be regarded as a disorder caused by hyperresolution of hyperinflammation in terms of a mirror-imaged counterregulation of SIRS. Of note, however, instead of a previously assumed biphasic inflammatory response consisting of an initial proinflammatory response and a subsequent compensatory antiinflammatory response, hyperresolving processes are now suggested to occur nearly in parallel with the hyperinflammatory response. There is presumably only a slight delay between initial hyperinflammation and subsequent hyperresolution that might be due to the excessive production of SAMPs by already DAMP-activated PRM-bearing innate immune cells. Nevertheless, there is a predominance of the initial hyperinflammatory phase, the scale of which may be preferentially determined by the amount of emitted DAMPs upon infectious or sterile injury as well as genetic factors. On the other hand, at the end of the hyperinflammatory state, the profound proresolving/immunosuppressive phase may still go on and make patients susceptible to secondary and/or nosocomial infections and consequential late-stage mortality (see Sect. 8.3.4 and Fig. 8.1).

5.4.3.2 Antiinflammatory/Immunosuppressive Mechanisms Involved in CARS

Remarkably, CARS is characterized by alterations in both the innate and the adaptive immune system that, on a cellular level, includes strong depletion of DCs, $CD4^+$ and $CD8^+$ T cells, and B cells, due to apoptosis. Beyond the loss of immune cells, a decreased cytokine response of monocytes to stimulation as well as expression of antiinflammatory cytokines such as IL-4, IL-10, IL-13, and TGF-β is typically associated with this disorder. In addition to the antiinflammatory response of the innate immune system, adaptive immune mechanisms are impaired. For example, MHC-II/HLA-DR expression on monocytes was shown to be persistently diminished associated with impaired antigen-presenting capabilities as a typical sign of sepsis-induced immunosuppression (for MHC-II-mediated direct presentation and cross-presentation of antigens, compare Vol. 1 [1], Part VIII, Sects. 31.3.4.1 and 31.3.6). Further, the $CD4^+$ T helper 1 cell (Th1)/Th2 cell ratio was observed to be imbalanced in terms of suppression of the Th1 response but enhancement of the Th2 response. Moreover, an increased frequency of Tregs has been found under septic conditions, mechanistically explained as a result of decreases in the effector populations of $CD4^{+}$ Th cells (for T helper cell responses, see Vol. 1 [1], Part VIII, Sects. 32.4 and 33.4). Besides Tregs, another population of suppressing cells, namely, myeloid-derived suppressor cells (MDSCs), is reportedly involved in CARS, mainly through stimulating the expansion of Tregs, and exertion of immunosuppressing effects on macrophages and DCs (for additional information compare also Vol. 1 [1], Part VIII, Sect. 33.4.8, p. 817). Finally, and of high interest, upregulation of coinhibitory receptors/checkpoint proteins was recently shown to contribute to post-sepsis immunosuppression. For example, upregulated expression of PD-1 and/or PD-L1 was demonstrated not only on adaptive immune cells such as T cells but also on innate immune cells including macrophages and neutrophils (for PD-1and PD-L1, see also Vol. 1 [1], Part VIII, Sect. 33.3.5 and Fig. 33.3). For more details of this emerging issue in sepsis research, the reader is referred to competent articles found in [99-106].

5.4.3.3 The Model of an Action of SAMPs in Hyperresolution

The model of SAMP-promoted resolution of inflammation has been outlined in Sect. 5.3.3. Logically, in reverse with the proinflammatory action of excessively emitted DAMPs in SIRS, production of SAMPs in excess should trigger hyperresolving pathways in CARS. More precisely expressed, given the parallelly running phases of promotion of inflammation and resolution of inflammation, the DAMPs:SAMPs ratio is low in that excessively emitted SAMPs outweigh (compare Fig. 5.2).

Indeed, the detection of PGE2 (a SAMP denoted as a IIIC-1 DAMP throughout this book) in in vitro and animal models of sepsis can be regarded as one of the first clues to SAMP-promoted proresolving processes involved in CARS (for informative articles, see also [107-112]). Also, the SAMP AnxA1 (a IIIC-3 DAMP) has been demonstrated to play a significant role in CARS, even in clinical studies. For example, in a subgroup of sepsis patients, the circulating level of AnxA1 was found to be elevated [113]. Moreover, in studies on sepsis in patients with severe trauma, the common promoter polymorphism *rs11666254* was shown to downregulate expression of the AnxA1-sensing FPR2 receptor and increase the risk of this dangerous disorder [114] (for FPRs, see Sect. 2.3.4.5 and Vol. 1 [1], Part II, Sect. 5.3.5.3). Recent experimental studies on animal models strongly confirmed these clinical findings [115, 116]). Also, experimental evidence has been reported suggesting that cAMP (a IIIC-2 DAMP), via activation of the protein kinase, may be involved in CARS [117, 118]. Moreover, there is also first evidence for a role of SPMs in CARS. Thus, as reported by Dalli et al. [119], lipid mediator profiles in human septic patients were observed to be correlated with outcome. Increases in plasma levels of selected SPMs including RvE2, LXB4, and RvD2 were found to associate with patients that survive for 28 days post admission to the medical intensive care unit.

Together, these experimental and clinical findings support the notion that the "resolving SAMP axis" (*PGE2 ↔ EP2/EP4 → cAMP → PKA → AnxA1 ↔ FPR2 → resolution*) and SPMs may be operating in septic patients, and for this reason, CARS may also be denoted as a "hyperresolution" syndrome (for resolving SAMP axis, compare also Vol. 1 [1], Part IV, Sect. 14.4.2.4 and Fig. 14.5).

Of note, besides these SAMPs mentioned, DAMPs acting as context-dependent SAMPs have been described. For example, in studies on 166 adult trauma patients, Timmermans et al. [120] observed an immunosuppressive effect of plasma nuclear DNA (nDNA) and HSP70 levels, higher concentrations of nDNA being found to be associated with infections (for more information, in particular, the puzzle of increased plasma levels of DAMPs associated with immunosuppression, see Sect. 8.3.5).

5.4.3.4 Concluding Remarks

According to modern trends in intensive care medicine, hyperresolution appears to be the most commonly used concept to qualify the immune status of patients with either sterile ("sepsis-like") or infectious SIRS. The definition of this critical septic complication as a form of immunosuppression is probably an oversimplification of the complex exaggerated antiinflammatory/proresolving response that is seen in patients dealing with a severe sterile or infectious insult. The central role of SAMPs in this life-threatening disorder is of great advantage and will certainly pave new ways to more successful therapeutic modalities in the near future.

5.4.4 Résumé

The clinical picture of SIRS and CARS has always been and still is a burning and challenging issue in intensive care medicine and, for this reason, has been tentatively chosen as examples for the description of the emerging model of DAMP-induced hyperinflammation and SAMP-promoted hyperresolution. As two sides of the same coin, both pathological conditions are subject to modern research in inflammation. In fact, researchers, together with intensive care clinicians, will have to explore novel therapeutic strategies aimed at balancing the two hyperreactive phases of one and the same life-threatening disease, that is, to reduce DAMP-induced hyperinflammation, on the one hand, and SAMP-promoted hyperresolution, on the other side. The topic will be resumed in Sect. 8.4.4.

5.5 Chronic Inflammation: A State of Nonresolving Inflammation

5.5.1 Introductory Remarks

Chronic inflammation—organ-specific or systemic—does underlie many chronic human diseases, perhaps even all of them, in one or the other form. Typical examples are pathogen-mediated, autoimmune, allergic, (neuro)degenerative, atherosclerotic, and malignant disorders. Chronic diseases, regardless of etiology and pathogenesis, adversely affect patients in terms of physical suffering and pain, impaired function, and diminished quality of life. In addition to the significant burden on patients and their families, chronic inflammatory diseases reflect a considerable burden on society due to high healthcare- and non-healthcare-related costs. Indeed, perhaps no single phenomenon contributes more to the medical burden in industrialized societies than nonresolving inflammation [121].

In Vol. 1 [1], Part VI, Sect. 22.2.4, the topic was already briefly addressed. Here, some fundamental aspects are touched again without going into detail. More information will be presented when dealing with single diseases in Chaps. 10 and 11.

5.5.2 The Role of DAMPs and SAMPs in Chronic Inflammation

Persistent or acute/chronic repetitive cell stress/tissue injury associated with various subroutines of RCD together with predisposing genetic factors (e.g., polymorphism of genes of the HLA system) is the prerequisite for chronic inflammatory responses. Modern notions in inflammation research now hold that chronic inflammation reflects a state of nonresolving inflammation fired and sustained by those insults (Fig. 5.3). The nature of these insults can vary depending on different causes such as:

– The presence of chronic infection in case of incomplete elimination of pathogens, e.g., *Mycobacterium tuberculosis*, methicillin-resistant *Staphylococcus aureus* in osteomyelitis; or in the form of persisting viral proteins in the absence of viral replication which may act as exogenously acquired, altered endogenous DAMPs

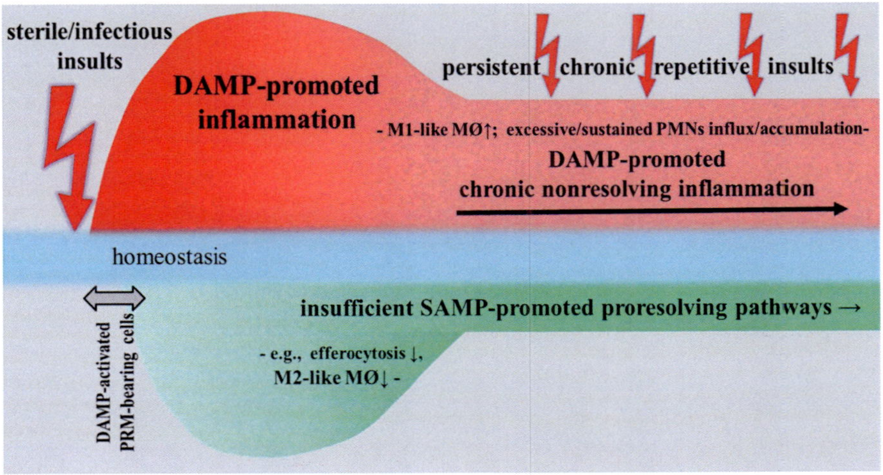

Fig. 5.3 Schematic diagram of a conceptual model illustrating a state of nonresolving inflammation, clinically manifested as chronic inflammation. Chronic nonresolving inflammation may be caused by either persistent or acute/chronic repetitive generation of high amounts of DAMPs that surpass the "normal" production of counterregulating SAMPs, or by defective proresolving mechanisms such as impaired efferocytosis, insufficient SAMPs emission, and a decreased number of M2-like macrophages. *MØ* macrophages, *PMNs* polymorphonuclear neutrophils, *PRM* pattern recognition molecule

- Disturbed metabolism, for example, due to chronic stress of the ER induced by accumulation of proinsulin
- Adaptive autoimmunity, as a result of the action of cytotoxic autoantibodies and autoreactive T lymphocytes
- Exposure to environmental chemicals/toxins (i.e., exogenous DAMPs, such as silica particles, air pollution particles, asbestos fibers, allergens)
- Continuous physical/traumatic forces, for example, tendonitis due to repetitive use or overuse of a certain area of the body
- Finally, the action of toxic ROS which may be secondarily generated in the course of inflammation

All these insults are intrinsically associated with the emission of more or less amounts of various classes of DAMPs. Accordingly, and in principle, chronic inflammation can be caused either by persistent or acute/chronic repetitive generation of such high amounts of DAMPs that surpass the "normal (homeostasis-striving)" production of counterregulatory SAMPs or by a (genetically determined) failure of the inflammation resolution response due to defective SAMPs emission, or even by both scenarios, when the DAMPs:SAMPs ratio is high in that DAMPs outweigh. For example, as reviewed [122], causes of inappropriate or inefficient resolving mechanisms can be found on a cellular or humoral level. Cellular roots mainly refer to the failure of neutrophils to undergo timely apoptosis, or failure of M2-like macrophages to clear those apoptotic neutrophils by efferocytosis [123], or an abnormal T-cell response, for instance, deficiency in Tregs. On the other hand, defective, that is, reduced or delayed, expression of soluble resolving factors such as SPMs or antiinflammatory cytokines may be the reason for ongoing inflammatory processes. For example, exudates from ongoing inflammation were shown to have a significant imbalance in the SPMs (SAMPs = IIIC-4 DAMPs) to proinflammatory leukotriene (IIIA-7 DAMPs) ratio compared with exudates from self-limited or resolving inflammation [124].

5.5.3 Résumé and Future Perspectives

Together, from a reductionist's point of view, chronic inflammation/frustrated resolution reflects a pathological alteration of the DAMPs:SAMPs ratio in favor of DAMP-promoted proinflammatory pathways. The real problem here is that chronic inflammatory processes can lead to further collateral tissue injury, thereby sustaining a vicious circle of inflammation. Are autoantigens involved, this scenario may even result in an autoimmune disease.

Clearly, nonresolving inflammation is by no means a primary cause of chronic inflammatory diseases such as atherosclerosis, obesity, cancer, COPD, asthma, inflammatory bowel disease, neurodegenerative disorders, or rheumatoid arthritis, but it contributes significantly to their pathogenesis. Further exploration of the function of DAMPs and SAMPs in such aggrieving diseases will undoubtedly help make proper therapeutic decisions as to whether and when to block DAMPs and administer SAMPs, with the aim to restore a "healthy/homeostatic" DAMP:SAMP ratio.

5.6 Epigenetics in Inflammation

5.6.1 Introductory Remarks

To prevent the potentially life-threatening destructive effects of efferent innate immune proinflammatory responses, the expression of inflammation-related genes is finely tuned and regulated at multiple levels, including transcription, mRNA processing, translation, PTMs, and degradation/ubiquitination (for additional information compare Vol. 1 [1], Part VI, Chpt. 24, p. 635). Transcriptional processes represent an essential, and often the most crucial, regulatory determinant of the inflammation process. As described in Vol. 1 [1], Part VI, Chpt. 22, many signaling pathways and transcription factors are involved in the inflammatory response, including NF-κB, MAPK, IRF, and JAK/STAT pathways, all factors controlling a large variety of inflammatory response genes. Upon activation by MAMPs and DAMPs or DAMPs, these pathways directly trigger and induce the expression of a limited set of transcription factors that promote the transcription of those inflammatory genes. However, these regulatory pathways are not sufficient enough to maintain and restore homeostasis in any situation. To fully guarantee homeostasis, the transcription of inflammatory genes must be finely controlled in the nucleus to ensure that each distinct gene is transcribed appropriately and at the "right" place at the "right" time.

Thus, all innate and adaptive immune cells involved in the regulation of inflammatory processes are confronted with the problem of controlling the requirement-dependent amounts and timing of expression of their various genes. Depending on the environmental circumstances, this control involves very short-term or relatively long-term but heritable modifications to the chromatin, albeit nonpermanent. Such modifications that do not change the DNA sequence are referred to as "epigenetic." The resulting epigenetic effects maintain the various patterns of gene expression in different cell types. Hence, expression of genes regulating innate immune processes such as pro-/antiinflammatory responses is not only controlled by MAMP-/DAMP-triggered transcriptional pathways but also by epigenetic modifications, which include DNA methylation, histone PTMs, and small noncoding RNA-associated regulation. In sum, the term "epigenetics" refers to the interaction of environmental factors, but also lifestyle and aging, with the genome that may result in heritable and modifiable gene expression or phenotype, which does not confer any changes in the DNA sequence itself.

Tremendous progress has been made in current research of epigenetics in various cellular processes, diseases, as well as behavior and sociality across the tree of life. The emerging impact of epigenetic regulations on innate immune events—that is, on acute/chronic inflammatory and fibrotic processes—has briefly been outlined in Vol. 1 [1], Part VI, Sect. 24.2 and Fig. 24.1. Each cell is equipped with the same DNA, yet what determines the phenotype and function of a cell is epigenetic. In fact, accumulating evidence has shown that innate immune cells, such as monocytes, macrophages, DCs, and NK cells, can be influenced by the encounters with injurious → inflammatory stimuli, undergoing functional reprogramming and developing changed responses to subsequent challenges [125]. And increasing evidence suggests—and this is the reason why the topic is presented in more detail here—that DAMPs may drive epigenetic modifications [126–128].

5.6.2 Some Basics of Epigenetic Modifications

5.6.2.1 General Remarks

To avoid uncomfortable turning back to Vol. 1 [1], Part VI, Sect. 24.2.2, at this point, a few basics of epigenetic modifications are briefly repeated here. In eukaryotic cells, DNA is packaged into chromatin, the basic repeating unit of which is a nucleosome. A nucleosome consists of 147 bp nucleotides wrapped around a histone octamer, which is composed of two copies each of histone H2A, H2B, H3, and H4. Nucleosomes are packaged into progressively higher-order structures to form chromosomes ultimately. Generally, such epigenetic changes can be categorized into several major biochemical mechanisms, including changes in (1) DNA methylation (primarily CpG cytosine-5 methylation); (2) covalent histone PTMs such as histone acetylation, methylation, phosphorylation, and ubiquitination (Fig. 5.4); and (3) RNA-based mechanisms (action of long and small noncoding RNAs) (Figs. 5.5 and 5.6).

5.6.2.2 Writers—Readers—Erasers—Epigenators

Importantly, these histone modifications lead to a change in the net charge of nucleosomes, relaxing interactions between histones and DNA. This directly affects the levels of chromatin compaction, creating condensed (closed) *heterochromatic* or more open *euchromatic* regions and thus restricting or allowing access of transcription factors to promoters or enhancers on DNA as well as DNA and RNA polymerases. Hence, all these modifications alter—as a key process—the accessibility of DNA to transcription machinery and therefore influence and regulate gene expression. In other words, chromatin exists in structural forms that provide access of DNA to transcription factors in responsive euchromatin and mask access to the transcriptional apparatus in compacted heterochromatin [129–135].

Proteins that carry out these DNA and histone tail modifications have been called either "writers" (histone-modifying enzymes), "readers" (acetyl- or methyl-binding proteins such as Bromo and Chromo), or "erasers" (histone-demodifying enzymes) [135–137]. Epigenetic writers catalyze the addition of chemical groups onto either histone tails or the DNA itself. These modifications are known as epigenetic marks. Epigenetic reader domains refer to effector proteins that recognize and are recruited to specific epigenetic marks, thereby aiding assembly of the appropriate transcriptional machinery at distinct sites of recognition. Notably, the histone modifications combinatorially and dynamically constitute "histone code," which accurately regulates not only a variety of DNA-templated processes but also chromosome segregation and DNA repair. Intriguingly, not only do histone modifications determine the accessibility of DNA but are also directly responsible for recruiting transcriptional machinery to specific loci. Also, it is worth noting that epigenetic marks are not

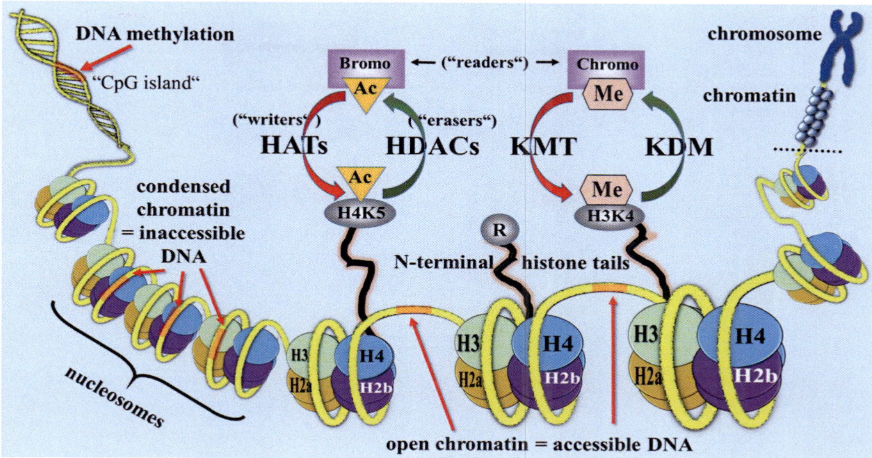

Fig. 5.4 Simplified schematic model of epigenetic modifications exemplified by DNA methylation, histone acetylation/deacetylation of H4 lysine 5, and histone methylation/demethylation of H3 lysine 4. The illustration shows the organization and packaging of genetic material. Each nucleosome is made of DNA wrapped around eight histone proteins that function like a spool and are called a histone octamer. Each histone octamer (here shown in four colored circles, one [H3] not visible) is composed of two copies each of the histone proteins H2A (brownish), H2B (violet), H3 (green), and H4 (blue). Histone modifications impact chromatin compaction, creating condensed (closed) heterochromatic or more open euchromatic regions and, thus, restricting or allowing access of transcription factors to promoters or enhancers on DNA as well as DNA and RNA polymerases. Hence, all these modifications change the accessibility of DNA to transcription machinery and therefore influence and regulate gene expression. Nucleosomes (eight-circle colored) are represented by DNA (yellow) wrapped around eight histone proteins, H2A, H2B, H3, and H4. N-terminal histone tails (black) are shown protruding from H3 and H4. DNA methylation occurs preferentially at CpG island. Covalent histone modifications are transduced by histone-modifying enzymes ("writers") and removed by antagonizing activities of enzymes ("erasers"). The type of enzyme action shown is acetylation and methylation. Protein domains with specific affinity for a histone tail modification are called "readers." *Ac* acetyl group, *Bromo* bromodomains, *Chromo* chromodomains, *CpG* cytosine phospho-bound guanosine, *HATs* histone acetyltransferases, *HDAC* histone deacetyltransferases, *K* lysine, *KDM* lysine demethylase, *KMT* lysine methyltransferase, *Me* methyl group, *R* arginine. (Sources: [135, 136, 156-158, 160, 174, 176, 179-182])

necessarily permanent modifications; by contrast, they can be removed by a group of enzymes known as "erasers" to reverse the influence of a given epigenetic mark on gene expression. Accordingly, such enzymes responsible for the addition/removal of these modifications include but are not limited to DNA methyltransferases (DNMTs) and demethylating *ten-eleven translocase* (TET); histone acetyltransferases (HATs) and histone deacetylases (HDACs); HMTs and histone demethylases (HDMs); as well as ubiquitin ligases/deubiquitinating enzymes (DUBs) (compare Fig. 5.4).

Of note, three categories of signals are proposed to operate in the establishment of a stably heritable epigenetic state [138]. An extracellular signal referred to as the "epigenator" originates from the environment and can trigger the start of the

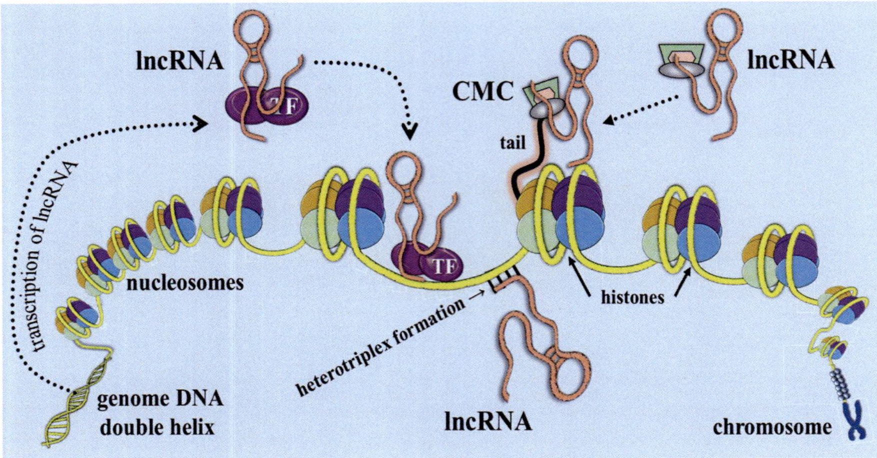

Fig. 5.5 Simplified schematic model of epigenetic modifications by long noncoding RNAs in terms of RNA↔DNA interactions, exemplified by their function as guides. By this mechanism, noncoding RNAs may act by binding active effector proteins such as chromatin modifiers and transcription factors, thereby serving to direct such proteins to sequence-specific DNA sites, resulting in either positive or negative regulation of gene transcription. In addition to these indirect mechanisms, lncRNA can interact with double-stranded DNA (RNA↔DNA↔DNA heterotriplex), thereby directly regulating gene expression. *CMC* chromatin-modifying complex, *lncRNA* long noncoding RNA, *TF* transcription factor. (Sources: [227, 228, 233, 235, 236])

epigenetic pathway. (In fact, it is tantalizing to speculate that, in the future, DAMPs will turn out to operate as those epigenators.) The *epigenetic initiator* receives the signal from the *epigenator* and is capable of determining the precise chromatin location and/or DNA environment for the establishment of the epigenetic pathway. The *epigenetic maintainer* functions to sustain the chromatin environment in the initial and succeeding generations. Persistence of the chromatin milieu may require collaboration between the *initiator* and the *maintainer.* Accordingly, epigenetic mechanisms are adaptable and can integrate environmental changes. They have the capability to respond to and be modified by environmental factors. The outcome of this interaction depends on the environmental stressor, for example, oxidative stress [139], and can be a normal physiological response or deregulation of the epigenome producing an abnormal phenotype.

Here, it is important to note that, although enzymes modify histones, resulting in changing chromatin, i.e., nucleosome structure, this itself is no epigenetic regulation [140]. Epigenetics needs a kind of memory, which is heritable, self-perpetuating, and reversible, and does not change the DNA sequence [141] (also compare "trained immunity," described in Vol. 1[1], Part VI, Sect. 24.2.4). Grounded on this fundamental prerequisite, epigenetic changes should persist over a more extended period of time. In line with this concept, the maintenance of the epigenome has been shown to overcome DNA replication and cell division. Indeed, recent findings demonstrated that accurate parental histone recycling preserves positional information and

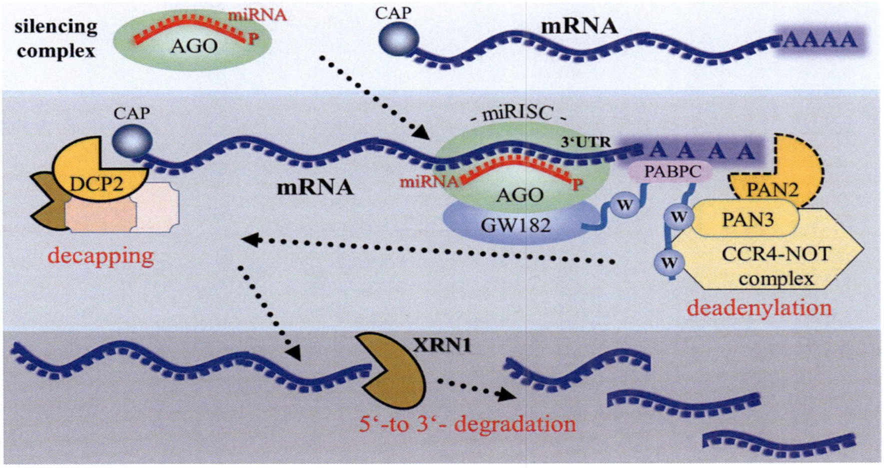

Fig. 5.6 Simplified schematic model of the degradation of target mRNA by noncoding microRNAs. The microRNA-induced silencing complex (miRISC) binds to a specific sequence at the three prime untranslated region (3′-UTR) of the target mRNA through "Watson-Crick" base pairing mechanisms. Next, GW182 family proteins, bound to Argonaute, provide the scaffolding required to recruit other effector proteins, such as the poly(A)-deadenylase complexes PAN2-PAN3 and CCR4-NOT, following miRNA↔target mRNA interaction. PAN2-PAN3 initiates deadenylation, while the CCR4-NOT complex completes the process. The interaction between the tryptophan (W)-repeats of GW182 and poly(A)-binding protein C promotes efficient deadenylation. Following deadenylation, cap removal (decapping) of the cap on target mRNA occurs facilitated by decapping protein 2 and associated proteins, followed by 5′–3′ degradation of the target mRNA by exoribonuclease 1. *A* adenine, *AAAA* poly(A) tail, *AGO* argonaute, *CCR4-NOT* carbon catabolite repressor 4- negative on TATA, *DCP2* decapping protein 2, *miRNA* microRNA, *miRISC* microRNA-induced silencing complex, *PABPC* poly(A)-binding protein C, *PAN2/3* poly(A)-nuclease 2/3, *UTR* untranslated region, *W* tryptophan, *XRN1* exoribonuclease 1. (Sources: [255, 256, 260-263, 285])

allows PTM transmission to daughter cells, while modification of new histones gives rise to complex epigenome fluctuations across the cell cycle that could underlie cell-to-cell heterogeneity [142, 143].

5.6.2.3 Trained Immunity: An Example of Epigenetic Modifications

As briefly introduced in Sect. 3.7 and in Vol. 1 [1], Part VI, Sect. 24.2.4, the concept of *trained immunity* holds that cells of the innate immune system can also establish a memory of past stimulation via a process of epigenetic reprogramming that allows modifying their response upon new injurious challenges such as infections. As discussed by Netea and van der Meer [144] (who first described this phenomenon [145]), "trained immunity is very likely an old biological process that evolved for protection of multicellular organisms lacking adaptive immune responses. Due to its beneficial effects for protection against infection, it was retained in vertebrates, and we see some of these effects mirrored in the non-specific protective effects induced by certain infections or vaccines."

The Emerging Role of DAMPs in Trained Immunity

The emerging role of DAMPs as critical inducers of epigenetic modifications governing processes in trained immunity was impressively and authentically reviewed by Crişan et al. [146]. Of note, in pioneering in vitro experiments on cultured human monocytes, oxLDL (a Subclass IIB-4 DAMP recognized by TLR2 and TLR4) was shown to train these innate immune cells to promote, through epigenetic histone modifications, a long-lasting proinflammatory phenotype with increased production of proinflammatory cytokines (including the inducible DAMP TNF) and chemokines, augmented foam cell formation, and increased production of MMPs [126]. In support of these findings are experiments on VSMCs, also demonstrating that oxLDL can induce sustained activation of VSMCs with enhanced secretion of inflammatory cytokines in response to restimulation [147]. More recently, the oligomeric S100A4 protein was also identified as a rheumatoid arthritis-relevant DAMP with the capacity to induce trained immunity [128].

Metabolic Induction of Trained Immunity

In Vol. 1 [1], Part VI, Sect. 24.4, it was briefly discussed that in addition to PRM-triggered signaling pathways, intracellular metabolic pathways such as OXPHOS and aerobic glycolysis (the Warburg effect) in innate immune cells can alter their function when getting activated to execute effector responses (for additional information compare also Fig. 24.3 in Vol. 1 [1], Part VI, Sect. 24.4, p. 650). Notably, in targeted studies on β-glucan-induced trained immunity, a shift from OXPHOS to aerobic glycolysis, regulated via the dectin-1→Akt/→mTOR→ hypoxia-inducible factor 1alpha (HIF1α) pathway, was identified as a central regulatory mechanism involved in this innate immune memory reaction [148] (for additional information about the Akt-mTOR pathway, see Vol. 1 [1], Part VI, Sect. 22.3.4.2, p. 494 and Fig. 22.5, p.495; for the CLR dectin-1 recognizing β-glucan, see Part II, Sect. 5.2.7.2, p. 62 and Fig. 5.6, p. 61). More recent studies now have specified these earlier observations and shown that glycolysis, glutaminolysis, and cholesterol synthesis are non-redundant metabolic pathways that are essential for trained immunity in monocytes and macrophages. Among the distinct metabolite changes, fumarate was identified as a key metabolite that induces trained immunity, an effect mediated at least partially by induction of histone modifications such as H3K4me3 and H3K27Ac [149, 150] (for H3K4 methylation and H3K acetylation, see below). The authors of these studies [150] who also investigated monocytes of patients with hyper-immunoglobulin D syndrome that are mevalonate kinase-deficient but accumulate mevalonate concluded that "Monocytes from patients with mevalonate accumulation acquire a trained immunity phenotype, characterized by an increased expression of cytokines and genes in the glycolysis pathway. Furthermore, inhibition of the cholesterol synthesis pathway by statins prevents the trained immunity phenotype. Statins could therefore be used as a treatment option for diseases that are mediated via trained immunity, until more specific drugs for inhibiting trained immunity are available."

As with all efferent innate immune responses, although beneficial in the context of recurrent infections, trained immunity—when uncontrolled—may eventually contribute to chronic immune-mediated diseases, such as atherosclerosis and autoimmune disease [151, 152]. This dangerous development may be at least in part due to the fact that one epigenetic mechanism can affect another one, and "feed-forward" loops can and do exist.

5.6.2.4 Concluding Remarks

Importantly, there is growing evidence suggesting that epigenetic pathways leading to epigenetic modifications are implicated in both acute inflammatory and chronic inflammatory/fibrotic disorders, as well as in processes of innate immune memory development, supporting the idea that these pathways are initiated by MAMPs and DAMPs or DAMPs. In the following, this burning topic is briefly sketched regarding modifications in acute inflammation and hyperinflammation, whereas this issue regarding fibrosis is alluded in Sect. 6.6.

5.6.3 Epigenetic Regulation of Inflammation by DNA Methylation and Histone Modifications

5.6.3.1 General Remarks

Some studies on epigenetic regulation of innate inflammatory responses have already briefly described in Vol. 1 [1], Part VI, Sect. 24.2.3. Innate immune cells, all equipped with a genome containing the same DNA sequence, serve as the body's "defenders" against environmental stress and injury. As described above, this function includes the initial establishment of a robust inflammatory response followed by an inflammation-resolving and, finally, tissue repairing response. To fulfill this task aimed at restoring homeostasis, the cells can change their phenotype, that is, their activation state upon an injurious insult. A typical example is the transition of "classically activated" M1-like macrophages to "alternatively activated" M2-like macrophages (for a recent review, see [153], and for further relevant papers, see [16, 154, 155]; also compare Vol. 1 [1], Part III, Sect. 8.2.2.3 and Fig. 8.2, Part VI, Sect. 22.2.3.2, and Part VIII, Fig. 36.1; also compare Fig. 3.4). This unique property is the result of cellular reprogramming to additional levels of regulation, for example, by epigenetic modifications. For instance, emerging findings from recent research have suggested the existence of new regulatory epigenetic-based macrophage polarization mechanisms of histones modifications in inflammation (reviewed in [16, 156]). Here, the topic is briefly sketched with respect to inflammatory scenarios; a similar example, the transition of fibroblasts to myofibroblasts in tissue repairing processes, is described in Sect. 6.6.3.

5.6.3.2 DNA Methylation in Inflammation

Methylation of DNA refers to a process by which the addition of a methyl group from S-adenosyl methionine, that is, the methyl donor transfers to a nucleotide of DNA. In eukaryotes, the methylation occurs on the carbon-C5 position of cytosine in the DNA and in *cytosine phospho-bound guanine dinucleotides* called CpG islands. This leads to the formation of 5-methylcytosine (5mC) [157, 158]. Around 70% of mammalian genes contain in their proximal promoter regions a (mostly unmethylated) CpG island [159, 160] (compare Fig. 5.4). The rest of the genomes are known to be CpG poor. The CpG-island methylation at the promoter region is usually associated with gene repression and silencing; however, when DNA methylation is within the gene body, it is associated with gene activation [160]. On the other hand, demethylation and hypomethylation of CpG island promoters are linked to increased gene expression/gene activation [157].

Typically, DNA methylation is reportedly enhanced and modulated by DNMTs that add a methyl group to cytosine bases, forming 5-methylcytosine, as well as methyl-binding proteins (MBPs) (reviewed in [161–163]). Demethylation is mediated by direct removal of 5mC or further modification of the cytosine bases, such as oxidation of 5mC to 5-hydroxymethylcytosine (5-hmC) catalyzed by TET. The TET enzymes were discovered to successively oxidize not only 5hmC but also 5-formylcytosine and 5-carboxylcytosine (reviewed in [164, 165]). According to their different functions in DNA methylation, DNMTs, MBPs, and TET have also be denoted as writers, readers, and erasers, respectively, referred to DNMTs, MBPs, and TET [166].

DNA Methylation in Inflammation

In inflammatory responses, DNA methylation has been already investigated though rather rare. Nevertheless, as shown in animal models, DNA methylation is obviously causally linked to macrophage polarization and chronic inflammation-associated disease [167, 168]. Interestingly, in studies on activated M1-like and alternatively activated M2-like macrophages, DNA methylation by DNMT1 was shown to play an important role in the regulation of macrophage polarization and inflammation [169]. The studies further demonstrated that myeloid DNMT1 deficiency results in decreased macrophage PPARγ1 promoter DNA methylation, increased alternative adipose tissue macrophage activation (i.e., activation of M2-like macrophages), and decreased adipose tissue macrophages-mediated inflammation, which results in improved insulin sensitivity in obese animals. In contrast, DNMT1-mediated PPARγ1 promoter DNA methylation in macrophages was found to be significantly enhanced by obesity-associated factors, such as saturated fatty acids and proinflammatory cytokines (for PPARs, see Box 5.1 and [170, 171]).

Box 5.1 Peroxisome Proliferator-Activated Receptors

Peroxisome proliferator-activated receptors (PPARs) are ligand-activated transcription factors of nuclear hormone receptor superfamily consisting of three subtypes: PPARα, PPARγ, and PPARβ/δ. Because they play a critical role in lipid and glucose homeostasis, they are also denoted as lipid and insulin sensors. Many natural and synthetic ligands influence the expression of these receptors that are expressed in many tissues, including adipocytes, hepatocytes, and endothelial cells. Activation of PPARα reduces triglyceride level and is implicated in regulation of energy homeostasis, while PPARγ is mostly involved in the regulation of the adipogenesis, energy balance, and lipid biosynthesis. Interestingly, PPARβ/δ is involved in fatty acid oxidation, mostly in skeletal and cardiac muscles, but it was also shown to regulate blood glucose and cholesterol levels. Their role in DNA methylation is described in Sect. 5.6.3.2.

For further reading, see [170, 171].

Other lines of studies on a mouse model with a macrophage-specific transgene of DNMT1 or PPARγ revealed the ectopic expression of DNMT1 in atherosclerosis-associated macrophages [172]. In these experiments, DNMT1 was demonstrated to promote the proinflammatory activation of atherosclerosis-associated macrophages and the progression of this disease in mouse models. The study also revealed that PPARγ was a target of DNMT1-regulated DNA methylation and was involved in DNMT1-mediated chronic inflammation and development of atherosclerosis. Together, therapeutically, DNMT inhibition could decrease the M1-like polarization in inflammation but promote an antiinflammatory M2-like macrophage phenotype.

In addition, as already briefly described in Vol.1 [1], Part VI, Sect. 24.2.3, in studies on DNMT3a-deleted macrophages, various specific enzymes or mediators have been shown to regulate inflammatory gene expression via controlling chromatin status. In the antiviral immunity, DNA methyltransferase DNMT3a was shown to upregulate HDAC9 via epigenetic mechanisms to deacetylase the kinase TBK1 for activation, contributing to enhanced IFN production [173]. These studies documented that DNMT3a did not directly regulate the transcription of genes encoding type I IFNs; instead, it increased their production through an epigenetic mechanism by maintaining high expression of the HDAC9. In turn, HDAC9 directly maintained the deacetylation status of the critical PRM-signaling molecule TBK1 and enhanced its kinase activity. The authors further discussed that these findings indicate that a chromatin regulator is capable of establishing a macrophage-specific function for rapid antiviral responses. The researchers concluded that their data add mechanistic insight into the cross talk between epigenetic modifications and PTMs in the regulation of PRM signaling and activation of antiviral innate immune responses [173].

5.6.3.3 Histone Acetylation and Deacetylation

Histone acetylation and deacetylation play a critical role in the regulation of inflammatory genes, and emerging evidence suggests that both epigenetic modifications are involved in multiple diseases, including inflammatory disorders. Without going into detail, they are cursorily discussed in this section.

Histone Acetylation

Histone acetylation is a process by which conserved lysine residues within the N-terminal tail, protruding from the histone core of the nucleosome, are acetylated by HATs as part of gene regulation. Specifically, the HATs transfer an acetyl group from acetyl CoA to form ε-N-acetyl-lysine, thereby contributing to DNA accessibility to transcriptional regulation proteins [174, 175]. For example, *H3K9ac* is an epigenetic histone mark, whereby an acetyl group is transferred to the lysine 9 residue on the histone H4 protein. Histone acetyltransferases such as CBP/p300, MOF, HBO1, or KAT6A mainly acetylate histones 3 (H3K9ac, H3K14ac, H3K18ac, H3K23ac, H3K27ac, H3K56ac) and histones 4 (H4K5ac, H4K8ac, H4K12ac, H4K16ac) [176]. Due to this fact, HATs are generally recognized as coactivators of transcription. The HATs play a major role in the epigenetic regulation of gene expression by triggering gene activation mechanisms.

Role of HATs in Inflammation

However, reports on a role of HATs in specific gene activation during inflammation are sparse. Nevertheless, as reviewed by Daskalaki et al. [156], positive histone marks H3K4me3 and H3K9/14ac, critical for rendering the promoter region accessible to *polymerase II* (Pol II) and transcription factors, were shown to be downregulated at the promoter region of proinflammatory mediator genes following stimulation [177, 178]. Further examples of HATs involved in macrophage activation not discussed here have been cited by Daskalaki et al. [156].

Histone Deacetylation

Acetylation of lysine residues on histones is highly reversible and can be removed by the process of histone deacetylation catalyzed by histone deacetylases (HDACs). These enzymes represent a complex family of gene transcription regulating proteins that are mainly responsible for removing the acetyl groups introduced on histones by HATs. In higher mammals, 18 HDACs have been identified and are grouped in four classes based on sequence similarities. The Class I proteins consist of HDAC1, HDAC2, HDAC3, and HDAC8; the Class II proteins are constituted of HDAC4, HDAC5, HDAC7, HDAC9 (Subclass IIa), and HDAC 6 and HDAC10 (Subclass IIb); Class III proteins include the sirtuins SIRT1, SIRT2, SIRT3, SIRT4, SIRT5, SIRT6, and SIRT7; and Class IV has just the only member HDAC11. To allow deacetylation of histones, HDACs must be in the nucleus, whereby some enzymes are reportedly mainly found in the nucleus to regulate signaling and gene expression, whereas some others shuttle between the cytosol and nucleus (for reviews, see [156, 179–182]).

Role of HDACs in Inflammation

Of note, HDACs have been identified as critical regulators of innate and adaptive immune responses by triggering mainly but not exclusively gene-silencing mechanisms (also reviewed in [156]). Regarding PRM-triggered innate immune pathways, Class I HDACs have been shown to modulate TLR- and IFN-regulated genes primarily [183], in the expression of TLR-induced gene possessing both negative and positive effects [184]. Evidence for a positive/proinflammatory regulation, for example, was provided by studies using HDAC inhibitors (trichostatin A, suberoylanilide hydroxamic acid, or valproic acid) that were demonstrated to suppress recruitment of the p65 subunit of NF-κB to inflammatory promoters following TLR-mediated activation in murine DCs and macrophages [185, 186] (also compare Vol. 1 [1], Part VI, Sect. 22.3.3.2 and Fig. 22.3). On the other hand, HDAC1 was found to act as a negative feedback/antiinflammatory regulator of innate immune responses as demonstrated by studies showing that it downregulates promoter activity of TLR-induced genes such as IL-12p40 [187] and type I IFN-β [188]. Together, although HDACs possess divergent roles, Class I HDACs are considered to be predominantly negative regulators of TLR-triggered signaling pathways [156].

Research on members of Class II HDACs found out that HDAC7 is upregulated in inflammatory macrophages, and only a specific HDAC7 isoform, HDAC7-u, could be documented to act as a positive regulator by promoting the expression of a subset of TLR-induced proinflammatory genes in a HIF1α-dependent mechanism [189]. In other lines of studies on a pre-B-cell line cellular transdifferentiation system, HDAC7 suppression was observed to inhibit transcriptional reprogramming during B cell precursors → macrophage transdifferentiation and acquisition of key proinflammatory phenotype [190]. Moreover, in in vitro experiments on murine and human macrophage cell lines, HDAC5 overexpression was shown to be associated with a significant increase of TNF and *monocyte chemoattractant protein-1* (MCP-1), paralleled by activation of the NF-κB pathway [191]. Conversely, in these studies, HDAC5 knockdown by small interfering RNA (siRNA) was observed to result in the suppression of cytokine production. According to the authors' conclusion, these findings support the concept that HDAC5 is directly involved in promoting inflammatory responses in both murine and human macrophages [191].

Sirtuins, that is, Class III HDACs, are a family of histone deacetylases that contain seven enzymatic activities in mammals and function to suppress gene transcription by epigenetic mechanisms. Nuclear sirtuins (SIRT1, 2, 6, and 7), in particular, may play an essential role in the regulation of inflammatory responses. As reviewed by Mendes et al. [192], SIRT1 reportedly suppresses inflammatory responses by interfering with NF-κB activity and inducible nitric oxide synthase (iNOS) production. Similar effects exert SIRT2 whose activity includes the deacetylation of p65 subunit of NF-κβ and RIP-1, while SIRT6 has been shown to interact with p65/RelA bound to the NF-κB promoter region and repress transcriptional activity. In addition, other sets of studies have shown that the absence of SIRT7 produced an increase in inflammation, demonstrating that SIRT7 also functioned to decrease inflammation. In line with these experimental observations on antiinflammatory effects of SIRT1 and SIRT2 are recent studies revealing that SIRT1 can negatively regulate the NLRP3 inflammasome in vascular cells [193]. In this study, evidence was also provided indicating that the molecule *cluster of differentiation 40* (CD40) may be involved in the regulation of NLRP3 inflammasome by SIRT1. The authors concluded among others that their results provide new mechanisms for understanding the potential role of SIRT1 in modulating NLRP3 inflammasome-related inflammation.

5.6.3.4 Histone Methylation in Inflammation

According to recently published evidence, modification of histones by methylation plays an emerging role not only in many biological processes but also in inflammatory diseases. Unlike acetylation, histone methylation can have both positive and negative effects on transcription, depending on the site of methylation. Histone methylation is mediated by HMTs and, depending on the histone and residue of modification, contributes to either active or repressive chromatin configurations. The HMTs are histone-modifying proteins that catalyze the addition of methyl groups on lysine and arginine histone residues.

Lysine Methylation

Lysine methylation is a process by which histone lysine (K) methyltransferases (KMTs) transfer one, two, or three methyl groups, respectively, from S-adenosyl-L-methionine to the ε-amino group of a lysine residue on histone proteins (compare Fig. 5.4). For example, *H3K4me3* is an epigenetic histone mark, whereby three methyl groups (trimethylation) are transferred to the lysine 4 residue on the histone H3 protein. All members of the KMT group contain an evolutionarily conserved SET (for *Su(var)3-9, enhancer-of-zeste, trithorax*) catalytic domain comprised of 130 amino acids except the non-SET domain KMT *Dot1p*. Today, more than 50 SET domain-containing proteins have been identified in humans, with a proven or predicted enzymatic role in performing lysine methylation on histone tails. The SET-containing KMTs are classified in six different subfamilies (EZH, SET1, SET2, SMYD, SUV39, PRDM) based on sequence homology within and around the catalytic SET domain and according to structural similarities in the SET domain. A number of SET-containing KMTs such as SUV4-20, SET8, and SET 7/9, however, do not fall into these subfamilies because of lacking sequences or conservation flanking their SET domains (for reviews, see [156, 194, 195]).

Role of KMTs in Inflammation

Lysine methyltransferases have been shown to regulate PRM-triggered innate immune responses via regulation of pro-/antiinflammatory signaling pathways. For example, in an in vitro model of SIRS, the NF-κB subunit RelB was shown to initiate facultative ("closed") heterochromatin formation by interacting with the histone H3 lysine methyltransferase G9a (catalyzing H3K9 dimethylation), which then mediates heterochromatin formation, thereby promoting gene silencing [196]. The authors concluded that "these data provide novel insight into how RelB initiates silencing in the phenotype associated with severe systemic inflammation in humans, a disease with major morbidity and mortality."

In other lines of in vitro and in vivo studies, the H3K4 methyltransferase SET7/9 was found to be a novel coactivator of NF-κB [197]. Specifically, the experiments revealed that gene silencing of SET7/9 with siRNAs in monocytes significantly inhibits TNF-induced (i.e., inducible DAMP-induced) inflammatory genes and histone H3-lysine 4 methylation on these promoters, as well as monocyte adhesion to ECs or VSMCs. Also, in these studies, inflammatory gene induction by the DAMP S100 B was found to be attenuated in SET7/9 knockdown monocytes (for S100B acting as a Subclass IA-1 DAMP, see Vol. 1 [1], Part IV, Sect. 12.2.4.2). Strikingly, these findings are in support of the notion that DAMPs may induce inflammatory responses not only by transcriptional mechanisms but also via activation of epigenetic modifications (compare Sect. 3.7.2).

Some data on histone methylation in macrophage polarization (M-like→M2-like) have also been reported (reviewed in [17]). Generally, HMTs promote polarization of macrophages toward the M2-like phenotype. For example, in studies on human M1 macrophages, trimethylation of the H3K9 by SETDB1 (a SUV39 family protein) was demonstrated to silence TNF transcription [198]. Other sets of studies on a *mycobacterium tuberculosis* infection model provided evidence for a role of SET8 in promoting the antiinflammatory M2-like macrophage phenotype [199]. On the other hand, some HMTs are associated with M1 macrophage polarization. For example, the expression of the H3K4-methyltransferase *mixed lineage leukemia* (MLL) was shown to be enhanced in M1 polarized human macrophages and to be responsible for H3K4 trimethylation of signature gene promoters [200]. These findings let the authors conclude that MLL can be regarded as a potential novel marker for M1 polarization.

Arginine Methylation

Protein arginine methylation is a common PTM in eukaryotes. Protein arginine (R) methyltransferases (PRMTs) catalyze the transfer of one or two methyl groups from S-adenosylmethionine to the guanidino nitrogen atoms of arginine in histones (but also non-histone proteins). This reaction results in the formation of S-adenosylhomocysteine and methylarginines. Three main forms of methylarginines have been identified in eukaryotes: ω-N^G-monomethylarginine (MMA), ω -N^G, N^G-asymmetric dimethylarginine (aDMA), and ω-N^G, N'^G-symmetric dimethylarginine (sDMA). For example, the asymmetric *H4R3me2a* is an epigenetic histone mark, whereby two methyl groups are transferred to the arginine 3 residue on the histone 4 protein. As another example of PRMT-mediated methylation, PRMT5 has been shown to catalyze the *H4R3me2s* mark, that is, the symmetrical dimethylation of the Arg-3 residue in H4 N-terminal tail, whereas PRMT1 can catalyze *H4R3me2a*, that is, the asymmetrical dimethylation of the same residue.

In humans, the PRMTs are grouped into in three categories according to their catalytic activity: type I (PRMT1, PRMT2, PRMT3, PRMT4, PRMT6, and PRMT8) and type II (PRMT5 and PRMT9) enzymes perform the formation of MMA as an intermediate before the establishment of aDMA or sDMA, respectively, whereas PRMT7 is a type III enzyme that catalyzes only the formation of MMA, and thus far, histones are its only known substrates.

Arginine methylation is known to play a major role in gene regulation because of the ability of the PRMTs to deposit key activating histone marks (histone H4R3me2a, H3R2me2s, H3R17me2a, H3R26me2a) or repressive histone marks (H3R2me2a, H3R8me2a, H3R8me2s, H4R3me2s) (for reviews, see [156, 194, 201, 202]).

Role of PRMTs in Inflammation

In addition to KMTs, PRMTs have also been shown to regulate innate immune responses via regulation of PRM-triggered pro-/antiinflammatory signaling pathways. At the time being, four PRMTs are discussed to be involved in regulation of PRM-triggered inflammatory responses: PRMT1, PRMT5, PRTM4 (also called *coactivator-associated arginine methyltransferase 1* [CARM1]), and PRMT6 (reviewed in [203]). For example, both biochemical and genetic evidence was provided showing that PRMT4 synergistically coactivates NF-κB-mediated transactivation, in concert with the transcriptional coactivators p300/CREB-binding protein and the p160 family of steroid receptor coactivators – identifying PRMT4 as a novel transcriptional coactivator of NF-κB [204] (CREB, for *cyclic AMP response element-binding protein*; p300 is a homolog of CREB-binding protein; for the p160 steroid receptor coactivator family, see [205]).

Similarly, PRMT1 is reportedly considered to regulate inflammatory pathways through control of NF-κB-dependent gene expression in collaboration with other coactivators. Thus, PRTM1 was demonstrated to form, under TNF stimulation, a nuclear complex with p65 and PARP1, whereby this methyltransferase is recruited to p65-containing complexes that are associated with promoters [206]. However, additional targeted experiments are required to fully understand how PRMT1 regulates NF-κB-dependent gene expression via collaboration with other cofactors. In addition, it is worth mentioning here that a series of elegant experiments, including examination of livers of patients suffering from cirrhosis, has revealed a role of PRMT1 in M2-like macrophage transdifferentiation [207]. Moreover, in studies in mice, first evidence has been elaborated on a role of PRMT5 and PRMT6 in NF-κB regulation [208, 209]. However, their exact mechanisms of activation of NF-κB-related gene expression are not entirely clear and are still being explored.

5.6.3.5 Histone Demethylation in Inflammation

According to recently published evidence, modification of histones by demethylation plays an emerging role not only in many biological processes but also in inflammatory diseases. Since recent studies have demonstrated that histone methylation is not an irreversible modification but can also be enzymatically reversed by HDMs, the interest of clinicians in this topic as a new therapeutic option has grown up considerably.

Two evolutionarily conserved families of histone lysine demethylases (KDMs), which utilize different reaction mechanisms to establish demethylation, have been identified, the lysine-specific demethylases (LSD1 and LSD2) and the Jumonji C (JmjC) demethylases (including KDM6B, KDM5A, KDM5B, KDM4A, KDM4B, and KDM2B) (compare Fig. 5.4) (for reviews, see [210-212]). LSD1 reportedly catalyzes demethylation of H3K4me1 and H3K4me2 and can also demethylate H3K9me1 and H3K9me2, whereas LSD2 has been shown to demethylate H3K4me1 and H3K4me2. Both LSD1 and LSD2 use a flavin adenine dinucleotide (FAD)-dependent amine oxidation reaction to catalyze the demethylation of their substrate. Members of the JmjC demethylase family (counting 30) possess the JmjC domain that confers demethylase activity and substrate specificity, whereby demethylases with activity toward H3K4, H3K9, H3K27, H3K36, and H4K20 have been identified. Notably, the demethylase reaction catalyzed by this family of proteins is a dioxygenase reaction that depends on Fe(II) and α-ketoglutarate.

Histone Demethylation in Inflammation

A growing body of evidence suggests emerging roles of KDMs in regulation of inflammation and immune functions (reviewed by Kang et al. in [213]). An earlier study in 2002 provided already the first clue to a role histone demethylation in inflammatory responses [214]. In this study, exposure of human monocyte-derived DCs to LPS (signaling through TLR4) led to rapid or delayed induction of various inflammatory cytokines. Among them, several genes encoding for the cytokines with delayed induction had transiently lost H3K9 methylation at the promoter regions during exposure to LPS. A subsequent study in LPS-stimulated macrophages identified KDM6B (= JmjD3) as the vital KDM involved in LPS-induced inflammatory responses [215]. Intriguingly, the KDM6B induction of KDM6B was shown to be dependent upon NF-κB.

Regarding macrophage polarization, KDM6B was found to be indispensable for M2 macrophage differentiation [216, 217]. For example, in studies on a mycobacterial infection model, KDM6B was shown to orchestrate the mycobacterial infection-induced generation of foamy macrophages [217]. Interestingly, the investigators could further demonstrate in their work that TLR2 is involved in the regulation of KDM6B expression. In accordance, in investigations of in blood leukocytes from patients with active pulmonary tuberculosis disease, KDM6B gene/protein expressions were found to be decreased (together with Histone H3K14 hypoacetylation and H3K27 hypermethylation along with HDAC1 upregulation) [218].

In sum, as with other epigenetic modifications, the discovery of enzymes involved in the histone demethylation process has emerged considerably over recent year and now plays an important role in the dynamic regulation of histone methylation and its crucial role in development and diseases [219–221].

5.6.3.6 Concluding Remarks

Collectively, there is ample evidence for a critical role of epigenetic modifications such as DNA methylation and histone modifications in innate immune defense responses. As an integral part of inflammatory responses, they take care of the homeostatic tasks of inflammatory processes. However, growing evidence has shown that aberrant profiles of these modifications contribute to the dysregulation of immune responses, resulting in the development of a variety of disorders, strikingly in autoimmune diseases. Research on this topic is on full tours but challenging. For example, further studies are required to break the distinct histone modification code, which is implicated in the pathogenesis of various diseases.

5.6.4 Regulation of Inflammatory Responses by Long Noncoding RNAs

5.6.4.1 General Remarks

Noncoding RNAs (ncRNAs) are a loosely classified group of RNA transcripts with no apparent protein-coding role. The different subclasses of ncRNAs include miRNAs, a class of short ncRNAs; and a variety of long ncRNAs (lncRNAs), such as circular RNAs (cirRNAs), long intervening noncoding RNAs (lincRNAs), and antisense RNAs. This group of RNAs controls, i.e., activates or represses specific gene expression programs by regulating transcriptional, posttranscriptional, and posttranslational processes.

During the past decade, mainly due to new achievements in more profound and more sensitive RNA sequencing, there has been an explosion of new discoveries of epigenomic regulatory lncRNAs. Also referred to as epi-lncRNAs, these RNA transcripts are widely expressed in all tissues. Estimated to exceed the number of 58,000 in the human genome, lncRNAs are found in every branch of life, and, even more importantly, their overexpression, deficiency, or mutation have been implicated in numerous human diseases. However, although some lncRNAs such as *metastasis-associated lung adenocarcinoma transcript 1* (MALAT1) and *nuclear enriched abundant transcript 1* (NEAT1) are highly expressed, many (or most) lncRNAs are expressed only weakly, and thus the information on lncRNAs obtained from transcriptome-wide studies is usually too limited to drive functional investigation of lncRNAs.

Unlike several functionally and structurally well-defined species of noncoding RNAs, such as miRNA, the definition of lncRNAs remains arbitrary. Thus, to distinguish them from short noncoding RNAs, the sequence-length of lncRNA transcripts is defined to consist of more than 200 nucleotides, transcribed by RNA Pol II, but not translated into proteins. In Vol. 1 [1], Part IV, Sect. 24.2.3.3, the theme was briefly introduced. Here, some features of lncRNAs in relation to inflammation are resumed without going into details (for competent reviews, see [222-229]).

5.6.4.2 The Nature of Long Noncoding RNAs

Plausibly, the expression of lncRNAs is tightly regulated, given their vital role in cell functions. Recent work has revealed that certain transcription factors and chromatin remodeling enzymes are responsible for regulation of their expression. Notably, similar to mRNA, the majority of lncRNA classes are pre-lncRNAs and thus processed to mature lncRNAs in the form of capping, splicing, and polyadenylation (for capping, splicing, polyadenylation, see Box 5.2, and [230–232]). Like proteins, lncRNA functionality is dependent on proper subcellular localization. Interestingly, lncRNA transcripts can localize in many different places within the cell, including the chromatin, nucleus, cytoplasm, and exosomes. However, they are more enriched in the nucleus relative to the cytoplasm, and within the nucleus, they occupy the chromatin fraction.

Box 5.2 Capping, Splicing, and Polyadenylation

Capping All eukaryotic mRNA contains a cap structure, that is, N7-methylated guanosine linked to the first nucleotide of the RNA via a reverse 5′ to 5′ triphosphate linkage. In addition to its vital role of cap-dependent initiation of protein synthesis, the messenger RNA (mRNA) cap also functions as a protective group from 5′ to 3′ exonuclease cleavage and a unique identifier for recruiting protein factors for pre-mRNA splicing, polyadenylation, and nuclear export. The cap also acts as the anchor for the recruitment of initiation factors that initiate protein synthesis and the 5′ to 3′ looping of mRNA during translation.

Splicing In molecular biology, splicing is a modification of an RNA after transcription in which introns are removed, and exons are joined. Thus, an intron is any noncoding nucleotide sequence within a gene that is removed by RNA splicing during maturation of the final RNA product; an exon is any part of a gene that encodes a part of the final mature RNA produced by that gene after introns have been removed by RNA splicing. This process is needed for the typical eukaryotic messenger RNA before it can be used to produce a correct protein through translation. For many eukaryotic introns, splicing is done in a series of reactions catalyzed by the spliceosome, a complex of small nuclear ribonucleoproteins (snRNPs), but there are also self-splicing introns.

Polyadenylation Polyadenylation is the addition of a long chain of adenine nucleotides (poly[A] tail) to an mRNA. A long chain of adenine nucleotides (poly[A]) tail is found at the 3′ end of nearly every fully processed eukaryotic mRNA and has been suggested to influence virtually all aspects of mRNA metabolism. Its proposed functions include conferring mRNA stability, promoting an mRNA's translational efficiency, and having a role in transport of processed mRNA from the nucleus to the cytoplasm

For further reading, see [230-232].

5.6.4.3 Biological Mechanisms of Long Noncoding RNAs

The lncRNA biological mechanisms converge on establishing intermolecular interactions with other biomolecules, such as DNA, other RNAs, and proteins. Thus, mechanistically, their functions are preferentially discussed based on those RNA↔DNA, RNA↔RNA, and RNA↔protein interactions they engage (reviewed by Chen et al. [228], Li et al. [233], and Qian et al. [234]). A critical biological mechanism of function is their interaction with DNA. In fact, most lncRNAs function by modulating the transcription of target downstream genomic loci in "cis" (i.e., in the vicinity of the structural portion of genes) or in "trans" (remotely located genes) via tethering with target DNA through the recognition of specific chromatin features or as an RNA↔DNA heteroduplex. In spite of the high number of lncRNAs discovered and the wide variety of effector proteins with which they can interact, four common molecular mechanisms have been proposed. First, lncRNAs can function as molecular signals in response to unique stimuli, serving as an indicator of transcriptional activity. Second, they can act as a decoy by binding their targets, without producing any further effect, the main function of decoy lncRNAs being to limit the availability of specific regulatory factors by acting as a molecular disposer. Third, lncRNAs may act as guides by binding regulatory or enzymatically active effector proteins, such as chromatin modifiers and transcription factors, thereby serving to direct such proteins to sequence-specific sites, resulting in either positive or negative regulation of gene transcription (Fig. 5.5). For example, lncRNA can act as a guide to promote the gene expression via recruiting transcription factors to the region of the gene promoter. Also, lncRNAs can function as dynamic scaffolds by bringing effector proteins together in a spatiotemporal fashion. As such scaffolds, they play a structural role by providing a central platform for the transient assembly of multiple enzymatic complexes such as histone-modifying complexes and other regulatory cofactors. Finally, besides RNA forming base pairs with single-stranded DNA through Watson-Crick interactions (duplex, i.e., [guanine ↔ cytosine and adenine ↔ thymine]), it can interact with dsDNA by inserting into the major groove of the duplex structure with sequence specificity (= RNA↔DNA↔DNA heterotriplex), thereby directly regulating gene expression (Fig. 5.5) (reviewed in [228, 233, 235, 236]). Interestingly, the transcription of lncRNA itself was shown to lead to local chromatin changes that are not mediated by the noncoding transcript per se. In a study by Engreitz et al. [237] analyzing the mechanisms of local gene regulation mediated by twelve lncRNAs, five were found to regulate the expression of their neighboring genes in cis. However, as surprisingly observed by the investigators, none of those cis regulators required the lncRNA transcripts themselves but instead depended on processes associated with their transcription.

Notably, several classes of lncRNAs function through RNA↔RNA interactions that can be generally classified into two groups: interactions mediated by proteins or those effected by direct RNA base pairing. For example, such an RNA binding is a significant mechanism deployed by circRNAs to modulate gene expression. In this case, lncRNAs contain structural domains that can sense and bind other RNAs via complementary base pairing. As reviewed [228], the versatility of the interaction confers multiple roles to RNA↔RNA hybrids, from control of RNA biogenesis to competition for common targets.

Furthermore, lncRNAs have been reported to function through RNA↔protein interactions. Thus, an essential mechanism of lncRNA function is the modular pairing of DNA binding and protein interaction to recruit chromatin-modifying proteins/enzymes that regulate gene regulation via the chemical modification of histones [238, 239] (see also the previous section). For example, the lncRNA *HOXA distal transcript antisense RNA* (HOTTIP) was shown to maintain gene transcription by tethering with the adaptor *WD repeat-containing protein 5* (WDR5), a core subunit of the histone H3K4-methyltransferase complex [240].

Finally, it should be noted that, mechanistically, the function of lncRNA is much more complex and complicated than outlined here. For further details of lncRNA interactions, the reader is referred to competent articles found under [228, 233, 234, 239, 241].

5.6.4.4 Long Noncoding RNAs in the Regulation of Innate Immune Inflammatory Responses

A growing body of evidence for the role of lncRNAs in the regulation of inflammatory responses has recently been published. This is not a surprising observation since lncRNAs are known to be expressed in innate immune cells such as macrophages, DCs, neutrophils, and NK cells, but also in T and B lymphocytes. Indeed, several studies have identified critical functions for lncRNAs in PRM-triggered innate immune responses at the level of gene transcription, posttranscriptional protein modification, and chromatin accessibility (reviewed by Mathy and Chen [227] and Chen et al. [228]). Moreover, as reported by Murphy and Medvedev in their review on lncRNAs as regulators of TLR signaling [242], accumulating evidence indicates that lncRNAs regulate TLR4-driven expression of inflammatory genes by multiple mechanisms, by interactions with transcription factors (e.g., NF-κB, IRF3) or their regulators (e.g., IκBα) (for TLR4 signaling, compare Vol. 1 [1], Part VI, Sect. 22.3.2.2 and Fig. 22.3).

Among such signal-specific lncRNAs, the expression of lincRNA- COX-2 has already been touched in Vol. 1 [1], Part VI, Sect. 24.2.3.3. In studies on bone marrow-derived macrophages and DCs, Carpenter et al. [243] could demonstrate that lincRNA-COX-2 is induced more than 1,000-fold following activation of the TLRs (TLR1, TLR2, TLR7, TLR8). Interestingly, in their studies, the authors further showed that transcription of lincRNA-COX-2 is dependent on signaling through the TLR adaptor MyD88 and the transcription factor NF-κB. In conclusion on these findings and other data not cited here, the authors proposed a model "whereby TLR signaling induces lncRNAs, such as lincRNA-Cox2, that serve as repressors and activators of genes through their physical interactions with various regulatory complexes. As such, lncRNAs represent a novel component of the innate immune response that can restrain and promote aspects of inflammatory signaling."

Another example of a lncRNA shown to regulate innate immune pathways is THRIL (for *TNF And HNRNPL Related Immunoregulatory Long Noncoding RNA*). This lncRNA was found to regulate the expression of the inducible DAMP TNF in Pam3CSK4-activated THP1 macrophages (THP1: a human monocyte cell line) [244]. Notably, the molecule Pam3CSK4 is a synthetic lipopeptide that acts as a TLR2/TLR1 heterodimer agonist, that is, as a DAMP. Based on their results, the authors found THRIL to function through forming an RNA/protein complex with the *heterogeneous nuclear ribonucleoprotein L* (hnRNPL, a protein involved in the stress response), the complex regulating transcription of the TNF gene by binding to its promoter [244]. Together, these data may point to a specific action of THRIL in recruiting hnRNPL to a specific genomic locus, where it can contribute to DAMP→TLR-stimulated gene transcription.

Intriguingly, lncRNAs have also been discussed to be involved in coordinated changes in gene expression associated with the polarization state of macrophages, that is, the switch from M1-like to M2-like macrophages [227]. For example, studies on human monocyte-derived macrophages revealed a differentiated lncRNA expression profile depending on either activation toward M1-like macrophages or M2-like macrophages [245]. Specifically, the lncRNA *TCONS_00019715* was detected to be strongly upregulated under M1-like-polarizing conditions but downregulated in M2-like macrophages. Of note, several recently reported studies have added other distinct lncRNAs to the emerging list of lncRNAs that demonstrate a crucial regulatory role in macrophage polarization, among them *lncRNA-MM2P* [246], MALAT1 [247], and *TUC339* [248]. For example, MALAT1 was found to be involved in M1 activation, whereas inhibition by knockdown augments the M2 phenotype in macrophage [247].

It should also be noted that lncRNAs have been discovered that restrict inflammatory responses. One example is the lncRNA *lincRNA erythroid prosurvival* (lincRNA-EPS) that is expressed in innate immune cells such as macrophages and DCs [249]. In studies on bone-marrow-derived macrophages exposed to TLR2, TLR3, and TLR4 agonists (including the double-stranded RNA analog *polyinosinic-polycytydilic acid* [poly I:C]), the expression of lincRNA-EPS was observed to be downregulated in response to all three TLR ligands in a time-dependent manner. Also, TLR4-mediated suppression of lincRNA-EPS was observed in DCs. The study further revealed that lincRNA-EPS specifically repress the expression of interferon genes in TLR-activated macrophages cells, thereby restraining inflammation in vivo. Mechanistically, lincRNA-EPS was shown to function at least in part through its interaction with *hnRNP* supposed to be critically involved in the transcriptional regulation of gene expression (compare above, the role of THRIL in recruiting hnRNPL). However, the mechanism whereby lincRNA-EPS specifically localizes to the genomic loci of interferon genes to mediate gene repression remains to be fully defined. The authors conclude [249] that "that the precise regulation of lincRNA-EPS expression in macrophages is essential to control inflammatory responses by suppressing the transcription of key immune genes. lincRNA-EPS, therefore, acts as an important component of the molecular circuitry to prevent spontaneous activation of immune genes, chronic inflammation, and immune pathologies."

5.6.4.5 Concluding Remarks

Together, it has been recognized that lncRNAs play a critical role in the regulation of gene transcription during innate immune defense responses. They achieve this fine regulation by acting as signals, decoys, guides, or scaffolds and even by direct interaction with genomic DNA. Moreover, and of major interest from the perspective of this book, an increasing number of clinical studies has revealed that dysregulation of lncRNAs is associated with a panoply of human diseases. Growing knowledge about the precise function of lncRNAs function in the regulation of efferent innate immune responses is expected to pave the way for the development of new therapeutic strategies for many inflammatory/autoimmune diseases.

5.6.5 Small Noncoding RNAs (MicroRNAs) in Regulation of Gene Expression

5.6.5.1 General Remarks

Typical small noncoding RNAs are miRNAs and small nucleolar RNAs (snoRNAs), both of which play critical roles in regulating gene expression [250, 251]. Here, the miRNAs are briefly addressed, although they are not directly implicated in chromatin state-related epigenetics but have effects on the epigenetic machinery, and their expression is controlled by epigenetic mechanisms.

The miRNAs are short (~22 nt) noncoding RNAs that were discovered in 1993 in studies on *Caenorhabditis elegans* [252, 253] and, after that, have revolutionized the field of molecular biology. Soon, miRNAs were detected in all animal model systems, and some were shown to be highly conserved across species. Between 50 and 80% of miRNAs are encoded within introns of host mRNA genes (gene introns: noncoding regions). New miRNAs are still being discovered, and their roles in gene regulation are well recognized. In humans, hundreds of different miRNAs have been identified, many of which are conserved in other animals, and these conserved miRNAs have preferentially conserved interactions with most human mRNAs [254]. This inferred regulation of most human mRNAs suggests that miRNAs—besides their global role in biology—influence virtually all diseases (note: comprehensive information about miRNAs have recently been published by O'Brien et al. [255] and Bartel [256]).

5.6.5.2 Biogenesis and Mode of Action of MicroRNAs

MicroRNAs are transcribed in the nucleus, at first by RNA Pol II, in the form of long primary transcripts (called pri-miRNAs), and then processed to precursory miRNAs (pre-miRNAs). Thus, pri-miRNAs are further processed into pre-miRNAs by the microprocessor complex, consisting of an RNA binding protein *DiGeorge Syndrome Critical Region 8* (DGCR8) and a ribonuclease III enzyme, called Drosha. The pre-miRNA is exported to the cytoplasm in a so-called *Exportin 5/RanGTP*-dependent manner (hereto compare [257]) and processed by the RNase III endonuclease *Dicer* to produce the mature mdiRNA duplex consisting of 20–25 base pairs in length. Finally, either the 5′ or 3′ strands of the mature miRNA duplex is loaded into the Argonaute (AGO) family of proteins to form a *miRNA-induced silencing complex* (miRISC) [258, 259] (for the various terms, see Box 5.3). The mature miRNAs then posttranscriptionally silence target mRNAs by base pairing. Notably, the biogenesis of miRNA is classified into canonical and noncanonical, whereby the canonical biogenesis pathway is the dominant pathway by which miRNAs are processed. By contrast, multiple noncanonical miRNA biogenesis pathways make use of different combinations of the proteins involved in the canonical pathway, mainly Drosha, Dicer, exportin 5, and AGO2 (for details, see reviews by O'Brien et al. and Bartel under [255, 256]).

Box 5.3 Terms Helpful for Mechanism of miRNAs Function

5' and 3' mean "five prime" and "three prime," which indicate the carbon numbers in the DNA's sugar backbone. The 5' carbon has a phosphate group attached to it and the 3' carbon a hydroxyl (-OH) group.

RanGTP (Ran, for Ras-related nuclear protein, also known as GTP-binding nuclear protein Ran). The small GTPase Ran regulates the interaction of transport receptors with a number of cellular cargo proteins. The high-affinity binding of the GTP-bound form of Ran to import receptors promotes cargo release, whereas its binding to export receptors stabilizes their interaction with the cargo. The RanGTP system has moonlighting functions exerting a spatial control over protein interactions that drive specific functions depending on the cellular context.

Dicer is an enzyme that is well-known for its role as a riboendonuclease in the small RNA pathway. In this canonical role, Dicer is a critical regulator of the biogenesis of microRNA and small interfering RNA, an endonuclease that processes double-stranded RNA and precursor microRNAs into small interfering RNAs and microRNAs, respectively. Emerging evidence demonstrates that Dicer's endonuclease role extends beyond the generation of small RNAs; it is also involved in processing additional endogenous and exogenous substrates and is becoming increasingly implicated in regulating a variety of other cellular processes, outside of its endonuclease function.

RISC (RNA-induced silencing complex-loading complex) is a protein complex containing Dicer, a double-stranded RNA-binding protein, Argonaute, heat shock protein 90, and potentially other proteins that is required for loading small RNAs onto the Argonaute protein.

Argonaute Proteins Argonaute proteins (AGO proteins) are key players in all small RNA-guided gene-silencing processes. They are highly conserved, and family members are found in nearly all eukaryotes. The eukaryotic Argonaute family can be divided into AGO proteins and so-called PIWI proteins (an abbreviation of *P-element Induced WImpy testis in Drosophila*), which are homologous to *Drosophila melanogaster* Piwi. AGO proteins mainly interact with microRNAs or short interfering RNAs and are involved in cytoplasmic posttranscriptional gene-silencing processes.

GW 182 Proteins GW182 proteins are denoted according to their molecular weight and the presence of glycine and tryptophan repeats (either GW, WG, or GWG motifs). GW182-containing foci became known as GW bodies (GWBs). According to studies, GWBs coincide with mRNA-processing bodies or P-bodies. GW182 family proteins are essential for microRNA-mediated gene silencing in animal cells. They are recruited to miRNA targets through direct interactions with Argonaute proteins and promote target silencing. They do so by repressing translation and enhancing mRNA turnover. Although the precise mechanism of action of GW182 proteins is not fully understood, these proteins have been demonstrated to interact with the cytoplasmic *poly(A)-binding protein* (PABP) and with the *poly(A)-nuclease 2* (PAN2)-PAN3 and CCR4-NOT (*carbon catabolite repressor 4- negative on TATA*), deadenylase complexes. These data provide evidence suggesting that GW182 proteins function as scaffold proteins for the assembly of the multiprotein complex that silences miRNA targets.

For further reading, see [255, 256]).

Mechanism of Action

Although context-dependent upregulation of gene expression by miRNAs has been reported, most studies have been focused on how miRNAs inhibit gene expression—as emphasized here. In fact, miRNAs are involved in negative epigenetic regulation by—simply explained—binding to a specific sequence at the three prime untranslated region (3′-UTR) of the target mRNA using the "seed" sequence in the miRNA through "Watson-Crick" base pairing mechanisms (3'-UTR is the untranslated section of the mRNA that immediately follows the translation termination codon). This mode of gene silencing leads to breakdown of the target mRNA and/or blocking of protein translation. However, functionally, this mode of interaction is much more complex and involves the miRISC (for details, see reviews by Jonas and Izaurralde [260], O'Brien et al. [255], and Bartel [256]). In brief (see Fig. 5.6), the formation of a silencing miRISC complex begins with the recruitment of the GW182 proteins which provide the scaffolding required to recruit other effector proteins, such as the poly(A)-nuclease (PAN) deadenylation complexes PAN2-PAN3 and CCR4-NOT (for *carbon catabolite repressor 4- negative on TATA*), following miRNA↔target mRNA interaction. Degradation of the mRNA target is initiated by deadenylation, which is followed by decapping and 5′-to-3′ exonucleolytic decay in consecutive steps: target mRNA poly(A)-deadenylation is instigated by PAN2/3 and completed by the CCR4-NOT complex. The interaction between the tryptophan (W)-repeats of GW182 and *poly(A)-binding protein C* (PABPC) promotes efficient deadenylation. Following, decapping occurs facilitated by decapping protein 2 (DCP2) and associated proteins, followed by 5′−3′ degradation by exoribonuclease 1 (XRN1) (Fig. 5.6) (for original articles, see also [261-263]). Of note, these processes take place in the cytoplasm after formation of the miRISC complex; however, they have been shown to occur also in the nucleus, though the intranuclear function of miRNA is still unclear.

Extracellular Release of miRNAs

Numerous studies have demonstrated that miRNAs can be released into extracellular fluids and thus have been detected in biological fluids, such as plasma and serum, cerebrospinal fluid, saliva, breast milk, urine, tears, colostrum, peritoneal fluid, bronchial lavage, seminal fluid, and ovarian follicular fluid (reviewed in [255]). Encounter of extracellular miRNA—now operating as putative inducible DAMPs—with PRM-bearing cells then may result in TLR7 (TLR8 in humans)-triggered efferent innate immune responses, but this is another story [264] (for additional information compare Vol. 1 [1], Part VI, Sect. 22.3.3.3, p. 492 and Fig. 22.4, p. 490). The mechanisms of extracellular miRNA uptake are not well understood. It has been suggested that vesicle-associated extracellular miRNAs (compare Sect. 3.5.3.2) may be engulfed via endocytosis, phagocytosis, or direct fusion with the plasma membranes, while vesicle-free secreted miRNAs may be taken up by specific receptors on the cell surface [265] (for additional information compare also Vol.1[1], Part VI, Sects. 22.6.2, p. 557 and 22.6.3, p. 560 and Figs. 22.14, p. 558 and 22.15, p. 561).

5.6.5.3 MicroRNAs in the Regulation of Innate Immune Inflammatory Responses

The role of noncoding miRNAs in inflammation is more precisely defined compared to lncRNAs. Numerous miRNAs have been described to be involved in DAMP-triggered innate immune responses. In particular, the function of PRM-bearing mobile cells such as macrophages and DCs are governed by strict miRNA regulation. Importantly, an appropriately orchestrated inflammatory response, including DC activation, is also critical for the subsequent activation of T cells and development of specific adaptive immunity. Depending upon the target mRNAs, miRNAs may either promote or suppress inflammation. However, in general, they appear to function mainly in the downregulation of inflammatory pathways; in particular, many miRNAs reportedly suppress NF-κB signaling, the homeostatic aim being to keep inflammatory processes under control and prevent excessive hyperinflammation. Also, to fulfill these tasks, miRNAs must control—either positively or negatively – every step of the DAMP↔PRM-triggered inflammatory pathways (for reviews, see [266-272]; for the various PRM (e.g., TLR)-triggered pathways see Vol. 1 [1], Part VI, Subchapter Sects. 22.3 and Figs. 22.3, 22.4, and 22.6).

The list of such miRNAs (= miR-n) that regulate innate immune responses is long and includes miR-21, miR-125b, miR-146, miR-147, miR-511, miR-155, miR-181b, miR-187, and miR-223. It is beyond the scope of this section to describe them all. Instead, here, only a few examples will be presented in abbreviated form only.

- miR-21 is a negative regulator of TLR4 signaling by targeting the *programmed cell death 4* (PDCD4), thereby dampening NF-κB activation and IL-6 expression, but enhancing IL-10 expression. Notably, recent studies have revealed an essential role for miR-21 in the resolution of inflammation
- miR-124 is a negative regulator of inflammation by targeting several pathways such as STAT and TLRs. Interestingly, miR-124, like miR-155 and miR-223, has been identified to regulate both M1 and M2 macrophage polarization
- miR-146 consists of two genes, miR-146a and miR-146b, which are expressed in response to proinflammatory stimuli as negative feedback to control excessive inflammation. Both miR-146a and miR-146b were shown to control the inflammatory process by directly targeting TLR signaling on the level of IRAK1 and *tumor necrosis factor receptor-associated factor 6* (TRAF6)
- miR-155 exhibits both anti- and proinflammatory functions, depending on the stimulating MAMP/DAMP involved. This miRNA was demonstrated to target *TGF-β activated kinase 1 binding protein 2* (TAB2) and Pellino-1, that is, adaptors in the signaling complex that activates IKKβ. On the one hand, upregulation of this miRNA was found to result in mitigation of inflammatory pathways. On the other hand, its proinflammatory effect presumably takes place via downregulation of negative downstream regulators of inflammation, including *suppressor of cytokine signaling 1* (SOCS1)
- miR-181 family members were found to have a central role in vascular inflammation by regulating critical signaling pathways, such as downstream NF-κB signaling. For example, miR-181b was shown to exert an antiinflammatory function in ECs
- miR-223 serves as a negative feedback mechanism controlling excessive innate immune responses. This miRNA, like miR-105, and miR-19 directly target TLR2, TLR3, or TLR4, thereby impacting the ability of immune cells to engage with TLR-binding agonists.

Together, miRNAs are critical regulators in gene expression and, importantly, were detected to play a crucial role in many human diseases, thereby representing emerging therapeutic targets. Thus, this topic will be resumed in the following chapters if and when appropriate.

5.6.5.4 Concluding Remarks

Like DNA methylation and histone modifications, miRNAs operate as essential regulators of gene expression as part of the epigenetic machinery. In addition to posttranscriptional gene silencing by miRNAs (compare Fig. 5.6), the epigenetic mechanisms also include DNA methylation, histone modifications, and their cross talk. As discussed above, epigenetic modifications reportedly play a critical role in the pathogenesis of many diseases and have been harnessed to explain several features of complex disorders. However, as outlined elsewhere, miRNAs not only function as a part of the epigenetic machinery but are also themselves epigenetically modified by DNA methylation and histone modification [273]. Moreover, there is a strong connection between the epigenome and the "miRNome," and any dysregulation of this complex system can result in various physiological conditions and pathologies. Indeed, > 60 miRNA genes are reportedly epigenetically regulated in association with >20 diseases [273].

And not to forget: it is now accepted that extracellular/circulating miRNAs can not only serve as biomarkers for diseases but also play significant roles as DAMPs in intercellular communication. For example, obviously, via TLR7-MyD88-dependent pathways, some murine miRNAs released into the blood during sepsis were found to contribute to the regulation of efferent innate immune responses such as complement activation, cytokine production, and leukocyte migration [264, 274].

5.6.6 Résumé

As a clinician, to learn the tremendous progress in specifying the impact of the epigenetic machinery on inflammatory diseases is a unique experience. Indeed, the field of epigenetics of human disorders has undergone a remarkable transition from earlier genome-wide association studies (GWAS) to epigenome-wide association studies (EWAS) [275, 276]. There have been numerous diseases, exposures, and lifestyle factors investigated with EWAS, with several significant associations now identified. Indeed, over the last decade, the design of GWAS has delivered a tremendously diverse set of discoveries in human genetics. As concluded by Visscher et al. [276], "it has delivered on its original aim of detecting associations between common DNA variants and human disease and disorders. It has led to a better understanding of the genetic architecture of complex traits and therefore of past natural selection on traits associated with fitness. It has led to the discovery of variants, genes, and biological pathways that play a role in specific diseases and disorders. It has led to new discoveries in disease epidemiology and to the discovery or repurposing of candidate therapeutics."

However, there was and still is increasing recognition that GWAS have only explained a minor portion of the heritability of human disorders. On the other hand, EWAS have revealed that, in some human disorders such as autoimmune diseases, epigenetic modifications represent an emerging link between genetic and environmental factors. While epigenetic modifications have been well characterized in diseases such as cancer and autoimmune diseases, knowledge on changes in inflammatory diseases is lagging behind with some disease-specific differences [277]. Nevertheless, as discussed elsewhere [278], recent evidence so far available indicates that studies of epigenetics are significantly advancing our knowledge of inflammatory conditions. Such progress is also supported by recent findings that have briefly been summarized in this subchapter. A striking example mentioned above is the epigenetic control of M1-like or M2-like activation states of macrophages – governing promotion and resolution of inflammation – that has been shown to rely on PTMs of histone proteins adjacent to inflammatory-related genes. DAMP:SAMP ratio-dependent changes in methylation and acetylation of histones by HATs, HDADs, HMTs, and HDMs can all impact how macrophage phenotypes are generated and, thus, how inflammation is resolved or not resolved, respectively.

Moreover, it is widely recognized that environmental insults implicated in the pathogenesis of human diseases promote emission and generation of DAMPs. Also, there is growing evidence suggesting that epigenetic modifications of PRM-bearing innate immune cells are promoted by MAMPs and DAMPs [18, 279–283] and even DAMPs alone (i.e., the TLR4 ligands S100A8 and S100A9) [284].

5.7 Outlook and Future Perspectives

The various facets of inflammatory responses described in this chapter, when getting uncontrolled and dysregulated, let intuit their enormous impact on future modern medicine. Nevertheless, most of these responses are complex and complicated such as the epigenetically modified processes, and, thus, their proper implementation by clinicians into innovative diagnostic and therapeutic procedures will be a challenge. For example, how to translate the new fundamental knowledge about DAMP-induced promotion of inflammation and SAMP-mediated resolution of inflammation into the development of new diagnostic and therapeutic modalities for diseases associated with inflammatory features? Further, how to determine precisely the moment when an ongoing proinflammatory response transitions into a proresolving response: questions over questions! As always in the long history of medicine, the proper answer to all these questions will come from clinical trials that are expected to be designed, conducted, and reported to the medical community in the near future. A first tentative approach to this emerging issue is attempted below in Chap. 7.

References

1. Land WG. Damage-associated molecular patterns in human diseases. In: Injury-induced innate immune responses, vol. 1. Cham: Springer International Publishing AG; 2018. https://www.springer.com/de/book/9783319786544.
2. Heil M, Land WG. Danger signals - damaged-self recognition across the tree of life. Front Plant Sci. 2014;5:578. http://www.ncbi.nlm.nih.gov/pubmed/25400647.

3. Savill J. Apoptosis in resolution of inflammation. J Leukoc Biol. 1997;61:375–80. http://www.ncbi.nlm.nih.gov/pubmed/9103222.
4. Fullerton JN, Gilroy DW. Resolution of inflammation: a new therapeutic frontier. Nat Rev Drug Discov. 2016;15:551–67. http://www.ncbi.nlm.nih.gov/pubmed/27020098.
5. Green DR, Oguin TH, Martinez J. The clearance of dying cells: table for two. Cell Death Differ. 2016;23:915–26. http://www.nature.com/articles/cdd2015172.
6. Elliott MR, Koster KM, Murphy PS. Efferocytosis signaling in the regulation of macrophage inflammatory responses. J Immunol. 2017;198:1387–94. http://www.ncbi.nlm.nih.gov/pubmed/28167649.
7. Greenlee-Wacker MC. Clearance of apoptotic neutrophils and resolution of inflammation. Immunol Rev. 2016;273:357–70. http://www.ncbi.nlm.nih.gov/pubmed/27558346.
8. Freeman GJ, Casasnovas JM, Umetsu DT, DeKruyff RH. TIM genes: a family of cell surface phosphatidylserine receptors that regulate innate and adaptive immunity. Immunol Rev. 2010;235:172–89. http://www.ncbi.nlm.nih.gov/pubmed/20536563.
9. Rothlin CV, Carrera-Silva EA, Bosurgi L, Ghosh S. TAM receptor signaling in immune homeostasis. Annu Rev Immunol. 2015;33:355–91. http://www.ncbi.nlm.nih.gov/pubmed/25594431.
10. A-González N, Castrillo A. Liver X receptors as regulators of macrophage inflammatory and metabolic pathways. Biochim Biophys Acta Mol Basis Dis. 1812;2011:982–94. http://linkinghub.elsevier.com/retrieve/pii/S0925443910002930.
11. Croasdell A, Duffney PF, Kim N, Lacy SH, Sime PJ, Phipps RP. PPARγ and the innate immune system mediate the resolution of inflammation. PPAR Res. 2015;2015:549691. http://www.ncbi.nlm.nih.gov/pubmed/26713087.
12. Biermann MHC, Podolska MJ, Knopf J, Reinwald C, Weidner D, Maueröder C, et al. Oxidative burst-dependent NETosis is implicated in the resolution of necrosis-associated sterile inflammation. Front Immunol. 2016;7:557. https://doi.org/10.3389/fimmu.2016.00557/full.
13. Murray PJ. Macrophage polarization. Annu Rev Physiol. 2017;79:541–66. https://doi.org/10.1146/annurev-physiol-022516-034339.
14. O'Neill LAJ, Artyomov MN. Itaconate: the poster child of metabolic reprogramming in macrophage function. Nat Rev Immunol. 2019;19:273–81. http://www.ncbi.nlm.nih.gov/pubmed/30705422.
15. Patel U, Rajasingh S, Samanta S, Cao T, Dawn B, Rajasingh J. Macrophage polarization in response to epigenetic modifiers during infection and inflammation. Drug Discov Today. 2017;22:186–93. http://www.ncbi.nlm.nih.gov/pubmed/27554801.
16. Zhou D, Yang K, Chen L, Zhang W, Xu Z, Zuo J, et al. Promising landscape for regulating macrophage polarization: epigenetic viewpoint. Oncotarget. 2017;8:57693–706. http://www.ncbi.nlm.nih.gov/pubmed/28915705.
17. Kapellos TS, Iqbal AJ. Epigenetic control of macrophage polarisation and soluble mediator gene expression during inflammation. Mediators Inflamm. 2016;2016:1–15. http://www.ncbi.nlm.nih.gov/pubmed/27143818.
18. Álvarez-Errico D, Vento-Tormo R, Sieweke M, Ballestar E. Epigenetic control of myeloid cell differentiation, identity and function. Nat Rev Immunol. 2015;15:7–17. http://www.nature.com/articles/nri3777.
19. Hallowell RW, Collins SL, Craig JM, Zhang Y, Oh M, Illei PB, et al. mTORC2 signalling regulates M2 macrophage differentiation in response to helminth infection and adaptive thermogenesis. Nat Commun. 2017;8:14208. https://doi.org/10.1038/ncomms14208.
20. Biswas SK, Gangi L, Paul S, Schioppa T, Saccani A, Sironi M, et al. A distinct and unique transcriptional program expressed by tumor-associated macrophages (defective NF-kappaB and enhanced IRF-3/STAT1 activation). Blood. 2006;107:2112–22. https://doi.org/10.1182/blood-2005-01-0428.
21. Fridlender ZG, Sun J, Kim S, Kapoor V, Cheng G, Ling L, et al. Polarization of tumor-associated neutrophil phenotype by TGF-β: "N1" versus "N2" TAN. Cancer Cell. 2009;16:183–94. https://linkinghub.elsevier.com/retrieve/pii/S1535610809002153.

22. Prame Kumar K, Nicholls AJ, Wong CHY. Partners in crime: neutrophils and monocytes/macrophages in inflammation and disease. Cell Tissue Res. 2018;371:551–65. https://doi.org/10.1007/s00441-017-2753-2.
23. O'Callaghan G, Houston A. Prostaglandin E2 and the EP receptors in malignancy: possible therapeutic targets? Br J Pharmacol. 2015;172:5239–50. http://www.ncbi.nlm.nih.gov/pubmed/26377664.
24. Kawahara K, Hohjoh H, Inazumi T, Tsuchiya S, Sugimoto Y. Prostaglandin E2-induced inflammation: relevance of prostaglandin E receptors. Biochim Biophys Acta Mol Cell Biol Lipids. 1851;2015:414–21. http://www.ncbi.nlm.nih.gov/pubmed/25038274.
25. Hangai S, Ao T, Kimura Y, Matsuki K, Kawamura T, Negishi H, et al. PGE2 induced in and released by dying cells functions as an inhibitory DAMP. Proc Natl Acad Sci U S A. 2016;113:3844–9. https://doi.org/10.1073/pnas.1602023113.
26. Koga K, Takaesu G, Yoshida R, Nakaya M, Kobayashi T, Kinjyo I, et al. Cyclic adenosine monophosphate suppresses the transcription of proinflammatory cytokines via the phosphorylated c-Fos protein. Immunity. 2009;30:372–83. http://www.ncbi.nlm.nih.gov/pubmed/19285436.
27. Sokolowska M, Chen L-Y, Liu Y, Martinez-Anton A, Qi H-Y, Logun C, et al. Prostaglandin E2 inhibits NLRP3 inflammasome activation through EP4 receptor and intracellular cyclic AMP in human macrophages. J Immunol. 2015;194:5472–87. https://doi.org/10.4049/jimmunol.1401343.
28. Lima KM, Vago JP, Caux TR, Negreiros-Lima GL, Sugimoto MA, Tavares LP, et al. The resolution of acute inflammation induced by cyclic AMP is dependent on annexin A1. J Biol Chem. 2017;292(33):13758–73. http://www.ncbi.nlm.nih.gov/pubmed/28655761.
29. Vourc'h M, Roquilly A, Asehnoune K. Trauma-induced damage-associated molecular patterns-mediated remote organ injury and immunosuppression in the acutely ill patient. Front Immunol. 2018;9:1330. https://doi.org/10.3389/fimmu.2018.01330/full.
30. Antonioli L, Fornai M, Blandizzi C, Pacher P, Haskó G. Adenosine signaling and the immune system: when a lot could be too much. Immunol Lett. 2019;205:9–15. http://www.ncbi.nlm.nih.gov/pubmed/29702147.
31. Perretti M, D'Acquisto F. Annexin A1 and glucocorticoids as effectors of the resolution of inflammation. Nat Rev Immunol. 2009;9:62–70. https://doi.org/10.1038/nri2470.
32. Gavins FNE, Hickey MJ. Annexin A1 and the regulation of innate and adaptive immunity. Front Immunol. 2012;3:354. http://www.ncbi.nlm.nih.gov/pubmed/23230437.
33. Sousa LP, Alessandri AL, Pinho V, Teixeira MM. Pharmacological strategies to resolve acute inflammation. Curr Opin Pharmacol. 2013;13:625–31. http://linkinghub.elsevier.com/retrieve/pii/S1471489213000416.
34. Sugimoto MA, Vago JP, Teixeira MM, Sousa LP. Annexin A1 and the resolution of inflammation: modulation of neutrophil recruitment, apoptosis, and clearance. J Immunol Res. 2016;2016:1–13. http://www.ncbi.nlm.nih.gov/pubmed/26885535.
35. Serhan CN. Pro-resolving lipid mediators are leads for resolution physiology. Nature. 2014;510:92–101. https://doi.org/10.1038/nature13479.
36. Basil MC, Levy BD. Specialized pro-resolving mediators: endogenous regulators of infection and inflammation. Nat Rev Immunol. 2015;16:51–67. http://www.ncbi.nlm.nih.gov/pubmed/26688348.
37. Serhan CN, Chiang N, Dalli J, Levy BD. Lipid mediators in the resolution of inflammation. Cold Spring Harb Perspect Biol. 2014;7:a016311. https://doi.org/10.1101/cshperspect.a016311.
38. Anderson HA, Maylock CA, Williams JA, Paweletz CP, Shu H, Shacter E. Serum-derived protein S binds to phosphatidylserine and stimulates the phagocytosis of apoptotic cells. Nat Immunol. 2003;4:87–91. https://doi.org/10.1038/ni871.
39. Frasch SC, Bratton DL. Emerging roles for lysophosphatidylserine in resolution of inflammation. Prog Lipid Res. 2012;51:199–207. http://www.ncbi.nlm.nih.gov/pubmed/22465125.
40. Frasch SC, Fernandez-Boyanapalli RF, Berry KAZ, Murphy RC, Leslie CC, Nick JA, et al. Neutrophils regulate tissue neutrophilia in inflammation via the oxidant-modified lipid

lysophosphatidylserine. J Biol Chem. 2013;288:4583–93. http://www.ncbi.nlm.nih.gov/pubmed/23293064.
41. Zagórska A, Través PG, Lew ED, Dransfield I, Lemke G. Diversification of TAM receptor tyrosine kinase function. Nat Immunol. 2014;15:920–8. http://www.ncbi.nlm.nih.gov/pubmed/25194421.
42. Franz S, Muñoz LE, Heyder P, Herrmann M, Schiller M. Unconventional apoptosis of polymorphonuclear neutrophils (PMN): staurosporine delays exposure of phosphatidylserine and prevents phagocytosis by MΦ-2 macrophages of PMN. Clin Exp Immunol. 2015;179:75–84. http://www.ncbi.nlm.nih.gov/pubmed/24995908.
43. Griffiths HR, Gao D, Pararasa C. Redox regulation in metabolic programming and inflammation. Redox Biol. 2017;12:50–7. http://www.ncbi.nlm.nih.gov/pubmed/28212523.
44. Lemke G. Phosphatidylserine is the signal for TAM receptors and their ligands. Trends Biochem Sci. 2017;42:738–48. http://www.ncbi.nlm.nih.gov/pubmed/28734578.
45. Dalli J, Serhan C. Macrophage proresolving mediators—the when and where. Microbiol Spectr. 2016;4. http://www.ncbi.nlm.nih.gov/pubmed/27337457.
46. Pirault J, Bäck M. Lipoxin and resolvin receptors transducing the resolution of inflammation in cardiovascular disease. Front Pharmacol. 2018;9:1273. https://doi.org/10.3389/fphar.2018.01273/full.
47. Leuti A, Maccarrone M, Chiurchiù V. Proresolving lipid mediators: endogenous modulators of oxidative stress. Oxid Med Cell Longev. 2019;2019:1–12. http://www.ncbi.nlm.nih.gov/pubmed/31316721.
48. Serhan CN, Levy BD. Resolvins in inflammation: emergence of the pro-resolving superfamily of mediators. J Clin Invest. 2018;128:2657–69. http://www.ncbi.nlm.nih.gov/pubmed/29757195.
49. Li Y, Cai L, Wang H, Wu P, Gu W, Chen Y, et al. Pleiotropic regulation of macrophage polarization and tumorigenesis by formyl peptide receptor-2. Oncogene. 2011;30:3887–99. http://www.nature.com/articles/onc2011112.
50. Titos E, Rius B, González-Périz A, López-Vicario C, Morán-Salvador E, Martínez-Clemente M, et al. Resolvin D1 and its precursor docosahexaenoic acid promote resolution of adipose tissue inflammation by eliciting macrophage polarization toward an M2-like phenotype. J Immunol. 2011;187:5408–18. https://doi.org/10.4049/jimmunol.1100225.
51. Dalli J, Zhu M, Vlasenko NA, Deng B, Haeggström JZ, Petasis NA, et al. The novel 13S,14S-epoxy-maresinis converted by human macrophages to maresin 1 (MaR1), inhibits leukotriene A4 hydrolase (LTA4H), and shifts macrophage phenotype. FASEB J. 2013;27:2573–83.
52. Rius B, Titos E, Morán-Salvador E, López-Vicario C, García-Alonso V, González-Périz A, et al. Resolvin D1 primes the resolution process initiated by calorie restriction in obesity-induced steatohepatitis. FASEB J. 2014;28:836–48. http://www.ncbi.nlm.nih.gov/pubmed/24249635.
53. Herová M, Schmid M, Gemperle C, Hersberger M. ChemR23, the receptor for chemerin and resolvin E1, is expressed and functional on M1 but not on M2 macrophages. J Immunol. 2015;194:2330–7. https://doi.org/10.4049/jimmunol.1402166.
54. Chiang N, Dalli J, Colas RA, Serhan CN. Identification of resolvin D2 receptor mediating resolution of infections and organ protection. J Exp Med. 2015;212:1203–17. https://doi.org/10.1084/jem.20150225.
55. Duffney PF, Falsetta ML, Rackow AR, Thatcher TH, Phipps RP, Sime PJ. Key roles for lipid mediators in the adaptive immune response. J Clin Invest. 2018;128:2724–31. http://www.ncbi.nlm.nih.gov/pubmed/30108196.
56. Lopategi A, Flores-Costa R, Rius B, López-Vicario C, Alcaraz-Quiles J, Titos E, et al. Frontline science: specialized proresolving lipid mediators inhibit the priming and activation of the macrophage NLRP3 inflammasome. J Leukoc Biol. 2019;105:25–36. https://doi.org/10.1002/JLB.3HI0517-206RR.
57. Barnig C, Cernadas M, Dutile S, Liu X, Perrella MA, Kazani S, et al. Lipoxin A4 regulates natural killer cell and type 2 innate lymphoid cell activation in asthma. Sci Transl Med. 2013;5:174ra26. https://doi.org/10.1126/scitranslmed.3004812.

58. Chiurchiù V, Leuti A, Dalli J, Jacobsson A, Battistini L, Maccarrone M, et al. Proresolving lipid mediators resolvin D1, resolvin D2, and maresin 1 are critical in modulating T cell responses. Sci Transl Med. 2016;8:353ra111. https://doi.org/10.1126/scitranslmed.aaf7483.
59. Krishnamoorthy N, Burkett PR, Dalli J, Abdulnour R-EE, Colas R, Ramon S, et al. Cutting edge: maresin-1 engages regulatory T cells to limit type 2 innate lymphoid cell activation and promote resolution of lung inflammation. J Immunol. 2015;194:863–7. https://doi.org/10.4049/jimmunol.1402534.
60. Serhan CN, de la Rosa X, Jouvene C. Novel mediators and mechanisms in the resolution of infectious inflammation: evidence for vagus regulation. J Intern Med. 2019;286(3):240–58. https://doi.org/10.1111/joim.12871.
61. Xu Z-Z, Zhang L, Liu T, Park JY, Berta T, Yang R, et al. Resolvins RvE1 and RvD1 attenuate inflammatory pain via central and peripheral actions. Nat Med. 2010;16:592–7, 1p following 597. http://www.nature.com/articles/nm.2123.
62. Ji R-R, Xu Z-Z, Strichartz G, Serhan CN. Emerging roles of resolvins in the resolution of inflammation and pain. Trends Neurosci. 2011;34:599–609. https://linkinghub.elsevier.com/retrieve/pii/S0166223611001391.
63. Park C-K, Xu Z-Z, Liu T, Lu N, Serhan CN, Ji R-R. Resolvin D2 is a potent endogenous inhibitor for transient receptor potential subtype V1/A1, inflammatory pain, and spinal cord synaptic plasticity in mice: distinct roles of resolvin D1, D2, and E1. J Neurosci. 2011;31:18433–8. https://doi.org/10.1523/JNEUROSCI.4192-11.2011.
64. Bone RC. The pathogenesis of sepsis. Ann Intern Med. 1991;115:457–69. http://www.ncbi.nlm.nih.gov/pubmed/1872494.
65. Hotchkiss RS, Karl IE. The pathophysiology and treatment of sepsis. N Engl J Med. 2003;348:138–50. http://www.ncbi.nlm.nih.gov/pubmed/12519925.
66. Bosmann M, Ward PA. The inflammatory response in sepsis. Trends Immunol. 2013;34:129–36. http://www.ncbi.nlm.nih.gov/pubmed/23036432.
67. Chousterman BG, Swirski FK, Weber GF. Cytokine storm and sepsis disease pathogenesis. Semin Immunopathol. 2017;39:517–28. http://www.ncbi.nlm.nih.gov/pubmed/28555385.
68. Bone RC, Balk RA, Cerra FB, Dellinger RP, Fein AM, Knaus WA, et al. Definitions for sepsis and organ failure and guidelines for the use of innovative therapies in sepsis. The ACCP/SCCM Consensus Conference Committee. American College of Chest Physicians/Society of Critical Care Medicine. Chest. 1992;101:1644–55. http://www.ncbi.nlm.nih.gov/pubmed/1303622.
69. Balk RA. Systemic inflammatory response syndrome (SIRS): where did it come from and is it still relevant today? Virulence. 2014;5:20–6. https://doi.org/10.4161/viru.27135.
70. Butcher NE, Balogh ZJ. Update on the definition of polytrauma. Eur J Trauma Emerg Surg. 2014;40:107–11. http://www.ncbi.nlm.nih.gov/pubmed/26815890.
71. Keel M, Trentz O. Pathophysiology of polytrauma. Injury. 2005;36:691–709. http://www.ncbi.nlm.nih.gov/pubmed/15910820.
72. Keel M, Eid K, Labler L, Seifert B, Trentz O, Ertel W. Influence of injury pattern on incidence and severity of posttraumatic inflammatory complications in severely injured patients. Eur J Trauma. 2006;32(4):387–95. https://core.ac.uk/download/pdf/159153545.pdf.
73. Devi Ramnath R, Weing S, He M, Sun J, Zhang H, Singh Bawa M, et al. Inflammatory mediators in sepsis: cytokines, chemokines, adhesion molecules and gases. J Organ Dysfunct. 2006;2:80–92. https://doi.org/10.1080/17471060500435662.
74. Aziz M, Jacob A, Yang W-L, Matsuda A, Wang P. Current trends in inflammatory and immunomodulatory mediators in sepsis. J Leukoc Biol. 2013;93:329–42. http://www.ncbi.nlm.nih.gov/pubmed/23136259.
75. Mosevoll KA, Skrede S, Markussen DL, Fanebust HR, Flaatten HK, Aßmus J, et al. Inflammatory mediator profiles differ in sepsis patients with and without bacteremia. Front Immunol. 2018;9:691. https://doi.org/10.3389/fimmu.2018.00691/full.
76. Almawash AM. The inflammatory mediators and sepsis. Int J Curr Microbiol App Sci. 2018;7:1763–76. https://www.ijcmas.com/abstractview.php?ID=7035&vol=7-3-2018&SNo=208.

77. Gotts JE, Matthay MA. Sepsis: pathophysiology and clinical management. BMJ. 2016;353:i1585. http://www.ncbi.nlm.nih.gov/pubmed/27217054.
78. Taeb AM, Hooper MH, Marik PE. Sepsis: current definition, pathophysiology, diagnosis, and management. Nutr Clin Pract. 2017;32:296–308. http://www.ncbi.nlm.nih.gov/pubmed/28537517.
79. Prauchner CA. Oxidative stress in sepsis: pathophysiological implications justifying antioxidant co-therapy. Burns. 2017;43:471–85. http://www.ncbi.nlm.nih.gov/pubmed/28034666.
80. Badeaux JE, Martin JB. Emerging adjunctive approach for the treatment of sepsis. Crit Care Nurs Clin North Am. 2018;30:343–51. http://www.ncbi.nlm.nih.gov/pubmed/30098738.
81. Erridge C. Endogenous ligands of TLR2 and TLR4: agonists or assistants? J Leukoc Biol. 2010;87:989–99. http://www.ncbi.nlm.nih.gov/pubmed/20179153.
82. Ward PA. New approaches to the study of sepsis. EMBO Mol Med. 2012;4:1234–43. https://doi.org/10.1002/emmm.201201375.
83. Wenceslau CF, McCarthy CG, Goulopoulou S, Szasz T, NeSmith EG, Webb RC. Mitochondrial-derived N-formyl peptides: novel links between trauma, vascular collapse and sepsis. Med Hypotheses. 2013;81:532–5. http://www.ncbi.nlm.nih.gov/pubmed/23890799.
84. Gentile LF, Moldawer LL. DAMPs, PAMPs, and the origins of SIRS in bacterial sepsis. Shock. 2013;39:113–4. http://www.ncbi.nlm.nih.gov/pubmed/23247128.
85. Kang J-W, Kim S-J, Cho H-I, Lee S-M. DAMPs activating innate immune responses in sepsis. Ageing Res Rev. 2015;24:54–65. https://linkinghub.elsevier.com/retrieve/pii/S1568163715000318.
86. Martin L, Koczera P, Zechendorf E, Schuerholz T. The endothelial glycocalyx: new diagnostic and therapeutic approaches in sepsis. Biomed Res Int. 2016;2016:1–8. http://www.ncbi.nlm.nih.gov/pubmed/27699168.
87. Timmermans K, Kox M, Scheffer GJ, Pickkers P. Danger in the intensive care unit. Shock. 2016;45:108–16. http://www.ncbi.nlm.nih.gov/pubmed/26513703.
88. Hauser CJ, Otterbein LE. Danger signals from mitochondrial DAMPS in trauma and post-injury sepsis. Eur J Trauma Emerg Surg. 2018;44:317–24. http://www.ncbi.nlm.nih.gov/pubmed/29797026.
89. Land WG. The role of damage-associated molecular patterns (DAMPs) in human diseases: part II: DAMPs as diagnostics, prognostics and therapeutics in clinical medicine. Sultan Qaboos Univ Med J. 2015;15:e157–70. http://www.ncbi.nlm.nih.gov/pubmed/26052447.
90. Parlato M, Cavaillon J-M. Host response biomarkers in the diagnosis of sepsis: a general overview. Methods Mol Biol. 2015;1237:149–211. https://doi.org/10.1007/978-1-4939-1776-1_15.
91. Kakihana Y, Ito T, Nakahara M, Yamaguchi K, Yasuda T. Sepsis-induced myocardial dysfunction: pathophysiology and management. J Intensive Care. 2016;4:22. http://www.ncbi.nlm.nih.gov/pubmed/27011791.
92. Armstrong BA, Betzold RD, May AK. Sepsis and septic shock strategies. Surg Clin North Am. 2017;97:1339–79. https://linkinghub.elsevier.com/retrieve/pii/S0039610917301135.
93. Raymond SL, Holden DC, Mira JC, Stortz JA, Loftus TJ, Mohr AM, et al. Microbial recognition and danger signals in sepsis and trauma. Biochim Biophys Acta Mol Basis Dis. 1863;2017:2564–73. https://linkinghub.elsevier.com/retrieve/pii/S0925443917300261.
94. Ward PA. The harmful role of C5a on innate immunity in sepsis. J Innate Immun. 2010;2:439–45. http://www.ncbi.nlm.nih.gov/pubmed/20588003.
95. Yan C, Gao H. New insights for C5a and C5a receptors in sepsis. Front Immunol. 2012;3:368. http://www.ncbi.nlm.nih.gov/pubmed/23233853.
96. Denning N-L, Aziz M, Gurien SD, Wang P. DAMPs and NETs in sepsis. Front Immunol. 2019;10:2536. http://www.ncbi.nlm.nih.gov/pubmed/31736963.
97. Freeman BD, Natanson C. Anti-inflammatory therapies in sepsis and septic shock. Expert Opin Investig Drugs. 2000;9:1651–63. https://doi.org/10.1517/13543784.9.7.1651.
98. Bone RC. Sir Isaac Newton, sepsis, SIRS, and CARS. Crit Care Med. 1996;24:1125–8. http://www.ncbi.nlm.nih.gov/pubmed/8674323.

99. Ward NS, Casserly B, Ayala A. The compensatory anti-inflammatory response syndrome (CARS) in critically ill patients. Clin Chest Med. 2008;29:617–25. http://www.ncbi.nlm.nih.gov/pubmed/18954697.
100. Hotchkiss RS, Monneret G, Payen D. Immunosuppression in sepsis: a novel understanding of the disorder and a new therapeutic approach. Lancet Infect Dis. 2013;13:260–8. https://linkinghub.elsevier.com/retrieve/pii/S147330991370001X.
101. Hotchkiss RS, Monneret G, Payen D. Sepsis-induced immunosuppression: from cellular dysfunctions to immunotherapy. Nat Rev Immunol. 2013;13:862–74. http://www.ncbi.nlm.nih.gov/pubmed/24232462.
102. Hamers L, Kox M, Pickkers P. Sepsis-induced immunoparalysis: mechanisms, markers, and treatment options. Minerva Anestesiol. 2015;81:426–39. http://www.ncbi.nlm.nih.gov/pubmed/24878876.
103. Delano MJ, Ward PA. The immune system's role in sepsis progression, resolution, and long-term outcome. Immunol Rev. 2016;274:330–53. https://doi.org/10.1111/imr.12499.
104. Andrassy M, Volz HC, Igwe JC, Funke B, Eichberger SN, Kaya Z, et al. High-mobility group box-1 in ischemia-reperfusion injury of the heart. Circulation. 2008;117:3216–26. https://doi.org/10.1161/CIRCULATIONAHA.108.769331.
105. van der Poll T. Myeloid-derived suppressor cells in sepsis. Am J Respir Crit Care Med. 2017;196:256–8. http://www.ncbi.nlm.nih.gov/pubmed/28762789.
106. Fallon EA, Biron-Girard BM, Chung C-S, Lomas-Neira J, Heffernan DS, Monaghan SF, et al. A novel role for coinhibitory receptors/checkpoint proteins in the immunopathology of sepsis. J Leukoc Biol. 2018;103:1151–64. http://www.ncbi.nlm.nih.gov/pubmed/29393983.
107. Haveman JW, Muller Kobold AC, Tervaert JW, van den Berg AP, Tulleken JE, Kallenberg CG, et al. The central role of monocytes in the pathogenesis of sepsis: consequences for immunomonitoring and treatment. Neth J Med. 1999;55:132–41. http://www.ncbi.nlm.nih.gov/pubmed/10509072.
108. Nicolete R, Lima KM, Júnior JMR, Jose PJ, Sanz M-J, Faccioli LH. Prostaglandin E2-loaded microspheres as strategy to inhibit phagocytosis and modulate inflammatory mediators release. Eur J Pharm Biopharm. 2008;70:784–90. http://www.ncbi.nlm.nih.gov/pubmed/18640269.
109. Németh K, Leelahavanichkul A, Yuen PST, Mayer B, Parmelee A, Doi K, et al. Bone marrow stromal cells attenuate sepsis via prostaglandin E2–dependent reprogramming of host macrophages to increase their interleukin-10 production. Nat Med. 2009;15:42–9. http://www.ncbi.nlm.nih.gov/pubmed/19098906.
110. Fullerton JN, O'Brien AJ, Gilroy DW. Pathways mediating resolution of inflammation: when enough is too much. J Pathol. 2013;231:8–20. https://doi.org/10.1002/path.4232.
111. Qiu G, Zheng G, Ge M, Huang L, Tong H, Chen P, et al. Adipose-derived mesenchymal stem cells modulate CD14++CD16+ expression on monocytes from sepsis patients in vitro via prostaglandin E2. Stem Cell Res Ther. 2017;8:97. http://www.ncbi.nlm.nih.gov/pubmed/28446249.
112. Chen I-J, Hee S-W, Liao C-H, Lin S-Y, Su L, Shun C-T, et al. Targeting the 15-keto-PGE2-PTGR2 axis modulates systemic inflammation and survival in experimental sepsis. Free Radic Biol Med. 2018;115:113–26. http://www.ncbi.nlm.nih.gov/pubmed/29175486.
113. Tsai W-H, Li I-T, Yu Y-B, Hsu H-C, Shih C-H. Serial changes in plasma annexin A1 and cortisol levels in sepsis patients. Chin J Physiol. 2014;57:1–7. http://www.airitilibrary.com/Publication/alDetailedMesh?DocID=03044920-201402-201403100001-201403100001-1-7.
114. Zhang H, Lu Y, Sun G, Teng F, Luo N, Jiang J, et al. The common promoter polymorphism rs11666254 downregulates FPR2/ALX expression and increases risk of sepsis in patients with severe trauma. Crit Care. 2017;21:171. http://www.ncbi.nlm.nih.gov/pubmed/28679406.
115. Huang P, Zhou Y, Liu Z, Zhang P. Interaction between ANXA1 and GATA-3 in Immunosuppression of CD4 + T Cells. Mediators Inflamm. 2016;2016:1–9. http://www.ncbi.nlm.nih.gov/pubmed/27833268.
116. Zhang L, Zheng Y, Hu R, Zhu L, Hu C, Cheng F, et al. Annexin A1 mimetic peptide AC2-26 inhibits sepsis-induced cardiomyocyte apoptosis through LXA4/PI3K/AKT signaling pathway. Curr Med Sci. 2018;38:997–1004. http://www.ncbi.nlm.nih.gov/pubmed/30536061.

117. Bao R, Shui X, Hou J, Li J, Deng X, Zhu X, et al. Adenosine and the adenosine A2A receptor agonist, CGS21680, upregulate CD39 and CD73 expression through E2F-1 and CREB in regulatory T cells isolated from septic mice. Int J Mol Med. 2016;38:969–75. http://www.ncbi.nlm.nih.gov/pubmed/27430240.
118. Escobar DA, Botero-Quintero AM, Kautza BC, Luciano J, Loughran P, Darwiche S, et al. Adenosine monophosphate-activated protein kinase activation protects against sepsis-induced organ injury and inflammation. J Surg Res. 2015;194:262–72. http://www.ncbi.nlm.nih.gov/pubmed/25456115.
119. Dalli J, Colas RA, Quintana C, Barragan-Bradford D, Hurwitz S, Levy BD, et al. Human sepsis eicosanoid and proresolving lipid mediator temporal profiles. Crit Care Med. 2017;45:58–68. http://www.ncbi.nlm.nih.gov/pubmed/27632672.
120. Timmermans K, Kox M, Vaneker M, van den Berg M, John A, van Laarhoven A, et al. Plasma levels of danger-associated molecular patterns are associated with immune suppression in trauma patients. Intensive Care Med. 2016;42:551–61. http://www.ncbi.nlm.nih.gov/pubmed/26912315.
121. Jacops P, Bissonnette R, Guenther LC. Socioeconomic burden of immune-mediated inflammatory diseases—focusing on work productivity and disability. J Rheumatol Suppl. 2011;88:55–61. http://www.ncbi.nlm.nih.gov/pubmed/22045980.
122. Nathan C, Ding A. Nonresolving inflammation. Cell. 2010;140:871–82. http://linkinghub.elsevier.com/retrieve/pii/S0092867410001820.
123. Novak ML, Thorp EB. Shedding light on impaired efferocytosis and nonresolving inflammation. Circ Res. 2013;113:9–12. http://www.ncbi.nlm.nih.gov/pubmed/23788501.
124. Fredman G, Li Y, Dalli J, Chiang N, Serhan CN. Self-limited versus delayed resolution of acute inflammation: temporal regulation of pro-resolving mediators and microRNA. Sci Rep. 2012;2:639. http://www.nature.com/articles/srep00639.
125. Dominguez-Andres J, Netea MG. Long-term reprogramming of the innate immune system. J Leukoc Biol. 2019;105:329–38. https://doi.org/10.1002/JLB.MR0318-104R.
126. Bekkering S, Quintin J, Joosten LAB, van der Meer JWM, Netea MG, Riksen NP. Oxidized low-density lipoprotein induces long-term proinflammatory cytokine production and foam cell formation via epigenetic reprogramming of monocytes. Arterioscler Thromb Vasc Biol. 2014;34:1731–8. https://doi.org/10.1161/ATVBAHA.114.303887.
127. van der Valk FM, Bekkering S, Kroon J, Yeang C, Van den Bossche J, van Buul JD, et al. Oxidized phospholipids on lipoprotein(a) elicit arterial wall inflammation and an inflammatory monocyte response in humans. Circulation. 2016;134:611–24. https://doi.org/10.1161/CIRCULATIONAHA.116.020838.
128. Neidhart M, Pajak A, Laskari K, Riksen NP, Joosten LAB, Netea MG, et al. Oligomeric S100A4 is associated with monocyte innate immune memory and bypass of tolerance to subsequent stimulation with lipopolysaccharides. Front Immunol. 2019;10:791. http://www.ncbi.nlm.nih.gov/pubmed/31037071.
129. Waterland RA. Epigenetic mechanisms and gastrointestinal development. J Pediatr. 2006;149:S137–42. http://linkinghub.elsevier.com/retrieve/pii/S002234760600624X.
130. Gibney ER, Nolan CM. Epigenetics and gene expression. Heredity (Edinb). 2010;105:4–13. http://www.ncbi.nlm.nih.gov/pubmed/20461105.
131. Kundaje A, Meuleman W, Ernst J, Bilenky M, Yen A, Heravi-Moussavi A, et al. Integrative analysis of 111 reference human epigenomes. Nature. 2015;518:317–30. http://www.ncbi.nlm.nih.gov/pubmed/25693563.
132. Rothbart SB, Strahl BD. Interpreting the language of histone and DNA modifications. Biochim Biophys Acta. 1839;2014:627–43. http://www.ncbi.nlm.nih.gov/pubmed/24631868.
133. Wei J-W, Huang K, Yang C, Kang C-S. Non-coding RNAs as regulators in epigenetics (review). Oncol Rep. 2016;37:3–9. http://www.ncbi.nlm.nih.gov/pubmed/27841002.
134. Moosavi A, Motevalizadeh AA. Role of epigenetics in biology and human diseases. Iran Biomed J. 2016;20:246–58. http://www.ncbi.nlm.nih.gov/pubmed/27377127.
135. Allis CD, Jenuwein T. The molecular hallmarks of epigenetic control. Nat Rev Genet. 2016;17:487–500. https://doi.org/10.1038/nrg.2016.59.

136. Torres IO, Fujimori DG. Functional coupling between writers, erasers and readers of histone and DNA methylation. Curr Opin Struct Biol. 2015;35:68–75. http://www.ncbi.nlm.nih.gov/pubmed/26496625.
137. Xu Y, Zhang S, Lin S, Guo Y, Deng W, Zhang Y, et al. WERAM: a database of writers, erasers and readers of histone acetylation and methylation in eukaryotes. Nucleic Acids Res. 2017;45:D264–70. https://doi.org/10.1093/nar/gkw1011.
138. Berger SL, Kouzarides T, Shiekhattar R, Shilatifard A. An operational definition of epigenetics. Genes Dev. 2009;23:781–3. https://doi.org/10.1101/gad.1787609.
139. Kreuz S, Fischle W. Oxidative stress signaling to chromatin in health and disease. Epigenomics. 2016;8:843–62. http://www.ncbi.nlm.nih.gov/pubmed/27319358.
140. Ptashne M. Epigenetics: core misconcept. Proc Natl Acad Sci U S A. 2013;110:7101–3. https://doi.org/10.1073/pnas.1305399110.
141. Riddihough G, Zahn LM. Epigenetics. What is epigenetics? Introduction. Science. 2010;330:611. https://doi.org/10.1126/science.330.6004.611.
142. Alabert C, Groth A. Chromatin replication and epigenome maintenance. Nat Rev Mol Cell Biol. 2012;13:153–67. http://www.ncbi.nlm.nih.gov/pubmed/22358331.
143. Reverón-Gómez N, González-Aguilera C, Stewart-Morgan KR, Petryk N, Flury V, Graziano S, et al. Accurate recycling of parental histones reproduces the histone modification landscape during DNA replication. Mol Cell. 2018;72:239–249.e5. http://www.ncbi.nlm.nih.gov/pubmed/30146316.
144. Netea MG, van der Meer JWM. Trained immunity: an ancient way of remembering. Cell Host Microbe. 2017;21:297–300. https://linkinghub.elsevier.com/retrieve/pii/S1931312817300653.
145. Netea MG, Quintin J, van der Meer JWM. Trained immunity: a memory for innate host defense. Cell Host Microbe. 2011;9:355–61. http://linkinghub.elsevier.com/retrieve/pii/S1931312811001284.
146. Crisan TO, Netea MG, Joosten LAB. Innate immune memory: implications for host responses to damage-associated molecular patterns. Eur J Immunol. 2016;46:817–8. https://doi.org/10.1002/eji.201545497.
147. Schnack L, Sohrabi Y, Lagache SMM, Kahles F, Bruemmer D, Waltenberger J, et al. Mechanisms of trained innate immunity in oxLDL primed human coronary smooth muscle cells. Front Immunol. 2019;10:13. http://www.ncbi.nlm.nih.gov/pubmed/30728822.
148. Cheng S-C, Quintin J, Cramer RA, Shepardson KM, Saeed S, Kumar V, et al. mTOR- and HIF-1 -mediated aerobic glycolysis as metabolic basis for trained immunity. Science (80-). 2014;345:1250684. http://www.ncbi.nlm.nih.gov/pubmed/25258083.
149. Arts RJW, Novakovic B, Ter Horst R, Carvalho A, Bekkering S, Lachmandas E, et al. Glutaminolysis and fumarate accumulation integrate immunometabolic and epigenetic programs in trained immunity. Cell Metab. 2016;24:807–19. https://linkinghub.elsevier.com/retrieve/pii/S1550413116305393.
150. Bekkering S, Arts RJW, Novakovic B, Kourtzelis I, van der Heijden CDCC, Li Y, et al. Metabolic induction of trained immunity through the mevalonate pathway. Cell. 2018;172:135–146.e9. http://www.ncbi.nlm.nih.gov/pubmed/29328908.
151. Arts RJW, Joosten LAB, Netea MG. The potential role of trained immunity in autoimmune and autoinflammatory disorders. Front Immunol. 2018;9:298. https://doi.org/10.3389/fimmu.2018.00298/full.
152. van der Heijden CDCC, Noz MP, Joosten LAB, Netea MG, Riksen NP, Keating ST. Epigenetics and trained immunity. Antioxid Redox Signal. 2018;29:1023–40. http://www.ncbi.nlm.nih.gov/pubmed/28978221.
153. Chen S, Yang J, Wei Y, Wei X. Epigenetic regulation of macrophages: from homeostasis maintenance to host defense. Cell Mol Immunol. 2019;7(1):36–49. http://www.ncbi.nlm.nih.gov/pubmed/31664225.
154. Chen L, Ge B, Casale FP, Vasquez L, Kwan T, Garrido-Martín D, et al. Genetic drivers of epigenetic and transcriptional variation in human immune cells. Cell. 2016;167:1398–1414.e24. http://www.ncbi.nlm.nih.gov/pubmed/27863251.

155. Aschenbrenner AC, Schultze JL. New “programmers” in tissue macrophage activation. Pflügers Arch Eur J Physiol. 2017;469:375–83. http://www.ncbi.nlm.nih.gov/pubmed/28185067.
156. Daskalaki MG, Tsatsanis C, Kampranis SC. Histone methylation and acetylation in macrophages as a mechanism for regulation of inflammatory responses. J Cell Physiol. 2018;233:6495–507. https://doi.org/10.1002/jcp.26497.
157. Marchal C, Miotto B. Emerging concept in DNA methylation: role of transcription factors in shaping DNA methylation patterns. J Cell Physiol. 2015;230:743–51. https://doi.org/10.1002/jcp.24836.
158. Schübeler D. Function and information content of DNA methylation. Nature. 2015;517:321–6. http://www.nature.com/articles/nature14192.
159. Estécio MRH, Issa J-PJ. Dissecting DNA hypermethylation in cancer. FEBS Lett. 2011;585:2078–86. https://doi.org/10.1016/j.febslet.2010.12.001.
160. Jones PA. Functions of DNA methylation: islands, start sites, gene bodies and beyond. Nat Rev Genet. 2012;13:484–92. http://www.nature.com/articles/nrg3230.
161. Jeltsch A, Broche J, Bashtrykov P. Molecular processes connecting DNA methylation patterns with DNA Methyltransferases and Histone Modifications in Mammalian Genomes. Genes (Basel). 2018;9:566. http://www.ncbi.nlm.nih.gov/pubmed/30469440.
162. Laisné M, Gupta N, Kirsh O, Pradhan S, Defossez P-A. Mechanisms of DNA methyltransferase recruitment in mammals. Genes (Basel). 2018;9:617. http://www.ncbi.nlm.nih.gov/pubmed/30544749.
163. Fournier A, Sasai N, Nakao M, Defossez P-A. The role of methyl-binding proteins in chromatin organization and epigenome maintenance. Brief Funct Genomics. 2012;11:251–64. http://www.ncbi.nlm.nih.gov/pubmed/22184333.
164. Yin X, Xu Y. Structure and function of TET enzymes. Adv Exp Med Biol. 2016;945:275–302. http://www.ncbi.nlm.nih.gov/pubmed/27826843.
165. Koivunen P, Laukka T. The TET enzymes. Cell Mol Life Sci. 2018;75:1339–48. http://www.ncbi.nlm.nih.gov/pubmed/29184981.
166. Du Q, Luu P-L, Stirzaker C, Clark SJ. Methyl-CpG-binding domain proteins: readers of the epigenome. Epigenomics. 2015;7:1051–73. https://doi.org/10.2217/epi.15.39.
167. Cao Q, Wang X, Jia L, Mondal AK, Diallo A, Hawkins GA, et al. Inhibiting DNA Methylation by 5-Aza-2’-deoxycytidine ameliorates atherosclerosis through suppressing macrophage inflammation. Endocrinology. 2014;155:4925–38. https://doi.org/10.1210/en.2014-1595.
168. Babu M, Durga Devi T, Mäkinen P, Kaikkonen M, Lesch HP, Junttila S, et al. Differential promoter methylation of macrophage genes is associated with impaired vascular growth in ischemic muscles of hyperlipidemic and type 2 diabetic mice: genome-wide promoter methylation study. Circ Res. 2015;117:289–99. https://doi.org/10.1161/CIRCRESAHA.115.306424.
169. Wang X, Cao Q, Yu L, Shi H, Xue B, Shi H. Epigenetic regulation of macrophage polarization and inflammation by DNA methylation in obesity. JCI Insight. 2016;1:e87748. http://www.ncbi.nlm.nih.gov/pubmed/27882346.
170. Grygiel-Górniak B. Peroxisome proliferator-activated receptors and their ligands: nutritional and clinical implications—a review. Nutr J. 2014;13:17. https://doi.org/10.1186/1475-2891-13-17.
171. Goto T. A review of the studies on food-derived factors which regulate energy metabolism via the modulation of lipid-sensing nuclear receptors. Biosci Biotechnol Biochem. 2018:1–10. http://www.ncbi.nlm.nih.gov/pubmed/30572788.
172. Yu J, Qiu Y, Yang J, Bian S, Chen G, Deng M, et al. DNMT1-PPARγ pathway in macrophages regulates chronic inflammation and atherosclerosis development in mice. Sci Rep. 2016;6:30053. http://www.ncbi.nlm.nih.gov/pubmed/27530451.
173. Li X, Zhang Q, Ding Y, Liu Y, Zhao D, Zhao K, et al. Methyltransferase Dnmt3a upregulates HDAC9 to deacetylate the kinase TBK1 for activation of antiviral innate immunity. Nat Immunol. 2016;17:806–15. http://www.ncbi.nlm.nih.gov/pubmed/27240213
174. Lee KK, Workman JL. Histone acetyltransferase complexes: one size doesn’t fit all. Nat Rev Mol Cell Biol. 2007;8:284–95. http://www.nature.com/articles/nrm2145.

175. Chypre M, Zaidi N, Smans K. ATP-citrate lyase: a mini-review. Biochem Biophys Res Commun. 2012;422:1–4. https://linkinghub.elsevier.com/retrieve/pii/S0006291X12008339.
176. Voss AK, Thomas T. Histone lysine and genomic targets of histone acetyltransferases in mammals. Bioessays. 2018;40:e1800078. https://doi.org/10.1002/bies.201800078.
177. Avvakumov N, Côté J. The MYST family of histone acetyltransferases and their intimate links to cancer. Oncogene. 2007;26:5395–407. http://www.nature.com/articles/1210608.
178. Chauhan A, Quenum FZ, Abbas A, Bradley DS, Nechaev S, Singh BB, et al. Epigenetic modulation of microglial inflammatory gene loci in helminth-induced immune suppression: implications for immune regulation in neurocysticercosis. ASN Neuro. 2015;7:175909141559212. https://doi.org/10.1177/1759091415592126.
179. Haberland M, Montgomery RL, Olson EN. The many roles of histone deacetylases in development and physiology: implications for disease and therapy. Nat Rev Genet. 2009;10:32–42. http://www.ncbi.nlm.nih.gov/pubmed/19065135.
180. Wang Z, Zang C, Cui K, Schones DE, Barski A, Peng W, et al. Genome-wide mapping of HATs and HDACs reveals distinct functions in active and inactive genes. Cell. 2009;138:1019–31. https://linkinghub.elsevier.com/retrieve/pii/S0092867409008411.
181. Seto E, Yoshida M. Erasers of histone acetylation: the histone deacetylase enzymes. Cold Spring Harb Perspect Biol. 2014;6:a018713. https://doi.org/10.1101/cshperspect.a018713.
182. Grabiec AM, Potempa J. Epigenetic regulation in bacterial infections: targeting histone deacetylases. Crit Rev Microbiol. 2018;44:336–50. http://www.ncbi.nlm.nih.gov/pubmed/28971711.
183. Shakespear MR, Halili MA, Irvine KM, Fairlie DP, Sweet MJ. Histone deacetylases as regulators of inflammation and immunity. Trends Immunol. 2011;32:335–43. https://linkinghub.elsevier.com/retrieve/pii/S1471490611000561.
184. Halili MA, Andrews MR, Labzin LI, Schroder K, Matthias G, Cao C, et al. Differential effects of selective HDAC inhibitors on macrophage inflammatory responses to the Toll-like receptor 4 agonist LPS. J Leukoc Biol. 2010;87:1103–14. https://doi.org/10.1189/jlb.0509363.
185. Bode KA, Schroder K, Hume DA, Ravasi T, Heeg K, Sweet MJ, et al. Histone deacetylase inhibitors decrease Toll-like receptor-mediated activation of proinflammatory gene expression by impairing transcription factor recruitment. Immunology. 2007;122:596–606. https://doi.org/10.1111/j.1365-2567.2007.02678.x.
186. Roger T, Lugrin J, Le Roy D, Goy G, Mombelli M, Koessler T, et al. Histone deacetylase inhibitors impair innate immune responses to Toll-like receptor agonists and to infection. Blood. 2011;117:1205–17. https://doi.org/10.1182/blood-2010-05-284711.
187. Lu J, Sun H, Wang X, Liu C, Xu X, Li F, et al. Interleukin-12 p40 promoter activity is regulated by the reversible acetylation mediated by HDAC1 and p300. Cytokine. 2005;31:46–51. http://linkinghub.elsevier.com/retrieve/pii/S1043466605001146.
188. Nusinzon I, Horvath CM. Positive and negative regulation of the innate antiviral response and beta interferon gene expression by deacetylation. Mol Cell Biol. 2006;26:3106–13. https://doi.org/10.1128/MCB.26.8.3106-3113.2006.
189. Shakespear MR, Hohenhaus DM, Kelly GM, Kamal NA, Gupta P, Labzin LI, et al. Histone deacetylase 7 promotes Toll-like receptor 4-dependent proinflammatory gene expression in macrophages. J Biol Chem. 2013;288:25362–74. http://www.ncbi.nlm.nih.gov/pubmed/23853092.
190. Barneda-Zahonero B, Román-González L, Collazo O, Rafati H, Islam ABMMK, Bussmann LH, et al. HDAC7 is a repressor of myeloid genes whose downregulation is required for transdifferentiation of pre-B cells into macrophages. PLoS Genet. 2013;9:e1003503. https://doi.org/10.1371/journal.pgen.1003503.
191. Poralla L, Stroh T, Erben U, Sittig M, Liebig S, Siegmund B, et al. Histone deacetylase 5 regulates the inflammatory response of macrophages. J Cell Mol Med. 2015;19:2162–71. https://doi.org/10.1111/jcmm.12595.
192. Mendes KL, de Lelis DF, Santos SHS. Nuclear sirtuins and inflammatory signaling pathways. Cytokine Growth Factor Rev. 2017;38:98–105. http://www.ncbi.nlm.nih.gov/pubmed/29132743.

193. Li Y, Yang X, He Y, Wang W, Zhang J, Zhang W, et al. Negative regulation of NLRP3 inflammasome by SIRT1 in vascular endothelial cells. Immunobiology. 2017;222:552–61. https://linkinghub.elsevier.com/retrieve/pii/S0171298516304302.
194. Cheng X. Structural and functional coordination of DNA and histone methylation. Cold Spring Harb Perspect Biol. 2014;6:a018747. https://doi.org/10.1101/cshperspect.a018747.
195. Deng P, Chen Q-M, Hong C, Wang C-Y. Histone methyltransferases and demethylases: regulators in balancing osteogenic and adipogenic differentiation of mesenchymal stem cells. Int J Oral Sci. 2015;7:197–204. http://www.nature.com/articles/ijos201541.
196. Chen X, El Gazzar M, Yoza BK, McCall CE. The NF-kappaB factor RelB and histone H3 lysine methyltransferase G9a directly interact to generate epigenetic silencing in endotoxin tolerance. J Biol Chem. 2009;284:27857–65. https://doi.org/10.1074/jbc.M109.000950.
197. Li Y, Reddy MA, Miao F, Shanmugam N, Yee J-K, Hawkins D, et al. Role of the histone H3 lysine 4 methyltransferase, SET7/9, in the regulation of NF-kappaB-dependent inflammatory genes. Relevance to diabetes and inflammation. J Biol Chem. 2008;283:26771–81. https://doi.org/10.1074/jbc.M802800200.
198. Eames HL, Saliba DG, Krausgruber T, Lanfrancotti A, Ryzhakov G, Udalova IA. KAP1/TRIM28: an inhibitor of IRF5 function in inflammatory macrophages. Immunobiology. 2012;217:1315–24. https://linkinghub.elsevier.com/retrieve/pii/S0171298512001908.
199. Singh V, Prakhar P, Rajmani RS, Mahadik K, Borbora SM, Balaji KN. Histone methyltransferase SET8 epigenetically reprograms host immune responses to assist mycobacterial survival. J Infect Dis. 2017;216:477–88. http://www.ncbi.nlm.nih.gov/pubmed/28931237.
200. Kittan NA, Allen RM, Dhaliwal A, Cavassani KA, Schaller M, Gallagher KA, et al. Cytokine induced phenotypic and epigenetic signatures are key to establishing specific macrophage phenotypes. PLoS One. 2013;8:e78045. https://doi.org/10.1371/journal.pone.0078045.
201. Bedford MT, Clarke SG. Protein arginine methylation in mammals: who, what, and why. Mol Cell. 2009;33:1–13. https://linkinghub.elsevier.com/retrieve/pii/S1097276508008563.
202. Blanc RS, Richard S. Arginine methylation: the coming of age. Mol Cell. 2017;65:8–24. https://linkinghub.elsevier.com/retrieve/pii/S1097276516307110.
203. Kim JH, Yoo BC, Yang WS, Kim E, Hong S, Cho JY. The role of protein arginine methyltransferases in inflammatory responses. Mediators Inflamm. 2016;2016:1–11. http://www.ncbi.nlm.nih.gov/pubmed/27041824.
204. Covic M, Hassa PO, Saccani S, Buerki C, Meier NI, Lombardi C, et al. Arginine methyltransferase CARM1 is a promoter-specific regulator of NF-κB-dependent gene expression. EMBO J. 2005;24:85–96. http://www.ncbi.nlm.nih.gov/pubmed/15616592.
205. Xu J, Li Q. Review of the in vivo functions of the p160 steroid receptor coactivator family. Mol Endocrinol. 2003;17:1681–92. http://www.ncbi.nlm.nih.gov/pubmed/12805412.
206. Hassa PO, Covic M, Bedford MT, Hottiger MO. Protein arginine methyltransferase 1 coactivates NF-kappaB-dependent gene expression synergistically with CARM1 and PARP1. J Mol Biol. 2008;377:668–78. https://linkinghub.elsevier.com/retrieve/pii/S0022283608000788.
207. Tikhanovich I, Zhao J, Bridges B, Kumer S, Roberts B, Weinman SA. Arginine methylation regulates c-Myc–dependent transcription by altering promoter recruitment of the acetyltransferase p300. J Biol Chem. 2017;292:13333–44. http://www.ncbi.nlm.nih.gov/pubmed/28652407.
208. Wei H, Wang B, Miyagi M, She Y, Gopalan B, Huang D-B, et al. PRMT5 dimethylates R30 of the p65 subunit to activate NF-κB. Proc Natl Acad Sci U S A. 2013;110:13516–21. https://doi.org/10.1073/pnas.1311784110.
209. Di Lorenzo A, Yang Y, Macaluso M, Bedford MT. A gain-of-function mouse model identifies PRMT6 as a NF-κB coactivator. Nucleic Acids Res. 2014;42:8297–309. http://www.ncbi.nlm.nih.gov/pubmed/24939901.
210. Pedersen MT, Helin K. Histone demethylases in development and disease. Trends Cell Biol. 2010;20:662–71. https://linkinghub.elsevier.com/retrieve/pii/S0962892410001790.
211. Kooistra SM, Helin K. Molecular mechanisms and potential functions of histone demethylases. Nat Rev Mol Cell Biol. 2012;13:297–311. http://www.nature.com/articles/nrm3327.

212. Dimitrova E, Turberfield AH, Klose RJ. Histone demethylases in chromatin biology and beyond. EMBO Rep. 2015;16:1620–39. http://www.ncbi.nlm.nih.gov/pubmed/26564907.
213. Kang M, Mehrazarin S, Park N-H, Wang C-Y. Epigenetic gene regulation by histone demethylases: emerging role in oncogenesis and inflammation. Oral Dis. 2017;23:709–20. http://www.ncbi.nlm.nih.gov/pubmed/27514027.
214. Saccani S, Natoli G. Dynamic changes in histone H3 Lys 9 methylation occurring at tightly regulated inducible inflammatory genes. Genes Dev. 2002;16:2219–24. https://doi.org/10.1101/gad.232502.
215. De Santa F, Narang V, Yap ZH, Tusi BK, Burgold T, Austenaa L, et al. Jmjd3 contributes to the control of gene expression in LPS-activated macrophages. EMBO J. 2009;28:3341–52. https://doi.org/10.1038/emboj.2009.271.
216. Satoh T, Takeuchi O, Vandenbon A, Yasuda K, Tanaka Y, Kumagai Y, et al. The Jmjd3-Irf4 axis regulates M2 macrophage polarization and host responses against helminth infection. Nat Immunol. 2010;11:936–44. http://www.nature.com/articles/ni.1920.
217. Holla S, Prakhar P, Singh V, Karnam A, Mukherjee T, Mahadik K, et al. MUSASHI-mediated expression of JMJD3, a H3K27me3 Demethylase, is involved in foamy macrophage generation during mycobacterial infection. PLoS Pathog. 2016;12:e1005814. https://doi.org/10.1371/journal.ppat.1005814.
218. Chen Y-C, Chao T-Y, Leung S-Y, Chen C-J, Wu C-C, Fang W-F, et al. Histone H3K14 hypoacetylation and H3K27 hypermethylation along with HDAC1 up-regulation and KDM6B down-regulation are associated with active pulmonary tuberculosis disease. Am J Transl Res. 2017;9:1943–55. http://www.ncbi.nlm.nih.gov/pubmed/28469799.
219. Hyun K, Jeon J, Park K, Kim J. Writing, erasing and reading histone lysine methylations. Exp Mol Med. 2017;49:e324. http://www.ncbi.nlm.nih.gov/pubmed/28450737.
220. Burchfield JS, Li Q, Wang HY, Wang R-F. JMJD3 as an epigenetic regulator in development and disease. Int J Biochem Cell Biol. 2015;67:148–57. http://www.ncbi.nlm.nih.gov/pubmed/26193001.
221. Chakraborty A, Viswanathan P. Methylation-demethylation dynamics: implications of changes in acute kidney injury. Anal Cell Pathol. 2018;2018:1–16. http://www.ncbi.nlm.nih.gov/pubmed/30073137.
222. Esteller M. Non-coding RNAs in human disease. Nat Rev Genet. 2011;12:861–74. http://www.nature.com/articles/nrg3074.
223. Iyer MK, Niknafs YS, Malik R, Singhal U, Sahu A, Hosono Y, et al. The landscape of long noncoding RNAs in the human transcriptome. Nat Genet. 2015;47:199–208. http://www.nature.com/articles/ng.3192.
224. Ulitsky I. Evolution to the rescue: using comparative genomics to understand long non-coding RNAs. Nat Rev Genet. 2016;17:601–14. http://www.nature.com/articles/nrg.2016.85.
225. Quinn JJ, Chang HY. Unique features of long non-coding RNA biogenesis and function. Nat Rev Genet. 2016;17:47–62. http://www.nature.com/articles/nrg.2015.10.
226. Beermann J, Piccoli M-T, Viereck J, Thum T. Non-coding RNAs in development and disease: background, mechanisms, and therapeutic approaches. Physiol Rev. 2016;96:1297–325. https://doi.org/10.1152/physrev.00041.2015.
227. Mathy NW, Chen X-M. Long non-coding RNAs (lncRNAs) and their transcriptional control of inflammatory responses. J Biol Chem. 2017;292:12375–82. http://www.ncbi.nlm.nih.gov/pubmed/28615453.
228. Chen YG, Satpathy AT, Chang HY. Gene regulation in the immune system by long noncoding RNAs. Nat Immunol. 2017;18:962–72. https://doi.org/10.1038/ni.3771.
229. Uszczynska-Ratajczak B, Lagarde J, Frankish A, Guigó R, Johnson R. Towards a complete map of the human long non-coding RNA transcriptome. Nat Rev Genet. 2018;19:535–48. http://www.nature.com/articles/s41576-018-0017-y.
230. Katahira J. Nuclear export of messenger RNA. Genes (Basel). 2015;6:163–84. http://www.ncbi.nlm.nih.gov/pubmed/25836925.
231. Kaida D. The reciprocal regulation between splicing and 3′-end processing. Wiley Interdiscip Rev RNA. 2016;7:499–511. http://www.ncbi.nlm.nih.gov/pubmed/27019070.

232. Stewart M. Polyadenylation and nuclear export of mRNAs. J Biol Chem. 2019;294(9): 2977–87. http://www.ncbi.nlm.nih.gov/pubmed/30683695.
233. Li Y, Syed J, Sugiyama H. RNA-DNA triplex formation by long noncoding RNAs. Cell Chem Biol. 2016;23:1325–33. https://linkinghub.elsevier.com/retrieve/pii/S2451945616303464.
234. Qian X, Zhao J, Yeung PY, Zhang QC, Kwok CK. Revealing lncRNA structures and interactions by sequencing-based approaches. Trends Biochem Sci. 2019;44:33–52. http://www.ncbi.nlm.nih.gov/pubmed/30459069.
235. Cao J. The functional role of long non-coding RNAs and epigenetics. Biol Proced Online. 2014;16:11. https://doi.org/10.1186/1480-9222-16-11.
236. Balas MM, Johnson AM. Exploring the mechanisms behind long noncoding RNAs and cancer. Noncoding RNA Res. 2018;3:108–17. https://linkinghub.elsevier.com/retrieve/pii/S2468054017300525.
237. Engreitz JM, Haines JE, Perez EM, Munson G, Chen J, Kane M, et al. Local regulation of gene expression by lncRNA promoters, transcription and splicing. Nature. 2016;539:452–5. http://www.nature.com/articles/nature20149.
238. Peschansky VJ, Wahlestedt C. Non-coding RNAs as direct and indirect modulators of epigenetic regulation. Epigenetics. 2014;9:3–12. https://doi.org/10.4161/epi.27473.
239. Ferrè F, Colantoni A, Helmer-Citterich M. Revealing protein–lncRNA interaction. Brief Bioinform. 2016;17:106–16. http://www.ncbi.nlm.nih.gov/pubmed/26041786.
240. Wang KC, Yang YW, Liu B, Sanyal A, Corces-Zimmerman R, Chen Y, et al. A long noncoding RNA maintains active chromatin to coordinate homeotic gene expression. Nature. 2011;472:120–4. http://www.nature.com/articles/nature09819.
241. Xiao Y, Zhang J, Deng L. Prediction of lncRNA-protein interactions using HeteSim scores based on heterogeneous networks. Sci Rep. 2017;7:3664. http://www.ncbi.nlm.nih.gov/pubmed/28623317.
242. Murphy MB, Medvedev AE. Long noncoding RNAs as regulators of Toll-like receptor signaling and innate immunity. J Leukoc Biol. 2016;99:839–50. http://www.ncbi.nlm.nih.gov/pubmed/26965636.
243. Carpenter S, Aiello D, Atianand MK, Ricci EP, Gandhi P, Hall LL, et al. A long noncoding RNA mediates both activation and repression of immune response genes. Science. 2013;341:789–92. https://doi.org/10.1126/science.1240925.
244. Li Z, Chao T-C, Chang K-Y, Lin N, Patil VS, Shimizu C, et al. The long noncoding RNA THRIL regulates TNFα expression through its interaction with hnRNPL. Proc Natl Acad Sci U S A. 2014;111:1002–7. https://doi.org/10.1073/pnas.1313768111.
245. Huang Z, Luo Q, Yao F, Qing C, Ye J, Deng Y, et al. Identification of differentially expressed long non-coding RNAs in polarized macrophages. Sci Rep. 2016;6:19705. http://www.nature.com/articles/srep19705.
246. Cao J, Dong R, Jiang L, Gong Y, Yuan M, You J, et al. LncRNA-MM2P identified as a modulator of macrophage M2 polarization. Cancer Immunol Res. 2019;7:292–305. http://www.ncbi.nlm.nih.gov/pubmed/30459152.
247. Cui H, Banerjee S, Guo S, Xie N, Ge J, Jiang D, et al. Long noncoding RNA Malat1 regulates differential activation of macrophage and response to lung injury. JCI Insight. 2019;4:e124522. http://www.ncbi.nlm.nih.gov/pubmed/30676324.
248. Li X, Lei Y, Wu M, Li N. Regulation of macrophage activation and polarization by HCC-derived exosomal lncRNA TUC339. Int J Mol Sci. 2018;19:2958. http://www.ncbi.nlm.nih.gov/pubmed/30274167.
249. Atianand MK, Hu W, Satpathy AT, Shen Y, Ricci EP, Alvarez-Dominguez JR, et al. A long noncoding RNA lincRNA-EPS acts as a transcriptional brake to restrain inflammation. Cell. 2016;165:1672–85. http://www.ncbi.nlm.nih.gov/pubmed/27315481.
250. Holley CL, Topkara VK. An introduction to small non-coding RNAs: miRNA and snoRNA. Cardiovasc Drugs Ther. 2011;25:151–9. http://www.ncbi.nlm.nih.gov/pubmed/21573765.

251. Huang C, Shi J, Guo Y, Huang W, Huang S, Ming S, et al. A snoRNA modulates mRNA 3' end processing and regulates the expression of a subset of mRNAs. Nucleic Acids Res. 2017;45:8647–60. http://academic.oup.com/nar/article/45/15/8647/4036314/A-snoRNA-modulates-mRNA-3-end-processing-and.
252. Lee RC, Feinbaum RL, Ambros V. The C. elegans heterochronic gene lin-4 encodes small RNAs with antisense complementarity to lin-14. Cell. 1993;75:843–54. http://www.ncbi.nlm.nih.gov/pubmed/8252621.
253. Wightman B, Ha I, Ruvkun G. Posttranscriptional regulation of the heterochronic gene lin-14 by lin-4 mediates temporal pattern formation in C. elegans. Cell. 1993;75:855–62. http://www.ncbi.nlm.nih.gov/pubmed/8252622.
254. Friedman RC, Farh KK-H, Burge CB, Bartel DP. Most mammalian mRNAs are conserved targets of microRNAs. Genome Res. 2009;19:92–105. https://doi.org/10.1101/gr.082701.108.
255. O'Brien J, Hayder H, Zayed Y, Peng C. Overview of microRNA biogenesis, mechanisms of actions, and circulation. Front Endocrinol (Lausanne). 2018;9:402. https://www.frontiersin.org/article/10.3389/fendo.2018.00402/full.
256. Bartel DP. Metazoan microRNAs. Cell. 2018;173:20–51. http://www.ncbi.nlm.nih.gov/pubmed/29570994.
257. Kawahara Y. Human diseases caused by germline and somatic abnormalities in microRNA and microRNA-related genes. Congenit Anom (Kyoto). 2014;54:12–21. https://doi.org/10.1111/cga.12043.
258. Kobayashi H, Tomari Y. RISC assembly: coordination between small RNAs and Argonaute proteins. Biochim Biophys Acta Gene Regul Mech. 1859;2016:71–81. http://www.ncbi.nlm.nih.gov/pubmed/26303205.
259. Nakanishi K. Anatomy of RISC: how do small RNAs and chaperones activate Argonaute proteins? Wiley Interdiscip Rev RNA. 2016;7:637–60. http://www.ncbi.nlm.nih.gov/pubmed/27184117.
260. Jonas S, Izaurralde E. Towards a molecular understanding of microRNA-mediated gene silencing. Nat Rev Genet. 2015;16:421–33. http://www.nature.com/articles/nrg3965.
261. Behm-Ansmant I, Rehwinkel J, Doerks T, Stark A, Bork P, Izaurralde E. mRNA degradation by miRNAs and GW182 requires both CCR4:NOT deadenylase and DCP1:DCP2 decapping complexes. Genes Dev. 2006;20:1885–98. https://doi.org/10.1101/gad.1424106.
262. Braun JE, Truffault V, Boland A, Huntzinger E, Chang C-T, Haas G, et al. A direct interaction between DCP1 and XRN1 couples mRNA decapping to 5' exonucleolytic degradation. Nat Struct Mol Biol. 2012;19:1324–31. http://www.nature.com/articles/nsmb.2413.
263. Christie M, Boland A, Huntzinger E, Weichenrieder O, Izaurralde E. Structure of the PAN3 pseudokinase reveals the basis for interactions with the PAN2 deadenylase and the GW182 proteins. Mol Cell. 2013;51:360–73. https://linkinghub.elsevier.com/retrieve/pii/S1097276513005108.
264. Feng Y, Zou L, Yan D, Chen H, Xu G, Jian W, et al. Extracellular microRNAs induce potent innate immune responses via TLR7/MyD88-dependent mechanisms. J Immunol. 2017;199:2106–17. http://www.ncbi.nlm.nih.gov/pubmed/28768728.
265. Chen X, Liang H, Zhang J, Zen K, Zhang C-Y. Secreted microRNAs: a new form of intercellular communication. Trends Cell Biol. 2012;22:125–32. https://linkinghub.elsevier.com/retrieve/pii/S0962892411002388.
266. Alam MM, O'Neill LA. MicroRNAs and the resolution phase of inflammation in macrophages. Eur J Immunol. 2011;41:2482–5. https://doi.org/10.1002/eji.201141740.
267. O'Connell RM, Rao DS, Baltimore D. microRNA regulation of inflammatory responses. Annu Rev Immunol. 2012;30:295–312. https://doi.org/10.1146/annurev-immunol-020711-075013.
268. Rebane A, Akdis CA. MicroRNAs: Essential players in the regulation of inflammation. J Allergy Clin Immunol. 2013;132:15–26. https://linkinghub.elsevier.com/retrieve/pii/S0091674913006039.
269. Liu G, Abraham E. MicroRNAs in immune response and macrophage polarization. Arterioscler Thromb Vasc Biol. 2013;33:170–7. http://www.ncbi.nlm.nih.gov/pubmed/23325473.

270. Li Y, Shi X. MicroRNAs in the regulation of TLR and RIG-I pathways. Cell Mol Immunol. 2013;10:65–71. http://www.nature.com/articles/cmi201255.
271. Tahamtan A, Teymoori-Rad M, Nakstad B, Salimi V. Anti-inflammatory microRNAs and their potential for inflammatory diseases treatment. Front Immunol. 2018;9:1377. http://www.ncbi.nlm.nih.gov/pubmed/29988529.
272. Garavelli S, De Rosa V, de Candia P. The multifaceted interface between cytokines and microRNAs: an ancient mechanism to regulate the good and the bad of inflammation. Front Immunol. 2018;9:3012. https://www.frontiersin.org/article/10.3389/fimmu.2018.03012/full.
273. Piletič K, Kunej T. MicroRNA epigenetic signatures in human disease. Arch Toxicol. 2016;90:2405–19. https://doi.org/10.1007/s00204-016-1815-7.
274. Xu J, Feng Y, Jeyaram A, Jay SM, Zou L, Chao W. Circulating plasma extracellular vesicles from septic mice induce inflammation via microRNA- and TLR7-dependent mechanisms. J Immunol. 2018;201:3392–400. http://www.ncbi.nlm.nih.gov/pubmed/30355788.
275. Flanagan JM. Epigenome-wide association studies (EWAS): past, present, and future. Methods Mol Biol. 2015;1238:51–63. http://www.ncbi.nlm.nih.gov/pubmed/25421654.
276. Visscher PM, Wray NR, Zhang Q, Sklar P, McCarthy MI, Brown MA, et al. 10 years of GWAS discovery: biology, function, and translation. Am J Hum Genet. 2017;101:5–22. http://www.ncbi.nlm.nih.gov/pubmed/28686856.
277. Fogel O, Richard-Miceli C, Tost J. Epigenetic changes in chronic inflammatory diseases. Adv Protein Chem Struct Biol. 2017;106:139–89. http://www.ncbi.nlm.nih.gov/pubmed/28057210.
278. Stylianou E. Epigenetics of chronic inflammatory diseases. J Inflamm Res. 2018;12:1–14. http://www.ncbi.nlm.nih.gov/pubmed/30588059.
279. Foster SL, Hargreaves DC, Medzhitov R. Gene-specific control of inflammation by TLR-induced chromatin modifications. Nature. 2007;447:972–8. http://www.nature.com/articles/nature05836.
280. Barski A, Cuddapah S, Cui K, Roh T-Y, Schones DE, Wang Z, et al. High-resolution profiling of histone methylations in the human genome. Cell. 2007;129:823–37. https://linkinghub.elsevier.com/retrieve/pii/S0092867407006009.
281. Escoubet-Lozach L, Benner C, Kaikkonen MU, Lozach J, Heinz S, Spann NJ, et al. Mechanisms establishing TLR4-responsive activation states of inflammatory response genes. PLoS Genet. 2011;7:e1002401. https://doi.org/10.1371/journal.pgen.1002401.
282. Saeed S, Quintin J, Kerstens HHD, Rao NA, Aghajanirefah A, Matarese F, et al. Epigenetic programming of monocyte-to-macrophage differentiation and trained innate immunity. Science. 2014;345:1251086. https://doi.org/10.1126/science.1251086.
283. Quintin J, Cheng S-C, van der Meer JWM, Netea MG. Innate immune memory: towards a better understanding of host defense mechanisms. Curr Opin Immunol. 2014;29:1–7. https://linkinghub.elsevier.com/retrieve/pii/S095279151400034X.
284. Ulas T, Pirr S, Fehlhaber B, Bickes MS, Loof TG, Vogl T, et al. S100-alarmin-induced innate immune programming protects newborn infants from sepsis. Nat Immunol. 2017;18:622–32. http://www.ncbi.nlm.nih.gov/pubmed/28459433.
285. Hayder H, O'Brien J, Nadeem U, Peng C. MicroRNAs: crucial regulators of placental development. Reproduction. 2018;155:R259–71. https://rep.bioscientifica.com/view/journals/rep/155/6/REP-17-0603.xml.

DAMP-Promoted Efferent Innate Immune Responses in Human Diseases: Fibrosis

6

6.1 Introduction

Normal wound healing is the classical work of DAMPs that promote repairing pathways leading to homeostatic, mainly myofibroblast-mediated formation of scar tissue at sites of tissue injury. Under normal conditions, this repairing response is terminated when the scar is appropriately established. Typically, this process is characterized by myofibroblast apoptosis as a fundamental mechanism during normal wound healing. During the resolution phase, this cell-specific apoptosis is triggered mainly by the extrinsic pathway [1–3] (for apoptosis, also compare Vol.1 [4], Part V, Sect. 19.2.2.3). However, when uncontrolled and dysregulated, the same repairing pathways can become detrimental, leading to tissue/organ fibrosis in terms of a failed resolution of the repair response.

In fact, failure to resolve inflammatory/repairing responses associated with failure of apoptotic fibroblast death, combined with DAMP-promoted uncontrolled overshooting repairing pathways, lead to tissue remodeling rather than normal wound healing. This pathological scenario has been cursorily introduced in Vol.1 [4], Part VIII, Sect. 36.4. Here, the topic is resumed and extended by discussing some fundamental aspects of interest for physicians from different disciplines who are daily confronted with patients suffering from various chronic fibrosis-based diseases. Indeed, the underlying innate immune and—eventually—adaptive immune, cellular, and molecular events of fibrotic diseases share many functional similarities, despite differences in etiology and clinical outcome.

Of note, organ fibrosis—as, for example, cardiac fibrosis—presents in two forms: (1) as a replacement, that is reparative fibrosis, or (2) interstitial, that is reactive fibrosis. Replacement fibrosis is activated by an injury and must be regarded as a controlled, self-limited reparative process in which dead cells are replaced with a collagen-based scar. Interstitial fibrosis refers to an uncontrolled chronically progressive expansion or intractable scarring of the interstitium in areas remote to the initial injury [5–7].

W. G. Land, *Damage-Associated Molecular Patterns in Human Diseases*,
https://doi.org/10.1007/978-3-030-53868-2_6

As outlined in Vol. 1, [4], Part VIII, Sect. 36.4.1, fibrosis is characterized by the aberrant accumulation of fibrous connective tissue consisting of components of the ECM around damaged or inflamed tissue, which can lead to permanent scarring as characterized by matrix cross-linking and organ malfunction. Characteristically, these changes are predominantly due to the function of PRM-bearing fibroblasts (in the liver: PRM-bearing hepatic stellate cells [HSCs]), which transdifferentiate into myofibroblasts upon tissue stress/injury. This process occurs via epigenetic modifications late in the proliferative phase and is also called activation of myofibroblasts. Doubtlessly, myofibroblasts can be seen as the key mediators of fibrosis. Believed to derive from various precursors, but mainly from resident fibroblasts, these innate immune cells represent a heterogeneous population of cells (for additional information also compare Fig. 9.1, p. 167, Vol. 1 [4], Part III, Sect. 9.3.2). Myofibroblasts are characterized by (1) upregulation of the expression of cytoskeletal proteins, including alpha-smooth muscle actin (α-SMA), which form contractile stress fibers, and by (2) acquired increased contractility. Via contraction of these fibers, myofibroblasts mediate the mechanoregulation of fibrotic matrix remodeling through the formation of so-called focal adhesions, which are integral proteins of integrin signaling (see below). Typically, these cells secrete abundant amounts of ECM molecules, including collagen (COL) I, extra-domain A and B containing fibronectin (FNIII EDA/FNIII EDB), and MMPs (for additional information also compare Vol. 1 [4], Part III, Sect. 9.3, p. 166). Other innate immune cells, such as neutrophils and macrophages, complete their detrimental effects in terms of a complicated network of molecular, cellular, and humoral innate immune processes.

As known to all physicians, fibrotic disorders represent a growing cause of morbidity and mortality worldwide. The reason for this can be seen in scar formation that is associated with organ dysfunction. A few examples of this scenario have been given by Hinz [8]: "skin scars do not contain glands and hair follicles, scar tissue stabilizing the heart after myocardial infarct does not beat, scarred lungs do not contribute to gas exchange, sclerotic kidneys do not filter, and collagen in the liver cannot perform hepatocyte functions. If normal acute repair is successful, it is the amount of remaining functional tissue that mostly decides whether we live or die."

As a typical feature of a wide range of chronic pathologies across multiple organ systems, fibrotic diseases that include cardiac, pulmonary and kidney fibrosis, liver cirrhosis, and systemic sclerosis account for at least one-third of deaths worldwide. Alone in the USA, fibrotic disorders have been estimated to contribute to 45% of all-cause mortality [9]; moreover, current therapies for fibrosis are few and of limited efficacy. Therefore, there is an urgent need to understand how fibrosis may regress and to identify potential therapeutic approaches. Deeper insights into mechanisms of DAMP-promoted fibrotic pathways may be helpful in reaching this goal: reason enough to start, in this section, with a more general overview of this topic in light of controlled homeostatic and uncontrolled pathological DAMP-triggered fibrotic responses.

6.2 The Role of the Extracellular Matrix in Homeostasis

6.2.1 Introductory Remarks

The ECM is a three-dimensional, non-cellular tissue structure that is vital for life. During the past decades, it has become clear that the function of the ECM is not restricted to physical support for tissue integrity and elasticity, guaranteeing the cohesion of our body. Far beyond this property, it is a dynamic structure that is remodeled constantly to regulate and control cell and tissue homeostasis. In mammals, the ECM comprises around 300 proteins, known as the "core matrisome," and includes proteins such as collagen, proteoglycans (PGs), glycosaminoglycans, and glycoproteins. Collagens are the main structural proteins and are classified into both fibrillar (COL I–III, V, and XI) and non-fibrillar forms. Collagen fibrils provide tensile strength to the ECM, limiting the distensibility of tissues. Also, there are large numbers of ECM-modifying enzymes, ECM-binding growth factors, and other ECM-associated proteins. Two main types of ECM can be distinguished that differ in their location and composition: the interstitial connective tissue matrix that surrounds cells and provides structural scaffolding for tissues as well as the basement membrane, which refers to a special form of ECM that separates the epithelium from the surrounding stroma (reviewed in [10-14]).

6.2.2 Breakdown of the Extracellular Matrix by Proteinases

As described in Vol. 1 [4], Part IV, Sect. 13.2, cleavage of ECM components is the main process during ECM remodeling and is mandatory for the release of class IIA DAMPs (see also Sect. 3.4.2 and Table 3.1). The cleavage process of ECM is executed by different families of proteinases. The main enzymes involved in such ECM degradation are the MMPs whose activity is low in normal conditions but increased during stress-/injury-induced tissue inflammation and repair. The MMPs are produced either as soluble or cell membrane-anchored proteinases and cleave ECM components with wide substrate specificities.

So far, 23 human MMPs have been identified. Most MMPs are secreted as zymogens and are subsequently activated in the extracellular space; however, some of them are also membrane-bound proteins. The enzymes are often secreted as an inactive pro-MMP form, which is cleaved to the active form by various proteinases, including other MMPs or by oxidative modification of the thiol group. Together, MMPs can degrade all ECM proteins, and their proteolytic actions on the ECM have crucial roles in tissue development, organogenesis, branching morphogenesis, innate immune inflammatory and repairing responses, as well as in a variety of diseases (for reviews, see [11, 15-17]).

Another group of ECM-cleaving enzymes refers to so-called adamalysins, which include ADAMs (a disintegrin and metalloproteinases) and ADAMTS (ADAMs with a thrombospondin motif) (reviewed in [11, 18]). So far, 22 ADAM genes have been identified in humans, but only 12 encode active proteinases. ADAMs are membrane-bound enzymes, capable of shedding a multitude of proteins from the surface of the cell. The structure and function of ADAMs are related to those of a family of snake venom metalloproteinases, which also possess a potential adhesion domain as well as a potential proteinase domain. Mammalian ADAMs are involved in various biological and disease-related processes, such as cell–cell fusion, adhesion, and intracellular signaling. A second group comprises the ADAMTS that are secreted proteinases with thrombospondin type I-like repeats in their carboxy-terminal sequences. The relevance of ADAMTS enzymes has become evident in patients with a deficiency in ADAMTS-13, a VWF-cleaving proteinase. These patients develop thrombotic thrombocytopenic purpura, a devastating thrombotic disorder caused by widespread microvascular thrombi composed of platelets and VWF. The function of other ADMTS is still elusive (for VWF acting as an inducible IIIA-4 DAMP, compare also Vol. 1 [4], Part IV, Sect. 14.2.5.3 and Fig. 14.2).

Notably, MMPs synthesis and proteolysis require tight regulation to avoid excessive and deleterious tissue degradation and guarantee tissue homeostasis. These processes are finely regulated at various levels, that is, gene expression, processing of mRNA, intracellular and extracellular activation, regulation by *tissue inhibitors of metalloproteinases* (TIMPs), and activation or inactivation by other proteinases [16, 19]. The TIMP family consists of four members (TIMP1–TIMP4) that reversibly inhibit the activity of MMPs, ADAMs, and ADAMTS. The MMP-to-TIMP ratios determine the overall proteolytic activity, and each TIMP displays preferential MMP-binding specificity. Interestingly, in healthy tissues, TIMPs appear to spare the ECM from degradation, and only following infectious/sterile injury do TIMPs appear to indirectly control ECM deposition (e.g., enhanced fibrosis observed in mice lacking TIMPs following injury) (reviewed in [19, 20]).

6.2.3 The Importance of the Extracellular Matrix Stiffness

As mentioned above, modern research in the field of ECM has revealed that the matrix is a dynamic structure that permanently regulates cell biology (e.g., cell migration, growth, differentiation, and survival) under steady-state conditions. Intriguingly, according to modern notions, this unique regulatory function of the ECM is not only based on biochemical interactions but also mediated by mechanical properties. The scenario has been descriptively outlined by Humphrey et al. [12] and Handorf et al. [21]. In vivo, cells reside in a highly organized microenvironment that consists of endogenous forces generated by the cells themselves (e.g., mediated by the cytoskeletal contractility), as well as exogenous forces that affect cells by the surrounding microenvironment. These exogenous environmental cues are permanently read by resident cells to respond and subsequently promote homeostasis. Generally, exogenous forces applied to cells exist in various forms, including gravity, shear stress, as well as tensile and compressive forces (note: for tensile forces and other terms of mechanobiology, see Box 6.1). These exogenous forces are received by cells through interaction with the ECM, and, importantly enough, the local stiffness of the ECM is a critical mechanical effector of these forces to influence subsequent cell behavior. Notably, the various stiffness-mediated forces are translated by cells into biochemical signaling cascades through the process of mechanotransduction, and evidence suggests that, reciprocally, cells play an active role in remodeling their matrix to maintain an ECM stress set point through a process known as "tensional homeostasis" [22]. It is this tensional homeostasis that appears to create a favorable mechanical environment for cell function. Collectively, it is this ECM-associated stiffness that enables cell ↔ ECM interactions to operate through an integrated set of sensors and effector pathways. Hence, these interactions use not only classical innate immune recognition molecules but also mechanosensors to trigger inflammatory and repairing signaling pathways.

Box 6.1 Terms Helpful in Mechanobiology

Strain refers to the deformation of material indicating changes in lengths or angles within a material, typically induced by applied stresses. Strain is positive if the material fibers are stretched and negative if they are compressed.

Stress is a measure of "force intensity," given as is force per unit area (i.e., typically reported in units of one newton per square meter (N/m^2), which is called a pascal (Pa)). Note that 1 nN/μm^2 = 1 kPa (where nN indicates a nanonewton and μm indicates a micron, viz., 1 nN = 10^{-9} N and 1 μm = 10^{-6} m), which shows equivalence between units used in molecular and cell/tissue level studies.

Tensile forces are pulling forces that act to lengthen a material in the direction of the applied force.

Tensile stress is the tensile force per unit area. Tensile stress applied to a material gives rise to tensile strain, which measures the lengthening (i.e., stretch) of a material. Tensile stress developed by a cell (due to myofilament or cytoskeletal contraction) will tend to cause compressive strain or shortening along the axis of tension development. During ventricular filling, acute diastolic tensile stress and strain are applied to the myocardium, while chronic left ventricular pressure overload will increase the tensile stress in the myocardium during systole.

Stiffness is the extent to which a material resists deformation in response to an applied force, literally how stress changes in response to strain; stiffness is the inverse of compliance. An ideal material possessing an infinite material stiffness is said to be rigid. In contrast, structural stiffness combines the effects of material stiffness and geometry. For example, a thin-walled tube composed of a stiff material can have the same structural stiffness as a thick-walled tube composed of a compliant material. Extracellular matrix stiffness is mainly determined by fibrillar collagens (collagen type I and III in the heart) and the degree of collagen cross-linking. Cell stiffness is largely determined by prestress.

Prestress is the stress remaining in the cell or tissue when external forces on the tissue are removed. Cellular prestress is often attributed to tension in stress fibers of the cytoskeleton balanced by compression in microtubules and/or cytoplasmic pressure (positive pressure is a negative, compressive stress). In tissue or cells adhered to ECM, these pulling forces are resisted by external tethers to the ECM. Prestress is modulated by cell stiffness and essential for cell differentiation. An increased prestress supports an increased initial stiffness, which in turn often affects cell phenotype.

Strength is a measure of resistance to material damage or failure; it is the maximum value of stresses that can be tolerated prior to failure. The terms hard and soft reflect a resistance to penetration or being scratched and thus particular aspects of strength.

Cell traction force is the tension exerted on the ECM and other cells via adhesion receptors (integrins and cadherins) as a result of cell shortening of the contracting cytoskeleton. It can be computed from measurements of the strains induced by cell contraction.

Compressive force is a pushing force; external forces that act to shorten the material in the direction of the applied force are compressive.

Shear tractions are tangential forces per unit area such as those due to friction or forces applied by a cell adhered to a matrix surface. In the heart, the torsional rotation of the ventricle during filling and ejection creates shearing stresses caused by the helical arrangement of myofibers in the wall. Transverse shearing stresses and strains also exist between myocardial laminar “sheets” during systole. In vascular biology, shear stress frequently refers to the forces of fluid flow on the surface of cells, e.g., due to blood flow. These shear stresses tend to be orders of magnitude lower than shear stresses due to cell interactions with solid matrix but are still biologically significant.

Further reading in [12, 31]

Together, the normal, and thus moderate, ECM stiffness is crucial for maintaining normal tissue homeostasis that is fundamental to cellular and tissue health. As detailed below, the mechanosensing process involves assessment of the mechanics of the matrix by the cells through integrins, cadherins, and the actomyosin cytoskeleton and is followed by a mechanoregulation process that includes the deposition, rearrangement, or removal of matrix to maintain overall form and function (for mechanosensors, compare also Sect. 2.4).

6.2.4 Résumé

In sum, it has become apparent that the ECM reflects a dynamic structure that is constantly remodeled to regulate and control cell and tissue homeostasis. However, when matrix mechanics become imbalanced, for example, due to chronically persistent or severe tissue injuries, excessive ECM production and deposition can occur that is associated with cross-linking of the existing matrix and fiber alignment. These processes result in an altered mechanical environment associated with increased ECM stiffness that—via mechanotransductive pathways—has been revealed as a powerful driver of progressive fibrosis (reviewed in [23, 24]). The scenario is briefly described in the next section.

6.3 From Extracellular Matrix to Cell Nucleus and Back: Mechanotransduction in Progressive Fibrosis

6.3.1 Introductory Remarks

The field of mechanobiology has profoundly emerged in the past two decades, greatly increasing our knowledge of how mechanical stimuli orchestrate cell behavior. The process of mechanosensing → mechanotransduction begins with the capability of cells to read the physical features of the microenvironment through adhesive proteins, mainly integrins, and to counterbalance extracellular forces by adjusting their own tensional state through actomyosin contractility and organization of the F-actin cytoskeleton for mechanosensors (also compare Sect. 2.4). Regarding involvement of mechanotransduction in relation to ECM stiffness in fibrogenesis, the molecular mechanisms that link the injury-altered mechanical microenvironment and activation of fibroblasts are of high interest. Current knowledge holds that this altered environment/mechanotransduction-caused activation of cells triggers intracellular signaling biochemical pathways that lead to changes in gene expression, cell phenotype, and function, for example, as reflected by transdifferentiation of fibroblasts to myofibroblasts. One of these mechanisms is related to one prominent feature of ECM in the fibrotic scar, namely, its high stiffness compared to the compliant texture of the surrounding normal ECM [25–27].

6.3.2 Integrins: Bi-directional "Inside-Out and Outside-In" Transmembrane Signaling Machines

6.3.2.1 General Remarks

The integrins in their role as mechanosensors have already briefly introduced in Sect. 2.4.4. From the perspective of this book, they are thought to be activated by putative cell-extrinsic dyshomeostatic DAMPs (see Sect. 3.4.3.3). These transmembrane proteins mediate interaction between the ECM and cells such as fibroblasts. Indeed, they can be regarded as bi-directional, that is, "inside-out and outside-in" transmembrane signaling machines that trigger mechanotransduction pathways through the ECM → integrin → focal adhesions → cytoskeleton → nucleus → mechanosensitive genes axis and back. Via this axis, ECM stiffness may contribute to activation of myofibroblasts, which in turn can promote profibrotic ECM stiffness. These sequelae of events can be regarded as the molecular backbone that drives activation of myofibroblasts as the central mediators of fibrosis (Fig. 6.1).

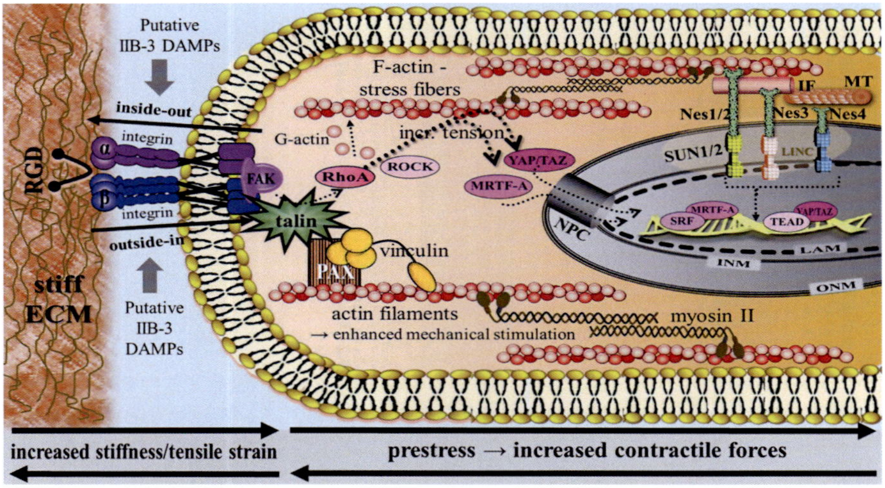

Fig. 6.1 Simplified narrative and conceptual model of transdifferentiation of a fibroblast into a myofibroblast via "outside-in" mechanotransduction pathways in a fibroblast linking the extracellular matrix to the nucleus and activating mechanosensitive genes. Mechanical cues arising from the stiff ECM in terms of putative cell-extrinsic IIB-3 DAMPs, mediated by RGD-activated integrins and perceived by the focal adhesions (here presented by FAK, talin, vinculin, PAX), are transmitted and propagated at the cytoskeleton level (shown as F-actin/stress fibers, microtubules, intermediate filaments, myosin II). Activation of the RhoA/ROCK signaling pathway by ECM-derived mechanical force (e.g., via FAK) promotes actin stress fiber assembly, thereby driving activation and nuclear translocation of transcriptional coactivators YAP/TAZ and MRTF-A. The two transcription coactivators form complexes with SRF and TEAD, respectively, to promote pro-fibrotic gene expression. Additionally, force transmission to the nucleus involves interaction of cytoskeletal elements (actin filaments, intermediate filaments, microtubules) with nesprin proteins on the outer nuclear membrane that transmit force through SUN domain proteins on the inner nuclear membrane to the nuclear lamina and interior/peripheral chromatin. The activated myofibroblast then may increase its contractile force (again reflecting putative cell-extrinsic IIB-3 DAMPs) that is ("inside-out") transmitted by (activated) integrins to contribute to ECM remodeling, and matrix assembly, thereby enhancing ECM stiffness: a fibrogenic vicious circle! *IIB-3 DAMPs* cell-extrinsic dyshomeostatic DAMPs, *ECM* extracellular matrix, *FAK* focal adhesion kinase, *incr.* increased, *INM* inner nuclear membrane, *IF* intermediate filaments, *LAM* nuclear lamina, *LINC* linker of nucleoskeleton and cytoskeleton complex, *MRTF-A* myocardin-related transcription factor A, *MT* microtubules, *Nes1/2,3,4* nesprin proteins 1,2,3,4, *NPC* nuclear pore complex, *ONM* outer nuclear membrane, *PAX* paxillin; *RGD* distinct amino acid sequence consisting of arginine, glycine, and aspartate, *Rho* Ras homolog gene family, member A, *ROCK* Rho-associated protein kinase, *SRF* serum response factor, *TAZ* transcriptional coactivator with PDZ-binding motif, *TEAD* TEA domain family members, *YAP* yes-associated protein. (Sources: [29-32, 55, 87, 220, 221])

6.3.2.2 Mechanisms of "Inside-Out and Outside-In" Signaling

The mechanisms involved are complex and complicated for a practicing clinician. Thus, for informative expertise on mechanistic details, the reader is referred to excellent review articles found in [8, 12, 28-34]. Here, the scenario is briefly sketched in a more oversimplified fashion.

On the ECM side, most integrins on fibroblasts bind to ECM components such as collagens, vitronectin, laminins, and fibronectin that serve as their ligands. The affinity of integrins for these ligands can be regulated within the cell in terms of an "inside-out signaling" or established by extracellular mechanical stimuli reflecting putative IIB-3 DAMPs (Fig. 6.1, also compare Sect. 3.4.3.3 and Fig. 3.3), which induce a high-affinity conformation change. Following such processes, integrins are activated, cluster, and reinforce molecular links at the ECM ↔ cell interface. Interestingly, many of these ECM ligands share a common integrin-binding motif, the "RGD" motif, a distinct amino acid sequence consisting of arginine, glycine, and aspartate (Arg-Gly-Asp). This motif, for example, is present in ECM fibronectin and fibrinogen that act as ligands of integrins.

On the cell side, integrins are connected with the cytoskeleton in a reciprocal feed-forward loop. Specifically, the cytoplasmic tail of integrin binds to integrin-associated, multimolecular complexes called focal adhesions, which are intracellularly located immediately beneath the cell membrane at the termini of cytoskeletal actin stress fibers, thereby spanning the ECM and the actomyosin cytoskeleton.

6.3.2.3 Integrins → Focal Adhesion-Mediated Signaling Pathways

As said, integrins have been identifying as molecular players that connect mechanical stimuli in terms of putative cell-extrinsic dyshomeostatic DAMPs that originated from the ECM stiffness to gene transcription and activation in adjacent cells. Numerous original and review articles have reported about this unique scenario (for informative articles covering also the following text, see [31, 34-43]). Since integrins, constituted by α and β subunits, have no intrinsic enzymatic activity, downstream signaling depends on intracellular interaction with enzymes and adaptor proteins through their cytoplasmic domain within the focal adhesions complex. Indeed, situated at the interface between the ECM and cytoskeleton, adhesions—operating as adaptor and signaling molecules—are superbly positioned to act in a variety of pathways that are triggered by force transmission between stresses generated within the ECM and the cytoskeleton (Fig. 6.1). Talin, for example, is such an adaptor protein, also called linker molecule. Talin forms the core of these complexes by linking the cytoplasmic tail of integrins directly to cytoskeletal actin and recruiting numerous proteins, including signaling molecules to focal adhesions in response to mechanical stimuli. In this regard, talin is considered the key force-sensing molecule, whereas another focal adhesion protein, vinculin, is one of the key mechanoeffectors [44].

6.3.2.4 Concluding Remarks

Together, putative cell-extrinsic dyshomeostatic DAMP-activated integrins are indeed highly dynamic regulators of cell function. They can drive wide-ranging fibrogenic cellular responses that contribute, for example, to homeostatic wound healing. In contrast, their aberrant function can lead to pathological events such as chronic fibrotic diseases, mirroring the Janus face of the innate immune system again.

6.3.3 Focal Adhesions: The Key Hub for Extracellular Matrix ↔ Cell Interaction

6.3.3.1 General Remarks

The focal adhesions can be regarded as the central hub for ECM ↔ cell interaction. They are comprised of more than 150 different proteins that are also collectively referred to as the "integrin adhesome" [39, 45]. The focal adhesion proteins—as structural proteins—respond to mechanical stimuli (e.g., talin, vinculin, α-actinin, integrin-linked kinase (ILK), PINCH, parvins, and p130Cas) or, as signaling proteins, mediate "outside-in" biochemical signaling (e.g., focal adhesion kinase (FAK), Cdc42, c-Abl tyrosine kinase, cortactin, Abl interactor-1(Abi-1) (compare Fig. 6.1)). Typically, cells adhering to rigid matrices such as stiff ECM reinforce their focal adhesions under load through mechanochemical feedback mechanisms; in other words, the nascent focal adhesions mature under high tension. Thus, high mechanical tension across integrin receptors, for example, caused by such increased ECM stiffness, results in (previously closed) partial talin unfolding and subsequent recruitment of and binding to vinculin as one of the main components of focal adhesions' inner core. Vinculin can interact with actin filaments, a process that is crucial to the strengthening of the focal adhesion and transmission/propagation of force to the actin cytoskeleton. Another focal adhesion scaffold/adaptor protein is paxillin (PAX) that contains different interacting domains (LIM, SH2, SH3, and LD). The mechanosensing properties of PAX lie in the coordinated recruitment of a network of other adhesomes and in its ability to bind activated vinculin, thus stabilizing focal adhesion ↔ cytoskeleton interaction (compare Fig. 6.1). Additionally, other LIM domain proteins are recruited to focal adhesions in response to increased mechanical tension (so-called LIM-domain-only proteins: multifunctional nuclear transcription coregulators that interacts with diverse proteins [46]).

Together, it is believed that many other proteins are also recruited to focal adhesions in a force-dependent manner; that is, they localize to those adhesions only when cell adhesion forces are high enough [47] (see also Ringer et al. [29]). In this way, increased stiffness of the ECM may contribute to myofibroblasts activation, promoting fibrogenesis/fibrosis (see below).

6.3.3.2 Signaling via the Focal Adhesion Complexes

Clustering of integrins—probably under the influence of talin, vinculin, and PAX—recruits and activates non-receptor protein tyrosine kinases such as FAK, Src, and Fyn in response to tension and ECM stiffness to form focal adhesion complexes (FACs). Recruitment of FAK is mediated through its *focal adhesion targeting* domain to integrin-associated proteins, including PAX. This triggers a conformational change of the FAK protein that releases the intramolecular inhibition leading to autophosphorylation, the first step in the activation of FAK associated with its binding to Src, which results in mutual activation of the kinase domains of both molecules (for conformational changes, see also Sect. 2.4.1.2). Focal adhesion kinase activation is essential for mechanotransduction of integrin signaling, for example, during myofibroblastic activation. The FAK induces a cascade of signaling events involving ERK1/2 and MAPKs, which, for instance, are known to induce myofibroblast differentiation and ECM production. Also, FAK, Src, and Fyn were shown to facilitate the activation of Rho GTPases through activating *guanine nucleotide exchange factors* (GEFs) and *GTPases-activating proteins* (GAPs) in response to increased tension. The small Rho GTPases have now expanded to contain 20 members and comprise a family of molecular switches that control signal transduction pathways in eukaryotic cells. A conformational change induced upon binding GTP promotes interaction with target (effector) proteins to generate a cellular response. A highly conserved function of Rho GTPases from yeast to humans is to control the actin cytoskeleton (reviewed in [48]).

Here, another focal adhesion protein, Hic-5, a PAX family member should briefly be noted that has been shown to play a crucial regulatory role in myofibroblast differentiation. The Hic-5 protein was found to shuttle between focal adhesions and the nucleus in a process at least partially dependent on cellular mechanical stress. Also, recent studies have shown that Hic-5 transcription is directly regulated by and enhances nuclear accumulation of a transcription factor, namely, *myocardin-related transcription factor A* (MRTF-A) that will be alluded to below (reviewed and reported in [34, 49-51]).

6.3.3.3 Role of the Rho/ROCK Pathway in Adjusting Cells' Prestress

The small Rho GTPases provide a functional linkage between mechanosensing through integrin-linked focal adhesions, on the one side, and, on the other side, the actomyosin cytoskeleton by generating traction forces reflecting prestress of a cell (for prestress, see Box 6.1). This function is largely exerted by the FAK signaling-stimulated Rho effector *Rho-associated coiled-coil containing protein kinase* (ROCK), which includes two isoforms: ROCK1 and ROCK2. These enzymes are important effectors of the *Ras homolog gene family, member A* (RhoA), which is a small GTPase protein in the Rho family (for informative articles, see [12, 52-56]). As reported, RhoA has several vital roles in cell behavior, including regulation of cell shape, transformation of cellular phenotypes, and actin cytoskeleton reorganization. Activation of the RhoA/ROCK2 signaling pathway by mechanical force was shown to mediate the biochemical alterations of the cells. Notably, in this way, the RhoA/ROCK pathway was found to regulate the strain-induced differentiation of fibroblast to myofibroblast [55].

Together, when cells are subjected to exogenous mechanical stress, the focal adhesion complexes sense and transmit mechanical stimulation to the cytoskeleton, which, besides others, stimulates ROCK-dependent actin remodeling and the formation of stress fibers [57]. This process subsequently affects nuclear translocation of transcription factors and thereby gene expression and regulation.

6.3.3.4 Concluding Remarks

In sum, focal adhesion proteins comprise a signaling network that plays a critical role in regulating the function of many cell types. However, this key hub for ECM $\leftrightarrow$ cell interaction has recently received attention as a potential mediator of fibrotic diseases. For example, evidence was reported showing that FAK is directly related to the activation of cardiac fibrosis in hypoxia condition and its pharmacological inhibition was found to decrease the fibrotic score, thereby preserving partial left ventricular function [58].

6.3.4 Cytoskeleton-Driven Mechanotransduction: Nuclear Translocation of Transcription Factors

6.3.4.1 General Remarks

The mechanical information arising from injury-induced modifications of the ECM, mediated by cell-extrinsic dyshomeostatic DAMP-activated integrins and perceived by the focal adhesions, are then propagated at the cytoskeleton level, whereby talin protein apparently mediates one of the first mechanical connections to the contractile actomyosin network (Fig. 6.1). The actomyosin cytoskeleton is a dynamic structure composed of filamentous polymers and regulatory cross-linking proteins that respond to external forces with a proportional cell-generated force. This occurs through assembly of an actomyosin contractile network and cytoskeletal remodeling. In other words, this unique system provides mechanical support to eukaryotic cells and regulates their motility, shape, and tension homeostasis. The cytoskeleton integrates the activity of a multitude of cytoplasmic proteins, whereby three main types of cytoskeletal polymer have to be highlighted: actin fibers/filaments (F-actin), microtubules (MTs), and intermediate filaments (IFs) (Fig. 6.1). Together, these polymers control the shape and mechanics of eukaryotic cells. All three polymers have crucial functions in arranging and maintaining the integrity of intracellular compartments, including (1) spatial organization of the contents of the cell; (2) physical and biochemical connection of the cell to the ECM; and (3) generation of contractile forces that enable the cell to move and—relevant from the perspective of this topic—change shape (for reviews see [59-61]).

Cytoskeleton contractility is generated by molecular nonmuscle myosin II (NMII) motors that work as chemo-mechanical transduction machines (compare Fig. 6.1). Nonmuscle myosin II is present in virtually all animal cell types and involved in numerous cell functions, including remodeling of the actin cytoskeleton. Three mammalian NMII heavy chain genes encode nonmuscle myosin heavy chain IIA (NMHIIA), NMHIIB, and NMHIIC, respectively. Despite the overall similarity, NMII paralogs exhibit significant differences in motor kinetics, structure, and dynamics of bipolar filaments and cellular functions. Thus, NMHIIA is responsible for generating traction force, whereas NMHIIB is better posed to stabilize focal adhesions in more central cellular regions. The function of NMHIIC is less understood but could involve either positive or negative regulation of cell adhesions.

Under increased tensile forces mediated by focal adhesions, NMII motors drive cell contraction by sliding movement of actin filaments along myosin molecules. F-actin and myosin II are held together by cross-linking proteins (e.g., α-actinin, fascin, filamin) in complex structures to form contractile bundles, called stress fibers (Fig. 6.1). Through these stress fibers, cells can exert further tensile forces that have been discussed to contribute to the assembly of both stress fibers themselves and their associated focal adhesions, thereby interrogating microenvironmental mechanics from the ECM to the cell and vice versa (for informative articles, see [61-66]).

6.3.4.2 Cytoskeleton-Driven Signaling Pathways: Role of Transcription Factors YAP/TAZ and MRTF-A/B

Finally, stiffness-induced ROCK-NMII-mediated contraction of actin stress fibers in fibroblasts drives nuclear translocation of two sets of Rho pathway effector transcriptional coactivators: (1) the Hippo pathway target, WW domain-containing proteins, YAP (*yes-associated protein*), and TAZ (WWTR1, *WW domain-containing transcription regulator protein 1*, also known *as transcriptional coactivator with PDZ-binding motif)* [30], and (2) MRTF-A (also known as MKL1, *megakaryoblastic leukemia 1*) and MRFT–B (also known as MKL2) [67]. Intriguingly, the regulation of the nuclear accumulation of TAZ/YAP and MRTF shows striking similarities: for example, nuclear translocation of both molecules is strongly promoted by increased ECM stiffness or cellular tension. In the following, they are briefly discussed.

6.3.4.3 The YAP and TAZ Pathway in Fibroblasts

The transcriptional coactivators YAP and its paralog TAZ have been identified as molecules at the nexus of multiple cellular inputs that are able to connect mechanical stimuli to gene transcription, thereby influencing cell behavior in homeostasis and diseases such as fibrosis. Here, guided by reviews of Dupont [30], Panciera et al. [68], and Totaro et al. [69], the scenario is briefly sketched by emphasizing that YAP and TAZ can sense mechanical cues from ECM and translate them into cell-specific transcriptional programs. The YAP/TAZ activity is regulated by the conformation and tension of the F-actin cytoskeleton, which in turn depends primarily on the substrate to which cells adhere. For example, YAP and TAZ are retained and localized in the cytoplasm in cells experiencing low levels of mechanical signaling, such as in fibroblasts attached to a soft ECM with low resistance associated with reduced maturation of focal adhesions and low actomyosin contractility. On the other hand, when perceiving high mechanical signaling from stiffer ECM causing integrin clustering associated with increased focal adhesion maturation and increased stress fiber tension/contractility, YAP and TAZ can be found in the nucleus. Mechanistically, Rho signaling is essential for YAP and TAZ activity (see above). Once activated, YAP/TAZ bind primarily to enhancer elements using so-called TEAD factors as DNA-binding platforms, an interaction originally described and functionally validated in *Drosophila melanogaster*. The TEAD factors (for *TEA domain family members*) are a family of DNA-binding transcription factors that cannot induce target gene transcription on their own and, thus, have to associate with YAP/TAZ.

Translocation of YAP and TAZ into the nucleus is triggered by and depends on the Hippo pathway (for the Hippo pathway, see [30, 69-71]; and Box 6.2). Thus, when Hippo signaling is absent, YAP and TAZ translocate to the nucleus to elicit their biological functions mainly by regulating gene transcription through their association with the DNA-binding TEAD 1–4 family members.

Box 6.2 The Hippo Pathway

The Hippo signaling pathway was initially identified in *Drosophila melanogaster* screens for tissue growth two decades ago and has been a subject extensively studied in both *Drosophila* and mammals in the last several years. The pathway takes its name from one of its key signaling components—the protein kinase *Hippo*. Mutations in this gene lead to tissue overgrowth or a "hippopotamus"-like phenotype. The core of the Hippo pathway consists of a kinase cascade, transcription coactivators, and DNA-binding partners. Together, the Hippo pathway consists of a complex signaling network with >30 components. This pathway is regulated by intrinsic cell machineries, such as cell-cell contact, cell polarity, and actin cytoskeleton, as well as a wide range of signals, including cellular energy status, mechanical cues, and hormonal signals that act through G protein-coupled receptors. The major role of the Hippo pathway has been defined to restrict tissue growth in adults and modulate cell proliferation, differentiation, and migration in developing organs. Pathologically, dysregulation of the Hippo pathway has been shown to result in aberrant cell growth and neoplasia.

Further reading in [30, 69-71]

Besides their functions as effectors of the Hippo and mechanotransduction pathways, YAP and TAZ are also biochemical and transcriptional mediators of Wnt signaling, providing a mechanistic link to the observed overlap between Wnt and YAP/TAZ biology in fibrogenesis [72] (for the Wnt pathway, see Sect. 2.3.4.7 and Box 2.1 and Sect. 6.5.3.4).

Importantly, YAP- and TAZ-mechanotransduction is emerging as a key player in human fibrotic disorders. Thus, nuclear localization of both molecules has been shown to induce myofibroblast differentiation in the liver [73], lung [74], and skin [75]. In addition, a link between chronic nonresolving inflammation, ECM stiffening, and altered YAP and TAZ signaling has recently been supposed (reviewed in [68]).

6.3.4.4 The MRTF-A and MRTF-B Pathway in Fibroblasts

Like YAP/TAZ, the transcriptional coactivators MRTF-A/B are liberated from the F-actin cytoskeleton by enhanced mechanical stimulation in case of increased ECM stiffness, whereas in soft matrix, they remain accumulated in the cytosol [76]. Specifically, G-actin assembles into F-actin polymers, thereby liberating MRTF from G-actin and allowing it to enter the nucleus. Once in the nucleus, MRTF binds serum response factor (SRF), and the complex drives expression of mechanosensitive genes [77–79]. Interestingly, RhoA activation was shown to promote MRTF-A translocation to the nucleus under strain status and SRF expression [55].

Mechanistically, nuclear shuttling of the mammalian homolog of Diaphanous 2 (mDia2) was proposed to play an important role in the control of MRTF subcellular localization, promotion of MRTF nuclear accumulation, and initiation of Rho signaling-mediated, MRTF-dependent gene expression [80]. Moreover, as touched already above, recent studies provided evidence suggesting that the focal protein Hic-5 is required for the nuclear accumulation of MRTF-A and the induction of cellular contractility, suggesting a crucial role for Hic-5 in myofibroblast differentiation [49]. Together, MRTF-A appears to be essential for fibroblast transdifferentiation into myofibroblast in response to mechanical cues.

Adding another level of complexity to the story, MRTF was demonstrated to associate with TAZ partly through a WW domain-dependent mechanism, thereby exhibiting multilevel crosstalk affecting each other's expression, transport, and transcriptional activity. Specifically, MRTF was shown to be essential for TAZ expression [81]. This scenario likely plays critical roles in the regulation of complex controlled and uncontrolled innate immune processes, including normal wound healing and fibrosis.

6.3.4.5 Concluding Remarks

Collectively, as stressed by Herum et al. in their excellent review [31], "these results demonstrate the importance of the cytoskeleton in regulating the profibrotic gene program by acting on nuclear translocation of transcription regulators."

6.3.5 Nuclear Mechanosensing: Mechanotransduction

Intriguingly, there is recent convincing evidence indicating that the nucleus itself can act as a mechanosensitive subcellular organelle that receives mechanical cues from the cell membrane to respond with changes in nuclear envelope structure and composition, chromatin organization, and gene expression (for reviews that served as sources for the following information, see also [31, 82-87]). The existence of such a connection between the cell membrane and the nucleus has been proven by studies revealing that the application of mechanical forces on integrin receptors at the cell membrane is followed shortly by nuclear structural reorganization and substantial deformation in the direction of the pulling force.

The structure of this largest and stiffest organelle in the cell allows proper function of such pathways: the nucleus consists roughly of the nuclear interior that contains chromatin and the surrounding nuclear envelope. The envelope is a continuous membrane system that comprises the outer and inner nuclear membranes and contains a large number of membrane-bound proteins, as well as nuclear pore complexes (NPCs) that serve as a gateway for large molecules to enter the nuclear interior (also compare Fig. 6.1). Beneath the inner membrane is the nuclear lamina localized, a filamentous protein network that consists of A-type, B-type, and A/C type lamins, and lamin-binding proteins, which provide structural stability to the nucleus.

The transmission of mechanical forces from the cell surface to the nucleus across the nuclear envelope is accomplished by specialized proteins as part of the *linker of the nucleoskeleton and cytoskeleton* (LINC) complex. The LINC complex consists of nesprin proteins (*nuclear envelope spectrin repeat protein*) that reside within the outer nuclear membrane and contain a C-terminal KASH (*Klarsicht, ANC-1, Syne homology*) domain, which interacts with SUN (*Sad1 Unc*) domain-containing proteins that protrude from the nuclear lumen into the perinuclear space between the inner and outer nuclear membranes (Fig. 6.1). The SUN proteins, in turn, bind to the nuclear lamina, nuclear pores, and chromatin. The nesprin proteins connect the cytoskeleton to the outer nuclear membrane through binding of actin (nesprin-1 and nesprin-2) and the intermediate filament (nesprin-3). In other words, force transmission to the nucleus involves interaction of cytoskeletal elements (actin filaments, intermediate filaments) with nesprin proteins on the outer nuclear membrane that transmits force through SUN domain proteins on the inner nuclear membrane to the nuclear lamina and interior. Also of importance is that SUN1 binds directly to lamin A and B of the nuclear lamina, thereby anchoring the LINC complex to the nucleoskeleton [88, 89]. It should also be noted here that, in studies on lamin A/C-deficient mice, lamin A/C was found to be critical for fibroblast activation and possibly differentiation into myofibroblasts [90] ("deficient" or "knockout" [KO] mice—also denoted with the symbol "-/-" are genetically modified mice in which researchers have inactivated, or "knocked out," an existing gene by replacing it or disrupting it with an artificial piece of DNA). In support of this observation are experiments on murine embryonic fibroblasts showing that lamin A/C and emerin (a protein of the inner nuclear membrane) can modulate actin dynamics regulating MRTF-A and SRF activity [91].

Intriguingly, there is recent evidence suggesting that the LINC complex regulates gene expression by modifying gene accessibility and chromatin packaging, a mechanism that would explain how the cell nucleus could respond directly to mechanical forces [87]. Indeed, SUN proteins were shown to bind directly to chromatin and are central for chromosome organization during mitosis, reflected in SUN1 KO mice being infertile due to the inability to implement cell division [92]. As concluded by the authors, these "results reveal that the inner nuclear membrane protein SUN1 is required for telomere attachment to the nuclear envelope during meiotic prophase I and demonstrate that telomere attachment to the nuclear envelop is essential for the efficient pairing/synapsis of homologous chromosomes and gametogenesis in mammals" [92]. On the other hand, the mechanism could also be of more indirect character, regulating gene expression as a result of altered nuclear structure, shape, and/or stiffness. Indeed, substrate stiffness has been found to be critical for LINC complex assembly [31, 93].

Collectively, as concluded by Kirby and Lammerding [87]: " It is now well-recognized that nuclear envelope proteins have an important role in the cellular response to mechanical stimuli, and that forces are transmitted from the cell surface and cytoskeleton to the interior of the nucleus. Findings suggest that the nucleus can act as a cellular mechanosensor. Nonetheless, many questions remain, including to what extent the nucleus itself responds to mechanical forces, where such nuclear mechanotransduction processes occur, and whether these nuclear processes complement or act in parallel or downstream of cytoplasmic signalling pathways."

6.3.6 Mechanosensitive Ion Channels in Fibroblasts

Before closing this section, it should not be unmentioned that other mechanosensors than integrins, that is, ion channels, have been discovered in fibroblasts although their role in regulating cell function is not as clear (for ion channels, see Sect. 2.4.2). For instance, cardiac and dermal myofibroblast differentiation in response to TGF-β and matrix stiffness was shown to be regulated by mechanosensitive ion channels, such as TRPs (TRP4 specifically), and involve downstream signaling of Akt, SMAD, and MRTF pathways [94–96]. The topic is briefly resumed further in Sect. 11.3.5.4.

6.3.7 Résumé

Modern research work in the field of ECM has revealed that the matrix is a dynamic structure that permanently regulates cell biology under steady-state conditions. Accordingly, in case of any exogenous force-induced disturbances of the ECM as reflected, for example, by a change of its stiffness, resident cells get informed to respond properly by triggering counteracting mechanotransductory and biochemical pathways. This response is usually associated with an adjustment of their behavior aimed at maintaining homeostasis. For example, myofibroblasts may become activated to increase their contractility or produce ECM components in case of abnormal ECM degradation.

In turn, resident cells such as fibroblasts continuously assess and control the structural integrity of the ECM to maintain its overall form, composition, and function that are vital for life. Thus, by using the integrin-mediated mechanotransductory ECM-nucleus axis reciprocally/retrogradely, these cells play an active role in remodeling their matrix to maintain an ECM stress set point through the process of "tensional homeostasis" that appears necessary to create a favorable mechanical environment for optimal cell function.

However, when this homeostatic balance of ECM ↔ cell interaction gets out of control, for example, in case of increased matrix stiffening due to severe or chronically persistent tissue injury, tissue fibrogenesis/fibrosis may be initiated or even progressing, for example, by promoting mechanoactivation of myofibroblasts through feed-forward loops. The activated cells then may produce further ECM components and increase their contractile force that is (inside-out) transmitted by (activated) integrins to the ECM, contributing to further ECM remodeling, thereby enhancing ECM stiffness: a fibrogenic vicious circle! In fact, the profibrotic role of increased ECM stiffness in the pathogenesis of many human diseases as an emerging research field of mechanobiology has gained increasing attention.

Nevertheless, as stressed by Humphrey et al. [12], several major outstanding questions remain: "How do tissues maintain normal matrix organization and tissue stiffness? What pathways mediate the negative feedback loop that prevents progression toward stiffer matrix and higher cell contractility? What governs the switch between these two states, the homeostatic one that maintains health versus the fibrotic one that compromises the function of many tissues? Lastly, can we devise treatments to break the fibrotic cycle and restore the homeostatic state? Understanding the regulatory pathways in detail and the factors that govern switching between these states is likely to be the best route forward."

Finally, another level of complexity of this scenario is added when looking at the role of DAMPs, in particular, the inducible DAMP TGF-β, in contributing to the self-perpetuating process of fibrosis, a burning issue that is intensely discussed in the following section.

6.4 The DAMP-Driven Self-Perpetuating Process of Fibrosis

6.4.1 Introductory Remarks

As mentioned, tissue injury-activated myofibroblasts secrete abundant amounts of ECM protein whose deposition culminates in the formation of stiff scar tissue that is not only dysfunctional but also ultimately inhibits tissue and organ function completely. Indeed, typical for the fibrotic scar developing in primarily soft organs is this feature of high stiffness compared to the compliant texture of the surrounding normal ECM [8, 97]. The fatality of this scenario is: once established, fibrosis can perpetuate itself through multiple feed-forward amplification loops that are generated as a consequence of chronic tissue injury.

Thus, while there is a consensus that myofibroblasts are the principal source of collagen and prominent mediators of fibrogenesis, the key danger signals and signaling pathways involved in their activation and persistence have been controversially discussed and are still subject of intense research.

Nonetheless, if one accepts the concept of fibrosis as a self-perpetuating process, driven by putative dyshomeostatic IIB-3 DAMP-activated integrins as transmembrane proteins mediating interaction between the ECM and fibroblasts, there should be other classes of DAMPs which initially induce the formation of ECM. Indeed, besides the new insights into mechanisms of mechanotransduction, recent work has been performed to reveal several biochemical DAMP-promoted signaling pathways that appear to orchestrate the process of activation of myofibroblasts as the main players in ECM formation. Some of them have already been presented as critical players in tissue repair in Vol. 1 [4], Part VIII, Sect. 36.3. Here, they are briefly re-addressed, this time in relation to fibrogenesis (for reviews, see [33, 34, 98-100]).

6.4.2 DAMP-Triggered Pathways Leading to Fibroblast Transdifferentiation into Myofibroblasts

Mechanisms of DAMP-induced activation of myofibroblasts promoting fibrogenesis have been introduced in Vol. 1 [4], Part VIII, Sect. 36.4.2.2. Of note, there is steadily growing evidence for a role of DAMPs in activating fibroblasts to develop into myofibroblasts [101–104]. For example, in studies on human dermal fibroblast [104], exogenous HMGB1was found to induce the proliferation of these cells and to act as a profibrotic molecule to produce collagen, decrease MMP-1, and increase

TIMP-1 mRNA expression. Moreover, in these studies, administration of HMGB1 was shown to increase the expression level of TGF-β1 and internal signaling molecules, such as Smad (for *similar to mothers against decapentaplegic)* 2 and 3, phosphorylated Smad 2/3 complex, ERK 1/2, Akt, and NF-κB. In other lines of studies on lung fibroblasts, HMGB1was shown to induce myofibroblast differentiation through NF-κB-mediated TGF-β1 release [103] (for these various signaling molecules, also compare Vol. 1 [4], Part VI, Sects. 22.3.3, 22.3.4.2, 22.3.9, and 22.5.9.3 and Fig. 22.13). In studies on dermal fibroblasts, S100A8 and S100A9 have been shown to promote fibroblast activation and fibrosis in the dermis [105]. Moreover, in experiments on necrotic myocardial cells containing multiple DAMPs, including HMGB1, S100A8, S100A9, GAL-3, and IL-1α, the necrotic cells were found to provoke a significant increase in fibroblast proliferation, α-SMA activation, and COL IA1 and IIIA1 mRNA expression [102]. Remarkably, eATP, in terms of an NLRP3-activating IA-2 DAMP, may also contribute to fibrosis via profibrotic pathways mediated by the activation of the NLRP3 inflammasome (for additional information compare Vol. 1 [4], Part VI, Subsection 22.4.2.2, p. 516). Indeed, studies on fibroblasts and different organs have demonstrated that the innate immune sensor NLRP3, mostly inflammasome-dependent [106, 107] but also inflammasome-independent [108], plays a crucial role in fibrogenesis and can orchestrate profibrotic innate immune responses under both infectious and sterile conditions. In fact, a large body of evidence suggests that the main products of the NLRP3 inflammasome, IL-1β, and IL-18 can exert profibrotic activities [109–113]. On the other hand, these reports are not without conflicts. For example, more recent studies on lung and dermal fibroblasts resulted in the conflicting observation that IL-1β attenuates myofibroblast formation and ECM production in fibroblasts exposed to TGF-β1 [114]. According to the authors' conclusion, these findings should give rise to reconsider the role of IL-1β in fibrosis. Thus, to date, the signaling pathways from the inflammasome to myofibroblast differentiation and continuous collagen synthesis have not been fully elucidated and await further clarification [115] (for TGF-β1 supposed to act context-dependently as a DAMP and SAMP, see Sect. 3.5.6.2).

Also, some class IIA DAMPs thought to be released from the injured ECM (e.g., mediated by mechanical forces) are reportedly involved in fibroblast activation. Thus, the FNIII EDA and TNC (both denoted as subclass IIA-3 DAMPs throughout the book, also compare Sect. 3.4.2 and Table 3.1.) were demonstrated to activate innate immune signaling in resident fibroblasts through TLR4 [99, 116]. Both DAMPs are glycoproteins that were shown to be produced locally by resident fibroblasts and promptly deposited in the ECM in response to tissue injury [117, 118] (for additional information compare Vol. 1 [4], Part IV, Sect. 13.2.4, p. 274). Indeed, as reviewed by Kelsh-Lasher et al. [119], FNIII EDA has been shown to contribute to prolonged inflammation and fibrosis in several mouse models of fibro-inflammatory disease. Moreover, keloid scars were found to have extensive amounts of this DAMP that can potentially contribute to the increased inflammation and collagen production associated with this disease.

As highlighted by Bhattacharyya et al. [99, 120], FNIII EDA and TNC were demonstrated to activate resident fibroblasts through TLR4. The authors outlined that FNIII EDA↔TLR4 triggers potent profibrotic responses, with enhanced synthesis of collagens and expression of the myofibroblast marker α-SMA. As further described [99], treatment of skin fibroblasts with TNC triggers TLR4-dependent profibrotic responses, including upregulation of TLR4 itself. Mice lacking TNC showed reduced skin and lung fibrosis in response to bleomycin.

6.4.3 Résumé

Together, one may discuss that the role of injury-induced constitutive DAMPs in fibrosis is primarily directed to transdifferentiate PRM-bearing fibroblasts into myofibroblasts. Once myofibroblasts are developed, they take the lead in fibrogenesis via a disastrous ECM/TGF-β-related self-activation process driven by positive feed-forward loops. Tragically, fibrotic tissues, in general, are associated with microvascular rarefication and diminished perfusion. As a result of decreased microvasculature, fibrotic tissues are often chronically hypoxic that may lead to cell death (apoptosis, necrosis), serving as a continuous source of DAMPs emission. For example, cell death has been reported to be associated with idiopathic pulmonary fibrosis [121], cardiac fibrosis [122, 123], and renal fibrosis [124, 125].

The role of DAMPs in activating fibroblasts and promoting fibrosis, as observed in various diseases, will be resumed in the following chapters when appropriate. Here, one of the main players in profibrotic feed-forward loops will be briefly highlighted, namely, the inducible DAMP TGF-β.

6.5 The Peculiar Role of the Inducible DAMP Transforming Growth Factor-Beta, Released from the Extracellular Matrix, in the Activation of Myofibroblasts

6.5.1 Introductory Remarks

In mammals, the TGF-β subfamily of cytokines consists of three isoforms, TGF-β1, TGF-β2, and TGF-β3, whereby TGF-β1 is the most abundantly secreted isoform by innate immune cells such as myofibroblasts (for additional information see also Vol. 1 [4], Part VI, Sect. 22.5.9, p. 547). As outlined in Sect. 3.5.6.2, this cytokine may be seen as an inducible context-dependent SAMP or DAMP that is secreted by DAMP-activated innate immune cells or released from the ECM by cell contractile forces that are transmitted by integrins. Here, regarding the pivotal role of this molecule in fibrogenesis, some crucial points are briefly resumed.

6.5.2 Release of TGF-Beta from the Extracellular Matrix to Operate as an Inducible DAMP

6.5.2.1 General Remarks

Secreted by activated cells, TGF-β is first stored as a large latent complex in the ECM waiting to be activated and to function. Two mechanisms have been discovered that can promote liberation of TGF-β from the ECM to operate as an inducible DAMP: cell traction-driven and proteinase-mediated release.

6.5.2.2 Cell Traction-Mediated Release of TGF-β from the Extracellular Matrix

In fibrogenesis/fibrosis, growing ECM straining and stiffening lower the threshold for TGF-β activation by increasing the mechanical resistance to cell pulling associated with increased tensile strain, that is, by enhancing the contractile force generated by myofibroblasts and needed to release TGF-β from the ECM (for reviews, see [8, 34, 126]). The transmission of the contractile force from myofibroblasts to the ECM is provided by integrins and primarily mediated by the formation of focal adhesions (inside-out signaling, see above).

The crucial point of TGF-β to be released from the ECM and to become critically involved in fibrogenesis must be seen in the presence of an RGD sequence consensus site for the binding of αv integrins (e.g., αvβ6 and αvβ8) in the LAP portion of latent TGF-β (see Fig. 6.2 and compare Sect. 3.5.6.2). In fact, numerous studies including single-molecule force spectroscopy and simulation studies have documented that integrin binding is the major prerequisite for latent TGF-β activation, in particular in conditions of inflammation and fibrosis (for informative articles, also related to the following text, see [127-143]). According to this model, actomyosin cytoskeleton-generated tensile cell contraction force (i.e., in terms of putative cell-extrinsic dyshomeostatic DAMPs) is transmitted to the (αv integrins—associated) RGD binding site in the ECM-anchored LAP portion and induces a putative conformational change that liberates the active TGF-β1 (Fig. 6.2). For this maneuver, the ECM binding site of LTBPs is sufficient and essential to allow latent TGF-β activation by αvβ6 integrin. Otherwise speaking, integrin pulling on LAP induces a conformational change that liberates the active TGF-β in a purely mechanical process, whereby the RGD-integrin attachment site in LAP lies in a perfect pulling axis opposite to the binding site of LAP to LTBP (Fig. 6.2). Accordingly, the forces applied to either site are predicted to release TGF-β from its LAP “straightjacket” in an all-or-nothing fashion (vividly described by Hinz [8]). In other words, as articulated by Lim et al. [144], when the ECM-tethered LTBP-LAP-TGF-β complex experiences tensional force via integrins present on the cell membrane, structural changes in LAP are induced, disrupting the LAP-TGF-β interaction and releasing the growth factor. In this way, the mechanical force can initiate conventional chemical ligand-mediated signaling events (also compare mechanosensing in Sect. 2.4).

Notably, there is accumulating evidence suggesting that TGF-β activation is controlled by the mechanical state of the ECM, whereby the ECM strain dependence of TGF-β1 activation establishes a mechanical checkpoint in the progression of tissue repair. As rationally argued by Hinz [8]: “During this gradual remodeling process, the ECM will eventually reach an organization degree that provides sufficient mechanical resistance for latent TGF-β1 activation by cell pulling. The available TGF-β1 will then contribute to the activation of fibroblasts into contractile myofibroblasts just when further remodeling of the strained and stiffened ECM requires stronger cell forces. At the tissue level, such subcellular contractions will induce gradual length changes in the associated ECM of several millimeters per week,

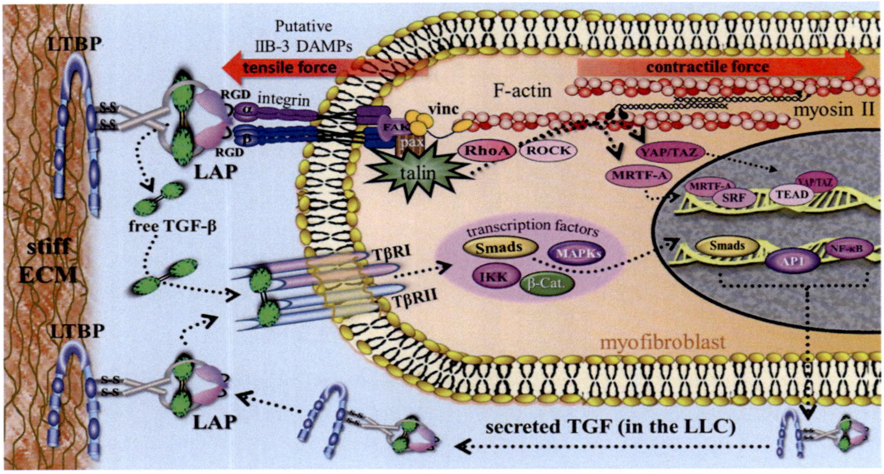

Fig. 6.2 Simplified schematic narrative model of a "feed-forward" loop in the maintenance of the myofibroblasts phenotype that enhances and aggravates tissue fibrosis. The loop consists of increasing ECM stiffening (on the left edge of the figure) that is associated with enhanced traction/tension force (reflecting integrin-activating IIB-3 DAMPs) that is generated by contractile myofibroblasts (e.g., via integrin ↔ focal adhesion proteins ↔ Rho-ROCK ↔ YAP/TAZ ↔ MRTF-A) (illustrated at the upper left corner of the figure). The consequent release from the LAP and availability of soluble TGF-β and its receptor (TβRI /TβRII) trigger signaling pathways (via transcription factors such as Smads), which contribute to transdifferentiation of fibroblasts into contractile myofibroblasts to secrete further ECM components and TGF-β (shown at the lower right corner) that is stored in the ECM as an LLC. In this way, integrin-mediated cell tensile force causes a steady release of the active TGF-β for receptor binding and formation of ligand-bound TβRI and TβRI complexes that trigger Smad-dependent and Smad-independent signaling pathways in other fibroblasts (here shown and exemplified in one cell) (see also next Fig. 6.3). *AP-1* activator protein-1, *β-Cat.* beta-catenin, *IIB-3 DAMPs* cell-extrinsic dyshomeostatic DAMPs, *ECM* extracellular matrix, *FAK* focal adhesion kinase, *IKK* IκB kinase, *LAP* latency-associated protein, *LLC* large latent complex, *LTBP* latent TGF-beta binding protein, *MAPKs* mitogen-activated protein kinases, *MRTF-A* myocardin-related transcription factor A, *NF-κB* nuclear factor–kappa B, *PAX* paxillin, *RGD* distinct amino acid sequence consisting of arginine, glycine, and aspartate, *Rho* Ras homolog gene family, member A, *ROCK* Rho-associated protein kinase, *Smad* similar to mothers against decapentaplegic, *SRF* serum response factor, *TAZ* transcriptional coactivator with PDZ-binding motif, *TβRI/TβRII* TGF-β receptor type I/II, *TEAD* TEA domain family members, *TGF-β* transforming growth factor-beta, *vinc* vinculin, *YAP* yes-associated protein. (Sources: [8, 34, 160])

consistent with the ECM remodeling in physiological repair over days and weeks, which can progress into contractures that develop over months and years in conditions of fibrosis."

Together, increasing ECM tensile strain/stiffening is (automatically) associated with enhanced traction force generated (e.g., via focal adhesion proteins → Rho-ROCK→ YAP/TAZ-MRTF-A) by contractile myofibroblasts. The consequent liberation and availability of TGF-β1 and its triggered signaling pathways contribute to transdifferentiation of fibroblasts into contractile myofibroblasts to secrete further ECM components, thereby creating a positive feed-forward loop that enhances and aggravates tissue fibrosis (Fig. 6.2).

6.5.2.3 Proteinase-Mediated Release of TGF-β from the Extracellular Matrix

Besides cell traction-driven activation of TGF-β, several proteinases are known to mediate the activation of this inducible DAMP as well (reviewed in [15, 34]). For example, the metalloproteinase MMP-14 has been reported to degrade LAP-1 but is dependent on simultaneous cell surface binding of the αvβ8 integrin to the RGD sequence of LAP [145]. Moreover, MMP-2 has been shown to directly cleave LAP-1 and LTBP-1 [146–148]. Also, the *bone morphogenetic protein-1* (BMP-1), a vertebrate metalloproteinase of the astacin family, has been shown to cleave LTBP-1 at two specific sites, liberating the LLC from ECM and resulting in activation of TGF-β1 after cleavage of LAP by non-BMP proteinases [146]. Serine proteinases, specifically plasmin, thrombin, elastase, chymase, trypsin, and kallikrein, complete mechanistic possibilities to cleave LTBP-1 and stimulate TGF-β1 activation [147, 149, 150]. However, the TGF-β1-activating mechanisms of these proteinases are still not well understood in vivo in the context of myofibroblast-mediated fibrosis. Finally, thrombospondin-1, a non-proteinase protein, is well-documented in vitro and in vivo for its critical role in activating TGF-β1 and promoting fibrosis [151]. For further factors that are involved in the transformation of latent TGF-β1 into an active form, the reader is referred to [8, 152, 153].

6.5.2.4 Concluding Remarks

In sum, the release of TGF-β from the anchored molecular complex on the ECM to operate as an inducible DAMP (at least as denoted in this book) is a complicated process that is elicited by several mechanisms. One may hypothesize that these mechanisms have evolved during evolution to prevent an accidental onset of fibrogenic pathologies. On the other hand, the growing understanding of those molecular mechanisms involved in the activation of this inducible DAMP may help develop novel therapeutic targets for suppressing fibrotic disorders.

6.5.3 Canonical and Noncanonical TGF-Beta-Triggered Signaling Pathways in Myofibroblast Activation

6.5.3.1 General Remarks

Compelling evidence indicates that the “uncaging” of TGF-β1 from the ECM is a crucial early step in driving myofibroblast activation (reviewed in [34, 153-155]). At the plasma membrane of the myofibroblast, the inducible DAMP binds to the TGF-β receptor complex to trigger canonical and noncanonical signaling pathways either through a Smad (Smad 2/3)-dependent or Smad-independent pathways (Fig. 6.3). Typically, these paths can crosstalk to each other (reviewed in [154, 156-160]; also compare Vol. 1 [4], Part VI, Sect. 22.5.9.3 and Fig. 22.13).

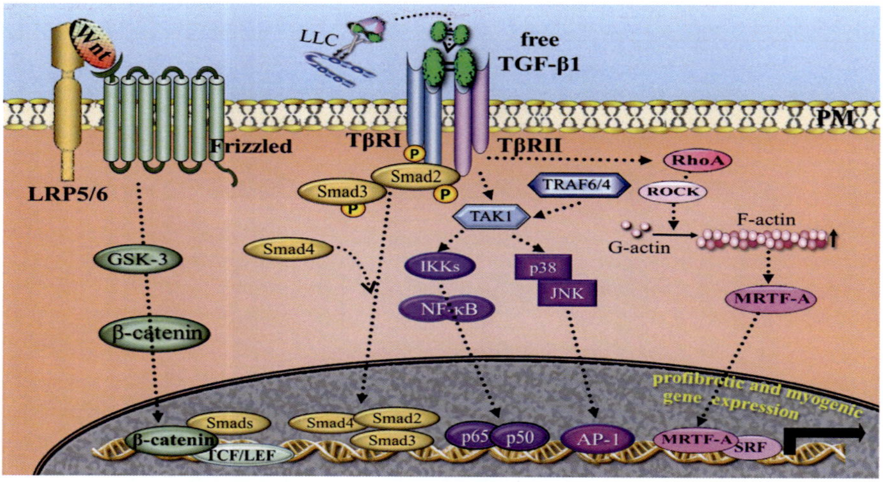

Fig. 6.3 Simplified schematic diagram of TGF-β-triggered Smad-dependent and Smad-independent pathways during fibroblast → myofibroblast differentiation. Once released from the latency-associated peptide (LAP)–latent TGF-β binding protein (LTBP) complex (see previous Fig. 6.2), the active homodimer form of TGF-β1 binds to TβRII that then recruits and activates TβRI. The active TβRI then activates (phosphorylates) Smad2 and Smad3, which complex with Smad4 to translocate to the nucleus. The Smad3 component of the complex binds directly to gene promoters to induce transcription of profibrotic molecules. TGF-β1 can interact with other signaling pathways, for example, and can activate the IKK →NF-κB and MAPKs (p38, JNK) in a Smad-independent manner. Also, TGF-β was found to induce cytoskeletal reorganization through RhoA → ROCK → MRTF-A signaling. The activation of RhoA and the ROCK-mediated actin fibrillation releases MRTF from its inactive, G-actin-bound state, allowing it to form transcriptional complexes with SRF that drive the full expression of myogenic proteins. MRTF-A/SRF-dependent gene expression appears to be essential for fibroblast transdifferentiation into myofibroblast in response to mechanical cues. Moreover, Wnt ligand-induced β-catenin stabilization can enable β-catenin to translocate to the nucleus and complex with Smad proteins and TCF/LEF, thereby enhancing gene transcription of profibrotic and myogenic molecules. Note: only a few noncanonical TGF-β-triggered signaling pathways are shown and very roughly depicted. *AP-1* activator protein-1, *GSK-3* a serine/threonine protein kinase, *IKKs* IκB kinases, *JNK* c-Jun-N-terminal protein kinase, *LAP* latency-associated protein, *LEF* lymphoid enhancer factor, *LLC* large latent complex, *LRP5/6* low-density lipoprotein receptor-related protein 5/6, *LTBP* latent TGF-beta binding protein, *MRTF-A* myocardin-related transcription factor A, *NF-κB* nuclear factor–kappa B, *P* phosphorylation, *PM* plasma membrane, *Rho* Ras homolog gene family, member A, *ROCK* Rho-associated protein kinase, *Smad* similar to mothers against decapentaplegic, *SRF* serum response factor, *TAK1* transforming growth factor-β-activated kinase 1, *TAZ* transcriptional coactivator with PDZ-binding motif, *TβRI/TβRII* TGF-β receptor type I/II, *TCF* T-cell factor, *TEAD* TEA domain family members, *TGF-β* transforming growth factor-beta, *TRAF6/4* tumor necrosis factor receptor-associated factor 6/4. (Sources: [154–160])

6.5.3.2 The Canonical TGF-Beta-Triggered Pathway in Myofibroblast Activation

In the canonical pathway, TGF-β1 triggers the TGF-β receptor complex (TβRI and TβRII) which in turn phosphorylates Smad2 and Smad3. These two signaling proteins then complex with Smad4 and translocate to the nucleus to initiate transcription of many genes. The Smad2/3 signaling is known to enhance the expression of ECM-remodeling proteins such as COL I and TIMP2—an important regulator of MMP activity (reviewed in [34, 102, 155]).

6.5.3.3 The Noncanonical TGF-Beta-Triggered Pathway in Myofibroblast Activation

Smad-independent pathways include the MAPK pathways leading to activation of JNK, ERK, and the small GTPases RhoA and Cdc42 as well as TGF-β1-promoted activation of the PI3K → Akt and JAK/STAT pathways (for both paths, also compare Vol. 1 [4], Part VI, Sects. 22.3.4.2 and 22.3.4.3, as well as Figs. 22.5 and 22.6). These non-Smad pathways carry out either stand-alone functions or converge back to Smads to modulate TGF-β signaling output (reviewed by Meng et al., Lu, and Zhang in [154, 157, 160]). The MAP kinases interact with TGF-β/Smad signaling at several levels, and these interactions are the most clearly established example of pathway crosstalk with TGF-β/Smad signaling (for details, see [154, 156, 157]).

Of note, there is evidence suggesting that TGF-β1 promotes activation of Rho → ROCK signaling [154, 161] that contributes to remodeling of the actin cytoskeleton as reflected by increased stress fiber formation [162]. In turn, RhoA → ROCK-upregulated cytoskeleton formation triggers nuclear translocation and accumulation of MRTF-A [163–165] (see also Fig. 6.2 and compare Fig. 6.3). As also mentioned above, this leads to MRTF-A/SRF-dependent gene expression that appears to be also essential for fibroblast transdifferentiation into myofibroblast in response to mechanical cues. That TGF-β1 plays a crucial role in such a mechanism of myofibroblast activation is supported by other lines of studies on organ fibrosis models showing that this inducible DAMP stimulates nuclear accumulation of MRTF-A [97, 166].

Moreover, YAP and TAZ were shown to interact with Smads to control Smad nucleocytoplasmic localization/shuttling, thereby contributing to TGF-β-induced cellular responses [157, 167, 168]. Reciprocally, active TGF-β signaling was observed to promote the nuclear accumulation of YAP/TAZ lending support to the concept of a crosstalk between the Hippo and the TGF-β signaling pathways [169]. As discussed elsewhere [155], these studies demonstrate how the control of phosphorylated Smad localization by YAP/TAZ represents one mechanism whereby increased ECM stiffness may increase the profibrotic effects of this inducible DAMP.

Another crosstalk between TGF-β and other signaling pathways refers to Smad proteins and the PI3K-Akt path that is of complex nature and can result in mutual activation or inhibition dependent on the cellular context and biological processes involved. In fibroblasts, TGF-β can reportedly activate PI3K directly and indirectly (for further reading see [154, 157, 170, 171]).

6.5.3.4 Interaction of TGF-Beta → Smads with Wnt → Beta-Catenin Signaling

One more crosstalk between Smad proteins and signaling pathways refers to the Wnt signaling pathway that can occur at multiple levels (for details, see again [154, 156, 157]). Notably, the Wnt proteins are a highly conserved family of secreted glycoproteins that play a vital role in tissue homeostasis (see also Box 2.1). The proteins are known to bind to the cell membrane co-receptors FZDs (for Wnt ↔FZDs, see Sect. 2.3.4.7) and LRP5/6 [172–174]. Upon binding to their receptors, Wnt proteins induce a cascade of intracellular downstream signaling events that involve several molecules and reactions. In the canonical pathway, Wnt signaling begins with binding to and the activation of FZDs together with LRP5/6 co-receptors. Upon binding to this complex, components of the steady degradation complex for β-catenin—such as glycogen synthase-kinase 3 (GSK-3, a serine/threonine-protein-kinase) and other co-proteins—are recruited to the receptor complex. Degradation of β-catenin is blocked and, thus, becomes stabilized to translocate to the nucleus, where it associates with TCF/LEF transcription factors and promotes the transcription of its target genes (Fig. 6.3) (for details, see [175-177]). Of note, interaction between β-catenin and TGF-β occurs at the gene level: thus, it could be demonstrated that β-catenin can be activated by TGF-β signaling to form a complex with phosphorylated Smad3 and the transcriptional coactivator CREB-bind protein [178, 179].

6.5.3.5 Concluding Remarks

Together, the interplay between TGF-β and Wnt-triggered signaling pathways exerts synergistic effects on myofibroblast differentiation, thereby promoting progressive fibrosis [159, 170, 180–182]. Moreover, besides an effect on myofibroblasts, Wnt5a was also shown to promote TGF-β1-mediated macrophage polarization and kidney fibrosis in mice by inducing the transcriptional regulators YAP/TAZ [183]. Plausibly, such experiments have aroused interest in using this pathway as a therapeutic target for protection against fibrotic diseases.

6.5.4 Support of TGF-Beta in Myoblast Activation: The Role of Extra Domain A Type III Repeat of Fibronectin

Obviously, however, strained ECM and activated TGF-β are not always sufficient for the full expression of the myofibroblastic phenotype, and other DAMP-triggered pathways are being discussed to contribute, for example, the FNIII EDA-triggered path. As mentioned above, FNIII EDA as a IIA-3 DAMP is recognized by TLR4. In addition, however, FNIII EDA is supposed to also serve as a ligand for the α4β1 integrin receptor. For example, FNIII EDA↔ α4β1 integrin interaction has been shown to contribute to the activation of myofibroblasts. In studies on human dermal fibroblast cultures, FNIII EDA↔ α4β1 integrin interaction was found to promote a contractile fibroblastic phenotype and an increase in fibronectin synthesis and deposition [184]. Of note, more recent studies of the group provided first evidence suggesting that both the α4 integrin and TLR4 on fibroblasts cooperatively regulate the NF-κB-dependent induction of fibro-inflammatory gene expression in response to FNIII EDA [119]. As concluded by the authors, these studies suggest a new role for integrins in DAMP-based signaling as ligand-binding TLR co-receptors required for TLR activation and downstream signaling in non-immune cells. Further—as argued by the authors [119]—these results suggest that the α4β1integrin specifically regulates the EDA-dependent synthesis of cytokines by human fibroblasts and further that cells adherent to FNIII EDA may be primed for a more robust inflammatory response to additional TLR4 ligands.

6.5.5 Résumé

Together, TGF-β that is actively released from the ECM by integrin-mediated cell tension and enzyme activities triggers various Smad-dependent and Smad-independent pathways leading to myofibroblast activation. Following, these cells respond with increased contractility and production of ECM components resulting in enhanced cell tension force and matrix stiffness. In addition, TGF-β-activated myofibroblasts secrete newly synthesized TGF-β that is stored in the ECM within the LLC. Enhanced integrin-mediated cell tensile force then causes another wave of active TGF-β release that promotes TβRI/TβRII-triggered Smad-dependent and Smad-independent signaling pathways: an impressive example of a self-perpetuating vicious cycle in the growth of ECM stiffness (compare Fig. 6.2).

Of note, this scenario of TGF-β-promoted self-perpetuating process of fibrogenesis may be aggravated by two other parallelly occurring mechanisms that also may contribute to self-perpetuating fibrogenesis, as mentioned already above. First, there is growing evidence suggesting that increasing ECM stiffness generates mechanical stimuli in terms of putative IIB-3 DAMPs, which activate integrins. These mechanosensitive sensors trigger mechanotransduction-mediated positive feed-forward loops that may contribute to activation of myofibroblasts, which, in turn, can promote profibrotic ECM stiffness. Second, fibrotic tissues, in general, are associated with microvascular rarefication and diminished perfusion. This leads to decreased microvasculature that is often associated with chronic hypoxia, which may result in RCD serving as a continuous source of DAMPs emission.

Together, these three DAMP-involving scenarios, the here mentioned TGF-β1-triggered pathways in conjunction with ECM stiffness↔myofibroblastic contraction-mediated mechanotransducing paths, as well as hypoxia-induced RCD in fibrous tissue, constitute self-perpetuating loops that potently propagate activation of myofibroblasts as the key cells in mediating fibrosis in a broad range of pathologies.

6.6 Epigenetics in Fibrosis

6.6.1 Introductory Remarks

A growing body of evidence has shown that epigenetics plays a crucial role in the pathogenesis of fibrosis (for a few basics of epigenetic modifications, see Sect. 5.6 and Figs. 5.4, 5.5, and 5.6, as well as Vol.1 [4], Part VI, Sect. 24.2.2, and Fig. 24.1). Indeed, epigenetics not only play a role in inflammation but also in fibrogenesis. Thus, not only can innate immune cells such as macrophages undergo functional reprogramming and develop changed responses to injurious challenges (M1-like → M2-like) [185, 186] but also the key cells in fibrogenesis, the fibroblasts, experience such epigenetic alterations. Accordingly, here, guided by the article of O'Reilly [187], a few remarks are added on the implication of epigenetic modifications in fibrosis by focusing on epigenetic regulation of stress-/injury-induced fibroblast activation. Clearly, changes in fibroblast gene expression associated with their transdifferentiation into myofibroblasts are central to the initiation and maintenance of a fibrotic response in fibrotic disorders regardless of etiology. Some aspects of this scenario are briefly touched in the following.

6.6.2 Epigenetic Mechanisms Involved in Fibrosis: Some Examples

6.6.2.1 General Remarks

There are three main epigenetic mechanisms involved in fibrosis: DNA methylation, histone modifications, and RNA interference, which can be triggered by environmental factors such as infectious/sterile tissue injury and hypoxic conditions. All three mechanisms have been implicated in the epigenetic control of fibrosis, whereby various overlapping and organ-specific mechanisms have been described to act in this scenario (Fig. 6.4). Indeed, there is evidence suggesting that DNA methylation and histone modifications are context-dependently interconnected in their regulation and promotion of gene silencing. Moreover, a bi-directional relationship has been described between histone modification and DNA methylation as well as ncRNAs and DNA methylation.

6.6.2.2 DNA Methylation in Fibrosis

Convincing evidence indicates that DNA methylation plays a vital role in the pathogenesis of organ fibrosis. Notably, aberrant DNA methylation can silence or activate gene expression patterns that drive the fibrosis process. In general, however, hypermethylation represses and hypomethylation activates gene expression (reviewed in [188-190]). For example, in studies on human cardiac fibroblast cells exposed to prolonged hypoxia, hypermethylation was found to be associated with heart fibrosis and mediated via DNMT enzymes [191]. Of striking importance is the DNA methylation process in the myofibroblast differentiation (see below).

6.6.2.3 Histone Acetyltransferases and Histone Acetylation

Aberrant levels of HATs are known to be associated with the development of several diseases. Among these writers, the p300 acetyltransferase plays a key role in fibrosis, and its availability governs the intensity of fibrotic responses (compare Fig. 5.4 and [187, 190]. For example, in studies on fibroblasts explanted from biopsies of lesional skin from patients with systemic sclerosis, P300 expression was shown to be elevated and positively regulated by TGF-β1 [192]. Further, this study revealed that increased p300 accumulation in TGF-β-treated fibroblasts is associated with histone hyperacetylation, whereas p300 depletion attenuated TGF-β-induced

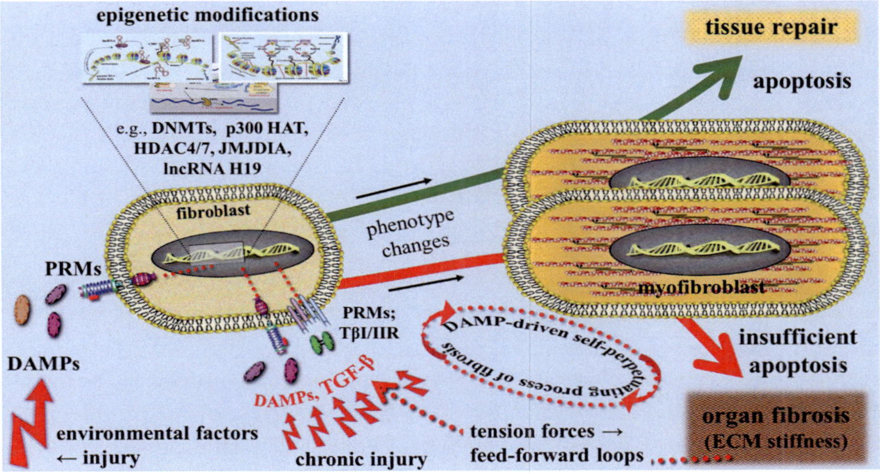

Fig. 6.4 Schematic diagram of a narrative model insinuating and illustrating the DAMP-driven, epigenetically and transcriptionally regulated self-perpetuating scenario of fibrogenesis. All three mechanisms (DNA methylation, histone modifications, and RNA interference) have been implicated in the epigenetic control of fibrosis, whereby various overlapping and organ-specific mechanisms have been described to act in this scenario. The key event is the DAMP-promoted transdifferentiation of fibroblasts into myofibroblasts. Under normal, non-pathological conditions, infectious/sterile injury-induced DAMPs trigger—via induction of epigenetic modifications (?)—activation of myofibroblasts to initiate tissue repair. After homeostatic tissue repair, myofibroblasts disappear through apoptosis (symbolized by green-colored arrow). In pathological situations, for example, in response to chronic infectious or sterile injury, or in case of dysregulated/overshooting emission of DAMPs including TGF-β, or both, myofibroblasts are insufficiently removed by apoptosis, their persistence leading to tissue remodeling and fibrosis. Moreover, myofibroblast/ECM stiffness-generated tension forces constitute positive feed-forward loops that potently propagate TGF-β-promoted activation of myofibroblasts (symbolized by red-colored arrows). *DNMTs* DNA methyltransferases, *ECM* extracellular matrix, *HATs* histone acetyltransferases, *HDAC* histone deacetyltransferases, *JMJD1A* jumonji domain-containing protein 1A, *lncRNA* long noncoding RNA, *PRM* pattern recognition molecule, *TβRI/TβRII* TGF-β receptor type I/II, *TGF-β* transforming growth factor-beta. (Sources: [192, 202, 214–217])

responses. Also, TGF-β was demonstrated to enhance both p300 recruitment and in vivo histone H4 acetylation at the *COL 11A2* locus. The authors of this study [192] concluded that their findings implicate p300-mediated histone acetylation as a fundamental epigenetic mechanism in fibrogenesis. Also of interest in this context are studies in mice showing that P300 acetyltransferase mediates stiffness-induced activation of HSCs into tumor-promoting myofibroblasts [193].

6.6.2.4 Histone Deacetylases and Deacetylation

Deacetylation by HDACs is associated with gene repression. Accordingly, dysregulation of HDACs has been observed in fibrotic diseases, for example, again in systemic sclerosis [194]. In addition, in studies on primary human idiopathic pulmonary fibrosis, fibroblasts, and a murine model of bleomycin-induced lung fibrosis, pulmonary fibrosis-derived fibroblasts (secreting high levels of collagen) pre-treated with an HDAC inhibitor were found to decrease collagen expression, associated with hyperacetylation levels in H3 and H4 in the lung fibroblasts [195]. There is also evidence for deregulation of liver HDACs involved in the development of liver fibrosis. For example, studies on an experimentally induced mouse liver fibrosis model provided evidence for the role of HDAC2 in HSC-T6 cell proliferation and TGF-β1-induced activation, suggesting that deregulation of HDACs may mechanistically be implicated in liver fibrosis [196].

6.6.2.5 Histone Methylation

Histone methylation by specific HMTs (KMTs, protein methyltransferases [PMTs]) can cause activation or repression of gene transcription depending on the recruitment of effector proteins (compare Fig. 5.4). For example, the histone lysine methyltransferase MML-1, which mediates histone lysine methylation, is upregulated in response to ethanol and leads to upregulation of multiple profibrotic genes and proteins [197]. In other lines of studies, TGF-β1 was shown to increase the expression of H3K4 methyltransferase SET7/9, and that subsequent H3K4 methylation plays a vital role in TGF-β1-induced promoter activation of fibrosis-associated genes [198]. Interestingly, age-related alterations in methylation have been detected. For instance, it could be demonstrated that the Thy-1(formerly called CD90) locus is hypermethylated in pulmonary fibrosis fibroblasts leading to its repression and subsequent activation of these cells (The Thy-1 gene encodes a cell surface glycoprotein). Also, Thy-1 is reportedly downregulated by hypoxia and the hypoxic environment in the lung of fibrosis patients, resulting in a hypoxia-induced downregulation of Thy-1 and enhanced TGF-β signaling leading to a profibrotic state (reviewed in [187]). This epigenetic "reader" is a crucial member of the methyl-CpG-binding protein family that binds methyl-DNA and recruits histone modifiers, including the histone methyltransferase EZH2, to suppress gene expression. In fact, MeCP2 was found to mediate downregulation of the expression of transcription factors PPARγ and IκBα in activated HSCs [190, 199]. On the other hand, histone methylation could be demonstrated to activate gene transcription. For example, the *absent, small, or homeotic disc 1* (ASH1) methyltransferase (targeting lysine 4 on histone H3) was identified as a positive regulator of multiple profibrogenic gene loci including TGF-β1, TIMP-1, and COL I [200].

6.6.2.6 Histone Demethylation

As touched in Sect. 5.6.3.5, a major group of KDMs are JmjC demethylases, which catalyze the removal of methyl groups from Nε-methylated lysyl residues on histone tails. A prominent member of this enzyme family is the *jumonji domain-containing protein 1A* (JMJD1A), also known as *jmjC domain-containing histone demethylation protein 2A* (JHDM2A). This enzyme is a recently characterized histone demethylase that catalyzes the removal of H3K9 mono- and dimethylation through iron- and α-ketoglutarate-dependent oxidative reactions [201]. This enzyme was recently shown to regulate liver fibrosis. Mechanistically, reduction of the demethylase enzyme was demonstrated to reinforce H3K9me2 marks in the PPARγ gene promoter, and this leads to repression of both PPARγ mRNA and protein levels [202] (for PPARγ, also compare Sect. 5.3.2.2). More recently, the histone demethylase JMJD2D (also called KDM4D) was reported to promote hepatic fibrogenesis via alteration of the methylation status of H3K9 by modulating the TLR4 signaling pathway [203]. The authors concluded that their "findings provide critical insights into the molecular mechanisms for the regulation of liver fibrosis in an epigenetic fashion"; and further that their data "highlight a previously unknown role for KDM4D, which shed light on how histone modification enzymes coordinate with transcription factors to regulate TLR4 expression and liver fibrosis. Thus, blockade of KDM4D-TLR4 signaling in HSCs may serve as a novel approach for the epigenetic interruption of liver fibrosis."

6.6.2.7 Long Noncoding RNAs and Noncoding MicroRNAs

Long noncoding RNAs and noncoding miRNAs are new epigenetic players involved in fibrotic processes. Given the increasing attention paid to their role in the regulation of fibrogenesis, they are briefly addressed here.

Noncoding MicroRNAs

Long noncoding RNAs have been shown to be implicated in fibrosis, including cardiac, pulmonary, hepatic, and renal fibrotic diseases (reviewed in [187, 204]; also compare Fig. 5.5). Thus, overexpression and knockdown of lncRNAs were demonstrated to alleviate or enhance the extent of fibrosis in vivo and in vitro. For example, H19, an imprinted gene transcribing a long noncoding RNA, was revealed to be involved in cardiac, pulmonary, hepatic, and renal fibrosis with a different mechanism, indicating that H19 probably serve as common therapeutic target for fibrosis. In cardiac fibrosis tissue treated with isoproterenol (a β-sympathomimetic isopropyl analog of epinephrine) and TGF-β1-treated cardiac fibroblasts, H19 was found to be significantly increased, while DUSP5 (a downstream target of p68 RNA helicase) was shown to be downregulated in this tissue and to activate cardiac fibroblasts [205]. In other lines of studies on liver fibrosis, the lncRNA *maternally expressed gene 3* (MEG3) was found to be reduced significantly and to be downregulated in HSCs by TGF-β1. Mechanistically, TGF-β1 mediated repression of MEG3 appears to be involved via hypermethylation of the gene and a subsequent increase in collagen [206].

Noncoding MicroRNAs

MicroRNAs complete the list of epigenetic modifiers implicated in fibrogenesis (compare Fig. 5.6). Indeed, in fibrotic diseases, miRNAs can regulate many of the molecules involved in fibrosis and in many different cell types, and they operate as either being pro- or antifibrotic molecules. Thus, abnormal expression of miRNAs was reported to be associated with cardiac, liver, lung, kidney, and systemic sclerosis (reviewed in [187, 190, 207]). Multiple miRNAs may simultaneously and synergistically be implicated in complex cellular processes such as epithelial-to-mesenchymal transition (EMT, also compare Fig. 9.1 in Vol. 1 [4], Part III, Sect. 9.3.2), and these miRNAs are supposed to play different roles in varying organs [208]. For example, a salient “fibromiRNA” [187] is miR-21 that has been shown to regulate ERK-MAP kinase signaling in cardiac fibroblasts [209] (for additional information also compare Vol. 1 [4], Part VI, Sect. 22.3.3.2, p. 490). Given their data, the authors suggested that “stimuli or procedures that induce cardiac stress result in miRNA-mediated activation of ERK–MAP kinase activity by means of an effect on SPRY1, which in turn positively regulates cardiac fibroblast survival, leading to fibrosis, hypertrophy, and cardiac dysfunction” (SPRY1 is the abbreviation of the protein-coding gene *protein sprouty homolog 1*, a potent inhibitor of the Ras/MEK/ERK pathway). This miRNA has further been shown to be elevated in pulmonary, hepatic, and renal fibrosis (reviewed in [187]). Of note, and critical regarding mechanisms of fibrogenesis, several miRNAs such as the profibrotic mi-R21 and miR-424 and the antifibrotic miR-101 and miR-153 are known to target many components of the TGF-β signaling pathway [210]. For example, in studies on a bleomycin-induced pulmonary fibrosis mouse model [211], miR-153 was shown to inhibit the fibrogenic activity of TGF-β1 and to diminish the contractile and migratory activities of pulmonary fibroblasts by directly targeting TβRII-3'UTR (for 3′UTR, also compare Fig. 5.6). Further, in vitro experiments of this study using the human pulmonary fibroblast line MRC-5 revealed that phosphorylation of Smad2/3 is significantly reduced when miR-153 is overexpressed, whereas the levels of total Smad2/3 remain unchanged (also compare Fig. 6.3).

6.6.2.8 Concluding Remarks

Together, pro- or antifibrotic histone-modifying enzymes and noncoding RNAs—as briefly touched in this section—induce critical epigenetic modifications, and the in vivo delivery of these enzymes and RNAs in the form of mimics or inhibitors have consequently been proposed as a promising therapeutic strategy for the treatment of organ fibrosis.

6.6.3 Epigenetic Regulation of Fibroblast → Myofibroblast Transition

6.6.3.1 General Remarks

As already stressed above, the central point of fibrogenesis is the transdifferentiation of fibroblasts into myofibroblasts. Changes in fibroblast gene expression are central to the initiation and maintenance of a fibrotic response. Thus, many studies have been published on the topic of fibroblast → myofibroblast transition, whereby most of them focused on the regulation of α-SMA gene expression (reviewed by Duong and Hagood [207] and Felisbino et al. [212].

6.6.3.2 DNA Methylation

Today, not much is known regarding TET protein involvement, nor about hydroxymethylation in fibrosis. Methylation abnormalities have recently been uncovered in fibrosis, both organ-specific and widespread fibrosis. Earlier findings already suggested that DNA methylation mediated by DNA methyltransferase is an important mechanism regulating the α-SMA gene expression during myofibroblast differentiation [213]. These findings are supported by recently published data demonstrating that DNA methylation regulates α-SMA expression during cardiac fibroblast differentiation [214]. Also, as already mentioned, studies on human cardiac fibroblast cells exposed to prolonged hypoxia reportedly resulted in a profibrotic state. These hypoxia-induced profibrotic changes were associated with global DNA hypermethylation and increased expression of DNMT enzymes that were found to lead ultimately to the development of a myofibroblast-like phenotype [191].

6.6.3.3 Histone Acetylation and Deacetylation

It was reported that the ECM protein COL I, a major contributor in organ fibrogenesis, is epigenetically regulated by the acetyltransferase p300 that, in subsequent studies, was shown to lead to an increased synthesis of collagen by TGF-β-activated myofibroblasts [215]. On the other side, as observed in experiments with cultured human skin fibroblasts, the histone deacetylase HDAC4 can most efficiently abrogate SMA expression and prevent TGF-β1-mediated morphological changes seen in myofibroblast differentiation. This HDAC was also found to upregulate expression of the *TGFβ-1 signaling pathway repressors 5′-TG-3c′-interacting factor* (TGIF) and TGIF2 homeoproteins [216]. The authors of this study concluded that HDAC4 is an essential epigenetic regulator of myofibroblasts differentiation. Interestingly, in studies on fibroblasts isolated from plaque tissue of Peyronie's disease, evidence was provided that HDAC7 promotes transdifferentiation of fibroblasts into myofibroblasts [217]. This evidence was deduced from experiments of siRNA-mediated knockdown of HDAC7 in these fibroblasts that was observed to attenuate TGF-β1-induced ECM production by inhibiting fibroblasts → myofibroblasts transition and by blocking activation of the Smad2/3 pathway.

6.6.3.4 Histone Methylation and Demethylation

As known, TGF-β1 upregulates the expression of a methyltransferase, specifically H3K4 methyltransferase SET7/9, that is responsible for the transcriptional activation of fibrotic genes [198]. From earlier reports, it was already known that several histone methyltransferases, including MLL1, MLL5, Set1, and KMT2H (ASH1), are highly upregulated during transdifferentiation of HSCs. All of these histone methyltransferases regulate methylation of H3K4, whereby ASH1 could be proven to orchestrate fibrogenic gene transcription during myofibroblast transdifferentiation [200]. More recently performed studies on human kidney fibroblasts revealed that the methyltransferase SET9—via interaction with Smad3—promotes expression of ECM proteins, collagen contractility, and myofibroblast differentiation [218] (compare Fig. 6.3). Data on the involvement of demethylating KDMs in fibroblast→ myofibroblast transition are also limited but have been shown in liver HSC activation to fibrotic myofibroblasts [202]. In these studies, the H3K9 demethylase JMJD1A was also demonstrated to be critical for myofibroblast differentiation of HSCs, because knockdown of JMJD1A led to increased expression of α-SMA [202].

6.6.3.5 Concluding Remarks

Collectively, DNA methylation and histone modifications are essential epigenetic regulators of myofibroblast differentiation, unveiling them as potential targets for treating myofibroblast-related disorders. However, this aim is, by far, not reached. As concluded by Duong and Hagood [207] in this context: "A more comprehensive understanding of the organ-specific epigenetic mechanisms involved in fibrosis, and of how to target them for therapeutic benefit without significant off-target effects, will facilitate the development of novel antifibrotic therapies."

6.6.4 Résumé

Together, one has to realize that epigenetics is critical in fibrogenesis, and intense research into this area is going on. Intriguingly, in fibrosis, there is a complex interaction between multiple cell types and signaling pathways that can all be affected by epigenetic modifications. And, as stressed by O'Reilly [187], one epigenetic mechanism is known to affect another one, and feed-forward-loops can and do operate. Nevertheless, the exact mechanisms responsible for fibrogenic changes in the epigenome remain incompletely understood. In particular, the provocative question of whether or not DAMPs are the leading players in inducing epigenetic modifications awaits urgent clarification.

6.7 Resolution of Fibrosis

Although fibrosis was previously thought to be irreversible, recent studies provided some evidence indicating that, under certain circumstances, the resolution of fibrosis is possible when the underlying causes of injury (i.e., emission of DAMPs) have been controlled. The mechanism of fibrosis resolution comprises degradation of the fibrotic ECM as well as elimination of fibrogenic myofibroblasts through their adaptation of various cell fates, including apoptosis, senescence, dedifferentiation, and reprogramming. Indeed, this topic is of high relevance for the development of novel effective therapeutic modalities. For example, further studies into genetic or pharmacological manipulations that can dictate specific myofibroblasts cell fate may help achieve new therapeutic options. This highly exciting topic is not further followed here. Instead, the reader is referred to the excellent review article of Jun and Lau [219].

6.8 Outlook and Future Perspectives

Recognizing that fibrotic processes are the underlying pathological feature of many therapy-resistant chronic diseases, experimental and clinical research on fibrotic processes is proceeding in full swing. Today, generally accepted notions hold that environmental parenchymal injury induces emission of DAMPs, which trigger an innate immune inflammatory/repairing response promoting wound healing. The vital event of this DAMP-promoted repairing process is seen in the transdifferentiation and proliferation of precursor fibroblasts from different origins into myofibroblasts. These cells produce abundant TGF-β and ECM proteins, including fibrillar collagens, which play a critical role in the different phases of wound healing, in particular, late-stage wound healing. Under normal conditions, this repairing response is terminated when the scar is appropriately established. Typically, this resolving process is characterized by myofibroblast apoptosis as a fundamental mechanism during healthy wound healing.

However, when uncontrolled and dysregulated, the same repairing pathways can become detrimental, leading to tissue/organ fibrosis in terms of a failed resolution of the repair response. In fact, failure to resolve inflammatory/repairing responses associated with failure of apoptotic fibroblast death, combined with DAMP-promoted uncontrolled overshooting repairing pathways, leads to tissue remodeling rather than normal wound healing.

Of note, there is a growing body of convincing evidence indicating that this DAMP-promoted complex scenario—particularly the transdifferentiation of precursor cells into myofibroblasts—is affected by epigenetic modifications. And it should be born in mind that one epigenetic mechanism can affect another one and feed-forward loops can and do exist [187]. The key question to raise at this point is: Are the DAMP-driven fibrotic processes due to DAMPs' properties to induce those epigenetic modifications as well? A tentative model of such a DAMP-driven, epigenetically regulated self-perpetuating scenario of fibrogenesis is insinuated Fig. 6.4.

References

1. Desmoulière A, Redard M, Darby I, Gabbiani G. Apoptosis mediates the decrease in cellularity during the transition between granulation tissue and scar. Am J Pathol. 1995;146:56–66. http://www.ncbi.nlm.nih.gov/pubmed/7856739.
2. Waring P, Müllbacher A. Cell death induced by the Fas/Fas ligand pathway and its role in pathology. Immunol Cell Biol. 1999;77:312–7. http://www.ncbi.nlm.nih.gov/pubmed/10457197.
3. Horowitz JC, Thannickal VJ. Mechanisms for the resolution of organ fibrosis. Physiology. 2019;34:43–55. http://www.ncbi.nlm.nih.gov/pubmed/30540232.
4. Land WG. Damage-associated molecular patterns in human diseases. In: Injury-induced innate immune responses, vol. 1. Cham: Springer International Publishing AG; 2018. https://www.springer.com/de/book/9783319786544.
5. Anderson KR, Sutton MG, Lie JT. Histopathological types of cardiac fibrosis in myocardial disease. J Pathol. 1979;128:79–85. https://doi.org/10.1002/path.1711280205.
6. Biernacka A, Frangogiannis NG. Aging and cardiac fibrosis. Aging Dis. 2011;2:158–73. http://www.ncbi.nlm.nih.gov/pubmed/21837283.
7. Shinde AV, Frangogiannis NG. Fibroblasts in myocardial infarction: a role in inflammation and repair. J Mol Cell Cardiol. 2014;70:74–82. https://linkinghub.elsevier.com/retrieve/pii/S0022282813003477.
8. Hinz B. The extracellular matrix and transforming growth factor-β1: tale of a strained relationship. Matrix Biol. 2015;47:54–65. https://linkinghub.elsevier.com/retrieve/pii/S0945053X15001055.

9. Wynn TA. Fibrotic disease and the T(H)1/T(H)2 paradigm. Nat Rev Immunol. 2004;4:583–94. https://doi.org/10.1038/nri1412.
10. Hynes RO, Naba A. Overview of the matrisome—an inventory of extracellular matrix constituents and functions. Cold Spring Harb Perspect Biol. 2012;4:a004903. https://doi.org/10.1101/cshperspect.a004903.
11. Bonnans C, Chou J, Werb Z. Remodelling the extracellular matrix in development and disease. Nat Rev Mol Cell Biol. 2014;15:786–801. http://www.ncbi.nlm.nih.gov/pubmed/25415508.
12. Humphrey JD, Dufresne ER, Schwartz MA. Mechanotransduction and extracellular matrix homeostasis. Nat Rev Mol Cell Biol. 2014;15:802–12. http://www.ncbi.nlm.nih.gov/pubmed/25355505.
13. Iozzo RV, Schaefer L. Proteoglycan form and function: a comprehensive nomenclature of proteoglycans. Matrix Biol. 2015;42:11–55. http://linkinghub.elsevier.com/retrieve/pii/S0945053X15000402.
14. Naba A, Clauser KR, Ding H, Whittaker CA, Carr SA, Hynes RO. The extracellular matrix: tools and insights for the "omics" era. Matrix Biol. 2016;49:10–24. http://www.ncbi.nlm.nih.gov/pubmed/26163349.
15. Kryczka J, Boncela J. Proteases revisited: roles and therapeutic implications in fibrosis. Mediators Inflamm. 2017;2017:1–14. https://www.hindawi.com/journals/mi/2017/2570154/.
16. Cui N, Hu M, Khalil RA. Biochemical and biological attributes of matrix metalloproteinases. Prog Mol Biol Transl Sci. 2017;147:1–73. http://www.ncbi.nlm.nih.gov/pubmed/28413025.
17. Herrera C, Escalante T, Rucavado A, Fox JW, Gutiérrez JM. Metalloproteinases in disease: identification of biomarkers of tissue damage through proteomics. Expert Rev Proteomics. 2018;15:967–82. http://www.ncbi.nlm.nih.gov/pubmed/30348024.
18. van Goor H, Melenhorst WB, Turner AJ, Holgate ST. Adamalysins in biology and disease. J Pathol. 2009;219:277–86. http://www.ncbi.nlm.nih.gov/pubmed/19662664.
19. Arpino V, Brock M, Gill SE. The role of TIMPs in regulation of extracellular matrix proteolysis. Matrix Biol. 2015;44–46:247–54. http://www.ncbi.nlm.nih.gov/pubmed/25805621.
20. Khokha R, Murthy A, Weiss A. Metalloproteinases and their natural inhibitors in inflammation and immunity. Nat Rev Immunol. 2013;13:649–65. http://www.nature.com/articles/nri3499.
21. Handorf AM, Zhou Y, Halanski MA, Li W-J. Tissue stiffness dictates development, homeostasis, and disease progression. Organogenesis. 2015;11:1–15. https://doi.org/10.1080/15476278.2015.1019687.
22. Tam SN, Smith ML, Stamenović D. Modeling tensional homeostasis in multicellular clusters. Int J Numer Method Biomed Eng. 2017;33:e02801. http://www.ncbi.nlm.nih.gov/pubmed/27163337.
23. Herrera J, Henke CA, Bitterman PB. Extracellular matrix as a driver of progressive fibrosis. J Clin Invest. 2018;128:45–53. https://www.jci.org/articles/view/93557.
24. Hinz B. Tissue stiffness, latent TGF-beta1 activation, and mechanical signal transduction: implications for the pathogenesis and treatment of fibrosis. Curr Rheumatol Rep. 2009;11:120–6. http://www.ncbi.nlm.nih.gov/pubmed/19296884.
25. Hinz B. Matrix mechanics and regulation of the fibroblast phenotype. Periodontol 2000. 2013;63:14–28. https://doi.org/10.1111/prd.12030.
26. Wells RG, Discher DE. Matrix elasticity, cytoskeletal tension, and TGF-beta: the insoluble and soluble meet. Sci Signal. 2008;1:pe13. https://doi.org/10.1126/stke.110pe13.
27. Engler AJ, Carag-Krieger C, Johnson CP, Raab M, Tang H-Y, Speicher DW, et al. Embryonic cardiomyocytes beat best on a matrix with heart-like elasticity: scar-like rigidity inhibits beating. J Cell Sci. 2008;121:3794–802. https://doi.org/10.1242/jcs.029678.
28. Jahed Z, Shams H, Mehrbod M, Mofrad MRK. Mechanotransduction pathways linking the extracellular matrix to the nucleus. Int Rev Cell Mol Biol. 2014;310:171–220. http://www.ncbi.nlm.nih.gov/pubmed/24725427.
29. Ringer P, Colo G, Fässler R, Grashoff C. Sensing the mechano-chemical properties of the extracellular matrix. Matrix Biol. 2017;64:6–16. http://www.ncbi.nlm.nih.gov/pubmed/28389162.

30. Dupont S. Role of YAP/TAZ in cell-matrix adhesion-mediated signalling and mechanotransduction. Exp Cell Res. 2016;343:42–53. http://www.ncbi.nlm.nih.gov/pubmed/26524510.
31. Herum KM, Lunde IG, McCulloch AD, Christensen G. The soft- and hard-heartedness of cardiac fibroblasts: mechanotransduction signaling pathways in fibrosis of the heart. J Clin Med. 2017;6:53. http://www.mdpi.com/2077-0383/6/5/53.
32. Martino F, Perestrelo AR, Vinarský V, Pagliari S, Forte G. Cellular mechanotransduction: from tension to function. Front Physiol. 2018;9:824. https://doi.org/10.3389/fphys.2018.00824/full.
33. Santos A, Lagares D. Matrix stiffness: the conductor of organ fibrosis. Curr Rheumatol Rep. 2018;20:2. http://www.ncbi.nlm.nih.gov/pubmed/29349703.
34. Zent J, Guo L-W. Signaling mechanisms of myofibroblastic activation: outside-in and inside-out. Cell Physiol Biochem. 2018;49:848–68. http://www.ncbi.nlm.nih.gov/pubmed/30184544.
35. Rossman KL, Der CJ, Sondek J. GEF means go: turning on RHO GTPases with guanine nucleotide-exchange factors. Nat Rev Mol Cell Biol. 2005;6:167–80. http://www.ncbi.nlm.nih.gov/pubmed/15688002.
36. Guilluy C, Swaminathan V, Garcia-Mata R, O'Brien ET, Superfine R, Burridge K. The Rho GEFs LARG and GEF-H1 regulate the mechanical response to force on integrins. Nat Cell Biol. 2011;13:722–7. http://www.nature.com/articles/ncb2254.
37. Hynes RO. Integrins: bidirectional, allosteric signaling machines. Cell. 2002;110:673–87. http://www.ncbi.nlm.nih.gov/pubmed/12297042.
38. Horton ER, Byron A, Askari JA, Ng DHJ, Millon-Frémillon A, Robertson J, et al. Definition of a consensus integrin adhesome and its dynamics during adhesion complex assembly and disassembly. Nat Cell Biol. 2015;17:1577–87. http://www.nature.com/articles/ncb3257.
39. Oakes PW, Gardel ML. Stressing the limits of focal adhesion mechanosensitivity. Curr Opin Cell Biol. 2014;30:68–73. https://linkinghub.elsevier.com/retrieve/pii/S095506741400074X.
40. Molkentin JD, Bugg D, Ghearing N, Dorn LE, Kim P, Sargent MA, et al. Fibroblast-specific genetic manipulation of p38 mitogen-activated protein kinase in vivo reveals its central regulatory role in fibrosis. Circulation. 2017;136:549–61. https://doi.org/10.1161/CIRCULATIONAHA.116.026238.
41. Hörner M, Chatelle C, Mühlhäuser WWD, Stocker DR, Coats M, Weber W, et al. Optogenetic control of focal adhesion kinase signaling. Cell Signal. 2018;42:176–83. http://www.ncbi.nlm.nih.gov/pubmed/29074139.
42. Zhao T, Li R, Tan X, Zhang J, Fan C, Zhao Q, et al. Simulated microgravity reduces focal adhesions and alters cytoskeleton and nuclear positioning leading to enhanced apoptosis via suppressing FAK/RhoA-mediated mTORC1/NF-κB and ERK1/2 pathways. Int J Mol Sci. 2018;19:1994. http://www.ncbi.nlm.nih.gov/pubmed/29986550.
43. Vogel V. Unraveling the mechanobiology of extracellular matrix. Annu Rev Physiol. 2018;80:353–87. http://www.ncbi.nlm.nih.gov/pubmed/29433414.
44. Klapholz B, Brown NH. Talin—the master of integrin adhesions. J Cell Sci. 2017;130:2435–46. http://www.ncbi.nlm.nih.gov/pubmed/28701514.
45. Zaidel-Bar R, Itzkovitz S, Ma'ayan A, Iyengar R, Geiger B. Functional atlas of the integrin adhesome. Nat Cell Biol. 2007;9:858–67. http://www.nature.com/articles/ncb0807-858.
46. Sang M, Ma L, Sang M, Zhou X, Gao W, Geng C. LIM-domain-only proteins: multifunctional nuclear transcription coregulators that interacts with diverse proteins. Mol Biol Rep. 2014;41:1067–73. http://www.ncbi.nlm.nih.gov/pubmed/24379077.
47. Schiller HB, Friedel CC, Boulegue C, Fässler R. Quantitative proteomics of the integrin adhesome show a myosin II-dependent recruitment of LIM domain proteins. EMBO Rep. 2011;12:259–66. https://doi.org/10.1038/embor.2011.5.
48. Hall A. Rho family GTPases. Biochem Soc Trans. 2012;40:1378–82. http://www.ncbi.nlm.nih.gov/pubmed/23176484.
49. Varney SD, Betts CB, Zheng R, Wu L, Hinz B, Zhou J, et al. Hic-5 is required for myofibroblast differentiation by regulating mechanically dependent MRTF-A nuclear accumulation. J Cell Sci. 2016;129:774–87. https://doi.org/10.1242/jcs.170589.

50. Shibanuma M, Kim-Kaneyama J, Ishino K, Sakamoto N, Hishiki T, Yamaguchi K, et al. Hic-5 communicates between focal adhesions and the nucleus through oxidant-sensitive nuclear export signal. Mol Biol Cell. 2003;14:1158–71. https://doi.org/10.1091/mbc.02-06-0099.
51. Kim-Kaneyama J, Suzuki W, Ichikawa K, Ohki T, Kohno Y, Sata M, et al. Uni-axial stretching regulates intracellular localization of Hic-5 expressed in smooth-muscle cells in vivo. J Cell Sci. 2005;118:937–49. https://doi.org/10.1242/jcs.01683.
52. Julian L, Olson MF. Rho-associated coiled-coil containing kinases (ROCK). Small GTPases. 2014;5:e29846. http://www.ncbi.nlm.nih.gov/pubmed/25010901.
53. Narumiya S, Thumkeo D. Rho signaling research: history, current status and future directions. FEBS Lett. 2018;592:1763–76. https://doi.org/10.1002/1873-3468.13087.
54. Boyle ST, Kular J, Nobis M, Ruszkiewicz A, Timpson P, Samuel MS. Acute compressive stress activates RHO/ROCK-mediated cellular processes. Small GTPases. 2018:1–17. http://www.ncbi.nlm.nih.gov/pubmed/29455593.
55. Yuan Y, Li M, To CH, Lam TC, Wang P, Yu Y, et al. The Role of the RhoA/ROCK signaling pathway in mechanical strain-induced scleral myofibroblast differentiation. Investig Opthalmol Vis Sci. 2018;59:3619. http://www.ncbi.nlm.nih.gov/pubmed/30029249.
56. Knipe RS, Probst CK, Lagares D, Franklin A, Spinney JJ, Brazee PL, et al. The Rho kinase isoforms ROCK1 and ROCK2 each contribute to the development of experimental pulmonary fibrosis. Am J Respir Cell Mol Biol. 2018;58:471–81. https://doi.org/10.1165/rcmb.2017-0075OC.
57. Amano M, Nakayama M, Kaibuchi K. Rho-kinase/ROCK: a key regulator of the cytoskeleton and cell polarity. Cytoskeleton (Hoboken). 2010;67:545–54. https://doi.org/10.1002/cm.20472.
58. Zhang J, Fan G, Zhao H, Wang Z, Li F, Zhang P, et al. Targeted inhibition of focal adhesion kinase attenuates cardiac fibrosis and preserves heart function in adverse cardiac remodeling. Sci Rep. 2017;7:43146. http://www.ncbi.nlm.nih.gov/pubmed/28225063.
59. Fletcher DA, Mullins RD. Cell mechanics and the cytoskeleton. Nature. 2010;463:485–92. http://www.ncbi.nlm.nih.gov/pubmed/20110992.
60. Chen T-J, Wu C-C, Tang M-J, Huang J-S, Su F-C. Complexity of the tensegrity structure for dynamic energy and force distribution of cytoskeleton during cell spreading. PLoS One. 2010;5:e14392. https://doi.org/10.1371/journal.pone.0014392.
61. Tang DD, Gerlach BD. The roles and regulation of the actin cytoskeleton, intermediate filaments and microtubules in smooth muscle cell migration. Respir Res. 2017;18:54. http://www.ncbi.nlm.nih.gov/pubmed/28390425.
62. Houdusse A, Sweeney HL. How Myosin Generates Force on Actin Filaments. Trends Biochem Sci. 2016;41:989–97. http://www.ncbi.nlm.nih.gov/pubmed/27717739
63. Koenderink GH, Paluch EK. Architecture shapes contractility in actomyosin networks. Curr Opin Cell Biol. 2018;50:79–85. http://www.ncbi.nlm.nih.gov/pubmed/29482169.
64. Lee S, Kumar S. Actomyosin stress fiber mechanosensing in 2D and 3D. F1000Research. 2016;5:2261. http://www.ncbi.nlm.nih.gov/pubmed/27635242.
65. Burridge K, Guilluy C. Focal adhesions, stress fibers and mechanical tension. Exp Cell Res. 2016;343:14–20. http://www.ncbi.nlm.nih.gov/pubmed/26519907.
66. Shutova MS, Svitkina TM. Mammalian nonmuscle myosin II comes in three flavors. Biochem Biophys Res Commun. 2018;506:394–402. http://www.ncbi.nlm.nih.gov/pubmed/29550471.
67. Parmacek MS. Myocardin-Related Transcription Factors. Circ Res. 2007;100:633–44. http://www.ncbi.nlm.nih.gov/pubmed/17363709
68. Panciera T, Azzolin L, Cordenonsi M, Piccolo S. Mechanobiology of YAP and TAZ in physiology and disease. Nat Rev Mol Cell Biol. 2017;18:758–70. http://www.ncbi.nlm.nih.gov/pubmed/28951564.
69. Totaro A, Panciera T, Piccolo S. YAP/TAZ upstream signals and downstream responses. Nat Cell Biol. 2018;20:888–99. http://www.nature.com/articles/s41556-018-0142-z.
70. Meng Z, Moroishi T, Guan K-L. Mechanisms of Hippo pathway regulation. Genes Dev. 2016;30:1–17. http://www.ncbi.nlm.nih.gov/pubmed/26728553.

71. Lin KC, Park HW, Guan K-L. Regulation of the Hippo pathway transcription factor TEAD. Trends Biochem Sci. 2017;42:862–72. http://www.ncbi.nlm.nih.gov/pubmed/28964625.
72. Piersma B, Bank RA, Boersema M. Signaling in fibrosis: TGF-β, WNT, and YAP/TAZ converge. Front Med. 2015;2:59. http://www.ncbi.nlm.nih.gov/pubmed/26389119.
73. Mannaerts I, Leite SB, Verhulst S, Claerhout S, Eysackers N, Thoen LFR, et al. The Hippo pathway effector YAP controls mouse hepatic stellate cell activation. J Hepatol. 2015;63:679–88. https://linkinghub.elsevier.com/retrieve/pii/S0168827815002949.
74. Liu F, Lagares D, Choi KM, Stopfer L, Marinković A, Vrbanac V, et al. Mechanosignaling through YAP and TAZ drives fibroblast activation and fibrosis. Am J Physiol Lung Cell Mol Physiol. 2015;308:L344–57. https://doi.org/10.1152/ajplung.00300.2014.
75. Piersma B, de Rond S, Werker PMN, Boo S, Hinz B, van Beuge MM, et al. YAP1 is a driver of myofibroblast differentiation in normal and diseased fibroblasts. Am J Pathol. 2015;185:3326–37. https://linkinghub.elsevier.com/retrieve/pii/S000294401500499X.
76. Johnson LA, Rodansky ES, Haak AJ, Larsen SD, Neubig RR, Higgins PDR. Novel Rho/MRTF/SRF inhibitors block matrix-stiffness and TGF-β-induced fibrogenesis in human colonic myofibroblasts. Inflamm Bowel Dis. 2014;20:154–65. https://academic.oup.com/ibdjournal/article/20/1/154-165/4578875.
77. Miralles F, Posern G, Zaromytidou A-I, Treisman R. Actin dynamics control SRF activity by regulation of its coactivator MAL. Cell. 2003;113:329–42. http://www.ncbi.nlm.nih.gov/pubmed/12732141.
78. Kuwahara K, Barrientos T, Pipes GCT, Li S, Olson EN. Muscle-specific signaling mechanism that links actin dynamics to serum response factor. Mol Cell Biol. 2005;25:3173–81. https://doi.org/10.1128/MCB.25.8.3173-3181.2005.
79. Mouilleron S, Langer CA, Guettler S, McDonald NQ, Treisman R. Structure of a pentavalent G-actin*MRTF-A complex reveals how G-actin controls nucleocytoplasmic shuttling of a transcriptional coactivator. Sci Signal. 2011;4:ra40. https://doi.org/10.1126/scisignal.2001750.
80. Staus DP, Weise-Cross L, Mangum KD, Medlin MD, Mangiante L, Taylor JM, et al. Nuclear RhoA signaling regulates MRTF-dependent SMC-specific transcription. Am J Physiol Heart Circ Physiol. 2014;307:H379–90. https://doi.org/10.1152/ajpheart.01002.2013.
81. Speight P, Kofler M, Szászi K, Kapus A. Context-dependent switch in chemo/mechanotransduction via multilevel crosstalk among cytoskeleton-regulated MRTF and TAZ and TGFβ-regulated Smad3. Nat Commun. 2016;7:11642. http://www.ncbi.nlm.nih.gov/pubmed/27189435.
82. Wang N, Tytell JD, Ingber DE. Mechanotransduction at a distance: mechanically coupling the extracellular matrix with the nucleus. Nat Rev Mol Cell Biol. 2009;10:75–82. http://www.nature.com/articles/nrm2594.
83. Chambliss AB, Khatau SB, Erdenberger N, Robinson DK, Hodzic D, Longmore GD, et al. The LINC-anchored actin cap connects the extracellular milieu to the nucleus for ultrafast mechanotransduction. Sci Rep. 2013;3:1087. http://www.nature.com/articles/srep01087.
84. Cho S, Irianto J, Discher DE. Mechanosensing by the nucleus: from pathways to scaling relationships. J Cell Biol. 2017;216:305–15. https://doi.org/10.1083/jcb.201610042.
85. Miroshnikova YA, Nava MM, Wickström SA. Emerging roles of mechanical forces in chromatin regulation. J Cell Sci. 2017;130:2243–50. https://doi.org/10.1242/jcs.202192.
86. Horn HF. LINC complex proteins in development and disease. Curr Top Dev Biol. 2014;109:287–321. https://linkinghub.elsevier.com/retrieve/pii/B9780123979209000044.
87. Kirby TJ, Lammerding J. Emerging views of the nucleus as a cellular mechanosensor. Nat Cell Biol. 2018;20:373–81. http://www.nature.com/articles/s41556-018-0038-y.
88. Haque F, Lloyd DJ, Smallwood DT, Dent CL, Shanahan CM, Fry AM, et al. SUN1 interacts with nuclear lamin A and cytoplasmic nesprins to provide a physical connection between the nuclear lamina and the cytoskeleton. Mol Cell Biol. 2006;26:3738–51. https://doi.org/10.1128/MCB.26.10.3738-3751.2006.

89. Nishioka Y, Imaizumi H, Imada J, Katahira J, Matsuura N, Hieda M. SUN1 splice variants, SUN1_888, SUN1_785, and predominant SUN1_916, variably function in directional cell migration. Nucleus. 2016;7:572–84. https://doi.org/10.1080/19491034.2016.1260802.
90. Nikolova V, Leimena C, McMahon AC, Tan JC, Chandar S, Jogia D, et al. Defects in nuclear structure and function promote dilated cardiomyopathy in lamin A/C-deficient mice. J Clin Invest. 2004;113:357–69. http://www.jci.org/articles/view/19448.
91. Ho CY, Jaalouk DE, Vartiainen MK, Lammerding J. Lamin A/C and emerin regulate MKL1-SRF activity by modulating actin dynamics. Nature. 2013;497:507–11. http://www.nature.com/articles/nature12105.
92. Ding X, Xu R, Yu J, Xu T, Zhuang Y, Han M. SUN1 is required for telomere attachment to nuclear envelope and gametogenesis in mice. Dev Cell. 2007;12:863–72. https://linkinghub.elsevier.com/retrieve/pii/S1534580707001189.
93. Stewart-Hutchinson PJ, Hale CM, Wirtz D, Hodzic D. Structural requirements for the assembly of LINC complexes and their function in cellular mechanical stiffness. Exp Cell Res. 2008;314:1892–905. https://linkinghub.elsevier.com/retrieve/pii/S0014482708001092.
94. Adapala RK, Thoppil RJ, Luther DJ, Paruchuri S, Meszaros JG, Chilian WM, et al. TRPV4 channels mediate cardiac fibroblast differentiation by integrating mechanical and soluble signals. J Mol Cell Cardiol. 2013;54:45–52. https://linkinghub.elsevier.com/retrieve/pii/S0022282812003987.
95. Numaga-Tomita T, Kitajima N, Kuroda T, Nishimura A, Miyano K, Yasuda S, et al. TRPC3-GEF-H1 axis mediates pressure overload-induced cardiac fibrosis. Sci Rep. 2016;6:39383. http://www.nature.com/articles/srep39383.
96. Sharma S, Goswami R, Merth M, Cohen J, Lei KY, Zhang DX, et al. TRPV4 ion channel is a novel regulator of dermal myofibroblast differentiation. Am J Physiol Cell Physiol. 2017;312:C562–72. https://doi.org/10.1152/ajpcell.00187.2016.
97. O'Connor JW, Riley PN, Nalluri SM, Ashar PK, Gomez EW. Matrix rigidity mediates TGFβ1-induced epithelial-myofibroblast transition by controlling cytoskeletal organization and MRTF-A localization. J Cell Physiol. 2015;230:1829–39. https://doi.org/10.1002/jcp.24895.
98. Turner NA. Inflammatory and fibrotic responses of cardiac fibroblasts to myocardial damage associated molecular patterns (DAMPs). J Mol Cell Cardiol. 2016;94:189–200. http://www.ncbi.nlm.nih.gov/pubmed/26542796.
99. Bhattacharyya S, Midwood KS, Yin H, Varga J. Toll-Like receptor-4 signaling drives persistent fibroblast activation and prevents fibrosis resolution in scleroderma. Adv Wound Care. 2017;6:356–69. https://doi.org/10.1089/wound.2017.0732.
100. Pakshir P, Hinz B. The big five in fibrosis: macrophages, myofibroblasts, matrix, mechanics, and miscommunication. Matrix Biol. 2018;68–69:81–93. https://linkinghub.elsevier.com/retrieve/pii/S0945053X18300349.
101. El-Karef A, Yoshida T, Gabazza EC, Nishioka T, Inada H, Sakakura T, et al. Deficiency of tenascin-C attenuates liver fibrosis in immune-mediated chronic hepatitis in mice. J Pathol. 2007;211:86–94. https://doi.org/10.1002/path.2099.
102. Zhang W, Lavine KJ, Epelman S, Evans SA, Weinheimer CJ, Barger PM, et al. Necrotic myocardial cells release damage-associated molecular patterns that provoke fibroblast activation in vitro and trigger myocardial inflammation and fibrosis in Vivo. J Am Heart Assoc. 2015;4:e001993. http://www.ncbi.nlm.nih.gov/pubmed/26037082.
103. Wang Q, Wang J, Wang J, Hong S, Han F, Chen J, et al. HMGB1 induces lung fibroblast to myofibroblast differentiation through NF-κB-mediated TGF-β1 release. Mol Med Rep. 2017;15:3062–8. http://www.ncbi.nlm.nih.gov/pubmed/28339089.
104. Lee WJ, Song SY, Roh H, Ahn HM, Na Y, Kim J, et al. Profibrogenic effect of high-mobility group box protein-1 in human dermal fibroblasts and its excess in keloid tissues. Sci Rep. 2018;8:8434. http://www.ncbi.nlm.nih.gov/pubmed/29849053.
105. Zhong A, Xu W, Zhao J, Xie P, Jia S, Sun J, et al. S100A8 and S100A9 are induced by decreased hydration in the epidermis and promote fibroblast activation and fibrosis in the dermis. Am J Pathol. 2016;186:109–22. http://www.ncbi.nlm.nih.gov/pubmed/26597884.

106. Artlett CM. The role of the NLRP3 inflammasome in fibrosis. Open Rheumatol J. 2012;6:80–6. http://www.ncbi.nlm.nih.gov/pubmed/22802905.
107. Kawaguchi M, Takahashi M, Hata T, Kashima Y, Usui F, Morimoto H, et al. Inflammasome activation of cardiac fibroblasts is essential for myocardial ischemia/reperfusion injury. Circulation. 2011;123:594–604. http://www.ncbi.nlm.nih.gov/pubmed/21282498.
108. Wang W, Wang X, Chun J, Vilaysane A, Clark S, French G, et al. Inflammasome-independent NLRP3 augments TGF-β signaling in kidney epithelium. J Immunol. 2013;190:1239–49. http://www.ncbi.nlm.nih.gov/pubmed/23264657.
109. Chaudhuri V, Zhou L, Karasek M. Inflammatory cytokines induce the transformation of human dermal microvascular endothelial cells into myofibroblasts: a potential role in skin fibrogenesis. J Cutan Pathol. 2007;34:146–53. http://www.ncbi.nlm.nih.gov/pubmed/17244026.
110. Gasse P, Riteau N, Charron S, Girre S, Fick L, Pétrilli V, et al. Uric acid is a danger signal activating NALP3 inflammasome in lung injury inflammation and fibrosis. Am J Respir Crit Care Med. 2009;179:903–13. https://doi.org/10.1164/rccm.200808-1274OC.
111. Riteau N, Gasse P, Fauconnier L, Gombault A, Couegnat M, Fick L, et al. Extracellular ATP is a danger signal activating P2X7 receptor in lung inflammation and fibrosis. Am J Respir Crit Care Med. 2010;182:774–83. http://www.ncbi.nlm.nih.gov/pubmed/20522787.
112. Fix C, Bingham K, Carver W. Effects of interleukin-18 on cardiac fibroblast function and gene expression. Cytokine. 2011;53:19–28. http://www.ncbi.nlm.nih.gov/pubmed/21050772.
113. Boza P, Ayala P, Vivar R, Humeres C, Cáceres FT, Muñoz C, et al. Expression and function of toll-like receptor 4 and inflammasomes in cardiac fibroblasts and myofibroblasts: IL-1β synthesis, secretion, and degradation. Mol Immunol. 2016;74:96–105. http://www.ncbi.nlm.nih.gov/pubmed/27174187.
114. Mia MM, Boersema M, Bank RA. Interleukin-1β attenuates myofibroblast formation and extracellular matrix production in dermal and lung fibroblasts exposed to transforming growth factor-β1. PLoS One. 2014;9:e91559. http://www.ncbi.nlm.nih.gov/pubmed/24622053.
115. Artlett CM, Thacker JD. Molecular activation of the NLRP3 Inflammasome in fibrosis: common threads linking divergent fibrogenic diseases. Antioxid Redox Signal. 2015;22:1162–75. http://www.ncbi.nlm.nih.gov/pubmed/25329971.
116. Bhattacharyya S, Tamaki Z, Wang W, Hinchcliff M, Hoover P, Getsios S, et al. FibronectinEDA promotes chronic cutaneous fibrosis through Toll-like receptor signaling. Sci Transl Med. 2014;6:232ra50. https://doi.org/10.1126/scitranslmed.3008264.
117. George J, Wang SS, Sevcsik AM, Sanicola M, Cate RL, Koteliansky VE, et al. Transforming growth factor-beta initiates wound repair in rat liver through induction of the EIIIA-fibronectin splice isoform. Am J Pathol. 2000;156:115–24. http://www.ncbi.nlm.nih.gov/pubmed/10623659.
118. Liao Y-F, Gotwals PJ, Koteliansky VE, Sheppard D, Van De Water L. The EIIIA segment of fibronectin is a ligand for integrins alpha 9beta 1 and alpha 4beta 1 providing a novel mechanism for regulating cell adhesion by alternative splicing. J Biol Chem. 2002;277:14467–74. http://www.ncbi.nlm.nih.gov/pubmed/11839764.
119. Kelsh-Lasher RM, Ambesi A, Bertram C, McKeown-Longo PJ. Integrin α4β1 and TLR4 cooperate to induce fibrotic gene expression in response to fibronectin's EDA domain. J Invest Dermatol. 2017;137:2505–12. https://linkinghub.elsevier.com/retrieve/pii/S0022202X17327951.
120. Bhattacharyya S, Varga J. Endogenous ligands of TLR4 promote unresolving tissue fibrosis: implications for systemic sclerosis and its targeted therapy. Immunol Lett. 2018;195:9–17. http://www.ncbi.nlm.nih.gov/pubmed/28964818.
121. Sauler M, Bazan IS, Lee PJ. Cell death in the lung: the apoptosis–necroptosis axis. Annu Rev Physiol. 2019;81:375–402. http://www.ncbi.nlm.nih.gov/pubmed/30485762
122. Piek A, de Boer RA, Silljé HHW. The fibrosis-cell death axis in heart failure. Heart Fail Rev. 2016;21:199–211. http://www.ncbi.nlm.nih.gov/pubmed/26883434
123. Frangogiannis NG. Cardiac fibrosis: cell biological mechanisms, molecular pathways and therapeutic opportunities. Mol Aspects Med. 2019;65:70–99. https://linkinghub.elsevier.com/retrieve/pii/S0098299718300670.

124. Manucha W, Vallés PG. Apoptosis modulated by oxidative stress and inflammation during obstructive nephropathy. Inflamm Allergy Drug Targets. 2012;11:303–12. http://www.ncbi.nlm.nih.gov/pubmed/22533548.
125. Grynberg K, Ma FY, Nikolic-Paterson DJ. The JNK signaling pathway in renal fibrosis. Front Physiol. 2017;8:829. http://www.ncbi.nlm.nih.gov/pubmed/29114233.
126. Dong X, Zhao B, Iacob RE, Zhu J, Koksal AC, Lu C, et al. Force interacts with macromolecular structure in activation of TGF-β. Nature. 2017;542:55–9. http://www.nature.com/articles/nature21035.
127. Huang XZ, Wu JF, Cass D, Erle DJ, Corry D, Young SG, et al. Inactivation of the integrin beta 6 subunit gene reveals a role of epithelial integrins in regulating inflammation in the lung and skin. J Cell Biol. 1996;133:921–8. http://www.ncbi.nlm.nih.gov/pubmed/8666675.
128. Bader BL, Rayburn H, Crowley D, Hynes RO. Extensive vasculogenesis, angiogenesis, and organogenesis precede lethality in mice lacking all alpha v integrins. Cell. 1998;95:507–19. http://www.ncbi.nlm.nih.gov/pubmed/9827803.
129. Munger JS, Huang X, Kawakatsu H, Griffiths MJ, Dalton SL, Wu J, et al. The integrin alpha v beta 6 binds and activates latent TGF beta 1: a mechanism for regulating pulmonary inflammation and fibrosis. Cell. 1999;96:319–28. http://www.ncbi.nlm.nih.gov/pubmed/10025398.
130. Zhu J, Motejlek K, Wang D, Zang K, Schmidt A, Reichardt LF. beta8 integrins are required for vascular morphogenesis in mouse embryos. Development. 2002;129:2891–903. http://www.ncbi.nlm.nih.gov/pubmed/12050137.
131. Annes JP, Munger JS, Rifkin DB. Making sense of latent TGFbeta activation. J Cell Sci. 2003;116:217–24. http://www.ncbi.nlm.nih.gov/pubmed/12482908.
132. Annes JP, Chen Y, Munger JS, Rifkin DB. Integrin alphaVbeta6-mediated activation of latent TGF-beta requires the latent TGF-beta binding protein-1. J Cell Biol. 2004;165:723–34. https://doi.org/10.1083/jcb.200312172.
133. Keski-Oja J, Koli K, von Melchner H. TGF-beta activation by traction? Trends Cell Biol. 2004;14:657–9. http://linkinghub.elsevier.com/retrieve/pii/S096289240400282X.
134. Wipff P-J, Rifkin DB, Meister J-J, Hinz B. Myofibroblast contraction activates latent TGF-beta1 from the extracellular matrix. J Cell Biol. 2007;179:1311–23. https://doi.org/10.1083/jcb.200704042.
135. Yang Z, Mu Z, Dabovic B, Jurukovski V, Yu D, Sung J, et al. Absence of integrin-mediated TGFbeta1 activation in vivo recapitulates the phenotype of TGFbeta1-null mice. J Cell Biol. 2007;176:787–93. https://doi.org/10.1083/jcb.200611044.
136. Xu MY, Porte J, Knox AJ, Weinreb PH, Maher TM, Violette SM, et al. Lysophosphatidic acid induces alphavbeta6 integrin-mediated TGF-beta activation via the LPA2 receptor and the small G protein G alpha(q). Am J Pathol. 2009;174:1264–79. https://linkinghub.elsevier.com/retrieve/pii/S0002944010609856.
137. Nishimura SL. Integrin-mediated transforming growth factor-beta activation, a potential therapeutic target in fibrogenic disorders. Am J Pathol. 2009;175:1362–70. https://linkinghub.elsevier.com/retrieve/pii/S0002944010606475.
138. Tatler AL, John AE, Jolly L, Habgood A, Porte J, Brightling C, et al. Integrin αvβ5-mediated TGF-β activation by airway smooth muscle cells in asthma. J Immunol. 2011;187:6094–107. https://doi.org/10.4049/jimmunol.1003507.
139. Giacomini MM, Travis MA, Kudo M, Sheppard D. Epithelial cells utilize cortical actin/myosin to activate latent TGF-β through integrin α(v)β(6)-dependent physical force. Exp Cell Res. 2012;318:716–22. https://linkinghub.elsevier.com/retrieve/pii/S0014482712000419.
140. Henderson NC, Arnold TD, Katamura Y, Giacomini MM, Rodriguez JD, McCarty JH, et al. Targeting of αv integrin identifies a core molecular pathway that regulates fibrosis in several organs. Nat Med. 2013;19:1617–24. http://www.nature.com/articles/nm.3282.
141. Hinz B. It has to be the alphav: myofibroblast integrins activate latent TGF-β1. Nat Med. 2013;19:1567–8. http://www.nature.com/articles/nm.3421.
142. Travis MA, Sheppard D. TGF-β activation and function in immunity. Annu Rev Immunol. 2014;32:51–82. http://www.ncbi.nlm.nih.gov/pubmed/24313777.

143. Sun Z, Guo SS, Fässler R. Integrin-mediated mechanotransduction. J Cell Biol. 2016;215:45–56. http://www.ncbi.nlm.nih.gov/pubmed/27872252.
144. Lim C-G, Jang J, Kim C. Cellular machinery for sensing mechanical force. BMB Rep. 2018;51:623–9. http://www.ncbi.nlm.nih.gov/pubmed/30293551.
145. Mu D, Cambier S, Fjellbirkeland L, Baron JL, Munger JS, Kawakatsu H, et al. The integrin alpha(v)beta8 mediates epithelial homeostasis through MT1-MMP-dependent activation of TGF-beta1. J Cell Biol. 2002;157:493–507. https://doi.org/10.1083/jcb.200109100.
146. Ge G, Greenspan DS. BMP1 controls TGFbeta1 activation via cleavage of latent TGFbeta-binding protein. J Cell Biol. 2006;175:111–20. https://doi.org/10.1083/jcb.200606058.
147. Jenkins G. The role of proteases in transforming growth factor-β activation. Int J Biochem Cell Biol. 2008;40:1068–78. http://www.ncbi.nlm.nih.gov/pubmed/18243766.
148. Kobayashi T, Kim H, Liu X, Sugiura H, Kohyama T, Fang Q, et al. Matrix metalloproteinase-9 activates TGF-β and stimulates fibroblast contraction of collagen gels. Am J Physiol Lung Cell Mol Physiol. 2014;306:L1006–15. https://doi.org/10.1152/ajplung.00015.2014.
149. Saharinen J, Taipale J, Keski-Oja J. Association of the small latent transforming growth factor-beta with an eight cysteine repeat of its binding protein LTBP-1. EMBO J. 1996;15:245–53. http://www.ncbi.nlm.nih.gov/pubmed/8617200.
150. Dallas SL, Rosser JL, Mundy GR, Bonewald LF. Proteolysis of latent transforming growth factor-beta (TGF-beta)-binding protein-1 by osteoclasts. A cellular mechanism for release of TGF-beta from bone matrix. J Biol Chem. 2002;277:21352–60. https://doi.org/10.1074/jbc.M111663200.
151. Kim CW, Pokutta-Paskaleva A, Kumar S, Timmins LH, Morris AD, Kang D-W, et al. Disturbed flow promotes arterial stiffening through Thrombospondin-1. Circulation. 2017;136:1217–32. https://doi.org/10.1161/CIRCULATIONAHA.116.026361.
152. Hinz B. Myofibroblasts. Exp Eye Res. 2016;142:56–70. http://www.ncbi.nlm.nih.gov/pubmed/26192991.
153. Robertson IB, Rifkin DB. Regulation of the bioavailability of TGF-β and TGF-β-related proteins. Cold Spring Harb Perspect Biol. 2016;8:a021907. https://doi.org/10.1101/cshperspect.a021907.
154. Meng X, Nikolic-Paterson DJ, Lan HY. TGF-β: the master regulator of fibrosis. Nat Rev Nephrol. 2016;12:325–38. http://www.ncbi.nlm.nih.gov/pubmed/27108839.
155. Carthy JM. TGFβ signaling and the control of myofibroblast differentiation: implications for chronic inflammatory disorders. J Cell Physiol. 2018;233:98–106. https://doi.org/10.1002/jcp.25879.
156. Zhang YE. Non-smad signaling pathways of the TGF-β family. Cold Spring Harb Perspect Biol. 2017;9:a022129. http://www.ncbi.nlm.nih.gov/pubmed/27864313.
157. Luo K. Signaling Cross Talk between TGF-β/Smad and Other Signaling Pathways. Cold Spring Harb Perspect Biol. 2017;9:a022137. http://www.ncbi.nlm.nih.gov/pubmed/27836834
158. Ma Z-Y, Zhong Z-G, Qiu M-Y, Zhong Y-H, Zhang W-X. TGF-β1 activates the canonical NF-κB signaling to promote cell survival and proliferation in dystrophic muscle fibroblasts in vitro. Biochem Biophys Res Commun. 2016;471:576–81. http://www.ncbi.nlm.nih.gov/pubmed/26874278.
159. Działo E, Tkacz K, Błyszczuk P. Crosstalk between TGF-β and WNT signalling pathways during cardiac fibrogenesis. Acta Biochim Pol. 2018;65:341–9. http://www.ncbi.nlm.nih.gov/pubmed/30040870.
160. Zhang YE. Mechanistic insight into contextual TGF-β signaling. Curr Opin Cell Biol. 2018;51:1–7. http://www.ncbi.nlm.nih.gov/pubmed/29149681.
161. Bhowmick NA, Ghiassi M, Bakin A, Aakre M, Lundquist CA, Engel ME, et al. Transforming growth factor-beta1 mediates epithelial to mesenchymal transdifferentiation through a RhoA-dependent mechanism. Mol Biol Cell. 2001;12:27–36. https://doi.org/10.1091/mbc.12.1.27.
162. Pellegrin S, Mellor H. Actin stress fibres. J Cell Sci. 2007;120:3491–9. http://www.ncbi.nlm.nih.gov/pubmed/17928305.
163. Gasparics Á, Sebe A. MRTFs- master regulators of EMT. Dev Dyn. 2018;247:396–404. https://doi.org/10.1002/dvdy.24544.

164. Ge J, Burnier L, Adamopoulou M, Kwa MQ, Schaks M, Rottner K, et al. RhoA, Rac1, and Cdc42 differentially regulate αSMA and collagen I expression in mesenchymal stem cells. J Biol Chem. 2018;293:9358–69. https://doi.org/10.1074/jbc.RA117.001113.
165. Korol A, Taiyab A, West-Mays JA. RhoA/ROCK signaling regulates TGFβ-induced epithelial-mesenchymal transition of lens epithelial cells through MRTF-A. Mol Med. 2016;22:713–23. http://www.molmed.org/content/pdfstore/16_041_Korol.pdf.
166. Hinson JS, Medlin MD, Lockman K, Taylor JM, Mack CP. Smooth muscle cell-specific transcription is regulated by nuclear localization of the myocardin-related transcription factors. Am J Physiol Heart Circ Physiol. 2007;292:H1170–80. https://doi.org/10.1152/ajpheart.00864.2006.
167. Varelas X, Sakuma R, Samavarchi-Tehrani P, Peerani R, Rao BM, Dembowy J, et al. TAZ controls Smad nucleocytoplasmic shuttling and regulates human embryonic stem-cell self-renewal. Nat Cell Biol. 2008;10:837–48. http://www.nature.com/articles/ncb1748
168. Narimatsu M, Samavarchi-Tehrani P, Varelas X, Wrana JL. Distinct polarity cues direct Taz/Yap and TGFβ receptor localization to differentially control TGFβ-induced Smad signaling. Dev Cell. 2015;32:652–6. https://linkinghub.elsevier.com/retrieve/pii/S1534580715001379.
169. Grannas K, Arngården L, Lönn P, Mazurkiewicz M, Blokzijl A, Zieba A, et al. Crosstalk between Hippo and TGFβ: subcellular localization of YAP/TAZ/Smad complexes. J Mol Biol. 2015;427:3407–15. https://linkinghub.elsevier.com/retrieve/pii/S0022283615002697,
170. Vallée A, Lecarpentier Y, Guillevin R, Vallée J-N. Interactions between TGF-beta1; canonical WNT/beta -catenin pathway and PPAR gamma; in radiation-induced fibrosis. Oncotarget. 2017;8:90579–604. http://www.ncbi.nlm.nih.gov/pubmed/29163854.
171. Zhai X-X, Tang Z-M, Ding J-C, Lu X-L. Expression of TGF-β1/mTOR signaling pathway in pathological scar fibroblasts. Mol Med Rep. 2017;15:3467–72. http://www.ncbi.nlm.nih.gov/pubmed/28393182.
172. Wodarz A, Nusse R. Mechanisms of Wnt signaling in development. Annu Rev Cell Dev Biol. 1998;14:59–88. https://doi.org/10.1146/annurev.cellbio.14.1.59.
173. Macdonald BT, Semenov MV, He X. SnapShot: Wnt/beta-catenin signaling. Cell. 2007;131:1204. https://linkinghub.elsevier.com/retrieve/pii/S0092867407015395.
174. Huang H, He X. Wnt/beta-catenin signaling: new (and old) players and new insights. Curr Opin Cell Biol. 2008;20:119–25. https://linkinghub.elsevier.com/retrieve/pii/S0955067408000197.
175. Willert K, Nusse R. Wnt Proteins. Cold Spring Harb Perspect Biol. 2012;4:a007864. http://www.ncbi.nlm.nih.gov/pubmed/22952392.
176. Clevers H, Nusse R. Wnt/β-catenin signaling and disease. Cell. 2012;149:1192–205. http://www.ncbi.nlm.nih.gov/pubmed/22682243.
177. Nusse R, Clevers H. Wnt/β-catenin signaling, disease, and emerging therapeutic modalities. Cell. 2017;169:985–99. http://www.ncbi.nlm.nih.gov/pubmed/28575679.
178. Zhou B, Liu Y, Kahn M, Ann DK, Han A, Wang H, et al. Interactions between β-catenin and transforming growth factor-β signaling pathways mediate epithelial-mesenchymal transition and are dependent on the transcriptional co-activator cAMP-response element-binding protein (CREB)-binding protein (CBP). J Biol Chem. 2012;287:7026–38. https://doi.org/10.1074/jbc.M111.276311.
179. Enzo MV, Cattelan P, Rastrelli M, Tosi A, Rossi CR, Hladnik U, et al. Growth rate and myofibroblast differentiation of desmoid fibroblast-like cells are modulated by TGF-β signaling. Histochem Cell Biol. 2019;151:145–60. https://doi.org/10.1007/s00418-018-1718-1.
180. Shafer SL, Towler DA. Transcriptional regulation of SM22alpha by Wnt3a: convergence with TGFbeta(1)/Smad signaling at a novel regulatory element. J Mol Cell Cardiol. 2009;46:621–35. https://linkinghub.elsevier.com/retrieve/pii/S0022282809000182.
181. Chen J-H, Chen WLK, Sider KL, Yip CYY, Simmons CA. β-catenin mediates mechanically regulated, transforming growth factor-β1-induced myofibroblast differentiation of aortic valve interstitial cells. Arterioscler Thromb Vasc Biol. 2011;31:590–7. https://doi.org/10.1161/ATVBAHA.110.220061.

182. Akhmetshina A, Palumbo K, Dees C, Bergmann C, Venalis P, Zerr P, et al. Activation of canonical Wnt signalling is required for TGF-β-mediated fibrosis. Nat Commun. 2012;3:735. http://www.nature.com/articles/ncomms1734.
183. Feng Y, Liang Y, Zhu X, Wang M, Gui Y, Lu Q, et al. The signaling protein Wnt5a promotes TGFβ1-mediated macrophage polarization and kidney fibrosis by inducing the transcriptional regulators Yap/Taz. J Biol Chem. 2018;293:19290–302. http://www.ncbi.nlm.nih.gov/pubmed/30333225.
184. Shinde AV, Kelsh R, Peters JH, Sekiguchi K, Van De Water L, McKeown-Longo PJ. The α4β1 integrin and the EDA domain of fibronectin regulate a profibrotic phenotype in dermal fibroblasts. Matrix Biol. 2015;41:26–35. https://linkinghub.elsevier.com/retrieve/pii/S0945053X14002169.
185. Zhou D, Yang K, Chen L, Zhang W, Xu Z, Zuo J, et al. Promising landscape for regulating macrophage polarization: epigenetic viewpoint. Oncotarget. 2017;8:57693–706. http://www.ncbi.nlm.nih.gov/pubmed/28915705.
186. Dominguez-Andres J, Netea MG. Long-term reprogramming of the innate immune system. J Leukoc Biol. 2019;105:329–38. https://doi.org/10.1002/JLB.MR0318-104R.
187. O'Reilly S. Epigenetics in fibrosis. Mol Aspects Med. 2017;54:89–102. http://www.ncbi.nlm.nih.gov/pubmed/27720780.
188. Dowson C, O'Reilly S. DNA methylation in fibrosis. Eur J Cell Biol. 2016;95:323–30. https://linkinghub.elsevier.com/retrieve/pii/S0171933516300164.
189. Zhang X, Hu M, Lyu X, Li C, Thannickal VJ, Sanders YY. DNA methylation regulated gene expression in organ fibrosis. Biochim Biophys Acta Mol Basis Dis. 1863;2017:2389–97. http://www.ncbi.nlm.nih.gov/pubmed/28501566.
190. Massey V, Cabezas J, Bataller R. Epigenetics in liver fibrosis. Semin Liver Dis. 2017;37:219–30. https://doi.org/10.1055/s-0037-1605371.
191. Watson CJ, Collier P, Tea I, Neary R, Watson JA, Robinson C, et al. Hypoxia-induced epigenetic modifications are associated with cardiac tissue fibrosis and the development of a myofibroblast-like phenotype. Hum Mol Genet. 2014;23:2176–88. https://doi.org/10.1093/hmg/ddt614.
192. Ghosh AK, Bhattacharyya S, Lafyatis R, Farina G, Yu J, Thimmapaya B, et al. p300 is elevated in systemic sclerosis and its expression is positively regulated by TGF-β: epigenetic feed-forward amplification of fibrosis. J Invest Dermatol. 2013;133:1302–10. https://linkinghub.elsevier.com/retrieve/pii/S0022202X15362394.
193. Dou C, Liu Z, Tu K, Zhang H, Chen C, Yaqoob U, et al. P300 Acetyltransferase mediates stiffness-induced activation of hepatic stellate cells into tumor-promoting myofibroblasts. Gastroenterology. 2018;154:2209–2221.e14. http://www.ncbi.nlm.nih.gov/pubmed/29454793.
194. Hemmatazad H, Rodrigues HM, Maurer B, Brentano F, Pileckyte M, Distler JHW, et al. Histone deacetylase 7, a potential target for the antifibrotic treatment of systemic sclerosis. Arthritis Rheum. 2009;60:1519–29. https://doi.org/10.1002/art.24494.
195. Zhang X, Liu H, Hock T, Thannickal VJ, Sanders YY. Histone deacetylase inhibition downregulates collagen 3A1 in fibrotic lung fibroblasts. Int J Mol Sci. 2013;14:19605–17. http://www.mdpi.com/1422-0067/14/10/19605.
196. Li X, Wu X-Q, Xu T, Li X-F, Yang Y, Li W-X, et al. Role of histone deacetylases(HDACs) in progression and reversal of liver fibrosis. Toxicol Appl Pharmacol. 2016;306:58–68. http://www.ncbi.nlm.nih.gov/pubmed/27396813.
197. Page A, Paoli PP, Hill SJ, Howarth R, Wu R, Kweon S-M, et al. Alcohol directly stimulates epigenetic modifications in hepatic stellate cells. J Hepatol. 2015;62:388–97. https://linkinghub.elsevier.com/retrieve/pii/S0168827814007351.
198. Sun G, Reddy MA, Yuan H, Lanting L, Kato M, Natarajan R. Epigenetic histone methylation modulates fibrotic gene expression. J Am Soc Nephrol. 2010;21:2069–80. https://doi.org/10.1681/ASN.2010060633.
199. Mann J, Oakley F, Akiboye F, Elsharkawy A, Thorne AW, Mann DA. Regulation of myofibroblast transdifferentiation by DNA methylation and MeCP2: implications for wound healing and fibrogenesis. Cell Death Differ. 2007;14:275–85. http://www.nature.com/doifinder/10.1038/sj.cdd.4401979.

200. Perugorria MJ, Wilson CL, Zeybel M, Walsh M, Amin S, Robinson S, et al. Histone methyltransferase ASH1 orchestrates fibrogenic gene transcription during myofibroblast transdifferentiation. Hepatology. 2012;56:1129–39. https://doi.org/10.1002/hep.25754.
201. Yamane K, Toumazou C, Tsukada Y, Erdjument-Bromage H, Tempst P, Wong J, et al. JHDM2A, a JmjC-containing H3K9 demethylase, facilitates transcription activation by androgen receptor. Cell. 2006;125:483–95. https://linkinghub.elsevier.com/retrieve/pii/S0092867406003850.
202. Jiang Y, Wang S, Zhao Y, Lin C, Zhong F, Jin L, et al. Histone H3K9 demethylase JMJD1A modulates hepatic stellate cells activation and liver fibrosis by epigenetically regulating peroxisome proliferator-activated receptor γ. FASEB J. 2015;29:1830–41. http://www.ncbi.nlm.nih.gov/pubmed/25609425
203. Dong F, Jiang S, Li J, Wang Y, Zhu L, Huang Y, et al. The histone demethylase KDM4D promotes hepatic fibrogenesis by modulating Toll-like receptor 4 signaling pathway. EBioMedicine. 2019;39:472–83. https://linkinghub.elsevier.com/retrieve/pii/S2352396418305590.
204. Jiang X, Zhang F. Long noncoding RNA: a new contributor and potential therapeutic target in fibrosis. Epigenomics. 2017;9:1233–41. https://doi.org/10.2217/epi-2017-0020.
205. Tao H, Cao W, Yang J-J, Shi K-H, Zhou X, Liu L-P, et al. Long noncoding RNA H19 controls DUSP5/ERK1/2 axis in cardiac fibroblast proliferation and fibrosis. Cardiovasc Pathol. 2016;25:381–9. https://linkinghub.elsevier.com/retrieve/pii/S1054880716300333.
206. He Y, Wu Y-T, Huang C, Meng X-M, Ma T-T, Wu B-M, et al. Inhibitory effects of long noncoding RNA MEG3 on hepatic stellate cells activation and liver fibrogenesis. Biochim Biophys Acta. 1842;2014:2204–15. https://linkinghub.elsevier.com/retrieve/pii/S0925443914002683.
207. Duong TE, Hagood JS. Epigenetic regulation of myofibroblast phenotypes in fibrosis. Curr Pathobiol Rep. 2018;6:79–96. http://www.ncbi.nlm.nih.gov/pubmed/30271681.
208. Bergmann C, Distler JH. Epigenetic factors as drivers of fibrosis in systemic sclerosis. Epigenomics. 2017;9:463–77. https://doi.org/10.2217/epi-2016-0150.
209. Thum T, Gross C, Fiedler J, Fischer T, Kissler S, Bussen M, et al. MicroRNA-21 contributes to myocardial disease by stimulating MAP kinase signalling in fibroblasts. Nature. 2008;456:980–4. https://doi.org/10.1038/nature07511.
210. Kang H. Role of microRNAs in TGF-β signaling pathway-mediated pulmonary fibrosis. Int J Mol Sci. 2017;18:2527. http://www.mdpi.com/1422-0067/18/12/2527.
211. Liang C, Li X, Zhang L, Cui D, Quan X, Yang W. The anti-fibrotic effects of microRNA-153 by targeting TGFBR-2 in pulmonary fibrosis. Exp Mol Pathol. 2015;99:279–85. https://linkinghub.elsevier.com/retrieve/pii/S0014480015001598.
212. Felisbino MB, McKinsey TA. Epigenetics in cardiac fibrosis: emphasis on inflammation and fibroblast activation. JACC Basic Transl Sci. 2018;3:704–15. https://linkinghub.elsevier.com/retrieve/pii/S2452302X18301268
213. Hu B, Gharaee-Kermani M, Wu Z, Phan SH. Epigenetic regulation of myofibroblast differentiation by DNA methylation. Am J Pathol. 2010;177:21–8. http://www.ncbi.nlm.nih.gov/pubmed/20489138.
214. He Y, Ling S, Sun Y, Sheng Z, Chen Z, Pan X, et al. DNA methylation regulates α-smooth muscle actin expression during cardiac fibroblast differentiation. J Cell Physiol. 2019;234:7174–85. http://www.ncbi.nlm.nih.gov/pubmed/30362530.
215. Rai R, Sun T, Ramirez V, Lux E, Eren M, Vaughan DE, et al. Acetyltransferase p300 inhibitor reverses hypertension-induced cardiac fibrosis. J Cell Mol Med. 2019;23(4):3026–31. http://www.ncbi.nlm.nih.gov/pubmed/30710427.
216. Glenisson W, Castronovo V, Waltregny D. Histone deacetylase 4 is required for TGFbeta1-induced myofibroblastic differentiation. Biochim Biophys Acta. 1773;2007:1572–82. https://linkinghub.elsevier.com/retrieve/pii/S0167488907001449.
217. Kang DH, Yin GN, Choi M-J, Song K-M, Ghatak K, Minh NN, et al. Silencing histone deacetylase 7 alleviates transforming growth factor-β1-induced profibrotic responses in fibroblasts derived from Peyronie's plaque. World J Mens Health. 2018;36:139. http://www.ncbi.nlm.nih.gov/pubmed/29706035.

218. Shuttleworth VG, Gaughan L, Nawafa L, Mooney CA, Cobb SL, Sheerin NS, et al. The methyltransferase SET9 regulates TGFB1 activation of renal fibroblasts via interaction with SMAD3. J Cell Sci. 2018;131:jcs207761. http://www.ncbi.nlm.nih.gov/pubmed/29222115.
219. Jun J-I, Lau LF. Resolution of organ fibrosis. J Clin Invest. 2018;128:97–107. https://www.jci.org/articles/view/93563.
220. Cimmino C, Rossano L, Netti PA, Ventre M. Spatio-temporal control of cell adhesion: toward programmable platforms to manipulate cell functions and fate. Front Bioeng Biotechnol. 2018;6:190. https://doi.org/10.3389/fbioe.2018.00190/full.
221. Ventre M, Netti PA. Engineering cell instructive materials to control cell fate and functions through material cues and surface patterning. ACS Appl Mater Interfaces. 2016;8:14896–908. https://doi.org/10.1021/acsami.5b08658.

Part III

DAMPs and SAMPs in Traumatic Disorders, Atherosclerosis, and Cerebro-Cardiovascular Diseases

DAMPs and SAMPs as Molecular Biomarkers, Therapeutic Targets, and Therapeutics

7

7.1 Introduction

Biological markers have been initially defined by Hulka et al. [1] as "cellular, biochemical, or molecular alterations that are measurable in biological media such as human tissues, cells, or fluids." Subsequently, a biomarker was explained as "A characteristic that is objectively measured and evaluated as an indicator of normal biological processes, pathogenic processes, or pharmacologic responses to a therapeutic intervention" [2]. Following, as discussed by Naylor [3], the definition has been broadened to include biological characteristics that can be objectively measured and evaluated as an indicator of normal biological and pathogenic processes or pharmacological responses to a therapeutic intervention. In practice, biomarkers include tools and technologies that help make a proper diagnosis, understanding the prediction, progression, regression, or outcome of treatment of disease. In other words, biomarkers should assist a physician in a diagnosis based on a combination of the patients' medical history, physical examination, and laboratory data.

Moreover, a biomarker may be a phenotypic measure (e.g., demographics), a protein, a genetic characterization (e.g., genotype, single nucleotide polymorphisms), or any other measure related to an individual, or it may be a constellation of such measures (i.e., a biomarker signature). Nonetheless, independent from such distinctions, the application of these various biomarkers in the diagnosis and management of human disorders such as CVD, infections, immunological and genetic disorders, and cancer is well known. Together, these definitions and distinct features can qualify DAMPs and SAMPs to be included in the category of biomarkers.

However, the clinical application of DAMPs and SAMPs is not restricted to their use as biomarkers. Thus, growing evidence from targeted experimental and first clinical studies have revealed that these molecules play a critical role in the pathogenesis of many diseases in that, for example, excessive or prolonged production of DAMPs and/or impaired generation of SAMPs may promote chronic inflammation and hyperinflammation. Plausibly, this pathogenetic involvement qualifies them as relevant drug targets, as well. Indeed, experimental data are accumulating, showing

W. G. Land, *Damage-Associated Molecular Patterns in Human Diseases*,
https://doi.org/10.1007/978-3-030-53868-2_7

that inflammatory disorders can be successfully treated with the use of DAMP inhibitors. On the other hand, DAMPs may also be therapeutically administered in case of a desired enhancement of adaptive immune responses.

Collectively, both the constitutive DAMPs and inducible DAMPs/SAMPs appear to be highly suitable to serve as future ideal diagnostic and prognostic biomarkers as well as therapeutic targets or therapeutics in daily clinical practice. Hence, by focusing on some practical aspects, a few remarks on this emerging field in modern medicine are worthwhile to write down in this chapter—so to speak as an introduction to future use of these molecules clinically.

7.2 DAMPs and SAMPs in Diagnosis and Prognosis

7.2.1 Introductory Remarks

Though not generally accepted in current routine medicine, the use of DAMPs and SAMPs as biological markers should be seriously considered as a valuable enrichment of modern diagnostic modalities. This all the more as biomarkers are meanwhile considered part of modern medicine [4]. In fact, traditional empirical medicine has shifted to modern medicine that includes the application of criteria of personalized medicine or precision medicine (both terms often used synonymously) that strives for improvements in tailoring and timing of diagnostic, prognostic, preventive, and therapeutic measures. Personalized precision medicine is endeavoring to subdivide patients into different categories based on their "molecular make-up," that is, using biomarkers. In other words, personalized precision medicine most frequently refers to a "medical model" using biomarker profiling for tailoring the right therapeutic strategy for the right patient, the correct dose, and at the right time and/or to determine the predisposition to disease and/or to deliver timely and stratified prevention [5, 6].

7.2.2 DAMPs and SAMPs as Diagnostics

A diagnostic biomarker should allow the early detection of a disease in a noninvasive way. As a tool for improved diagnostics, molecular signatures can be used to increase diagnostic accuracy in the general population, at-risk populations, or those with suspicious clinical findings that require confirmation [7]. As a simple and routine procedure, diagnostic biomarkers can be measured in body fluids such as plasma, cerebrospinal liquor, exudates, amniotic fluid, synovial fluid, and serous fluids. Also, molecular imaging probes that serve in detecting diagnostic biomarkers in human diseases have rapidly gained considerable attention in medicine, especially in the era of personalized medicine. The procedure provides the visualization, characterization, and measurement of biological processes at the cellular, subcellular, or even molecular level (reviewed in [8, 9]).

Today, a reasonable number of imaging modalities for clinical settings has been developed, whereby the main imaging modalities can be generally arranged into two categories (for a comprehensive review, see the articles of Chen/Chen and Massoud et al. [8, 10]). First, some of the imaging modalities, such as ultrasound and computed tomography (CT), can provide anatomical information which is depended on anatomical alterations associated with the disorder. Second, some other imaging modalities can provide functional information about the disease. These modalities include positron emission tomography (PET), single-photon emission computed tomography (SPECT), optical bioluminescence/fluorescence imaging, molecular magnetic resonance imaging (mMRI), and magnetic resonance spectroscopy (MRS). PET and SPECT, in addition, offer the possibility of quantification of disease-associated biochemical processes. As further outlined [8, 10], among the various imaging modalities, some of them, such as PET and SPECT, require the injection of molecular probes in the tested subject in order to acquire the imaging signal, while the others, such as optical imaging and mMRI, can follow the disorder either through the exogenous molecular probes or through the endogenous molecules. Because of the pivotal role of imaging probes in the realization of the power of molecular imaging, the design and development of the biologically active probe are becoming one of the major subjects of molecular imaging [10–13].

The core of all these diagnostic procedures is the molecular imaging probe that is an agent used to visualize, characterize, and quantify biological processes in living systems (reviewed in [8, 10]). A molecular imaging probe typically comprises (1) a signal agent for the corresponding imaging modality, (2) a targeting moiety that senses the intended molecular/cellular target, and (3) a linker connecting the imaging signal agent with the targeting moiety. The signal agent usually produces a signal for imaging purposes. The applicability of imaging probe to imaging modality can be determined in terms of the physical property of the label moiety (reviewed in [8, 10]).

On the other hand, levels of DAMPs and SAMPs can be measured in body fluids (e.g., HMGB1 [14], S100B proteins [15], SPMs [16]). Accordingly, from the perspective of this book, DAMPs and SAMPs appear to be of high value in their function as diagnostic markers, since they contribute clinically relevant information in many medical disciplines beyond what has been available as stress-/injury-induced biomarkers to clinicians in the past. In particular, acutely high or chronically persistent plasma levels of DAMPs associated with insufficient levels of SAMPs will serve as sensitive disease biomarkers and may guide clinicians and practitioners in their daily decision-making. Moreover, determining the levels and distribution of DAMPs in target tissues and in the circulation might represent novel biomarkers for quantitating and monitoring fibrotic diseases, in particular, for identifying patient subpopulations likely to benefit from interventions targeting the innate immune branch of fibrogenesis. Plausibly, such a procedure will allow designing small molecules and antibodies to selectively interrupt and disrupt fibrotic responses without interfering with antimicrobial immunity.

7.2.3 DAMPs and SAMPs as Prognostic and Predictive Biomarkers

The terms "prognostic" and "predictive" have been used in numerous publications to describe relationships between biomarkers and clinical outcomes; however, these terms are not always appropriately defined and often used interchangeably. Here, and throughout the book, the two terms are used according to the definitions published by Ruberg and Chen [17]. Accordingly, a prognostic biomarker is a clinical or biological/molecular characteristic that provides information on the likely patient health outcome (e.g., course of a disease/ disease recurrence), irrespective of the treatment, that is, in the absence of treatment. Thus, a prognostic biomarker can be thought of as a measure of the natural history of the disease. For example, as explained by the authors [17], high blood glucose is a prognostic biomarker for a variety of negative outcomes including CVD, retinopathy, and nephropathy, and the presence of certain mutations in the *breast cancer gene 1 and 2* gene conveys an increased risk of breast and ovarian cancers.

On the other hand, a predictive biomarker indicates the likely benefit to the patient from the treatment, compared to their condition at baseline. Accordingly, as further outlined by Ruberg and Chen [17], predictive markers are used to identify and classify patients to predict an outcome of interest in response to a particular treatment, meaning that they are harnessed to predict the differential benefit or risk of a particular therapy.

However, as argued by Sechidis et al. [18], in reality, biomarkers will almost always have some degree of prognostic value, and some degree of predictive value, but will also likely be dominated by one or the other.

From the perspective of this book, DAMPs and SAMPs may be both prognostic and predictive. For example, in their function as prognostic biomarkers, extremely high levels of DAMPs in polytrauma patients measured immediately after the accident may announce the development of a threatening MODS or even MOF; rapid reduction of these blood levels during subsequent appropriate treatment may predict a positive treatment effect leading to a beneficial outcome. On the other hand, too long periods of SAMPs in high concentrations may indicate a dangerous immunosuppressive phase following trauma (see Sect. 8.3.4). Hence, their use in therapeutic monitoring is taking several forms; besides predicting treatment responses, they may be harnessed to monitor for side effects and applied as surrogate endpoints in clinical trials.

7.2.4 Résumé

This short excerpt is just a brief introductory description of one part of the book title. The topic of DAMPs as biomarkers in diagnosis and prognosis of diseases has meanwhile raised considerable interest as documented by a growing number of publications (e.g., [19–22]). In the future, it may turn out that the measurement of DAMPs alone does not fulfill the expectations of physicians to obtain the diagnostic and prognostic information they requested and needed. Probably more exact information will be provided by targeted exploration, definition, and interpretation of distinct disease-specific "DAMPs pattern" and "SAMPs pattern" and/or even by a distinct DAMPs:SAMPs ratio. Indeed, the measurement and interpretation of "DAMPs and SAMPs patterns" and a "DAMPs:SAMPs ratio" may ultimately become a standard routine procedure for physicians in their daily diagnostic, prognostic, and predictive decision-making processes.

Certainly, future work is needed to establish more robust assays to evaluate the functional bioactivity of DAMPs and SAMPs and their antagonists. For example, forthcoming clinical studies would benefit from a development of antibody-based assays to quantify DAMPs and SAMPs, presently assessed by enzyme-linked immunosorbent assay (ELISA), reverse transcription-polymerase chain reaction (RT-PCR), immunohistochemical analysis, and mass spectrometry methods. Nevertheless, the field is rapidly moving. For example, an optimized liquid chromatography-mass spectrometry (LC-MS) method for the detection of SPMs in biological samples was recently published [16].

Finally, and according to the title of Vol. 2 of this book, the topic will be intensely resumed at the end of Chaps. 8–11 when dealing with DAMPs and SAMPs as biomarkers in human diseases.

7.3 DAMPs and SAMPs in Therapy: A Draft of Possible Guidelines

7.3.1 Introductory Remarks

The fact that pathological production of DAMPs and/or SAMPs in the course of the disease may reflect their dysregulated increased or decreased emission upon infectious/sterile stress/injury implies that they can be used as therapeutic targets or therapeutics. Nevertheless, the routine therapeutic use of DAMPs and SAMPs in patients is a new challenge for the medical profession and, thus, requires a careful discussion of regulations, caveats, and adaptations to the novel therapeutic paradigm in inflammation. Some thoughts on this emerging hot topic in modern medicine have already been published [23] and are put down on paper in the following again.

7.3.2 Antiinflammation Versus Proresolution: What Is the Difference?

As reviewed by Fullerton and Gilroy [24], the concept that resolution processes do not only cause the termination of inflammation but also assist the shift from innate to adaptive immune responses affords additional opportunity to target diseases that involve inflammation or chronic nonresolving inflammation (compare Sect. 5.3). It has therefore been especially necessary to dissociate the meaning of antiinflammation from that of proresolution, although the two concepts may not necessarily be mutually exclusive. In fact, targeting resolution should involve modifying the course of an already established DAMP-driven inflammatory disease in a clinically relevant manner, by harnessing endogenous "off switches" that cause inflammation to resolve. In this context, one has to realize that many effective anti-inflammatory treatment regimens are on the market (including non-steroidal antiinflammatory drugs (NSAIDs), anti-cytokine therapies, and steroids), which neither do interfere with the acting DAMPs nor do switch off the underlying disease processes intrinsically. Therefore, as a new paradigm, diseases that are driven by hyper-inflammation or continuing inflammation (in case of infectious inflammation after successful antibiotic/antiviral elimination of the pathogen) should be considered to treat by assessing three options: (1) by inhibiting the DAMPs as therapeutic targets that have been identified to provoke inflammation and/or (2) by applying SAMPs as therapeutics in terms of activating proresolution pathways that might be pathologically silenced and/or (3) by agonizing functional proresolution pathways (as similarly discussed in [24]).

7.3.3 Controlled Inflammatory Response Upon Injury: A Reference Point for Identification of a "Homeostatic DAMPs: SAMPs Ratio" and a "Homeostatic Window" of DAMPs and SAMPs Concentrations

7.3.3.1 General Remarks

The new knowledge about a controlled, self-limited, protective inflammatory response upon injury refers to a DAMP-promoted proinflammatory crescendo → decrescendo that proceeds—slightly shifted but nearly in parallel—to a SAMP-promoted proresolving reversed crescendo → decrescendo (compare Fig. 5.1). So plausible and reasonable this definition may be in light of recent research work in inflammation, so difficult it will be to implement this new knowledge into safe clinical practice. Some personal thoughts about this challenge are portrayed here.

7.3.3.2 The "Homeostatic DAMPs:SAMPs Ratio"

When considering DAMPs and SAMPs as therapeutic targets or their use as therapeutics, and for safety reasons, one may design and apply the ratio of DAMPs and SAMPs as a reference point operating in the course of an infectious/sterile injury-induced controlled inflammatory response resulting in *restitutio ad integrum*. Such a "homeostatic DAMPs:SAMPs ratio" may also be called a "homeostatic DAMPs:SAMPs signature." According to such a model, injury-induced DAMPs are dominating during the initial proinflammatory phase reflecting a DAMPs:SAMPs ratio greater than 1 (>1); via an intermediate ratio of ±1, the DAMPs:SAMPs ratio then inverses during the resolving phase to less than 1 (<1), and the *restitutio ad integrum* is finally marked by zero (Fig. 7.1). This endeavor is even complicated by the fact that, usually, several key DAMPs and SAMPs are acting in a given

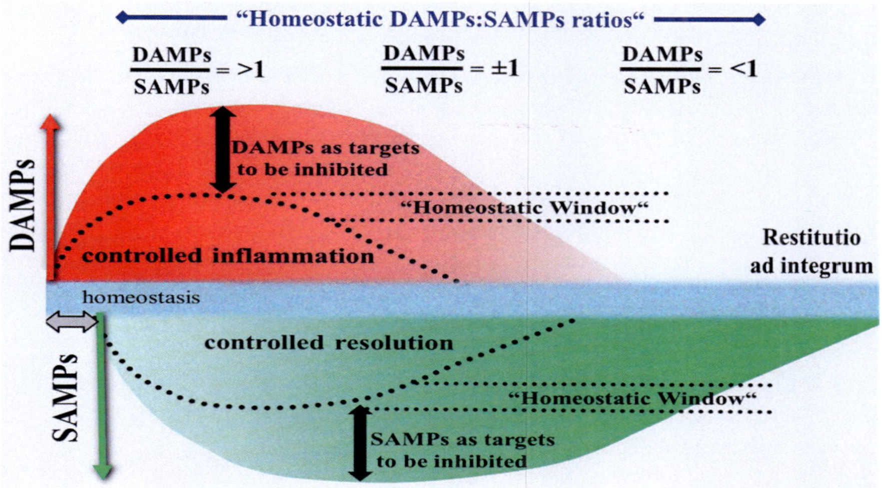

Fig. 7.1 Schematic diagram of the design of a narrative model illustrating a theoretical framework for a safe therapeutic strategy to inhibit excessive concentrations of DAMPs and SAMPs in hyperinflammation (e.g., systemic inflammatory response syndrome [SIRS]), followed by hyperresolution (e.g., compensatory antiinflammatory response syndrome [CARS]). The core of such as model is the a priori elaboration of an approximately "homeostatic DAMPs:SAMPs ratio" by choosing the model of an injury-induced controlled inflammatory response (compare Fig. 5.1) as a reference point for the identification of a such a ratio. Based on (1) such an elaborated "homeostatic DAMPs:SAMPs ratio" and (2) targeted clinical monitoring of adverse events, a "homeostatic window" of DAMPs and SAMPs concentrations is recommended to be defined. The window of DAMPs levels should not be exceeded because of increased risk of hyperinflammation-associated multiple organ failure; the window of SAMPs levels should not be exceeded because of increased risk of immunosuppression-associated life-threatening infections (also compare Fig. 8.3). (Source: This figure is a slightly modified figure published in Land WG. Use of DAMPs and SAMPs as therapeutic targets or therapeutics: a note of caution. Mol Diagn Ther 2020; http://www.ncbi.nlm.nih.gov/pubmed/32248387 [23])

inflammatory response (a so-called homeostatic DAMPs:SAMPs pattern ratio), the determination of their ratios given additional information.

7.3.3.3 The "Homeostatic Window" of DAMPs and SAMPs Concentrations

Importantly, before any considerations to choose DAMPs or SAMPs as therapeutic targets to be inhibited, their homeostatic concentrations (e.g., in body fluids) that are required to establish a *restitutio ad integrum* following injury have to be a priori identified aimed at defining a homeostatic DAMPs:SAMPs ratio in a given situation. More precisely, and for safety reasons, a "homeostatic window" for DAMPs and SAMPs concentrations must be worked out in orientating clinical trials (Fig. 7.1). The homeostatic window for DAMPs should not be exceeded because of increased risk of hyperinflammation and organ dysfunction but also not be undercut (deceeded) because of increased risk of compromised defensive repairing, that is, healing processes.

On the other hand, the homeostatic window for SAMPs should not be exceeded because of increased risk of hyperresolution and immunosuppression and not be deceeded because of increased risk of hyperinflammation and organ dysfunction. Plausibly, the final definition of such homeostatic windows in adherence to the homeostatic DAMPs:SAMPs ratio is a prerequisite—though not an easy one to explore—for any therapeutic intervention modality to be chosen. If an effective drug has been selected, for example, a blocking monoclonal antibody, the next step would be to define a therapeutic window for the drug's dosing that requires careful pharmacokinetic, pharmacodynamics, and pharmacogenomics studies.

7.3.3.4 Plasma Concentration of HMGB1, S100 Proteins, Circulating DNA, and Specialized Proresolving Mediators in Healthy Individuals (at a First Glance)

Plausibly, as a first reference point of defining a homeostatic window for DAMPs and SAMPs, their concentrations should be known as measured in healthy persons (i.e., baseline values)—clearly, a still white spot on the map. Nevertheless, first information is available about concentrations of the prominent DAMPs HMGB1, S100 proteins, and circulating DNA (i.e., nDNA and mtDNA) as found in healthy persons. Here, just for a first orientation, and not discussed in-depth, a few examples are briefly touched. For example, healthy individuals reportedly express plasma HMGB1 levels with a mean of 1.65 ± 0.04 ng/mL as assessed by standard ELISA methods, and the isoform of this constitutive HMGB1 pool is the fully reduced and non-acetylated molecule. For assessment of posttranslationally modified (hyper-acetylated) HMGB1, liquid chromatography-mass spectrometry is currently the only technology available [25, 26] (also compare comments to this issue in [27]; for additional information about the redox state of HMGB1, see Vol. 1 [28], Part IV, Sect. 12.2.2.5, p. 224, and Fig. 12.2, p. 225; for translationally modified secreted HMGB1, see Part IV, Sect. 14.3.3, p. 324, and Fig. 14.4, p. 326).

As for S100 proteins, the median plasma concentration of S100B proteins in healthy volunteers was estimated to be 0.052 μg/L [29]. In other studies, the median serum levels of S100A4 were found to be 11.8 (0–41.5) pg/mL, which was significantly lower than that in patients with acute myocardial infarction, found to be 89.6 (4.3–214.6) pg/mL. The cutoff value was set at 41.5 pg/mL (75th percentile of the S100A4 distribution in the controls) [30].

As for circulating DNA measured in healthy individuals, a median plasma concentration of nDNA and mtDNA of 1.64 × 103 and 8.32 × 107 copies/mL (measured by Q-PCR analysis technology), respectively, was found, corresponding to 5.43 and 1.36 ng/mL of plasma [31]. In other clinical studies in context with investigations on patients with acute cardiac diseases, healthy individuals were found to have plasma nDNA concentrations (measured by quantitative PCR) by 0.1683 ± 0.0254 ng/μL and mtDNA by 0.1517 ± 0.0924 ng/μL [32].

Plasma concentrations of SAMPs, here SPM profiles, have also been measured using liquid chromatography-tandem mass spectrometry (LC-MS) technology

[33, 34]. Of note, in a recently published evaluation of SPM profiles using an optimized LC-MS method for the detection of SPMs in biological samples, Kutzner et al. [16] concluded: "SPMs were generally not detectable/quantifiable in plasma and serum of healthy individuals, while good recovery rates were found in spiked samples. These results strongly support findings that circulating levels of SPMs are very low, i.e., <0.1 nM in healthy subjects. In samples from patients with end-stage renal disease (and peritonitis) or septic shock SPMs and precursors were detectable; however, not directly correlated with the health status and clinical outcome."

7.3.3.5 Concluding Remarks

It is not difficult to imagine that the workup of identifying and defining a context-dependent "homeostatic DAMPs:SAMPs ratio" and a homeostatic window of DAMPs and SAMPs concentrations to allow safe treatment options is a cumbersome task. On the other hand, this situation is not new and has been previously encountered when a new kind of treatment of targeting endogenous molecules was considered.

Future clinical studies will have to show whether such expensive and lavish investigations are worthwhile and make sense at all.

7.3.4 Caveats for Therapeutic Targeting of DAMPs and SAMPs in Hyperinflammation and Hyperresolution

Blockade/inhibition of DAMPs in hyperinflammatory processes (e.g., SIRS) should only be considered if their concentration exceeds the known "homeostatic window" in order not to jeopardize the proinflammatory protective defensive power of DAMPs. The same caveats have to be applied when considering blockade/inhibition of SAMPs in potential hyperresolving processes. Here, it is crucial not to interfere with the resolving processes required for optimal homeostatic healing (Fig. 7.1).

Probably, the main challenge of such a novel therapeutic maneuver in hyperinflammation lies in the fact of choosing an optimal time period suitable to block the action of DAMPs, on the one hand, and subsequently to inhibit the action of SAMPs, on the other side. This procedure must be well dosed and finely tuned. Otherwise, for example, in case of a too early blockade of DAMPs, potential pathogens may grow and spread out. On the other hand, too early inhibition of SAMPs may interfere with the beneficial repairing processes.

7.3.5 DAMPs as Therapeutic Targets and SAMPs as Therapeutics in Chronic Inflammation: The DAMPs: SAMPs Ratio as a Possible Guideline

As outlined in Sect. 5.5, chronic inflammation can be seen as a state of nonresolving inflammation.

Accordingly, two therapeutic options may be taken into account: inhibition of DAMPs as therapeutic targets or administration of SAMPs as therapeutics. Such a maneuver implies again that the ratio of DAMPs:SAMPs must be carefully measured at frequent intervals to allow proper tailor-made therapeutic decisions to be made. Maybe, at the end of the day (and when the pathogen in question is successfully controlled in case of infection), a context-dependent combination of all three concepts in moderate dosing might be the optimal therapeutic solution in chronic inflammation: (1) blocking the action of DAMPs, (2) applying/substituting SAMPs, and (3) administering antiinflammatory agents.

7.3.6 Résumé

Together, harnessing DAMPs and SAMPs as therapeutic targets and therapeutics are attractive novel therapeutic options, which will perhaps find their way into routine treatment modalities for many human diseases. Nevertheless, one has again to realize that the intrinsic nature of DAMPs and SAMPs is to maintain and restore homeostasis upon cell stress and tissue injury. A too drastic therapeutic manipulation of these molecules can result in dyshomeostasis, that is, pathologies and disorders. Thus, physicians and clinicians are confronted with a learning phase of how to handle any such therapeutic interventions. Besides others, strict monitoring of the DAMPs/SAMPs pattern within defined homeostatic windows during the whole course of the disease appears to be recommendable. Some more aspects are mentioned in the following.

7.4 DAMPs and SAMPs in Therapy: The Various Options in Practice

7.4.1 Introductory Remarks

Besides the various aspects of therapeutic caveats in harnessing DAMPs and SAMPs as therapeutic targets and therapeutics in diseases, they should be druggable molecules to allow therapeutic maneuvers with the use of certain effective agents. This other problem, arising at the horizon when considering such treatment options, is briefly addressed in the following.

7.4.2 DAMPs and SAMPs as Therapeutic Targets

For choosing DAMPs as therapeutics targets, DAMPs should be druggable molecules. Druggability is the property of a druggable molecule, that is, a biological target such as proteins and NA, by virtue of which they elicit a favorable clinical response when they contact a drug or a drug-like compound. Ideal drug targets should possess specific properties, including (1) binding with high affinity to a drug that must alter the function of the target with a therapeutic benefit to the patient, (2) differential expression across the body for specific targeting, and (3) the quality of a biomarker to monitor its efficacy and (4) freedom to operate, that is, lack of competitive binding [35–38]. DAMPs appear to fulfill these criteria.

The idea of choosing DAMPs, for example, HMGB1as therapeutic targets to inhibit innate immune responses with the use of monoclonal antibodies (mAbs) or biologicals, has already been proposed by Land in 2012 [39]. Today, several strategies are being discussed and applied to prevent DAMPs release or to inhibit their activities. Such therapeutic maneuvers are, for example, worth to consider in hyperinflammation (e.g., SIRS) and certain chronic inflammatory/autoimmune diseases. Current pharmacological strategies include the use of mAbs, peptides, decoy receptors, and small molecules but also absorption/adsorption procedures [40]. For example, plasma adsorption therapy was recently reported to adsorb HMGB1 efficiently [31]. In addition, as also discussed by Venereau et al. [41] and VanPatten and Al-Abed [42], in the future, the development of specific HMGB1 inhibitors such as specific small molecules may potentiate and fine-tune the pharmacological control of inflammation.

Indications to choose SAMPs as therapeutic targets may refer to situations of unwanted hyperresolution and/or immunosuppression, such as observed in CARS. Again, for choosing SAMPs as therapeutics targets in such cases, they should be druggable molecules.

7.4.3 SAMPs as Therapeutics in Chronic Inflammatory Processes

The concept of impaired resolution leading to chronic inflammatory disorders, autoimmune diseases like rheumatoid arthritis, and Crohn's disease, as well as contributing to allergic diseases such as asthma, has paved the way to consider SAMPs as therapeutics in activating inflammation-resolving processes. In principle, potential therapeutics include adenosine, AnxA1, and SPMs but also SPM derivatives, other synthetic small molecule agonists of SPM receptors, inhibitors of SPM-degrading enzymes (e.g., soluble epoxide hydrolase inhibitors), and modifiers of the SPM synthesis pathways. With the indications mentioned, SPMs have already proven potent proresolving actions in a range of disease models. Given their potency, many drug development opportunities are possible (for SPMs, see Sect. 5.3.3.2). As outlined by Serhan [43], aspirin and statins have a positive impact on these resolution pathways, producing epimeric forms of specific SPMs, whereas other drugs can disrupt timely resolution. As further outlined by this investigator [43], evidence from recent human and preclinical animal studies indicates that SPMs are physiologic mediators and pharmacologic agonists that stimulate resolution of inflammation and infection. This observation is reason enough to use them clinically as inhibitors and antagonists alone—and to develop immunoresolvents as agonists to test resolution pharmacology and their role in catabasis for their therapeutic potential [43]. Dalli [44] argues similarly when discussing the potential of resolution pharmacology-based approaches in developing new therapeutics for combatting infections that do not interfere with the immune response. This issue is also raised by Schett and Neurath [45] who discuss potential intervention strategies for fostering the resolution process and their implications for the therapy of inflammatory diseases.

Indeed, given the new concept of inflammation resolution as an essential part of inflammation biology and pathology (see Sect. 5.3), the development of SAMPs for clinical use is a dictate of the hour. As stated by Serhan in this context [43]: "The available evidence from extensive preclinical animal models, human SPM production in vivo, and the limited results of randomized clinical trials in humans suggest that it is indeed time to consider stimulating resolution in the 21st century as a new therapeutic direction for managing unwanted excessive inflammation and infection. Proresolution pharmacology can enhance the host innate response to expedite microbial clearance, limit collateral tissue damage, and stimulate tissue regeneration by enhancing endogenous resolution mechanisms that are programmed into the resolving exudates of the acute inflammatory response."

Indeed, not only SPMs but also other SAMPs could stimulate the development of novel therapeutic strategies encompassing a novel "resolution pharmacology" approach. The emerging topic will be sustainably resumed in the following chapters when and if appropriate.

7.4.4 DAMPs as Therapeutics to Boost Innate Resistance

7.4.4.1 General Remarks

The intrinsic evolution-determined nature of DAMPs is to promote adaptive immune defense responses via activation of antigen-presenting DCs (for additional information compare Vol. 1 [28], Part VIII, Chpt. 32, p. 749). This implies that they can be used as therapeutics in situations in which a robust immune defense response is desired, that is, to promote anti-pathogen-directed immune processes aimed at succeeding strong vaccination effects and to induce an ICD in cancer cells sought to instigate a potent antitumor immune response.

7.4.4.2 Administration of DAMPs in Vaccination Procedures

There is a wide indication field for the administration of DAMPs to boost short- and long-term innate resistance against pathogens and cancer cells. To remember: for a long time, adjuvants are used in vaccine formulations to induce potent adaptive (humoral!) immune responses that cannot be achieved with antigen alone [46]. Aluminum hydroxide (alum) is the most common adjuvant currently in clinical use [47, 48] that has been denoted as an exogenous DAMP in this book (for additional information compare Vol. 1 [28], Part IV, Sect. 15.2.2, p. 354). Of note, in studies in mice, alum was found to cause cell death associated with the subsequent release of host cell DNA identified by the authors as a DAMP [49]. However, one has to realize that—according to current knowledge—cell death leads to large amounts of other DAMPs as well, which all mediate adjuvanticity. Thus, it is not a surprise that the ongoing development of novel vaccines intends to incorporate the combination of DAMP-inducing adjuvants and PAMP adjuvants [50]. And in this context, it is tantalizing to speculate that, mechanistically, DAMPs mediate the positive health effects of dry sauna bathing as a form of whole-body thermotherapy. As postulated, frequent dry sauna bathing improves a variety of subjective and objective health criteria and appears to be associated with improved outcomes such as reduced overall mortality and reduced incidence of cardiovascular events and dementia, at least in men [51, 52].

7.4.4.3 Induction of DAMPs in Antitumor Therapy

The induction of an ICD aimed at promoting a robust antitumor immune response is currently an emerging topic in oncology. Fired by the danger/injury model in Immunology, a conceptual revolution in oncology has emerged in that cancer is considered as entities that can be detected and destroyed by the immune system under certain circumstances. The core of this new concept refers to the phenomenon of ICD. Of note, however, only a few lethal stimuli are intrinsically endowed with the ability to instigate ICD, including certain chemotherapeutics, radiotherapy, certain oncolytic viruses, and photodynamic therapy [53]. They are called "ICD inducers" [54]. There is accumulating evidence indicating that these therapeutic inducers cause ICD through ER stress associated with or induced by ROS [55]. Typically, ICD is associated with emission of a series of DAMPs that are generated in a precise spatiotemporally defined configuration. This coordinated emission of DAMPs then allows elicitation of a robust antitumor immune response that is associated with the establishment of immunological memory.

7.4.4.4 Concluding Remark

The clinical use of DAMPs as therapeutics aimed at promoting adaptive immune responses is emerging but probably not restricted to vaccination and antitumor therapy. Other fields of indication may be considered. For example, it may be imaginable to add certain DAMPs to antibiotic treatment in case of intractable infections, such as observed in infectious disorders caused by antibiotic-resistant pathogens.

7.4.5 Résumé

Here, some principles of DAMPs and SAMPs as therapeutic targets and therapeutics have been tentatively introduced. To implement these tasks clinically in the future, agonists to these molecules have to be developed, knowing that some are already available. For example, as reviewed by Venereau et al. [41] and Andersson et al. [27], there are reports on the successful use of polyclonal or mouse/rat anti-HMGB1 mAbs in a number of experimental inflammatory models. To enable development of HMGB1-targeted therapy for clinical use, humanized anti-HMGB1 mAbs have been worked out, for example, a partly humanized, chimeric mAb targeting HMGB1 with preserved functionality compared to the parental mouse anti-HMGB1 mAb [56].

Thus, removing or neutralizing extracellular HMGB1 in infectious or sterile inflammation would be a plausible approach to ameliorate human diseases concerned. However, up to now, there is only limited clinical evidence for therapeutic agents that target extracellular HMGB1, but several promising candidates are in preclinical or clinical development. As concluded in this context by Andersson et al. [27]: "Blocking excessive amounts of extracellular HMGB1, particularly the disulfide isoform, offers an attractive clinical opportunity to ameliorate systemic inflammatory diseases. Therapeutic interventions to regulate intracellular HMGB1 biology must still await a deeper understanding of intracellular HMGB1 functions. Future work is needed to create more robust assays to evaluate functional bioactivity of HMGB1 antagonists. Forthcoming clinical studies would also greatly benefit from a development of antibody-based assays to quantify HMGB1 redox isoforms, presently assessed by mass spectrometry methods".... "Together, we believe that HMGB1-specific antagonists should be tested in multiple parallel clinical studies of inflammatory disease syndromes to reveal whether blocking extracellular HMGB1 will benefit patients."

Certainly, such opinions, statements, and conclusions must be uttered for antagonists of all the other critical DAMPs and SAMPs. As imaginable, this research field—including the activities of the pharmaceutical industry—is currently in full swing, and many highly exciting reports can be expected in the near future, providing a promising expansion of the therapeutic spectrum to treat human diseases. Nevertheless, the crucial key question has not yet been answered satisfactorily: Is it feasible to achieve a lasting therapeutic effect by inhibiting only *one* DAMP or SAMP, or do we always have to inhibit a cocktail of key DAMPs or SAMPs according to distinct determined DAMPs or SAMPs patterns?

7.5 Outlook and Future Perspectives

The topic addressed in this chapter opens new avenues for modern medicine. Introduction of DAMPs and SAMPs as biomarkers in everyday clinical life will certainly enrich the diagnostic and prognostic options of clinicians and may allow better risk stratification of life-threatening diseases.

Beyond these positive aspects, and according to the opinion of the author of this book, DAMPs as biomarkers should play an increasing role in future environmental research. Thus, strikingly, the environment has now been recognized to be the major contributor to the global disease burden [57, 58]. Notably, 80–85% of human disease is reportedly linked to environmental exposures [59]. However, quantifying and specifying the myriad of environmental and lifestyle risk factors such as smoking, exposure to hazardous chemicals, and pathogenic microorganisms turned out to be very complex and difficult to manage [57, 60]. For example, persons can be exposed to a complex mixture of chemical and biological contaminants, with multiple sources, for varying durations across their life course.

To find a way out of this dilemma, the continuous endeavor of environmental research was intensified and culminated in the development of the "environmental health paradigm" [61]. This approach tries to integrate the knowledge of exposures and environmental health sciences by exploring the causal links between environmental exposure and adverse disease effects. Two prominent models emerged as a result of intense interdisciplinary discussions on the environmental health paradigm, called the *exposome* and the *adverse outcome pathway* concepts. The model of the environmental health paradigm—academically covered by the new field of *exposure science* [62]—has worldwide intensified efforts of modern environmental research to study adverse effects of environmental agents on humans and animals. The main subject of such cross-disciplinary studies is the search for new tools to specify and assess the risk of adverse health outcomes caused by harmful environmental factors. Indeed, the field of environmental research is flourishing, as reflected by the establishment of an interdisciplinary area of environmental health sciences and public health.

Excitingly, there is accumulating evidence in support of the notion that both exogenous DAMPs (i.e., presented as harmful environmental factors) and endogenous DAMPs (i.e., caused by harmful environmental factors) represent an important integrating momentum of both concepts. Though not perfect, such an approach should represent a first step to integrate these unique molecules and their pathology-mediating functions into these two environmental health research paradigms. This even more so, as this momentum may give rise to an interesting tautological discussion on the question: Is research on exogenous/endogenous DAMP-induced innate immune pathways and DAMP-shaped adaptive immune processes just a special part of environmental health research or even the same topic?! The final future aim of this approach certainly is to develop innovative DAMP-based in vitro tests for cumulative risk assessment, thereby allowing avoidance of the use of costly and (potentially) ethically flawed animal experiments.

Similarly, the introduction of DAMPs and SAMPs as therapeutic targets and therapeutics will certainly enrich the therapeutic options of clinicians and physicians and may allow new sophisticated and efficient treatment modalities indicated for all those disorders that are characterized by currently untreatable, dysregulated inflammatory responses. In all these therapeutic efforts, however, it should not be forgotten that these molecules are responsible for the daily defense against any stress or injury. Also, here, the "Hippocratic Oath" counts "primum non nocere."

References

1. Hulka B. Overview of biological markers. In: Hulka BS, Wilcosky TC, Griffith JD, editors. Biological markers in epidemiology. New York: Oxford University Press; 1990. ISBN 978-0195059847.
2. Biomarkers Definitions Working Group. Biomarkers and surrogate endpoints: preferred definitions and conceptual framework. Clin Pharmacol Ther. 2001;69:89–95. https://doi.org/10.1067/mcp.2001.113989.
3. Naylor S. Biomarkers: current perspectives and future prospects. Expert Rev Mol Diagn. 2003;3:525–9. https://doi.org/10.1586/14737159.3.5.525.
4. Foroutan B. Personalized medicine: a review with regard to biomarkers. J Bioequiv Availab. 2015;7:244–56. https://www.omicsonline.org/open-access/personalized-medicine-a-review-with-regard-to-biomarkers-jbb-1000248.php?aid=60613.

5. The Academy of Medical Sciences. Realising the potential of stratified medicine. 2013. https://acmedsci.ac.uk/viewFile/51e915f9f09fb.pdf.
6. Seyhan AA, Carini C. Are innovation and new technologies in precision medicine paving a new era in patients centric care? J Transl Med. 2019;17:114. https://doi.org/10.1186/s12967-019-1864-9.
7. Selleck MJ, Senthil M, Wall NR. Making meaningful clinical use of biomarkers. Biomark Insights. 2017;12:117727191771523. http://www.ncbi.nlm.nih.gov/pubmed/28659713.
8. Chen K, Chen X. Design and development of molecular imaging probes. Curr Top Med Chem. 2010;10:1227–36. http://www.ncbi.nlm.nih.gov/pubmed/20388106.
9. Zeng Y, Zhu J, Wang J, Parasuraman P, Busi S, Nauli SM, et al. Functional probes for cardiovascular molecular imaging. Quant Imaging Med Surg. 2018;8:838–52. http://www.ncbi.nlm.nih.gov/pubmed/30306063.
10. Massoud TF, Gambhir SS. Molecular imaging in living subjects: seeing fundamental biological processes in a new light. Genes Dev. 2003;17:545–80. https://doi.org/10.1101/gad.1047403.
11. Gambhir SS. Molecular imaging of cancer with positron emission tomography. Nat Rev Cancer. 2002;2:683–93. http://www.ncbi.nlm.nih.gov/pubmed/12209157.
12. Weissleder R. Molecular imaging in cancer. Science (80-). 2006;312:1168–71. http://www.ncbi.nlm.nih.gov/pubmed/16728630.
13. Weissleder R, Schwaiger MC, Gambhir SS, Hricak H. Imaging approaches to optimize molecular therapies. Sci Transl Med. 2016;8:355ps16. http://www.ncbi.nlm.nih.gov/pubmed/27605550.
14. Lehner J, Wittwer C, Fersching D, Siegele B, Holdenrieder S, Stoetzer OJ. Methodological and preanalytical evaluation of an HMGB1 immunoassay. Anticancer Res. 2012;32:2059–62. http://www.ncbi.nlm.nih.gov/pubmed/22593488.
15. Heizmann CW. S100B protein in clinical diagnostics: assay specificity. Clin Chem. 2004;50:249–51. http://www.ncbi.nlm.nih.gov/pubmed/14709667.
16. Kutzner L, Rund KM, Ostermann AI, Hartung NM, Galano J-M, Balas L, et al. Development of an optimized LC-MS method for the detection of specialized pro-resolving mediators in biological samples. Front Pharmacol. 2019;10:169. http://www.ncbi.nlm.nih.gov/pubmed/30899221.
17. Ruberg SJ, Shen L. Personalized medicine: four perspectives of tailored medicine. Stat Biopharm Res. 2015;7:214–29. https://doi.org/10.1080/19466315.2015.1059354.
18. Sechidis K, Papangelou K, Metcalfe PD, Svensson D, Weatherall J, Brown G. Distinguishing prognostic and predictive biomarkers: an information theoretic approach. Wren J, editor. Bioinformatics. 2018;34:3365–76. http://www.ncbi.nlm.nih.gov/pubmed/29726967.
19. Rzepka R, Dołęgowska B, Rajewska A, Kwiatkowski S. On the significance of new biochemical markers for the diagnosis of premature labour. Mediators Inflamm. 2014;2014:1–8. http://www.ncbi.nlm.nih.gov/pubmed/25548433,
20. Pilzweger C, Holdenrieder S. Circulating HMGB1 and RAGE as clinical biomarkers in malignant and autoimmune diseases. Diagnostics. 2015;5:219–53. http://www.ncbi.nlm.nih.gov/pubmed/26854151
21. Fucikova J, Moserova I, Urbanova L, Bezu L, Kepp O, Cremer I, et al. Prognostic and predictive value of DAMPs and DAMP-associated processes in Cancer. Front Immunol. 2015;6:402. http://www.ncbi.nlm.nih.gov/pubmed/26300886
22. Santos Samary C, Pelosi P, Leme Silva P, Rieken Macedo Rocco P. Immunomodulation after ischemic stroke: potential mechanisms and implications for therapy. Crit Care. 2016;20:391. http://www.ncbi.nlm.nih.gov/pubmed/27923376.
23. Land WG. Use of DAMPs and SAMPs as therapeutic targets or therapeutics: a note of caution. Mol Diagn Ther. 2020;24:251. http://www.ncbi.nlm.nih.gov/pubmed/32248387.
24. Fullerton JN, Gilroy DW. Resolution of inflammation: a new therapeutic frontier. Nat Rev Drug Discov. 2016;15:551–67. http://www.ncbi.nlm.nih.gov/pubmed/27020098.
25. Fukami A, Adachi H, Yamagishi S, Matsui T, Ueda S, Nakamura K, et al. Factors associated with serum high mobility group box 1 (HMGB1) levels in a general population. Metabolism. 2009;58:1688–93. https://linkinghub.elsevier.com/retrieve/pii/S002604950900225X.

26. Tang Y, Zhao X, Antoine D, Xiao X, Wang H, Andersson U, et al. Regulation of post-translational modifications of HMGB1 during immune responses. Antioxid Redox Signal. 2016;24:620–34. https://doi.org/10.1089/ars.2015.6409.
27. Andersson U, Yang H, Harris H. Extracellular HMGB1 as a therapeutic target in inflammatory diseases. Expert Opin Ther Targets. 2018;22:263–77. http://www.ncbi.nlm.nih.gov/pubmed/29447008.
28. Land WG. Damage-associated molecular patterns in human diseases. In: Injury-induced innate immune responses, vol. 1. Cham: Springer International Publishing AG; 2018. https://www.springer.com/de/book/9783319786544.
29. Wiesmann M, Missler U, Gottmann D, Gehring S. Plasma S-100b protein concentration in healthy adults is age- and sex-independent. Clin Chem. 1998;44:1056–8. http://www.ncbi.nlm.nih.gov/pubmed/9590385.
30. Gong X-J, Song X-Y, Wei H, Wang J, Niu M. Serum S100A4 levels as a novel biomarker for detection of acute myocardial infarction. Eur Rev Med Pharmacol Sci. 2015;19:2221–5. http://www.ncbi.nlm.nih.gov/pubmed/26166646.
31. Meddeb R, Dache ZAA, Thezenas S, Otandault A, Tanos R, Pastor B, et al. Quantifying circulating cell-free DNA in humans. Sci Rep. 2019;9:5220. http://www.ncbi.nlm.nih.gov/pubmed/30914716.
32. Wang L, Xie L, Zhang Q, Cai X, Tang Y, Wang L, et al. Plasma nuclear and mitochondrial DNA levels in acute myocardial infarction patients. Coron Artery Dis. 2015;26:296–300. http://www.ncbi.nlm.nih.gov/pubmed/25714070.
33. Dalli J, Colas RA, Serhan CN. Novel n-3 immunoresolvents: structures and actions. Sci Rep. 2013;3:1940. http://www.ncbi.nlm.nih.gov/pubmed/23736886.
34. Fosshaug LE, Colas RA, Anstensrud AK, Gregersen I, Nymo S, Sagen EL, et al. Early increase of specialized pro-resolving lipid mediators in patients with ST-elevation myocardial infarction. EBioMedicine. 2019;46:264–73. http://www.ncbi.nlm.nih.gov/pubmed/31345784,
35. Imming P, Sinning C, Meyer A. Drugs, their targets and the nature and number of drug targets. Nat Rev Drug Discov. 2006;5:821–34. http://www.nature.com/articles/nrd2132.
36. Davidson BL, McCray PB. Current prospects for RNA interference-based therapies. Nat Rev Genet. 2011;12:329–40. http://www.nature.com/articles/nrg2968.
37. Gashaw I, Ellinghaus P, Sommer A, Asadullah K. What makes a good drug target? Drug Discov Today. 2012;17:S24–30. http://www.ncbi.nlm.nih.gov/pubmed/22155646.
38. Zheng CJ, Han LY, Yap CW, Ji ZL, Cao ZW, Chen YZ. Therapeutic targets: progress of their exploration and investigation of their characteristics. Pharmacol Rev. 2006;58:259–79. https://doi.org/10.1124/pr.58.2.4.
39. Land WG. Emerging role of innate immunity in organ transplantation part III: the quest for transplant tolerance via prevention of oxidative allograft injury and its consequences. Transplant Rev (Orlando). 2012;26:88–102. https://linkinghub.elsevier.com/retrieve/pii/S0955470X11000565.
40. Gruda MC, Ruggeberg K-G, O'Sullivan P, Guliashvili T, Scheirer AR, Golobish TD, et al. Broad adsorption of sepsis-related PAMP and DAMP molecules, mycotoxins, and cytokines from whole blood using CytoSorb® sorbent porous polymer beads. PLoS One. 2018;13:e0191676. http://www.ncbi.nlm.nih.gov/pubmed/29370247.
41. Venereau E, De Leo F, Mezzapelle R, Careccia G, Musco G, Bianchi ME. HMGB1 as biomarker and drug target. Pharmacol Res. 2016;111:534–44. https://linkinghub.elsevier.com/retrieve/pii/S104366181630487X.
42. VanPatten S, Al-Abed Y. High mobility group Box-1 (HMGb1): current wisdom and advancement as a potential drug target. J Med Chem. 2018;61:5093–107. http://www.ncbi.nlm.nih.gov/pubmed/29268019.
43. Serhan CN. Treating inflammation and infection in the 21st century: new hints from decoding resolution mediators and mechanisms. FASEB J. 2017;31:1273–88. https://doi.org/10.1096/fj.201601222R.
44. Dalli J. Does promoting resolution instead of inhibiting inflammation represent the new paradigm in treating infections? Mol Aspects Med. 2017;58:12–20. http://www.ncbi.nlm.nih.gov/pubmed/28365269.

45. Schett G, Neurath MF. Resolution of chronic inflammatory disease: universal and tissue-specific concepts. Nat Commun. 2018;9:3261. http://www.ncbi.nlm.nih.gov/pubmed/30111884.
46. Desmet CJ, Ishii KJ. Nucleic acid sensing at the interface between innate and adaptive immunity in vaccination. Nat Rev Immunol. 2012;12:479–91. http://www.nature.com/articles/nri3247.
47. He P, Zou Y, Hu Z. Advances in aluminum hydroxide-based adjuvant research and its mechanism. Hum Vaccin Immunother. 2015;11:477–88. http://www.ncbi.nlm.nih.gov/pubmed/25692535.
48. Powell BS, Andrianov AK, Fusco PC. Polyionic vaccine adjuvants: another look at aluminum salts and polyelectrolytes. Clin Exp Vaccine Res. 2015;4:23. http://www.ncbi.nlm.nih.gov/pubmed/25648619.
49. Marichal T, Ohata K, Bedoret D, Mesnil C, Sabatel C, Kobiyama K, et al. DNA released from dying host cells mediates aluminum adjuvant activity. Nat Med. 2011;17:996–1002. http://www.nature.com/articles/nm.2403.
50. Hayashi T, Momota M, Kuroda E, Kusakabe T, Kobari S, Makisaka K, et al. DAMP-inducing adjuvant and PAMP adjuvants Parallelly enhance protective Type-2 and Type-1 immune responses to influenza Split vaccination. Front Immunol. 2018;9:2619. http://www.ncbi.nlm.nih.gov/pubmed/30515151.
51. Laukkanen T, Khan H, Zaccardi F, Laukkanen JA. Association between sauna bathing and fatal cardiovascular and all-cause mortality events. JAMA Intern Med. 2015;175:542. http://www.ncbi.nlm.nih.gov/pubmed/25705824.
52. Laukkanen T, Kunutsor S, Kauhanen J, Laukkanen JA. Sauna bathing is inversely associated with dementia and Alzheimer's disease in middle-aged Finnish men. Age Ageing. 2017;46:245–49. https://doi.org/10.1093/ageing/afw212.
53. Garg AD, Galluzzi L, Apetoh L, Baert T, Birge RBRB, Bravo-San Pedro JMJM, et al. Molecular and translational classifications of DAMPs in immunogenic cell death. Front Immunol. 2015;6:588. http://www.ncbi.nlm.nih.gov/pubmed/26635802.
54. Garg AD, Dudek-Peric AM, Romano E, Agostinis P. Immunogenic cell death. Int J Dev Biol. 2015;59:131–40. http://www.ncbi.nlm.nih.gov/pubmed/26374534.
55. Garg AD, Krysko DV, Vandenabeele P, Agostinis P. The emergence of phox-ER stress induced immunogenic apoptosis. Onco Targets Ther. 2012;1:786–8. http://www.ncbi.nlm.nih.gov/pubmed/22934283.
56. Lundbäck P, Lea JD, Sowinska A, Ottosson L, Fürst CM, Steen J, et al. A novel high mobility group box 1 neutralizing chimeric antibody attenuates drug-induced liver injury and postinjury inflammation in mice. Hepatology. 2016;64:1699–710. https://doi.org/10.1002/hep.28736.
57. Rappaport SM, Smith MT, Vandamme P, De Brandt E, Pot B, Foligné B, et al. Environment and disease risks. Science. 2010;330:460–1. http://www.ncbi.nlm.nih.gov/pubmed/20966241.
58. Manrai AK, Cui Y, Bushel PR, Hall M, Karakitsios S, Mattingly CJ, et al. Informatics and data analytics to support Exposome-based discovery for public health. Annu Rev Public Health. 2017;38:279–94. https://doi.org/10.1146/annurev-publhealth-082516-012737.
59. Uppal K, Walker DI, Liu K, Li S, Go Y-M, Jones DP. Computational metabolomics: a framework for the million metabolome. Chem Res Toxicol. 2016;29:1956–75. http://www.ncbi.nlm.nih.gov/pubmed/27629808.
60. Willett WC. Balancing life-style and genomics research for disease prevention. Science. 2002;296:695–8. https://doi.org/10.1126/science.1071055.
61. Wilson SH, Schwartz DA. Disease-first: a new paradigm for environmental health science research. Environ Health Perspect. 2006;114:A398. http://www.ncbi.nlm.nih.gov/pubmed/16835037.
62. Lioy PJ, Smith KR. A discussion of exposure science in the 21st century: a vision and a strategy. Environ Health Perspect. 2013;121:405–9. http://www.ncbi.nlm.nih.gov/pubmed/23380895.

8 DAMP-Controlled and Uncontrolled Responses to Trauma: Wound Healing and Polytrauma

8.1 Introduction

8.1.1 The Change of Medical Thinking in Traumatic Diseases

In trauma, mechanical tissue injuries and blood loss, associated with shock and secondary events, including IRI, hypothermia, hypoxia, coagulopathy, or neuroendocrine disorders, lead to cell stress and cell death [1]. Of particular note in this respect is the IRI of the individual's organism following successful resuscitation after severe trauma-associated shock. As typical for this event, generation of ROS leads to a heavy secondary boost of systemic injury affecting every organ and eliciting an organismal innate immune response [2, 3].

Historically,—as partially discussed in Vol. 1 [4], Part VI, Chpt. 22 and wonderfully reviewed by Hauser and Otterbein [5]—medical thinking in traumatic diseases has changed over time and reached a new dimension with the discovery of DAMPs.

Indeed, in the late 1980s/early 1990s, common medical knowledge was based on the notion that patients who had survived major trauma often developed a "sepsis-like" syndrome, where there was no sign of infection at all and all clinical cultures remained sterile. Some of these patients went on to die of MOF. Intensive care physicians assumed that such life-threatening febrile illnesses in injured patients represent the result of severe infection [6, 7]. This general concept was so carved in surgery that a hypothesis evolved postulating that shock leads to "bacterial translocation" through an otherwise intact gut mucosa [8–10]. As quoted from a paper by Baker et al. in 1988 [11]: "Hemorrhagic shock injured the gut mucosa and caused subepithelial edema and focal areas of necrosis. Thus, hemorrhagic shock followed by reinfusion of shed blood disrupts the gut barrier and allows indigenous bacteria normally contained within the gut to cause systemic infections." Together, bacteria and bacterial products entering the portal bloodstream were presumed at that time to cause the sepsis-like clinical picture in polytraumatized patients. Of note, it was already during that time, namely, in 1992, that this clinical febrile sepsis-like picture seen after injury was defined by *Bone* [12] as a SIRS. In fact, the definition of

W. G. Land, *Damage-Associated Molecular Patterns in Human Diseases*,
https://doi.org/10.1007/978-3-030-53868-2_8

SIRS—present in more than half of all intensive care unit (ICU) patients—referred to a combination of fever, leukocytosis, tachycardia, and tachypnea that could reflect a clinical inflammatory response to illness of any source [5].

During that same period—as published by Faist et al. in 1994 [13]—it became clear that, in the setting of major trauma and consecutively associated infectious complications, multiple cytokines could link injury and infection to a (dysregulated) state of hyperinflammation which ultimately may result in MODS or even MOF. A few years later, in 1997, it was shown that sterile tissue injuries were essential sources of cytokines [14], that is, a new concept was borne to recognizing that the immediate source of hyperinflammatory responses in trauma patients was cytokine synthesis at the sites of tissue injury per se. But there was no clear-cut reason at that time why cells at injury sites produce cytokines [5]. The years after the first description of DAMPs in 2003/2004 [15, 16] then paved the way to recognize and accept that any cell stress/tissue injury—may they be of infective or sterile origin—leads to the emission of DAMPs. For example, already in 2008, Flohé et al. [17] published a review article on the role of danger signals in traumatic injury, including burn injury by describing the involvement of HMGB1 and HSPs in trauma-induced tissue damage. More recently, this new model also led to studies of the Hauser group published in 2010 [18], demonstrating the release of mitochondrial DAMPs in trauma (also see below).

Today, the modern concept based on the danger/injury model in Immunology holds that infective/sterile injury leads to the emission of MAMPs and DAMPs or DAMPs, which trigger PRM-mediated innate immune inflammatory effector responses. However, when DAMPs are emitted uncontrolled and in excess and distributed systemically in an organism, they promote hyperinflammatory responses such as SIRS, a process that can end up with the catastrophe of MOF. Curiously, eventual death in the course of this protection-intended scenario may be compared with the suicide of an organism. Of note, in both clinical settings—as already pointed out in Sect. 5.4.3 and Fig. 5.2—a CARS is concomitantly initiated. In both SIRS and CARS, the exacerbated production of pro- or antiinflammatory mediators allows their detection in biological fluids and particularly within the bloodstream. Paradoxically, but typically, DAMP-induced robust innate immune responses in SIRS in terms of dysregulated overshooting hyperinflammation are accompanied by the development of long-lasting immunosuppression in terms of dysregulated overshooting antiinflammation, or still better "over-resolving" inflammation. This event that might be explained by the unproven possibility of DAMP-induced epigenetic modifications is logically associated with increased susceptibility to bacterial and viral infections (more details of this scenario are presented in Vol. 1 [4], Part VI, Sect. 22.2. and Fig. 22.1, and Sect. 5.4).

8.1.2 The Two Possible Outcomes of Any Trauma: Death or Survival

Trauma has been one of the leading health problems in the world for a long time. According to the *Global Burden of Disease Study 2013* report [19], in 2013, 973 million people approximately sustained but survived injuries that warranted some type of healthcare, and 4.8 million people died from injuries. Major causes of injury death were road injury (29.1%), self-harm (17.6%), falls (11.6%), and interpersonal violence (8.5%). Of the people who sustained injuries that warranted some type of healthcare, 5.8% warranted inpatient care, of whom 38.5% sustained fractures. Of the patients who warranted outpatient care, 75.2% sustained minor injuries. Those people who did not die from the lesions owed their survival functioning DAMP-promoted wound healing processes.

The two possible outcomes of any trauma, death and survival, impressively reflect the inherently ambivalent role of injury-induced DAMPs in medicine: their uncontrolled detrimental action in case of severe trauma/polytrauma that can lead to the deadly catastrophe of a SIRS associated with MOF [20], on the one hand; and, on the other hand, their controlled beneficial function that instigates the whole machinery of inflammation-/fibrosis-mediated wound healing following any kind of small or moderate trauma [21].

Consequently, in the following, the topic of wound healing will be briefly described first before moving to the main sections dealing with polytrauma.

8.2 DAMP-Promoted Wound Healing

8.2.1 Introductory Remarks

Wound healing is a highly dynamic and tightly coordinated innate immunity-driven process to achieve restoration of tissue integrity after infectious and/or traumatic tissue injuries. Basically, this process can be graded into four overlapping but distinct phases: (1) hemostasis, (2) inflammation, (3) proliferation, and (4) scar formation/remodeling → maturation [22–24]. The ECM performs central functions at all stages, both as a reinforcing material and cell instructor (for ECM, see Sect. 6.2, and also [25, 26]).

During hemostasis/inflammation, the wound is provisionally closed by a blood clot consisting of a platelet plug and a fibrin matrix, and recruitment of inflammatory cells, predominantly neutrophils and macrophages, is instigated. The hemostasis phase is promoted by DAMPs which were shown to contribute to thrombin generation via triggering tissue factor (TF) expression on monocytes and NET released by neutrophils [27] (for NETosis, see Sect. 4.3.6 and Vol. 1 [4], Part V, Sect. 19.3.6). The following proliferative phase is characterized by declining proinflammatory signals and cell proliferation initiated by local growth factors, including TGF-β1, platelet-derived growth factor (PDGF), TNF, and IL-13. During the final phase of wound healing, the scaring remodeling phase and processes such as wound reorganization, repair, and regeneration processes occur to restructure the damaged tissue [22, 23, 28].

What is important here to remember is that usual proper skin wound healing becomes obvious when our body's innate immune repair mechanisms fail, resulting in either nonhealing (subchronic inflammatory) wounds or excessive profibrotic repair as described in Chap. 6. For example, chronic wounds are difficult to treat and imply a tremendous burden for patients and global healthcare systems. In other words, the function of the myofibroblasts has to be kept in balance! Thus, controlled emission of DAMPs promotes activation of myofibroblasts that are the main producers and organizers of ECM, which is required to restore tissue integrity after injury. However, as also addressed above, too many myofibroblasts working for too long cause tissue contractures that ultimately obstruct organ function. On the other hand, insufficient myofibroblast activation and activities prevent normal wound healing (also compare [29, 30]).

Today, there is growing evidence in support of the notion that—like fibrogenesis—the whole wound healing scenario is the work of DAMPs. Typically, the generation of DAMPs correlates with the degree of severity of accidental insults in traumatic diseases ranging from small cuts to blunt-force trauma and bone fractures or severe large-scale physical or thermal injuries [31]. Following all these injurious lesions, DAMPs such as HMGB1 and HSPs not only induce an acute inflammatory response but are also responsible for subsequent tissue repair. Inflammation after tissue injury is undoubtedly a critical component of wound repair. Innate immune inflammatory cells migrate to the wound and promote tissue regeneration by removing cellular debris, killing and phagocytozing potential invading pathogens, and producing cytokines that promote collagen production, cellular migration, wound epithelialization, controlled "homeostatic" fibrogenesis, and angiogenesis. More specifically, these PRM-bearing cells include mobile inflammatory monocytes and tissue-resident macrophages [32–34], as well as fibroblasts/myofibroblasts [35–37], vascular cells including bone marrow-derived endothelial progenitor cells [38–41], EpCs such as keratinocytes [42] and tubular cells [43], HSCs [44], and, last but not least, stem cells, particularly, mesenchymal stem cells (MSCs) [45, 46]. In fact, any post-injury inflammatory, profibrotic, and angiogenic response, for example, after surgery or accidental trauma, is mediated by these DAMP-activated PRM-expressing innate immune cells [47, 48]. It is the DAMPs and their triggered pathways, together with the surrounding cytokine and growth factor milieu, that ultimately determine whether or not these post-injury innate cellular responses cause mild acute inflammation and wound healing [47, 49] or promote subchronic ongoing inflammation and fibrosis [50] (also compare Chaps. 5 and 6).

Details of this scenario have been outlined in Vol. 1 [4], Part VIII, Chpt. 36. Here, for quick understanding, and to spare the reader troublesome turning the leaves of the other book, parts of this chapter are rewritten.

8.2.2 DAMP-Induced Controlled Tissue Healing After Trauma

8.2.2.1 General Remarks

The crucial role of DAMPs in posttraumatic wound healing is increasingly appreciated and has also recently been reviewed elsewhere [51, 52]. Apparently, DAMPs can be considered critical players in tissue regeneration and repair. Regarding the first step of regeneration, the highly organized phagocyte-mediated resolution of innate immune inflammation, DAMPs drive the mechanism of efferocytosis as a critical process in efficient clearance of cellular debris and dead cells by phagocytes [53]. Another example refers to the observation that the Subclass IIA-3 DAMP FNIII EDA, through TLR signaling, is a potent stimulus for collagen production, myofibroblast differentiation, and wound healing in vitro [54] (for IIA-3 DAMPs, compare Table 3.1; and see Vol.1 [4], Part IV, Sect. 13.2.4.2, and Sect. 3.4.2). Further examples point to HMGB1 that was shown (1) to induce lung fibroblasts' differentiation into myofibroblasts and enhanced cell migration [55]; (2) to promote 3T3 fibroblast wound healing by inducing cell proliferation and migration [56] (3T3 fibroblast, a specialized standard fibroblast cell line); (3) to play a role in skeletal muscle regeneration modulating, in an autocrine–paracrine manner, myofibroblast and EC functions [57]; (4) to enhance proliferation of pulmonary arterial VSMCs and human arterial ECs [58]; and (5) to activate fibrogenic HSCs in vitro [59].

Moreover, DAMPs were found to activate circulating bone marrow-derived stromal stem cells that facilitate repairing processes. Thus, DAMPs were demonstrated to promote both proliferation and trafficking of MSCs, identifying HMGB1 as an essential factor in the regulation of these processes [60–62]. Other DAMPs refer to S100A4 proteins and uric acid that both have been shown dose-dependently to induce chemotaxis of MSCs with synergistic effects when combined [63]. In a more recent study, mitochondria released from dying cells were found to act as a critical environmental cue that controls the cytoprotective function of MSCs [64].

Another repairing mechanism refers to VSMC proliferation upon vascular injury, that is, the key event in the development of intimal hyperplasia leading to atherosclerosis [65]. Equipped with multiple PRMs, VSMCs have been shown to sense MAMPs and DAMPs [66, 67].

And not to forget is the process of autophagy that plays an essential role in regulating cell viability during tissue repair [68]. Indeed, as outlined in Sect. 4.2.2 and Vol. 1 [4], Part V, Sect. 18.2.5.3, autophagy is triggered and regulated by DAMPs [69, 70].

Together, there is increasing evidence indicating a crucial role of DAMPs in repair and regeneration. Since HMGB1, S100 proteins, eATP, and IL-33 represent the most investigated DAMPs in this burning field of regeneration mechanisms (as also reviewed elsewhere in [51, 52]), some more details are added in the following by focusing on the critical events of homeostatic fibrogenesis, angiogenesis, and reepithelialization.

8.2.2.2 High Mobility Group Box 1 and S100 Proteins

Besides its ability to promote MSCs migration and proliferation [60–62], HMGB1 was also shown in studies on skin grafting to operate as a chemoattractant by inducing accumulation of bone marrow-derived epithelial progenitors in skin grafts, promoting inflammatory suppression in the grafts, and subsequent epithelial tissue regeneration [71]. Another line of more recent studies provided evidence suggesting that HMGB1 enhances the secretion of various cytokines by MSCs and promotes osteogenic differentiation via the MAPK signaling pathway [72]. Growing interest is currently focused on the DAMP-triggered inflammatory response in myocardial injury, repair, and remodeling [73]. For example, in studies in a model of acute MI in transgenic mice exhibiting the cardiac-specific overexpression of HMGB1, the molecule in cardiac cells or its local administration provided first in vivo evidence that this DAMP induces myocardial regeneration by enhancing angiogenesis, restoring cardiac function, and improving survival after MI [74].

In complementation of such studies by examining murine necrotic myocardial cells, DAMPs (including HMGB1, GAL-3, S100β, S100A8, and S100A9) were shown (1) to provoke a significant increase in fibroblast proliferation, α-SMA activation, and COLIA1 and COLIIIA1 mRNA expression, and (2) to significantly increase fibroblast motility in a cell-wounding assay in a TLR4- and RAGE-dependent manner [75]. The profibrogenic role of HMGB1 could also be demonstrated in a study on a model of liver fibrogenesis [76]. These experiments revealed that HMGB1 dose-dependently stimulates proliferation of HSCs, upregulates de novo synthesis of COLI and α-SMA, and triggers Smad2 phosphorylation and its nuclear translocation through a TGF-β1-independent mechanism.

Besides contributing to fibrogenesis, HMGB1 was observed in other lines of studies to promote angiogenesis. Indeed, as reviewed [48], numerous studies have identified HMGB1 as a critical proangiogenic factor. In brief, HMGB1 plays a significant role in neovascularization of ischemic areas by recruiting endothelial progenitor cells through activation of integrins and inducing the migration and sprouting of ECs in a RAGE-dependent manner [77, 78]. Of note, the critical role of RAGE in regenerative pathways was also underlined by recent studies showing that this receptor is clearly involved in corneal reepithelialization, most probably mediated by signaling via S100 proteins [79].

Also, HMGB1 was found to stimulate ECs and macrophages to release proangiogenic cytokines such as *vascular endothelial growth factors* (VEGFs), TNF, and IL-8 [80]. Moreover, HMGB1 secreted by leukocytes was shown to be essential for the skeletal muscle to react to hypoxia and initiate angiogenesis in response to injury [81]. Accordingly, a recent report (again from studies on transgenic mice exhibiting the cardiac-specific overexpression of HMGB1) provided evidence that HMGB1 promotes angiogenesis and is capable of reducing the size of MI by facilitating (1) the mobilization and differentiation of bone marrow cells to endothelial progenitor cells, (2) their migration to the border zones of the infarction areas, and (3) engraftment as vascular ECs in new capillaries or arterioles in the infarcted heart [82]. In similar studies in mice, HMGB1, via signaling through IL-6, was demonstrated to be involved in angiogenesis and functional recovery after ischemic stroke [83].

Notably, recent experiments also provide first clues for a role of HMGB1 in kidney regeneration. Thus, as demonstrated in studies on prostate tumor cells [84], HMGB1 induces activation of the chaperone-like protein clusterin (Clu) that in other sets of studies on CluKO mice was shown to be required for renal tissue regeneration in the kidney repair phase after IRI associated with promotion of tubular cell proliferation [85] and fibrogenesis [86]. Moreover, HMGB1 has recently been proposed to be involved in human airway EpC repair and restitution via multiple pathways mediated by TLR4 and RAGE, that is, findings that underpin increased ECM synthesis and modulation of cell matrix adhesion [87].

Last but not least, HMGB1 has been found to promote VSMC proliferation associated with the development of intimal hyperplasia that, in turn, can lead to arterial occlusion [88]. In this study, HMGB1-triggered TLR4 signaling was demonstrated to stimulate VSMCs to migrate and producing monocyte chemotactic protein 1/ CCL2. Further, in this experiment, macrophages were found to produce VSMC mitogens in response to HMGB1 and this in a TLR4 → MyD88/TRIF → signaling-dependent manner. Similarly, as documented by a growing number of reports, extracellular S100 proteins contribute to VSMC proliferation [89–91].

In conclusion, HMGB1 released by injured cells promotes tissue repair by promoting fibrogenesis, angiogenesis, and reepithelialization. In fact, to denote HMGB1 as a prototypic DAMP responsible for regeneration may alone be already explained by the observation that increased HMGB1 serum concentrations have been measured immediately after nonprofessional marathon running that returned to baseline levels during the recovery week [92].

8.2.2.3 Extracellular Adenosine Triphosphate and Other Nucleotides

There is increasing evidence suggesting that nucleotides participate actively in the three phases of regeneration by interacting with purinergic receptors on different cell types, that is, involvement in resolution of inflammation, proliferation of cells, and reepithelialization processes. Indeed, as already mentioned in Vol. 1 [4], Part II, Sect. 5.3.4, the two families of P2Rs appear to have separate roles: P2XRs are involved in defense mechanisms and cell death, whereas P2YRs participate in wound healing [93]. For example, as shown in different models of tissue regeneration, both ATP and UTP released by apoptotic cells in a caspase-1-dependent manner act as "find-me" signals that recruit macrophages through P2Y2R, thereby promoting phagocytic clearance and, thus, facilitating the resolution phase [94] (for "find-me" signals, see Vol. 1 [4], Part IV, Sect. 12.2.5.2 and Fig. 12.4). Human neutrophils, also involved in the resolution phase, were found to release ATP that, in turn, guides their chemotaxis by feedback through P2Y2 receptors [95]. Moreover, both ATP and UTP were demonstrated to promote migration of VSMCs through binding of P2Y2R to the actin-binding protein filamin A that participates in the anchoring of membrane proteins for the actin cytoskeleton [96] (for actin cytoskeleton, also compare Fig. 6.1 in Chap. 6). Further, stimulation of P2Y receptors by nucleotides revealed a mitogenic effect on multiple cell types such as cardiac ECs [97], and fibroblasts [98]. Moreover, as recently reported, uridine adenosine tetraphosphate, a dinucleotide that exerts vascular influence via purinergic receptors, acts as a proangiogenic factor in vitro through purinergic P2Y receptors [99]. Together, these findings provide evidence for a role of nucleotides as proangiogenic DAMPs in tissue repair and angiogenesis.

Of note, studies have already been published in support of a critical function of eATP in regenerative and profibrotic processes. For example, evidence was provided indicating an early release by degenerating neurons of eATP that contributes to the activation of a series of intracellular pathways within Schwann cells that are crucial for nerve regeneration [100]. As concluded by the authors, these results contribute to defining the cross talk taking place among degenerating nerve terminals and perisynaptic Schwann cells, involved in the functional recovery of the neuromuscular junctions. In other sets of studies in rats, nucleotide release from dying cells after acute kidney injury (AKI) was found to promote proliferation of neighboring tubular cells, thus promoting wound closure via the downstream activation of Akt [101]. Again in other lines of studies on a rat liver model, eATP released after partial hepatectomy from hepatocytes and Kupffer cells was found to contribute to liver regeneration by activating cell cycle progression in hepatocytes [102]. Recent studies on a hepatectomy model in wild-type mice confirmed these findings by showing that treatment with ATP also promotes liver regeneration in this species. As an underlying mechanism, activation by eATP of the NLRP3 inflammasome could be demonstrated [103]. Remarkably, eATP, in terms of an NLRP3-activating IA-2 DAMP, may also contribute to tissue repair via profibrotic pathways mediated by the activation of the NLRP3 inflammasome (for additional information compare Vol. 1 [4], Part VI, Sect. 22.4.2.2, p. 516). Indeed, studies on fibroblasts and different organs have demonstrated that the innate immune sensor NLRP3, mostly inflammasome-dependent [104, 105], but also inflammasome-independent [106], plays a crucial role in fibrogenesis and can orchestrate profibrotic innate immune responses under both infectious and sterile conditions. In fact, a large body of evidence suggests that the principal products of the NLRP3 inflammasome, IL-1β and IL-18, can exert profibrotic activities [107–111] (for NLRP3 inflammasome, also compare Sect. 2.2.5). On the other hand, these reports are not without conflicts. For example, more recent studies on lung and dermal fibroblasts resulted in the conflicting observation that IL-1β attenuates myofibroblast formation and ECM production in fibroblasts exposed to TGF-β1 [112]. According to the authors' conclusion, these findings should give rise to reconsider the role of IL-1β in fibrosis. Thus, to date, the signaling pathways from the inflammasome to myofibroblast differentiation and chronic collagen synthesis have not been fully elucidated and await further clarification [113].

8.2.2.4 Interleukin-33

With IL-33, a constitutive/inducible DAMP has been reported to contribute to the wound healing process (for IL-33, see Vol. 1 [4], Part IV, Sects. 12.2.4.5 and 14.2.4.2; for IL-33 operating context-dependently as a DAMP or SAMP, see Sect. 3.5.6.3). As reviewed by Wilgus [52], multiple studies have demonstrated that IL-33 regulates the activity of cell types involved in cutaneous wound healing, and a physiological role for IL-33 in wound healing has been shown using several different genetically modified mouse strains in various wound healing models. For example, besides evidence for IL-33 to function in the cutaneous vasculature (angiogenesis), other sets of studies could show a role for this cytokine in regulating keratinocyte function and wound closure rates. These experiments revealed that IL-33 expression levels are upregulated in the skin after injury, particularly in keratinocytes. Thus, in one paper, a crucial role for IL-33 in the recruitment of ILC2s during skin repair, in particular, reepithelialization, was reported [114]. Interestingly, these data indicate that IL-33-responsive-ILC2s are an important link between the cutaneous epithelium and the innate immune system, acting to promote the restoration of skin integrity after injury (for ILC2, see Vol. 1 [4], Part III, Sect. 8.4.2.2). In another study on a murine wounding model, the elaborated experimental findings indicated that the nuclear IL-33 as a constitutive DAMP, but not secreted IL-33 as an inducible DAMP, promotes wound healing, probably by suppressing NF-κB to inhibit excessive inflammation and by maintaining keratinocyte proliferation or migration for epithelialization [115].

8.2.2.5 Concluding Remarks

Doubtlessly, there is an increasing interest of researchers and clinicians in the role of constitutive and inducible DAMPs in tissue regeneration and repair, and further publications on this issue can be expected soon. In fact, in regenerative medicine, strategies based on stem cells and growth factors have not yet proven broadly effective in the clinic. The hope, therefore, is that DAMP-induced innate immune-mediated mechanisms of tissue repair and regeneration may support existing regenerative strategies or could be even an alternative to using stem cells and growth factors.

Nonetheless, a particular role has still to be attributed to MSCs, all the more, as they express PRMs such as TLRs [116], thereby enabling them to sense DAMPs. Indeed, therapies with the use of MSCs are promising options to support organ and tissue regeneration. Yet, the application of MSCs requires MSCs with maximum regenerative capacity, and the question to be raised, therefore, is whether the most effective capacity of the MSC-based therapeutic potential can be achieved by direct DAMP-induced activation of MSCs before their application. And in fact and excitingly, a beneficial enhancing healing effect of the combination of stem cells with HMGB1 has recently been reported in models of fracture healing [117, 118] (for fracture healing, see below). Further support for such a therapeutic modality comes from so-called preconditioning strategies. Indeed, in vitro pretreatment in terms of preconditioning strategies has been shown to enhance survival, engraftment, and paracrine properties of MSCs and, therefore, optimize their reparative and regenerative capacity. However, when carefully looking at the different technologies of MSC preconditioning (including modulation of culture atmosphere {hypoxic or anoxic, addition of trophic factors, growth factors, cytokines, or hormones}) and pharmacological agents such as ROS inducers (reviewed in [119]), one can assume that they all are associated with the emission of DAMPs. Together, transplantation of DAMP-activated MSCs has a promising future in therapeutic strategies to accelerate tissue/fracture healing.

8.2.3 DAMP-Induced Controlled Bone Fracture Healing

8.2.3.1 General Remarks

Doubtlessly, fractures are the most common large-organ, traumatic injuries to humans. The process of fracture healing is highly complex and, in many respects, poorly understood. Several fundamental principles governing bone regeneration have, however, been well established and are briefly discussed here.

8.2.3.2 Repair of Bone Fractures

The repair of bone fractures is a postnatal regenerative innate immune process that recapitulates many of the ontological events of embryonic skeletal development (for reviews, see [120–122]). Typically, fracture healing and skeletal tissue repair involve an initial anabolic phase characterized by an increase in tissue volume related to the de novo recruitment and differentiation of MSCs cells that form skeletal and vascular tissues. This phase is followed by a catabolic phase that is characterized by a reduction in the volume of the callus tissues. Notably, in most fractures, a certain amount of mechanical instability leads to interfragmentary movement and, thus, to secondary fracture healing. Obviously, an optimal "window" of interfragmentary motion seems to be needed to activate innate immune cells to be enabled to develop sufficient calluses and to bridge a fracture stably (this is a plausible observation given the fact that any innate immune cell needs an injury, i.e., DAMPs, to get activated for functioning).

Of note, this fracture healing process reflects both innate and adaptive immune processes that are essential during the anabolic and catabolic phases. In the initial inflammatory stage after injury, PRM-bearing innate immune cells function to remove necrotic tissues, promote angiogenesis, initiate proliferative and remodeling repair processes resulting in reconstruction of bone. The inflammatory phase is instigated when disruption of the vasculature leads to a hematoma around the fracture site. The fibrin network of the hematoma serves as the first provisional matrix for the influx of PRM-bearing inflammatory cells that are attracted by platelet-derived factors, complement fragments, as well as multiple DAMPs released from necrotic cells and damaged ECM. The infiltrating cells include neutrophils and macrophages (removing the provisional fibrin matrix and necrotic cells via phagocytosis) but also adaptive immune T and B cells, which are also involved in controlling fracture healing. At different stages of fracture healing, the innate immune cells produce cytokines including IL-1β, TNF, IL-6, IL-17F, and IL-23 as well as chemokines such as CCL2 which convey different effects (for cytokines and chemokines, also compare Vol. 1 [4], Part VI, Sect. 22.5, and Table 22.1).

The inflammatory phase is followed by the proliferative phase, which involves a combination of intramembranous and endochondral ossification processes. Endochondral ossification reportedly involves the CCL2-driven recruitment of fibroblasts and osteoprogenitor cells as well as recruitment, proliferation, and differentiation of undifferentiated PRM-bearing MSCs into chondroblasts that form avascular cartilage. Along with accompanying fibrotic tissues, this cartilage tissue, commonly known as soft callus, provides initial mechanical stability for the fracture and serves as the scaffold for endochondral bone formation. The conversion of cartilage to bone is stimulated by progression of hypertrophy of PRM-expressing chondrocytes, which cause calcification of cartilage matrix and concurrent angiogenesis.

The final stage of fracture repair consists of the remodeling of the woven bone into the original laminar bone configuration by PRM-bearing osteoclasts (resorbing necrotic bone fragments and the necrotic ends of the fractured bone) that first create erosive pits on the bone surface, on which new bone is then laid down by PRM-bearing osteoblasts.

There is growing evidence suggesting that, like in wound healing, constitutive and inducible DAMPs are also involved in physiological bone fracture healing, for example, in the stimulation of osteogenic differentiation of MSCs. Indeed, a role of HMGB1 in bilateral femur fracture healing was already suggested in 2008 [123]. Some years later, the group around Huber-Lang demonstrated the role of complement in fracture healing [124, 125]. In these studies, besides others, the inducible IIIB-3 DAMP C5a was suggested to induce the migration and inflammatory response of osteoblasts and directly and indirectly regulates osteoclast formation, thereby contributing to a balanced fracture healing.

8.2.3.3 Concluding Remarks

In sum, there is growing evidence in support of the notion that DAMP-promoted innate immune inflammatory and repairing responses are essential for fracture healing. On the other hand, there is also recent evidence for the concept that overshooting emission and subsequent systemic distribution of fracture-associated DAMPs can cause remote organ dysfunction, a topic that will be addressed below. Further studies are required to investigate the therapeutic options with the use of DAMPs, that is, administration of certain DAMPs in poor fracture healing to prevent pseudarthrosis and, on the other hand, to suppress systemically circulating DAMPs to prevent remote organ disorders.

8.2.4 Aberrant Hyper- and Hyporeactive Wound Healing

Aberrant dysregulated wound healing can consist of either DAMP-promoted hyperreactive or hyporeactive innate immune processes. The hyperreactive version—that is, keloids—can be caused by cutaneous injury and irritation, including trauma, burns, surgery, and herpes zoster infection. Genetically determined susceptibility to the disease is suggested. As a locally aggressive fibroproliferative disorder of the skin, keloid is frequently accompanied by discomfort, contracture, and disfigurement and (reviewed in [126]). In surgery, this complication is greatly feared by plastic surgeons and their patients. By contrast, wound dehiscence may reflect an insufficient action of DAMPs.

Though the exact pathogenesis of keloid has not been fully elucidated, persistent and histologically localized inflammation is considered one of the main causes. This constant infiltration of immune cells during prolonged and intense inflammation contributes to the continuous growth of keloid lesions. In fact, the reticular layer of keloids contains inflammatory cells, increased numbers of fibroblasts, newly formed blood vessels, and collagen deposits [126, 127]. Moreover, proinflammatory cytokines, such as IL-1α, IL-1β, IL-6, and TNF, are upregulated in keloid tissues, suggested to promote chronic inflammation, which in turn may cause the invasive growth of keloids [128, 129].

Quite expectedly, DAMPs appear to be involved in this abnormal cutaneous wound healing. Thus, in a study recently reported by Lee et al. [130], HMGB1 and its cognate PRMs (TLRs, RAGE) were demonstrated to be actively expressed in keloid tissues. Also, in this series of experiments, exogenous HMGB1 treatment was shown to increase the expression level of COLI and COLIII, elastin, and fibronectin in dermal spheroid cultures, suggesting HMGB1 to have a vital pathogenetic role in keloid formation.

The hyporeactive version of wound healing refers to poorly and slowly healing of wounds. For example, poorly healing wounds in diabetic patients [131] and pressure ulcer formation in individuals with spinal cord injury [132, 133] are well-known phenomena for all physicians. Such wounds represent major healthcare problems, and current treatment methods are only partially effective. Also, such wounds are prone to get infected, which can lead to amputation and further disability.

Clearly, further studies are needed to investigate the potential therapeutic options with the use of DAMPs as therapeutic targets or therapeutics, that is, inhibition of DAMPs in case of an impending keloid formation and administration of certain DAMPs in case of poorly healing wounds, respectively (see Sect. 8.4.3).

8.2.5 Résumé

DAMP-promoted wound healing as a complex, highly regulated process can be regarded as a classical function of the innate immune system aimed at restoring homeostasis. However, the cascade of DAMP/SAMP-promoted events involved in homeostatic wound healing can be disturbed, leading to either keloid formation or chronic, nonhealing wounds that subject the patient to significant discomfort and distress. The healing of a superficial wound requires the orchestration of many efferent innate immune responses to provide an optimal outcome. Nonetheless, as discussed elsewhere [134], even optimally, wound tissue never reaches its pre-injured strength, and multiple aberrant healing states can result in chronic nonhealing wounds.

8.3 Polytrauma

8.3.1 Introductory Remarks

Trauma has been one of the leading health problems in the world for a long time. Doubtlessly, the severest form of damage to an individual can be seen in a polytrauma. The diagnosis of polytrauma is made when a severe injury has affected two or more body systems or organs. Usually, in polytrauma patients, the admitting physician of the emergency department diagnoses a traumatic brain injury (TBI) and identifies at least one of the injuries to be potentially life-threatening in severity. The multiply injured patient intensely treated in the ICU may die or, in case of survival, may suffer from impairments in physical, cognitive, psychological, or psychosocial functioning [135–139].

Immediate and early trauma deaths are generally due to primary TBI, acute blood loss, and hemorrhagic shock [140]. Whereas in earlier times, most patients have abruptly died from these lesions, today, they survive as a result of significant improvements in the management strategies. The life-saving actions are mainly owed to improved standards of trauma care due to defined algorithms of pre- and in-hospital trauma care (e.g., control and correction of massive blood loss to achieve hemodynamic stability), which have been established in most industrialized and developing countries. Nevertheless, patients who survive experience subsequent mortality in the ICU that is mainly a consequence of MOF, often accompanied by infection-induced sepsis [141, 142].

8.3.2 Pathophysiology and Pathogenesis of Polytrauma

8.3.2.1 General Remarks

The typical pathophysiological course of survivors under intensive care treatment is characterized by a systemic defense response to severe injury that begins within 30 min following trauma and involves interactions across the hemostatic, inflammatory, endocrine, and neurological systems. Modern notions hold that this clinical syndrome reflects an uncontrolled overshooting systemic innate immune response caused by polytrauma-induced emission of large amounts of DAMPs, which—like in infection-induced sepsis [143]—circulate systemically to affect the whole body of the patient. And it is the DAMPs that lead to the catastrophe of the sterile hyperinflammatory, sepsis-like, life-threatening SIRS most often associated with MODS or MOF. There are several hypotheses reported about the initiators and drivers of MODS including barrier failure, electrophysiological alterations, microcirculatory disturbances, inflammation-induced cell dysfunction, protein alterations, and microbiome shifts (for competent articles and further reading, see [1, 18, 31, 144–149]; for SIRS, compare also Sect. 5.4.2).

Typically, this DAMP-induced, systemic cytokine/chemokine-mediated hyperinflammatory response to severe trauma is associated with an intense and long-lasting counterbalancing CARS, resulting in posttraumatic immunosuppression [150–153]. As discussed in Sect. 5.4.3, CARS can be regarded as a disorder caused by hyperresolution of hyperinflammation in terms of a mirror-imaged counterregulation of SIRS (also see Relja and Land [154], and compare Fig. 5.2, and see Fig. 8.1). However, as mentioned above, instead of a previously assumed biphasic inflammatory response consisting of an initial proinflammatory response followed by a subsequent counterbalancing antiinflammatory response, hyperresolving processes are now considered to occur nearly in parallel with the hyperinflammatory response. This usually observed course of a polytrauma is briefly sketched here.

8.3.2.2 Systemic Inflammatory Response Syndrome

Accumulating evidence indicates that lethal SIRS associated with MOF is the result of traumatic injury-induced cell death in the form of ACD and RCD such as apoptosis, necroptosis, and ferroptosis [155–159] serving as robust sources for emission of large amounts of DAMPs. As outlined in Sect. 4.3, and in Vol. 1 [4], Part V, Chap. 20, these various subroutines of RCD, in particular, in the form of RN may trigger several waves of constitutive and inducible DAMPs resulting in the "horror of an injury-induced avalanche of DAMPs" leading to SIRS and MOF (for additional

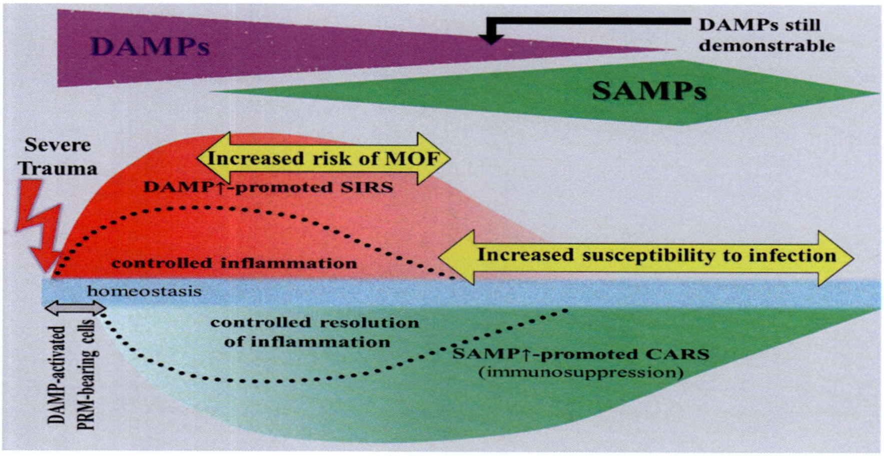

Fig. 8.1 Schematic diagram of a conceptual model illustrating the posttraumatic uncontrolled overshooting hyperinflammatory response observed in SIRS that is induced by excessive production of DAMPs. This DAMP-induced hyperinflammatory response proceeds in parallel to a long-lasting hyperresolution response observed in CARS that is induced by production of counterbalancing SAMPs in excess (the controlled homeostatic proinflammatory and resolving responses are faded in, separated by dotted lines). The short delay of the beginning of the hyperresolving response should symbolize that SAMPs in terms of inducible suppressing DAMPs are secreted by DAMP-activated PRM-expressing innate immune cells. The initial hyperinflammatory phase is associated with an increased risk of multiple organ failure, whereas the long-lasting hyperresolution phase is characterized by a state of immunosuppression that is associated with increased susceptibility of patients to infections. Note: The overlapping hyperinflammatory and hyperresolution responses allow to still measuring DAMPs in the hyperresolving phase characterized by increased susceptibility of patients to infections. *CARS* compensatory antiinflammatory response syndrome, *MOF* multiple organ failure, *PRM* pattern recognition molecule, *SIRS* systemic inflammatory response syndrome. (Sources: [1, 18, 31, 144, 146–148, 150–153]. Note: This figure is slightly modified from Fig. 1 published in [154]: Relja B, Land WG. Damage-associated molecular patterns in trauma. Eur J Trauma Emerg Surg. 2019 Oct 14. doi: 10.1007/s00068-019-01235-w)

information compare also Vol. 1 [4], Part V, Chap. 20, p. 467 and Fig. 20.1, p. 469). Experimental support for such a scenario model comes from studies on a rat model of MODS using fracture trauma followed by hemorrhage [160]. The results from these experiments suggested that necroptosis is heavily involved in the pathology of MODS.

Clinically, as partially mentioned above, SIRS is characterized by local and systemic release of proinflammatory cytokines produced by DAMP-activated innate immune cells including IL-1β (reflecting activated inflammasomes), TNF and IL-6, AA metabolites, proteins of the contact phase and coagulation systems, and complement factors as well as hormonal mediators [140, 161–164] (for global DAMP-induced inflammatory responses, also compare Vol. 1, [4], Part VI, Sects. 22.2.4 and 22.2.5). Proinflammatory cytokines also activate the coagulation pathways, whereby enhanced thrombin formation increases fibrinogen cleavage and reduces fibrin monomers from polymerizing to form stable fibrin clots (hypercoagulability), which is why fibrinogen depletion is observed. Additionally, DAMP-induced endothelial expression of adhesion molecules facilitates leukocyte adhesion, which promotes extravasation into damaged tissue that is controlled by vascular endothelial cadherin [165, 166]. Also, EC damage, accumulation of leukocytes, disseminated intravascular coagulation (DIC), and microcirculatory disturbances lead finally to apoptosis and necrosis of parenchymal cells, with the development of MODS or MOF. Importantly, DAMPs emitted in excess were shown to trigger DIC (reviewed in [27, 167–169]). Thus, HMGB1 levels are elevated in patients with sepsis and/or DIC, and extracellular HMGB1 was found to stimulate TF expression on monocytes, inhibit protein C activation, and promote microvascular thrombosis development [170, 171]. Moreover, other DAMPs such as histones and extracellular DNA involved in NETosis formation are suggested to mediate immunothrombosis in DIC (for NETosis, see Vol. 1 [4], Part V, Sect. 19.3.6). Mechanistically, DAMPs (like MAMPs) were demonstrated to trigger TF expression on NET release by neutrophils, promoting immunothrombosis [172–174]. Although TF-mediated and NET-mediated immunothrombosis play a role in early host defense against bacterial dissemination, uncontrolled immunothrombosis may lead to DIC. As known, Factor VII (FVII) can bind to TF. Tissue factor subsequently facilitates the activation of FVII into activated FVII (FVIIa), thereby initiating the extrinsic coagulation pathway followed by the activation of FX and thrombin formation.

Pathophysiology of Burn Injury

Thermal injury following burns—like traumatic events in all insulted tissues—is also typically associated with a pronounced innate immune inflammatory response that, in its most severe form, can typically develop into a SIRS, acute respiratory distress syndrome (ARDS) and/or MOF [175–178]. The complex pathophysiological mechanisms operating in burn injury have recently been reviewed [179, 180]. Current notions hold that burn wounds include three zones of injury: zone of coagulation, zone of stasis, and zone of hyperemia [181]. The region of coagulation represents necrotic tissue that was damaged at the time of injury. As outlined elsewhere [182], this area is surrounded by a zone of stasis, with inflammation and low levels of perfusion. Outside the zone of stasis is a zone of hyperemia, where microvascular perfusion is not impaired. Often, the area of stasis will progress and become necrotic within the first 48 h following thermal injury. As a result, the initial burn expands in area and depth.

The initial phase in burn injury is dominated by the formation of ROS and RNS and secretion/release of proinflammatory cytokines such as TNF and IL-6, mainly produced by macrophages [183–185]. For example, in a murine burn injury model, TNF levels were shown to be increased as early as 3 h postburn and remained elevated up to 24 h. The IL-6 level was also significantly increased at the early time point of 3 h post-injury and was demonstrated to be further elevated by 24 h after burns as compared with that of sham mice. At 3 and 7 days post-injury, all cytokine levels had returned to normal or were not detectable [186].

Besides others, these inflammatory mediators, along with the increase of vascular hydrostatic pressure caused by vessel dilation, are the major reasons for systemic microvascular leakage observed in burns. Furthermore, severe epidermal burn injury often triggers significant apoptotic cell death. Also, as discussed elsewhere

[187], ACD and RN, such as necroptosis, can be assumed to occur in severe burn injuries, though not thoroughly investigated so far. Typically, during this early stage, severe burn injury may also lead to SIRS and MOF (reviewed in [180]).

8.3.2.3 Compensatory Antiinflammatory Response Syndrome

As briefly introduced above, the clinical manifestation of severe multiple tissue injury, including burn damage, is characterized by pathognomonic overlapping innate immune responses. The above sketched systemic cytokine/chemokine-induced hyperinflammatory response resulting in SIRS is followed—before it ends (!)—by an intense and long-lasting CARS associated with posttraumatic immunosuppression that predisposes patients to infectious sepsis and MOF [151–153, 183, 185]. For example, in a murine burn injury model, IL-10 levels were significantly increased at the early time point of 3 h post-injury and were observed to be further elevated by 24 h after burns as compared with that of sham mice [186]. Of note, accumulating evidence suggests that this greatly feared complication associated with high susceptibility of the patient to secondary bacterial, fungal, and viral infection is mediated by suppressing Class IIIC–DAMPs, that is, SAMPs which control homeostasis following injury (compare Table 3.1, and for additional information see Vol. 1 [4], Part IV, Sect. 14.4, p. 330, and Sect. 3.5.5).

8.3.2.4 Concluding Remarks

Remarkably, the new insights into the contribution of DAMPs and SAMPs to the sepsis-like inflammation and immune paralysis-like states observed in severely injured patients may be helpful in further specifying the clinical picture presented by a polytrauma. Starting with the definition of SIRS and CARS and proceeding to the terms *mixed antagonist response syndrome* (MARS) and *persistent inflammation, immunosuppression, and catabolism syndrome* (PICS), the role of these injury-induced activating and suppressing molecules marks the preliminary endpoint of this exciting development. Thus, in the following, a closer look is taken at these two—obviously dissonant—scenarios, whereby the potential action of DAMPs and tentative role of SAMPs in the two phases are highlighted.

8.3.3 DAMP-Triggered Hyperinflammatory Pathways in Polytrauma

8.3.3.1 General Remarks

The crucial role of DAMPs in the pathology of severe trauma has already been addressed above. Traumatic conditions can be provoked during various scenarios, including:

1. Mechanical trauma to any portion of the body from a blow, crush, penetrating wound, or surgical procedures, that is, complications which are usually related to fracture, hemorrhage, and infection

2. Thermal trauma, that is, any tissue insult due to the application of heat in any form to the external or internal body surfaces
3. Metabolic trauma such as promoted by IRI, acidosis and hypoxia/hypoxemia

All these dangerous scenarios can result in a critical care illness, a life-threatening disorder associated with excessive release of DAMPs.

Theoretically, in polytrauma, all subclasses of constitutive and inducible DAMPs may be induced by traumatic cell stress/tissue injury, but IA-1 and IA-2 DAMPs released from necrotic cells undergoing ACD and/or RCD, as well as inducible DAMPs actively secreted/released from stressed or dying cells, can be regarded as the critical danger signals (defined in Vol. 1 [4], Part IV, Chaps. 12–14). Accordingly, these DAMPs trigger various PRMs including inflammasome-activating receptors such as NLRP3 to promote innate immune effector responses, for example, proinflammatory and antiinflammatory processes (for a narrative description of PRMs and their triggered effector pathways, see Vol. 1 [4], Part II and Part VI, Chaps. 22–24). Some of those trauma-induced DAMPs have already been detected and are briefly described here.

8.3.3.2 High Mobility Group Box I, Heat Shock Proteins, and S100 Proteins

As could be expected, the well-known "classical" DAMPs such as HMGB1, HSPs, and S100 proteins have been measured in critically ill patients as well as in experimental trauma models. Indeed, their future use as diagnostic/prognostic markers and therapeutic targets represents an attractive goal of research. In the following, a brief overview of observational human studies and animal intervention studies relevant to intensive care-related conditions is neatly provided.

High Mobility Group Box I

Early animal studies had already revealed a role of the HMGB1→TLR4 pathway in the initiation of systemic inflammation and end-organ injury following isolated peripheral tissue injury [188]. Additionally, other sets of studies on a murine hemorrhagic shock model could demonstrate that treatment with anti-HMGB1 antibody improved survival at 24 h after hemorrhagic shock, suggesting that anti-HMGB1 antibodies might be used as a therapeutic to ameliorate the morbidity of hemorrhagic shock in trauma patient [189]. In subsequent experiments on a hemorrhagic shock/resuscitation (HS/R) model in mice, HMGB1 levels in the lungs, liver, and serum were observed to be increased as early as 2 h after HS/R [190]. Further, in a murine burn injury model, HMGB1 levels were shown to be elevated ~tenfold at 24 h after injury but at no other times after injury [186]. In subsequent clinical studies in severe trauma patients, HMGB1 was found to be systemically released within 30–60 min, peaking 2 to 6 h after injury (for release and secretion of HMGB1 and its cognate PRMs, see Vol. 1 [4], Part IV, Sects. 12.2.2 and 14.3.3). Remarkably, patients who develop organ dysfunction and nonsurvivors of severe trauma have reportedly very high levels of this IA-1 DAMP. Moreover, HMGB1 levels were found to be predictive of the outcome of traumatic lesions, as shown, for example, in patients with TBI [191–193] (see also below). Interestingly, in this context, in patients with acute liver failure due to severe liver cell injury from a variety of causes, high concentrations of circulating HMGB1—together with histones—were found to contribute to SIRS associated with MOF [194].

Furthermore, as also sketched in Vol. 1 [4], Part IV, Sect. 12.2.2.5 and Fig. 12.2, the variations of redox conditions influence HMGB1 activity. During severe trauma, excessive production of ROS enhances oxidative stress and leads to multiple redox reactions, thereby promoting the proinflammatory function of HMGB1 [195]. On the other hand, the reduced form rather enhances chemotactic signaling.

Heat Shock Proteins

So far, only a few studies have investigated the relation of HSPs to trauma-induced tissue damage (reviewed in [196]). In an early clinical study conducted in 2001—at a time when the term "DAMPs" was not even borne—the expression of HSPs, that is, HSP27, HSP60, HSP70, and HSP90 in PBMCs of septic trauma patients, was found to be significantly increased compared to healthy volunteers [197]. In a subsequent clinical study on severely traumatized patients, HSP72 was already detected in the serum within 30 min after injury [198]. The authors observed that elevated initial serum levels of HSP72 are associated with survival after severe trauma, but are not related to the incidence or severity of the post-injury inflammatory response or organ dysfunction (for release and secretion of HSPs, see Vol. 1 [4], Part IV, Sects. 12.2.3 and 14.2.2.2). Other earlier studies also reported HSPs to be released into the extracellular compartment after trauma [199, 200]. More recently, Timmermans et al. [201] resumed the measurement of HSPs in trauma patients and found that plasma levels of HSP70 were profoundly increased immediately following trauma and remained elevated for 10 days. Notably, the authors noticed that HSP70 (as nuclear DNA and S100 protein) was associated with a suppressed state of the immune system, a puzzle that is discussed in Sect. 8.3.5.

S100A Proteins

Only a few reports are available, demonstrating the role of S100A proteins in severe trauma. In a clinical study on polytrauma and burn trauma patients, serum concentrations of S100A8 and S100A9 proteins were found to be increased in a biphasic manner with the early peak at initial presentation representing the innate response to injury [202] (for release and secretion of S100A proteins, see Vol. 1 [4], Part IV, Sects. 12.2.4.2 and 14.2.2.4). Notably, the investigators observed that survivors showed significantly lower S100A8 and S100A9 concentrations than non-survivors. Also, in a study on human trauma victims, human blunt trauma survivors were seen to produce higher levels of S100A8/S100A9 than non-survivors, and a preliminary screen suggested that IFN-γ-inducible protein 10 (CXCL10) was significantly increased in monocytes/macrophages stimulated with S100A8/S100A9 [203]. Thus, like HSP70, S100A8/S100A9 DAMPs appear to exert a protective role after trauma.

8.3.3.3 Mitochondria-Derived DAMPs

During severe trauma associated with ACD and/or forms of RN, not only HMGB1, HSPs, and S100A proteins but also other DAMPs derived from the nucleus and, most importantly, from the mitochondria are locally released and can enter the bloodstream to become systemically distributed (reviewed in [20, 204, 205]). This category of DAMPs mainly includes circular DNA strands containing CpG DNA repeats, N-formylated peptides, and mtDNA itself.

Mitochondrial DNA

Of note, in extensive trauma, increasing attention has been devoted to the crucial role of DAMPs originating from mitochondria which are evolutionarily derived from bacteria (comprehensively reviewed by Hauser and Ottenbein in [5], also mentioned in [204, 206, 207]). These DAMPs have been detected in the form of mtDNA fragments, mtDNA in microparticles/vesicles (compare Sect. 3.5.3.2), and cell-free mitochondria.

Mitochondrial DNA, which has been best investigated DAMP so far, triggers the activation of multiple PRMs, including TLR9-, NLRP3-, and cGAS→STING-triggered pathways (for additional information compare Vol. 1 [4], Part VI, Sects. 22.3.3.3, p. 492 and 22.3.7.3, p. 507). Intriguingly, the plasma levels of DNA were observed to increase parallel to the severity of the trauma, and clinical studies in massively injured human subjects provided the first observational evidence that plasma mtDNA are associated—mainly via activation of PMNs—with the evolution of SIRS, MOF, and mortality [208, 209]. One of the most interesting reported findings was that a determination of mtDNA levels made within 8 h of hospital admission allowed differentiation between survivors and non-survivors [208].

Interestingly, in earlier studies, it has already been found that mtDNA, observed to activate neutrophils directly in terms of a IA-1 DAMP, is *extracellularly* released not only during polytrauma but also under various traumatic conditions including hemorrhagic shock and severe TBI (for TBI, see Sect. 9.2) [210, 211]). The extracellular release of mtDNA could also strikingly be documented in SIRS patients with AKI when the investigators found this DAMP in the urine of the patients and could observe that its concentration correlated with severity of renal dysfunction [212]. On the other hand, when mtDNA is released *within* cells, for example, in the course of stress-induced mitochondrial dysfunction, it may act as a IIC-2 DAMP to activate the cGAS→STING pathway leading to increased expression of type I IFNs operating as inducible DAMPs (for additional information compare Vol. 1 [4], Part VI, Sect. 22.3.7, p. 505, and Fig. 22.8, p. 508). Moreover, as further outlined [5], mtDNA can also be released passively along with mitochondria during cell death, actively either emitted in exosomes or extruded from neutrophils in the production of NETs. Notably, in all situation of passive release into the extracellular environment, mtDNA is taken up by phagocytosing innate immune cells to be recognized by TLR9 located at the endosomal membrane (for additional information see Vol. 1 [4], Part VI, Sect. 22.3.3.3, p. 492, and Fig. 22.4, p. 490). Also, when mtDNA is intracellularly released into the cytosol, it can activate the NLRP3 inflammasome that in turn recruits and activates caspase-1 to resulting in GSDMD pore-induced pyroptosis associated with release of IL-1β acting as an inducible DAMP [213] (for NLRP3 inflammasome, see Sect. 2.2.5.3 and Fig. 2.1; for additional information see Vol. 1 [4], Part VI, Sect. 22.4.2.2, p. 516, and Fig. 22.11, p. 517; for additional information about GSDMD pore-induced pyroptosis, compare Vol. 1 [4], Part V, Sect. 19.3.4.2, p. 447, and Fig. 19.7, p. 448).

Also worthwhile to mention here are studies showing that mtDNA and ROS—in terms of a cross talk—are often released from damaged mitochondria together to form oxidized mtDNA [214–216]. In turn, oxidized mtDNA has been shown to activate the NLRP3 inflammasome [217], now known to be associated with the release of IL-1β and constitutive DAMPs from pyroptotic cells.

Other Mitochondria-Derived DAMPs: Formyl Peptides, Heme, and Cytochrome C

Other mitochondria-derived DAMPs include mitochondrial formyl peptides (mtFPs), heme, and cytochrome C (Cyt C) (also reviewed by Hauser and Otterbein in [5]). Of the > thousands of proteins in mitochondria, only 13 mtFPs are actually synthesized in the mitochondria, with all these hydrophobic peptides beginning with N-formylmethionine (fMet). The fMet is a derivative of the amino acid methionine in which a formyl group has been added to the amino group) (reviewed in [218, 219]). Mitochondrial formyl peptides, operating as IA-1 DAMPs are recognized by FPRs, which—as described in Vol. 1 [4], Part II, Sect. 5.3.5.3, and Part IV, Sect.12.2.4.6—belong to the family of GPCRs (for review see [220]; also compare Sect. 2.3.4.5). A few such peptides (i.e., five) released in the systemic circulation after clinical trauma were found to have inflammatory activities and to attract PMNs to trauma sites while suppressing PMN responses to other chemoattractants [221].

Heme—a tetrapyrrole containing a central iron ion and synthesized in the mitochondria—is a versatile signaling molecule controlling the activities of diverse regulators ranging from transcription factors to MAP kinases [222] (for heme as a IA-1 DAMP, see also Vol. 1 [4], Part IV, Sect. 12.2.4.8). Upon severe trauma, this DAMP was shown to bind to TLR4 and trigger several downstream stress response pathways and was suggested to play a central role in the pathogenesis of severe sepsis [223].

Finally, Cyt C—a IA-1 DAMP as described in Vol. 1 [4], Part IV, Sect. 12.2.4.6—is also released from dying cells during cellular trauma and can act as a danger signal in the extracellular space. For example, in experiments on rabbits, oxidative injury to mitochondria was demonstrated to be associated with high mitochondrial expression of Cyt C [224]. In studies on a burn model in mice, circulating Cyt C levels were found to be elevated eightfold as early as 3 h post-injury and remained elevated at 24 h. At 3 days post-injury, they returned to sham levels [186] (see also below).

8.3.3.4 Histones

Another critical member of IA-1 DAMPs refers to the circulating extracellular histones, which reportedly act as clinically relevant mediators of multiple organ injuries [225, 226]. As briefly outlined in Vol. 1 [4], Part IV, Sect. 12.2.4.4, histones and nucleosomes are critical nuclear proteins that contribute to the structural organization and stability of chromatin (for histones and nucleosomes, also compare Fig. 5.4 in Sect. 5.6.2.2). When released from dying cells (succumbing to ACD or RCD such as NETosis) into the extracellular space, histones (free histones), DNA-bound histones (nucleosomes), or part of NETs, have been recognized as candidates of the DAMP family, and as such all three can be detected in serum after significant cellular death such as occurring in infective or sterile SIRS. Besides their immunostimulatory capacities in inducing TLR2- and TLR4-mediated inflammatory responses, extracellular histones were shown to cause direct TLR-independent cytotoxicity to epithelial and endothelial tissue. In fact, histones were found to elicit—in terms of two progressive stages—primary injury on ECs via charge interaction, resulting in the release of another wave of DAMPs which induce secondary tissue injuries [225–228]. The exact mechanism of this unique cytotoxic effect is not entirely clear. However, current theories suggest that extracellular histone binds to phospholipid–phosphodiester bonds, similar to their DNA-binding sites, an effect that alters membrane permeability and instigates calcium ion influx (reviewed in [226]). As such, extracellular histones have a central role in necroinflammation [229].

Due to their proinflammatory and cytotoxic effects, extracellular histones have been shown to contribute to excessive and overwhelming cell damage and death, thus contributing to the pathogenesis of both sepsis and ARDS, which may be associated with MOF [230]. Of note, together with HMGB1, histones were recently shown to play a significant role in inducing SIRS and MOF in acute liver failure [194].

8.3.3.5 Complement Fragments (C3a, C5a) and Neoantigens

Expectedly, the humoral part of the innate immune system, which is likely to be induced by class IIB-1 DAMPs in terms of injury-induced neoantigens and other DAMPs such as fragments of the complement system, is activated immediately after trauma as well. Activation of complement in trauma patients has been verified by detection of elevated plasma C3a, C5a (i.e., inducible IIIB-3 DAMPs) and C5b-9 levels which correlate with disease severity (for further reading, see [144, 161, 231–236]).

8.3.3.6 Concluding Remarks

The list of DAMPs involved in severe trauma as addressed here is certainly not complete and will be extended soon (also reviewed by Relja et al. [237] and Relja and Land [154]). Importantly, however, all of these injury-promoted pathways are supposed to converge into release of large amounts of DAMPs, that is, "an avalanche" of DAMPs leading to the well-known sterile hyperinflammatory state associated with SIRS and potential MOF. At this point, it should be already noted that the emission of large amounts of DAMPs as observed in the hyperinflammatory phase overlaps the nearly concomitantly running SAMP-promoting hyperresolving phase characterized by increased susceptibility of patients to infections. In other words, DAMPs can still be measured in the hyperresolution phase when patients are already prone to infections (more of this obviously puzzling finding in Sect. 8.3.5).

8.3.4 SAMP-Triggered Posttraumatic Antiinflammatory/Proresolving and Immunosuppressive Processes

8.3.4.1 General Remarks

Intensive care clinicians are well aware of the phenomenon that severe trauma does not only elicit a SIRS but most often also results in the subsequent development of a so-called immunoparalysis or immunosuppression phase, rendering patients in the ICU prone to secondary infections. In fact, this dangerous phase after severe sepsis remains the leading cause of mortality [26]. Indeed, more patients die in the immunosuppression phase where the risk of a secondary infection increases (for reviews, see [153, 201, 205, 238, 239]). Notably, a considerable number of studies provided evidence for the development of a post-trauma immunosuppressive state. For example, antigen-presenting DCs were found to acquire reduced responsiveness to bacterial components within few hours after trauma hemorrhage [240]. In this murine study, these "professionals" among APCs were found to secrete reduced levels of TNF and IL-12 upon stimulation with LPS and to be less potent in inducing T-cell proliferation in comparison to DCs from sham mice. This observation was associated with decreased expression of MHC-II and IFN-γ. The phenomenon of decreased expression of MHC-II molecules/HLA-DR appears to be a typical feature of immunosuppression in polytraumatic patients as well [241] (for MHC-II molecules, also compare Vol. 1 [4], Part VIII, Sects. 31.3.4.1, 31.3.4.2, and 31.3.6). In fact, modern notions now hold that, in infectious/sterile injury-induced sepsis, both proinflammatory and hypoinflammatory/immunosuppressive responses occur early and nearly simultaneously, although the net initial effect of these competing processes is typically manifested by an early dominant hyperinflammatory phase characterized by shock, fever, and hypermetabolism (Fig. 8.1) (also compare [242–244]).

Accordingly, antiinflammatory/proresolving therapy could theoretically improve the survival rate of polytraumatized patients in the early hyperinflammatory status, while it may be deleterious if applied subsequently during the trauma-induced immunosuppressive phase [245]. Mechanistically, current notions hold that a posttraumatic immunosuppressive response—besides the action of innate immune-mediated antiinflammatory cytokines such as IL-10 and IL-4 and TGF-β—involves a shift away from adaptive immune Th1 responses toward Th2 responses [246, 247]. Moreover, in severe postburn injury, growing supportive evidence reportedly suggests an immunopathogenic role of Th2, Th17 cells, and γδT cells [185, 248–250]. Also, as observed in septic shock patients, increased levels of circulating Tregs have been described, appearing immediately after the onset of sepsis but persisting only in those septic patients who subsequently died [251] (also compare Fig. 5.1). These results were further extended and modified by demonstrating that this relative increase is due to a decrease in effector T-cell numbers rather than changes in absolute numbers of Tregs [252] (for Th1, Th2, Th17 cells, see Vol. 1 [4], Part VIII, Sect. 32.4; for Tregs Sect. 33.4; for γδT cells, Part VII, Sect. 28.4).

Interestingly, more recent studies on sera from septic patients have suggested a new mechanism through which sepsis may mediate immunoparalysis. Thus, sera from septic patients were found to suppress IL-1β production in macrophages stimulated with eATP, likely by antagonizing upstream NLRP3 or proinflammatory pathways [253]. This suppressive effect peaked on day 3 after admission and persisted until day 7 among patients who did not survive but was lost by day 7 among patients who survived.

Together, this scenario of post-trauma (innate immune) antiinflammatory/proresolving and (adaptive immune) immunosuppressive processes is not a surprising one for DAMP researchers because—as outlined in Vol. 1 [4] Part IV, Sect. 14.4, and in Sect. 5.3.3—accumulating evidence now indicates that, besides activating DAMPs (i.e., agonists), suppressing DAMPs, that is, SAMPs (i.e., antagonists) are emitted upon stress and injury, which, in parallel to proinflammatory responses, convey antiinflammatory and proresolving processes, as well as shape immunosuppressive responses aimed at maintaining tissue homeostasis.

8.3.4.2 The Model of Uncontrolled Overshooting Generation of SAMPs

In polytrauma, there is tentative (still unproven) evidence of a model suggesting that simultaneously or somewhat retardedly with uncontrolled overshooting emission of proinflammatory DAMPs in excess (resulting in hyperinflammatory SIRS and MOF), uncontrolled overshooting generation/emission of SAMPs (i.e., class IIIC DAMPs) in excess takes place.

These counterbalancing "suppressing molecules" are supposed to lead to exaggerated and long-lasting CARS associated with a stage of immunosuppression—still aimed at maintaining tissue homeostasis (Fig. 8.1). Regarding such a scenario, one may discuss that the desperate attempt of the innate immune defense system to reach homeostasis via emission of SAMPs in case of severe injury-induced SIRS tragically ends up with the counterregulating creation of an overshooting antiinflammatory/proresolving and immunosuppressive milieu rendering the patient susceptible to secondary life-threatening, often lethal infections. Indeed, there are already some first reports in the international literature dedicated to this hot topic.

As already briefly mentioned in Sect. 3.5.5, and here resumed, as SAMPs, particular molecules such as PGE2, cAMP, extracellular adenosine, AnxA1, and, most importantly, SPMs have been identified (for additional information also compare Vol. 1 [4], Part IV, Sect. 14.4, p. 330). Regarding the effects of SAMPs, antiinflammatory and proresolving properties have to be distinguished (also compare Sect. 7.3.2). The different meanings are stressed by Levy and Serhan [254]: "Antiinflammatory actions decrease granulocyte recruitment and activation, resulting in a predisposition to infection... Mediators with antiinflammatory properties lead to decreased leukocyte: endothelial cell interactions, platelet aggregation, vascular permeability and leukocyte generation of reactive oxygen species. In sharp contrast, proresolving actions activate tissue-resident cells to decrease vascular and tissue inflammation to restore organ function—a process termed catabasis to represent a return from the battle of inflammation…. Mediators with proresolving properties stimulate endothelial nitric oxide and prostacyclin release, mucosal epithelial expression of anti-microbial peptides and macrophage phagocytosis, including efferocytosis, microbial clearance, removal of cellular debris and noxious stimuli (e.g., antigen) and their cellular efflux to lymph nodes. These 'proresolving' actions increase tissue host defense either directly or indirectly via restoration of tissue homeostasis."

8.3.4.3 Prostaglandin E2

Prostaglandin E2 is an endogenous lipid mediator produced from the metabolism of AA. The various biological functions governed by PGE2 are mediated through its four distinct prostaglandin E receptors (EPs), designated as EP1, EP2, EP3, and EP4. The lipid mediator is generated during the onset phase of inflammation and mediates antiinflammation/proresolution effects during the late stage of inflammation [255] (for PGE2, also see Vol. 1 [4] Part IV, Sect. 14.4.2.2). Upon generation, PGE2 is then inactivated via an oxidation reaction catalyzed by NAD^+-dependent *15-hydroxyprostaglandin dehydrogenase* to generate 15k-PGE2 [256].

Of note, Flohé et al. [17], in 2008, emphasized already the potential role of PGE2 in posttraumatic hypoinflammation/immunosuppression by quoting studies performed by Ertel et al. [257], reporting on the detection of PGE2 in the circulation after hemorrhage. In fact, the authors of this study had demonstrated that PGE2 is directly involved in the suppression of different macrophage functions after hemorrhage. They wrote: "In vivo blockade of PGE2 production by ibuprofen following hemorrhage significantly improved macrophage functions and did not affect the hemodynamic response to resuscitation. Therefore the cyclooxygenase inhibitor ibuprofen represents a safe and potent agent in the therapy of hemorrhage-induced immunosuppression " [257]. Notably, some years before, Faist et al. [258] had reported on high PGE2 levels found in patients with major trauma and peaked on days 5 and 7 post-trauma. Interestingly, the authors already suggested that the suppression of IL-2 synthesis post-trauma is partially caused by this excessive PGE2 output. These early clinical findings could experimentally be confirmed by data from a study in an animal model of MOF in rabbits, suggesting that an excessive generation and release of PGE2 may be involved in the pathogenesis of immunosuppression and MOF following hemorrhage and resuscitation [259].

More recently performed studies on experimental sepsis models confirmed these early clinical and experimental observations showing that the production of PGE2 is involved in severe sepsis-induced immunosuppression [185, 260–262]. In one such experimental series [260], ketoprofen treatment was found to inhibit PGE2 production, thereby qualifying this agent as an attractive target to prevent secondary infections in immunocompromised septic patients. In another model of sepsis-induced AKI in mice [261], tenuigenin, a natural product isolated from *Polygala tenuifolia* root, was also found to inhibit the production PGE2. In more recent experiments, targeting the 15-keto-PGE2- prostaglandin reductase 2 (PTGR2) axis was demonstrated to mitigate systemic inflammation and improve survival of septic mice (15-keto-PGE2 is a PGE2 metabolite, whose further processing is catalyzed by PTGR2).

8.3.4.4 Annexin A1

The SAMP AnxA1 has briefly been outlined in Vol. 1 [4], Part IV, Sect. 14.4.3. To repeat, within peripheral blood cells, under homeostatic conditions, AnxA1 is mainly expressed and stored in subcellular granules of neutrophils, eosinophils, and monocytes, with small amounts expressed in specific subsets of lymphocytes. In activated or apoptotic cells [263, 264], AnxA1 is released from its storage site and translocates to the membrane, where—as a leaderless protein like members of the IL-1 family—it is secreted via different unconventional secretory pathways (for unconventional pathways, also see Vol. 1 [4], Part IV, Sect. 11.2.4.3). The biological actions of this antiinflammatory, proresolving, and immunosuppressive molecule—like most SPMs—are mediated though the ALX/FPR2 receptor. As outlined in Sect. 2.3.4.5, and Vol. 1 [4], Part II, Sect. 5.3.5.3, the FPRs are GPCRs that usually transduce chemotactic signals mainly in phagocytes. The FPR2 receptor is shared by a variety of other DAMPs, mediating diverse biological functions of relevance for host innate immune defense.

Although the level of AnxA1 in the peripheral blood of polytraumatized patients has not been determined, some data from critically ill patients suffering from infectious sepsis are available. Thus, in a Chinese study on a relatively small number of sepsis patients, the AnxA1 level was found to be elevated in 56% of patients over the 7-day observation period. However, the daily levels of the patients over time were not significantly different from the levels of the control individuals [265]. The authors discussed that the observed elevation of AnxA1 level in their patients is likely due to the release of AnxA1—in either free form or wrapped in microparticles—by activated neutrophils or monocytes/macrophages in response to the infectious insults as reported from other studies [264, 266–268].

Nevertheless, though the data is still sparse, an immunosuppressive effect of this SAMP is understandable as AnxA1 has been proposed to interact with GATA-protein binding 3 (GATA3) to influence T-cell differentiation in $CD4^+$ T cells [269] (Fig. 8.2) (for GATA3, compare Vol. 1 [4], Part VIII, Sect. 32.4.4, and Fig. 32.4). Of interest in this context to mention is that, in a murine model of endotoxemia, AnxA1 and FPR2 were demonstrated to have a critical role in the manifestation of adrenal insufficiency known to contribute to morbidity and mortality in a high proportion of patients with sepsis [270].

8.3.4.5 Adenosine

The function of intracellular cAMP and extracellular adenosine as inducible SAMPs has been cursorily outlined in Sects. 3.5.5.3 and 3.5.5.4. Here, their role in critically ill patients is briefly touched.

Intense studies on the role of cAMP in sepsis are sparse. Interestingly, however, in a survey of effects of the SPM MaR1 on mitochondrial function in experimentally induced sepsis in mice and sepsis patients, cAMP concentration was observed to be upregulated by treatment with MaR1, with the outcome of decreased lung injury in septic mice [271]. In these studies, the investigators could demonstrate that MaR1 protects the experimentally induced sepsis in vivo and in vitro and sepsis patients through the ALX→ cAMP→ ROS pathway. Furthermore, the studies also showed that MaR1 induces increases in the levels of cAMP, suggesting that the beneficial MaR1 response is associated with an action of cAMP.

In other lines of studies reviewed by Vourc'h et al. [205], extracellular adenosine was shown to promote protective Th2 immunity, a critical component of posttraumatic immunosuppression observed in CARS. Indeed, when binding to GPCR, extracellular adenosine is suggested to activate DCs to promote the production of

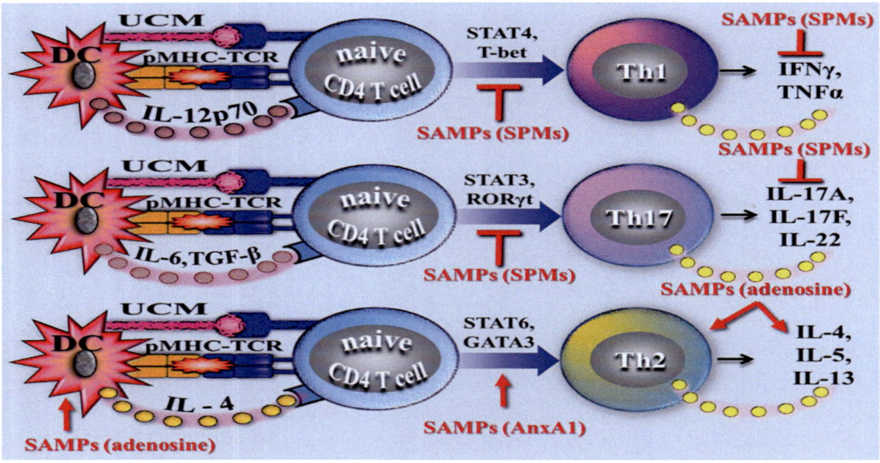

Fig. 8.2 Schematic diagram of a model illustrating the role of SAMPs in suppressing destructive Th1 and Th17 adaptive immune responses but promoting a protective Th2 response. SPMs in their function as SAMPs reduce lineage-specific cytokine production by activated Th1 (i.e., IFN-γ) and Th17 cells (i.e., IL-17) by downregulating their signature transcription factors T-bet and RORγt. By contrast, adenosine in its function as a SAMP is suggested to activate DCs to promote the production of the antiinflammatory cytokines IL-4 by Th2 cells, and AnxA1 has been proposed to interact with the transcription factor GATA3 to influence T-cell differentiation in CD4+ T cells. Note: The figure corresponds to Fig. 32.4 in Vol. 1 [4], Part VIII, Sect. 32.4. *DC* dendritic cell, *GATA3* GATA-protein binding 3, *IFNγ* interferon gamma, *IL* interleukin, *pMHC* peptide/major histocompatibility complex molecule, *RORγt* retinoic acid receptor-related orphan receptor gamma t, *STAT* signal transducer and activator of transcription, *TCR* T-cell receptor, *TGF-β* transforming growth factor-beta, *TNF* tumor necrosis factor, *UCM* up-regulated costimulatory molecules. (Sources: [205, 269, 272, 274, 275])

the antiinflammatory cytokines IL-4 and IL-13 by CD4+ Th2 cells (Fig. 8.2). The findings were supported by other lines of studies on a model of worm infection in mice [272], suggesting that A2AAR initiates a protective Th2 immune response. In this model, A2AAR was found to induce expression of IL-33, which subsequently triggered ILC2 and Th2 cell activation and production of IL-4 and IL-13, that is, cytokines which are known to participate in posttraumatic immunosuppression (here, IL-33 is denoted as an inducible SAMP, for IL-33 acting as a DAMP, see also Sect. 3.5.6.3 and Vol. 1 [4], Part IV, Sect. 14.2.4.2; for ILC2, see Vol. 1 [4], Part III, Sect. 8.4.2.2).

8.3.4.6 Specialized Proresolving Mediators Involved in Posttraumatic Immunosuppression

Of note, as reported by Dalli et al. [273], the lipid mediator profiles in human septic patients are correlated with outcome. Intriguingly, in sepsis non-survivors, the authors found significantly higher inflammation-initiating mediators, including prostaglandin F2α (PGF2α) and chemoattractant LTB4 (= an inducible DAMP, see Sect. 3.5.3.3), and SPMs including RvE1, RvD5, and 17R-PdD1 than was observed in surviving sepsis subjects. This signature was present at ICU admission and persisted for 7 days. Further analysis revealed an increased respiratory failure in non-survivors. Higher inflammation-initiating mediators (including PGF2α) and selected proresolving pathways were associated with the development of ARDS, while other traditional clinical indices were not predictive of ARDS development. Since the primary objective of this study was not to correlate SPMs levels with infections, a possible immunosuppressive effect was not investigated.

On the other hand, first evidence from other lines of studies has already been published reporting an effect of several SPMs in shaping, that is, suppressing adaptive immune responses. As previously mentioned in Sect. 3.5.5.5, in a series of in vitro experiments performed by Chiurchiu et al. [274], the SPMs RvD1, RvD2, and MaR1 were shown to modulate adaptive immune responses in human peripheral blood lymphocytes (see also review by Duffney et al. [275]). For example, the SPMs reportedly regulate DC activation markers, including suppression of cytokine production and expression of MHC molecules and costimulatory markers that promote a return to homeostasis following an acute inflammatory response. Moreover, these lipid mediators were found to sharply reduce lineage-specific cytokine production by activated $CD4^+$ Th1 (i.e., IFN-γ) and $CD4^+$ Th17 cells (i.e., IL-17) as well as $CD8^+$ T cells (i.e., TNF, IFN-γ), but not to modulate T-cell inhibitory receptors (e.g., PD-1 and CTLA-4) or abrogate their capacity to proliferate (for PD-1 and CTLA-4, compare Vol. 1 [4], Part VIII, Sect. 33.3.5 and Fig. 33.3). Further targeted in vitro experiments revealed that the tested SPMs can prevent naïve $CD4^+$ T-cell differentiation into Th1 and Th17 by downregulating their signature transcription factors, T-bet and RORγt [274] (see Fig. 8.2; for these transcription factors, for additional information see also Vol. 1 [4], Part VIII, Sect. 32.4, p. 765, and Fig. 32.4, p. 766). This mechanism was found to be mediated by members of the GPCR family, namely, GPR32 and ALX/FPR2 (for GPCRs and GPCR signaling, for additional information compare Vol. 1 [4], Part II, Sect. 5.3.5.3, p. 80, Fig. 5.11, p. 79, and Part VI, Sect. 22.3.10, p. 513). In these studies reported by Chiurchiu et al. [274], the authors could also show that SPMs—concomitantly with Th1 and Th17 downregulation—enhance de novo generation and function of iTregs via the GPR32 receptor (for additional information about iTregs, see Vol. 1 [4], Part VIII, Sect. 33.4.3.3, p. 813 and Fig. 33.4, p. 801). These findings are supported by another study on the property of the SPM MaR1 [276]. In these in vitro experiments, MaR1—together with TGF-β—was found to promote the generation of iTregs. Of note, these findings provide another explanation for the increased susceptibility to infections as observed in polytraumatized patients: bacteria or viruses, under the influence of SPMs, might induce bacterial or viral antigen-specific iTregs associated with immunotolerance of those pathogens.

8.3.4.7 Concluding Remarks: The Model of SAMP-Promoted Hyperresolution in CARS

Though the data from SAMPs involved in polytrauma is sparse and though the various suppressing molecules are not systemically investigated, there is preliminary evidence suggesting a role of this class of suppressing DAMPs in posttraumatic inflammation. Future more targeted studies, including clinical trials, should reveal whether or not such a model is of any value for developing SAMP-reducing therapeutic strategies.

8.3.5 The Puzzle of Increased Plasma Levels of DAMPs Associated with Post-Trauma Immunosuppression

8.3.5.1 General Remarks

In Vol. 1 [4], Part VI, Sect 22.2.5, I discussed: "Paradoxically, DAMP-induced robust innate immune responses in SIRS in terms of dysregulated overshooting hyperinflammation are *accompanied* by development of long-lasting immunosuppression in terms of dysregulated overshooting anti-inflammation/"over-resolving" inflammation. This event is logically associated with an increased susceptibility to infections and might be explained by DAMP-induced epigenetic modifications". In Fig. 22.1 (Vol. 1 [4], Part VI), the epigenetic programming ("e.g., M1 → M2 macrophages; AnxA1, PGE2, SPMs [others]) is ascribed to SAMPs (for additional information also compare Vol. 1 [4], Part VI, Sect. 24.2, p. 636).

However, science is moving fast, and, thus, in Chap. 5, in particular Sect. 5.4.3.3 and Figs. 5.1 and 5.2, this model has been a bit more specified by emphasizing that DAMP-promoted SIRS and SAMP-promoted CARS are now considered to occur nearly in parallel (that is, a new meaning of *accompanied*). As stressed above, there is only a slight delay between initial hyperinflammation and subsequent hyperresolution due to the production of SAMPs by already DAMP-activated PRM-bearing innate immune cells. Such a model may reasonably explain that DAMPs are still demonstrable and measurable in the SAMP-promoted hyperresolution phase characterized by increased susceptibility to infection (illustrated in Fig. 8.1). This said ahead, the reports on this topic are briefly quoted in the following.

8.3.5.2 First Report on a Role of DAMPs in Posttraumatic Immunosuppression

One of the first narrative reports on a possible role of DAMPs involved in posttraumatic immunosuppression was published by Timmermans et al. [201]. In 166 adult trauma patients, the authors determined circulating levels of DAMPs and cytokines and evaluated an immunosuppressive effect by determination of HLA–DRA gene expression and ex vivo LPS-stimulated cytokine production. The researchers found that plasma nDNA and HSP70 levels but not mtDNA were profoundly increased post-trauma immediately and remained elevated for 10 days. Further, plasma nDNA and HSP70 levels were shown to correlate negatively with HLA–DRA expression. Moreover, ex vivo cytokine production revealed an antiinflammatory phenotype already at the trauma scene that persisted in the following days, characterized by attenuated proinflammatory cytokines TNF and IL-6, and increased antiinflammatory IL-10 production. Notably, higher concentrations of nDNA and a further decrease of HLA–DRA expression was observed to be associated with infections. Intriguingly, by interpreting their clinical findings, the authors [201] concluded "that trauma results in release of DAMPs and that this is associated with an acute predominantly antiinflammatory response and a suppressed state of the immune system. In trauma patients, these events take place already before hospital admission, and the observed immune suppressed state is not preceded or accompanied by a pronounced proinflammatory phase. Aggravated immune suppression, as indicated by further decrease of HLA-DRA expression, is associated with the development of nosocomial infections in this patient population".

8.3.5.3 Recent Findings on Increased Plasma Levels of DAMPs Associated with Immunosuppression

The findings published by Timmermans et al. [201] were supported by recent studies on patients undergoing cytoreductive surgery (CRS) combined with hyperthermic intraperitoneal chemotherapy (HIPEC) [277]. The investigators found plasma levels of DAMPs (HSP70, HMGB1, S100A8/S100A9, S100A12, and nDNA) to be profoundly increased following this therapeutic maneuver. Evidence of immune suppression was observed to be already apparent during the procedure, illustrated by a decrease of HLA–DR expression. The authors concluded that CRS–HIPEC is associated with profound DAMP release and immune suppression. In this context, that is, in a recent review on inflammasomes in tissue damages and immune disorders after trauma, a possible impairment of inflammasome functions as a component of trauma-induced immunosuppression is also discussed [163].

8.3.5.4 Concluding Remarks

The potential role of DAMPs and SAMPs in trauma-induced immunosuppression remains an essential issue in experimental and clinical trauma research because the clarification of their function will provide critical clues for future therapeutic strategies in polytrauma patients. Further studies in this burning research field should reveal whether trauma-induced immunosuppression is the work of SAMPs and/or certain DAMPs that may have acquired distinct "SAMP traits" (compare Sect. 3.5.6). Maybe, both, SAMPs and certain DAMPs, have to be determined to assess the overall risk and outcome for patients who have suffered trauma.

8.3.6 Résumé

There is growing evidence in support of the model that, in severe multiple trauma, massive numbers of dying cells lead to excessive emission of both constitutive and inducible DAMPs, which dominate the clinical picture of SIRS and MOF. In terms of a counterreaction—desperately but vainly aimed at reaching homeostasis—DAMP- activated innate immune cells, mainly macrophages and neutrophils, are suggested to produce excessive amounts of inducible suppressing DAMPs, that is, SAMPs to elicit anti-/hypoinflammatory immunosuppressive processes. Tragically, this attempt to restore homeostasis leads to increased susceptibility of polytraumatized patients to secondary life-threatening nosocomial infections. This designed scenario represents a considerable challenge for making a proper prognostic assessment that is crucial for the stratification of patients that are at high risk for post-trauma complications or adverse outcomes. Also, this scenario would call for effective therapeutic strategies that have to take into account the new paradigm of overlapping hyperinflammatory and hyperresolving responses (Fig. 8.1). One approach to tackle this complex scenario would be to measure continuously, from hospital admission onward, the ratio of the DAMP pattern/SAMP pattern and to determine the exact point of time when the (assumed) DAMP > SAMP ratio may shift to an (assumed) SAMP > DAMP ratio (compare Sect. 7.3.3).

As will be resumed below, this may be helpful in adjusting the therapeutic strategy to the actual innate immune state of the patient, that is, to block (1) DAMPs during the hyperinflammatory phase of the disease when a ratio of DAMPs > SAMPs is measured and (2) SAMPs during the hyperresolving period at the very moment, when there is a shift to the ratio of SAMPs > DAMPs.

However, this scenario of generation and emission of DAMPs and SAMPs is not an event restricted to severe multiple injuries leading to SIRS and MOF and CARS but is also encountered locally—though in moderate amounts—to provoke an acute isolated organ or soft tissue injury. Consequently, in the following Chap. 9, some classical acute organ injuries are briefly described.

8.4 DAMPs and SAMPs as Diagnostics, Prognostics, Therapeutics, and Therapeutic Targets in Dysregulated Wound Healing and Polytrauma

8.4.1 Introductory Remarks

Currently, the use of DAMPs and SAMPs as diagnostics and therapeutics in wound healing is a marginal theme and, therefore, not an important issue. However, one should not lose sight of this option. For example, in poorly healing wounds, local application of DAMPs might be an effective treatment. On the other hand, there is an increasing piece of evidence from recent literature strongly recommending the use of DAMPs (less SAMPs) as diagnostics and therapeutic targets in patients with severe traumatic diseases. Indeed, rapid risk stratification of patients with an acute systemic or organ-specific traumatic injury would allow making proper ad hoc management decisions and prognostications, followed by the development of straightforward therapeutic strategies. Some of those topics were already briefly or partly touched in the running text. Here, the literature concerned and currently available is briefly reviewed—knowing full well that this is just the beginning of the development of a new era of monitoring in traumatic diseases.

8.4.2 DAMPs and SAMPs as Diagnostic and Prognostic Biomarkers in Trauma Patients

8.4.2.1 General Remarks

In polytraumatized patients, DAMPs and SAMPs can be seen as the origins of both SIRS and CARS and are therefore promising targets as biomarkers for patient stratification and as therapeutic targets. Though still to assess as a model, the application of DAMPs and SAMPs as biomarkers can be expected to improve the speed of clinical decision-making, in particular, in designing and executing trauma-tailored and patient-individualized treatment strategies.

8.4.2.2 DAMPs as Biomarkers in Polytrauma

There are already first reports about clinical studies on the use of DAMPs as critical biomarkers in polytrauma. The overall objective of such studies was to explore and understand the association of early DAMP release in trauma with the development of MOF and its potential for therapeutic modulation. Accordingly, the focus of these studies was directed on the prognostic value of these injury-induced variables in predicting outcomes in traumatized patients, thereby allowing to develop strategies for the stratification of trauma patients into cohorts at risk for outcomes thought to be significant to early and late outcomes after injury. This type of stratification could be critically useful in the design of clinical trials targeting efferent innate immune pathways early after injury (also compare [278]).

High Mobility Group Box 1

In earlier studies on severe trauma in humans, HMGB1 was already found to be systemically released within 30–60 min, peaking 2 to 6 h after injury. Remarkably, patients who develop organ dysfunction and non-survivors of severe trauma were observed to have very high levels of this DAMP. Moreover, HMGB1 levels were found to be predictive of outcome of traumatic lesions, as shown, for example, in patients with TBI [191–193]. In a more recently performed clinical study, all patients with multiple trauma showed markedly high HMGB1 circulating levels in all time points evaluated [279]. Moreover, the investigators found a significant association between HMGB1 expression, both mRNA and protein, and the *Injury Severity Score* (ISS), supporting the prognostic role of HMGB1 in multiple trauma patients. Also, as a result of this study, enhanced HMGB1 levels were shown to be associated with a poor prognosis, and patients with highest levels died few days after trauma.

Heat Shock Protein 70

In another clinical study on trauma patients, levels of HSP70 were observed to be elevated significantly after trauma, and the magnitude of the increase was related to the severity of the injury [280]. Interestingly, the serum HSP70 levels were found to be increased in patients with not only severe but minor and moderate injuries as well, when compared to healthy controls. Furthermore, in this analysis, HSP70 levels were shown to continue to rise in cases of infection.

Mitochondria-Derived DAMPs

Moreover, in extensive trauma, increasing attention has been devoted to the crucial role of mitochondria-derived DAMPs, since they have been shown—as mentioned in Sect. 8.3.3.3—to be markedly elevated in severely injured patients [18]. This category of DAMPs mainly includes circular DNA strands containing CpG DNA repeats, N-formylated peptides, and mtDNA itself [281]. Interestingly, it has been found that mtDNA, observed to activate neutrophils after binding to TLR9 directly, is released under various traumatic conditions, including shock and severe TBI [210, 211]. Recent clinical studies in massively injured human subjects provided the first observational evidence that plasma mtDNA DAMPs are associated with the evolution of SIRS, MOF, and mortality [208]. One of the most interesting reported findings was that a determination of mtDNA DAMP levels made within 8 h of hospital admission allowed the differentiation between survivors and non-survivors [208]. Also, in more recent studies on mtDNA levels in 139 trauma patients, subjects who developed MODS were demonstrated to have significantly higher concentrations of mtDNA in their circulation at only 2 h following injury [282]. Moreover, in this clinical study, isolated tissue injury, without shock, was found to result in a dose-dependent increase in mtDNA release, whereas the combination of severe shock and severe trauma was observed to lead to a substantial rise in circulating mtDNA. Given their data, the authors suggested that mtDNA release into the circulation occurs as a result of mechanical tissue injury and cellular injury, related to hypoperfusion [282].

Notably, a recently systematic review was conducted to assess circulating cell-free mtDNA as a biomarker of mortality in critically ill patients [283]. After having reviewed 40 studies accounting for 3450 critically ill patients, the authors came to the conclusion that "most studies are small, lack validation cohorts, and utilize different protocols to measure mtDNA." And the proposed: "Standardization of mtDNA protocols and the completion of a large, prospective, multicenter trial may be warranted to firmly establish the clinical usefulness of mtDNA."

Complement Fragments

Interestingly, the humoral part of the innate immune system, which is also likely to be induced by Subclass IIB-1 DAMPs in terms of injury-induced neoantigens, namely, the complement system, is activated immediately after trauma as well. Indeed, severe, sterile, injury-induced, systemic intravascular activation of the complement cascade (in particular, the mannose-binding lectin {MBL}-mediated pathway) reportedly can promote MOF by contributing to a fulminant inflammatory response associated with DIC and comprised microcirculation [124, 284].

Of note, within minutes after polytrauma, a significant increase in circulating complement activation products has been observed, including the inducible IIIB-3 DAMPs C3a and C5a, but also the membrane attack complex (MAC) sC5b-9 (reviewed by Karasu et al. [236]). In particular, an enhanced C3a/C3 ratio in plasma early after trauma was found to be prognostic for lethal outcome [231]. In other sets of studies, enhanced C3a levels were shown to act as an indicator for MODS [285] (for C3a and C5a, see Vol. 1 [4], Part IV, Sect. 14.3.4, and for the complement system, see Part VI, Sect. 23.2 and Fig. 23.1).

8.4.2.3 SAMPs as Biomarkers in Polytrauma

To our knowledge, no reports on the monitoring of SAMPs in polytrauma patients have been published so far. However, Dalli et al. [273] investigated the SPM profiles in infectious sepsis patients that may serve as first information about their profiles in polytrauma patients. In their clinical analysis, the investigators demonstrated that sepsis non-survivors show significantly higher SPMs, including RvE1, RvD5, and 17R-PD-1 as compared to surviving sepsis subjects. Interestingly, this signature was observed at ICU admission and found to persist for 7 days. Further analysis of the authors revealed an increased respiratory failure in non-survivors. Higher select proresolving pathways were shown to be associated with the development of ARDS, while other traditional clinical indices were not predictive of ARDS development. Similar investigations on SAMPs in trauma patients can, therefore, be expected with exciting attention.

8.4.2.4 Concluding Remarks

The few selected examples of DAMPs in their role as biomarkers, as described here, can be regarded as the beginning of a new era in monitoring systemic traumatic diseases. In principle, every DAMP documented to play a critical pathogenetic role in trauma can be harnessed as a diagnostic/predictive/prognostic biomarker. However, instead of concentrating on one DAMP as a biomarker, a distinct pattern of several DAMPs will probably turn out to be more reliable and instructive in predicting the outcome of traumatic diseases in different types of patients. This endeavor presupposes, however, that typical DAMP patterns in different patient categories must first be explored. However, as progress in this research field moves forward, SAMPs (still better "SAMPs patterns") are supposed to accompany the DAMPs as biomarkers soon or later. More precisely, and as already recommended in Chap. 7, Sect. 7.3.3 and Fig. 7.1, the determination of a DAMP/SAMP ratio in terms of a DAMP/SAMP signature appears to be the most accurate parameter to monitor the course and the outcome of a trauma. Indeed, continuous tracing of the DAMP/SAMP ratio may turn out to emerge to a crucial future parameter in reflecting the patient status in critically ill subjects and, thus, may set the stage as a novel approach for evaluating outcomes and modulating treatment responses in patients with traumatic diseases.

Finally, one has to state—and this applies to all following chapter sections on the use of DAMPs as biomarkers—that standardization of DAMP protocols and the completion of large, prospective, multicenter trials may be warranted to firmly establish the clinical usefulness of DAMPs as biomarkers in general.

8.4.3 DAMPs and SAMPs as Therapeutics in Dysregulated Wound Healing

Before starting with the therapeutic use of DAMPs and SAMPs as therapeutic options in trauma patients, a few words are devoted to their potential therapeutic benefit in dysregulated wound healing. For example, poorly healing wounds in diabetics and pressure ulcer formation in individuals with spinal cord injury are well-known phenomena for all physicians. Such wounds represent major healthcare problems, and current treatment methods are only partially effective. Also, such wounds are prone to get infected, which can lead to amputation and further disability. In sum, such wounds appear to be an indication for local application of DAMPs known to be critical players in tissue regeneration and repair (for additional information compare Vol. 1 [4], Part VIII, Sect. 36.3, p. 847).

As was to be expected, the prototypical DAMP HMGB1 known to have a pronounced tissue repairing potential was already documented to accelerate the physiological regenerative response to various injuries, in part via targeting endogenous stem cells. For example, in studies on a rat tibial osteotomy model, the combination of HMGB1 gelatin sponges with MSC sheets was demonstrated to increase bone formation resulting in acceleration of fracture healing [117]. The authors concluded that commercially available natural gelatin sponges may be used as carriers accelerating fracture healing. In other lines of studies, fully reduced HMGB1 was shown to accelerate the regeneration of multiple tissues by transitioning stem cells to G_{Alert} [118]. Besides others, these experiments revealed that HMGB1 is released following fracture in both humans and mice, forms a heterocomplex with CXCL12, and acts via CXCR4 to accelerate skeletal, hematopoietic, and muscle regeneration in vivo. In view of their findings (including others not quoted here), the authors [118] proposed a model "in which a highly conserved injury signal, HMGB1, acts via a well-established maintenance-signaling pathway, CXCL12–CXCR4, to ultimately promote tissue regeneration. Potentially this pathway may be targeted to accelerate healing in any tissue that relies on repair by cells that express CXCR4 and can transition to GAlert. In the clinic, we envisage that FR-HMGB1 would be administered as a single dose either locally or systemically soon after injury or even up to 2 wk beforehand to accelerate healing."

On the other hand, at least theoretically, the local use of SAMPs as therapeutics may be an option in treating unwanted keloid formation and hypertrophic scars, which represent an aberrant response to the wound healing process (reviewed in [286]).

It will be of great interest to follow the literature on this topic in the near future. It seems at least imaginable that the local use of DAMPs in precise temporal order, together with the application of stem cells, might become a satisfactory therapeutic option in treating poorly healing wounds successfully.

8.4.4 DAMPs and SAMPs as Therapeutic Targets in Polytrauma: A Theoretical Framework

8.4.4.1 General Remarks

In principle, the therapeutic application of DAMPs or SAMPs in traumatic diseases is to prevent the pathological consequences (e.g., hyperinflammation, chronic inflammation) without interfering with the homeostatic healing processes leading to *restitutio ad integrum*. Thus, in the case of polytrauma, the therapeutic aim is to inhibit the development of life-threatening SIRS, eventually resulting in MOF, as well as to prevent the development of CARS associated with increased susceptibility to infections.

Here, given the lack of substantial clinical experience, only some theoretical aspects of a proposal are designed and presented by choosing the model of a DAMP/SAMP ratio as a guide in tailoring treatment modalities. Indeed, as already outlined in Chap. 7, Sects. 7.3.3 and 7.3.4, for future optimal treatment modalities, the exact status of the DAMP/SAMP ratio could be determined in each patient. This concept would allow precise and timely intervention after trauma or during infectious sepsis, either by inhibiting DAMPs (e.g., in the initial phase of SIRS) or blocking SAMPs (e.g., in the subsequent stage of CARS) to rebalance the immune response.

On the basis of preclinical studies on suitable experimental models, proposals of harnessing DAMPs as future therapeutic targets in traumatic diseases are increasingly published, both in polytrauma and isolated acute organ injury. Moreover, first clinical studies have already been tackled.

8.4.4.2 Antagonists of DAMPs in Development for Clinical Use

Regarding the nature of the development of polytrauma-associated SIRS, the elimination/blockade of DAMPs or the administration of SAMPs (or their inducers) may represent key strategic treatment options. While antagonists against every DAMP potentially involved in polytrauma are not available yet, HMGB1 is currently the DAMP that has been the focus of such therapeutic strategies and, thus, deserves a few more words.

In fact, there are already reports on successful use of polyclonal or mouse/rat anti-HMGB1 monoclonal antibodies, investigated in many experimental inflammatory models [287, 288]. However, antagonists of HMGB1 that could presumably be administered to patients—provided approval by regulatory authorities—have been reviewed by Andersson et al. [289]. So far, two different humanized anti-HMGB1 monoclonal antibodies have been reported to be worked out [290, 291]. Moreover, *Affibody* molecules targeting HMGB1 have been investigated in different preclinical ischemic stroke models (Affibody molecules are small (6.5-kDa) affinity proteins based on a three-helix bundle domain framework and act as mimics with a favorable tissue distribution). According to a final report summary on these experiments (https://cordis.europa.eu/project/rcn/110068/reporting/en), HMGB1 blockage by these *Affibody* molecules as a treatment for stroke was not successful. As outlined in this report: "The negative results above could have several explanations. The two most likely are either the inability of the selected Affibody molecules in the selected doses to neutralize HMGB1 released during stroke and the second is the redundancy in the inflammatory mechanisms activated after a stroke. In that scenario, neutralization of HMGB1 alone is not sufficient to impact inflammation ensuing ischemic stroke."

Also, in a very recent publication (see [292]), anti-HMGB1 mAb, recombinant HMGB1 antagonist box A protein (that is one of the two DNA-binding domains in HMGB1), acetylcholine, GTS-21, and the dynamin-specific inhibitor of endocytosis were reported to inhibit internalization of HMGB1 or HMGB1–LPS complexes in cultured macrophages. These agents were shown to prevent macrophage activation in response to HMGB1 and/or HMGB1–LPS complexes. The authors concluded that these results demonstrate that therapies based on HMGB1 antagonists and the cholinergic antiinflammatory pathway share a previously unrecognized molecular mechanism of substantial clinical relevance.

In addition, recombinant box A protein was found to act as a potent HMGB1 antagonist in many other preclinical studies of inflammatory conditions. However, several reasons have so far precluded further clinical development (also reviewed in [289]). Nevertheless, publications of clinical trials in this field can be expected soon.

8.4.4.3 Elimination/Blockade of DAMPs in the Hyperinflammatory Phase of Severe Trauma

As mentioned in Sect. 7.4.2, plasma adsorption therapy was recently reported to adsorb HMGB1 [290] efficiently. In addition, as also discussed by Venereau et al. [288], VanPatten and Al-Abed [293], and Andersson et al. [289], in the future, the development of specific HMGB1 inhibitors/antagonists such as specific small molecules may potentiate and fine-tune the pharmacological control of inflammation.

The correctness of the thought that such therapeutic approaches may provide a much-needed treatment in critically injured trauma patients show recently reported studies. One such experiment was performed by Black et al. [294] in swine using a trauma model of hemorrhage and IRI that was accompanied by accumulation of mtDNA in plasma. Pretreatment of traumatized animals with an experimental PI3K inhibitor (supposed to prevent release of mtDNA in plasma) was observed to prevent organ and bioenergetics dysfunction and to be associated with a significant decrease in plasma mtDNA to the levels of control animals. The authors argued that these findings may comprise a new pharmacologic strategy to prevent mtDNA damage and DAMP release and prevent or treat trauma-related MODS.

Similar observations were made by Aswani et al. [282] in studies on a rat model of severe trauma hemorrhage shock. According to the authors, this trauma model is associated with cellular stress, failure of mitophagy, and autophagy, increasing degrees of oxidative stress, translocation of mtDNA to the cytosol, and activation of apoptotic cell death pathways [295, 296]. This study aimed to determine whether neutralizing mtDNA with the NA scavenging polymer, hexadimethrine bromide (HDMBr), at a clinically relevant time point in vivo would reduce the severity of organ injury in this model. Hexadimethrine bromide has been shown to prevent the activation of TLRs in a CpG DNA-dependent toxic shock murine model and improve survival [297]. Indeed, as described by the investigators [282], the use of HDMBr was found to cause a significant reduction in circulating mtDNA by about 50%. Also, HDMBr scavenging of circulating mtDNA (and nDNA) was shown to be associated with rescue from severe multiple organ injury. In particular, treatment of the trauma hemorrhage shock in rats with HDMBr was demonstrated to improve lung histological appearances suggesting that this NA scavenging polymer possesses definite lung protective properties. Given their data, the authors [282] suggested that HDMBr could have utility in rescue from human trauma-induced MODS.

Complement Cascade Intervention Strategies

In the context of trauma, hemorrhagic shock, and sepsis, a few preclinical complement-targeting studies reportedly showed promising results (reviewed by

Karasu et al. [236]). On the other hand, complement-interfering drugs have been evaluated in other clinical settings so far. Thus, as discussed by Karasu et al. [236], studies to block the complement cascade in polytraumatized patients are urgently demanded. However, for several logistic reasons, innovative studies early after polytrauma addressing the complement cascade are somewhat rare and have not been performed on the C3 or C5 level yet. Thus, as concluded by the authors [236], "further scientific knowledge and translational efforts are demanded for targeting complement pathways in the setting of trauma, hemorrhagic shock, and sepsis with the aim to offer causal therapy and improved outcome."

Together, the so far published preclinical studies aimed at treating severe systemic trauma are promising. Thus, regarding the clinical situation, one can firmly conclude that removal of proinflammatory DAMPs from circulation is an unmet need in the treatment of critically ill patients (compare in this context also [226, 298]). However, as outlined previously (Sect. 7.3.3), before such a therapeutic concept becomes part of routine treatment, a homeostatic window of concentrations of the DAMPs involved is recommended to be worked out in clinical studies in order not to compromise the DAMP-promoting repairing/regenerative processes. Also, prospective continuous monitoring of the DAMP/SAMP ratio in critically ill patients is supposed to be helpful for intensive care clinicians to assess the strength and the nature of the trauma-induced innate immune response in each patient. Such assessments based on a given DAMP/SAMP signature would then allow intensive care clinicians to make proper tailor-made therapeutic decisions.

Finally, another conceivable option to treat the hyperinflammatory phase should not remain unmentioned, namely, the administration of SAMPs. Nevertheless, this option carries a certain risk in that it may even foster the development of CARS.

8.4.4.4 Elimination/Blockade of SAMPs in Polytrauma-Associated CARS: A Future Therapeutic Option?

If the model of CARS as an expression of overshooting SAMPs is correct, blockade or elimination of SAMPs, especially SMPs, under strict observance of the DAMP/SAMP ratio in relation to the homeostatic window could theoretically be considered. However, such clinical trials have not been designed so far, but they may become a clinical reality in the near future. Nevertheless, in this context, it appears at least worth mentioning that, in one experimental series on a model for sepsis induction in Balb/c and C57BL/6 mice (cecal ligation and puncture) [260], ketoprofen treatment was found to inhibit the production of the SAMP PGE2, thereby qualifying this agent as an attractive target to prevent secondary infections in the immunocompromised septic patients.

In another model of sepsis-induced AKI in mice [261], tenuigenin, a natural product isolated from *Polygala tenuifolia* root, was also shown to inhibit the production PGE2. In more recent experiments, targeting the 15-keto-PGE2-PTGR2 axis was demonstrated to mitigate systemic inflammation and improve survival of septic mice (nota bene: 15-keto-PGE2 is a PGE2 metabolite, whose further processing is catalyzed by PTGR2). Another supportive experiment documenting the detrimental role of SAMPs in sepsis refers to a study in which the effects of the AnxA1 mimetic peptide AC2-26 on sepsis-induced cardiomyocyte apoptosis were explored [299]. The investigators of these experiments could show that this mimetic peptide was able to inhibit sepsis-induced cardiomyocyte apoptosis in vitro and in vivo through the LXA4/PI3K/AKT signaling pathway.

8.4.4.5 Concluding Remarks

Together, as reflected by some select examples from the literature as addressed here, the preclinical evidence for the efficacy of targeting DAMPs in systemic traumatic diseases is convincing. Therefore, time appears to be mature to design and test DAMP-specific antagonists in both systemic and organ-specific traumatic diseases (see next chapter), with the aim to explore whether or not blocking DAMPs will benefit patients. On the other hand, testing SAMP-specific antagonists remains obviously reserved for CARS as a typical complication of polytrauma. Nevertheless, there is growing evidence for a successful use of SAMPs, in particular, SPMs as therapeutics to be administered in acute organ injuries. Thus, it can be assumed that first clinical trials in this exciting field of modern therapeutic possibilities will be reported soon.

8.4.5 Résumé: The Use of the "Homeostatic Window" of DAMP and SAMP Concentrations in Exploiting DAMPs and SAMPs as Therapeutic Targets

According to the reports quoted in this chapter, one can conceivably assume that DAMPs and fewer SAMPs (?) will soon find their way into clinical routine as diagnostic, prognostic, and predictive biomarkers in traumatic diseases.

Much more different, that is, more difficult to assess is their future routine use as therapeutic targets and therapeutics, respectively. Undoubtedly, treatment modalities based on inhibitors/antagonists, specifically targeting DAMPs, have provided encouraging results in many preclinical models of infectious and sterile injury-induced inflammatory responses. And one does not need to be a prophet to predict that clinical trials will be designed and conducted soon to explore whether blocking DAMPs and SAMPs in SIRS and CARS will benefit patients.

However, before starting such trials, the possible risks of future therapeutic exploitation of DAMPs and SAMPs have to be clearly defined and solidly assessed. First of all, and to repeat possible safety guidelines outlined in Sect. 7.3.3, the DAMP/SAMP ratio in plasma (and body fluids if applicable) is proposed to be determined by choosing, for example, measurement of key DAMPs such as HMGB1 and mtDNA as well as key SAMPs such as SPMs. For such studies, and also to select and recruit patients that might benefit from such interventions, there is a need to develop assays for plasma DAMP and SAMP assessments providing rapid information about the continuously monitored DAMP/SAMP ratio. Further, in adherence to this ratio, the "homeostatic windows" for DAMP and SAMP concentrations that are required to establish a *restitutio ad integrum* following injury have to be taken into account, in particular, when the course of the disease prompts the clinician to decide at what point to start the treatment (compare Fig. 8.3). Regarding

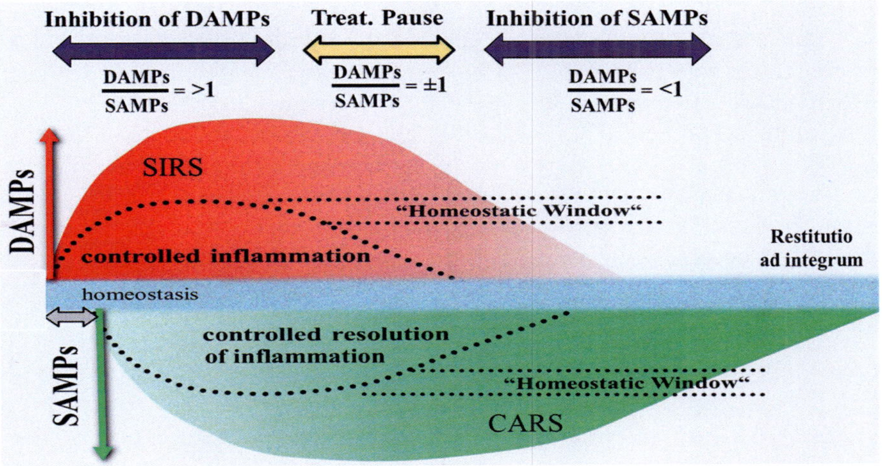

Fig. 8.3 This figure is the same as Fig. 7.1 in Sect. 7.3.3 but this time ideally designed to help the intensive care clinician decide to exploit DAMPs and SAMPs as therapeutic targets in the post-polytrauma period. According to this conceptual model, and guided by continuous monitoring of DAMP and SAMP levels, excessive DAMP levels should be decreased to homeostatic levels in the initial hyperinflammatory phase to prevent MOF; in the hyperresolving phase, excessive SAMPs levels should be decreased to homeostatic levels to prevent immunosuppression-promoted susceptibility to infection. The timely weaning and application of the inhibiting agents depend on the continuously measured DAMP and SAMP levels, which should be in the "homeostatic window," that is, adjusted to levels that were previously determined in controlled inflammatory and resolving responses as explored in clinical trials. *CARS* compensatory antiinflammatory response syndrome, *SIRS* systemic inflammatory response syndrome, *Treat* treatment

severe traumatic injuries, laboratory values of DAMPs above the "homeostatic window" may signal an increased risk of hyperinflammation and organ dysfunction, and laboratory values below the window pose the risk of compromised defensive repairing, that is, healing processes. On the other hand, values of SAMPs above the "homeostatic window" may carry an increased risk of hyperresolution and immunosuppression, whereas values below the window may signal an increased risk of hyperinflammation and organ dysfunction.

When such precautions have been put in place to ensure the patient's safety and when an effective drug (or a "drug cocktail") has been selected, for example, a blocking monoclonal antibody, the next step would be to define a therapeutic window for the drug's dosing that requires careful pharmacokinetic, pharmacodynamics, and pharmacogenomics studies.

Certainly, the development of therapeutic agents to neutralize/block/inhibit the DAMP-promoted hyperinflammatory effects holds promise for a drastic enrichment of trauma management. However, there is a major problem left that may also apply for SAMP-promoted hyperresolving responses. Given so many DAMPs emitted in traumatic diseases, the critical question is: does the therapeutic use of one blocking drug against one distinct DAMP have any beneficial effect at all? In other words, it is doubtful—given the redundancy in DAMP-promoted inflammatory mechanisms—whether blocking of one DAMP alone is sufficient to impact injury-induced hyperinflammation. This dilemma would call for the administration of a cocktail of antagonists against a DAMP pattern, at least, against a pattern of key DAMPs that has been determined and defined in a given trauma patient.

After all, and at the end of the day, the therapeutic use of DAMPs and SAMPs may turn out to be obsolete because of the enormous redundancy in DAMP-promoted inflammatory and SAMP-promoted resolving mechanisms. What would stay in the future as a better therapeutic option would be to prevent subroutines of RN such as necroptosis, pyroptosis, and ferroptosis. For such novel therapeutic strategies, however, suitable drugs such as necrostatin-1 and ferrostatin-1 have yet to be clinically developed (compare Sect. 3.3).

8.5 Outlook and Future Perspectives

In this chapter, data and observations are collected and presented, which are in support of the two proposed models of excessive levels of DAMPs promoting hyperinflammation (i.e., SIRS) and excessive levels of SAMPs promoting hyperresolution (i.e., CARS) (Fig. 8.1). Certainly, future clinical trials, as well as growing clinical expertise and experience will show whether or not the concept is right or wrong, at least in part. If correct in principle, however, both models are supposed to be modified in one way or another.

Irrespective of these restrictive remarks, measurement of both DAMPs and SAMPs in severely injured or infection-related sepsis patients will soon find its way in routine intensive care medicine. For example, at the patient's hospital admission, the determination of DAMPs in bodily fluids may allow a first assessment of further diagnostic procedures, risk stratification, and, most importantly, urgent therapeutic decisions. Further determination of a distinct DAMP pattern may add valuable information about the course of subsequent hyperinflammatory complications, for instance, the interactive crosstalk between musculoskeletal trauma and remote organ injury. In addition, immediate and continuous parallel measurement of SAMPs and determination of a distinct SAMP pattern may provide valid information about an imminent counterbalancing hyperresolution (= resolution of hyperinflammation) syndrome, clinically manifest as immunosuppression-caused increased susceptibility to infections.

Given the proposed conceptual models are correct, at least in part, the proper exploitation of DAMPs and SAMPs as therapeutic targets may prove to be a real therapeutic challenge. As outlined in Sect. 8.4.5 and illustrated in Fig. 8.3, there are possible risks associated with those maneuvers in that excessive inhibition of DAMPs may pose the risk of compromised repairing events, that is, healing processes, and excessive inhibition of SAMPs may carry an increased risk of hyperinflammation-associated organ dysfunction. Given such imponderabilities, it is proposed for future therapeutic strategies to comply with certain safety precautions, for example, to adhere to a "homeostatic window" for DAMP and SAMP concentrations that are required to establish a *restitutio ad integrum* following a severe traumatic injury.

References

1. Lord JM, Midwinter MJ, Chen Y-F, Belli A, Brohi K, Kovacs EJ, et al. The systemic immune response to trauma: an overview of pathophysiology and treatment. Lancet. 2014;384:1455–65. http://www.ncbi.nlm.nih.gov/pubmed/25390327.
2. Dorweiler B, Pruefer D, Andrasi TB, Maksan SM, Schmiedt W, Neufang A, et al. Ischemia-reperfusion injury. Eur J Trauma Emerg Surg. 2007;33:600–12. http://www.ncbi.nlm.nih.gov/pubmed/26815087.
3. Land WG. Emerging role of innate immunity in organ transplantation: part I: evolution of innate immunity and oxidative allograft injury. Transplant Rev (Orlando). 2012;26:60–72. http://www.ncbi.nlm.nih.gov/pubmed/22000662.
4. Land WG. Damage-associated molecular patterns in human diseases. In: Injury-induced innate immune responses, vol. 1. Cham: Springer International Publishing AG; 2018. https://www.springer.com/de/book/9783319786544.
5. Hauser CJ, Otterbein LE. Danger signals from mitochondrial DAMPS in trauma and post-injury sepsis. Eur J Trauma Emerg Surg. 2018;44:317–24. http://www.ncbi.nlm.nih.gov/pubmed/29797026.
6. Faist E, Baue AE, Dittmer H, Heberer G. Multiple organ failure in polytrauma patients. J Trauma. 1983;23:775–87. http://www.ncbi.nlm.nih.gov/pubmed/6620431.
7. Stillwell M, Caplan ES. The septic multiple-trauma patient. Crit Care Clin. 1988;4:345–73. http://www.ncbi.nlm.nih.gov/pubmed/3048591.
8. Schlag G, Redl H, Hallström S. The cell in shock: the origin of multiple organ failure. Resuscitation. 1991;21:137–80. http://www.ncbi.nlm.nih.gov/pubmed/1650020.
9. Schweinburg FB, Seligman AM, Fine J. Transmural migration of intestinal bacteria; a study based on the use of radioactive Escherichia coli. N Engl J Med. 1950;242:747–51. https://doi.org/10.1056/NEJM195005112421903.
10. Van Leeuwen PA, Boermeester MA, Houdijk AP, Ferwerda CC, Cuesta MA, Meyer S, et al. Clinical significance of translocation. Gut. 1994;35:S28–34. http://www.ncbi.nlm.nih.gov/pubmed/8125386.
11. Baker JW, Deitch EA, Li M, Berg RD, Specian RD. Hemorrhagic shock induces bacterial translocation from the gut. J Trauma. 1988;28:896–906. http://www.ncbi.nlm.nih.gov/pubmed/3294427.
12. Bone RC. Toward an epidemiology and natural history of SIRS (systemic inflammatory response syndrome). JAMA. 1992;268:3452–5. http://www.ncbi.nlm.nih.gov/pubmed/1460735.
13. Faist E, Hartl WH, Baue AE. Immune mechanisms of post-traumatic hyperinflammation and sepsis. Immun Infekt. 1994;22:203–13. http://www.ncbi.nlm.nih.gov/pubmed/7821950.
14. Hauser CJ, Zhou X, Joshi P, Cuchens MA, Kregor P, Devidas M, et al. The immune microenvironment of human fracture/soft-tissue hematomas and its relationship to systemic immunity. J Trauma. 1997;42:895–903; discussion 903-4. http://www.ncbi.nlm.nih.gov/pubmed/9191672.
15. Land W. Allograft injury mediated by reactive oxygen species: from conserved proteins of drosophila to acute and chronic rejection of human transplants. Part III: Interaction of (oxidative) stress-induced heat shock proteins with Toll-like receptor-bearing cells. Transplant Rev. 2003;17:67–86. http://linkinghub.elsevier.com/retrieve/pii/S0955470X0380006X.
16. Seong S-Y, Matzinger P. Hydrophobicity: an ancient damage-associated molecular pattern that initiates innate immune responses. Nat Rev Immunol. 2004;4:469–78. http://www.ncbi.nlm.nih.gov/pubmed/15173835.
17. Flohé SB, Flohé S, Schade FU. Invited review: deterioration of the immune system after trauma: signals and cellular mechanisms. Innate Immun. 2008;14:333–44. https://doi.org/10.1177/1753425908100016.
18. Zhang Q, Raoof M, Chen Y, Sumi Y, Sursal T, Junger W, et al. Circulating mitochondrial DAMPs cause inflammatory responses to injury. Nature. 2010;464:104–7. http://www.nature.com/articles/nature08780.

19. Haagsma JA, Graetz N, Bolliger I, Naghavi M, Higashi H, Mullany EC, et al. The global burden of injury: incidence, mortality, disability-adjusted life years and time trends from the Global Burden of Disease study 2013. Inj Prev. 2016;22:3–18. http://www.ncbi.nlm.nih.gov/pubmed/26635210.
20. Land WG. The role of damage-associated molecular patterns (DAMPs) in human diseases: part II: DAMPs as diagnostics, prognostics and therapeutics in clinical medicine. Sultan Qaboos Univ Med J. 2015;15:e157–70. http://www.ncbi.nlm.nih.gov/pubmed/26052447.
21. Wynn TA, Ramalingam TR. Mechanisms of fibrosis: therapeutic translation for fibrotic disease. Nat Med. 2012;18:1028–40. https://doi.org/10.1038/nm.2807.
22. Martin P. Wound healing—aiming for perfect skin regeneration. Science. 1997;276:75–81. http://www.ncbi.nlm.nih.gov/pubmed/9082989.
23. Singer AJ, Clark RAF. Cutaneous wound healing. N Engl J Med. 1999;341:738–46. http://www.ncbi.nlm.nih.gov/pubmed/10471461.
24. Chester D, Brown AC. The role of biophysical properties of provisional matrix proteins in wound repair. Matrix Biol. 2017;60–61:124–40. https://linkinghub.elsevier.com/retrieve/pii/S0945053X16301858.
25. Velnar T, Bailey T, Smrkolj V. The wound healing process: an overview of the cellular and molecular mechanisms. J Int Med Res. 2009;37:1528–42. https://doi.org/10.1177/147323000903700531.
26. Volk SW, Iqbal SA, Bayat A. Interactions of the extracellular matrix and progenitor cells in cutaneous wound healing. Adv Wound Care. 2013;2:261–72. http://www.ncbi.nlm.nih.gov/pubmed/24527348.
27. Ito T. PAMPs and DAMPs as triggers for DIC. J Intensive Care. 2014;2:65. http://www.ncbi.nlm.nih.gov/pubmed/25705424.
28. Sun BK, Siprashvili Z, Khavari PA. Advances in skin grafting and treatment of cutaneous wounds. Science. 2014;346:941–5. https://doi.org/10.1126/science.1253836.
29. Bochaton-Piallat M-L, Gabbiani G, Hinz B. The myofibroblast in wound healing and fibrosis: answered and unanswered questions. F1000Research. 2016;5:752. http://www.ncbi.nlm.nih.gov/pubmed/27158462.
30. Hinz B. The role of myofibroblasts in wound healing. Curr Res Transl Med. 2016;64:171–7. http://www.ncbi.nlm.nih.gov/pubmed/27939455.
31. Stoecklein VM, Osuka A, Lederer JA. Trauma equals danger—damage control by the immune system. J Leukoc Biol. 2012;92:539–51. https://doi.org/10.1189/jlb.0212072.
32. Wynn TA, Vannella KM. Macrophages in tissue repair, regeneration, and fibrosis. Immunity. 2016;44:450–62. http://www.ncbi.nlm.nih.gov/pubmed/26982353.
33. Meng X-M, Tang PM-K, Li J, Lan HY. Macrophage phenotype in kidney injury and repair. Kidney Dis (Basel, Switzerland). 2015;1:138–46. http://www.ncbi.nlm.nih.gov/pubmed/27536674.
34. Sun Y-Y, Li X-F, Meng X-M, Huang C, Zhang L, Li J. Macrophage phenotype in liver injury and repair. Scand J Immunol. 2017;85:166–74. http://www.ncbi.nlm.nih.gov/pubmed/27491503.
35. Klingberg F, Hinz B, White ES. The myofibroblast matrix: implications for tissue repair and fibrosis. J Pathol. 2013;229:298–309. http://www.ncbi.nlm.nih.gov/pubmed/22996908.
36. Micera A, Balzamino BO, Di Zazzo A, Biamonte F, Sica G, Bonini S. Toll-like receptors and tissue remodeling: the pro/cons recent findings. J Cell Physiol. 2016;231:531–44. http://www.ncbi.nlm.nih.gov/pubmed/26248215.
37. Darby IA, Zakuan N, Billet F, Desmoulière A. The myofibroblast, a key cell in normal and pathological tissue repair. Cell Mol Life Sci. 2016;73:1145–57. http://www.ncbi.nlm.nih.gov/pubmed/26681260.
38. He J, Xiao Z, Chen X, Chen M, Fang L, Yang M, et al. The expression of functional Toll-like receptor 4 is associated with proliferation and maintenance of stem cell phenotype in endothelial progenitor cells (EPCs). J Cell Biochem. 2010;111:179–86. http://www.ncbi.nlm.nih.gov/pubmed/20506307.

39. Wanjare M, Kusuma S, Gerecht S. Perivascular cells in blood vessel regeneration. Biotechnol J. 2013;8:434–47. http://www.ncbi.nlm.nih.gov/pubmed/23554249.
40. Psaltis PJ, Simari RD. Vascular wall progenitor cells in health and disease. Circ Res. 2015;116:1392–412. http://www.ncbi.nlm.nih.gov/pubmed/25858065.
41. Salvador B, Arranz A, Francisco S, Córdoba L, Punzón C, Llamas MÁ, et al. Modulation of endothelial function by Toll like receptors. Pharmacol Res. 2016;108:46–56. http://www.ncbi.nlm.nih.gov/pubmed/27073018.
42. Portou MJJ, Baker D, Abraham D, Tsui J. The innate immune system, toll-like receptors and dermal wound healing: a review. Vascul Pharmacol. 2015;71:31–6. http://www.ncbi.nlm.nih.gov/pubmed/25869514.
43. Hato T, El-Achkar TM, Dagher PC. Sisters in arms: myeloid and tubular epithelial cells shape renal innate immunity. Am J Physiol Renal Physiol. 2013;304:F1243–51. http://www.ncbi.nlm.nih.gov/pubmed/23515715.
44. Weiskirchen R, Tacke F. Cellular and molecular functions of hepatic stellate cells in inflammatory responses and liver immunology. Hepatobiliary Surg Nutr. 2014;3:344–63. http://www.ncbi.nlm.nih.gov/pubmed/25568859.
45. Hwa Cho H, Bae YC, Jung JS. Role of toll-like receptors on human adipose-derived stromal cells. Stem Cells. 2006;24:2744–52. http://www.ncbi.nlm.nih.gov/pubmed/16902195.
46. Delarosa O, Dalemans W, Lombardo E. Toll-like receptors as modulators of mesenchymal stem cells. Front Immunol. 2012;3:182. http://www.ncbi.nlm.nih.gov/pubmed/22783256.
47. Straino S, Di Carlo A, Mangoni A, De Mori R, Guerra L, Maurelli R, et al. High-mobility group box 1 protein in human and murine skin: involvement in wound healing. J Invest Dermatol. 2008;128:1545–53. http://linkinghub.elsevier.com/retrieve/pii/S0022202X15339099.
48. Yang S, Xu L, Yang T, Wang F. High-mobility group box-1 and its role in angiogenesis. J Leukoc Biol. 2014;95:563–74. http://www.ncbi.nlm.nih.gov/pubmed/24453275.
49. Zampell JC, Yan A, Avraham T, Andrade V, Malliaris S, Aschen S, et al. Temporal and spatial patterns of endogenous danger signal expression after wound healing and in response to lymphedema. Am J Physiol Cell Physiol. 2011;300:C1107–21. https://doi.org/10.1152/ajpcell.00378.2010.
50. Duffield JS, Lupher M, Thannickal VJ, Wynn TA. Host responses in tissue repair and fibrosis. Annu Rev Pathol. 2013;8:241–76. https://doi.org/10.1146/annurev-pathol-020712-163930.
51. Vénéreau E, Ceriotti C, Bianchi ME. DAMPs from cell death to new life. Front Immunol. 2015;6:422. http://www.ncbi.nlm.nih.gov/pubmed/26347745.
52. Wilgus TA. Alerting the body to tissue injury: the role of Alarmins and DAMPs in cutaneous wound healing. Curr Pathobiol Rep. 2018;6:55–60. http://www.ncbi.nlm.nih.gov/pubmed/29862143.
53. Arandjelovic S, Ravichandran KS. Phagocytosis of apoptotic cells in homeostasis. Nat Immunol. 2015;16:907–17. http://www.ncbi.nlm.nih.gov/pubmed/26287597.
54. Bhattacharyya S, Tamaki Z, Wang W, Hinchcliff M, Hoover P, Getsios S, et al. Fibronectin EDA promotes chronic cutaneous fibrosis through Toll-like receptor signaling. Sci Transl Med. 2014;6:232ra50. http://www.ncbi.nlm.nih.gov/pubmed/24739758.
55. Lee C-C, Wang C-N, Lee Y-L, Tsai Y-R, Liu J-J. High mobility group box 1 induced human lung myofibroblasts differentiation and enhanced migration by activation of MMP-9. PLoS One. 2015;10:e0116393. http://www.ncbi.nlm.nih.gov/pubmed/25692286.
56. Ranzato E, Patrone M, Pedrazzi M, Burlando B. Hmgb1 promotes wound healing of 3T3 mouse fibroblasts via RAGE-dependent ERK1/2 activation. Cell Biochem Biophys. 2010;57:9–17. http://www.ncbi.nlm.nih.gov/pubmed/20361273.
57. De Mori R, Straino S, Di Carlo A, Mangoni A, Pompilio G, Palumbo R, et al. Multiple effects of high mobility group box protein 1 in skeletal muscle regeneration. Arterioscler Thromb Vasc Biol. 2007;27:2377–83. http://www.ncbi.nlm.nih.gov/pubmed/17872450.
58. Zabini D, Crnkovic S, Xu H, Tscherner M, Ghanim B, Klepetko W, et al. High-mobility group box-1 induces vascular remodelling processes via c-Jun activation. J Cell Mol Med. 2015;19:1151–61. http://www.ncbi.nlm.nih.gov/pubmed/25726846.

59. Kao Y-H, Jawan B, Goto S, Hung C-T, Lin Y-C, Nakano T, et al. High-mobility group box 1 protein activates hepatic stellate cells in vitro. Transplant Proc. 2008;40:2704–5. http://www.ncbi.nlm.nih.gov/pubmed/18929840.
60. Pistoia V, Raffaghello L. Damage-associated molecular patterns (DAMPs) and mesenchymal stem cells: a matter of attraction and excitement. Eur J Immunol. 2011;41:1828–31. http://www.ncbi.nlm.nih.gov/pubmed/21706488.
61. Lotfi R, Eisenbacher J, Solgi G, Fuchs K, Yildiz T, Nienhaus C, et al. Human mesenchymal stem cells respond to native but not oxidized damage associated molecular pattern molecules from necrotic (tumor) material. Eur J Immunol. 2011;41:2021–8. http://www.ncbi.nlm.nih.gov/pubmed/21538978.
62. Prockop DJ, Oh JY. Mesenchymal stem/stromal cells (MSCs): role as guardians of inflammation. Mol Ther. 2012;20:14–20. http://www.ncbi.nlm.nih.gov/pubmed/22008910.
63. Eisenbacher JL, Schrezenmeier H, Jahrsdörfer B, Kaltenmeier C, Rojewski MT, Yildiz T, et al. S100A4 and uric acid promote mesenchymal stromal cell induction of IL-10+/IDO+ lymphocytes. J Immunol. 2014;192:6102–10. http://www.ncbi.nlm.nih.gov/pubmed/24795458.
64. Mahrouf-Yorgov M, Augeul L, Da Silva CC, Jourdan M, Rigolet M, Manin S, et al. Mesenchymal stem cells sense mitochondria released from damaged cells as danger signals to activate their rescue properties. Cell Death Differ. 2017;24:1224–38. http://www.ncbi.nlm.nih.gov/pubmed/28524859.
65. Bennett MR, Sinha S, Owens GK. Vascular smooth muscle cells in atherosclerosis. Circ Res. 2016;118:692–702. http://www.ncbi.nlm.nih.gov/pubmed/26892967.
66. Lim S, Park S. Role of vascular smooth muscle cell in the inflammation of atherosclerosis. BMB Rep. 2014;47:1–7. http://www.ncbi.nlm.nih.gov/pubmed/24388105.
67. Rai V, Agrawal DK. The role of DAMPs and PAMPs in inflammation-mediated vulnerability of atherosclerotic plaques. Can J Physiol Pharmacol. 2017;95(10):1245–53. http://www.ncbi.nlm.nih.gov/pubmed/28746820.
68. Duann P, Lianos EA, Ma J, Lin P-H. Autophagy, innate immunity and tissue repair in acute kidney injury. Int J Mol Sci. 2016;17:662. http://www.ncbi.nlm.nih.gov/pubmed/27153058.
69. Hou W, Zhang Q, Yan Z, Chen R, Zeh Iii HJ, Kang R, et al. Strange attractors: DAMPs and autophagy link tumor cell death and immunity. Cell Death Dis. 2013;4:e966. http://www.ncbi.nlm.nih.gov/pubmed/24336086.
70. Li G, Tang D, Lotze MT. Ménage à Trois in stress: DAMPs, redox and autophagy. Semin Cancer Biol. 2013;23:380–90. http://www.ncbi.nlm.nih.gov/pubmed/23994764.
71. Tamai K, Yamazaki T, Chino T, Ishii M, Otsuru S, Kikuchi Y, et al. PDGFRalpha-positive cells in bone marrow are mobilized by high mobility group box 1 (HMGB1) to regenerate injured epithelia. Proc Natl Acad Sci U S A. 2011;108:6609–14. http://www.ncbi.nlm.nih.gov/pubmed/21464317.
72. Feng L, Xue D, Chen E, Zhang W, Gao X, Yu J, et al. HMGB1 promotes the secretion of multiple cytokines and potentiates the osteogenic differentiation of mesenchymal stem cells through the Ras/MAPK signaling pathway. Exp Ther Med. 2016;12:3941–7. http://www.ncbi.nlm.nih.gov/pubmed/28105126.
73. Frangogiannis NG. The inflammatory response in myocardial injury, repair, and remodelling. Nat Rev Cardiol. 2014;11:255–65. http://www.ncbi.nlm.nih.gov/pubmed/24663091.
74. Kitahara T, Takeishi Y, Harada M, Niizeki T, Suzuki S, Sasaki T, et al. High-mobility group box 1 restores cardiac function after myocardial infarction in transgenic mice. Cardiovasc Res. 2008;80:40–6. http://www.ncbi.nlm.nih.gov/pubmed/18558628.
75. Zhang W, Lavine KJ, Epelman S, Evans SA, Weinheimer CJ, Barger PM, et al. Necrotic myocardial cells release damage-associated molecular patterns that provoke fibroblast activation in vitro and trigger myocardial inflammation and fibrosis in vivo. J Am Heart Assoc. 2015;4:e001993. http://www.ncbi.nlm.nih.gov/pubmed/26037082.
76. Kao Y-H, Lin Y-C, Tsai M-S, Sun C-K, Yuan S-S, Chang C-Y, et al. Involvement of the nuclear high mobility group B1 peptides released from injured hepatocytes in murine hepatic fibrogenesis. Biochim Biophys Acta. 1842;2014:1720–32. http://www.ncbi.nlm.nih.gov/pubmed/24970745.

77. Chavakis E, Hain A, Vinci M, Carmona G, Bianchi ME, Vajkoczy P, et al. High-mobility group box 1 activates integrin-dependent homing of endothelial progenitor cells. Circ Res. 2007;100:204–12. http://www.ncbi.nlm.nih.gov/pubmed/17218606.
78. Mitola S, Belleri M, Urbinati C, Coltrini D, Sparatore B, Pedrazzi M, et al. Cutting edge: extracellular high mobility group box-1 protein is a proangiogenic cytokine. J Immunol. 2006;176:12–5. http://www.ncbi.nlm.nih.gov/pubmed/16365390.
79. Nass N, Trau S, Paulsen F, Kaiser D, Kalinski T, Sel S. The receptor for advanced glycation end products RAGE is involved in corneal healing. Ann Anat. 2017;211:13–20. http://www.ncbi.nlm.nih.gov/pubmed/28163201.
80. van Beijnum JR, Nowak-Sliwinska P, van den Boezem E, Hautvast P, Buurman WA, Griffioen AW. Tumor angiogenesis is enforced by autocrine regulation of high-mobility group box 1. Oncogene. 2013;32:363–74. http://www.ncbi.nlm.nih.gov/pubmed/22391561.
81. Campana L, Santarella F, Esposito A, Maugeri N, Rigamonti E, Monno A, et al. Leukocyte HMGB1 is required for vessel remodeling in regenerating muscles. J Immunol. 2014;192:5257–64. http://www.ncbi.nlm.nih.gov/pubmed/24752445.
82. Nakamura Y, Suzuki S, Shimizu T, Miyata M, Shishido T, Ikeda K, et al. High mobility group box 1 promotes angiogenesis from bone marrow-derived endothelial progenitor cells after myocardial infarction. J Atheroscler Thromb. 2015;22:570–81. http://www.ncbi.nlm.nih.gov/pubmed/25735431.
83. Chen J-Y, Yu Y, Yuan Y, Zhang Y-J, Fan X-P, Yuan S-Y, et al. Enriched housing promotes post-stroke functional recovery through astrocytic HMGB1-IL-6-mediated angiogenesis. Cell Death Discov. 2017;3:17054. http://www.ncbi.nlm.nih.gov/pubmed/28845299.
84. Zhou J, Chen X, Gilvary DL, Tejera MM, Eksioglu EA, Wei S, et al. HMGB1 induction of clusterin creates a chemoresistant niche in human prostate tumor cells. Sci Rep. 2015;5:15085. http://www.ncbi.nlm.nih.gov/pubmed/26469759.
85. Nguan CYC, Guan Q, Gleave ME, Du C. Promotion of cell proliferation by clusterin in the renal tissue repair phase after ischemia-reperfusion injury. Am J Physiol Renal Physiol. 2014;306:F724–33. http://www.ncbi.nlm.nih.gov/pubmed/24477687.
86. Guo J, Guan Q, Liu X, Wang H, Gleave ME, Nguan CYC, et al. Relationship of clusterin with renal inflammation and fibrosis after the recovery phase of ischemia-reperfusion injury. BMC Nephrol. 2016;17:133. http://www.ncbi.nlm.nih.gov/pubmed/27649757.
87. Ojo OO, Ryu MH, Jha A, Unruh H, Halayko AJ. High-mobility group box 1 promotes extracellular matrix synthesis and wound repair in human bronchial epithelial cells. Am J Physiol Lung Cell Mol Physiol. 2015;309:L1354–66. http://www.ncbi.nlm.nih.gov/pubmed/26432865.
88. Cai J, Yuan H, Wang Q, Yang H, Al-Abed Y, Hua Z, et al. HMGB1-driven inflammation and intimal hyperplasia after arterial injury involves cell-specific actions mediated by TLR4 significance. Arterioscler Thromb Vasc Biol. 2015;35:2579–93. http://www.ncbi.nlm.nih.gov/pubmed/26515416.
89. Donato R, Cannon BR, Sorci G, Riuzzi F, Hsu K, Weber DJ, et al. Functions of S100 proteins. Curr Mol Med. 2013;13:24–57. http://www.ncbi.nlm.nih.gov/pubmed/22834835.
90. Reimann S, Fink L, Wilhelm J, Hoffmann J, Bednorz M, Seimetz M, et al. Increased S100A4 expression in the vasculature of human COPD lungs and murine model of smoke-induced emphysema. Respir Res. 2015;16:127. http://www.ncbi.nlm.nih.gov/pubmed/26483185.
91. Choe N, Kwon D-H, Shin S, Kim YS, Kim Y-K, Kim J, et al. The microRNA miR-124 inhibits vascular smooth muscle cell proliferation by targeting S100 calcium-binding protein A4 (S100A4). FEBS Lett. 2017;591:1041–52. http://www.ncbi.nlm.nih.gov/pubmed/28235243.
92. Bekos C, Zimmermann M, Unger L, Janik S, Hacker P, Mitterbauer A, et al. Non-professional marathon running: RAGE axis and ST2 family changes in relation to open-window effect, inflammation and renal function. Sci Rep. 2016;6:32315. http://www.ncbi.nlm.nih.gov/pubmed/27653273.
93. Idzko M, Ferrari D, Eltzschig HK. Nucleotide signalling during inflammation. Nature. 2014;509:310–7. http://www.ncbi.nlm.nih.gov/pubmed/24828189.

94. Elliott MR, Chekeni FB, Trampont PC, Lazarowski ER, Kadl A, Walk SF, et al. Nucleotides released by apoptotic cells act as a find-me signal to promote phagocytic clearance. Nature. 2009;461:282–6. http://www.ncbi.nlm.nih.gov/pubmed/19741708.
95. Chen Y, Corriden R, Inoue Y, Yip L, Hashiguchi N, Zinkernagel A, et al. ATP release guides neutrophil chemotaxis via P2Y2 and A3 receptors. Science. 2006;314:1792–5. http://www.ncbi.nlm.nih.gov/pubmed/17170310.
96. Yu N, Erb L, Shivaji R, Weisman GA, Seye CI. Binding of the P2Y2 nucleotide receptor to filamin A regulates migration of vascular smooth muscle cells. Circ Res. 2008;102:581–8. http://www.ncbi.nlm.nih.gov/pubmed/18202316.
97. Satterwhite CM, Farrelly AM, Bradley ME. Chemotactic, mitogenic, and angiogenic actions of UTP on vascular endothelial cells. Am J Physiol. 1999;276:H1091–7. http://www.ncbi.nlm.nih.gov/pubmed/10070096.
98. Jin H, Seo J, Eun SY, Joo YN, Park SW, Lee JH, et al. P2Y2 R activation by nucleotides promotes skin wound-healing process. Exp Dermatol. 2014;23:480–5. http://www.ncbi.nlm.nih.gov/pubmed/24816122.
99. Zhou Z, Chrifi I, Xu Y, Pernow J, Duncker DJ, Merkus D, et al. Uridine adenosine tetraphosphate acts as a proangiogenic factor in vitro through purinergic P2Y receptors. Am J Physiol Heart Circ Physiol. 2016;311:H299–309. http://www.ncbi.nlm.nih.gov/pubmed/27233766.
100. Negro S, Bergamin E, Rodella U, Duregotti E, Scorzeto M, Jalink K, et al. ATP released by injured neurons activates Schwann cells. Front Cell Neurosci. 2016;10:134. http://www.ncbi.nlm.nih.gov/pubmed/27242443.
101. Nakagawa S, Omura T, Yonezawa A, Yano I, Nakagawa T, Matsubara K. Extracellular nucleotides from dying cells act as molecular signals to promote wound repair in renal tubular injury. Am J Physiol Renal Physiol. 2014;307:F1404–11. http://www.ncbi.nlm.nih.gov/pubmed/25354940.
102. Gonzales E, Julien B, Serrière-Lanneau V, Nicou A, Doignon I, Lagoudakis L, et al. ATP release after partial hepatectomy regulates liver regeneration in the rat. J Hepatol. 2010;52:54–62. http://www.ncbi.nlm.nih.gov/pubmed/19914731.
103. Ando T, Ito H, Kanbe A, Hara A, Seishima M. Deficiency of NALP3 signaling impairs liver regeneration after partial hepatectomy. Inflammation. 2017;40:1717–25. http://www.ncbi.nlm.nih.gov/pubmed/28656530.
104. Artlett CM. The role of the NLRP3 inflammasome in fibrosis. Open Rheumatol J. 2012;6:80–6. http://www.ncbi.nlm.nih.gov/pubmed/22802905.
105. Kawaguchi M, Takahashi M, Hata T, Kashima Y, Usui F, Morimoto H, et al. Inflammasome activation of cardiac fibroblasts is essential for myocardial ischemia/reperfusion injury. Circulation. 2011;123:594–604. http://www.ncbi.nlm.nih.gov/pubmed/21282498.
106. Wang W, Wang X, Chun J, Vilaysane A, Clark S, French G, et al. Inflammasome-independent NLRP3 augments TGF-β signaling in kidney epithelium. J Immunol. 2013;190:1239–49. http://www.ncbi.nlm.nih.gov/pubmed/23264657.
107. Chaudhuri V, Zhou L, Karasek M. Inflammatory cytokines induce the transformation of human dermal microvascular endothelial cells into myofibroblasts: a potential role in skin fibrogenesis. J Cutan Pathol. 2007;34:146–53. http://www.ncbi.nlm.nih.gov/pubmed/17244026.
108. Gasse P, Riteau N, Charron S, Girre S, Fick L, Pétrilli V, et al. Uric acid is a danger signal activating NALP3 inflammasome in lung injury inflammation and fibrosis. Am J Respir Crit Care Med. 2009;179:903–13. https://doi.org/10.1164/rccm.200808-1274OC.
109. Riteau N, Gasse P, Fauconnier L, Gombault A, Couegnat M, Fick L, et al. Extracellular ATP is a danger signal activating P2X7 receptor in lung inflammation and fibrosis. Am J Respir Crit Care Med. 2010;182:774–83. http://www.ncbi.nlm.nih.gov/pubmed/20522787.
110. Fix C, Bingham K, Carver W. Effects of interleukin-18 on cardiac fibroblast function and gene expression. Cytokine. 2011;53:19–28. http://www.ncbi.nlm.nih.gov/pubmed/21050772.
111. Boza P, Ayala P, Vivar R, Humeres C, Cáceres FT, Muñoz C, et al. Expression and function of toll-like receptor 4 and inflammasomes in cardiac fibroblasts and myofibroblasts: IL-1β synthesis, secretion, and degradation. Mol Immunol. 2016;74:96–105. http://www.ncbi.nlm.nih.gov/pubmed/27174187.

112. Mia MM, Boersema M, Bank RA. Interleukin-1β attenuates myofibroblast formation and extracellular matrix production in dermal and lung fibroblasts exposed to transforming growth factor-β1. PLoS One. 2014;9:e91559. http://www.ncbi.nlm.nih.gov/pubmed/24622053.
113. Artlett CM, Thacker JD. Molecular activation of the NLRP3 inflammasome in fibrosis: common threads linking divergent fibrogenic diseases. Antioxid Redox Signal. 2015;22:1162–75. http://www.ncbi.nlm.nih.gov/pubmed/25329971.
114. Rak GD, Osborne LC, Siracusa MC, Kim BS, Wang K, Bayat A, et al. IL-33-dependent group 2 innate lymphoid cells promote cutaneous wound healing. J Invest Dermatol. 2016;136:487–96. https://linkinghub.elsevier.com/retrieve/pii/S0022202X15000469.
115. Oshio T, Komine M, Tsuda H, Tominaga S-I, Saito H, Nakae S, et al. Nuclear expression of IL-33 in epidermal keratinocytes promotes wound healing in mice. J Dermatol Sci. 2017;85:106–14. https://linkinghub.elsevier.com/retrieve/pii/S0923181116308805.
116. Shirjang S, Mansoori B, Solali S, Hagh MF, Shamsasenjan K. Toll-like receptors as a key regulator of mesenchymal stem cell function: an up-to-date review. Cell Immunol. 2017;315:1–10. http://www.ncbi.nlm.nih.gov/pubmed/28284487.
117. Xue D, Zhang W, Chen E, Gao X, Liu L, Ye C, et al. Local delivery of HMGB1 in gelatin sponge scaffolds combined with mesenchymal stem cell sheets to accelerate fracture healing. Oncotarget. 2017;8:42098–115. http://www.ncbi.nlm.nih.gov/pubmed/28431400.
118. Lee G, Espirito Santo AI, Zwingenberger S, Cai L, Vogl T, Feldmann M, et al. Fully reduced HMGB1 accelerates the regeneration of multiple tissues by transitioning stem cells to G Alert. Proc Natl Acad Sci. 2018;115:E4463–72. http://www.ncbi.nlm.nih.gov/pubmed/29674451.
119. Schäfer R, Spohn G, Baer PC. Mesenchymal stem/stromal cells in regenerative medicine: can preconditioning strategies improve therapeutic efficacy? Transfus Med Hemother. 2016;43:256–67. https://doi.org/10.1159/000447458.
120. Bastian O, Pillay J, Alblas J, Leenen L, Koenderman L, Blokhuis T. Systemic inflammation and fracture healing. J Leukoc Biol. 2011;89:669–73. http://www.ncbi.nlm.nih.gov/pubmed/21208896.
121. Loi F, Córdova LA, Pajarinen J, Lin T, Yao Z, Goodman SB. Inflammation, fracture and bone repair. Bone. 2016;86:119–30. https://linkinghub.elsevier.com/retrieve/pii/S8756328216300540.
122. Einhorn TA, Gerstenfeld LC. Fracture healing: mechanisms and interventions. Nat Rev Rheumatol. 2015;11:45–54. http://www.ncbi.nlm.nih.gov/pubmed/25266456.
123. Kaczorowski DJ, Mollen KP, Edmonds R, Billiar TR. Early events in the recognition of danger signals after tissue injury. J Leukoc Biol. 2008;83:546–52. http://www.ncbi.nlm.nih.gov/pubmed/18032691.
124. Huber-Lang M, Kovtun A, Ignatius A. The role of complement in trauma and fracture healing. Semin Immunol. 2013;25:73–8. http://linkinghub.elsevier.com/retrieve/pii/S1044532313000353.
125. Ehrnthaller C, Huber-Lang M, Nilsson P, Bindl R, Redeker S, Recknagel S, et al. Complement C3 and C5 deficiency affects fracture healing. PLoS One. 2013;8:e81341. http://www.ncbi.nlm.nih.gov/pubmed/24260573.
126. Ogawa R. Keloid and hypertrophic scars are the result of chronic inflammation in the reticular dermis. Int J Mol Sci. 2017;18:606. http://www.mdpi.com/1422-0067/18/3/606.
127. Bran GM, Goessler UR, Hormann K, Riedel F, Sadick H. Keloids: current concepts of pathogenesis (review). Int J Mol Med. 2009;24:283–93. http://www.ncbi.nlm.nih.gov/pubmed/19639219.
128. Chen W, Fu X, Sun X, Sun T, Zhao Z, Sheng Z. Analysis of differentially expressed genes in keloids and normal skin with cDNA microarray. J Surg Res. 2003;113:208–16. http://www.ncbi.nlm.nih.gov/pubmed/12957131.
129. Dong X, Mao S, Wen H. Upregulation of proinflammatory genes in skin lesions may be the cause of keloid formation (Review). Biomed Rep. 2013;1:833–6. https://doi.org/10.3892/br.2013.169.

130. Lee WJ, Song SY, Roh H, Ahn HM, Na Y, Kim J, et al. Profibrogenic effect of high-mobility group box protein-1 in human dermal fibroblasts and its excess in keloid tissues. Sci Rep. 2018;8:8434. http://www.ncbi.nlm.nih.gov/pubmed/29849053.
131. Baltzis D, Eleftheriadou I, Veves A. Pathogenesis and treatment of impaired wound healing in diabetes mellitus: new insights. Adv Ther. 2014;31:817–36. http://www.ncbi.nlm.nih.gov/pubmed/25069580.
132. Groah SL, Schladen M, Pineda CG, Hsieh C-HJ. Prevention of pressure ulcers among people with spinal cord injury: a systematic review. PM&R. 2015;7:613–36. http://www.ncbi.nlm.nih.gov/pubmed/25529614.
133. Grigorian A, Sugimoto M, Joe V, Schubl S, Lekawa M, Dolich M, et al. Pressure ulcer in trauma patients: a higher spinal cord injury level leads to higher risk. J Am Coll Clin Wound Spec. 2017;9:24–31.e1. http://www.ncbi.nlm.nih.gov/pubmed/30591898.
134. Han G, Ceilley R. Chronic wound healing: a review of current management and treatments. Adv Ther. 2017;34:599–610. http://www.ncbi.nlm.nih.gov/pubmed/28108895.
135. Dewar D, Moore FA, Moore EE, Balogh Z. Postinjury multiple organ failure. Injury. 2009;40:912–8. http://linkinghub.elsevier.com/retrieve/pii/S0020138309002824.
136. Gironda RJ, Clark ME, Ruff RL, Chait S, Craine M, Walker R, et al. Traumatic brain injury, polytrauma, and pain: challenges and treatment strategies for the polytrauma rehabilitation. Rehabil Psychol. 2009;54:247–58. https://doi.org/10.1037/a0016906.
137. Paffrath T, Lefering R, Flohé S, TraumaRegister DGU. How to define severely injured patients?—an Injury Severity Score (ISS) based approach alone is not sufficient. Injury. 2014;45:S64–9. http://www.ncbi.nlm.nih.gov/pubmed/25284238.
138. Charters E, Gillett L, Simpson GK. Efficacy of electronic portable assistive devices for people with acquired brain injury: a systematic review. Neuropsychol Rehabil. 2015;25:82–121. https://doi.org/10.1080/09602011.2014.942672.
139. Bridgeland HJ, Hartenberger KE, Poppen AN, Zobrist KC, Steinwedel C. Polytrauma in veterans: what does it mean for the medical-surgical nurse? Medsurg Nurs. 2014;23:213–37. http://www.ncbi.nlm.nih.gov/pubmed/25318333.
140. Keel M, Trentz O. Pathophysiology of polytrauma. Injury. 2005;36:691–709. http://www.ncbi.nlm.nih.gov/pubmed/15910820.
141. Wafaisade A, Lefering R, Bouillon B, Sakka SG, Thamm OC, Paffrath T, et al. Epidemiology and risk factors of sepsis after multiple trauma: an analysis of 29,829 patients from the Trauma Registry of the German Society for Trauma Surgery. Crit Care Med. 2011;39:621–8. https://insights.ovid.com/crossref?an=00003246-201104000-00002.
142. Fröhlich M, Lefering R, Probst C, Paffrath T, Schneider MM, Maegele M, et al. Epidemiology and risk factors of multiple-organ failure after multiple trauma. J Trauma Acute Care Surg. 2014;76:921–8. http://www.ncbi.nlm.nih.gov/pubmed/24662853.
143. Denning N-L, Aziz M, Gurien SD, Wang P. DAMPs and NETs in sepsis. Front Immunol. 2019;10:2536. http://www.ncbi.nlm.nih.gov/pubmed/31736963.
144. Huber-Lang M, Lambris JD, Ward PA. Innate immune responses to trauma. Nat Immunol. 2018;19:327–41. http://www.nature.com/articles/s41590-018-0064-8.
145. Howard BM, Kornblith LZ, Christie SA, Conroy AS, Nelson MF, Campion EM, et al. Characterizing the gut microbiome in trauma: significant changes in microbial diversity occur early after severe injury. Trauma Surg Acute Care Open. 2017;2:e000108. https://doi.org/10.1136/tsaco-2017-000108.
146. Gebhard F, Huber-Lang M. Polytrauma—pathophysiology and management principles. Langenbecks Arch Surg. 2008;393:825–31. http://www.ncbi.nlm.nih.gov/pubmed/18431593.
147. Hirsiger S, Simmen H-P, Werner CML, Wanner GA, Rittirsch D. Danger signals activating the immune response after trauma. Mediators Inflamm. 2012;2012:315941. http://www.hindawi.com/journals/mi/2012/315941/.
148. Timmermans K, Kox M, Scheffer GJ, Pickkers P. Danger in the intensive care unit. Shock. 2016;45:108–16. http://www.ncbi.nlm.nih.gov/pubmed/26513703.

149. Messerer DAC, Denk S, Föhr KJ, Halbgebauer R, Braun CK, Hönes F, et al. Complement C5a alters the membrane potential of neutrophils during hemorrhagic shock. Mediators Inflamm. 2018;2018:2052356. https://www.hindawi.com/journals/mi/2018/2052356/.
150. Osuchowski MF, Welch K, Siddiqui J, Remick DG. Circulating cytokine/inhibitor profiles reshape the understanding of the SIRS/CARS continuum in sepsis and predict mortality. J Immunol. 2006;177:1967–74. http://www.ncbi.nlm.nih.gov/pubmed/16849510.
151. Xiao W, Mindrinos MN, Seok J, Cuschieri J, Cuenca AG, Gao H, et al. A genomic storm in critically injured humans. J Exp Med. 2011;208:2581–90. https://doi.org/10.1084/jem.20111354.
152. Asehnoune K, Roquilly A, Abraham E. Innate immune dysfunction in trauma patients: from pathophysiology to treatment. Anesthesiology. 2012;117:411–6. https://doi.org/10.1097/ALN.0b013e31825f018d.
153. Hotchkiss RS, Monneret G, Payen D. Immunosuppression in sepsis: a novel understanding of the disorder and a new therapeutic approach. Lancet Infect Dis. 2013;13:260–8. https://linkinghub.elsevier.com/retrieve/pii/S147330991370001X.
154. Relja B, Land WG. Damage-associated molecular patterns in trauma. Eur J Trauma Emerg Surg. 2019. http://www.ncbi.nlm.nih.gov/pubmed/31612270.
155. Duprez L, Takahashi N, Van Hauwermeiren F, Vandendriessche B, Goossens V, Vanden Berghe T, et al. RIP kinase-dependent necrosis drives lethal systemic inflammatory response syndrome. Immunity. 2011;35:908–18. http://linkinghub.elsevier.com/retrieve/pii/S1074761311005085.
156. Ofengeim D, Yuan J. Regulation of RIP1 kinase signalling at the crossroads of inflammation and cell death. Nat Rev Mol Cell Biol. 2013;14:727–36. http://www.nature.com/articles/nrm3683.
157. Pasparakis M, Vandenabeele P. Necroptosis and its role in inflammation. Nature. 2015;517:311–20. http://www.nature.com/articles/nature14191.
158. Newton K, Manning G. Necroptosis and inflammation. Annu Rev Biochem. 2016;85:743–63. https://doi.org/10.1146/annurev-biochem-060815-014830.
159. Magtanong L, Dixon SJ. Ferroptosis and brain injury. Dev Neurosci. 2018;40:382–95. http://www.ncbi.nlm.nih.gov/pubmed/30820017.
160. Cui Y-L, Qiu L-H, Zhou S-Y, Li L-F, Qian Z-Z, Liu X-M, et al. Necroptosis as a potential therapeutic target in multiple organ dysfunction syndrome. Oncotarget. 2017;8:56980–90. http://www.oncotarget.com/fulltext/18252.
161. Burk A-M, Martin M, Flierl MA, Rittirsch D, Helm M, Lampl L, et al. Early complementopathy after multiple injuries in humans. Shock. 2012;37:348–54. http://content.wkhealth.com/linkback/openurl?sid=WKPTLP:landingpage&an=00024382-201204000-00002.
162. Cauwels A, Rogge E, Vandendriessche B, Shiva S, Brouckaert P. Extracellular ATP drives systemic inflammation, tissue damage and mortality. Cell Death Dis. 2017;5:e1102. http://www.ncbi.nlm.nih.gov/pubmed/24603330.
163. Bortolotti P, Faure E, Kipnis E. Inflammasomes in tissue damages and immune disorders after trauma. Front Immunol. 2018;9:1900. https://doi.org/10.3389/fimmu.2018.01900/full.
164. Guisasola MC, Ortiz A, Chana F, Alonso B, Vaquero J. Early inflammatory response in polytraumatized patients: cytokines and heat shock proteins. A pilot study. Orthop Traumatol Surg Res. 2015;101:607–11. https://linkinghub.elsevier.com/retrieve/pii/S1877056815001073.
165. Sun S, Sursal T, Adibnia Y, Zhao C, Zheng Y, Li H, et al. Mitochondrial DAMPs increase endothelial permeability through neutrophil dependent and independent pathways. PLoS One. 2013;8:e59989. http://www.ncbi.nlm.nih.gov/pubmed/23527291.
166. Vestweber D. How leukocytes cross the vascular endothelium. Nat Rev Immunol. 2015;15:692–704. http://www.ncbi.nlm.nih.gov/pubmed/26471775.
167. Toh C-H, Alhamdi Y, Abrams ST. Current pathological and laboratory considerations in the diagnosis of disseminated intravascular coagulation. Ann Lab Med. 2016;36:505. http://www.ncbi.nlm.nih.gov/pubmed/27578502.

168. Liaw PC, Ito T, Iba T, Thachil J, Zeerleder S. DAMP and DIC: the role of extracellular DNA and DNA-binding proteins in the pathogenesis of DIC. Blood Rev. 2016;30:257–61. http://www.ncbi.nlm.nih.gov/pubmed/26776504.
169. Levi M. Pathogenesis and diagnosis of disseminated intravascular coagulation. Int J Lab Hematol. 2018;40:15–20. http://www.ncbi.nlm.nih.gov/pubmed/29741245.
170. Hatada T, Wada H, Nobori T, Okabayashi K, Maruyama K, Abe Y, et al. Plasma concentrations and importance of High Mobility Group Box protein in the prognosis of organ failure in patients with disseminated intravascular coagulation. Thromb Haemost. 2005;94:975–9. http://www.schattauer.de/index.php?id=1214&doi=10.1160/TH05-05-0316&no_cache=1.
171. Ito T, Kawahara K, Nakamura T, Yamada S, Nakamura T, Abeyama K, et al. High-mobility group box 1 protein promotes development of microvascular thrombosis in rats. J Thromb Haemost. 2007;5:109–16. https://doi.org/10.1111/j.1538-7836.2006.02255.x.
172. Tilley R, Mackman N. Tissue factor in hemostasis and thrombosis. Semin Thromb Hemost. 2006;32:005–10. http://www.ncbi.nlm.nih.gov/pubmed/16479457.
173. Zelaya H, Rothmeier A, Ruf W. Tissue Factor at the crossroad of coagulation and cell signaling. J Thromb Haemost. 2018;16:1941–52. http://www.ncbi.nlm.nih.gov/pubmed/30030891.
174. Grover SP, Mackman N. Tissue factor. Arterioscler Thromb Vasc Biol. 2018;38:709–25. http://www.ncbi.nlm.nih.gov/pubmed/29437578.
175. Nguyen TT, Gilpin DA, Meyer NA, Herndon DN. Current treatment of severely burned patients. Ann Surg. 1996;223:14–25. http://www.ncbi.nlm.nih.gov/pubmed/8554414.
176. Baue AE, Durham R, Faist E. Systemic inflammatory response syndrome (SIRS), multiple organ dysfunction syndrome (MODS), multiple organ failure (MOF): are we winning the battle? Shock. 1998;10:79–89. http://www.ncbi.nlm.nih.gov/pubmed/9721973.
177. Dahiya P. Burns as a model of SIRS. Front Biosci. 2009;14:4962–7. http://www.ncbi.nlm.nih.gov/pubmed/19482598.
178. Raoof M, Zhang Q, Itagaki K, Hauser CJ. Mitochondrial peptides are potent immune activators that activate human neutrophils Via FPR-1. J Trauma Inj Infect Crit Care. 2010;68:1328–34. https://insights.ovid.com/crossref?an=00005373-201006000-00009.
179. Kaddoura I, Abu-Sittah G, Ibrahim A, Karamanoukian R, Papazian N. Burn injury: review of pathophysiology and therapeutic modalities in major burns. Ann Burns Fire Disasters. 2017;30:95–102. http://www.ncbi.nlm.nih.gov/pubmed/29021720.
180. Nielson CB, Duethman NC, Howard JM, Moncure M, Wood JG. Burns. J Burn Care Res. 2017;38:e469–81. http://www.ncbi.nlm.nih.gov/pubmed/27183443.
181. Hussain A, Dunn KW. Predicting length of stay in thermal burns: a systematic review of prognostic factors. Burns. 2013;39:1331–40. http://linkinghub.elsevier.com/retrieve/pii/S0305417913001472.
182. Bohr S, Patel SJ, Shen K, Vitalo AG, Brines M, Cerami A, et al. Alternative erythropoietin-mediated signaling prevents secondary microvascular thrombosis and inflammation within cutaneous burns. Proc Natl Acad Sci U S A. 2013;110:3513–8. https://doi.org/10.1073/pnas.1214099110.
183. Schwacha MG. Macrophages and post-burn immune dysfunction. Burns. 2003;29:1–14. http://www.ncbi.nlm.nih.gov/pubmed/12543039.
184. Sehirli O, Sener E, Sener G, Cetinel S, Erzik C, Yeğen BC. Ghrelin improves burn-induced multiple organ injury by depressing neutrophil infiltration and the release of pro-inflammatory cytokines. Peptides. 2008;29:1231–40. http://linkinghub.elsevier.com/retrieve/pii/S0196978108000843.
185. Ravat F, Payre J, Peslages P, Fontaine M, Sens N. Burn: an inflammatory process. Pathol Biol (Paris). 2011;59:e63–72. http://linkinghub.elsevier.com/retrieve/pii/S0369811409002326.
186. Rani M, Nicholson SE, Zhang Q, Schwacha MG. Damage-associated molecular patterns (DAMPs) released after burn are associated with inflammation and monocyte activation. Burns. 2017;43:297–303. http://www.ncbi.nlm.nih.gov/pubmed/28341255.
187. Reddy AS, Abraham A, McClain SA, Clark RAF, Ralen P, Sandoval S, et al. The role of necroptosis in burn injury progression in a rat comb burn model. Acad Emerg Med. 2015;22:1181–6. http://www.ncbi.nlm.nih.gov/pubmed/26375585.

188. Levy RM, Mollen KP, Prince JM, Kaczorowski DJ, Vallabhaneni R, Liu S, et al. Systemic inflammation and remote organ injury following trauma require HMGB1. Am J Physiol Regul Integr Comp Physiol. 2007;293:R1538–44. https://doi.org/10.1152/ajpregu.00272.2007.
189. Yang R, Harada T, Mollen KP, Prince JM, Levy RM, Englert JA, et al. Anti-HMGB1 neutralizing antibody ameliorates gut barrier dysfunction and improves survival after hemorrhagic shock. Mol Med. 2006;12:105–14. http://www.molmed.org/content/pdfstore/article-3154.pdf.
190. Fan J, Li Y, Levy RM, Fan JJ, Hackam DJ, Vodovotz Y, et al. Hemorrhagic shock induces NAD(P)H oxidase activation in neutrophils: role of HMGB1-TLR4 signaling. J Immunol. 2007;178:6573–80. http://www.ncbi.nlm.nih.gov/pubmed/17475888.
191. Cohen MJ, Brohi K, Calfee CS, Rahn P, Chesebro BB, Christiaans SC, et al. Early release of high mobility group box nuclear protein 1 after severe trauma in humans: role of injury severity and tissue hypoperfusion. Crit Care. 2009;13:R174. https://doi.org/10.1186/cc8152.
192. Peltz ED, Moore EE, Eckels PC, Damle SS, Tsuruta Y, Johnson JL, et al. HMGB1 is markedly elevated within 6 hours of mechanical trauma in humans. Shock. 2009;32:17–22. http://www.ncbi.nlm.nih.gov/pubmed/19533845.
193. Wang K-Y, Yu G-F, Zhang Z-Y, Huang Q, Dong X-Q. Plasma high-mobility group box 1 levels and prediction of outcome in patients with traumatic brain injury. Clin Chim Acta. 2012;413:1737–41. http://linkinghub.elsevier.com/retrieve/pii/S0009898112003415.
194. Yang R, Zou X, Tenhunen J, Tønnessen TI. HMGB1 and extracellular histones significantly contribute to systemic inflammation and multiple organ failure in acute liver failure. Mediators Inflamm. 2017;2017:5928078. https://www.hindawi.com/journals/mi/2017/5928078/.
195. Venereau E, Casalgrandi M, Schiraldi M, Antoine DJ, Cattaneo A, De Marchis F, et al. Mutually exclusive redox forms of HMGB1 promote cell recruitment or proinflammatory cytokine release. J Exp Med. 2012;209:1519–28. https://doi.org/10.1084/jem.20120189.
196. Guisasola MC, Alonso B, Bravo B, Vaquero J, Chana F. An overview of cytokines and heat shock response in polytraumatized patients. Cell Stress Chaperones. 2018;23:483–9. http://www.ncbi.nlm.nih.gov/pubmed/29101529.
197. Hashiguchi N, Ogura H, Tanaka H, Koh T, Nakamori Y, Noborio M, et al. Enhanced expression of heat shock proteins in activated polymorphonuclear leukocytes in patients with sepsis. J Trauma. 2001;51:1104–9. http://www.ncbi.nlm.nih.gov/pubmed/11740261.
198. Pittet J-F, Lee H, Morabito D, Howard MB, Welch WJ, Mackersie RC. Serum levels of Hsp 72 measured early after trauma correlate with survival. J Trauma. 2002;52:611–7. http://www.ncbi.nlm.nih.gov/pubmed/11956372.
199. Pockley AG, Shepherd J, Corton JM. Detection of heat shock protein 70 (Hsp70) and anti-Hsp70 antibodies in the serum of normal individuals. Immunol Invest. 1998;27:367–77. http://www.ncbi.nlm.nih.gov/pubmed/9845422.
200. Aneja R, Odoms K, Dunsmore K, Shanley TP, Wong HR. Extracellular heat shock protein-70 induces endotoxin tolerance in THP-1 cells. J Immunol. 2006;177:7184–92. http://www.ncbi.nlm.nih.gov/pubmed/17082636.
201. Timmermans K, Kox M, Vaneker M, van den Berg M, John A, van Laarhoven A, et al. Plasma levels of danger-associated molecular patterns are associated with immune suppression in trauma patients. Intensive Care Med. 2016;42:551–61. http://www.ncbi.nlm.nih.gov/pubmed/26912315.
202. Austermann J, Friesenhagen J, Fassl SK, Petersen B, Ortkras T, Burgmann J, et al. Alarmins MRP8 and MRP14 induce stress tolerance in phagocytes under sterile inflammatory conditions. Cell Rep. 2014;9:2112–23. http://linkinghub.elsevier.com/retrieve/pii/S2211124714009747.
203. Wang J, Vodovotz Y, Fan L, Li Y, Liu Z, Namas R, et al. Injury-induced MRP8/MRP14 stimulates IP-10/CXCL10 in monocytes/macrophages. FASEB J. 2015;29:250–62. https://doi.org/10.1096/fj.14-255992.
204. Thurairajah K, Briggs GD, Balogh ZJ. The source of cell-free mitochondrial DNA in trauma and potential therapeutic strategies. Eur J Trauma Emerg Surg. 2018;44:325–34. http://www.ncbi.nlm.nih.gov/pubmed/29633007.

205. Vourc'h M, Roquilly A, Asehnoune K. Trauma-induced damage-associated molecular patterns-mediated remote organ injury and immunosuppression in the acutely ill patient. Front Immunol. 2018;9:1330. https://doi.org/10.3389/fimmu.2018.01330/full.
206. Harrington JS, Choi AMK, Nakahira K. Mitochondrial DNA in sepsis. Curr Opin Crit Care. 2017;23:284–90. http://www.ncbi.nlm.nih.gov/pubmed/28562385.
207. Grazioli S, Pugin J. Mitochondrial damage-associated molecular patterns: from inflammatory signaling to human diseases. Front Immunol. 2018;9:832. http://www.ncbi.nlm.nih.gov/pubmed/29780380.
208. Simmons JD, Lee Y-L, Mulekar S, Kuck JL, Brevard SB, Gonzalez RP, et al. Elevated levels of plasma mitochondrial DNA DAMPs are linked to clinical outcome in severely injured human subjects. Ann Surg. 2013;258:591–6; discussion 596–8. http://content.wkhealth.com/linkback/openurl?sid=WKPTLP:landingpage&an=00000658-900000000-98352.
209. Gu X, Yao Y, Wu G, Lv T, Luo L, Song Y. The plasma mitochondrial DNA is an independent predictor for post-traumatic systemic inflammatory response syndrome. PLoS One. 2013;8:e72834. https://doi.org/10.1371/journal.pone.0072834.
210. Zhang Q, Itagaki K, Hauser CJ. Mitochondrial DNA is released by shock and activates neutrophils via p38 map kinase. Shock. 2010;34:55–9. http://content.wkhealth.com/linkback/openurl?sid=WKPTLP:landingpage&an=00024382-201007000-00010.
211. Walko TD, Bola RA, Hong JD, Au AK, Bell MJ, Kochanek PM, et al. Cerebrospinal fluid mitochondrial DNA: a novel DAMP in pediatric traumatic brain injury. Shock. 2014;41:499–503. http://content.wkhealth.com/linkback/openurl?sid=WKPTLP:landingpage&an=00024382-201406000-00005.
212. Jansen MPB, Pulskens WP, Butter LM, Florquin S, Juffermans NP, Roelofs JJTH, et al. Mitochondrial DNA is released in urine of sirs patients with acute kidney injury and correlates with severity of renal dysfunction. Shock. 2018;49:301–10. http://www.ncbi.nlm.nih.gov/pubmed/28837526.
213. Fang C, Wei X, Wei Y. Mitochondrial DNA in the regulation of innate immune responses. Protein Cell. 2016;7:11–6. https://doi.org/10.1007/s13238-015-0222-9.
214. Collins LV, Hajizadeh S, Holme E, Jonsson I-M, Tarkowski A. Endogenously oxidized mitochondrial DNA induces in vivo and in vitro inflammatory responses. J Leukoc Biol. 2004;75:995–1000. http://www.ncbi.nlm.nih.gov/pubmed/14982943.
215. Giorgi C, Marchi S, Simoes ICM, Ren Z, Morciano G, Perrone M, et al. Mitochondria and reactive oxygen species in aging and age-related diseases. Int Rev Cell Mol Biol. 2018;340:209–344. http://www.ncbi.nlm.nih.gov/pubmed/30072092.
216. Muftuoglu M, Mori MP, de Souza-Pinto NC. Formation and repair of oxidative damage in the mitochondrial DNA. Mitochondrion. 2014;17:164–81. http://www.ncbi.nlm.nih.gov/pubmed/24704805.
217. Shimada K, Crother TR, Karlin J, Dagvadorj J, Chiba N, Chen S, et al. Oxidized mitochondrial DNA activates the NLRP3 inflammasome during apoptosis. Immunity. 2012;36:401–14. http://www.ncbi.nlm.nih.gov/pubmed/22342844.
218. Carp H. Mitochondrial N-formylmethionyl proteins as chemoattractants for neutrophils. J Exp Med. 1982;155:264–75. http://www.ncbi.nlm.nih.gov/pubmed/6274994.
219. He H-Q, Ye R. The Formyl peptide receptors: diversity of ligands and mechanism for recognition. Molecules. 2017;22:455. http://www.ncbi.nlm.nih.gov/pubmed/28335409.
220. Chen K, Bao Z, Gong W, Tang P, Yoshimura T, Wang JM. Regulation of inflammation by members of the formyl-peptide receptor family. J Autoimmun. 2017;85:64–77. http://www.ncbi.nlm.nih.gov/pubmed/28689639.
221. Kaczmarek E, Hauser CJ, Kwon WY, Rica I, Chen L, Sandler N, et al. A subset of five human mitochondrial formyl peptides mimics bacterial peptides and functionally deactivates human neuetrophils. J Trauma Acute Care Surg. 2018;85:936–43. http://www.ncbi.nlm.nih.gov/pubmed/29787548.
222. Mense SM, Zhang L. Heme: a versatile signaling molecule controlling the activities of diverse regulators ranging from transcription factors to MAP kinases. Cell Res. 2006;16:681–92. http://www.nature.com/articles/7310086.

223. Larsen R, Gozzelino R, Jeney V, Tokaji L, Bozza FA, Japiassú AM, et al. A central role for free heme in the pathogenesis of severe sepsis. Sci Transl Med. 2010;2:51ra71. https://doi.org/10.1126/scitranslmed.3001118.
224. Li W, Zhao S, Cheng F, Rao T, Yu W, Ruan Y, et al. Oxidative damage and mitochondrial injuries differ following pneumoperitoneum pressure in rabbit models of varying degrees of hydronephrosis. Mol Med Rep. 2018;17:6819–27. http://www.ncbi.nlm.nih.gov/pubmed/29512718.
225. Kawai C, Kotani H, Miyao M, Ishida T, Jemail L, Abiru H, et al. Circulating extracellular histones are clinically relevant mediators of multiple organ injury. Am J Pathol. 2016;186:829–43. http://www.ncbi.nlm.nih.gov/pubmed/26878212.
226. Silk E, Zhao H, Weng H, Ma D. The role of extracellular histone in organ injury. Cell Death Dis. 2017;8:e2812. http://www.ncbi.nlm.nih.gov/pubmed/28542146.
227. Xu J, Zhang X, Monestier M, Esmon NL, Esmon CT. Extracellular histones are mediators of death through TLR2 and TLR4 in mouse fatal liver injury. J Immunol. 2011;187:2626–31. http://www.ncbi.nlm.nih.gov/pubmed/21784973.
228. Allam R, Scherbaum CR, Darisipudi MN, Mulay SR, Hagele H, Lichtnekert J, et al. Histones from dying renal cells aggravate kidney injury via TLR2 and TLR4. J Am Soc Nephrol. 2012;23:1375–88. https://doi.org/10.1681/ASN.2011111077.
229. Linkermann A, Stockwell BR, Krautwald S, Anders H-J. Regulated cell death and inflammation: an auto-amplification loop causes organ failure. Nat Rev Immunol. 2014;14:759–67. http://www.nature.com/articles/nri3743.
230. Xu J, Zhang X, Pelayo R, Monestier M, Ammollo CT, Semeraro F, et al. Extracellular histones are major mediators of death in sepsis. Nat Med. 2009;15:1318–21. http://www.ncbi.nlm.nih.gov/pubmed/19855397.
231. Hecke F, Schmidt U, Kola A, Bautsch W, Klos A, Köhl J. Circulating complement proteins in multiple trauma patients—correlation with injury severity, development of sepsis, and outcome. Crit Care Med. 1997;25:2015–24. http://www.ncbi.nlm.nih.gov/pubmed/9403752.
232. Ganter MT, Brohi K, Cohen MJ, Shaffer LA, Walsh MC, Stahl GL, et al. Role of the alternative pathway in the early complement activation following major trauma. Shock. 2007;28:29–34. https://insights.ovid.com/crossref?an=00024382-200707000-00005.
233. Rittirsch D, Redl H, Huber-Lang M. Role of complement in multiorgan failure. Clin Dev Immunol. 2012;2012:1–10. http://www.ncbi.nlm.nih.gov/pubmed/23320021.
234. Paredes RM, Reyna S, Vernon P, Tadaki DK, Dallelucca JJ, Sheppard F. Generation of complement molecular complex C5b-9 (C5b-9) in response to poly-traumatic hemorrhagic shock and evaluation of C5 cleavage inhibitors in non-human primates. Int Immunopharmacol. 2018;54:221–5. https://linkinghub.elsevier.com/retrieve/pii/S1567576917304204.
235. Li Y, Yang Z, Chavko M, Liu B, Aderemi OA, Simovic MO, et al. Complement inhibition ameliorates blast-induced acute lung injury in rats: potential role of complement in intracellular HMGB1-mediated inflammation. PLoS One. 2018;13:e0202594. http://www.ncbi.nlm.nih.gov/pubmed/30133517.
236. Karasu E, Nilsson B, Köhl J, Lambris JD, Huber-Lang M. Targeting complement pathways in polytrauma- and sepsis-induced multiple-organ dysfunction. Front Immunol. 2019;10:543. https://doi.org/10.3389/fimmu.2019.00543/full.
237. Relja B, Mörs K, Marzi I. Danger signals in trauma. Eur J Trauma Emerg Surg. 2018;44:301–16. http://www.ncbi.nlm.nih.gov/pubmed/29728738.
238. Tschoeke SK, Ertel W. Immunoparalysis after multiple trauma. Injury. 2007;38:1346–57. http://linkinghub.elsevier.com/retrieve/pii/S0020138307004019.
239. Angus DC, Linde-Zwirble WT, Lidicker J, Clermont G, Carcillo J, Pinsky MR. Epidemiology of severe sepsis in the United States: analysis of incidence, outcome, and associated costs of care. Crit Care Med. 2001;29:1303–10. http://www.ncbi.nlm.nih.gov/pubmed/11445675.
240. Kawasaki T, Fujimi S, Lederer JA, Hubbard WJ, Choudhry MA, Schwacha MG, et al. Trauma-hemorrhage induces depressed splenic dendritic cell functions in mice. J Immunol. 2006;177:4514–20. http://www.ncbi.nlm.nih.gov/pubmed/16982888.

241. Vester H, Dargatz P, Huber-Wagner S, Biberthaler P, van Griensven M. HLA-DR expression on monocytes is decreased in polytraumatized patients. Eur J Med Res. 2015;20:84. http://www.eurjmedres.com/content/20/1/84.
242. Hotchkiss RS, Monneret G, Payen D. Sepsis-induced immunosuppression: from cellular dysfunctions to immunotherapy. Nat Rev Immunol. 2013;13:862–74. http://www.ncbi.nlm.nih.gov/pubmed/24232462.
243. Leentjens J, Kox M, van der Hoeven JG, Netea MG, Pickkers P. Immunotherapy for the adjunctive treatment of sepsis: from immunosuppression to immunostimulation. Time for a paradigm change? Am J Respir Crit Care Med. 2013;187:1287–93. https://doi.org/10.1164/rccm.201301-0036CP.
244. Islam MN, Bradley BA, Ceredig R. Sterile post-traumatic immunosuppression. Clin Transl Immunol. 2016;5:e77. http://www.ncbi.nlm.nih.gov/pubmed/27195120.
245. Pugin J. Sepsis and the immune response. Intensive Care Med. 1999;25:1027–8. http://www.ncbi.nlm.nih.gov/pubmed/10501766.
246. Spolarics Z, Siddiqi M, Siegel JH, Garcia ZC, Stein DS, Denny T, et al. Depressed interleukin-12-producing activity by monocytes correlates with adverse clinical course and a shift toward Th2-type lymphocyte pattern in severely injured male trauma patients. Crit Care Med. 2003;31:1722–9. https://insights.ovid.com/crossref?an=00003246-200306000-00019.
247. Marik PE, Flemmer M. The immune response to surgery and trauma. J Trauma Acute Care Surg. 2012;73:801–8. http://www.ncbi.nlm.nih.gov/pubmed/22976420.
248. Rendon JL, Choudhry MA. Th17 cells: critical mediators of host responses to burn injury and sepsis. J Leukoc Biol. 2012;92:529–38. http://www.ncbi.nlm.nih.gov/pubmed/22753950.
249. Kim A, Lang T, Xue M, Wijewardana A, Jackson C, Vandervord J. The role of Th-17 cells and γδ T-cells in modulating the systemic inflammatory response to severe burn injury. Int J Mol Sci. 2017;18:758. http://www.ncbi.nlm.nih.gov/pubmed/28368347.
250. Rani M, Schwacha MG. The composition of T-cell subsets are altered in the burn wound early after injury. PLoS One. 2017;12:e0179015. http://www.ncbi.nlm.nih.gov/pubmed/28575063.
251. Monneret G, Debard A-L, Venet F, Bohe J, Hequet O, Bienvenu J, et al. Marked elevation of human circulating CD4+CD25+ regulatory T cells in sepsis-induced immunoparalysis. Crit Care Med. 2003;31:2068–71. https://insights.ovid.com/crossref?an=00003246-200307000-00027
252. Venet F, Pachot A, Debard A-L, Bohé J, Bienvenu J, Lepape A, et al. Increased percentage of CD4+CD25+ regulatory T cells during septic shock is due to the decrease of CD4+CD25- lymphocytes. Crit Care Med. 2004;32:2329–31. http://www.ncbi.nlm.nih.gov/pubmed/15640650
253. Ho VM, Hirohashi N, Kong W-S, Yun G, Ota K, Itai J, et al. Sera from septic patients contain the inhibiting activity of the extracellular ATP-dependent inflammasome pathway. Tohoku J Exp Med. 2018;245:193–204. https://www.jstage.jst.go.jp/article/tjem/245/3/245_193/_article.
254. Levy BD, Serhan CN. Resolution of acute inflammation in the lung. Annu Rev Physiol. 2014;76:467–92. http://www.ncbi.nlm.nih.gov/pubmed/24313723.
255. Fink MP. Prostaglandins and sepsis: still a fascinating topic despite almost 40 years of research. Am J Physiol Lung Cell Mol Physiol. 2001;281:L534–6. https://doi.org/10.1152/ajplung.2001.281.3.L534.
256. Tai H-H, Ensor CM, Tong M, Zhou H, Yan F. Prostaglandin catabolizing enzymes. Prostaglandins Other Lipid Mediat. 2002;68–69:483–93. http://www.ncbi.nlm.nih.gov/pubmed/12432938.
257. Ertel W, Morrison MH, Ayala A, Perrin MM, Chaudry IH. Blockade of prostaglandin production increases cachectin synthesis and prevents depression of macrophage functions after hemorrhagic shock. Ann Surg. 1991;213:265–71. http://www.ncbi.nlm.nih.gov/pubmed/1998408.
258. Faist E, Mewes A, Baker CC, Strasser T, Alkan SS, Rieber P, et al. Prostaglandin E2 (PGE2)-dependent suppression of interleukin alpha (IL-2) production in patients with major trauma. J Trauma. 1987;27:837–48. http://www.ncbi.nlm.nih.gov/pubmed/2956432.

259. Yao YM, Wang YP, Tian HM, Yu Y, Chang GY, Shi ZG, et al. Reduction of circulating prostaglandin E2 level by antiserum against core lipopolysaccharide in a rabbit model of multiple organ failure. J Trauma. 1996;40:270–7. http://www.ncbi.nlm.nih.gov/pubmed/8637078.
260. Brogliato AR, Antunes CA, Carvalho RS, Monteiro APT, Tinoco RF, Bozza MT, et al. Ketoprofen impairs immunosuppression induced by severe sepsis and reveals an important role for Prostaglandin E2. Shock. 2012;38:620–9. http://www.ncbi.nlm.nih.gov/pubmed/23143054.
261. Xu Y, Jiang Y, Gai W, Yu B. Protective role of tenuigenin on sepsis-induced acute kidney injury in mice. Exp Ther Med. 2017;14:5051–6. http://www.ncbi.nlm.nih.gov/pubmed/29201213.
262. Chen I-J, Hee S-W, Liao C-H, Lin S-Y, Su L, Shun C-T, et al. Targeting the 15-keto-PGE2-PTGR2 axis modulates systemic inflammation and survival in experimental sepsis. Free Radic Biol Med. 2018;115:113–26. http://www.ncbi.nlm.nih.gov/pubmed/29175486.
263. Gavins FNE, Hickey MJ. Annexin A1 and the regulation of innate and adaptive immunity. Front Immunol. 2012;3:354. http://www.ncbi.nlm.nih.gov/pubmed/23230437.
264. Pupjalis D, Goetsch J, Kottas DJ, Gerke V, Rescher U. Annexin A1 released from apoptotic cells acts through formyl peptide receptors to dampen inflammatory monocyte activation via JAK/STAT/SOCS signalling. EMBO Mol Med. 2011;3:102–14. https://doi.org/10.1002/emmm.201000113.
265. Tsai W-H, Li I-T, Yu Y-B, Hsu H-C, Shih C-H. Serial changes in plasma annexin A1 and cortisol levels in sepsis patients. Chin J Physiol. 2014;57:1–7. http://www.airitilibrary.com/Publication/alDetailedMesh?DocID=03044920-201402-201403100001-201403100001-1-7.
266. Dalli J, Norling LV, Renshaw D, Cooper D, Leung K-Y, Perretti M. Annexin 1 mediates the rapid anti-inflammatory effects of neutrophil-derived microparticles. Blood. 2008;112:2512–9. https://doi.org/10.1182/blood-2008-02-140533.
267. Perretti M, Christian H, Wheller SK, Aiello I, Mugridge KG, Morris JF, et al. Annexin I is stored within gelatinase granules of human neutrophil and mobilized on the cell surface upon adhesion but not phagocytosis. Cell Biol Int. 2000;24:163–74. https://doi.org/10.1006/cbir.1999.0468.
268. Tsai W-H, Chien H-Y, Shih C-H, Lai S-L, Li I-T, Hsu S-C, et al. Annexin A1 mediates the anti-inflammatory effects during the granulocytic differentiation process in all-trans retinoic acid-treated acute promyelocytic leukemic cells. J Cell Physiol. 2012;227:3661–9. https://doi.org/10.1002/jcp.24073.
269. Huang P, Zhou Y, Liu Z, Zhang P. Interaction between ANXA1 and GATA-3 in immunosuppression of CD4 + T cells. Mediators Inflamm. 2016;2016:1–9. http://www.ncbi.nlm.nih.gov/pubmed/27833268.
270. Buss NAPS, Gavins FNE, Cover PO, Terron A, Buckingham JC. Targeting the annexin 1-formyl peptide receptor 2/ALX pathway affords protection against bacterial LPS-induced pathologic changes in the murine adrenal cortex. FASEB J. 2015;29:2930–42. http://www.ncbi.nlm.nih.gov/pubmed/25818588.
271. Gu J, Luo L, Wang Q, Yan S, Lin J, Li D, et al. Maresin 1 attenuates mitochondrial dysfunction through the ALX/cAMP/ROS pathway in the cecal ligation and puncture mouse model and sepsis patients. Lab Invest. 2018;98:715–33. http://www.ncbi.nlm.nih.gov/pubmed/29467458.
272. Patel N, Wu W, Mishra PK, Chen F, Millman A, Csóka B, et al. A2B adenosine receptor induces protective antihelminth type 2 immune responses. Cell Host Microbe. 2014;15:339–50. http://linkinghub.elsevier.com/retrieve/pii/S1931312814000596.
273. Dalli J, Colas RA, Quintana C, Barragan-Bradford D, Hurwitz S, Levy BD, et al. Human sepsis eicosanoid and proresolving lipid mediator temporal profiles. Crit Care Med. 2017;45:58–68. http://www.ncbi.nlm.nih.gov/pubmed/27632672.
274. Chiurchiù V, Leuti A, Dalli J, Jacobsson A, Battistini L, Maccarrone M, et al. Proresolving lipid mediators resolvin D1, resolvin D2, and maresin 1 are critical in modulating T cell responses. Sci Transl Med. 2016;8:353ra111. https://doi.org/10.1126/scitranslmed.aaf7483.

275. Duffney PF, Falsetta ML, Rackow AR, Thatcher TH, Phipps RP, Sime PJ. Key roles for lipid mediators in the adaptive immune response. J Clin Invest. 2018;128:2724–31. http://www.ncbi.nlm.nih.gov/pubmed/30108196.
276. Krishnamoorthy N, Burkett PR, Dalli J, Abdulnour R-EE, Colas R, Ramon S, et al. Cutting edge: maresin-1 engages regulatory T cells to limit type 2 innate lymphoid cell activation and promote resolution of lung inflammation. J Immunol. 2015;194:863–7. https://doi.org/10.4049/jimmunol.1402534.
277. Leijte GP, Custers H, Gerretsen J, Heijne A, Roth J, Vogl T, et al. Increased plasma levels of danger-associated molecular patterns are associated with immune suppression and postoperative infections in patients undergoing cytoreductive surgery and hyperthermic intraperitoneal chemotherapy. Front Immunol. 2018;9:663. http://www.ncbi.nlm.nih.gov/pubmed/29675023.
278. Lamparello AJ, Namas RA, Constantine G, McKinley TO, Elster E, Vodovotz Y, et al. A conceptual time window-based model for the early stratification of trauma patients. J Intern Med. 2019. http://www.ncbi.nlm.nih.gov/pubmed/30623510.
279. Polito F, Cicciu M, Aguennouz M, Cucinotta M, Cristani M, Lauritano F, et al. Prognostic value of HMGB1 and oxidative stress markers in multiple trauma patients: a single-centre prospective study. Int J Immunopathol Pharmacol. 2016;29:504–9. http://www.ncbi.nlm.nih.gov/pubmed/27343243.
280. Ren B, Zou G, Huang Y, Xu G, Xu F, He J, et al. Serum levels of HSP70 and other DAMP proteins can aid in patient diagnosis after traumatic injury. Cell Stress Chaperones. 2016;21:677–86. https://doi.org/10.1007/s12192-016-0694-4.
281. Krysko DV, Agostinis P, Krysko O, Garg AD, Bachert C, Lambrecht BN, et al. Emerging role of damage-associated molecular patterns derived from mitochondria in inflammation. Trends Immunol. 2011;32:157–64. http://www.ncbi.nlm.nih.gov/pubmed/21334975.
282. Aswani A, Manson J, Itagaki K, Chiazza F, Collino M, Wupeng WL, et al. Scavenging circulating mitochondrial DNA as a potential therapeutic option for multiple organ dysfunction in trauma hemorrhage. Front Immunol. 2018;9:891. http://www.ncbi.nlm.nih.gov/pubmed/29867926.
283. Harrington JS, Huh J-W, Schenck EJ, Nakahira EK, Siempos II, Choi AMK. Circulating mitochondrial DNA as predictor of mortality in critically ill patients. Chest. 2019;156(6):1120–36. http://www.ncbi.nlm.nih.gov/pubmed/31381882.
284. Huber-Lang M, Ignatius A, Brenner RE. Role of complement on broken surfaces after trauma. Adv Exp Med Biol. 2015;865:43–55. http://www.ncbi.nlm.nih.gov/pubmed/26306442.
285. Roumen RM, Redl H, Schlag G, Zilow G, Sandtner W, Koller W, et al. Inflammatory mediators in relation to the development of multiple organ failure in patients after severe blunt trauma. Crit Care Med. 1995;23:474–80. http://www.ncbi.nlm.nih.gov/pubmed/7874897.
286. Berman B, Maderal A, Raphael B. Keloids and hypertrophic scars. Dermatol Surg. 2017;43:S3–18. http://www.ncbi.nlm.nih.gov/pubmed/27347634.
287. Andersson U, Tracey KJ. HMGB1 is a therapeutic target for sterile inflammation and infection. Annu Rev Immunol. 2011;29:139–62. https://doi.org/10.1146/annurev-immunol-030409-101323.
288. Venereau E, De Leo F, Mezzapelle R, Careccia G, Musco G, Bianchi ME. HMGB1 as biomarker and drug target. Pharmacol Res. 2016;111:534–44. https://linkinghub.elsevier.com/retrieve/pii/S104366181630487X.
289. Andersson U, Yang H, Harris H. Extracellular HMGB1 as a therapeutic target in inflammatory diseases. Expert Opin Ther Targets. 2018;22:263–77. http://www.ncbi.nlm.nih.gov/pubmed/29447008.
290. Lundbäck P, Lea JD, Sowinska A, Ottosson L, Fürst CM, Steen J, et al. A novel high mobility group box 1 neutralizing chimeric antibody attenuates drug-induced liver injury and postinjury inflammation in mice. Hepatology. 2016;64:1699–710. https://doi.org/10.1002/hep.28736.
291. Nishibori M. Anti-HMGB1 humanized monoclonal antibody. Abstract at the 8th International DAMPs and Alarmins Symposium. Cold Spring Harbour, NY; 2017.

292. Yang H, Liu H, Zeng Q, Imperato GH, Addorisio ME, Li J, et al. Inhibition of HMGB1/RAGE-mediated endocytosis by HMGB1 antagonist box A, anti-HMGB1 antibodies, and cholinergic agonists suppresses inflammation. Mol Med. 2019;25:13. http://doi/10.1186/s10020-019-0081-6.
293. VanPatten S, Al-Abed Y. High mobility group box-1 (HMGb1): current wisdom and advancement as a potential drug target. J Med Chem. 2018;61:5093–107. http://www.ncbi.nlm.nih.gov/pubmed/29268019.
294. Black GE, Sokol KK, Moe DM, Simmons JD, Muscat D, Pastukh V, et al. Impact of a novel phosphoinositol-3 kinase inhibitor in preventing mitochondrial DNA damage and damage-associated molecular pattern accumulation. J Trauma Acute Care Surg. 2017;83:683–9. http://www.ncbi.nlm.nih.gov/pubmed/28930961.
295. Kepp O, Galluzzi L, Kroemer G. Mitochondrial control of the NLRP3 inflammasome. Nat Immunol. 2011;12:199–200. http://www.nature.com/articles/ni0311-199.
296. Oka T, Hikoso S, Yamaguchi O, Taneike M, Takeda T, Tamai T, et al. Mitochondrial DNA that escapes from autophagy causes inflammation and heart failure. Nature. 2012;485:251–5. https://doi.org/10.1038/nature10992.
297. Pisetsky DS, Lee J, Leong KW, Sullenger BA. Nucleic acid-binding polymers as anti-inflammatory agents: reducing the danger of nuclear attack. Expert Rev Clin Immunol. 2012;8:1–3. http://www.ncbi.nlm.nih.gov/pubmed/22149331.
298. Eppensteiner J, Davis RP, Barbas AS, Kwun J, Lee J. Immunothrombotic activity of damage-associated molecular patterns and extracellular vesicles in secondary organ failure induced by trauma and sterile insults. Front Immunol. 2018;9:190. http://www.ncbi.nlm.nih.gov/pubmed/29472928.
299. Zhang L, Zheng Y, Hu R, Zhu L, Hu C, Cheng F, et al. Annexin A1 mimetic peptide AC2-26 inhibits sepsis-induced cardiomyocyte apoptosis through LXA4/PI3K/AKT signaling pathway. Curr Med Sci. 2018;38:997–1004. http://www.ncbi.nlm.nih.gov/pubmed/30536061.

Solid Organ Injury

9

9.1 Introduction

This chapter is a continuation of Chap. 8 focusing not only on traumatic but also on nontraumatic solid organ injuries, including drug-induced organ toxicity and intoxications, all of which are known to be associated with the emission of pathogenetic DAMPs. These molecules—in case of an infectious injury together with MAMPs—can trigger acute uncontrolled/dysregulated proinflammatory processes, clinically manifested as an acute organ-specific disease. Eventually, in case of acute repetitive or persistent injuries, tissue inflammation transitions—via chronic nonresolving inflammation and under involvement of MAMP/DAMP-promoted profibrotic pathways—into chronic organ fibrosis, often clinically manifested as chronic organ failure (for global DAMP-induced inflammatory and fibrotic responses, also compare Vol. 1, [1], Part VI, Sects. 22.2.4 and 22.2.5, and Part VIII, Sect. 36.4). Here, some major organ-specific injuries have been selected, restricted to the brain, lung, kidney, liver, pancreas, and musculoskeletal system but all emphasized in light of the danger/injury model in Immunology.

In addition, given some peculiarities of intoxications per se and excessive alcohol consumption as a global healthcare problem, in particular, the alcoholic intoxication has been chosen as a typical acute injury affecting many tissues and organs, including the brain, liver, and pancreas. From the perspective of the book, a few aspects are touched to this kind of organ damage by highlighting the role of DAMPs again.

9.2 Brain Injury

9.2.1 Introductory Remarks

Neuroinflammation is defined as the homeostatic or dysregulated innate immune response of the CNS against cell stress and tissue injury. The neuroinflammatory

W. G. Land, *Damage-Associated Molecular Patterns in Human Diseases*,
https://doi.org/10.1007/978-3-030-53868-2_9

response presents shared characteristics with peripheral inflammation but also retains specific features, such as the existence of the blood–brain barrier (BBB) and the cerebrospinal fluid (CSF), or the activation of PRM-bearing glial cells. Etiologically, several brain injuries are known to induce neuroinflammation, including TBI, cerebral stroke, bacterial and viral infections, and alcoholic intoxication. Here, a few remarks are made restricted to TBI and alcohol intoxication.

9.2.2 Traumatic Brain Injury

Etiologically, the most important variants of neuroinflammation-inducing injury are traumatically acquired brain injuries that are clinically grouped by severity: mild, moderate, and severe injuries [2]. The severe acute TBI—a leading cause of death and disability worldwide—is a heterogeneous disorder resulting from an external force applied to the head. The TBI triggers a focal immune response that is initiated within minutes after the primary injury. This focal brain inflammation involves both brain-resident and peripheral immune cells with complicated interactions. Typically, the development of cerebral edema (CE) plays a central role in the evolution of this particular injury and is closely associated with pathoneurological outcomes (for reviews, see [3, 4]). Current notions hold that TBI promotes a robust innate immune response induced by DAMPs that are also denoted as immunological stressors elsewhere [5, 6]. In the following, the emerging evidence and features of focal brain inflammation after TBI are briefly outlined by highlighting the pathogenetic role of DAMPs.

9.2.3 Regulated Cell Death in Traumatic Brain Injury

As experimentally shown, various subroutines of RCD reportedly occur in TBI including apoptosis [7], necroptosis [8–10], ferroptosis [11–15], and pyroptosis [16, 17] (for RCD, see Sect. 4.3 and Vol. 1 [1], Part V, Chap. 19).

The subroutine of ferroptosis has been uncovered to play a vital role in TBI. In fact, besides nonenzymatic oxidation mechanisms contributing to the overall oxidative burden immediately following brain injury, subsequent action of upregulated enzymes causing lipid peroxidation has recently been described, including members of the COX family, LOX family, and cytochrome P450 [18–20] (for mechanisms of lipid peroxidation-associated ferroptosis (compare Sect. 4.3.4.2 and Vol. 1 [1], Part V, Sect. 19.3.3 and Fig. 19.6).

Given the impact of these pro-oxidative processes in TBI (also see below), the detection of ferroptotically dying neurons is not surprising. For example, in a pediatric rat controlled cortical impact model of TBI, elevated levels of oxidized polyunsaturated PE lipid species could be detected at early time points (1–4 h) post-injury, consistent with the loss of GPX4 function and initiation of ferroptotic cell death [21]. In other studies on a controlled cortical impact model of TBI in mice, a loss of iron-positive cells and morphological evidence consistent with ferroptosis (i.e., shrunken mitochondria) were observed at or near the injury site [14]. Moreover, in these experiments, cell death and the associated long-term motor and cognitive dysfunction were reduced by co-treatment with ferrostatin-1, an inhibitor of ferroptosis, administered at the time of injury directly into the cerebral ventricles.

In sum, these first observations suggest RCD to serve as critical sources of DAMPs, which trigger necro-neuroinflammatory responses involved in the pathogenesis of TBI, although the underlying molecular mechanisms are still not fully understood.

9.2.4 Pathogenesis of Traumatic Brain Injury (in Brief)

9.2.4.1 General Remarks

The pathophysiology of TBI is dominated by a complex dynamic process that initiates a multitude of cascades of pathological pathways, including alterations in cerebral perfusion, activation of inflammatory cytokines, and excitotoxicity (i.e., overactivations of receptors for the excitatory neurotransmitter glutamate, such as the *N-methyl*-d-*aspartate* [NMDA] receptor and *α-amino-3-hydroxy-5-methyl-4-isoxazolepropionic acid* [AMPA] receptor). Its symptomatic presentation varies with each individual, injury type, injury severity, age, and gender. The complexity of the process results from primary and secondary brain injuries that result in temporary or permanent neurological deficits. The primary injury of TBI causes direct damage to neural tissue and refers to insults incurred from external mechanical forces of trauma that are regarded as the major factor determining the patients' outcomes. Focal intracranial hemorrhage, epidural and subdural hematoma, brain contusion, and direct axonal damage are all examples of primary lesions that reflect primary sources of constitutive and inducible DAMPs (for pathologies induced by primary brain injury in TBI, see also [22]). Subsequently, a cascade of secondary injury processes (i.e., delayed nonmechanical damages) is initiated at the time of the insult and develops posttraumatically—from minutes to days from the primary impact.

9.2.4.2 Main DAMP-Triggered Pro-oxidative and Proinflammatory Processes Involved in the Pathophysiology of Traumatic Brain Injury

The subsequent injury is of essential pathophysiological importance. This injury is caused by multiple interconnected molecular pathways including but not limited to alterations in cerebral perfusion, ion/fluid imbalance such as calcium and iron perturbations, ROS-mediated oxidative stress, disruption of the BBB, mitochondrial dysfunction, excitotoxicity, and a neuroinflammatory response comprised of local and systemic immune activation (for in-depth articles, see [4, 23–30]). Oxidative stress is of particular relevance. As emphasized [31], excessive glutamate at the synaptic junction, which in turn activates its NMDA and AMPA receptors, facilitates excessive calcium influx into the neuronal cells and promotes oxidative stress

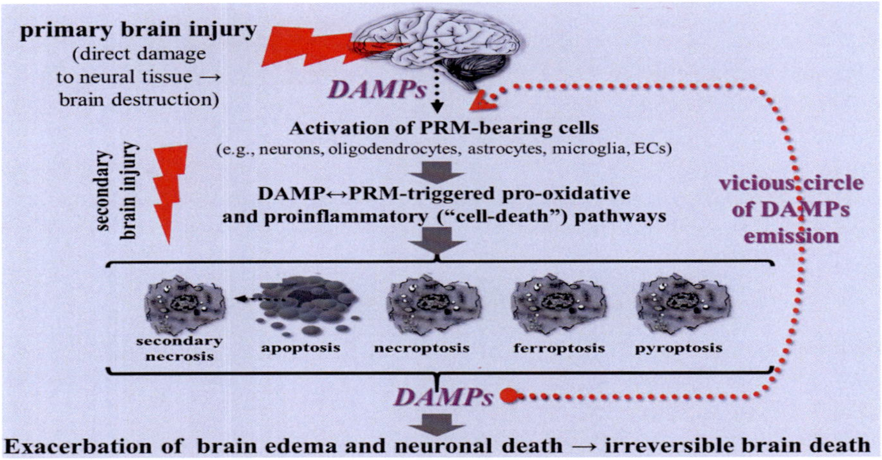

Fig. 9.1 Simplified schematic diagram of a conceptual model illustrating emission of constitutive and inducible DAMPs during primary and secondary brain injury in TBI. Emission of DAMPs as a cause of external mechanical forces of the initial trauma promotes innate immune pro-oxidative and proinflammatory processes, which converge to and culminate in cell death pathways resulting in various subroutines of regulated necrosis (apoptosis → secondary necrosis, necroptosis, pyroptosis, ferroptosis). These various forms of regulated necrosis serve as secondary sources of emission of constitutive and inducible DAMPs, which, again, promote cell death pathways resulting in subroutines of regulated necrosis (i.e., a vicious circle of DAMPs emission). In severe trauma, these processes may lead to irreversible brain death. Note: compare also Sect. 4.3 and Fig. 4.2a, b and also Vol. 1 [1], Part V, Sect. 19.3, and Figs. 19.2, 19.4, 19.6, and 19.7. *PRM* pattern recognition molecules. (Sources: [4, 7–14, 16, 17, 23–30])

that further leads to mitochondrial dysfunction, oxidation of lipids, proteins, and DNA.

All these pro-oxidative and proinflammatory processes converge to and culminate in cell death pathways resulting in death of cerebral cells (Fig. 9.1). These cells are all susceptible to traumatic injury, with neurons being the most sensitive to direct injury, followed by oligodendrocytes, astrocytes, microglia, and ECs being particularly resistant to damage. As experimentally shown, various forms of cell death may occur, executed either directly via ACD or indirectly through RCD, as mentioned above. With the discovery of these subroutines of RCD, the critical sources of secondarily emitted DAMPs in TBI became evident, that is, DAMPs that are released from the damaged meninges, glial limitans, and parenchyma. Indeed, there is growing evidence in support of the notion that the emission of DAMPs that is associated with the various forms of TBI-induced neuronal cell death not only initiate but also perpetuate innate immune "cell death" pathways involved in the pathophysiology of TBI [25, 32, 33] (Fig. 9.1). These DAMP-promoted innate immune inflammatory responses, including complement activation, lead—or at least contribute—to CE that (1) plays a vital role in the evolution of injury following brain trauma, (2) is closely associated with neurologic outcomes, and, most importantly, (3) can lead to intracranial hypertension. Indeed, it is this intracranial hypertension that can compromise cerebral perfusion pressure and cerebral blood flow, which can eventually cause irreversible brain injury, herniation, and death (for reviews, see [27, 34–36]).

9.2.4.3 SAMP-Promoted Inflammation-Resolving Processes in Traumatic Brain Injury

A resolution phase of the inflammatory response has been reported but does not always occur following TBI, and, thus, chronic inflammation can persist. Indeed, monocytes were shown to convert into macrophages that have the ability to produce neuroprotective cytokines (IL-10, TGF-β) in response to DAMPs. These macrophages are implicated in the cleanup of debris and damaged cells. Studies have also shown other beneficial aspects of cerebral immunity following brain injuries, besides resolution of inflammation, preservation of barrier function, and the release of trophic factors (for review, see Jassam et al. [27]). However, little is known regarding the role SAMPs in the resolving phase after TBI; nevertheless, a few SAMPs such as LXs, Rvs, and Pds have been described and will be briefly touched below.

9.2.4.4 Concluding Remarks

Together, modern insights into pathogenetic mechanisms of TBI have revealed a pivotal role of DAMPs that are implicated in various brain injury-induced neurological pathologies, including excitotoxicity, development of edema, and neuroinflammatory activities. Of note, in addition to focal brain inflammation, accumulating evidence obtained from patients and animal models suggests that brain inflammation after TBI is not restricted to the lesions but instead disseminates to areas remote from the lesions. Furthermore, the disseminated brain inflammation may be persistent and impact brain pathology, causing progressive neurodegeneration [30].

Histopathologically, various DAMPs reportedly induce proinflammatory activation in microglia, astrocytes, and neurons [37–40]: a topic that will be further explored below.

9.2.5 Alcohol-Related Brain Injury

Excessive, acute repetitive, and chronic alcohol consumptions are associated with the induction of a neuroinflammatory response in the brain that may contribute to neurodegeneration. Of note, as seen in other forms of injury, heavy alcohol intake, such as binge drinking, was observed to induce necrosis associated with neurodegeneration. Most commonly, long-standing heavy alcohol abuse leads to disproportionate loss of cerebral white matter and impairments in executive function (for reviews, see [41–44]).

Acute effects of alcohol on the CNS are mainly caused by injurious alcohol poisoning leading to encephalopathy, whereas chronic alcohol abuse is known to have long-lasting adverse effects on brain function and produce deficits ranging from mild cognitive impairment to dementia. The spectrum of dementias encompasses

Wernicke–Korsakoff syndrome, Marchiafava–Bignami, and acquired hepatocerebral degeneration. Also, alcoholics often sustain TBI and can secondarily develop debilitating or fatal CNS diseases [45, 46].

Various pathophysiological mechanisms of alcohol-induced injury have been described, including inflammation, impaired anabolic signaling, upregulation of catabolic processes, and dysregulation in lipid metabolism. Current notions hold that alcohol-related metabolic encephalopathy is mediated by a self-perpetuating injury loop initiated by astrocyte swelling, which leads to oxidative and nitrosative stress, impaired intracellular signaling, PTMs of proteins, and gene expression (reviewed in [44, 47, 48]).

9.2.6 DAMPs in Brain Injury

9.2.6.1 General Remarks

As reported, both primary and secondary injury in TBI results in the release of DAMPs such as HMGB1, DNA and RNA, S100 proteins, ATP, uric acid, LPLs (i.e., inducible IIIB-5 DAMPs, a major phospholipid component of OxLDL), and lipid peroxidation-derived carbonyl adducts of proteins. Other critical sources of DAMPs refer to simultaneously occurring extracerebral organ injuries. For example, in studies in mice, bone fracture-stimulated emission of HMGB1 was shown to contribute to the development of secondary TBI [49]. Subsequently, DAMP-activated innate immune cells such as glial cells, neurons, leukocytes, and ECs produce inducible DAMPs including TNF and IL-1β which drive and expand early posttraumatic neuroinflammation (reported in [26, 27, 50–53]). Of note, the proinflammatory TNF was demonstrated to be linked to brain edema, BBB disruption, and recruitment of leukocytes, whereas the antiinflammatory IL-10 was assumed to possess neuroprotective properties [26, 54].

9.2.6.2 High Mobility Group Box 1

High mobility group box 1 has been described in Vol. 1 [1], Part IV, Sect. 12.2.2, denoted as a constitutive IA-1 DAMP, and Sect. 14.3.3, denoted as an inducible IIIB-2 DAMP (compare Table 3.1). The role of HMGB1 in TBI has recently been reviewed by Parker et al. [55]. So far, six studies have assessed the role of HMGB1 in TBI using mouse or rat models [56–61]. In sum, HMGB1—suggested to be released by injured necrotic neurons into the extracellular space—was shown to be involved in both early and later stages after TBI [57], and experimental inhibition of this IA-1 DAMP expression proved to be beneficial.

For example, in studies in rats, administration of an anti-HMGB1 mAb after TBI was shown to remarkably inhibit fluid percussion-induced brain edema [56] (for details, see Sect. 9.9.3.2). In contrast, intravenous injection of recombinant HMGB1 dose-dependently produced the opposite effects. Further experiments suggested the involvement of RAGE as the predominant receptor for HMGB1. In other lines of studies, ethyl pyruvate was shown to have protective effects on the development of CE following TBI in rats suggested by the authors to be mediated by the reduction of HMGB1-triggered TLR4 → NF-κB signaling pathway [58]. In support of these findings were other lines of studies on a murine TBI model demonstrating that HMGB1 promotes CE via activation of TLR4 [59]. In two separate studies exploring potential therapeutic options, the neuroprotective agent glycyrrhizin was observed to (1) reduce CE significantly, (2) suppress the increase in BBB permeability and impairment of motor functions, and (3) improve outcomes in rats following TBI by downregulation of HMGB1-triggered, TLR4 or RAGE → NF-κB-mediated inflammatory responses in the injured rat brain [60, 61]. Together, these experimental studies in rodents significantly show that, following TBI, HMGB1 is released from damaged and necrotic neurons to trigger efferent innate immune pathways contributing to CE and other typical pathological features of this life-threatening organ injury.

Of note, there are a few reports on a role of DAMPs, in particular, HMGB1, in mounting a neuroinflammatory milieu in alcohol-induced brain injury (also compare [62]). For example, in rats, alcohol exposure during adolescence was found to activate HMGB1 → TLR4 signaling in the brain, and this activation was observed to persist into adulthood correlating with adult neurocognitive dysfunction [63]. In other lines of studies on mice, chronic alcohol treatment was shown to increase HMGB1 in cortex and cerebellum [64]. Also, as demonstrated by experiments in rats exposed to intragastric binge ethanol administrations, HMGB1 was found to be upregulated in the frontal cortex of the animals. In support of such findings are in vitro experiments on human and rat neurons, showing that ethanol can directly induce HMGB1 release in neuronal cells, associated with *nicotinamide adenine dinucleotide phosphate-dependent oxidase* 2 (NOX2)/NLRP1 inflammasome signaling [65].

The impressive findings of a pathogenetic role of HMGB1 in experimental TBI are reflected by clinical observations too. So far, four reports of investigating this DAMP in patients with TBI have been published [57, 59, 66, 67]. As competently summarized by Parker et al. [55], immunohistochemical examination of HMGB1 expression in brain tissue taken postmortem from patients with TBI showed immunoreactivity to be either lost or translocalized to the cytoplasm of intralesional cells up to 1 day following injury. In cases resulting in death between 2 and 20 days post-TBI, HMGB1 was localized in the cytoplasm of infiltrating phagocytic microglia.

Importantly, levels of HMGB1 could be measured in the CSF of adult patients with TBI [59] whereas, in pediatric patients, the CSF levels of HMGB1 were found to be even predictive for outcome [67]. Indeed, the detection of HMGB1 in the CSF indicates that this DAMP is released from injured neurons following TBI in humans. Moreover, an observational clinical study in patients with severe TBI revealed that the plasma HMGB1 concentration can be successfully used as a novel biomarker for significantly predicting 1-year mortality and unfavorable outcome of TBI [66].

Of interest in this context are clinical studies providing similar data in individuals with excessive alcohol consumption. Thus, young female regular alcohol binge drinkers reportedly show elevated HMGB1 in plasma [68], and—as revealed by postmortem brain studies on human alcoholic patients, who averaged over ten drinks per day with lifetime consumption of over 500 kg of alcohol—the expression of HMGB1 was found to be increased in the frontal cortex of those patients [64]. Moreover, in similar analyses of human postmortem samples of the orbitofrontal cortex, the RAGE receptor was found to be upregulated in the postmortem human alcoholic orbitofrontal cortex, and an earlier age of drinking onset could be demonstrated to be correlated with increased RAGE, TLR4, and HMGB1 expression [69]. Given these data (and other data not quoted here), the authors concluded that "these data reveal that early life insults exert long-lasting neuroimmune changes in the developing CNS that might contribute to increased risk of developing alcohol dependence and other psychopathologies."

Together, these clinical studies demonstrate increased circulating levels of HMGB1 in plasma or CSF of patients with TBI or increased alcohol consumption, suggesting this IA-1 DAMP to contribute to the pathogenesis of TBI and alcoholic brain diseases including Wernicke–Korsakoff syndrome and alcoholic dementia.

9.2.6.3 Mitochondrial DNA

Mitochondrial DNA has been described in Vol. 1 [1], Part IV, Sect. 13.4.3.2, denoted as IIC-2 DAMPs. The critical role of mtDNA in severe trauma has been outlined in Sect. 8.3.3.3. The involvement of this DAMP in TBI could be demonstrated in investigations on the CSF of pediatric patients [70]. As reported, the mean CSF mtDNA in pediatric TBI was increased in comparison to controls. Remarkably, the CSF mtDNA concentration in pediatric patients who later died or had a severe disability was significantly higher than that of the survivors. Moreover, the authors found a significant correlation between CSF mtDNA and HMGB1, indicating that both DAMPs are increased in the CSF following TBI in pediatric patients.

9.2.6.4 S100 Proteins

S100 proteins have been described in Vol. 1 [1], Part IV, Sect. 12.2.4.2, denoted as constitutive IA-1 DAMPs, and Sect. 14.2.2.4, denoted as inducible IIIA-1 DAMPs. Out of the family of S100 proteins, S100 B proteins have been reported as classical serum biomarkers in TBI, first published already in 1995 [71], and now regarded as a critical DAMP. Similar to other DAMP levels such as HMGB1, the protein was found to be increased in the bloodstream in the acute phase of the trauma and assessed as one of the strongest single predictors of unfavorable TBI outcome [72]. Studies in patients with TBI revealed a primary peak of S100B level during the time of the initial injury, followed by a secondary peak resulting from the second injury predicting an unfavorable outcome [73]. In an analysis of serum levels of S100B proteins in pediatric patients with TBI, median serum levels of S100B at admission were shown to decrease significantly 1 week after TBI [74]. Follow-up of these patients revealed that serum S100B levels 1 week after injury in patients with unfavorable 6-month outcomes were significantly higher than levels 1 week after injury in patients with favorable outcomes. The authors concluded that serial measurements of serum S100B may help to assess brain damage and clinical outcome of pediatric patients with TBI.

A role of S100 proteins has also been investigated in white matter damage after TBI. As reviewed [5], acutely elevated serum levels of S100B were associated with patient mortality and poor acute and chronic outcomes after severe TBI and were predictive of cognitive function at 4 months after pediatric mild TBI.

9.2.6.5 Oxidation-Specific Epitopes

Membrane-bound OSEs (denoted as IIB-1 DAMPs) have been described in Vol. 1 [1], Part IV, Sect. 13.3.2, and briefly resumed in Sect. 3.4.3.2. They include molecules such as PS, OxPLs containing OxCL, PC, or PE headgroups, as well as 4-HNE, MDA, and oxidized phosphatidylethanolamine (OxPE), all of which are sensed by a broad range of cellular and humoral PRMs (compare also Vol. 1 [1], Part IV, Sect. 13.3.2.2. and Fig. 13.1). Of note, in studies of lipid peroxidation in TBI, these OSEs were already detected (reviewed by Bayır's group in [13]). For example, increased 4-HNE or HNE-modified proteins have been found in brain tissue using various experimental models of TBI, and an increase of MDA was observed in plasma or CSF in patients following severe TBI [75–77].

Intriguingly, first studies provided evidence for a role of OSEs such as oxygenated PE and oxygenated PL in triggering RCD. Thus, as recently reported [78], oxygenated PEs, especially those containing omega-6 fatty acids such as AA and adrenic acid, were shown to trigger ferroptosis, thereby providing a source for emission of large amounts of further DAMPs. By contrast, oxidation of CL to OxCL—also generated in the injured brain [12]—was demonstrated to be a required step in the execution of apoptosis [79, 80]. Indeed, the temporal profile of CL oxidation in the injured brain was found to indicate the initiation of apoptosis 3 h following TBI [81].

In sum, evidence is accumulating that redox signaling in ferroptosis and apoptosis is based on specific engagement of two different classes of phospholipids; however, in TBI, both ferroptosis and apoptosis (when transforming to secondary necrosis) may serve as a source of emission of DAMPs: again an impressive example of a "DAMPs axis" operating in acute organ injury.

9.2.6.6 Concluding Remarks

There is an increasing number of reports on DAMPs in TBI—less in alcohol-related brain injury—which document the growing pathogenetic role of these molecules in acute brain injury. It has become evident—like in all kinds of organ injuries and given the complexity of pathophysiological processes in TBI—that there are various DAMPs released from cells succumbing RN in the traumatically injured brain. Recognized by PRM-bearing cells such as microglial cells, astrocytes, and neurons, they trigger intracerebral life-threatening proinflammatory signaling pathways that may culminate in brain death. Certainly, as potential therapeutic targets, the list of these molecules mentioned here will be supplemented soon.

9.2.7 SAMPs in Brain Injury

To date, only a few studies on the inflammation-resolving function of SAMPs in TBI have been published. As discussed above, at later stages after injury, SAMPs such as LXs, Rvs, and Pds reportedly contribute to the resolution of inflammation. In this context, oxidized PtdSer has been discussed as a potential SAMP involved in TBI. However, "To date, no studies have directly connected PS oxidation and coagulation status in TBI, but it is possible that oxidized PS may prevent injury propagation through an unexplored role in promotion of coagulation" [13]. Interestingly, in an investigation of the effect of SPMs on posttraumatic sleep and functional outcome following diffuse TBI in mice, the resolvins AT-D1 and E1 were found to differentially impact the functional outcome, posttraumatic sleep, and microglial activation following diffuse brain injury in the mouse [82].

Of great interest is the role of the SAMP extracellular adenosine in brain injuries. Indeed, TBI is known to be associated with increased brain levels of extracellular adenosine (reviewed in [83]). For example, in studies in pediatric patients with severe TBI, CSF adenosine concentration was observed to be increased in a time- and severity-dependent manner in infants and children after severe head injury [84]. The authors argued that the association between CSF adenosine and glutamate concentrations may reflect an endogenous attempt at neuroprotection against excitotoxicity after severe TBI. In subsequent studies on mice undergoing experimental TBI, this early adenosine release response was shown—via activation of purine A1 receptors—to suppress seizures [85] and microglial response-mediated brain inflammation [86]. Intriguingly, the authors concluded [86] that the activated A1 receptor "is an endogenous inhibitor of the microglial response to TBI, likely via inhibition of proliferation, and this may represent a therapeutic avenue to modulate microglia after TBI"—a recommendation that was echoed by Jackson et al. [83]: "Developing therapeutics that recruit astrocytes to produce/release adenosine could have beneficial effects in TBI" (for purinergic receptors, compare Sect. 2.3.3, and Vol. 1 [1], Part II, Sect. 5.3.4).

Another SAMP, PGE2, was also observed to contribute to the therapeutic efficacy of MSCs in experimental TBI [87]. In this study on mice, among the immunomodulatory factors assessed, the therapeutic benefit of MSCs was observed to correlate with the secretion of PGE2 by MSCs before treatment.

Also of interest in this context is a report on AnxA1 in BBB protection after experimental intracerebral hemorrhage [88]. This study on an experimental intracerebral hemorrhage model in rats provided evidence suggesting that the proresolving effect of AnxA1 may also participate in a protective effect on intracerebral hemorrhage-induced secondary brain injury.

Together, the beneficial function of some SAMPs in TBI has been documented; however, more targeted studies, in particular, with the use of SPMs, are needed to confirm their protective abilities in TBI.

9.2.8 Résumé

Although there is a lack of effective treatment for TBI recovery today, the efforts for developing therapeutic strategies on TBI recovery have been continuously made over the past several decades. Besides improvement of standard medical and surgical interventions, attention should also be paid to the use of DAMPs inhibitors and administration of SAMPs or their derivates. Indeed, a growing number of reports on DAMPs released from injured cells and tissue during TBI have confirmed their pivotal role in the initiation and regulation of inflammatory responses, which induce the damage cascade leading to secondary brain damage. Nevertheless, future studies are needed to define the role of SAMPs in brain injury. It can be expected that results from such future studies, in particular, with the use of SPMs in brain trauma will provide new TBI treatments by controlling resolution and downstream mechanisms of neuroinflammatory responses.

Also, subroutines of RN emerge as future therapeutic targets for protecting the injured brain. As mentioned above, the occurrence of necroptosis, pyroptosis, and ferroptosis in an animal model of TBI has already been described. Administration of distinct RN inhibitors has to be taken into consideration aimed at preventing a priori emission of DAMPs. For example, in studies on a murine TBI model, application of ferrostatin-1 (a ferroptosis inhibitor, also known as Fer-1) by cerebral ventricular injection was recently demonstrated to significantly reduce neuronal cell death and improve long-term cognitive and motor function [14]. Further studies in this field are now required to determine the therapeutic window of such inhibitors and develop clinically feasible drugs.

9.3 Acute and Chronic Lung Injury

9.3.1 Introductory Remarks

Acute lung injury is an acute inflammatory disorder with substantial morbidity that can develop into a complex pulmonary process first officially described as ARDS in 1967 [89]. This life-threatening—in about 40% of patients lethal—disorder develops in most cases within 2–5 days of hospitalization and is usually diagnosed clinico-radiographically. Of note, if the timely homeostatic resolution of acute lung inflammation is unrestrained, or if exposure to toxic environmental factors turns out to be acute repetitive or persistent, a COPD can develop. Again, this COPD is a life-threatening disorder that is associated with high morbidity and mortality and, thus, creates enormous challenges for healthcare systems. Here, both diseases are examined in more detail in light of the danger/injury model.

9.3.2 Acute Lung Injury → Acute Respiratory Distress Syndrome

As touched, ALI, when proceeding to ARDS, is associated with high mortality and morbidity rates that increase with disease severity (for reviews, see [90–96]). In the earlier periods, there were some difficulties with an accurate assessment of the clinical symptomology of ARDS. Then, in 2012, the Berlin definition was published stressing the mutually exclusive categories of the disease: mild, moderate, and severe—as based on the degree of hypoxemia and four ancillary variables for severe ARDS. These are radiographic severity, respiratory system compliance, positive end-expiratory pressure, and corrected expired volume per minute (these variables were later removed because they did not contribute to the predictive validity of severe ARDS for mortality) [97].

In light of new insights into mechanisms of controlled and uncontrolled DAMP-promoted efferent innate immune responses, mild ALI-induced pulmonary inflammation (i.e., pneumonia) resulting in resolution of the inflammatory response may reflect a controlled protective innate immune response, whereas ALI→ARDS represents a typical dysregulated overshooting efferent response caused by emission of DAMPs in excess.

9.3.3 Regulated Cell Death and Necroinflammation in Acute Lung Injury

Recently, the event of RCD in ARDS has been well appreciated and is of growing particular importance (for subroutines of RCD, see Sect. 4.3 and also Vol. 1 [1], Part V, Chpt. 19). Besides apoptosis of cells of the distal pulmonary epithelium and the endothelium [98, 99], necroptosis is discussed as another emerging subroutine of RCD. Thus, in experiments on mice, RIP3-mediated necroptosis of alveolar wall EpCs and macrophage-like cells was demonstrated to be a significant mechanism of enhanced inflammation and lung tissue injury in high dose LPS-induced severe ARDS [100] (compare Fig. 9.2). Moreover, in an experimental rat model of ARDS, necroptosis could be

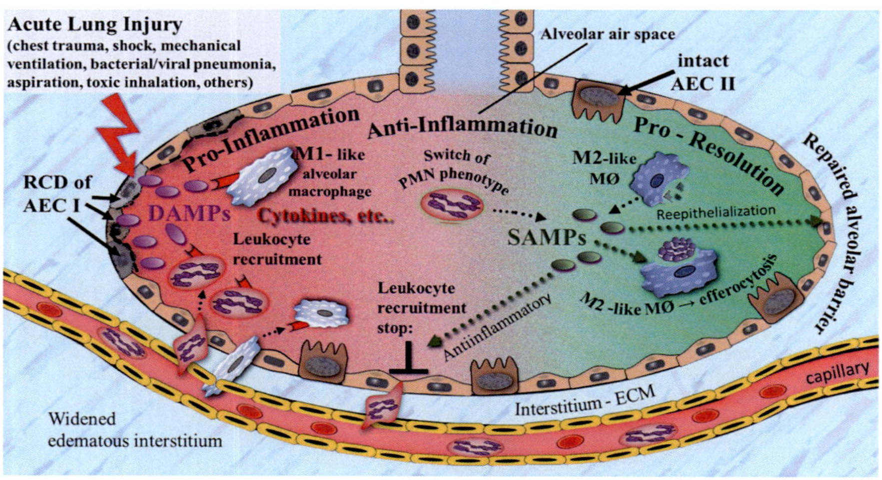

Fig. 9.2 Simplified schematic diagram of a narrative model of the action of DAMPs and SAMPs in acute lung injury. Injury-induced DAMPs (e.g., released from type I alveolar epithelial cells succumbing to RCD) activate innate immune cells such as polymorphonuclear leukocytes and M1-like macrophages that in turn promote acute pulmonary inflammation via secretion of proinflammatory mediator substances (e.g., cytokines). SAMPs mainly secreted by injury-activated M2-like macrophages contribute to resolution of alveolar inflammation via promotion of antiinflammatory mechanisms (e.g., production of IL-10), efferocytosis, and reepithelialization—the end result being repair of the alveolar barrier. *AECI* type I alveolar epithelial cells, *AECII* type II alveolar epithelial cells, *ECM* extracellular matrix, *MØ* macrophage, *PMN* polymorphonuclear leukocytes, *RCD* regulated cell death. (Sources: [110–113, 164, 455])

induced by oleic acid, also suggesting that the pathogenesis of this disease may involve necroptosis [101]. These first experimental findings are supported by a clinical study showing that blood transfusion-related ALI enhances the susceptibility to ARDS in critically ill transfused patients and mice through necroptosis of lung ECs [102]. Of note, besides necroptosis of alveolar cells, initial emerging evidence suggested that necroptosis and pyroptosis of alveolar macrophages may also play essential roles in the progression of lung inflammation resulting in ARDS [101, 103]. Nevertheless, the role of necroptosis and pyroptosis (and probably also ferroptosis) in the development of ARDS is to be determined more solidly by further targeted studies.

Importantly, a role of NETs/NETosis in the pathogenesis of ARDS has also been reported. Based on an analysis of bronchial aspirates from ARDS patients showing NETs to be significantly correlated with the degree of ARDS, a *hydrochloric acid (HCL) aspiration-induced* ALI model was developed in mice to assess whether NETs are pathogenetic and whether targeting NETs is protective [104]. Indeed, with the use of this experimental model, the authors were successful in demonstrating that HCl aspiration causes severe lung injury, together with significantly increased levels of NETs, which are correlated with the severity of ALI → ARDS.

Together, these first observations point to subroutines of RCD as critical sources of DAMPs, which trigger necro-hyperinflammatory responses involved in the pathogenesis of ARDS. Nevertheless, the molecular mechanisms responsible for the development of these ARDS-associated conditions—though increasingly learned—are still not fully understood, but there is growing evidence in support of the notion that the DAMPs play a vital role in these pathologies.

9.3.4 Pathogenesis of Acute Lung Injury → Acute Respiratory Distress Syndrome (in Brief)

9.3.4.1 General Remarks

Development of ALI → ARDS is a classical complication after major trauma with shock, but other numerous acute alveolar injury-causing insults have been described including but not limited to infection, mechanical ventilation, acute bacterial or viral pneumonia, burns, aspiration of gastric contents, immunologically mediated pulmonary hemorrhage, and vasculitis. Predisposing clinical factors that may contribute to that kind of an overshooting innate immune response include acute pancreatitis, blood transfusions, drug overdose reactions, and cigarette smoke or toxic gas inhalation. Moreover, genetic polymorphisms that predispose individuals to the injurious effects of specific bacteria or viruses may also influence the development of ALI and ARDS (for competent papers, see [90, 92, 96, 105, 106]).

9.3.4.2 MAMP/DAMP-Driven Promotion of Lung Inflammation in Acute Lung Injury → Acute Respiratory Distress Syndrome

Despite many years of experimental and clinical studies, the exact molecular mechanisms governing pathogenesis of ALI → ARDS remained unclear until it became evident that MAMP/DAMP-triggered innate immune responses play a crucial role in this peculiar organ injury as well (additional involvement of MAMPs refer to pathogen-mediated ALI).

The typical pathophysiological scenario observed in ALI and ARDS is based on an initial acute pulmonary inflammatory response due to direct or indirect lung injury caused by those factors listed above. The severe uncontrolled inflammatory responses are the result of secretion/release of cytokines (e.g., TNF, IL-1β, IL-6, IL-8) and histamine by MAMP/DAMP- or DAMP-activated pulmonary PRM-bearing cells such as resident alveolar M1-like macrophages, alveolar epithelial, and vascular cells. These cells—in terms of an amplifying inflammatory response and associated with increased vascular permeability—recruit further mobile PRM-expressing cells such as neutrophils, monocytes, macrophages, platelets, and DCs to the lung. Excessive neutrophilic influx into the alveolar space leads to the generation of ROS and further proinflammatory factors, which could aggravate the disruption of the alveolar–capillary barrier (compare Fig. 9.2).

Notably, in the case of pathogen-induced ALI, T and B lymphocyte as cells of the pathogen-specific adaptive immune response join the family of infiltrating cells. Arrived in the lung, the mobile immune cells, in turn, get activated to produce further cytokines and chemokines as well as cytotoxic mediators such as ROS and proteolytic enzymes (proteases) and granular enzymes. Additionally, recruited dying neutrophils produce NETs. These products at the efferent arm of the innate immune response (in case of infection, plus adaptive immune T and B cells) mediate vascular endothelial and alveolar epithelial cell damage that leads to disruption of the alveolar endothelial and epithelial barriers (for in-depth articles, see [90, 95, 107, 108]). It is this alveolar epithelium that can be regarded as a critical target of the innate immune attacks. It is composed of two types of cells, which, under homeostatic conditions, form a natural barrier. Type I cells, which make up 90% of the alveolar epithelium, are sensitive to toxins and oxidative stress and are prone to necrosis. They are easily injured compared to PRM-expressing type II cells, which make up 10% of the alveolar surface area and—as a defender of the alveolus—are involved in surfactant production and sodium transport, as well as induce proliferation and differentiation to type I cells contributing to alveolar epithelial repair [109] (compare Fig. 9.2, and also Vol. 1 [1], Part III, Sect. 9.2.4). The interaction between the epithelial barrier and the other barrier, that is, the microvascular endothelium plays a crucial role in controlling fluid accumulation in the alveolar space. The various inflammatory and cytotoxic mediators mentioned above promote RCD of both alveolar type I and II EpCs and ECs (apoptosis, necroptosis) leading to disruption of the barriers associated with hyperpermeability, resulting in pulmonary edema, intrapulmonary hemorrhage, severely impaired gas exchange, decreased lung compliance, and increased pulmonary arterial pressure. Further, the injury of alveolar epithelium impairs active fluid transport mechanisms in the lung, preventing reabsorption of edema fluid from the alveolar space, which is a key step in the resolution of ALI → ARDS (reviewed in [90, 95, 98, 107, 108]).

9.3.4.3 SAMP-Mediated Protection of Pulmonary Function in Acute Lung Injury

Finally, in those patients with ALI who do not proceed to or survive ARDS, a resolution of inflammation can be observed characterized by fluid clearance and solute reabsorption from the alveolus [110, 111]. Several mechanisms central to controlling the resolution of lung inflammation and injury have been discussed, including enhanced efferocytosis of apoptotic neutrophils/eosinophils performed by antiinflammatory and/or proresolving macrophages. In particular, a shift from M1-like to M2-like macrophages appears to be the principal mechanism involved in this resolution of inflammation stage (compare Fig. 9.2). The M2-like macrophages promote alveolar epithelial cell transition and fibrosis formation mainly by release of TGF-β and IL-10 [110, 112, 113] (for M1-like and M2-like macrophages, see Sect. 5.3.2.3 and also Vol. 1 [1], Part III, Sects. 8.2.2.2 and 8.2.2.3 and Fig. 8.2).

9.3.4.4 Pathohistological Stages in Acute Lung Injury

The sequelae of the efferent innate immune pathways in ALI are reflected by typical pathohistological stages. The early initial scenario is the exudative stage characterized by diffuse alveolar damage; a subsequent second stage of proliferation is manifested by resolution of pulmonary edema, proliferation of type II alveolar cells, squamous metaplasia, and early deposition of collagen; the third stage of fibrosis is characterized by obliteration of normal lung architecture, diffuse fibrosis, and cyst formation [95, 114, 115]. For patients who survive ARDS, a fourth stage can be distinguished: the resolution stage that usually remains with minimal lung damage [112].

9.3.4.5 Concluding Remarks

There is growing evidence for a critical role of DAMPs in the pathogenesis of both pathogen- and sterile injury-mediated ARDS, its pathophysiologic hallmark being disruption of the alveolar–capillary barrier. As observed in other acute organ injuries, subtypes of RCD have been discovered to serve as a crucial source of DAMP emission. Of equal importance, however, are recent studies showing that SAMPs are involved in the resolution stage of ARDS. The following sections should add some more details to these new pathogenetic perspectives in this life-threatening acute lung disease.

9.3.5 DAMPs in Acute Lung Injury

9.3.5.1 General Remarks: Emission of DAMPs upon Sterile and Infectious Lung Injury

An increasing number of articles are devoted to a pathogenetic role of intrapulmonary DAMPs emission in ALI → ARDS, including sepsis-induced ARDS, among them reviews published by Tolle and Standiford [116] and Englert et al. [117].

Also, a function of DAMPs in (massive) transfusion-related acute lung injury (TRALI) resulting in ARDS has been already discussed [118, 119]. On the other hand, other extrapulmonary sources of DAMPs may also aggravate ALI. For example, in studies on rats, release of mtDNA associated with hip fracture was found to promote lung injury [120].

Here, it should be particularly stressed that DAMPs have also been demonstrated in severe infections associated with ALI → ARDS, an observation that underlines the correctness of the danger/injury model in Immunology, namely, that a robust pathogen-induced inflammatory defense response is mainly provoked by the emission of DAMPs upon pathogen-mediated tissue injury. When this response is uncontrolled and exaggerated, it can lead to a life-threatening disease such as ARDS. This topic has been thoroughly reviewed by Kang et al. [121] discussing the demonstration of organ-specific DAMPs as involved in pathogen-induced sepsis, often associated with ARDS. For example, remarkably high levels of HMGB1 have been found in the pulmonary epithelial lining fluid of patients with sepsis [122]. Moreover, host-derived DAMPs, such as OxPLs and HMGB1, were shown to be generated during influenza virus infection and causing ALI [123].

Thus, given the growing attention paid to DAMPs as potential therapeutic targets in this life-threatening lung disease, they deserve a few more words.

9.3.5.2 High Mobility Group Box 1

Already before the term DAMPs was coined, in a study in mice, HMGB1 was shown to mediate acute inflammatory lung injury [124]. In this study, HMGB1 given intratracheally was observed to promote an acute inflammatory response to the lungs, with neutrophil influx and accumulation, the development of alveolar edema, and increased pulmonary release of IL-1β, and secretion of TNF. Histological investigation revealed diffuse alveolar damage identical to the pathological findings in ALI → ARDS [124]. In other sets of experiments in rats, intratracheal instillation of HMGB1 was found to provoke persistently exacerbated acute lung inflammation, induction of inducible nitric oxide synthase (iNOS) in alveolar macrophages, and increased lung nitric oxide production [125]. The authors concluded that iNOS expressed by alveolar macrophages facilitates the development of HMGB1-induced ALI.

Interestingly, in a murine hemorrhage model associated with ALI, neutrophils expressing HMGB1was detected in the lungs after hemorrhage [126]. The intrapulmonary expression of HMGB1 was found to be increased within 4 h of hemorrhage and then remained elevated for more than 72 h after blood loss. The authors argued that these results demonstrate that hemorrhage leads to increased HMGB1 expression in the lungs, primarily through neutrophil sources, and that this IA-1 DAMP participates in hemorrhage-induced ALI.

In more recent studies on an adult mouse model, inhibition of extracellular HMGB1 was shown to mitigate hyperoxia-induced inflammatory ALI [127]. In other lines of studies in rats, inhibition of HMGB1 by the antiinflammatory agent *ketamine* was demonstrated to alleviate LPS-induced ALI [128]. In a subsequent similar study in rats, inhibition of HMGB1 by paeonol (the main active component of *Paeonia suffruticosa*, which has been used to inhibit the inflammatory response in traditional Chinese medicine), was found to attenuate LPS-induced ALI as well [129].

Again, in other sets of experiments in rodents, blocking of HMGB1 with an anti-HMGB1 antibody was found to mitigate ALI. Thus, in one study on a ventilator-induced lung injury model in rabbits, intratracheal instillation of such an antibody improved oxygenation, limited microvascular permeability and neutrophil influx into the alveolar lumen, as well as decreased concentrations of TNF in bronchoalveolar lavage fluid [130]. In studies on a murine model of *Pseudomonas aeruginosa* pneumonia, exposure to hyperoxia reportedly led to a significant elevation in concentrations of airway HMGB1 and increased mortality in infected mice [131]. Treatment of these mice with a neutralizing anti-HMGB1 monoclonal antibody resulted in a reduction in bacterial counts, injury, and numbers of neutrophils in the lungs, as well as an increase in leukocyte phagocytic activity compared with mice receiving a control antibody. This improved phagocytic function was observed by the investigators to be associated with reduced concentrations of airway HMGB1 [131].

Intense clinical studies on HMGB1 in patients with ALI → ARDS are still limited, though—according to an early clinical observation already in 1999—high HMGB1 levels were already found to be associated with increased mortality in subjects with severe sepsis [132]. Further, one small study of 21 patients with sepsis-induced ALI revealed that HMGB1 levels were higher in epithelial lung fluid and plasma compared to controls. Interestingly, these findings could be observed persistently during both the acute and subacute phases of ARDS [133]. In subsequent investigations, HMGB1 levels were determined in bronchoalveolar lavage fluid of trauma patients during mechanical ventilation and ventilator-associated pneumonia [134]. The authors reported that long-term mechanical ventilation is associated with increased HMGB1 levels that are elevated during ventilator-associated pneumonia compared with healthy volunteers. In a more recent study on patients with severe pneumonia and ARDS requiring mechanical ventilation [135], the investigators remarkably observed the day 1 HMGB1 concentration to be a critical, independent biomarker for ICU mortality.

9.3.5.3 Heat Shock Proteins

The function of HSPs in ALI → ARDS has not been investigated systematically. In a series of experimental studies on the role of HSP72 in lung inflammation, in vitro assays showed that extracellular HSP72 can induce a dose-dependent increase in IL-8 expression and activation of NF-κB in bronchial EpCs [136]. In subsequent in vivo experiments in mice, the investigator group observed that intratracheal installation of HSP72 can induce upregulation of chemokine and TNF levels, and increase neutrophil influx in bronchoalveolar lavage fluid. Further studies on this model using TLR4 mutant mice revealed an essential role of TLR4 in HSP-mediated lung inflammation [136]. In a previously performed clinical analysis, the presence of extracellular HSP72 was reportedly demonstrated in bronchoalveolar lavage fluid and plasma of patients suffering from ALI [137].

9.3.5.4 Nucleic Acids

Mitochondrial DNA

A pathogenetic role of mtDNA in ALI → ARDS has been reported as well. In one of the first studies, Sun et al. [138] could show that mitochondrial DAMPs including mtDNA, but also mFPs, can essentially trigger endothelial permeability changes as observed in ALI → ARDS (compare Sect. 8.3.3.3). Subsequent studies used several models to confirm the pathogenetic role of mtDNA in this life-threatening syndrome. Thus, in a model of *Pseudomonas aeruginosa*-induced vascular injury in perfused isolated rat lungs, mtDNA (originating from the mammalian mitochondrial genome) was demonstrated to accumulate in the perfusion medium substantially [139]. In studies on a murine endotoxemia model, several experiments were performed to prove an effect of mtDNA on ALI [140]. In a first series of experiments using this model, mtDNA was found to be released in the plasma following intraperitoneal injection of LPS. In a second series of experiments, intraperitoneal administration of mtDNA was demonstrated to cause apparent ALI and systemic inflammation associated with increased IL-1β and IL-6 levels. Accompanying analyses provided evidence that the LPS-induced mtDNA release occurred in a TLR4-dependent manner, whereas mtDNA-induced ALI and systemic inflammation happened in a TLR9-dependent but TLR4-independent mode [140]. Subsequent studies on a rat model of full-thickness thermal injury produced similar results by demonstrating increased mtDNA plasma concentrations and—as revealed by related experiments—mtDNA administration-caused severe ARDS. The critical pathogenetic role of mtDNA in the development of ALI → ARDS could be documented by another recent study on a rat intratracheal *Pseudomonas aeruginosa* model [141].

Of note, in a clinical study on patients with suspected ventilator-associated pneumonia, higher levels of mtDNA were detected in the bronchoalveolar lavage fluid [142]. In another clinical study conducted by the same group, mtDNA in transfusion products was suggested to contribute to the development of ARDS after multiple transfusions [119], thereby confirming the first proposal of the "work of DAMPs" operating in TRALI [118]. In these clinical investigations, detectable levels of mtDNA were found in packed red blood cells, fresh frozen plasma, and platelets, with the latter two transfusion products containing significant amounts of mtDNA fragments. Also, the investigators observed a linear relationship between the mtDNA given during transfusion and the serum concentration of mtDNA fragments. Even more remarkably, the quantity of mtDNA in serum measured at 24 h after transfusion predicted the occurrence of ARDS. According to the authors' conclusion, these findings support the idea that mtDNA DAMPs in transfusion products significantly contribute to the incidence of ARDS after massive transfusions.

Interestingly, apart from mtDNA, mitochondrial peptides—via FPR-1 → MAPKs/AKT signaling—were recently shown to activate type II alveolar EpCs to induce pulmonary inflammation, thereby possibly contributing to ARDS [143].

Histones

Besides nuclear NAs, nuclear proteins, that is, histones have been identified as DAMPs to contribute to ALI. As outlined in Vol. 1 [1], Part IV, Sect. 12.2.4.4 and reviewed by Silk et al. [103], histones may be released into the extracellular space in three forms: freely, as a DNA-bound nucleosome, or as part of NETs; but all three forms can be detected in serum after significant cellular death caused by various injuries. As reported in patients with an acute history of severe blunt trauma [144], circulating histones increase to toxic levels within 4 h and correlate with the severity of ALI. The high levels were significantly associated with markers of endothelial damage and coagulation activation. In in vitro systems, used in parallel to the clinical observation, histones were observed to damage ECs, stimulate cytokine release, and promote NET formation and myeloperoxidase release. In murine trauma models, cytokines and markers for endothelial damage and coagulation activation were shown to increase immediately after trauma or histone infusion significantly. Pathological examinations showed that the lungs were the predominantly affected organ with edema, hemorrhage, microvascular thrombosis, and neutrophil congestion [144].

In another clinical study on patients with ARDS, extracellular histone levels in plasma and bronchoalveolar lavage fluid were also found to be excessively increased and associated with ARDS severity and mortality [145]. In ex vivo investigations, the authors could demonstrate that ARDS patients' bronchoalveolar lavage fluid induces epithelial and endothelial cell damage remarkably and stimulates cytokine production in the supernatant of the model cell line U937 (a human macrophage cell line).

Together, there is increasing experimental and clinical evidence for a critical pathogenetic role of extracellular histones in the development and progression of ARDS.

9.3.5.5 S100A Proteins

The role of S100 proteins such as S100A8 and S100A9 in ALI has already been thoroughly reviewed elsewhere [146–148]. The function of these DAMPs—either passively released from necrotic cells or actively secreted by activated immune cells—is mediated via their cognate PRMs TLR4 or RAGE, although other receptors are also implicated in S100A9 function (for additional information also compare Vol. 1 [1], Part IV, Sects. 12.2.4.2, p. 229 and 14.2.2.4, p. 310). Of note, the role of these DAMPs in ALI is ambivalent in that S100A8 operates as a DAMP exerting proinflammatory effects while S100A8/S100A9 and S100A9 slip into a "SAMP-like" function to convey antiinflammatory properties.

Collectively, the involvement of S100A proteins in ALI has been well documented both in experimental and clinical studies. For example, in studies in rats and mice, S100A9 mRNA was shown to be upregulated in lungs undergoing injurious mechanical ventilation [149, 150]. In patients with ARDS, upregulation of neutrophil-derived S100A12 (and its receptor RAGE) expression in lung tissue and bronchoalveolar lavage fluid was reportedly significantly higher when compared with healthy controls [146, 151]. Also, S100A8/A9 protein levels were found to be elevated in the bronchoalveolar lavage fluid of ARDS patients [146].

A proinflammatory function of S100A proteins was described by Chakraborty et al. [147], referring to studies on in vitro cultured alveolar EpCs and an in vivo murine model of lung injury. The authors could demonstrate that S100A8 drives lung inflammation via activation of alveolar EpCs in a TLR4-dependent manner, as documented by release of cytokines and chemokines [147]. Further, in these studies, the investigators demonstrated that inhaled endogenous S100A8 directly induces neutrophil recruitment into the bronchoalveolar lavage fluid. According to the authors' conclusion, this observation confirms the significance of this DAMP in inflammation-related neutrophil immigration, knowing that one of the key features of ALI is infiltration of neutrophils into the lungs.

By contrast to the proinflammatory effect of S100A8, an antiinflammatory function of S100A proteins could be demonstrated by Hiroshima et al. in studies in mice [148]. Again in experiments on a murine lung model using S100A protein inhalation, the authors showed critical functional differences of S100A8/A9 and S100A9 that distinguish them from S100A8. Thus, unlike S100A8, S100A9 was found to promote mild neutrophil and lymphocyte influx, possibly mediated in part by increased mast cell degranulation and selective upregulation of some chemokine genes. Moreover, the S100 proteins did not significantly induce proinflammatory mediators, including TNF, IL-1β, or IL-6. Furthermore, compared to the marked increase induced by S100A8, S100A8/A9 or S100A9 did not alter substantially basal IL-10 mRNA over the time course tested. Also, like S100A8, S100A9 and S100A8/A9 were shown to reduce neutrophil influx in ALI provoked by LPS challenge but were somewhat less inhibitory, possibly, because of differential effects on expression of some chemokines.

Together, the studies on S100A proteins published by Chakraborty et al. [147] and Hiroshima et al. [148]—here briefly reviewed—suggest a proinflammatory role of S100A8 and an antiinflammatory protective role of S100A8/A9 or S100A9 in lung injury. Accordingly, in their conclusion, the authors proposed [148], "that their secretion by infiltrating myeloid cells, and induction in macrophages and EpCs by particular agonists, may contribute to normal lung homeostasis and protection against excessive fulminant inflammation" (in this context, also compare Sect. 3.5.6).

9.3.5.6 DAMPs Activating the NLRP3 Inflammasome

There are some reports in the literature suggesting that MAMPs/DAMPs (i.e., IA-2 DAMPs) contribute to ALI → ARDS via activation of the NLRP3 inflammasome, that is, probably via induction of pyroptosis [152, 153]. In support of this concept are, for example, experimental studies demonstrating that eATP is released during injurious mechanical ventilation, thereby contributing to pulmonary inflammation and lung edema [154, 155]; that is, studies that let suggest a role of this DAMPs in the activation of the NLRP3 inflammasome.

Another IA-2 DAMP, uric acid, was also reported to be involved in ALI mediated by the NLRP3 inflammasome [156]. In these studies, local uric acid levels were found to be increased in patients with ALI; in experiments in mice performed in parallel, allopurinol and uricase were documented to attenuate ventilator-induced alveolar barrier dysfunction. Also, this DAMP was demonstrated to accumulate intrapulmonarily in a bleomycin-induced lung injury model and to promote lung inflammation [157]. The investigators also could show that local administration of exogenous uric acid crystals recapitulates lung inflammation.

9.3.5.7 Extracellular Matrix-Derived Proteins

Increased ECM turnover is a characteristic feature of tissue injury in ARDS. DAMPs released from the ECM in the form of proteolytically cleaved fragments (Class IIA

DAMPs) can reportedly contribute to ALI → ARDS (for class IIA DAMPs, see Sect. 3.4.2 and also Vol. 1 [1], Part IV, Sect. 13.2). Such a DAMP is hyaluronan (HA), or fragment of hyaluronan (fHA) that was shown to be associated with organ dysfunction in ARDS (for HA, see Vol. 1 [1], Part IV, Sect. 13.2.3.2). As reviewed by Esposito et al. [158], increased fHA deposition has been demonstrated in the lung tissue of rats with bleomycin-induced lung injury and in humans suffering from ARDS; also, increased HA synthesis has been observed in nonhuman primates with ARDS. Notably, in a clinical study on ARDS patients [158], increasing circulating and alveolar fHA levels were demonstrated to be associated with the severity of ALI. Moreover, the investigators noticed that alveolar fHA was apparently related to respiratory organ dysfunction rather than systemic organ dysfunction, while circulating fHA was found to be related to systemic organ dysfunction. Given these observations, the authors suggested compartmentalized effects of fHA in ARDS. Mechanistically, they discussed the possibility that—besides others—fHA may initiate inflammatory responses via TLRs [158]. In this context, it is worth mentioning another clinical study on ARDS patients providing evidence that some urinary glycosaminoglycans (GAGs), including fHA, can be used as predictive biomarkers in ARDS [159].

9.3.5.8 Concluding Remarks

Collectively, these data reinforce the concept that DAMPs play a pivotal pathogenetic role in the development of infectious and sterile lung inflammation. Their primary homeostatic function is to initiate a protective innate immune defense response as clinically manifested by a mild ALI symptomatology. However, when emitted in excess, they drive an uncontrolled exaggerated inflammatory response culminating in the life-threatening ARDS [121–123]. And, again, it should be stressed that such an exaggerated potentially lethal DAMPs response occurs in defense against infections—initially intended to rescue the host but, tragically, may even kill the patient: in a way, a kind of suicide.

9.3.6 SAMPs in Acute Lung Injury

9.3.6.1 General Remarks

Homeostatic timely resolution of acute lung inflammation is mandatory: if unrestrained, ARDS can develop; if it becomes chronic, then COPD can develop. In the first place, restitution of barrier integrity is of utmost importance to relieve alveolar edema leading to hypoxemia. Thus, lung-specific proresolving events include clearance of edema and transitional matrix, reepithelialization of the airways, and restoration of pulmonary surfactants. It is the task of SAMPs, in particular, SPMs, to execute these events. In fact, as emphasized by Levy and Serhan [160], restitution of barrier integrity, recruitment of monocytoid cells, as well as promotion of M2-like macrophage-mediated clearance of dead cells and tissue debris are all proresolving responses orchestrated by SPMs (compare Fig. 9.2).

9.3.6.2 Specialized Proresolving Mediators

Previous experimental studies have already demonstrated that SPMs such as LXA4 and RvD1 could regulate the alveolar fluid clearance in ARDS to protect the lung function [161–163]. As recently reviewed by Wang et al. [164], further studies have extended evidence in support of the notion that SPMs might enhance the alveolar epithelium repair, inhibit the proinflammatory cytokines, and upregulate the ion channel activity and protein expression in a receptor-dependent manner to increase the alveolar fluid clearance, thereby contributing to ALI → ARDS resolution [164]. Plausibly, these recent findings have been considered to serve as promising agents for the treatment of ARDS.

9.3.6.3 Adenosine–Prostaglandin E2–Annexin A1

Earlier studies had already identified extracellular adenosine as a protective molecule in inflammatory lung conditions, including acute and chronic lung diseases [90, 165, 166]. In more recent in vitro and in vivo experiments on cell lines and mice [167], the authors reevaluated the role of adenosine kinase during ALI (the adenosine kinase inhibits elevated extracellular adenosine levels). They found that adenosine kinase is repressed during inflammation, both in vitro and in vivo. This repression reportedly translates into a protective response during pulmonary inflammation, as observed in animal experiments involving genetic repression of adenosine kinase. Moreover, the investigators could demonstrate in pharmacological studies that the in vivo inhibition of adenosine kinase (associated with elevated adenosine) mitigates tissue injury during pulmonary inflammation. According to the authors' conclusion, these data show that adenosine kinase is a valuable target for reducing the inflammatory changes associated with lung injury and should be pursued as a therapeutic option [167].

In a systematic review and meta-analysis, a beneficial effect of inhaled prostaglandins in patients with ARDS was explored [168]. The meta-analysis could demonstrate that inhaled prostaglandins improve oxygenation and decrease pulmonary artery pressures and may be associated with adverse events. However, as concluded by the authors, the use of inhaled prostaglandins in ARDS requires further targeted experiments. More targeted studies on the role of PGE2 in ALI → ARDS are still lacking.

Also, in a recent study evaluating the role of AnxA1 in the treatment of acute radiation-induced lung injury, this SAMP was found to reduce the expression of IL-6 and inhibit the release of myeloperoxidase from monocytes and macrophages [169]. The authors argued that this antiinflammatory effect may underscore the mechanism by which AnxA1 in the plasma of patients with this type of lung injury is associated with treatment outcome.

9.3.6.4 Concluding Remarks

As can be seen from the current literature available, the detection and function of SAMPs in ALI → ARDS is still a poorly explored, however, emerging research field. On the other hand, resolution of inflammation in this disease is an appreciated typical feature, documented by many experimental studies, and a failure to resolve ongoing inflammation is well-known to increase mortality and prolong morbidity in survivors. Thus, in the course of the currently noticed "high season" of this research discipline, relevant reports on this topic can be expected soon.

9.3.7 Acute Repetitive or Persistent Lung Injury → Chronic Obstructive Pulmonary Disease

9.3.7.1 General Remarks

As already touched above, acute repetitive or persistent lung injury can lead to COPD that is a heterogeneous and complex pulmonary disease, causing significant healthcare burdens worldwide. Thus, the incidence of COPD has increased in the past few decades and has become a major public health problem and will remain a challenge for clinicians within the twenty-first century. Worldwide, COPD is in the spotlight, since its high prevalence, morbidity, and mortality create enormous challenges for healthcare systems (reviewed in [170, 171]). The development of COPD is mainly the result of continued exposure to various environmental risk factors, although genetic host factors have a role in determining disease susceptibility and pathogenesis (reviewed in [172, 173]). Among the environmental factors, cigarette smoking is a significant risk factor for COPD, but environmental tobacco smoking also contributes to its development. Occupational exposure to vapor, dust, gas, and fumes, as well as outdoor air pollution, is another important risk factor for disease exacerbation and mortality.

9.3.7.2 Pathogenesis of Chronic Obstructive Pulmonary Disease (in Brief)

The clinical features of COPD encompass emphysema, chronic bronchitis, obstruction and destruction of the small airways, and enlargement/disorganization of alveoli, that is, loss of alveolar tissue associated with emphysema. Peribronchiolar fibrosis surrounding the small airways contributes to the obstructive pathophysiology in COPD (for reviews, see [171, 174–176]). The chronic inflammatory course of the disease is aggravated by episodes of acute exacerbations.

Characterization of Chronic Nonresolving Airway Inflammation

Typically, chronic nonresolving airway inflammation in COPD is characterized by activation of the innate immune system, involving neutrophils, macrophages, ILCs, and activated DCs, located in the lung tissue and the airway lumen. Also, the adaptive (auto)immune system is activated in COPD, as documented by lung infiltration of Th1, Th17, and B cells, along with a decrease in Tregs in the airways. Moreover, an impact of the lung microbiome on COPD progression and risk of exacerbation has been described. And not to forget are epigenetic modifications that have been reported in patients with COPD to be sometimes linked to disease severity and susceptibility. Together, all these processes result in this typical heterogeneous and complex pulmonary disease (for reviews, see [175–182]). Importantly, as reviewed by Poh et al. [183], COPD can "overlap" with other respiratory diseases, including bronchiectasis, fibrosis, and obstructive sleep apnea. While COPD alone confers morbidity and mortality, common features with contrasting clinical outcomes can occur in COPD "overlap syndromes," such as asthma-COPD, bronchiectasis-COPD, and fibrosis-COPD.

Pathogenetic Mechanisms of Environmental Factors in Promoting Action of DAMPs

Environmental factors, as mentioned above, include inhaled toxic/noxious substances such as cigarette smoke, which were shown to cause subroutines of bronchial RCD such as autophagic cell death, necroptosis, parthanatos, and ferroptosis [184–188]. As outlined in Sect. 4.3 and Vol. 1 [1], Part V, Sect. 19.3, these forms of RCD are associated with release of endogenous DAMPs. Usually, these DAMPs trigger inflammasome-independent proinflammatory responses.

In addition, other environmental factors may operate directly as exogenous DAMPs such as inhaled pathogenic air pollutants, including asbestos, crystalline silica, and airborne particulate matter (see Sect. 3.6). This category of IVA-4 DAMPs triggers inflammasome-dependent proinflammatory processes predominantly.

Pathogenetically, DAMP-promoted chronic nonresolving inflammatory, fibrogenic, and adaptive (auto)immune pathways are involved in the development of this heterogeneous and complex pulmonary disease that causes—as already mentioned—significant healthcare burden (morbidity and mortality) worldwide (for DAMP-promoted innate and adaptive immune pathways, see Vol. 1 [1], Part VI, Chpt. 22 and Part VIII, Chpt. 32; for DAMP-promoted self-perpetuating fibrotic pathways, see Sects. 6.4 and 6.5).

9.3.7.3 DAMPs and SAMPS in Chronic Obstructive Pulmonary Disease

There are already reports about the potential pathogenetic role of endogenous DAMPs in COPD (reviewed in [189–191]). Indeed, several clinical studies could demonstrate the presence of DAMPs (e.g., HMGB1, HSPs, S100A proteins, eATP, and GALs) in the serum and extracellular lung fluids, including bronchoalveolar lavage, epithelial lining fluid, and sputum of COPD patients.

First Evidence for Exogenous DAMPs in COPD

Early reports on the contribution of exogenous IVA-4 DAMPs to the pathogenesis of COPD have also been published. Thus, in studies on RAW 264.7 cells (a murine macrophage cell line) and ex vivo lung tissue explants obtained from elastase-induced emphysema animal models, diesel exhaust particles and a cigarette smoking extract were shown to activate the NLRP3 inflammasome [192], known to contribute to proinflammatory and profibrotic processes [193]. These experimental findings are in agreement with (1) epidemiologic studies pointing to a role of air pollutants in the increase in respiratory symptoms and mortality rate in COPD patients [27] and (2) the direct demonstration of inflammasome activation in the lung tissues from patients with COPD at acute exacerbation [194] (for activation of the NLRP3 inflammasome via exogenous DAMPs, e.g., particles, see Sects. 2.2.5.3

and 3.6; also compare Vol. 1 [1], Part II, Sect. 12.2.5.4, Part IV, Sect. 15.2, and Part VI, Sect. 22.4.2.2).

First Evidence for SAMPs in COPD

According to the new view of COPD as a state of nonresolving bronchial inflammation, there is emerging preclinical and clinical evidence suggesting COPD be pathogenetically linked to insufficient levels or activity of SAMPs, in particular, SPMs (reviewed and discussed in [195–197]). Thus, in vitro and preclinical in vivo studies could show that SPMs have bronchoprotective proresolving effects. For example, RvD1 was demonstrated to reduce significantly neutrophilic lung inflammation and proinflammatory cytokine production caused by smoke exposure and promote differentiation of M2-like macrophages associated with enhanced capacity for neutrophil efferocytosis [198]. Also, in this study, RvD1 was found to accelerate the resolution of lung inflammation when given after the final smoke exposure. Clinically, patients suffering from moderate to severe COPD were observed to have reduced levels of LXA4 and LXB4 in exhaled breath condensates [199, 200].

9.3.7.4 Concluding Remarks

Together, these studies again prove the concept of the action of agonist ↔ antagonist, that is, DAMPs ↔ SAMPs in the pathogenesis of diseases, and further highlight essential mechanisms by which DAMPs and SAMPs can positively and negatively influence promotion and resolution of inflammation, thereby contributing pathogenetically to a chronic inflammatory disease, here chronic lung inflammation manifested as COPD. In addition to these insights into lung physiology and disease pathogenesis provided by measuring the presence of DAMPs and SAMPs, monitoring of a DAMP/SAMP signature would be an additional option to improve current therapeutic modalities. This concept would allow us to define and design an appropriate and individualized strategy for the treatment of COPD patients (DAMPs as therapeutic targets and SAMPs as therapeutics; see Sect. 9.9.3), without risking the untoward side effects (i.e., immunosuppression), mediated by traditional antiinflammatory medications.

9.3.8 Résumé

Research work on DAMPs in ALI → ARDS has undoubtedly contributed to understanding its pathogenesis/pathophysiology. In particular, the recognition that DAMPs are emitted during the very treatment aimed to reduce mortality, that is, therapeutic mechanical ventilation, has opened new ways of therapeutic strategies. Additionally, by understanding the role of DAMPs as biomarkers in the pathophysiology of ALI → ARDS, a new category of rational therapeutic targets has gained considerable attention. Moreover, the new mechanistic insights into the process of transition from DAMP-promoted inflammation to SAMP-driven resolution of inflammation are now appreciated as a critical prerequisite to survive the hyperinflammatory and subsequent fibroproliferative stages of ALI → ARDS. Plausibly, in case of progressive therapy-resistant ALI → ARDS (that might eventually proceed to COPD), administration of SAMPs would be a stringent therapeutic option to implement soon clinically (see Sect. 9.9.3.3). Certainly, to reach this goal, further targeted studies on experimental animal models of ALI are needed. In particular, sophisticated determination of DAMPs and SAMPs, including monitoring the DAMP/SAMP signature, during different phases of ARDS would be necessary to identify those patients in whom such a therapeutic intervention could be beneficial. Similar concluding remarks can be made for DAMPs involved in COPD. Current studies so far available demonstrate that DAMPs occur in both lung microenvironment and serum. Nevertheless, further exploration of DAMPs in their capacity to influence COPD progression is needed. In particular, that is, in the burning interest of current environmental research and public health, it is time for urgent health studies on the pathogenetic role of air pollutants operating as exogenous DAMPs in COPD.

9.4 Acute and Chronic Kidney Injury

9.4.1 Introductory Remarks

Acute kidney injury is a common life-threatening inflammatory disorder, with reported mortality rates up to 50% with the most severe diseases [201–203]. Of note, AKI, in case of a failure of inflammation resolution associated with incomplete recovery from the acute disorder, can transit to chronic kidney disease (CKD), resulting in severe fibrosis clinically manifested by end-stage renal failure. Besides AKI, acute repetitive or persistent insults to the renal parenchyma associated with chronic inflammation in terms of nonresolving inflammation can also result in permanent fibrosis and renal dysfunction, which, if left untreated, may progress to CKD. Both diseases are briefly addressed in the following.

9.4.2 Acute Kidney Injury → Acute Renal Failure

Acute kidney injury as caused by local and systemic stimuli including ischemia reperfusion, nephrotoxic insult, renal hypoperfusion, volume depletion, hypotension, infection/sepsis, and major surgery is characterized by an abrupt decrease in glomerular filtration rate, clinically manifested as a rapid decline of kidney function. This organ-specific acute injury is further characterized by damage to tubular EpCs and ECs and robust inflammatory responses including intrarenal infiltration of inflammatory cells (e.g., leukocytes, macrophages), as well as upregulation of chemokines and cytokines (reviewed in [204–206]).

Acute renal injury is dangerous and costly, affecting around one in five patients' emergency admissions to the hospital. The organ-specific injury, formerly known as "acute renal failure (ARF)," has been traditionally described as a rapid decrease (ranging from hours to weeks to less than 3 months) in kidney function as measured by increases in serum creatinine. A variant, acute traumatic AKI, is a serious complication and is usually induced by trauma-associated severe hypotension linked to blood loss leading to renal ischemia/secondary IRI as well as crush injuries and rhabdomyolysis.

Another mostly preventable cause of AKI refers to nephrotoxicity induced by drugs such as calcineurin inhibitors and specific anticancer agents (e.g., cisplatin) reportedly. Although nephrotoxicity is most commonly associated with injury in the tubulointerstitial compartment as either acute tubular necrosis or acute interstitial nephritis [207], a growing body of literature has also highlighted the potential for drug-induced glomerular lesions [208]. Several mechanisms are likely to induce nephrotoxicity, including direct damage to DNA and induction of oxidative stress, mitochondrial dysfunction, as well as apoptotic and necrotic renal cell death, all of which known to lead to an extensive inflammatory response (reviewed in [209, 210]).

Together, AKI carries a high rate of unacceptably, long-term morbidity and mortality. As treatment options, renal replacement therapies such as chronic dialysis and kidney transplantation are available.

9.4.3 Regulated Cell Death and Necroinflammation in Acute Kidney Injury

Typically, ischemic renal damage such as drug-induced nephrotoxicity is characterized by subroutines of RCD such as apoptosis, necroptosis, pyroptosis, ferroptosis, NETosis, and *mitochondrial permeability transition* (MPT)-driven RN, all serving as critical sources of DAMPs [211–214] (see Box 4.1, and also compare Vol. 1 [1], Part V, Chap. 19). Consequently, the DAMPs activate mobile and sessile innate immune cells, including leukocytes, macrophages, and tubular EpCs and ECs to produce proinflammatory cytokines, chemokines, and other inflammatory mediator substances. These cytokines, partly in terms of inducible DAMPs such as TNF, promote further forms of RCD, which may contribute to intrarenal necroinflammation in terms of an autoamplification loop between cell necrosis and the inflammatory response [215, 216]) (for additional information also compare Vol. 1 [1], Part V, Chpt. 20, p. 467 and Fig. 20.1, p. 469). Repeatedly acute or persistent insults to the renal parenchyma associated with chronic inflammation in terms of nonresolving inflammation can result in permanent fibrosis and renal dysfunction, which, if left untreated, may progress to CKD (see below). Of note, there is growing evidence suggesting that both acute renal necroinflammation and kidney fibrosis reflect the work of DAMPs (for further literature, see [211, 215–223]).

9.4.4 Pathogenesis of Acute Kidney Injury → Acute Renal Failure (in Brief)

9.4.4.1 General Remarks

The pathogenesis of the acute disorder exemplified by ischemic AKI has been thoroughly reviewed [224–226] and is predominantly characterized by severe cytoskeletal changes of innate PRM-bearing resident cells such as EpCs and ECs as well as recruitment of innate PRM-expressing mobile cells including leukocytes and macrophages (Fig. 9.3). As typical for efferent innate immune responses, numerous interactions between these cells have been described (for cells of the innate immune system, also compare Vol. 1 [1], Part III).

Thus, following a reduction in effective kidney perfusion, EpCs are unable to maintain adequate intracellular ATP, and its depletion results in various forms of DAMP-emitting RCD. During an ischemic insult, all segments of the nephron can be affected, but the most commonly injured EpC is the proximal tubular cell. Additionally, the other major EpCs of the nephron involved in the pathophysiology of ischemic AKI are those of the medullary thick ascending limb, located distally. As a typical consequence of hemodynamic disturbances and ischemia-promoted

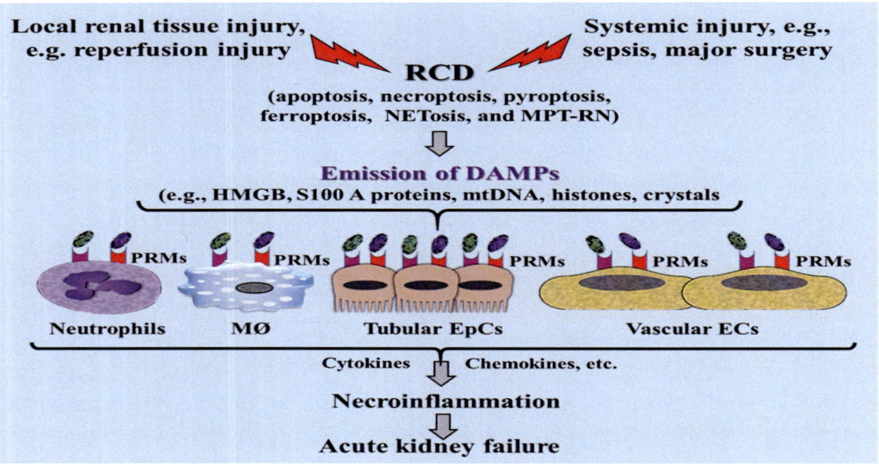

Fig. 9.3 Simplified schematic diagram of a model illustrating DAMP-promoted renal necroinflammation that may lead to acute kidney failure. Acute kidney injury, caused by local and systemic injurious stimuli, results in various injury-induced subroutines of RCD providing productive sources for the emission of DAMPs. Intrarenal PRM-bearing cells such as leukocytes, macrophages, tubular EpCs, and ECs, following recognition of DAMPs, trigger pathways leading to necroinflammation. In case of insufficient resolution of inflammation, the processes may result in acute kidney failure. *EC* endothelial cells, *EpCs* epithelial cells, *HMGB1* high mobility group box 1, *MPT-RN* mitochondrial permeability transition-driven necrosis, *mtDNA* mitochondrial DNA, *MØ* macrophage, *NETosis* formation of neutrophil extracellular traps (NETs) by neutrophils, *PRMs* pattern recognition molecules, *RCD* regulated cell death. (Sources: [204–206, 211–214, 223])

ATP depletion, disruption of the actin cytoskeleton occurs that is associated with the loss of tight junctions and adheren junctions resulting in decline of function and decrease in glomerular filtration rate.

9.4.4.2 DAMP-Driven Promotion of Innate Immune Responses in Acute Kidney Injury

Of note, in parallel, DAMP-activated PRM-bearing epithelial proximal tubular cells produce necroinflammatory cytokines, such as TNF, IL-6, IL-1β, IL-8, and TGF-β, as well as chemokines such as CCL2 and CCL5 [227, 228] (for chemokines, see also Vol. 1 [1], Part VI, Sect. 22.5.11, and Tables 22.1 and 22.2). Inflammation is a critical trigger for further forms of RN (e.g., necroptosis), whereby both events can drive the autoamplification loop of necroinflammation [223]. Mechanistically, cytokines operating as inducible DAMPs may be discussed to trigger secondary RN (e.g., TNF in necroptosis).

Moreover, the PRM-expressing ECs and VSMCs of the microcirculation play critical roles in the pathophysiology of AKI. Thus, ischemia has reportedly profound effects on the renal endothelium, resulting in microvascular dysregulation and continued ischemia and further injury, especially in the outer stripe of the kidney. Importantly, the initial ischemic insult is aggravated by a number of factors, including activation of the clotting cascade, the formation of microthrombi within the vascular lumen, and impaired vascular reactivity. A characteristic feature of the latter is increased vasoconstriction and decreased vasodilatation, promoted by vasoactive mediators including the inducible IIIA-8 DAMP ET-1 [225] (for ET-1, compare Sect. 3.5.3.6, and Vol. 1 [1], Part IV, Sect. 14.2.5.3, and Fig. 14.2). Notably, like DAMP-activated EpCs, DAMP-activated renal ECs also secrete necroinflammatory cytokines that are so important in the pathogenesis of ischemic AKI.

9.4.4.3 SAMP-Promoted Resolution of Inflammation in Acute Kidney Injury

Amazingly, only a few studies have been published regarding the process of resolution of inflammation in AKI. In principle, however, one can assume that the same mechanisms govern this active innate immune process as observed in other models on examining resolving inflammatory pathways. Such an assumption is supported by recent studies showing that polarization of macrophages into the M2-like type contributes to resolution of inflammation in AKI (reviewed in [229], also compare Sect. 5.3.2).

Interestingly, the cold-shock protein Y-box-binding protein-1(YB-1)—a transcriptional and translational factor, which regulates many cellular processes including cell proliferation, DNA repair, and cellular stress response—has recently been reported to orchestrate onset and resolution of renal inflammation via IL-10 gene regulation [230, 231]. However, these preliminary findings suggest that YB-1 is an antiinflammatory molecule rather than an inflammation-resolving factor, i.e., a SAMP. Further publications of exciting data from this research field can be expected.

9.4.4.4 Pathohistological Features in Acute Kidney Injury

Histopathologically, these effects are manifested by vascular congestion, edema formation, reduced microvascular blood flow, and margination and adhesion of PRM-bearing innate immune cells to the endothelium, leading to the expansion phase of AKI. Moreover, these AKI-associated vascular changes lead to increased microvascular permeability that is likely to be caused by a combination of factors, including disruption of the endothelial monolayer, alterations in contacts between ECs, and upregulated leukocyte ↔ endothelial interactions (for additional information also compare Vol.1 [1], Part VI, Sect. 22.2.2.2, p. 478, and Fig. 22.2, p. 479). Together, the microvascular function is compromised, leading to DIC and microvascular thrombosis, as well as contributing to decreased local tissue perfusion and organ dysfunction or failure. Expectedly, initial intrarenal DAMP ↔ PRM-triggered, EpC- and EC-secreted chemokines and cytokines—via the phenomenon of leukocyte ↔ endothelial interaction—attract mobile innate PRM-bearing cells such as leukocytes and macrophages to infiltrating the kidney and contributing to amplification of necroinflammation via secretion of further cytokines and chemokines.

9.4.4.5 Concluding Remarks

Together, accumulating evidence suggests that the pathogenesis of AKI is dominated by necroinflammatory pathways triggered by DAMPs derived from various subroutines of RCD (Fig. 9.3). If not stopped at an early stage via inflammation-resolving processes, necroinflammation can lead to ARF or even systemic inflammation and remote organ injury. As with other organ-specific inflammatory processes, renal necroinflammation is the consequence of the emission of DAMPs, which are addressed in the following section.

9.4.5 DAMPs in Acute Kidney Injury

9.4.5.1 General Remarks

There is accumulating evidence in support of the notion that the pathophysiological scenario, as briefly outlined above, is the work of AKI-induced DAMPs. Although, at the time being, research in the role of DAMPs in various causes of AKI is in full swing, not all relevant DAMPs have been fully elucidated so far, whereas most data are available from studies on IRI models. In the following, a few reports about this topic are quoted.

9.4.5.2 High Mobility Group Box 1

The DAMP HMGB1 has been studied in some renal (allograft) IRI models of AKI. For example, in studies on a murine IRI model, HMGB1 was found to be expressed/upregulated, and its blockade was shown to reduce renal IRI by dampening the inflammatory response [232]. In other lines of studies on a murine IRI/AKI model, ischemia alone was found to be associated with release of HMGB1. Subsequent postischemic reperfusion appeared to induce localization of HMGB1 to renal tubules, peritubular capillaries, and glomeruli, where the renal cells might be more susceptible to ischemic insult [233]. In this study, administration of blocking antibody to HMGB1 was shown to be associated with a reduction in tubular apoptosis and inflammation in situ and in vivo with preservation of renal function. In view of these findings, the authors suggested that released HMGB1 by ischemic renal parenchyma cells may act as an essential early mediator in delayed inflammatory response during IRI, and targeting HMGB1 may represent a potential therapeutic approach in the prevention of clinical IRI associated with kidney transplantation. In support of these findings is a more recently published report showing that preconditioning with recombinant HMGB1 affords significant protection from TLR4-dependent kidney IRI, indicating therapeutic potential [234].

Of note, production of HMGB1 via tubular cells upstream of TLR4 activation was also demonstrated to be promoted by the nephrotoxic calcineurin inhibitor ciclosporin [235]. Moreover, in other lines of studies, neutralizing HMGB1 with an anti-HMGB1 antibody was shown to ameliorate chronic CsA nephrotoxicity via inhibition of the TLR4 signaling pathway [236]. Also, in studies on chemotherapy drugs against cancer, cisplatin-induced poly(ADP-ribose) polymerase activation was found to contribute to HMGB1 release from kidney proximal tubular cells, resulting in the promotion of inflammation during cisplatin nephrotoxicity [237]. However, the research area of DAMPs in drug-induced nephrotoxicity is poorly explored. On the other hand, these molecules may serve as valuable biomarkers in view of the fact that currently used routine biomarkers such as serum creatinine and blood urea nitrogen increase late in the course of injury and only after substantial kidney injury occurs, when the damage may be irreversible. Thus, clinical work is desired to see if DAMPs prove useful in clinical trials with nephrotoxic drugs and can be translated to the clinic for standard patient care (also compare Sect. 9.9.2).

9.4.5.3 S100 Proteins

S100 proteins also belong to the group of DAMPs already studied in models of AKI. For example, in studies on a murine IRI model, S100B was observed to be expressed following postischemic reperfusion of the kidney [232]. In other sets of studies on a renal model of contrast-induced AKI, the S100A8/A9-TLR4-NLRP3 inflammasome pathway was found to be involved in this kind of injury [238]. In a recently reported clinical study on pediatric patients suffering from AKI, S100A8/S100A9 was detected in the urine and proposed by the authors to use as a biomarker for the prediction of adverse outcome of AKI requiring renal replacement therapy [239]. A similar proposal of applying S100A8/S100A9 as a diagnostic and prognostic biomarker in intrinsic AKI was also made elsewhere [240].

9.4.5.4 Mitochondrial DNA

Early pathological changes of mitochondria, including a reduction in abundance, organelle swelling, and fragmentation, have also been observed in the renal tubular epithelium in AKI of different etiologies [241, 242]. Additionally, during renal injury, damaged mitochondria have been reported to release mtDNA [243, 244].

Also, in a clinical study on patients with AKI, mtDNA was measured in the urine, the severity of the disease was quantified, and patients were followed for 90 days [242]. As reported from the authors, the measured urinary mtDNA levels turned out to be a marker of AKI severity, as reflected by its significant correlation with the peak serum creatinine level, duration of hospital stay, and probably the need for temporary dialysis. Again, like other DAMPs, urinary mtDNA has also the potential to serve as a biomarker of AKI.

9.4.5.5 Histones

The role of extracellular histones in AKI has been thoroughly investigated by the Anders group (Allam et al. [245]) (for histones, also compare Vol. 1 [1], Part IV, Sect.12.2.4.4). The authors showed that dying tubular EpCs release histones into the extracellular space that directly interact with TLR2 and TLR4 to induce MyD88, NF-κB, and MAPK signaling. They further demonstrated that these DAMPs also had directly toxic effects on renal ECs and tubular EpCs in vitro. In addition, the investigators could show that direct injection of histones into the renal arteries of mice results in induction of leukocyte recruitment, microvascular vascular leakage, renal inflammation, and structural features of AKI in a TLR2/TLR4-dependent manner. Extended experiments of the group revealed that neutralizing anti-histone IgG can suppress intrarenal inflammation, neutrophil infiltration, and tubular cell necrosis and improve renal excretory function. Notably, in recently extended studies, the Anders group could demonstrate that histones and NETs enhance tubular necrosis and remote organ injury in ischemic AKI [246]. In sum, and also discussed elsewhere [247, 248], the release of histones from dying cells—like other DAMPs described here—support the concept that renal damage-triggered emission of DAMPs elicits a robust efferent innate immune response, which contributes to the pathogenesis of AKI.

9.4.5.6 Uromodulin

Uromodulin is a kidney-specific extracellular inducible DAMP and has been denoted as a IIIA-4 DAMP in this book (for additional information see Vol. 1 [1], Part IV, Sect. 14.2.5.4, p. 318). Uromodulin is selectively produced by the cells of the thick ascending limb and secreted into urine from the apical cell membrane. The function of uromodulin remains elusive, but the available data suggest that this protein might regulate salt transport, protect against urinary tract infection and kidney stones, and have roles in kidney injury and innate immunity (reviewed in [249]). As outlined by Anders and Schaefer [250], under homeostatic conditions, uromodulin is immunologically inert inside the tubular lumen. However, injury to tubular cells enables uromodulin to leak into the interstitial compartment, where it turns into a DAMP that activates interstitial TLR4-bearing DCs [251]. Notably, other lines of studies have demonstrated that uromodulin can trigger activation of the NLRP3 inflammasome resulting in the release of IL-1β [252]. This inducible DAMP has gained increasing attention and recently been proposed to serve as a biomarker in the urinary tract [253].

9.4.5.7 DAMPs Activating the NLRP3 Inflammasome: Crystals

The list of DAMPs involved in AKI has recently been extended by the description of crystals. For example, as outlined [254], the glomerular ultrafiltrate can be enriched with minerals, proteins, or drug metabolites, especially in states of volume depletion promoting supersaturation. This acute condition can induce a sudden onset of crystal formation, resulting in acute episodes of crystal-induced tubular cell injury, interstitial inflammation, and impairment of renal function. Supersaturation of urine leads to crystallization of solutes in renal tubules. Subsequently, these crystallized deposits contribute to kidney injury by inducing direct and indirect cytotoxicity as well as by setting up an autoamplification loop of necroinflammation. Whereas direct cytotoxicity is associated with emission of various DAMPs, indirect cytotoxicity can be mediated via crystal-induced activation of the NLRP3 inflammasome resulting in pyroptosis [255] (for crystals as DAMPs, NLRP3, and pyroptosis, compare also Vol. 1 [1], Part IV, Sect. 12.2.5, and Part V, Sect. 19.3.4).

9.4.5.8 Concluding Remarks

Together, the pathogenetic role of DAMPs in AKI is well-established. So, it is worth to recall the local demonstration of DAMPs in infections again, contributing to a robust pathogen-induced inflammatory defense response to infectious damage [121]. When this response is uncontrolled and exaggerated, for example, in infectious sepsis-induced AKI, it might lead to that feared abrupt decline of kidney function (compare Fig. 9.3).

Consequently, in a first clinical trial on sepsis patients, removal of circulating DAMPs (mtDNA, nDNA, HSP70, HMGB1) during continuous veno-venous hemofiltration therapy was attempted aimed at monitoring the outcome in the patients [256]. Interestingly, the investigators could demonstrate a partial beneficial effect of this therapeutic maneuver by observing a reduction of urinary DAMPs and removal of plasma DAMPs. However, the higher clearance rate of DAMPs, especially HSP70 and HMGB1, was significantly associated with immune disorders (immunosuppression!) and poor prognosis. The unsatisfactory outcome of the study is difficult to explain. At least it may be a warning sign not to interfere therapeutically with DAMP concentrations without strict monitoring of the homeostatic DAMP/SAMP ratio (compare Sect. 7.3.3).

9.4.6 SAMPs in Acute Kidney Injury

The principle of involvement of SAMPs in resolution of inflammation appears to apply for AKI as well though reports on this topic have been published only sporadically. Nevertheless, in various AKI models, including IRI and drug-induced nephrotoxicity, AnxA1, or an AnxA1 mimetic was shown to possess protective properties against renal injury [257–259]. In other lines of studies in mice [260], *microsomal prostaglandin E2 synthase-1* (mPGES-1)—an inducible enzyme that converts prostaglandin H2 to PGE2—was observed to exert potentially protective effect against renal fibrosis and inflammation induced by unilateral ureteral obstruction. Also, as revealed by studies on various AKI models, there is accumulating direct and indirect evidence for a protective role of extracellular adenosine in renal injury-induced inflammation and fibrosis. The topic has been thoroughly reviewed by Bauerle et al. [261]. The authors concluded: "Extracellular adenosine is a central signaling molecule involved in modulation of inflammatory events and mediating adaptation to hypoxia. Adenosine signaling helps alleviate ischemic injury in other organs, and more recently, experimental studies show promising results in AKI as well. Such studies highlight pharmacologic strategies to enhance extracellular adenosine signaling or the targeting of individual adenosine receptors, particularly, the A1, A2A, or A2BAR are effective in preventing or treating AKI from ischemia in murine models."

Together, there is an emerging role of SAMPs such as AnxA1, PGE2, and extracellular adenosine in promoting resolving inflammatory pathways in AKI, thereby potentially preventing renal fibrosis. Thus, one can expect further progress in this research field when SPMs have been investigated as well.

9.4.7 Acute Repetitive or Chronic Kidney Injury → Chronic Kidney Disease

9.4.7.1 General Remarks

Of note, acute renal injury can transit to CKD in case of incomplete recovery from AKI, leading to long-term functional deficits that are severe and progressive in subpopulations of patients with pre-existing CKD. Indeed, the kidneys from patients recovering from AKI were shown to exhibit chronic dysfunction, tubule atrophy, and interstitial fibrosis [262]. Besides AKI, acute repetitive or persistent insults to the renal parenchyma associated with chronic inflammation in terms of nonresolving inflammation can result in permanent fibrosis and renal dysfunction, which, if left untreated, may progress to CKD. Chronic kidney disease is defined by structural abnormalities or impaired excretory renal function, suggestive of a loss of functional nephrons. Risk factors for the development and progression of CKD include low nephron number at birth, nephron loss due to increasing age, and—as addressed here—acute or chronic kidney injuries caused by toxic exposures or diseases, for example, hypertension, obesity, and T2DM (for review, see [263]).

9.4.7.2 Pathogenesis of Chronic Kidney Disease: Renal Fibrosis (in Brief)

Renal fibrosis, irrespective of its etiology, is a final common stage of almost all CKDs chronic kidney diseases. The progression of CKD associated with chronic inflammation in terms of nonresolving inflammation is characterized by the constant loss of renal cells and their replacement by overshooting repairing responses. Thus, one of the consequences of CKD is glomerulosclerosis and tubulointerstitial fibrosis caused by an imbalance between excessive synthesis and reduced breakdown of the ECM [263, 264]. Typically, as with fibrosis in other organs, renal interstitial fibrosis results from activation and proliferation of fibroblasts to myofibroblasts, secretion and accumulation of ECM, and displacement of normal renal tubules. Profibrotic factors such as DAMPs are released/secreted by injured tubular epithelial and infiltrated inflammatory cells such as macrophages to promote complex cascades of signaling events leading to this myofibroblastic activation, proliferation, and ECM production [265–267] (see Sects. 6.4 and 6.5; for additional information see also Vol. 1 [1], Part VIII, Sect. 36.4, p. 851).

Notably, the scenario of fibrogenesis is much more complex, and current notions about the fibrotic pathways as described in detail in Chap. 6 include the process of mechanosensing → mechanotransduction mediated by integrins-driven bi-directional "inside-out and outside-in" transmembrane signaling (Sect. 6.3.2, Fig. 6.1); the role of focal adhesions as the key hub for ECM ↔ cell interaction (Sect. 6.3.3, Fig. 6.1); as well as mechanisms of cytoskeleton-driven and nuclear mechanotransduction (Sects. 6.3.4 and 6.3.5, Fig. 6.1).

9.4.7.3 DAMPs and SAMPs in Kidney Fibrosis

Of note, there is growing evidence suggesting that not only acute renal necroinflammation but also kidney fibrosis reflect the work of DAMPs (compare again [211, 215–220, 222, 223]; for fibrosis, see Chap. 6 and Vol. 1 [1], Part VIII, Sect. 36.4). As outlined and argued in Sect. 6.4, fibrosis can be considered a DAMP-driven self-perpetuating process: once myofibroblasts are developed, they take the lead in fibrogenesis via a disastrous ECM/TGF-β-related self-activation process driven by positive feed-forward loops (compare Fig. 6.2).

DAMPs Promoting Renal Fibrosis

As outlined in Sect. 6.4.2, several DAMPs such as HMGB1, S100A8, S100A9, and GAL-3, as well as, in particular, TGF-β (denoted as an inducible DAMP in this book) have been reported to drive fibrogenesis. First direct or indirect evidence for the role of DAMPs in CKD-associated renal fibrosis has already been published. For example, in studies on a murine IRI model, an inhibitor of HMGB1 release, the *grape seed proanthocyanidin extract* was shown to attenuate IRI-induced chronic renal fibrosis [268]. In other lines of studies on a model of immune-mediated EMT established in human proximal tubular EpCs, human recombinant HMGB1 treatment was shown to induce alterations in epithelial morphology consistent with EMT, thereby indicating a potentially crucial DAMP in the development of renal fibrosis [269]. Again in other sets of studies on a murine model of unilateral ureteral obstruction-mediated renal fibrosis under ER stress, indirect evidence was provided showing that HMGB1 is implicated in the pathogenesis of renal fibrosis [270]. Interestingly, in studies on the same murine fibrosis model, S100A8/A9 DAMPs were demonstrated to promote renal fibrosis in obstructive nephropathy [271].

Importantly, inflammasomes (e.g., the NLRP3 and AIM2 inflammasome) have been shown to be implicated in CKD (reviewed in [272]) indicating that, besides the DAMPs mentioned, other DAMPs that indirectly activate the NLRP3 inflammasome (Subclass IA-2 DAMPs) may be pathogenetically involved in renal fibrogenesis, found in many chronic renal disorders. As such DAMPs, crystals such as calcium oxalates have already been demonstrated to contribute to renal inflammation in nephrocalcinosis, leading to renal fibrosis (see Mulay and Anders [273]). Interestingly, there is evidence for a pathogenetic role of ASC specks in this scenario, that is, an inducible DAMP as denoted from the perspective of this book (see Sects. 2.2.5.4 and 3.5.4.2). For instance, in studies on the murine unilateral ureteral obstruction model of CKD, ASC speck deficiency was found to significantly reduce inflammatory cell infiltration and cytokine expression and improve subsequent renal fibrosis [274]. Also, in these studies, ASC was observed to be specifically upregulated in collecting duct EpCs. In this context, it is worthwhile mentioning an experiment showing that macrophage uptake of necrotic cell DNA activates the AIM2 inflammasome to regulate a proinflammatory phenotype in CKD [275] (for AIM2 inflammasome, see Sect. 2.2.8).

SAMPs Mitigating Kidney Fibrosis

Also, again, one may discuss the unproven possibility that the process of nonresolving inflammation proceeding to renal fibrosis is pathogenetically linked to insufficient levels or activity of SAMPs. Indeed, initial evidence in support of such a concept has already been published, for example, by Higashi et al. [265] who reported on analysis studies on gene expression patterns among fibroblast populations at different stages of injury or repair. The investigators could demonstrate that inherent gene expression changes in activated fibroblasts accompany the transition from AKI to repair and regeneration. However, in chronic models, activated fibroblasts were found to be resistant to the antifibrotic effects of the SAMP PGE2 due to suppression of a subset of PGE receptors. Also, there is preliminary evidence for the SAMP AnxA1 to have protective effects in renal fibrosis. For instance, in studies on a rat fibrosis model, activation of AnxA1 signaling in renal fibroblasts was demonstrated to exert antifibrotic effects [276].

In other studies on rats with CKD, microRNA-206 overexpression was observed to inhibit EMT of renal tubular EpCs and glomerulosclerosis by inactivating the JAK/STAT signaling pathway via downregulation of AnxA1 [277].

9.4.7.4 Concluding Remarks

Collectively, there is an emerging role of DAMPs and SAMPs involved in acute or chronic injury-promoted kidney fibrosis: a development that raises the pathogenetic mechanisms traditionally known in CKD to another level of complexity. Whereas the impact of DAMPs in renal fibrosis appears to be well-established, the role of SAMPs is still elusive. Thus, harnessing DAMPs as therapeutic targets in renal fibrosis is promising. On the other hand, also under consideration of the emerging role of SAMPs in the pathogenesis of AKI as mentioned above, similar studies to use SAMPs as therapeutics in fibrosis are urgently needed. The justification of this endeavor will be to see if such therapeutic approaches are of any benefit for patients with progressive CKD (compare also below the section on the use of DAMPs as future therapeutic targets and SAMPs as future therapeutics).

9.4.8 Résumé

Today, the pathogenetic role of DAMPs in AKI and CKD is well-established, whereas the contribution of SAMPs to their pathogenesis can be assumed but needs further studies to come to a final assessment and conclusion. Nevertheless, the exact molecular mechanisms for the development of AKI and renal fibrosis have not been fully explored. Notably, recent advances in epigenetic research have also raised interest in the role of epigenetic modifications in acute renal inflammation and fibrosis. In fact, there is already first evidence of activation of epigenetic regulatory mechanisms in both acute renal disease and susceptibility to CKD [266, 278–281]. Should the concept of DAMP-promoted epigenetic modifications once been confirmed, novel therapeutic modalities for AKI and CKD may be provided (compare here also Sect. 6.6; for additional information see Vol.1 [1], Part VI, Sect. 24.2.4.4, p. 644: DAMP-Induced Trained Immunity, as also briefly described in Sect. 3.7). Such a therapeutic approach is even more desirable regarding the potential AKI-to-CKD transition or the acute repetitive/persistent injury-mediated kidney fibrosis mentioned above. Here, the proposal for future continuous monitoring of a DAMP/SAMP signature may help make therapeutic decisions on when to use DAMPs as therapeutic targets and SAMPs as therapeutics.

9.5 Acute and Chronic Liver Injury

9.5.1 Introductory Remarks

Acute liver injury may lead to acute liver failure (ALF), which is an uncommon but severe disease. With an incidence of fewer than ten cases per million persons per year in the developed world, ALF is seen most often in previously healthy adults in their 30s and presents unique challenges in clinical management [282–284]. Acute liver failure can proceed to chronic hepatic failure called "acute-on-chronic liver failure" (ACLF) [285, 286]. On the other hand, acute repetitive or persistent hepatic injuries such as excessive alcohol consumption or viral hepatitis can result in various chronic liver diseases, histopathologically characterized by hepatic fibrosis that proceeds to cirrhosis [287]. These various injury-promoted diseases are briefly addressed here in light of the danger/injury hypothesis.

9.5.2 Acute Liver Injury → Acute Liver Failure

Acute liver injury → ALF is defined as a clinical syndrome characterized by significant liver dysfunction, coagulopathy, and hepatic encephalopathy. The definition includes the fact that it occurs in a patient without pre-existing liver disease and duration of illness in a limited period of time (in about 8 weeks or less). Notably, earlier stages of acute liver injury are usually diagnosed by hepatic dysfunction and significant coagulopathy (reduced clotting factors) and edema (low albumin), while discernible encephalopathy is still lacking. The etiology varies with geography. Apart from traumatic liver injury, hepatotrophic viruses are the most common cause of ALF in developing countries, whereas hepatotoxic drugs are the most common cause of ALF in the western industrialized nations [288].

Acetaminophen (APAP) (also known as paracetamol) hepatotoxicity is a global issue. The intoxication is responsible for nearly half of the ALF cases in the USA and remains the leading cause of liver transplantation. According to information provided by the *American National Poison Data System* (NPDS), paracetamol is one of the 25 drugs associated with the largest number of pathological fatalities, either alone or in combination with other agents [289].

The mortality of ALF is high and the cause of death is often sepsis/SIRS with MOF. However, timely liver transplantation may save the life of patients. As said, acute liver injury → liver failure is most frequently caused by severe viral infections and hepatotoxic drugs but can also result from prolonged periods of trauma-associated shock followed by hepatic IRI. Accordingly, the proper management of hepatic trauma by clinicians—may it be nonoperative or require hepatic resection in severe cases—should always include the mandatory option of treating hepatic IRI (for further readings, see [283, 284, 290–294]).

9.5.3 Regulated Cell Death and Necroinflammation in Acute Liver Injury

Acute liver injury → ALF is characterized by massive hepatocyte necrosis associated with extensive loss of parenchyma. Today, there is accumulating evidence indicating that hepatocytes succumb mainly from various subroutines of insult-induced RCD, which serve as productive sources of DAMPs emission to trigger hepatic necroinflammatory pathways. Indeed, the hepatocytes can be regarded as the targets of any injury since they have been shown to succumb from apoptosis, necroptosis, ferroptosis, and pyroptosis [295–299].

The various forms of RCD have been best investigated in drug-induced hepatic cell death (reviewed by Iorga et al. [300, 301]). Interestingly, it is not APAP itself that causes hepatotoxicity but rather a reactive metabolite, the *N-acetyl-p-benzoquinone imine* (NAPQI). Under normal circumstances, NAPQI is rapidly converted to nontoxic metabolites by GSH. However, in situations of GSH depletion, such as APAP overdose, chronic alcohol ingestion, and malnutrition, NAPQI persists and leads to liver injury that induces severe liver cell damage and results in inflammation and hepatocyte cell death. Mechanistically, several damaging effects of NAPQI are discussed, including formation of protein adducts by reacting with sulfhydryl groups resulting in mitochondrial dysfunction and cell death (for further reading, see the relevant articles [300, 302–304]).

Notably, there is already first evidence for a role of subroutines of RN in APAP hepatotoxicity, including necroptosis, ferroptosis, and pyroptosis [304–307]. As a possible vital injurious factor, excessive ROS-mediated oxidative stress has been identified to occur during APAP hepatotoxicity resulting in cell necrosis [308]. This observation let suggest that, besides necroptosis, ferroptotic cell death may also occur in APAP hepatotoxicity (for ferroptosis, see Sect. 4.3.4, and compare Vol. 1 [1], Part V, Sect. 19.3.3). Indeed, and remarkably, in earlier studies, this subroutine of RCD has already been described to be involved in APAP-induced cell death [309]. Together, the description of the various subroutines of RN in APAP hepatotoxicity strongly suggests a dominating role of DAMPs in mediating innate immune local and lethal systemic necroinflammation in APAP-induced hepatotoxicity.

9.5.4 Pathogenesis of Acute Liver Injury → Acute Liver Failure (in Brief)

9.5.4.1 General Remarks

As observed in other acute organ injuries, the various liver insults result in DAMP-promoted necroinflammatory pathways in PRM-bearing hepatic cells, which mount the typical inflammatory milieu via secretion of the inflammatory mediators (including cytokines such as TNF and IL-1β, denoted as inducible DAMPs in this book).

In this proinflammatory scenario, the dominating innate immune cells are the Kupffer cells that serve as sentinels for liver homeostasis. Indeed, Kupffer cells, the most abundant tissue resident macrophage population, are key for the maintenance of liver integrity and its restoration after infectious or sterile injury, as well as the local initiation and resolution of innate and adaptive immunity [297, 310]. Notably, the mechanism of resolution of hepatic inflammation is poorly investigated. Nevertheless, in case of insufficient inflammation-resolving processes, acute liver injury can proceed to ALF.

9.5.4.2 DAMP-Governed Innate Immune Responses in Acute Liver Failure

According to current notions, the pathological changes in ALF are the result of innate immune-mediated pathophysiological processes, whereby MAMP/DAMP-governed pathways predominate in ALF caused by hepatotropic viruses, and DAMP-triggered responses are more critical in toxic etiologies.

Regarding pathological features, hepatocyte necrosis occurs due to ATP depletion causing cellular swelling and cell membrane disruption. Although not specifically quantitatively defined, severe liver injury patterns are identified as diffuse, massive, and zonal with massive hepatic necrosis, with near-complete parenchymal necrosis associated with variable inflammation and ductular reaction as the most severe pathologic presentation of ALF [284, 311]. The systemic pathology of ALF at autopsy is generally that of multiorgan system failure. All organ systems can be affected, but most clinically relevant is the development of encephalopathy. Moreover, hemorrhagic complications related to coagulopathy and possible ensuing DIC are common.

9.5.4.3 SAMP-Promoted Resolution of Inflammation in Acute Liver Injury

Interestingly, as reviewed [312], following the acute proinflammatory stage, cytokines and chemokines secreted by activated Kupffer cells further attract the homing and transmigration of protective neutrophils and macrophages to facilitate hepatic inflammation resolution, regeneration, and repair. In more recent studies on an APAP-induced liver injury model in support of this concept, improvement of resolution and liver regeneration was found to be mainly mediated by M2-like macrophages. Mechanistically, the investigators [312] could show that the chemokine CCL5 can facilitate M1-like macrophage polarization and impede M2-like polarization. Similar observations were made in studies on another experimental model of acute hepatic injury in mice, suggesting that polarization of macrophages from the M1-like phenotype to the M2-like phenotype is implicated in amelioration of liver injury and accelerated hepatic regeneration [313]. So far, however, there are only a few reports on the demonstration of SAMPs in acute liver injury, as briefly touched below.

9.5.4.4 Concluding Remarks

Acute liver injury has been observed to mediate remote organ damage, such as brain injury. The pathophysiology of cerebral edema and hepatic encephalopathy, as seen in acute liver injury → ALF, is multifactorial and includes altered BBB secondary to inflammatory mediators leading to microglial activation, accumulation of glutamine secondary to ammonia crossing the BBB, and subsequent oxidative stress leading to depletion of ATP and GTP. These pathogenetic changes ultimately lead to astrocyte swelling and cerebral edema (also compare [314]).

9.5.5 DAMPs in Acute Liver Injury

9.5.5.1 General Remarks

As in AKI, there is increasing evidence for a pathogenetic role of DAMPs in acute liver injury, including drug-triggered hepatotoxicity, which are also supposed to mediate systemic complications. According to studies on liver IRI models and drug-triggered hepatotoxicity, subroutines of hepatic RCD may serve as sources of DAMPs, the subroutines including apoptosis and RN, with recently reported evidence for necroptosis, ferroptosis, pyroptosis, and NETosis [300, 301, 315–320] (for RCD, again compare Sect. 4.3, and Vol. 1 [1], Part V, Chap. 19). Those DAMPs subsequently activate PRM-bearing Kupffer cells. In turn, activated Kupffer cells promote hepatic necroinflammatory pathways via release of cytokines and chemokines that recruit further inflammation-promoting neutrophils and monocytes. Additionally, the DAMPs activate HSCs as the key drivers of hepatic fibrosis (for reviews, see [302, 321–323]). Here, some DAMPs shown to be involved in acute hepatic injury are briefly touched.

9.5.5.2 High Mobility Group Box 1

The participation of HMGB1 in the pathogenesis of acute liver injury has recently been reviewed by Yang et al. [324]. Earlier studies on a murine IRI already demonstrated HMGB1 to act as an early mediator of injury and inflammation in liver IRI, implicating TLR4 as one of the receptors that is involved in the process [325]. A subsequent experiment on a liver IRI model did not only confirm these findings but could also show that HMGB1 (and also histones (see below)) promote NET formation through the TLR signaling pathway. Development of NETs subsequently exacerbates organ damage and initiates inflammatory responses during liver IRI [326]. First clinical studies confirmed these experimental findings by demonstrating increased HMGB1 levels in sera from ALF patients, which correlated with the associated SIRS symptomatology [327].

Also, there is convincing experimental evidence indicating that HMGB1 significantly contributes to drug hepatotoxicity at both the early inflammatory phase and the late regeneration phase [328]. For example, in a lethal APAP overdose model in mice, HMGB1 was found to impair hepatocyte regeneration markedly, and blockade of HMGB1 was observed to enhance the late-phase liver structure recovery significantly [329]. In other experiments on a murine APAP-induced acute liver injury model, neutralization of HMGB1 with a chimeric antibody was shown to attenuate the early phase of post-injury inflammation [330]. Also, in other lines of experiments on APAP-challenged hepatocytes in vivo and in vitro [331], release of HMGB1 was significantly detected in both liver perfusate from APAP-treated mice and culture supernatant of APAP-challenged hepatocytes.

Excitingly, HMGB1 is reportedly also involved in clinical APAP hepatotoxicity. In fact, acetaminophen intoxication is currently known to be one of the best characterized HMGB1-dependent clinical condition in patients. Remarkably, hepatocytes contain more HMGB1 than most other cell types, and hepatocyte-specific conditional hepatocyte-specific HMGB1 knockout has established the crucial role of HMGB1 in drug-induced liver injury but also other liver diseases [332, 333] .

For example, HMGB1was demonstrated to be elevated in the sera of APAP overdose patients with liver injury compared to overdose patients without liver injury [334]. Interestingly, the investigators observed that this DAMP correlated with alanine aminotransferase activity and the prothrombin time. Further, increased total and acetylated HMGB1 was found to be associated with worse prognosis or observed in patients that died or required a liver transplant, compared to spontaneous survivors. The authors concluded from their data that acetylated HMGB1 is a better predictor of outcome than the other markers of cell death.

Consequently, given all this information from targeted studies, HMGB1 has been proposed to be a promising therapeutic target for acute liver injury → liver failure [335].

9.5.5.3 Histones and Extracellular DNA

The role of histones in acute liver injury has been reviewed by Silk et al. [247] and Yang et al. [324]. In experiments on mice, circulating histones (i.e., H3) were found to exacerbate inflammation with ALF; on the other hand, blockade of these DAMPs with an anti-H3 antibody showed potent protective effects as reflected by reduction in the risk of mortality, suggesting a potential therapeutic strategy for ALF [336, 337]. Moreover, in studies on a hepatic IRI model, histones were observed to activate the NLRP3 inflammasome in Kupffer cells through binding to TLR9 [338].

Clinically, and in agreement with experimental data, circulating histones have been detected in patients with ALF, demonstrating that these DAMPs operate as critical mediators of systemic inflammation and cellular damage in this human liver disease [339]. Notably, these data could be confirmed by a more recent study on ICU patients with acute liver injury showing that the levels of extracellular histones were significantly and independently associated with the presence of acute injury [340]. The authors argued that increased histones may contribute to the development of this organ injury in ICU patients, although many other mechanisms may also play crucial roles in its development.

Of note, there is also first experimental evidence for a role of histones in APAP-induced hepatotoxicity. Thus, in a murine model of APAP-induced hepatotoxicity, blockade of histones was shown to attenuate acute fatal liver injury, suggesting that extracellular histones are the major mediators of death in acute fatal liver injury [337].

Excitingly, first evidence was provided to suggest also a contribution of extracellular DNA to APAP-induced liver injury. Thus, in clinical studies—accompanied by parallel studies in mice—nDNA fragments and mtDNA were shown to be released into the plasma of patients and mice after APAP overdose [341]. The authors discussed that "in patients, the release of DAMPs, such as nuclear DNA fragments and mtDNA during the injury phase, contributes to activation of innate immune cells, which are involved in the removal of necrotic cell debris and thus contribute to the recovery as observed in mice." The authors concluded that their findings provide strong support for the hypothesis "that mitochondrial dysfunction and DNA damage are critical events in the mechanism of cell necrosis after APAP overdose in patients." Subsequent experiments in mice confirmed this conclusion by demonstrating that treatment with APAP is associated with DNA release into the hepatocyte cytoplasm, which occurred in parallel with cell death in vitro [342].

9.5.5.4 Uric Acid and Extracellular ATP

DAMPs indirectly activating the NLRP3 inflammasome (Subclass IA-2DAMPs) such as uric acid (i.e., monosodium urate [MSU] crystals) and eATP have been identified to mediate APAP-induced hepatotoxicity as well (for IA-2DAMPs and NLRP3 inflammasome, see Sect. 2.2.5.3 and Vol. 1 [1], Part IV, Sect. 12.2.5, and Part VI, Sect. 22.4.2.2). In earlier studies on an APAP-induced liver injury model, uric acid was already suggested to trigger a cell death-induced inflammatory response [343]. Information about eATP as a critical DAMP involved in APAP hepatotoxicity was documented in experiments on mice genetically deficient in the purinoreceptor P2X7. These studies demonstrated that exposure to this DAMP (and nicotinamide adenine dinucleotide), as well as the P2X7 receptor, is required for manifestations of APAP-induced hepatotoxicity [344] (for P2X7 receptor, see Sect. 2.3.3 and Vol. 1 [1], Part II, Sect. 5.3.4.3); for the mechanism of NLRP3 inflammasome activation via eATP ↔ P2X7 receptor binding, compare Fig. 2.1 and Vol. 1 [1], Part VI, Fig. 22.11). Other sets of experiments on a murine model of APAP poisoning revealed remarkable changes in the liver environment during APAP overdose that were dependent on eATP signaling [345]. Consequently, inhibition of ATP action was shown to reduce the liver damage significantly. Moreover, in these studies, primary mouse hepatocytes also developed hyperresponsiveness to eATP following APAP exposure, which was prevented by a P2 purine receptor blocker. Also, human-derived cells cultivated in vitro were shown to be protected from these toxic effects when the same blockage strategy was employed. The authors of this study [345] postulated that ATP released from necrotic cells may cause cell death or accelerate APAP-induced cell death. However, subsequently published data, demonstrated in four different types of hepatocytes (human and mouse), could not confirm this concept [346]. Today, one may discuss the unproven possibility that eATP may contribute to APAP-induced cell death via promotion of pyroptotic cell death.

9.5.5.5 Concluding Remarks

Today, the necroinflammation-inducing role of DAMPs in acute liver injury, including drug-induced hepatotoxicity, is well-established. Further investigation is necessary to elucidate precisely the pathogenetic role of DAMPs and their impact on prognosis in this clinical organ injury. Of considerable interest would also be to extend the spectrum of DAMPs that are involved in ALF. Doubtlessly, there are many more DAMPs operating in this fatal disorder than described until today.

9.5.6 SAMPs in Acute Liver Injury

There are only a few reports on the demonstration of SAMPs in acute liver injury. Studies on a model of nonalcoholic steatohepatitis in wild-type and KO mice revealed that macrophage-derived AnxA1 plays a functional role in mitigating hepatic inflammation and fibrogenesis during progression of this disease [347]. Notably, in this study, the authors observed consistently that in vitro addition of recombinant AnxA1 to macrophages isolated from nonalcoholic steatohepatitis livers downmodulates M1 polarization through stimulation of IL-10 production.

Also, the cytoprotective effect of PGE2 on the liver has been known for a long time [348]. More recent studies on a model of bile duct ligation in rats showed partial PGE2-mediated immune suppression [349]. Moreover, findings from experiments on a model of acute liver inflammation and injury in transgenic mice suggested that 15-keto-PGE2 from hepatocytes can inhibit inflammatory cytokine production in Kupffer cells and that this paracrine mechanism negatively regulates LPS-induced necroinflammatory response in the liver [350]. In addition, in other lines of studies on a model of LPS/D-galactosamine-induced hepatitis [351], injection of an analog of the SAMP cAMP 1 h before hepatotoxic agents was found to exert a liver-protective effect, as indicated by an increased survival of mice and a significant decrease of plasma alanine aminotransferase level (for cAMP acting as a SAMP, see Sect.

3.5.5.3 and Vol. 1 [1], Part IV, Sect. 14.4.2.3, and Fig. 14.5). A protective effect of SPMs on acute liver injury has also been reported. Thus, in a murine model of hepatic IRI, RvD1 was found to attenuate IRI-induced hepatocellular damage and the proinflammatory response [352].

Intriguingly, first evidence for the protective action of SAMPs in drug-induced hepatotoxicity has already been reported. Indeed, studies in mice provided first in vivo evidence for a beneficial role of the SAMP PGE2 released upon APAP-induced liver injury [353]. In other lines of studies on thioacetamide-primed rats, hepatic overexpression of the SAMP Anx1 was observed to inhibit APAP-induced expansion of liver injury [354]. Further experiments in this study showed that inhibition of the biosynthesis of this SAMP abolishes this protective effect.

In addition, in studies on mice [355], another SAMP, namely, extracellular adenosine, was also demonstrated to exert a significant protective effect against APAP-induce hepatotoxicity. Plausibly, given these first reports, further studies on SAMPs in APAP-induce liver injury are highly desired.

Together, there is initial evidence for a protective role of SAMPs such as AnxA1, PGE2, cAMP, and SPMs on acute liver injury. Further progress can be expected when SPMs have been investigated in more extensive studies in this research field.

9.5.7 Acute Repetitive or Persistent Liver Injury → Chronic Liver Disease/Failure

9.5.7.1 General Remarks

Various chronic liver diseases, triggered by acute repetitive or persistent, infectious or sterile hepatic injuries, can lead—via DAMPs-promoted chronic inflammation in terms of nonresolving inflammatory pathways—to hepatic fibrosis that proceeds to cirrhosis as the final histopathological picture. As a considerable medical burden, various forms of liver fibrosis are known to cause severe morbidity and mortality worldwide. Etiologically, hepatic fibrosis → cirrhosis can arise in consequence of liver-damaging exogenous/toxic, infectious, toxic/allergic, immunopathological/autoimmune, or vascular processes or an inborn error of metabolism, including alcoholic steatohepatitis, nonalcoholic steatohepatitis, nonalcoholic fatty liver disease, chronic hepatitis B or C virus infection, and chronic cholangiopathies (for reviews, see [321, 356]).

9.5.7.2 Acute-on-Chronic Liver Failure

A special form of chronic liver diseases is ACLF. This chronic disorder is defined as the acute deterioration of pre-existing chronic liver disease, usually related to an acute precipitating event in terms of an acute infectious or sterile liver injury [285, 286]. Typically, ACLF is observed in patients suffering from cirrhosis that undergoes acute decompensation. The epidemiology, diagnostic criteria, characteristics, clinical course, and prognosis of ACLF have recently been detailed in the CANONIC study, an extensive multicenter European prospective observational investigation in >1000 patients treated for acute decompensation of cirrhosis [357]. Of note, pathogenetically, ACLF develops in the setting of an exacerbated systemic inflammatory response to initial infectious or sterile acute liver damage, that is, hepatic injuries associated with the emission of MAMPs and DAMPs or DAMPs. As also observed in SIRS associated, for instance, with polytrauma (see Sects. 5.4.2.2 and 8.3.2.2), this hyperinflammatory response is associated with MOF resulting in a high short-term mortality rate [358, 359].

Until to date, the pathogenetic role of MAMPs and DAMPs or DAMPs in ACLF is not firmly proven but intensely proposed and discussed [358, 360]. However, given their documentation in SIRS (see Sects. 5.4.2.3 and 8.3.3), they operate in this acute liver disease most likely and will undoubtedly be described in more detail soon.

9.5.7.3 Pathogenesis of Chronic Liver Disease: Hepatic Fibrosis/Cirrhosis (in Brief)

There is accumulating evidence suggesting that acute repetitive or persistent insults to the hepatic parenchyma, associated with chronic inflammation in terms of nonresolving inflammation, can result in permanent liver fibrosis → cirrhosis. As outlined in Vol. 1 [1], Part VI, Chpt. 22, and in Sects. 5.5, 6.3, and 6.4, the scenario of inflammation proceeding to fibrosis is orchestrated by multiple cell types, mostly PRM-bearing innate immune cells such as leukocytes, macrophages, and fibroblasts, all of them committed to contributing to the pathogenesis of inflammatory/fibrotic diseases. In the pathogenesis of liver fibrosis → cirrhosis, these cells refer to parenchymal cells, the hepatocytes; the Kupffer cells, i.e., the resident "macrophages" in the liver; and the HSCs, the hepatic "fibroblasts" (Fig. 9.4).

As mentioned above, the hepatocytes and Kupffer cells can be regarded as the targets of any injury since they have been shown to succumb from apoptosis, necroptosis, ferroptosis, and pyroptosis [295–299], that is, subroutines of hepatic insult-induced RCD that serve as productive sources of DAMPs emission.

DAMPs—together with MAMPs in infectious injury—are sensed by PRM-expressing resident Kupffer cells, which trigger NLRP3 inflammasome-dependent and inflammasome-independent signaling pathways to mount an intrahepatic proinflammatory milieu (including secretion/release of cytokines, chemokines, and adhesion molecules; also compare [295–297, 361–363]). Besides Kupffer cells, other cells such as profibrotic macrophages, neutrophils, DCs, and T/B lymphocytes also contribute to chronic hepatic inflammation—today interpreted as nonresolving inflammation—that is considered to lead to fibrogenesis/fibrosis.

Together, constitutive DAMPs released from cells undergoing RCD as well as inducible DAMPs secreted by activated inflammatory cells (e.g., TGF-β, IL-1β (see below))—together with MAMPs in case of infectious injury—activate PRM-bearing HSCs which transdifferentiate into myofibroblasts (reviewed in [321, 322, 364]). These activated HSCs then, via both serving as the major source of ECM production and interacting with the ECM, drive the mechanisms resulting in liver fibrosis/cirrhosis (Fig. 9.4). This process occurs via epigenetic modifications late in the proliferative phase and is also called activation of myofibroblasts (for details of transdifferentiation into myofibroblasts and epigenetic modifications, see Sects. 6.4, 6.5, and 6.6).

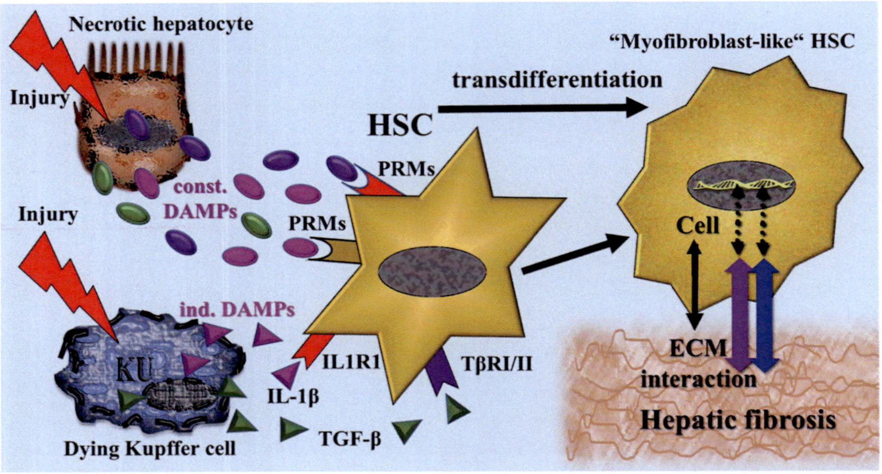

Fig. 9.4 Simplified diagrammatic model of the pathogenetic role of DAMPs in promoting activation of PRM-bearing HSCs to "myofibroblast-like" HSCs serving as the major source of ECM production and interacting with the ECM to drive liver fibrosis. Constitutive DAMPs are released from necrotic hepatocytes and Kupffer cells, whereas inducible DAMPs are either released from pyroptotic Kupffer cells (IL-1β) or secreted by these cells (TGF-β). Interaction of "myofibroblast-like" HSCs with ECM through integrin-mediated bi-directional "inside-out and outside-in" transmembrane mechanotransduction (symbolized by the two blue/violet-colored bi-directional arrows) leads to progressive liver fibrosis (compare Sect. 6.3 and Fig. 6.1). *Constit* constitutional, *ECM* extracellular matrix, *HSC* hepatic stellate cell, *IL-1β* interleukin-1 beta, *IL1R1* interleukin-1 receptor type I, *ind* inducible, *TGF-β* transforming growth factor-beta, *TβRI/II* transforming growth factor-beta receptor I/II. (Sources: [295–297, 302, 321–323, 361–363])

Of note, although HSCs are known as the primary cells responsible for liver fibrogenesis, studies have shown contributing roles for other cells, pathways, and molecules in the development of fibrosis depending on the etiology of liver fibrosis [364–366]. Indeed, the current notions about the complex scenario of fibrogenesis are presented in detail in Chap. 6, including the process of mechanosensing → mechanotransduction mediated by integrins-driven bi-directional "inside-out and outside-in" transmembrane signaling (Sect. 6.3.2, Fig. 6.1); the role of focal adhesions as the critical hub for ECM ↔ cell interaction (Sect. 6.3.3, Fig. 6.1); as well as mechanisms of cytoskeleton-driven and nuclear mechanotransduction (Sects. 6.3.4 and 6.3.5, Fig. 6.1).

9.5.7.4 DAMPs and SAMPs in Liver Fibrosis

The progression of chronic liver diseases involves chronic parenchymal injury associated with constant RCD-mediated emission of DAMPs, which trigger persistently proinflammatory, profibrotic, and overshooting repairing responses. As outlined in Sect. 6.4.2, several DAMPs such as HMGB1, S100A8, S100A9, and GAL-3, as well as, in particular, TGF-β (denoted as an inducible DAMP in this book) have been reported to drive fibrogenesis. Moreover, the DAMP-driven self-perpetuating process in fibrosis has been detailed in Sects. 6.4 and 6.5: once MAMP/DAMP-activated myofibroblasts are developed, they take the lead in fibrogenesis via a disastrous ECM/TGF-β-related self-activation process driven by positive feed-forward loops (compare Fig. 6.2).

Constitutive and Inducible DAMPs in Promoting Hepatic Inflammation → Liver Fibrosis

Some distinct constitutive DAMPs involved in liver fibrosis have already been identified and are selectively mentioned here. For example, early in vitro experiments provided already evidence for HMGB1 to activate HSCs [367]. In the context of chronic liver disease, HMGB1 has reportedly been implicated in nonalcoholic steatohepatitis, alcoholic liver disease (ALD), and liver fibrosis (reviewed in [368]). Of interest is the clinical observation that liver HMGB1 protein expression correlates with fibrosis stage in patients with chronic hepatitis C virus infection and primary biliary cirrhosis [369]. Serum levels of HMGB1 were also found to be increased in these patients compared to healthy controls, suggesting secretion of this DAMP. Also, in studies on mice, S100A4 was found to be secreted by a subpopulation of macrophages and to promote the development of liver fibrosis [370]. The authors could show that this DAMP activates HSCs and accumulates in the liver during the progression of liver fibrosis. Further, in studies on mice, the NLRP3-activating IA-2DAMP eATP was shown to potentiate HSC activation (and thus ECM deposition), dependent on P2X7R-mediated NLRP3 inflammasome activation [371] (for NLRP3 inflammasome activation, compare Sect. 2.2.5). Inducible DAMPs have also been reported to activate HSCs. For instance, IL-1β was shown to promote the proliferation of rat HSCs, whereby IL-1 type I receptor (IL1R1), JNK, and AP-1 pathways were observed to be involved in this process [372]. Last but not least, the inducible DAMP TGF-β1 was shown to play a critical role in the development of hepatic fibrosis by triggering the Smad (Smad2, Smad3, Smad4) signaling pathway (known to operate in HSCs) [373] (Fig. 9.4; also compare Fig. 6.3).

SAMPs in Mitigating Hepatic Inflammation → Liver Fibrosis

According to the model of SAMP-promoted resolution of inflammation, the development of liver fibrosis should be decelerated or even prevented by the emission of SAMPs. Indeed, preclinical and clinical evidence suggesting SPMs being able to enhance nonalcoholic steatohepatitis and fibrosis resolution has already recently been reviewed [374]. Although the concept is still not validly proven, preliminary supportive data in this research field were already reported. For example, in studies on the murine model of hepatic IRI mentioned above [352], the interesting finding was observed that RvD1 modulates macrophage polarization in that it attenuates the IRI-induced increase of proinflammatory M1 marker genes in Kupffer cells, associated with a decrease of M2 marker genes. As also observed by the investigators, RvD1 markedly augments the efferocytic activity of Kupffer cells. Together, these findings indicated antiinflammatory and proresolving actions of RvD1, suggesting that this SAMP might interfere with the development of liver fibrosis. A similar concept can be discussed when looking at the studies on a murine model of nonalcoholic steatohepatitis also mentioned above [347]. In these studies, the authors observed that in vitro addition of recombinant AnxA1 to macrophages isolated from nonalcoholic steatohepatitis livers downmodulates M1 polarization through stimulation of IL-10 production; again a clue that administration of SAMPs might interfere with the development of liver fibrosis.

9.5.7.5 Concluding Remarks

Together, research on DAMPs and SAMPs impacting development of liver fibrosis is still in its infancy. Progress in this field, however, is of great interest because DAMPs as therapeutic targets or SAMPs as therapeutics may be a new therapeutic approach to interfere with the development of liver fibrosis → cirrhosis. This is all the more so, as many experimental data have provided evidence of the reversibility of liver fibrosis [375]. In particular, identification of key DAMPs found to activate/transdifferentiate HSCs as the major drivers of liver fibrogenesis may serve as a potential target of antifibrotic therapy. A future use of SAMPs as therapeutics might also be an option but has still to be proven by appropriate targeted experiments.

9.5.8 Alcohol-Related Liver Injury → Alcoholic Liver Disease

9.5.8.1 General Remarks

Here, the alcohol-related liver injury leading to the development of ALD is separately highlighted because excessive alcohol consumption is a global healthcare problem with enormous social, economic, and clinical consequences. According to the 2018 report of the World Health Organization (WHO) [376], the harmful use of alcohol resulted in an estimated three million deaths (5.3% of all deaths) globally in 2016; these estimates incorporate both the detrimental and beneficial health effects of alcohol consumption. The effects of alcohol consumption on mortality are higher than those of tuberculosis (2.3%), human immunodeficiency virus/acquired immune deficiency syndrome (HIV/AIDS) (1.8%), diabetes (2.8%), hypertension (1.6%), digestive diseases (4.5%), road injuries (2.5%), and violence (0.8%). As known, excessive drinking over decades injures nearly every organ in the body. However, the liver sustains the earliest and the highest degree of tissue injury from excessive drinking because this substance of abuse is mainly metabolized by liver cells, which express high levels of two major alcohol oxidizing enzymes, alcohol dehydrogenase, and cytochrome P450 2E1 (CYP2 E1) (reviewed in [377, 378]).

Alcoholic liver disease is a major cause of morbidity and mortality from heavy alcohol use and is the leading cause of death from chronic alcohol consumption [379]. The disorder is known as a metabolic liver disease in which pathological progression is largely driven by inflammatory responses. Chronic consumption of alcohol dramatically alters liver function at multiple levels in all liver cell types. As with all other inflammatory diseases, infiltration of PRM-bearing neutrophils is regarded as a hallmark of alcoholic steatohepatitis; however, ALD is also associated with infiltration of many other types of PRM-bearing inflammatory cells including Kupffer cells and natural killer T (NKT) cells (for NKT cells, see Vol. 1 [1], Part III, Sect. 8.5.2).

9.5.8.2 Pathogenesis of Alcoholic Liver Disease (in Brief)

Various pathophysiological mechanisms of alcohol-induced tissue and organ injury have been described, including oxidative stress, inflammation, PTMs of proteins, impaired anabolic signaling, upregulation of catabolic processes, and dysregulation in lipid metabolism (reviewed in [47, 48]). Indeed, the pathogenesis of ALD is complex as comprehensively reviewed by Orna et al. [378]; but here only briefly outlined.

The alcohol-induced changes result in a spectrum of liver abnormalities, usually starting with the earliest initiator stage of steatosis, characterized by the deposition of fat in hepatocytes (fatty liver). Beyond fatty liver, ALD consists of a continuum of partly overlapping liver pathologies with variable degrees of (obviously nonresolving) inflammation (steatohepatitis) and progressive fibrosis, associated with excessive deposition of ECM. The fibrotic response begins with active pericellular fibrosis, which may progress to cirrhosis, characterized by excessive liver scarring, vascular alterations, and eventual liver failure. As already stressed above, PRM-bearing Kupffer cells and HSCs have been identified again as the dominating cells in promoting alcohol-induced inflammatory changes and progression to fibrosis and cirrhosis.

While steatosis and inflammation are treatable and reversible upon abstinence, severe alcoholic steatohepatitis and decompensating cirrhosis have a grave prognosis. The pathological progression of ALD is overwhelmingly driven by DAMP-promoted inflammatory processes. Also, as a typical feature of ALD, MAMPs derived from gut microbes, which translocate to the mesenteric lymphatic system and portal circulation, contribute in concert with DAMPs to the establishment of hepatic inflammation (for reviews, see [48, 380]). Moreover, intestinal dysbiotic microbiota and impaired intestinal barrier integrity are additional critical players in the pathophysiology of acute alcoholic steatohepatitis. Such involvement of MAMPs in innate immune inflammatory pathways is facilitated by increased gut permeability, caused by chronic alcohol consumption. This scenario is known to result in higher amounts of LPS in portal and systemic blood of patients with ALD [381, 382] (for the function of LPS as a possible microbe-derived exogenous DAMP in triggering innate immune inflammatory pathways, compare also Sect. 3.2.2 and Vol.1 [1], Part IV, Sect. 11.3). In sum, gut dysbiosis can be considered a critical upstream causal event and an example of organ crosstalk in the pathogenesis of ALD (also compare [383, 384]).

Pathogenetic Role of Regulated Cell Death in Alcoholic Liver Disease

As already described in this chapter, organ injuries usually induce subroutines of RCD that are the main sources of DAMPs emission. This scenario has also been observed in alcohol-related liver injury. Thus, during chronic ethanol consumption, hepatocytes were shown to undergo RCD, including apoptosis, necroptosis, ferroptosis, and pyroptosis (reviewed in [299, 385–387]), which serve as rich sources of

DAMPs in ALD as well. Of interest in this context are recent studies in mice [388], showing that overexpression of the adipose-specific lipin-1 (an enzyme involved in the generation of diacylglycerol during synthesis of phospholipids and triglycerides) can cause lipid peroxidation and promote ferroptotic liver damage after ethanol administration.

9.5.8.3 DAMPs in Alcoholic Liver Damage

The prototype danger signal HMGB1 is again the most investigated DAMP in ALD, all the more, as liver biopsies from patients with this disorder showed a marked increase in HMGB1 expression and translocation, which correlated with disease stage, compared with healthy explants [389]. In this earlier study, the investigators further demonstrated that HMGB1 increases both in liver and serum from patients with acute alcoholic steatohepatitis superimposed on ALD and cirrhosis and that there is a correlation among the progressive increase in HMGB1 expression, translocation, and secretion with ALD stage in humans. Moreover, in parallel-conducted mouse models of alcohol-induced liver injury, they found that alcohol intake facilitates hepatic and serum HMGB1 expression, translocation from the nucleus to the cytoplasm, and secretion in these animals similar to what they observed in humans [389]. In a clinical study in patients with acute alcoholic hepatitis aimed to identify potential predictive biomarkers (together with MAMPs) for disease severity and clinical outcomes, HMGB1 was evaluated as a potential indicator of disease severity [390]. In this study, the investigators found HMGB1 to be increased in the acute phase of the disease and positively correlated with *model for end-stage liver disease* (MELD) score (a MELD score is a number that ranges from 6 to 40, based on laboratory tests to assess the urgency for a liver transplant, see [391]). There is also first evidence suggesting a role of the inflammasome in promoting the progression of ALD [392]. This initial suggestion was supported by studies in mice showing that deficiency of NLRP3 prevents the development of alcohol-induced liver inflammation and significantly ameliorates liver damage and steatosis [393]. Further data from this study indicated that ethanol-damaged hepatocytes release uric acid, and eATP, that is, inflammasome-activating IA-2 DAMPs, which are recognized by liver immune cells as inflammatory signals. The authors argued that "the final common pathway of this signaling is most likely represented by the activation of inflammasome, which is required for processing and activation of IL-1β, a key inflammatory cytokine involved in the pathogenesis of alcoholic steatohepatitis…" [393]. More recently conducted studies on alcoholic hepatitis human and animal liver samples and hepatocytes provided evidence demonstrating that alcohol induces pyroptosis of hepatocytes by activating the NLRP3 inflammasome mediated by TXNIP overexpression [394] (for TXNIP, denoted as a metabolic DAMP in this book, acting in NLRP3 inflammasome, see Vol. 1 [1], Part IV, Sect. 13.4.6.3, and Part VI, Sect. 22.4.2.2).

9.5.8.4 Concluding Remarks

Together, ALD comprises a broad spectrum of disease ranging from asymptomatic fatty liver to alcoholic steatohepatitis, progressive fibrosis, and cirrhosis. Again, as reviewed elsewhere [395] and as also underlined by the tenor of this book, ALD-associated fibrosis reflects an uncontrolled wound healing response to ethanol-promoted liver damage, which is characterized by excessive accumulation of collagen and other ECM proteins. As a pivotal event to develop liver fibrosis, activation of HSCs leads to production of ECM proteins; different cell types such as portal fibroblasts and bone marrow-derived myofibroblasts are also supposed to contribute but to a lesser extent (also compare Sect. 6.2). Together, one can assume that development of liver fibrosis transitioning to cirrhosis represents the work of DAMPs again. Indeed, as comprehensively described in Sects. 6.4 and 6.5, modern notions hold that fibrosis can be regarded as a DAMP-driven self-perpetuating process.

9.5.9 Résumé

Today, the pathogenetic role of DAMPs in acute liver injury → ALF and chronic injury-promoted liver fibrosis is well documented, whereas the role of SAMPs has still to be investigated more precisely to draw firm conclusions. Also, preclinical and clinical studies have clearly revealed a critical role of DAMPs in ethanol-induced injury to the liver. Moreover, it should not be forgotten to mention here that, besides alcohol, intoxications can be caused by poisons. An impressive example is the mushroom poisoning of the liver that can lead to acute liver injury and ALF [396]. Identification of DAMPs involved in this disease and their use as therapeutic targets will undoubtedly extend the therapeutic armamentarium to be applied in this potentially life-threatening liver injury.

Indeed, for clinicians working in ICUs, the routine measurement of DAMPs and SAMPs as diagnostic and prognostic biomarkers in those patients may become an exciting option soon. Intense clinical studies examining the pattern of DAMP and SAMP emission and tentatively defining a homeostatic DAMP/SAMP signature in those patients may not only assist in predictive risk modeling and reduction in morbidity and mortality but might also be helpful in making the right and reasonable therapeutic decision. The questions to get correctly answered are at what exact stage of a severe liver damage to start and to stop inhibition of DAMPs, and when to begin and discontinue application of SAMPs, questions that also apply to patients with a different solid organ injury.

9.6 Acute and Chronic Pancreas Injury

9.6.1 Introductory Remarks

Pancreatic injuries are well-known to abdominal surgeons as an acute traumatic injury and to gastroenterologists as an acute or chronic alcohol-related injury. Traumatic injuries to the pancreas are rare and difficult to diagnose. They are usually subtle to identify by different diagnostic imaging modalities, and these injuries are often overlooked in cases with extensive multiorgan trauma. The most evident findings of pancreatic injury are posttraumatic pancreatitis with blood, edema, and soft tissue infiltration of the anterior pararenal space (reviewed in [397]). However, this is not the theme of this section. Instead, here, focus is directed on alcohol-related pancreatic injury, which is one of the most common causes of both acute and chronic pancreatitis (comprehensively reviewed by Klochkov and Sun in [398]).

9.6.2 Acute Alcohol-Related Pancreatic Injury → Acute Pancreatitis

9.6.2.1 General Remarks

Acute injury-induced pancreatitis is a necroinflammatory disease resulting from exocrine cell destruction by infiltrating inflammatory cells. Acute pancreatic inflammation will either resolve with the pancreas fully regenerating, lead to transient organ failure, or progress to cause systemic inflammation and MOF. Although commonly associated with pancreatitis, alcohol alone is unable to trigger pancreatitis. Instead, alcohol and its metabolic byproducts are supposed to predispose the pancreas to injuries from agents that generally do not (or only mildly) cause pancreatitis (for reviews, see [398–400]).

9.6.2.2 Pathogenesis of Acute Pancreatitis (in Brief)

As reviewed [398, 400], the complete pathogenesis of this disease is not entirely known but is supposed to originate from alcohol's effects on the small pancreatic ducts and acinar cells. The pancreas uses oxidative and non-oxidative metabolism to process alcohol. The oxidative pathway leads to the formation of acetaldehyde that causes detrimental effects in acinar cells through activation of stellate cells and increased expression of proinflammatory cytokines. The non-oxidative path requires the formation of fatty acid ethyl ester synthase, which leads to activation of key transcription factors, sustained increases in intracellular calcium, and inhibition of ECM, finally resulting in further cell injury. Moreover, alcohol also promotes premature activation of trypsinogen and other digestive and lysosomal enzymes within the acinar cells, thereby promoting the pancreatic tissue to auto-digest. The whole scenario contributes to aggravation of pancreatic inflammation. Another contributing mechanism is intra-acinar activation of NF-κB that further drives the inflammatory response. The NF-κB-mediated inflammatory response appears to be typically associated with acute pancreatitis, as well as the potentially fatal SIRS as the worst outcome of this disease. In other words and from the perspective of this book, the scenario of alcohol-induced pancreatitis reflects the work of local emission of DAMPs which might systemically be released in case of SIRS/MOF (a topic that "cries for proving determinations"!).

9.6.2.3 Concluding Remarks

The incidence of acute pancreatitis is increasing, and alcohol is still recognized as one of the most common causes. A tremendous amount of work has provided evidence of several mechanisms by which ethanol and both its oxidative and non-oxidative metabolites damage pancreatic cells. In this context, Clemens et al. [400] concluded: "By understanding the mechanisms by which ethanol alter the normal physiology of the pancreas, we have uncovered potential targets for therapeutic intervention. Further experimental work and clinical studies are required to determine the utility of these targets in treating alcoholic pancreatitis." Again, it can be expected that the measurement of ethanol-induced emission of DAMPs will contribute to progress in this therapy.

9.6.3 Acute Repetitive or Chronic Alcohol-Related Pancreatic Injury → Chronic Pancreatitis

Chronic pancreatitis is believed to result from recurrent attacks of acute pancreatitis. Although alcoholic pancreatitis can remain an acute disorder, in many cases, this acute disease progresses to chronic alcoholic pancreatitis. Notably, it was reported that such a progression from acute to chronic pancreatitis is most common in habitual alcohol abusers, indicating that excessive alcohol consumption is involved in acute pancreatitis progressing to a chronic fibrotic disorder (reviewed in [400]).

Typically, chronic pancreatitis is a syndrome characterized by chronic progressive pancreatic inflammation (obviously in terms of nonresolving inflammation) that progresses to fibrosis and scarring, resulting in loss of exocrine (acinar), endocrine (islet cells), and ductal cells [401]. The pathogenesis of chronic alcoholic pancreatitis is poorly understood, but current notions hold that chronic alcohol consumption sensitizes the acinar cell to injury by interfering with mechanisms that protect against ER stress. The alcohol injury-induced complex chronic inflammatory disorder that is linked to genetic, metabolic, and environmental factors leads to the development of pancreatic insufficiency, steatorrhea, diabetes, pancreatic calcification, and fibrosis (reviewed in [402]).

9.6.4 DAMPs in Alcohol-Induced Pancreatitis

Of note, the emission of DAMPs has already been observed in experimental alcoholic pancreatitis. In earlier experiments on a rat model of acute alcohol-induced pancreatitis, nuclear release of HMGB1 was seen as a feature of necrotic cell death [403]. In similar experiments on alcohol-fed rats, tissue release of HMGB1 was found to be correlated well with the systemic necrosis marker lactate dehydrogenase [404]. Also, in investigations on ethanol-induced pancreatic injury using a mouse model of binge ethanol exposure, the authors detected release of HMGB1 from necrotic cells [405]. Certainly, the list of DAMPs involved in this disease is still small but can be expected to increase shortly. In fact, regarding the role of DAMPs in other forms of acute pancreatitis [406], their pathogenetic role in this (sometimes life-threatening) disorder cannot be overestimated.

9.6.5 Résumé

In summary, preclinical and clinical studies have revealed a critical role of DAMPs not only in ethanol-induced injury to the brain and liver but also—as briefly touched here—to the pancreas. Thus, this research field appears to require broader clinical and practical attention. For example, in the case of acute severe alcoholic pancreatitis, inhibition of DAMPs involved may even help save the patient's life. It can be expected that, in the future, gastroenterologists will get familiar with the new approach of treating this excessive alcohol consumption-induced disorder.

9.7 Traumatic Musculoskeletal Injury Affecting Remote Organs

9.7.1 Introductory Remarks

As any organ injury, severe musculoskeletal trauma can trigger an inflammatory response, and an excessive hyperinflammatory response is known to result in SIRS and MOF, an exciting observation that deserves to be briefly addressed in this chapter.

A peculiar feature of musculoskeletal trauma is the historical observation that it can lead to a "secondary injury" affecting distant organs, also referred to as the secondary injury model. As reviewed [407], this pathophysiological model was originally developed more than 40 years ago. In this model, acute trauma is denoted as the primary injury, "whereas secondary injury refers to damage to otherwise uninjured cells that was a direct consequence of the physiologic response to primary injury. In the original model, mechanisms for secondary injury were hypothesized based on then-contemporary understandings of Immunology and cellular pathology." Today, this model can be easily explained by systemic release of locally emitted DAMPs into the blood circulation. In the following, a few examples of this phenomenon are addressed by choosing bone fracture and soft tissue injury, promoting remote organ injuries.

9.7.2 Bone Fractures and DAMP-Promoted Remote Organ Injuries

9.7.2.1 General Remarks

Early studies already showed that bone fractures, eventually associated with soft tissue injury, play a pivotal role in the induction of systemic inflammation and remote organ dysfunction after fracture. For example, experiments using a murine model of bilateral femur fracture alone or in combination with soft tissue injury affecting the thighs revealed that each injury promoted systemic inflammation, but the combination of both injuries was required to induce marked remote liver dysfunction associated with systemic inflammation [408]. Intrinsically, any bone fracture leads to emission of bona fide DAMPs, which initiate a healing efferent innate immune response. Again, there is a double role of DAMPs in case of bone fracture: local emission promotes fracture healing (see Sect. 8.2.3 [409]), and massive emission and systemic distribution may lead to remote organ injuries such as TBI and ALI. Indeed, earlier experimental studies have already demonstrated an increase in cytokines within human fracture site hematomas, as well as in the systemic circulation of patients sustaining fracture [410]. Research in this field of traumatic lesions is at the beginning. However, a few reports have been published which are briefly quoted here.

9.7.2.2 Pathophysiology of Bone Fractures (in Brief)

Under homeostatic conditions, bone fracture heals up in the course of a DAMP-promoted physiological inflammatory innate immune process. However, in massive multiple fractures often associated with soft tissue damage, pathophysiological mechanisms in terms of systemic inflammation and remote organ injuries, associated with cytokine release, have been described [411–414]. Current knowledge now holds that delivery of large amounts of DAMPs in the blood circulation promotes systemic inflammation by affecting susceptible organs such as the brain and the lung. In the following, this topic is briefly reviewed by describing selected DAMPs involved in this process.

9.7.2.3 DAMPs Emission in Bone Fractures

Though only a limited number of DAMPs in this research field has been investigated, the data of the published studies are convincing and have contributed to more knowledge of the pathophysiology of TBI and ALI, especially in the understanding of the cascade of their complications.

High Mobility Group Box 1

In a model of bilateral femur fracture in TLR4 wild-type mice, treatment with antibodies to HMGB1 was found to cause a suppression of circulating IL-6 and IL-10 and lower serum alanine aminotransferase levels, indicating a pathogenetic role of HMGB1 in this model of trauma-induced inflammation [415]. According to the authors' conclusion, these data demonstrate a critical role for an HMGB1 → TLR4 pathway in the initiation of systemic inflammation and end-organ injury following isolated peripheral tissue injury. More recent experiments on a model of closed fracture musculoskeletal injury in mice supported these data by demonstrating that the upregulated expression of HMGB1 mRNA after injury—indicating infliction of sterile inflammation—could be significantly decreased by intravenous injection of lidocaine [416]. In other sets of studies on a murine model of tibia bone fracture one day after experimental stroke induction, intraperitoneal injection of neutralizing anti-HMGB1antibodies was found to attenuate the bone fracture-mediated inflammatory effects on the cerebrum [417]. According to the authors' conclusion, these findings suggest that bone fracture shortly after stroke enhances stroke injury via augmented inflammation through HMGB1. These experimental observations could be confirmed by further studies on a bone fracture/TBI model in mice (already mentioned above), demonstrating that bone fracture can stimulate the inflammatory cytokines releases and exacerbate TBI symptoms [49]. Notably, HMGB1 was dramatically elevated by bone fracture, and the severity of TBI was reduced after blocking HMGB1. Given these data, the authors suggested that HMGB1-mediated inflammation may have a substantial impact on the secondary TBI.

Mitochondrial DNA

Mitochondrial DNA belongs to the few DAMPs investigated in the context of fracture-mediated remote organ injury. Thus, in studies on a model of hip fracture in rats mentioned above, mtDNA was found to induce ALI [120]. In the first part of the experiments, the effects of hip fracture were investigated; in the second part, the impact of intravenously injected mtDNA on the animals. The experimentally set fracture resulted in significant mtDNA release, TLR9 → NF-κB expression, and lung injury, whereas the mtDNA injection could indirectly induce pulmonary damage. The investigators concluded that these results suggest the lung injury to be induced by hip fracture, probably under involvement of the mtDNA → TLR9 → NF-κB pathway.

9.7.3 Soft Tissue Injury Promoting Remote Organ Injuries

A severe form of soft tissue injury is exemplified by rhabdomyolysis that can be caused by direct traumatic injury as a result of drugs, toxins, infections, muscle ischemia, electrolyte, and metabolic disorders. The disease is a complex medical condition involving the rapid dissolution of damaged or injured skeletal muscle. Of note, rhabdomyolysis is reportedly associated with high morbidity and mortality when subsequently promoting the development of AKI in the days following initial presentation and develops in 33% of patients. It is well accepted that AKI is the result of an accumulation of myoglobin, which is nephrotoxic. Hypovolemia is another associated factor that leads to renal hypoperfusion (reviewed in [418, 419]). Notably, there is first evidence suggesting myoglobin may contribute to rhabdomyolysis-induced AKI via the TLR4 → NF-κB pathways [420]. However, whether myoglobin acts as a DAMP in this scenario to be sensed by TLR4 has still to be confirmed in other targeted experiments.

9.7.4 Résumé

In a chapter on the role of DAMPs in solid organ injuries, the topic of musculoskeletal injuries affecting remote organs is of high interest. Indeed, the documentation of locally emitted DAMPs to promote remote organ injuries is an impressive example of the property of these molecules—when released into the blood circulation—to spread out systemically and function in any part of the body. As outlined above (Sect. 8.3.3), this scenario can culminate in SIRS when DAMPs are produced in excess.

Of note, this phenomenon is not restricted to the two examples mentioned here and appears to be a general fundamental event. For instance, another similar scenario refers to postoperative remote lung injury (e.g., ARDS) that has been observed to occur following various surgeries and is associated with short- and long-term morbidity and mortality [421]. Here again, the release of DAMPs may trigger a systemic inflammatory response, which ultimately results in organ injury, including lung injury: undoubtedly, another field of using DAMPs as biomarkers and therapeutic targets!

9.8 Biomechanical Injury to Articular Cartilage → Osteoarthritis

9.8.1 Introductory Remarks

More in terms of an appendix and in passing, injury-induced (sterile) osteoarthritis (OA) should be added to the list of solid organ injuries, addressed in this chapter. Biomechanical injuries to articular cartilage are thought to be pathogenetically involved in this degenerative bone/joint inflammatory process. Indeed, the articular cartilage resides in a complex and dynamic mechanical environment in vivo, characterized by compressive and shear stresses along multiple axes and hydrostatic and osmotic pressures throughout (reviewed in [422, 423]).

The chronic arthropathy, characterized by progressive destruction of articular cartilage, remodeling of the underlying bone, formation of ectopic bone, hypertrophy of the joint capsule, and inflammation of the synovial lining, is a common disease that can affect joints from any part of the body, in particular, the knee, hip, and shoulder, and represents a major cause of disability and joint pain worldwide. As known to every physician, female gender, elderly people, and obese individuals show high susceptibility to this joint disease [424–426].

9.8.2 Regulated Cell Death

It is soundly imaginable that aberrant acute repetitive or chronic articular cartilage load may lead to any form of RCD. And indeed, for example, apoptosis has been reported to occur in osteoarthritic cartilage, whereby, however, the relative contribution of chondrocyte apoptosis in the pathogenesis of OA was challenging to evaluate, and contradictory reports exist on the rate of apoptotic chondrocytes in osteoarthritic cartilage [427].

On the other hand, convincing evidence from studies on a cartilage trauma model has been provided for the involvement of necroptosis in OA disease [428]. Moreover, in this study, the investigators found a possible link between cartilage injury and necroptotic processes, depending on oxidative stress and cytokine release.

Also, other lines of studies revealed a vital role of synovial fibroblast pyroptosis in the onset and development of knee OA. An orienting study on fibroblast-like synoviocytes provided already first evidence for a pathogenetic role of NLRP3 inflammasome-related pyroptosis in knee OA [429]. In a subsequent study on a knee OA model in rats, the same investigator group provided evidence for synovial macrophage pyroptosis to participating in the pathological process [430].

Although ferroptosis has not been described to occur in OA so far, one may assume that this subroutine of RN also takes place given the knowledge that oxidative stress and lipid peroxidation are pathogenetically involved in this disorder [431, 432].

Together, there is first evidence indicating involvement of various subroutines of RCD in the pathogenesis of OA, which—as definitely documented in other injury-promoted inflammatory disorders—may serve as sources of DAMPs emission.

9.8.3 Pathogenesis of Osteoarthritis (in Brief)

Accumulating evidence suggests OA to reflecting a multifactorial disorder in which low-grade, chronic inflammation in terms of nonresolving inflammation—and not chronic degenerative processes as previously thought—plays a central role, whereby the synovitis is characterized by infiltration of inflammatory cells into the synovium. In the inflamed joint tissues and fluids, the full palette of inflammatory mediators has been identified, including cytokines, chemokines, and growth factors. These mediators can be produced by different cell types within the joint such as macrophages, fibroblast-like synoviocytes, chondrocytes, and resident or infiltrating immune cells.

Moreover, there is also increasing evidence for joint injury-emitted DAMPs to promote these sterile inflammatory processes (reviewed in [425, 433, 434]).

9.8.4 DAMPs in Osteoarthritis

Already very early, a first report on the role of DAMPs in OA was published by Sokolove and Lepus [435]. In their review, the authors discussed ECM-derived DAMPs (biglycan, fibronectin, HA, TNC), HMGB1 and S100 proteins, and crystals released from cartilage. In a subsequent review [436], the scenario of DAMP-activated macrophages in OA was highlighted. Among others, the authors discussed that the damage caused to chondrocytes by activated macrophages would lead to the release of more DAMPs, creating a positive feedback loop that leads to the continued destruction of cartilage. More precise knowledge about OA-associated DAMPs was added by more recent studies. For example, in experiments on human monocyte-derived macrophages, it could be demonstrated that basic calcium phosphate crystals can polarize primary human macrophages toward an M1-like phenotype sustaining proinflammatory processes [437].

9.8.5 Résumé

Together, there is no doubt that DAMPs are heavily involved in the pathogenesis of OA and may even explain the pathogenetic complexity of the inflammatory mechanisms discovered in this disorder. Future work is needed to fully define the

DAMP-triggered molecular pathways mediating the low-grade inflammation in OA and, even more important, to uncover a potential insufficient role of SAMPs that may contribute to the nonresolving nature of this inflammation. If such data are available, the value of using intra-articular DAMPs as therapeutic targets or administering SAMPs intra-articularly could be evaluated as future therapeutic approaches in OA.

9.9 DAMPs and SAMPs as Diagnostics, Prognostics, Therapeutics, and Therapeutic Targets in Solid Organ Injury

9.9.1 Introductory Remarks

During recent times, as already known for polytrauma, an increased interest in the use of DAMPs and SAMPs as biomarkers and therapeutic targets for specific organ injuries can be noted. As discussed in the previous chapter, in polytraumatized patients, DAMPs and SAMPs can be seen as the origin of the development of both SIRS and CARS and are therefore promising molecules as biomarkers for patient stratification and as therapeutic targets and therapeutics. By contrast, in patients suffering from organ-specific injuries, for example, TBI, the determination of DAMPs and SAMPs will give individual information about the severity of the injury, their possible remote effects, and early signs of either controlled healing or uncontrolled disease-causing processes. Also, identification of such biomarkers could allow improved understanding of the pathological processes involved in organ-specific injury and may be helpful in diagnosis, prognostication, and development of novel therapies. In fact, the application of DAMPs and SAMPs as biomarkers is expected to improve the speed of clinical decision-making, in particular, in designing and executing patient-individualized treatment strategies.

Some of those topics were already briefly or partly touched in the running text. Here, the published literature is reviewed—well aware that this is just the begin of the development of a new era of monitoring in solid organ injuries.

9.9.2 DAMPs and SAMPs as Diagnostic and Prognostic Biomarkers

9.9.2.1 General Remarks

As said, monitoring of DAMPs and SAMPs in organ-specific injury has gained increasing attention regarding their function as valuable biomarkers. Indeed, currently used routine biochemical biomarkers of organ damage mostly inform physicians in a delayed fashion, when the organ-specific damage is too advanced or even irreversible. Such traditional biomarkers include glial fibrillary acidic protein for brain injury; serum creatinine and kidney injury marker-1 for kidney injury; serum glutamic oxaloacetic transaminase and serum glutamic pyruvic transaminase for liver injury; cardiac troponin for heart damage; intestinal-type fatty acid-binding protein for gut injury; and D-dimer for coagulopathy (compare also review in [408]).

The routine sequential determination of DAMPs and SAMPs, however, may represent an early prognostic sign as to whether a given acute infectious or sterile organ injury will result in a normal healing, inflammation-promoting → inflammation-resolving response or may proceed—via nonresolving inflammatory/fibrotic processes—to acute and/or chronic organ failure. Accordingly, the use of DAMPs in addition to such "familiar" biomarkers may contribute to a sophisticated application of criteria of personalized medicine that strives for improvements in tailoring and timing of diagnostic, prognostic, preventive, and therapeutic measures.

9.9.2.2 Traumatic Brain Injury

Most work on DAMPs in their function as biomarkers in TBI has been reported regarding S100 proteins. For example, as already mentioned above, in an analysis of serum levels of S100B proteins in pediatric patients with TBI, median serum levels of S100B at admission were shown to decrease significantly 1 week after TBI [74]. Follow-up of these patients revealed that serum levels of this DAMP 1 week after injury in patients with unfavorable 6-month outcomes were substantially higher than levels 1 week after injury in patients with favorable outcomes. The authors concluded that serial measurements of serum S100B may help assess brain damage and clinical outcome of pediatric patients with TBI. The increasing importance of S100B proteins acting as biomarkers in TBI has also been discussed and reviewed elsewhere (see [438–440]).

Additionally, as already mentioned earlier, levels of HMGB1 could be measured in the CSF of adult patients with TBI [59] whereas, in pediatric patients, the CSF levels of HMGB1 were found to be even predictive for outcome [67]. Moreover, an observational clinical study in patients with severe TBI revealed that the plasma HMGB1 concentration can be successfully used as a novel biomarker for significantly predicting 1-year mortality and unfavorable outcome of TBI [66]. These findings were confirmed by recent reports on the role of HMGB1 as a viable biomarker in TBI, as published elsewhere [55, 441]. There is agreement among the authors that HMGB1 is a promising prospective candidate for future studies, which should explore the predictive value of this DAMP in TBI.

Also, as already touched above [70], mtDNA measured in the CSF of children with severe TBI has been proposed to be a useful biomarker that correlates with neurological outcome after TBI.

Interestingly, time seems to be mature for SAMPs to join the scene. Thus, an experimental study on a model of TBI in mice provided initial evidence for SPMs, to be used as biomarkers [82] (see below under SAMPs as therapeutics).

9.9.2.3 Acute Lung Injury

As already mentioned in Sect. 8.3.5, DAMPs have reportedly also been explored as promising biomarkers in ALI [132–135]. Thus, informative HMGB1 levels could be measured in bronchoalveolar lavage fluid of trauma patients during mechanical ventilation and ventilator-associated pneumonia [134]. In a more recent study on patients with severe pneumonia and ARDS requiring mechanical ventilation [135], the investigators remarkably observed the day 1 HMGB1 concentration to be a critical, independent biomarker for ICU mortality. Other DAMPs were also explored. For example, in studies on ARDS patients, plasma and bronchoalveolar lavage fluid extracellular histone levels were found to be much higher in ARDS patients than in healthy controls [145]. The extended analysis of the clinical data revealed a significant association between extracellular histones and ARDS severity and mortality. Also, extracellular histones were shown to be correlated with an evident systemic inflammation detected in ARDS patients. The authors concluded [145] that "extracellular histones in ARDS patients are excessively increased and may contribute to disease aggravation by inducing cellular damage and promoting systemic inflammation."

Moreover, as already mentioned in Sect. 9.3.5.4, in a clinical study on patients with suspected ventilator-associated pneumonia, higher levels of mtDNA were detected in the bronchoalveolar lavage fluid [142]. In another clinical study conducted by the same group, mtDNA in transfusion products was suggested to contribute to the development of ARDS after multiple transfusions [119]. These findings certainly enrich the list of DAMPs to be harnessed as biomarkers in ALI. The authors of this study concluded [119]: "Finally, to determine the true value of serum mtDNA DAMP measurements as predictive biomarkers for the evolution of ARDS and MODS in the setting of severe injury, it will ultimately be necessary to standardize means for measuring and reporting mtDNA abundance and apply these to a substantial patient cohort."

9.9.2.4 Acute Kidney Injury

In a recently reported clinical study on pediatric patients suffering from AKI, S100A8/S100A9 was detected in the urine and proposed by the authors to use as a biomarker for the prediction of adverse outcome requiring renal replacement therapy [239]. A similar proposal for applying S100A8/S100A9 as a diagnostic and prognostic biomarker in intrinsic AKI was made elsewhere [240]. Also, in a clinical study on patients with AKI, mtDNA was measured in the urine, the severity of the disease was quantified, and patients were followed for 90 days [242]. As reported from the authors, the measured urinary mtDNA levels turned out to be a marker of AKI severity, as reflected by its significant correlation with the peak serum creatinine level, duration of hospital stay, and probably the need for temporary dialysis. Thus, like other DAMPs, urinary mtDNA has also the potential to serve as an essential biomarker of AKI. In similar clinical studies on surgical critically ill patients [442], elevated urinary mtDNA levels could identify newly developed AKI and predict renal replacement therapy or hospital mortality in those patients. Finally, the use of urinary mtDNA as a biomarker of renal dysfunction could be confirmed in patients with AKI following cardiac surgery [443]. Postoperatively, the investigators found that urinary mtDNA was associated with increased risk of worsening AKI following initial sample collection and that this DAMP predicts AKI progression by *receiver operator characteristic* analysis.

9.9.2.5 Acute Liver Injury

DAMPs such as HMGB1, nDNA, and mtDNA have already been used as biomarkers in APAP intoxication/hepatotoxicity and showed a good correlation with the course of this acute liver disease [304]. Remarkably, as a typical result of clinical studies, measurement of plasma levels of HMGB1 reportedly surpasses all other biomarkers to predict clinical outcome for APAP-overdosed patients [333, 444]. Importantly, the systemic HMGB1 release from the APAP-induced liver injury was observed to be biphasic. One may discuss that this observation nicely documents the initial injury-induced passive release of HMGB1 as a constitutively expresses IA-1 DAMP, followed by active secretion of acetylated, disulfide HMGB1 as an inducible IIIB-2 DAMP via DAMP-activated innate immune cells (see also Table 3.1 and Vol. 1 [1], Part IV, Sect. 11.2). In this context, it is worth mentioning even a report on a significant increase in plasma HMGB1 in patients with acute alcoholic hepatitis [390] that was appreciated by the authors as a potential biomarker that will improve the prediction of disease progression and survival in ALD.

9.9.2.6 Concluding Remarks

The few selected examples of DAMPs in their role as biomarkers, as described here, can be regarded as the beginning of a new era in monitoring injury-induced organ-specific diseases. In principle, every DAMP documented to play a critical pathogenetic role in solid organ injury can be harnessed as a diagnostic/predictive/prognostic biomarker. However, as already stressed in Sect. 8.4.2.4, instead of concentrating on one DAMP as a biomarker, a distinct pattern of several DAMPs will probably turn out to be more instructive in predicting the outcome of organ injury in different types of patients. This endeavor presupposes, however, that typical DAMP patterns in different patient categories must first be explored.

However, as progress in this research field moves forward, SAMPs (still better "SAMP patterns") are supposed to accompany the DAMPs as biomarkers sooner or later. The first evidence for such a concept is already available. For example, in studies in pediatric patients with severe TBI, the concentration of the SAMP adenosine in CSF was observed to be increased in a time- and severity-dependent manner in infants and children after severe head injury [84]. More precisely, and as already stressed in Sect. 7.3.3 and Fig. 7.1, the determination of a DAMP/SAMP ratio in terms of a DAMP/SAMP signature appears to be the most accurate parameter to monitor the course and the outcome of an individual organ injury. Indeed, one is tempted to speculate that each organ-specific injury is marked by a specific DAMPs/SAMPs pattern. Accordingly, continuous tracing of the DAMP/SAMP ratio might turn out to emerge to an essential future parameter in reflecting the status of injured organs.

9.9.3 DAMPs as Therapeutic Targets and SAMPs as Therapeutics

9.9.3.1 General Remarks

In principle, the therapeutic application of DAMPs or SAMPs in solid organ injuries is to prevent the pathological consequences (e.g., hyperinflammatory, chronic inflammatory → fibrotic responses) without interfering with the homeostatic healing processes. In the case of isolated organ injury, this means to prevent the development of a potentially life-threatening organ-specific acute disease such as ARDS (acute organ failure) or a chronic inflammatory/nonresolving → fibrotic disease (chronic organ failure).

Again, for future optimal treatment modalities, the exact status of the DAMP/SAMP ratio as a guide in tailoring treatment options might be necessary to be determined for each organ injury (e.g., a priori to be established by targeted studies and increasing experience in large cohorts of patients). This would allow precise and timely intervention after the onset of the disorder, that is, appropriate inhibition of DAMPs and administration of SAMPS, aimed at reaching full restitutio ad integrum.

On the basis of preclinical studies on suitable experimental models, initial proposals of harnessing DAMPs (less SAMPs) as future therapeutic targets in isolated acute organ injury have already been communicated. Also, antagonists of DAMPs are in development for clinical use, as previously addressed in Sect. 8.4.4.2. Here, some recent publications on their use in solid organ injuries are briefly cited.

9.9.3.2 Blockade of DAMPs in Acute Organ Injuries

The theoretical background of interventions in acute isolated organ injuries differs from that as outlined for interventions in polytrauma in that a hyperresolving/immunosuppressive phase is not relevant. Instead, the therapeutic imperative strives for the prevention of an injury-induced hyperinflammatory state that may lead to acute organ dysfunction or even failure. Accordingly, a blockade/elimination of DAMPs or administration of SAMPs has to be taken into consideration.

Blockade of DAMPs in Traumatic Brain Injury

The blockade of HMGB1 has been successfully applied in several models of acute organ injury. In studies on rats already mentioned above, administration of an anti-HMGB1 mAb after TBI was shown to remarkably inhibit fluid percussion-induced brain edema [56]. This effect was associated with inhibition of HMGB1 translocation, protection of BBB integrity, suppression of inflammatory molecule expression, and improvement of motor function. Also, in a murine TBI model, blockade of HMGB1 by an *HMGB1 A-box fragment* (an antagonist competing with full-length HMGB1 for receptor binding) was shown to reverse brain damages in the mice following TBI [445]. The experiments further revealed that the antagonist could significantly reduce brain edema by protecting the integrity of the BBB, ameliorate cell degeneration, and decrease expression of proinflammatory cytokines released in the injured brain after TBI. These cellular and molecular effects were accompanied by improved behavioral performance in TBI mice. The authors of these experiments suggested from their data [445] that HMGB1 A-box may have therapeutic potential for the secondary brain damages in TBI. In another study on a murine model of olfactory nerve transection, injection of an anti-HMGB1 antibody was shown to be associated with significantly smaller areas of injury-associated tissue, fewer astrocytes and macrophages/microglia, and an increase in regenerating nerve fibers [446]. Given these findings, the investigators proposed that inhibition of HMGB1 could provide a new therapeutic strategy for the treatment of olfactory dysfunction following head injuries. Also, as documented by other lines of studies on a rat TBI model [447], intravenous injection of an anti-HMGB1 mAb can attenuate accumulation of activated microglia in the rat cortex in the ipsilateral hemisphere after TBI. Moreover, these experiments showed that anti-HMGB1 mAb inhibits HMGB1 translocation, suppresses impairment of motor function, and has positive effects on electroencephalography activity. In their conclusion, the investigators argued that anti-HMGB1 mAb may prevent cognitive dysfunction after TBI. In the context of these reports, a study on glycyrrhizin, an inhibitor of HMGB1, is also of interest [448]. In these experiments, glycyrrhizin was used to investigate whether the inhibition of this DAMP could modulate microglia/macrophage polarization after TBI. The results obtained showed that treatment with this inhibitor ameliorates the neurological function recovery, reduces the lesion volume, and inhibits the release and expression of HMGB1 after TBI. Further, the investigators observed that the administration of this substance could suppress M1 phenotype activation and promoted M2 phenotype activation of microglia/macrophages. Given their interesting findings, the authors suggested that glycyrrhizin mitigates TBI by inhibiting M1 phenotype while promoting M2 phenotype activation of microglia/macrophages, at least partly through inhibiting HMGB1 [448].

Blockade of DAMPs in Acute Lung Injury

As outlined in Sect. 8.3.5.2, several experiments have convincingly proven a beneficial effect of HMGB1 inhibition in mitigating ALI [127–131]. In one of those cited studies on a mouse model of hyperoxic inflammatory lung injury [127], inhibition of HMGB1 by neutralizing anti-HMGB1 antibodies, administrated before or after onset of the hyperoxic exposure, was found to mitigate pulmonary edema and inflammatory responses significantly. The authors concluded that—if these results could be translated to humans—"they suggest that HMGB1 inhibitors provide treatment regimens for oxidative inflammatory lung injury in patients receiving hyperoxia through mechanical ventilation." Similar observations were made in studies on a paraquat-induced ALI, in which blocking of HMGB1 signaling by glycyrrhizin was shown to dramatically inhibit the infiltration of neutrophils and attenuate lung injury [449]. In this context, studies on a rat model of crush injury are of interest showing that intravenous administration of anti-HMGB1 antibody was associated with amelioration of histological findings of lung damage [450].

Blockade of DAMPs in Acute Kidney Injury

As also mentioned above, neutralizing HMGB1 with an anti-HMGB1 antibody was shown to ameliorate chronic CsA nephrotoxicity via inhibition of the TLR4 signaling pathway [236]. Moreover, the mitigating effect of the functional HMGB1 inhibitor glycyrrhizin on TBI could also be demonstrated in AKI. In an experimental model of renal IRI [451], glycyrrhizic acid was shown to reduce the hypoxia-induced death of tubular EpCs. The authors discussed that inhibition of the interaction of HMGB1 with tubular EpCs through this substance may represent a therapeutic strategy for the attenuation of renal injury following renal IRI. In other sets of studies on the model of folic acid-induced renal damage [452], melatonin pretreatment was shown to improve cell cycle arrest of tubular EpCs. Notably, this protective function of melatonin was observed to be closely related to the inhibition of nucleocytoplasmic translocation of HMGB1 in tubular EpCs. Further, as already touched above, extended experiments of the Anders group on AKI models revealed that neutralizing anti-histone IgG can suppress intrarenal inflammation, neutrophil infiltration, and tubular cell necrosis and improve renal excretory function [245].

Blockade of DAMPs in Acute Liver Injury

A beneficial effect of HMGB1 inhibition could also be shown in models of acute liver injury. For example, in studies on a mouse model of APAP overdose, blockade of HMGB1 by an anti-HMGB1 antibody was found to significantly improve hepatocyte regeneration, associated with decreased serum transaminases, reduced number of hepatic infiltrating inflammatory cells, and restored liver structure [329]. In similar studies on the same model, blockade of HMGB1 by a partly humanized mouse anti-HMGB1 mAb was found to mitigate APAP-induced serum elevations of alanine aminotransferase significantly and abrogate markers of APAP-induced inflammation completely [330]. The authors concluded: "This is the first report describing the generation of a partly humanized HMGB1-neutralizing antibody with validated therapeutic efficacy and with a prolonged therapeutic window, as compared to NAC, in APAP-ALI. The therapeutic effect was mediated by HMGB1 neutralization and attenuation of postinjury inflammation. These results represent important progress toward clinical implementation of HMGB1-specific therapy as a means to treat APAP-ALI and other inflammatory conditions" [330].

Besides blocking HMGB1, the inhibition of other DAMPs can be assumed to have a beneficial effect on acute liver injury. For example, as briefly touched above, in studies on the model of APAP overdose, blockade of histones by anti-histone Abs was demonstrated to be protective [337, 339].

9.9.3.3 Administration of SAMPs in Acute Organ Injuries

The theoretical background of administering SAMPs in acute organ injuries is grounded on their ability to regulate host innate immune host responses, such as inhibiting the production of proinflammatory cytokines, stopping recruitment of neutrophils in inflammatory tissues, and stimulating polarization of M2-like macrophages to promote phagocytosis of apoptotic cells (efferocytosis) and cellular debris (compare Sect. 5.3.3). In other words, these properties of SAMPs could be therapeutically harnessed to prevent DAMP-promoted dyshomeostatic progression of inflammation that may result in acute and/or chronic organ dysfunction or even failure.

Protective Effect of SAMPs on Traumatic Brain Injury

Excitingly, a study on a model of TBI in mice (mentioned above [82]) provided initial evidence for SAMPs to mitigate the neuroinflammatory response following acute brain injury. One SAMP, the SPM RvD1, showed significant efficacy in ameliorating the motor and cognitive deficits resulting from diffuse TBI. The other SAMP, RvE1, elicited a dramatic increase in posttraumatic sleep and tempered microglia activation without significantly influencing behavioral outcome compared to saline treatment.

The divergence in histological (microglial activation) and physiological (sleep activity) outcomes from functional (motor and cognitive performance) outcomes was interpreted by the investigators in suggesting that microglial reactivity may contribute to posttraumatic sleep and that RvD1 may achieve therapeutic efficacy through means other than inflammation resolution alone. Given their observations, the authors argued [82] that SPMs demonstrate proof of principle as a therapeutic approach for diffuse brain injury, where additional studies are warranted.

In other lines of studies on a model of focal brain injury, RvD1 was observed to halt remote neuroinflammation and improve functional recovery after focal brain damage via ALX/FPR2 receptor-regulated miRNAs [453]. In these experiments, the in vivo administration of RvD1 promoted functional recovery and neuroprotection by reducing the activation of microglia and astrocytes as well as by impairing inflammatory-induced neuronal cell death in remote regions. In view of their findings, the authors proposed "that innovative therapies based on RvD1-ALX/FPR2 axis could be exploited to curtail remote damage and enable neuroprotective effects after acute focal brain damage."

Protective Effect of SAMPs on Acute Lung Injury and Acute Respiratory Distress Syndrome

Initial studies on a potential beneficial effect of SAMPs administration on ALI and ARDS have also been reported. For example, inhibition of adenosine kinase, an enzyme that is known to inhibit elevated levels of the SAMP extracellular adenosine, was demonstrated to reduce the inflammatory changes associated with lung injury [167]. The therapeutic effect of active inhibition of adenosine kinase is interpreted as a consequence of increased adenosine levels, that is, a finding that indirectly reflects a protective effect of extracellular adenosine on ALI.

Earlier studies have already demonstrated that SPMs (i.e., LxA4, RvD1) can regulate the clearance of alveolar fluids in ARDS to protect the lung function [161–163]. Specifically, intravenous administration of RvD1 was demonstrated to stimulate clearance of alveolar fluid clearance through a mechanism partly depending on alveolar epithelial sodium channel and Na, K-ATPase activation via the FPR2 (also called ALX) → cAMP → PI3K signaling pathway [163]. Also, in other sets of experiments on a rat model of IRI-induced ALI [454], administration of the active N-terminal peptide of AnxA1 was shown to attenuate increased lung edema, neutrophil infiltration, inflammatory cytokine production, oxidative stress, and tissue damage. These improvements were shown to be attributed to FPR activation (for AnxA1, FPR2, and cAMP in SAMP-triggered resolution pathways, also compare Vol. 1 [1], Part IV, Sects. 14.4.2 and 14.4.3 and Fig. 14.5).

These promising experimental findings prompted Wang et al. [164] to write a review on this topic. The authors concluded: "The present review discusses a novel mechanism for pulmonary edema fluid reabsorption. SPMs might provide new opportunities to design "reabsorption-targeted" therapies with high degrees of precision in controlling ALI/ARDS."

Protective Effect of SAMPs on Acute Liver Injury

There are also first clues to a protective role of SAMPs in acute liver injury. As already mentioned above, preclinical and clinical evidence suggesting SPMs being able to enhance nonalcoholic steatohepatitis and fibrosis resolution has already recently been reviewed [374]. Moreover, in studies on a model of nonalcoholic steatohepatitis in mice [347], hepatic AnxA1 was observed to be increased in parallel with progression of liver injury. In extension of this experiment, in vitro addition of recombinant AnxA1 to macrophages isolated from nonalcoholic steatohepatitis livers were found to downmodulate M1 polarization through stimulation of IL-10 production. Furthermore, the investigators could demonstrate that the degree of hepatic fibrosis was enhanced in methionine–choline-deficient-fed AnxA1KO mice. Given their observations [347], the authors concluded that macrophage-derived AnxA1 plays a functional role in modulating hepatic inflammation and fibrogenesis during progression of nonalcoholic steatohepatitis.

9.9.3.4 Concluding Remarks

Together, as reflected by some selected examples from the literature as addressed here, the preclinical evidence for the efficacy of targeting DAMPs in organ-specific injuries is convincing. Therefore, time appears to be mature to develop, design, and test DAMP-specific antagonists in these acute diseases to explore whether or not blocking DAMPs will benefit patients. Further, there is initial evidence for the successful use of SAMPs, in particular, SPMs as therapeutics to be administered in acute organ injuries. Thus, it can be cautiously assumed that first clinical trials in this exciting field of new therapeutic options will be reported soon.

9.9.4 Résumé

According to the reports quoted in this chapter, one can conceivably assume that DAMPs, fewer SAMPs (?) will soon find their way into clinical routine as diagnostic, prognostic, and predictive biomarkers in injury-induced organ diseases. However, as already discussed for polytrauma (Sect. 8.4.5), much more different, that is, more difficult to assess is their future routine use as therapeutic targets and therapeutics in solid organ injuries. Undoubtedly, treatment modalities based on inhibitors/antagonists, specifically targeting DAMPs, have provided encouraging results in several preclinical models of injury-induced inflammatory responses. However, before starting such trials, the possible risks of future therapeutic exploitation of DAMPs and SAMPs have to be clearly defined, as outlined in detail in Sect. 8.4.5. Nevertheless, as typical for current therapeutic achievements in medicine, clinical trials will give us the final answer to all these imponderabilities—in case they will be designed and conducted at all.

9.10 Outlook and Future Perspectives

This chapter should reflect the emerging role of DAMPs and SAMPs in injury-induced organ-specific diseases. In particular, the impact of DAMPs on promotion of organ-specific hyperinflammation, chronic nonresolving inflammation, and fibrosis, as well as the potential properties of SAMPs in resolving organ-specific inflammation are highlighted. To understand these complex scenarios, one may reduce the various cellular and molecular pathways involved to a fundamental sequence of injury-induced events. The "pathogenetic matrix" of such events—that could also be applied to other organ injuries not mentioned here—can be designed in the form of two axes (Fig. 9.5): acute or chronic organ injury → RCD → emission of DAMPs and SAMPS → necroinflammation → resolution of inflammation (restitutio ad integrum), or nonresolving hyperinflammation (acute organ failure), or nonresolving chronic inflammation transitioning to progressive fibrosis (chronic organ failure).

Regarding a final evaluation of the weight of using DAMPs and SAMPs as biomarkers, therapeutic targets, and therapeutics in injury-induced, organ-specific diseases, one has to wait for robust real-world data provided by future well-targeted clinical trials. It will be essential to design and conduct such studies under combination of molecular and clinical methods to ensure a high probability of reliable information that will enable safe decision-making in day-to-day clinical practice in the future.

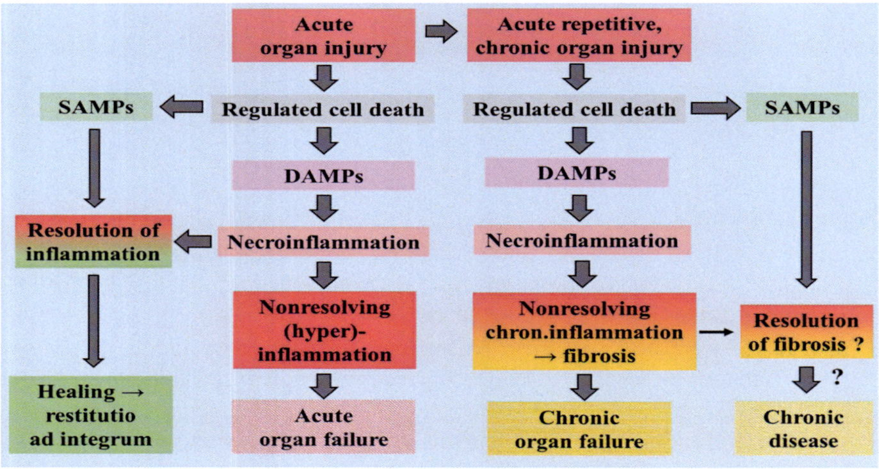

Fig. 9.5 Model of a fundamental pathogenetic matrix of a sequence of acute or chronic organ injury-induced cellular/molecular pathways as generally observed in acute or chronic organ-specific diseases resulting in acute or chronic organ failure

References

1. Land WG. Damage-associated molecular patterns in human diseases; Vol. 1: Injury-induced innate immune responses. Cham: Springer International Publishing AG; 2018. https://www.springer.com/de/book/9783319786544.
2. Blennow K, Brody DL, Kochanek PM, Levin H, McKee A, Ribbers GM, et al. Traumatic brain injuries. Nat Rev Dis Primers. 2016;2:16084. http://www.ncbi.nlm.nih.gov/pubmed/27853132.
3. Mayer AR, Quinn DK, Master CL. The spectrum of mild traumatic brain injury. Neurology. 2017;89:623–32. http://www.ncbi.nlm.nih.gov/pubmed/28701496.
4. Galgano M, Toshkezi G, Qiu X, Russell T, Chin L, Zhao L-R. Traumatic brain injury. Cell Transplant. 2017;26:1118–30. http://www.ncbi.nlm.nih.gov/pubmed/28933211.
5. Braun M, Vaibhav K, Saad NM, Fatima S, Vender JR, Baban B, et al. White matter damage after traumatic brain injury: a role for damage associated molecular patterns. Biochim Biophys Acta - Mol Basis Dis. 1863;2017:2614–26. http://www.ncbi.nlm.nih.gov/pubmed/28533056.
6. Sun M, McDonald SJ, Brady RD, O'Brien TJ, Shultz SR. The influence of immunological stressors on traumatic brain injury. Brain Behav Immun. 2018;69:618–28. http://www.ncbi.nlm.nih.gov/pubmed/29355823.
7. Stoica BA, Faden AI. Cell death mechanisms and modulation in traumatic brain injury. Neurotherapeutics. 2010;7:3–12. http://www.ncbi.nlm.nih.gov/pubmed/20129492.
8. Liu T, Zhao D, Cui H, Chen L, Bao Y, Wang Y, et al. Therapeutic hypothermia attenuates tissue damage and cytokine expression after traumatic brain injury by inhibiting necroptosis in the rat. Sci Rep. 2016;6:24547. http://www.ncbi.nlm.nih.gov/pubmed/27080932.
9. Liu Z-M, Chen Q-X, Chen Z-B, Tian D-F, Li M-C, Wang J-M, et al. RIP3 deficiency protects against traumatic brain injury (TBI) through suppressing oxidative stress, inflammation and apoptosis: dependent on AMPK pathway. Biochem Biophys Res Commun. 2018;499:112–9. http://linkinghub.elsevier.com/retrieve/pii/S0006291X18303875.
10. Zhang H-B, Cheng S-X, Tu Y, Zhang S, Hou S-K, Yang Z. Protective effect of mild-induced hypothermia against moderate traumatic brain injury in rats involved in necroptotic and apoptotic pathways. Brain Inj. 2017;31:406–15. http://www.ncbi.nlm.nih.gov/pubmed/28140659.
11. Stockwell BR, Friedmann Angeli JP, Bayir H, Bush AI, Conrad M, Dixon SJ, et al. Ferroptosis: a regulated cell death nexus linking metabolism, redox biology, and disease. Cell. 2017;171:273–85. http://www.ncbi.nlm.nih.gov/pubmed/28985560.
12. Ji J, Kline AE, Amoscato A, Samhan-Arias AK, Sparvero LJ, Tyurin VA, et al. Lipidomics identifies cardiolipin oxidation as a mitochondrial target for redox therapy of brain injury. Nat Neurosci. 2012;15:1407–13. http://www.nature.com/articles/nn.3195.
13. Anthonymuthu TS, Kenny EM, Lamade AM, Kagan VE, Bayır H. Oxidized phospholipid signaling in traumatic brain injury. Free Radic Biol Med. 2018;124:493–503. https://linkinghub.elsevier.com/retrieve/pii/S0891584918311420.
14. Xie B, Wang Y, Lin Y, Mao Q, Feng J, Gao G, et al. Inhibition of ferroptosis attenuates tissue damage and improves long-term outcomes after traumatic brain injury in mice. CNS Neurosci Ther. 2019;25:465–75. http://www.ncbi.nlm.nih.gov/pubmed/30264934.
15. Magtanong L, Dixon SJ. Ferroptosis and brain injury. Dev Neurosci. 2018;40:382–95. http://www.ncbi.nlm.nih.gov/pubmed/30820017.
16. Adamczak SE, de Rivero Vaccari JP, Dale G, Brand FJ, Nonner D, Bullock MR, et al. Pyroptotic neuronal cell death mediated by the AIM2 inflammasome. J Cereb Blood Flow Metab. 2014;34:621–9. http://journals.sagepub.com/doi/10.1038/jcbfm.2013.236.
17. Lee SW, de Rivero Vaccari JP, Truettner JS, Dietrich WD, Keane RW. The role of microglial inflammasome activation in pyroptotic cell death following penetrating traumatic brain injury. J Neuroinflammation. 2019;16:27. https://jneuroinflammation.biomedcentral.com/articles/10.1186/s12974-019-1423-6.
18. Hickey RW, Adelson PD, Johnnides MJ, Davis DS, Yu Z, Rose ME, et al. Cyclooxygenase-2 activity following traumatic brain injury in the developing rat. Pediatr Res. 2007;62:271–6. http://www.nature.com/doifinder/10.1203/PDR.0b013e3180db2902.

19. Zhang L, Zhang W-P, Hu H, Wang M-L, Sheng W-W, Yao H-T, et al. Expression patterns of 5-lipoxygenase in human brain with traumatic injury and astrocytoma. Neuropathology. 2006;26:99–106. http://www.ncbi.nlm.nih.gov/pubmed/16708542.
20. Harris LK, Black RT, Golden KM, Reeves TM, Povlishock JT, Phillips LL. Traumatic brain injury-induced changes in gene expression and functional activity of mitochondrial cytochrome C oxidase. J Neurotrauma. 2001;18:993–1009. http://www.liebertpub.com/doi/10.1089/08977150152693692.
21. Wenzel SE, Tyurina YY, Zhao J, St Croix CM, Dar HH, Mao G, et al. PEBP1 Wardens Ferroptosis by enabling lipoxygenase generation of lipid death signals. Cell. 2017;171:628–641.e26. https://linkinghub.elsevier.com/retrieve/pii/S0092867417311388.
22. Maas AIR, Stocchetti N, Bullock R. Moderate and severe traumatic brain injury in adults. Lancet Neurol. 2008;7:728–41. https://linkinghub.elsevier.com/retrieve/pii/S1474442208701649.
23. Werner C, Engelhard K. Pathophysiology of traumatic brain injury. Br J Anaesth. 2007;99:4–9. http://www.ncbi.nlm.nih.gov/pubmed/17573392.
24. Prins M, Greco T, Alexander D, Giza CC. The pathophysiology of traumatic brain injury at a glance. Dis Model Mech. 2013;6:1307–15. http://dmm.biologists.org/cgi/doi/10.1242/dmm.011585.
25. Quillinan N, Herson PS, Traystman RJ. Neuropathophysiology of brain injury. Anesthesiol Clin. 2016;34:453–64. http://www.ncbi.nlm.nih.gov/pubmed/27521191.
26. Simon DW, McGeachy MJ, Bayır H, Clark RSB, Loane DJ, Kochanek PM. The far-reaching scope of neuroinflammation after traumatic brain injury. Nat Rev Neurol. 2017;13:171–91. http://www.ncbi.nlm.nih.gov/pubmed/28186177.
27. Jassam YN, Izzy S, Whalen M, McGavern DB, El Khoury J. Neuroimmunology of traumatic brain injury: time for a paradigm shift. Neuron. 2017;95:1246–65. http://linkinghub.elsevier.com/retrieve/pii/S0896627317306128.
28. Zhang L, Wang H. Targetinsg the NF-E2-related factor 2 pathway: a novel strategy for traumatic brain injury. Mol Neurobiol. 2018;55:1773–85. http://link.springer.com/10.1007/s12035-017-0456-z.
29. O'leary RA, Nichol AD. Pathophysiology of severe traumatic brain injury overview. J Neurosurg Sci. 2018;62:542–8. http://www.ncbi.nlm.nih.gov/pubmed/29790727.
30. Shi K, Zhang J, Dong J-F, Shi F-D. Dissemination of brain inflammation in traumatic brain injury. Cell Mol Immunol. 2019;16:523–30. http://www.nature.com/articles/s41423-019-0213-5.
31. Khatri N, Thakur M, Pareek V, Kumar S, Sharma S, Datusalia AK. Oxidative stress: major threat in traumatic brain injury. CNS Neurol Disord Drug Targets. 2018;17:689–95. http://www.eurekaselect.com/163257/article.
32. Shi H, Hua X, Kong D, Stein D, Hua F. Role of Toll-like receptor mediated signaling in traumatic brain injury. Neuropharmacology. 2019;145:259–67. https://linkinghub.elsevier.com/retrieve/pii/S0028390818304003.
33. Puntambekar SS, Saber M, Lamb BT, Kokiko-Cochran ON. Cellular players that shape evolving pathology and neurodegeneration following traumatic brain injury. Brain Behav Immun. 2018;71:9–17. http://www.ncbi.nlm.nih.gov/pubmed/29601944.
34. Stocchetti N, Maas AIR. Traumatic intracranial hypertension. N Engl J Med. 2014;370:2121–30. http://www.ncbi.nlm.nih.gov/pubmed/24869722.
35. Winkler EA, Minter D, Yue JK, Manley GT. Cerebral edema in traumatic brain injury. Neurosurg Clin N Am. 2016;27:473–88. http://www.ncbi.nlm.nih.gov/pubmed/27637397.
36. Jha RM, Kochanek PM, Simard JM. Pathophysiology and treatment of cerebral edema in traumatic brain injury. Neuropharmacology. 2019;145:230–46. http://www.ncbi.nlm.nih.gov/pubmed/30086289.
37. Farina C, Aloisi F, Meinl E. Astrocytes are active players in cerebral innate immunity. Trends Immunol. 2007;28:138–45. https://linkinghub.elsevier.com/retrieve/pii/S1471490607000245.

38. Rivest S. Regulation of innate immune responses in the brain. Nat Rev Immunol. 2009;9:429–39. http://www.ncbi.nlm.nih.gov/pubmed/19461673.
39. Lehnardt S. Innate immunity and neuroinflammation in the CNS: the role of microglia in Toll-like receptor-mediated neuronal injury. Glia. 2010;58:253–63. http://doi.wiley.com/10.1002/glia.20928.
40. Liesz A, Dalpke A, Mracsko E, Antoine DJ, Roth S, Zhou W, et al. DAMP signaling is a key pathway inducing immune modulation after brain injury. J Neurosci. 2015;35:583–98. http://www.jneurosci.org/cgi/doi/10.1523/JNEUROSCI.2439-14.2015.
41. Kelley KW, Dantzer R. Alcoholism and inflammation: neuroimmunology of behavioral and mood disorders. Brain Behav Immun. 2011;25:S13–20. https://linkinghub.elsevier.com/retrieve/pii/S0889159110005866.
42. Orio L, Alen F, Pavón FJ, Serrano A, García-Bueno B. Oleoylethanolamide, neuroinflammation, and alcohol abuse. Front Mol Neurosci. 2019;11:490. http://www.ncbi.nlm.nih.gov/pubmed/30687006.
43. Obernier JA, Bouldin TW, Crews FT. Binge ethanol exposure in adult rats causes necrotic cell death. Alcohol Clin Exp Res. 2002;26:547–57. http://www.ncbi.nlm.nih.gov/pubmed/11981132.
44. de la Monte SM, Kril JJ. Human alcohol-related neuropathology. Acta Neuropathol. 2014;127:71–90. http://www.ncbi.nlm.nih.gov/pubmed/24370929.
45. Charness ME. Brain lesions in alcoholics. Alcohol Clin Exp Res. 1993;17:2–11. http://www.ncbi.nlm.nih.gov/pubmed/8452204.
46. Victor M. Alcoholic dementia. Can J Neurol Sci. 1994;21:88–99. http://www.ncbi.nlm.nih.gov/pubmed/8087744.
47. Osna NA, Kharbanda KK. Multi-organ alcohol-related damage: mechanisms and treatment. Biomolecules. 2016;6:20. http://www.mdpi.com/2218-273X/6/2/20.
48. Souza-Smith FM, Lang CH, Nagy LE, Bailey SM, Parsons LH, Murray GJ. Physiological processes underlying organ injury in alcohol abuse. Am J Physiol Metab. 2016;311:E605–19. http://www.ncbi.nlm.nih.gov/pubmed/27436613.
49. Yang L, Guo Y, Wen D, Yang L, Chen Y, Zhang G, et al. Bone fracture enhances trauma brain injury. Scand J Immunol. 2016;83:26–32. http://www.ncbi.nlm.nih.gov/pubmed/26448486.
50. Corps KN, Roth TL, McGavern DB. Inflammation and neuroprotection in traumatic brain injury. JAMA Neurol. 2015;72:355–62. http://archneur.jamanetwork.com/article.aspx?doi=10.1001/jamaneurol.2014.3558.
51. Sheikh AM, Nagai A, Ryu JK, McLarnon JG, Kim SU, Masuda J. Lysophosphatidylcholine induces glial cell activation: role of rho kinase. Glia. 2009;57:898–907. http://doi.wiley.com/10.1002/glia.20815.
52. Uchida K. Redox-derived damage-associated molecular patterns: ligand function of lipid peroxidation adducts. Redox Biol. 2013;1:94–6. http://linkinghub.elsevier.com/retrieve/pii/S2213231712000201.
53. Ransohoff RM, Brown MA. Innate immunity in the central nervous system. J Clin Invest. 2012;122:1164–71. http://www.jci.org/articles/view/58644.
54. Ziebell JM, Morganti-Kossmann MC. Involvement of pro- and anti-inflammatory cytokines and chemokines in the pathophysiology of traumatic brain injury. Neurotherapeutics. 2010;7:22–30. http://link.springer.com/10.1016/j.nurt.2009.10.016.
55. Parker TM, Nguyen AH, Rabang JR, Patil A-A, Agrawal DK. The danger zone: systematic review of the role of HMGB1 danger signalling in traumatic brain injury. Brain Inj. 2017;31:2–8. http://www.ncbi.nlm.nih.gov/pubmed/27819487.
56. Okuma Y, Liu K, Wake H, Zhang J, Maruo T, Date I, et al. Anti-high mobility group box-1 antibody therapy for traumatic brain injury. Ann Neurol. 2012;72:373–84. http://doi.wiley.com/10.1002/ana.23602.
57. Gao T-L, Yuan X-T, Yang D, Dai H-L, Wang W-J, Peng X, et al. Expression of HMGB1 and RAGE in rat and human brains after traumatic brain injury. J Trauma Acute Care Surg. 2012;72:643–9. https://insights.ovid.com/crossref?an=01586154-201203000-00014.

58. Su X, Wang H, Zhao J, Pan H, Mao L. Beneficial effects of ethyl pyruvate through inhibiting high-mobility group box 1 expression and TLR4/NF-κB pathway after traumatic brain injury in the rat. Mediators Inflamm. 2011;2011:807142. http://www.hindawi.com/journals/mi/2011/807142/.
59. Laird MD, Shields JS, Sukumari-Ramesh S, Kimbler DE, Fessler RD, Shakir B, et al. High mobility group box protein-1 promotes cerebral edema after traumatic brain injury via activation of toll-like receptor 4. Glia. 2014;62:26–38. http://doi.wiley.com/10.1002/glia.22581.
60. Gu X-J, Xu J, Ma B-Y, Chen G, Gu P-Y, Wei D, et al. Effect of glycyrrhizin on traumatic brain injury in rats and its mechanism. Chin J Traumatol. 2014;17:1–7. http://www.ncbi.nlm.nih.gov/pubmed/24506915.
61. Okuma Y, Liu K, Wake H, Liu R, Nishimura Y, Hui Z, et al. Glycyrrhizin inhibits traumatic brain injury by reducing HMGB1-RAGE interaction. Neuropharmacology. 2014;85:18–26. http://linkinghub.elsevier.com/retrieve/pii/S0028390814001749.
62. Szabo G, Lippai D. Converging actions of alcohol on liver and brain immune signaling. Int Rev Neurobiol. 2014;118:359–80. https://linkinghub.elsevier.com/retrieve/pii/B9780128012840000117.
63. Vetreno RP, Crews FT. Adolescent binge drinking increases expression of the danger signal receptor agonist HMGB1 and Toll-like receptors in the adult prefrontal cortex. Neuroscience. 2012;226:475–88. https://linkinghub.elsevier.com/retrieve/pii/S0306452212008809.
64. Crews FT, Qin L, Sheedy D, Vetreno RP, Zou J. High mobility group box 1/Toll-like receptor danger signaling increases brain neuroimmune activation in alcohol dependence. Biol Psychiatry. 2013;73:602–12. https://linkinghub.elsevier.com/retrieve/pii/S000632231200889X.
65. Wang X, Chu G, Yang Z, Sun Y, Zhou H, Li M, et al. Ethanol directly induced HMGB1 release through NOX2/NLRP1 inflammasome in neuronal cells. Toxicology. 2015;334:104–10. http://www.ncbi.nlm.nih.gov/pubmed/26079697.
66. Wang K-Y, Yu G-F, Zhang Z-Y, Huang Q, Dong X-Q. Plasma high-mobility group box 1 levels and prediction of outcome in patients with traumatic brain injury. Clin Chim Acta. 2012;413:1737–41. http://linkinghub.elsevier.com/retrieve/pii/S0009898112003415.
67. Au AK, Aneja RK, Bell MJ, Bayir H, Feldman K, Adelson PD, et al. Cerebrospinal fluid levels of high-mobility group box 1 and cytochrome C predict outcome after pediatric traumatic brain injury. J Neurotrauma. 2012;29:2013–21. http://www.liebertpub.com/doi/10.1089/neu.2011.2171.
68. Antón M, Rodríguez-González A, Rodríguez-Rojo IC, Pastor A, Correas Á, Serrano A, et al. Increased plasma oleoylethanolamide and palmitoleoylethanolamide levels correlate with inflammatory changes in alcohol binge drinkers: the case of HMGB1 in women. Addict Biol. 2018;23:1242–50. http://doi.wiley.com/10.1111/adb.12580.
69. Vetreno RP, Qin L, Crews FT. Increased receptor for advanced glycation end product expression in the human alcoholic prefrontal cortex is linked to adolescent drinking. Neurobiol Dis. 2013;59:52–62. https://linkinghub.elsevier.com/retrieve/pii/S0969996113001964
70. Walko TD, Bola RA, Hong JD, Au AK, Bell MJ, Kochanek PM, et al. Cerebrospinal fluid mitochondrial DNA: a novel DAMP in pediatric traumatic brain injury. Shock. 2014;41:499–503. http://content.wkhealth.com/linkback/openurl?sid=WKPTLP:landingpage&an=00024382-201406000-00005.
71. Ingebrigtsen T, Romner B, Kongstad P, Langbakk B. Increased serum concentrations of protein S-100 after minor head injury: a biochemical serum marker with prognostic value? J Neurol Neurosurg Psychiatry. 1995;59:103–4. http://www.ncbi.nlm.nih.gov/pubmed/7608699.
72. Vos PE, Jacobs B, Andriessen TMJC, Lamers KJB, Borm GF, Beems T, et al. GFAP and S100B are biomarkers of traumatic brain injury: an observational cohort study. Neurology. 2010;75:1786–93. http://www.neurology.org/cgi/doi/10.1212/WNL.0b013e3181fd62d2.
73. Thelin EP, Nelson DW, Bellander B-M. A review of the clinical utility of serum S100B protein levels in the assessment of traumatic brain injury. Acta Neurochir. 2017;159:209–25. http://www.ncbi.nlm.nih.gov/pubmed/27957604.

74. Park S-H, Hwang S-K. Prognostic value of serum levels of S100 calcium-binding protein B, neuron-specific enolase, and interleukin-6 in pediatric patients with traumatic brain injury. World Neurosurg. 2018;118:e534–42. http://www.ncbi.nlm.nih.gov/pubmed/30257306.
75. Bayir H, Marion DW, Puccio AM, Wisniewski SR, Janesko KL, Clark RSB, et al. Marked gender effect on lipid peroxidation after severe traumatic brain injury in adult patients. J Neurotrauma. 2004;21:1–8. http://www.liebertpub.com/doi/10.1089/089771504772695896.
76. Cristofori L, Tavazzi B, Gambin R, Vagnozzi R, Signoretti S, Amorini AM, et al. Biochemical analysis of the cerebrospinal fluid: evidence for catastrophic energy failure and oxidative damage preceding brain death in severe head injury: a case report. Clin Biochem. 2005;38:97–100. http://linkinghub.elsevier.com/retrieve/pii/S0009912004002516.
77. Lorente L, Martín MM, Abreu-González P, Ramos L, Argueso M, Cáceres JJ, et al. Association between serum malondialdehyde levels and mortality in patients with severe brain trauma injury. J Neurotrauma. 2015;32:1–6. http://www.ncbi.nlm.nih.gov/pubmed/25054973.
78. Kagan VE, Mao G, Qu F, Angeli JPF, Doll S, Croix CS, et al. Oxidized arachidonic and adrenic PEs navigate cells to ferroptosis. Nat Chem Biol. 2017;13:81–90. http://www.nature.com/articles/nchembio.2238.
79. Orrenius S, Zhivotovsky B. Cardiolipin oxidation sets cytochrome C free. Nat Chem Biol. 2005;1:188–9. http://www.nature.com/doifinder/10.1038/nchembio0905-188.
80. Kagan VE, Tyurin VA, Jiang J, Tyurina YY, Ritov VB, Amoscato AA, et al. Cytochrome C acts as a cardiolipin oxygenase required for release of proapoptotic factors. Nat Chem Biol. 2005;1:223–32. http://www.nature.com/doifinder/10.1038/nchembio727.
81. Bayir H, Tyurin VA, Tyurina YY, Viner R, Ritov V, Amoscato AA, et al. Selective early cardiolipin peroxidation after traumatic brain injury: an oxidative lipidomics analysis. Ann Neurol. 2007;62:154–69. http://doi.wiley.com/10.1002/ana.21168.
82. Harrison JL, Rowe RK, Ellis TW, Yee NS, O'Hara BF, Adelson PD, et al. Resolvins AT-D1 and E1 differentially impact functional outcome, post-traumatic sleep, and microglial activation following diffuse brain injury in the mouse. Brain Behav Immun. 2015;47:131–40. http://www.ncbi.nlm.nih.gov/pubmed/25585137.
83. Jackson EK, Kotermanski SE, Menshikova EV, Dubey RK, Jackson TC, Kochanek PM. Adenosine production by brain cells. J Neurochem. 2017;141:676–93. http://www.ncbi.nlm.nih.gov/pubmed/28294336.
84. Robertson CL, Bell MJ, Kochanek PM, Adelson PD, Ruppel RA, Carcillo JA, et al. Increased adenosine in cerebrospinal fluid after severe traumatic brain injury in infants and children: association with severity of injury and excitotoxicity. Crit Care Med. 2001;29:2287–93. http://www.ncbi.nlm.nih.gov/pubmed/11801827.
85. Kochanek PM, Vagni VA, Janesko KL, Washington CB, Crumrine PK, Garman RH, et al. Adenosine A1 receptor knockout mice develop lethal status epilepticus after experimental traumatic brain injury. J Cereb Blood Flow Metab. 2006;26:565–75. http://www.ncbi.nlm.nih.gov/pubmed/16121125.
86. Haselkorn ML, Shellington DK, Jackson EK, Vagni VA, Janesko-Feldman K, Dubey RK, et al. Adenosine A1 receptor activation as a brake on the microglial response after experimental traumatic brain injury in mice. J Neurotrauma. 2010;27:901–10. http://www.ncbi.nlm.nih.gov/pubmed/20121416.
87. Kota DJ, Prabhakara KS, Toledano-Furman N, Bhattarai D, Chen Q, DiCarlo B, et al. Prostaglandin E2 indicates therapeutic efficacy of mesenchymal stem cells in experimental traumatic brain injury. Stem Cells. 2017;35:1416–30. http://www.ncbi.nlm.nih.gov/pubmed/28233425.
88. Wang Z, Chen Z, Yang J, Yang Z, Yin J, Zuo G, et al. Identification of two phosphorylation sites essential for annexin A1 in blood–brain barrier protection after experimental intracerebral hemorrhage in rats. J Cereb Blood Flow Metab. 2017;37:2509–25. http://www.ncbi.nlm.nih.gov/pubmed/27634935.
89. Ashbaugh DG, Bigelow DB, Petty TL, Levine BE. Acute respiratory distress in adults. Lancet (London, England). 1967;2:319–23. http://www.ncbi.nlm.nih.gov/pubmed/4143721.

90. Matthay MA, Ware LB, Zimmerman GA. The acute respiratory distress syndrome. J Clin Invest. 2012;122:2731–40. http://www.ncbi.nlm.nih.gov/pubmed/22850883.
91. Johnson ER, Matthay MA. Acute lung injury: epidemiology, pathogenesis, and treatment. J Aerosol Med Pulm Drug Deliv. 2010;23:243–52. http://www.ncbi.nlm.nih.gov/pubmed/20073554.
92. Butt Y, Kurdowska A, Allen TC. Acute lung injury: a clinical and molecular review. Arch Pathol Lab Med. 2016 [cited 2019 Sep 14];140:345–50. http://www.ncbi.nlm.nih.gov/pubmed/27028393.
93. Komiya K, Akaba T, Kozaki Y, Kadota J-I, Rubin BK. A systematic review of diagnostic methods to differentiate acute lung injury/acute respiratory distress syndrome from cardiogenic pulmonary edema. Crit Care. 2017;21:228. http://ccforum.biomedcentral.com/articles/10.1186/s13054-017-1809-8.
94. Bellani G, Laffey JG, Pham T, Fan E, Brochard L, Esteban A, et al. Epidemiology, patterns of care, and mortality for patients with acute respiratory distress syndrome in intensive care units in 50 countries. JAMA. 2016;315:788–800. http://jama.jamanetwork.com/article.aspx?doi=10.1001/jama.2016.0291.
95. Rawal G, Yadav S, Kumar R. Acute respiratory distress syndrome: an update and review. J Transl Intern Med. 2018;6:74–7. http://www.ncbi.nlm.nih.gov/pubmed/29984201.
96. Confalonieri M, Salton F, Fabiano F. Acute respiratory distress syndrome. Eur Respir Rev. 2017;26:160116. http://err.ersjournals.com/lookup/doi/10.1183/16000617.0116-2016.
97. ARDS Definition Task Force, Ranieri VM, Rubenfeld GD, Thompson BT, Ferguson ND, Caldwell E, et al. Acute respiratory distress syndrome: the Berlin definition. JAMA. 2012;307:2526–33. http://jama.jamanetwork.com/article.aspx?doi=10.1001/jama.2012.5669.
98. Matute-Bello G, Liles WC, Steinberg KP, Kiener PA, Mongovin S, Chi EY, et al. Soluble Fas ligand induces epithelial cell apoptosis in humans with acute lung injury (ARDS). J Immunol. 1999;163:2217–25. http://www.ncbi.nlm.nih.gov/pubmed/10438964.
99. Chambers E, Rounds S, Lu Q. Pulmonary endothelial cell apoptosis in emphysema and acute lung injury. Adv Anat Embryol Cell Biol. 2018;228:63–86. http://www.ncbi.nlm.nih.gov/pubmed/29288386.
100. Wang L, Wang T, Li H, Liu Q, Zhang Z, Xie W, et al. Receptor interacting protein 3-mediated necroptosis promotes lipopolysaccharide-induced inflammation and acute respiratory distress syndrome in mice. Ahmad S, editor. PLoS One. 2016;11:e0155723. http://www.ncbi.nlm.nih.gov/pubmed/27195494.
101. Pan L, Yao D-C, Yu Y-Z, Chen B-J, Li S-J, Hu G-H, et al. Activation of necroptosis in a rat model of acute respiratory distress syndrome induced by oleic acid. Sheng Li Xue Bao. 2016;68:661–8. http://www.ncbi.nlm.nih.gov/pubmed/27778032.
102. Qing DY, Conegliano D, Shashaty MGS, Seo J, Reilly JP, Worthen GS, et al. Red blood cells induce necroptosis of lung endothelial cells and increase susceptibility to lung inflammation. Am J Respir Crit Care Med. 2014;190:1243–54. http://www.atsjournals.org/doi/abs/10.1164/rccm.201406-1095OC.
103. Fan EKY, Fan J. Regulation of alveolar macrophage death in acute lung inflammation. Respir Res. 2018;19:50. http://www.ncbi.nlm.nih.gov/pubmed/29587748.
104. Li H, Zhou X, Tan H, Hu Y, Zhang L, Liu S, et al. Neutrophil extracellular traps contribute to the pathogenesis of acid-aspiration-induced ALI/ARDS. Oncotarget. 2018;9:1772–84. http://www.ncbi.nlm.nih.gov/pubmed/29416730.
105. Bersten AD, Edibam C, Hunt T, Moran J, Australian and New Zealand Intensive Care Society Clinical Trials Group. Incidence and mortality of acute lung injury and the acute respiratory distress syndrome in three Australian States. Am J Respir Crit Care Med. 2002;165:443–8. http://www.ncbi.nlm.nih.gov/pubmed/11850334.
106. Epelbaum O, Aronow WS. Mechanical ventilation in the acute respiratory distress syndrome. Hosp Pract. 2017;45:88–98. http://www.ncbi.nlm.nih.gov/pubmed/28510501.
107. Lee K-Y. Pneumonia, acute respiratory distress syndrome, and early immune-modulator therapy. Int J Mol Sci. 2017;18:388. http://www.mdpi.com/1422-0067/18/2/388.

108. Yang C-Y, Chen C-S, Yiang G-T, Cheng Y-L, Yong S-B, Wu M-Y, et al. New insights into the immune molecular regulation of the pathogenesis of acute respiratory distress syndrome. Int J Mol Sci. 2018;19:588. http://www.ncbi.nlm.nih.gov/pubmed/29462936.
109. Ware LB, Matthay MA. The acute respiratory distress syndrome. N Engl J Med. 2000;342:1334–49. http://www.nejm.org/doi/abs/10.1056/NEJM200005043421806.
110. Herold S, Mayer K, Lohmeyer J. Acute lung injury: how macrophages orchestrate resolution of inflammation and tissue repair. Front Immunol. 2011;2:65. http://journal.frontiersin.org/article/10.3389/fimmu.2011.00065/abstract.
111. Matthay MA, Ware LB. Resolution of alveolar edema in acute respiratory distress syndrome. Physiology and biology. Am J Respir Crit Care Med. 2015;192:124–5. http://www.ncbi.nlm.nih.gov/pubmed/26177166.
112. Aggarwal NR, King LS, D'Alessio FR. Diverse macrophage populations mediate acute lung inflammation and resolution. Am J Physiol Cell Mol Physiol. 2014;306:L709–25. http://www.ncbi.nlm.nih.gov/pubmed/24508730.
113. Robb CT, Regan KH, Dorward DA, Rossi AG. Key mechanisms governing resolution of lung inflammation. Semin Immunopathol. 2016;38:425–48. http://www.ncbi.nlm.nih.gov/pubmed/27116944.
114. Matthay MA, Zemans RL. The acute respiratory distress syndrome: pathogenesis and treatment. Annu Rev Pathol. 2011;6:147–63. http://www.annualreviews.org/doi/10.1146/annurev-pathol-011110-130158.
115. Katzenstein A-L. Acute lung injury patterns: diffuse alveolar damage and bronchiolitis obliterans organizing pneumonia. In: Katzenstein A-L, editor. Katzenstein and Askin's surgical pathology of non-neoplastic lung disease. Philadelphia: Elsevier Saunders; 2006, ISBN-13:978-0721600413.
116. Tolle LB, Standiford TJ. Danger-associated molecular patterns (DAMPs) in acute lung injury. J Pathol. 2013;229:145–56. http://www.ncbi.nlm.nih.gov/pubmed/23097158.
117. Englert JA, Bobba C, Baron RM. Integrating molecular pathogenesis and clinical translation in sepsis-induced acute respiratory distress syndrome. JCI Insight. 2019;4(2):e124061. http://www.ncbi.nlm.nih.gov/pubmed/30674720.
118. Land WG. Transfusion-related acute lung injury: the work of DAMPs. Transfus Med Hemother. 2013;40:3–13. https://www.karger.com/Article/FullText/345688.
119. Simmons JD, Lee Y-LL, Pastukh VM, Capley G, Muscat CA, Muscat DC, et al. Potential contribution of mitochondrial DNA damage associated molecular patterns in transfusion products to the development of acute respiratory distress syndrome after multiple transfusions. J Trauma Acute Care Surg. 2017;82:1023–9. http://insights.ovid.com/crossref?an=01586154-201706000-00007.
120. Gan L, Chen X, Sun T, Li Q, Zhang R, Zhang J, et al. Significance of serum mtDNA concentration in lung injury induced by hip fracture. Shock. 2015;44:52–7. http://content.wkhealth.com/linkback/openurl?sid=WKPTLP:landingpage&an=00024382-201507000-00008.
121. Kang J-W, Kim S-J, Cho H-I, Lee S-M. DAMPs activating innate immune responses in sepsis. Ageing Res Rev. 2015;24:54–65. https://linkinghub.elsevier.com/retrieve/pii/S1568163715000318.
122. Ueno T, Ikeda T, Ikeda K, Taniuchi H, Suda S, Yeung MY, et al. HMGB-1 as a useful prognostic biomarker in sepsis-induced organ failure in patients undergoing PMX-DHP. J Surg Res. 2011;171:183–90. https://linkinghub.elsevier.com/retrieve/pii/S0022480409012669.
123. Patel MC, Shirey KA, Boukhvalova MS, Vogel SN, Blanco JCG. Serum high-mobility-group box 1 as a biomarker and a therapeutic target during respiratory virus infections. Sher A, editor. MBio. 2018;9(2):e00246-18. http://mbio.asm.org/lookup/doi/10.1128/mBio.00246-18.
124. Abraham E, Arcaroli J, Carmody A, Wang H, Tracey KJ. HMG-1 as a mediator of acute lung inflammation. J Immunol. 2000;165:2950–4. http://www.ncbi.nlm.nih.gov/pubmed/10975801.
125. Ren D, Sun R, Wang S. Role of inducible nitric oxide synthase expressed by alveolar macrophages in high mobility group box 1-induced acute lung injury. Inflamm Res. 2006;55:207–15. http://link.springer.com/10.1007/s00011-006-0072-2.

126. Kim JY, Park JS, Strassheim D, Douglas I, Diaz del Valle F, Asehnoune K, et al. HMGB1 contributes to the development of acute lung injury after hemorrhage. Am J Physiol Lung Cell Mol Physiol. 2005;288:L958–65. http://www.physiology.org/doi/10.1152/ajplung.00359.2004.
127. Entezari M, Javdan M, Antoine DJ, Morrow DMP, Sitapara RA, Patel V, et al. Inhibition of extracellular HMGB1 attenuates hyperoxia-induced inflammatory acute lung injury. Redox Biol. 2014;2:314–22. http://www.ncbi.nlm.nih.gov/pubmed/24563849.
128. Qin M-Z, Gu Q-H, Tao J, Song X-Y, Gan G-S, Luo Z-B, et al. Ketamine effect on HMGB1 and TLR4 expression in rats with acute lung injury. Int J Clin Exp Pathol. 2015;8:12943–8. http://www.ncbi.nlm.nih.gov/pubmed/26722488.
129. Liu X, Xu Q, Mei L, Lei H, Wen Q, Miao J, et al. Paeonol attenuates acute lung injury by inhibiting HMGB1 in lipopolysaccharide-induced shock rats. Int Immunopharmacol. 2018;61:169–77. http://www.ncbi.nlm.nih.gov/pubmed/29883962.
130. Ogawa EN, Ishizaka A, Tasaka S, Koh H, Ueno H, Amaya F, et al. Contribution of high-mobility group box-1 to the development of ventilator-induced lung injury. Am J Respir Crit Care Med. 2006;174:400–7. http://www.atsjournals.org/doi/abs/10.1164/rccm.200605-699OC.
131. Patel VS, Sitapara RA, Gore A, Phan B, Sharma L, Sampat V, et al. High mobility group box-1 mediates hyperoxia-induced impairment of Pseudomonas aeruginosa clearance and inflammatory lung injury in mice. Am J Respir Cell Mol Biol. 2013;48:280–7. http://www.atsjournals.org/doi/abs/10.1165/rcmb.2012-0279OC.
132. Wang H, Bloom O, Zhang M, Vishnubhakat JM, Ombrellino M, Che J, et al. HMG-1 as a late mediator of endotoxin lethality in mice. Science. 1999;285:248–51. http://www.ncbi.nlm.nih.gov/pubmed/10398600.
133. Ueno H, Matsuda T, Hashimoto S, Amaya F, Kitamura Y, Tanaka M, et al. Contributions of high mobility group box protein in experimental and clinical acute lung injury. Am J Respir Crit Care Med. 2004;170:1310–6. http://www.atsjournals.org/doi/abs/10.1164/rccm.200402-188OC.
134. van Zoelen MAD, Ishizaka A, Wolthuls EK, Choi G, van der Poll T, Schultz MJ. Pulmonary levels of high-mobility group box 1 during mechanical ventilation and ventilator-associated pneumonia. Shock. 2008;29:441–5. http://insights.ovid.com/crossref?an=00024382-200804000-00003.
135. Tseng C-C, Fang W-F, Leung S-Y, Chen H-C, Chang Y-C, Wang C-C, et al. Impact of serum biomarkers and clinical factors on intensive care unit mortality and 6-month outcome in relatively healthy patients with severe pneumonia and acute respiratory distress syndrome. Dis Markers. 2014;2014:1–9. http://www.ncbi.nlm.nih.gov/pubmed/24723739.
136. Chase MA, Wheeler DS, Lierl KM, Hughes VS, Wong HR, Page K. Hsp72 induces inflammation and regulates cytokine production in airway epithelium through a TLR4- and NF-kappaB-dependent mechanism. J Immunol. 2007;179:6318–24. http://www.ncbi.nlm.nih.gov/pubmed/17947709.
137. Ganter MT, Ware LB, Howard M, Roux J, Gartland B, Matthay MA, et al. Extracellular heat shock protein 72 is a marker of the stress protein response in acute lung injury. Am J Physiol Lung Cell Mol Physiol. 2006;291:L354–61. http://www.physiology.org/doi/10.1152/ajplung.00405.2005.
138. Sun S, Sursal T, Adibnia Y, Zhao C, Zheng Y, Li H, et al. Mitochondrial DAMPs increase endothelial permeability through neutrophil dependent and independent pathways. Zhao Y-Y, editor. PLoS One. 2013;8:e59989. http://www.ncbi.nlm.nih.gov/pubmed/23527291.
139. Kuck JL, Obiako BO, Gorodnya OM, Pastukh VM, Kua J, Simmons JD, et al. Mitochondrial DNA damage-associated molecular patterns mediate a feed-forward cycle of bacteria-induced vascular injury in perfused rat lungs. Am J Physiol Lung Cell Mol Physiol. 2015;308:L1078–85. http://www.physiology.org/doi/10.1152/ajplung.00015.2015.
140. Zhang L, Deng S, Zhao S, Ai Y, Zhang L, Pan P, et al. Intra-peritoneal administration of mitochondrial DNA provokes acute lung injury and systemic inflammation via Toll-like receptor 9. Int J Mol Sci. 2016;17:1425. http://www.mdpi.com/1422-0067/17/9/1425.
141. Lee Y-L, Obiako B, Gorodnya OM, Ruchko MV, Kuck JL, Pastukh VM, et al. Mitochondrial DNA damage initiates acute lung injury and multi-organ system failure evoked in rats by

intra-tracheal Pseudomonas aeruginosa. Shock. 2017;48:54–60. http://insights.ovid.com/crossref?an=00024382-201707000-00008.
142. Simmons JD, Freno DR, Muscat CA, Obiako B, Lee Y-LL, Pastukh VM, et al. Mitochondrial DNA damage associated molecular patterns in ventilator-associated pneumonia: prevention and reversal by intratracheal DNase I. J Trauma Acute Care Surg. 2017;82:120–5. http://content.wkhealth.com/linkback/openurl?sid=WKPTLP:landingpage&an=01586154-201701000-00016.
143. Zhang X, Wang T, Yuan Z-C, Dai L-Q, Zeng N, Wang H, et al. Mitochondrial peptides cause proinflammatory responses in the alveolar epithelium via FPR-1, MAPKs, and AKT: a potential mechanism involved in acute lung injury. Am J Physiol Lung Cell Mol Physiol. 2018;315:L775–86. https://www.physiology.org/doi/10.1152/ajplung.00466.2017.
144. Abrams ST, Zhang N, Manson J, Liu T, Dart C, Baluwa F, et al. Circulating histones are mediators of trauma-associated lung injury. Am J Respir Crit Care Med. 2013;187:160–9. http://www.atsjournals.org/doi/abs/10.1164/rccm.201206-1037OC.
145. Lv X, Wen T, Song J, Xie D, Wu L, Jiang X, et al. Extracellular histones are clinically relevant mediators in the pathogenesis of acute respiratory distress syndrome. Respir Res. 2017;18:165. http://www.ncbi.nlm.nih.gov/pubmed/28865478.
146. Lorenz E, Muhlebach MS, Tessier PA, Alexis NE, Duncan Hite R, Seeds MC, et al. Different expression ratio of S100A8/A9 and S100A12 in acute and chronic lung diseases. Respir Med. 2008;102:567–73. http://linkinghub.elsevier.com/retrieve/pii/S0954611107004714.
147. Chakraborty D, Zenker S, Rossaint J, Hölscher A, Pohlen M, Zarbock A, et al. Alarmin S100A8 activates alveolar epithelial cells in the context of acute lung injury in a TLR4-dependent manner. Front Immunol. 2017;8:1493. http://journal.frontiersin.org/article/10.3389/fimmu.2017.01493/full.
148. Hiroshima Y, Hsu K, Tedla N, Wong SW, Chow S, Kawaguchi N, et al. S100A8/A9 and S100A9 reduce acute lung injury. Immunol Cell Biol. 2017;95:461–72. http://www.ncbi.nlm.nih.gov/pubmed/28074060.
149. Copland IB, Kavanagh BP, Engelberts D, McKerlie C, Belik J, Post M. Early changes in lung gene expression due to high tidal volume. Am J Respir Crit Care Med. 2003;168:1051–9. http://www.atsjournals.org/doi/abs/10.1164/rccm.200208-964OC.
150. Altemeier WA, Matute-Bello G, Gharib SA, Glenny RW, Martin TR, Liles WC. Modulation of lipopolysaccharide-induced gene transcription and promotion of lung injury by mechanical ventilation. J Immunol. 2005;175:3369–76. http://www.ncbi.nlm.nih.gov/pubmed/16116230.
151. Wittkowski H, Sturrock A, van Zoelen MAD, Viemann D, van der Poll T, Hoidal JR, et al. Neutrophil-derived S100A12 in acute lung injury and respiratory distress syndrome. Crit Care Med. 2007;35:1369–75. https://insights.ovid.com/crossref?an=00003246-200705000-00024.
152. Feng Z, Qi S, Zhang Y, Qi Z, Yan L, Zhou J, et al. Ly6G+ neutrophil-derived miR-223 inhibits the NLRP3 inflammasome in mitochondrial DAMP-induced acute lung injury. Cell Death Dis. 2017;8:e3170. http://www.ncbi.nlm.nih.gov/pubmed/29144508.
153. Li D, Ren W, Jiang Z, Zhu L. Regulation of the NLRP3 inflammasome and macrophage pyroptosis by the p38 MAPK signaling pathway in a mouse model of acute lung injury. Mol Med Rep. 2018;18:4399–409. http://www.ncbi.nlm.nih.gov/pubmed/30152849.
154. Rich PB, Douillet CD, Mahler SA, Husain SA, Boucher RC. Adenosine triphosphate is released during injurious mechanical ventilation and contributes to lung edema. J Trauma. 2003;55:290–7. https://insights.ovid.com/crossref?an=00005373-200308000-00014.
155. Matsuyama H, Amaya F, Hashimoto S, Ueno H, Beppu S, Mizuta M, et al. Acute lung inflammation and ventilator-induced lung injury caused by ATP via the P2Y receptors: an experimental study. Respir Res. 2008;9:79. http://respiratory-research.biomedcentral.com/articles/10.1186/1465-9921-9-79.
156. Kuipers MT, Aslami H, Vlaar APJ, Juffermans NP, Tuip-de Boer AM, Hegeman MA, et al. Pre-treatment with allopurinol or uricase attenuates barrier dysfunction but not inflammation during murine ventilator-induced lung injury. Ryffel B, editor. PLoS One. 2012;7:e50559. https://dx.plos.org/10.1371/journal.pone.0050559.

157. Gasse P, Riteau N, Charron S, Girre S, Fick L, Pétrilli V, et al. Uric acid is a danger signal activating NALP3 inflammasome in lung injury inflammation and fibrosis. Am J Respir Crit Care Med. 2009;179:903–13. http://www.atsjournals.org/doi/abs/10.1164/rccm.200808-1274OC.
158. Esposito AJ, Bhatraju PK, Stapleton RD, Wurfel MM, Mikacenic C. Hyaluronic acid is associated with organ dysfunction in acute respiratory distress syndrome. Crit Care. 2017;21:304. http://www.ncbi.nlm.nih.gov/pubmed/29237497.
159. Schmidt EP, Overdier KH, Sun X, Lin L, Liu X, Yang Y, et al. Urinary glycosaminoglycans predict outcomes in septic shock and acute respiratory distress syndrome. Am J Respir Crit Care Med. 2016;194:439–49. http://www.atsjournals.org/doi/10.1164/rccm.201511-2281OC.
160. Levy BD, Serhan CN. Resolution of acute inflammation in the lung. Annu Rev Physiol. 2014;76:467–92. http://www.ncbi.nlm.nih.gov/pubmed/24313723.
161. Wang Q, Lian Q-Q, Li R, Ying B-Y, He Q, Chen F, et al. Lipoxin A(4) activates alveolar epithelial sodium channel, Na,K-ATPase, and increases alveolar fluid clearance. Am J Respir Cell Mol Biol. 2013;48:610–8. http://www.atsjournals.org/doi/abs/10.1165/rcmb.2012-0274OC.
162. Yang Y, Cheng Y, Lian Q-Q, Yang L, Qi W, Wu D-R, et al. Contribution of CFTR to alveolar fluid clearance by lipoxin A4 via PI3K/Akt pathway in LPS-induced acute lung injury. Mediators Inflamm. 2013;2013:862628. http://www.hindawi.com/journals/mi/2013/862628/.
163. Wang Q, Zheng X, Cheng Y, Zhang Y-L, Wen H-X, Tao Z, et al. Resolvin D1 stimulates alveolar fluid clearance through alveolar epithelial sodium channel, Na,K-ATPase via ALX/cAMP/PI3K pathway in lipopolysaccharide-induced acute lung injury. J Immunol. 2014;192:3765–77. http://www.jimmunol.org/cgi/doi/10.4049/jimmunol.1302421.
164. Wang Q, Yan S-F, Hao Y, Jin S-W. Specialized pro-resolving mediators regulate alveolar fluid clearance during acute respiratory distress syndrome. Chin Med J (Engl). 2018;131:982. http://www.ncbi.nlm.nih.gov/pubmed/29664060.
165. Morote-Garcia JC, Rosenberger P, Kuhlicke J, Eltzschig HK. HIF-1-dependent repression of adenosine kinase attenuates hypoxia-induced vascular leak. Blood. 2008;111:5571–80. http://www.bloodjournal.org/cgi/doi/10.1182/blood-2007-11-126763.
166. Morote-Garcia JC, Köhler D, Roth JM, Mirakaj V, Eldh T, Eltzschig HK, et al. Repression of the equilibrative nucleoside transporters dampens inflammatory lung injury. Am J Respir Cell Mol Biol. 2013;49:296–305. http://www.atsjournals.org/doi/abs/10.1165/rcmb.2012-0457OC.
167. Köhler D, Streißenberger A, Morote-García JC, Granja TF, Schneider M, Straub A, et al. Inhibition of adenosine kinase attenuates acute lung injury. Crit Care Med. 2016;44:e181–9. http://content.wkhealth.com/linkback/openurl?sid=WKPTLP:landingpage&an=00003246-900000000-97119.
168. Fuller BM, Mohr NM, Skrupky L, Fowler S, Kollef MH, Carpenter CR. The use of inhaled prostaglandins in patients with ARDS. Chest. 2015;147:1510–22. http://www.ncbi.nlm.nih.gov/pubmed/25742022.
169. Han G, Lu K, Xu W, Zhang S, Huang J, Dai C, et al. Annexin A1-mediated inhibition of inflammatory cytokines may facilitate the resolution of inflammation in acute radiation-induced lung injury. Oncol Lett Spandidos Publications. 2019;18:321–9.
170. López-Campos JL, Tan W, Soriano JB. Global burden of COPD. Respirology. 2016;21:14–23. http://www.ncbi.nlm.nih.gov/pubmed/26494423.
171. GOLD Report. Global initiative for chronic obstructive lung diseases (GOLD). 2019. https://goldcopd.org/wp-content/uploads/2018/11/GOLD-2019-v1.7-FINAL-14Nov2018-WMS.pdf.
172. Kim WJ, Lee CY. Environmental exposures and chronic obstructive pulmonary disease. Mol Cell Toxicol. 2017;13:251–5. http://link.springer.com/10.1007/s13273-017-0027-4.
173. Qiao D, Ameli A, Prokopenko D, Chen H, Kho AT, Parker MM, et al. Whole exome sequencing analysis in severe chronic obstructive pulmonary disease. Hum Mol Genet. 2018;27:3801–12. https://academic.oup.com/hmg/article/27/21/3801/5060721.
174. Postma DS, Timens W. Remodeling in asthma and chronic obstructive pulmonary disease. Proc Am Thorac Soc. 2006;3:434–9. http://www.ncbi.nlm.nih.gov/pubmed/16799088.

175. Bagdonas E, Raudoniute J, Bruzauskaite I, Aldonyte R. Novel aspects of pathogenesis and regeneration mechanisms in COPD. Int J Chron Obstruct Pulmon Dis. 2015;10:995. http://www.ncbi.nlm.nih.gov/pubmed/26082624.
176. Rabe KF, Watz H. Chronic obstructive pulmonary disease. Lancet. 2017;389:1931–40. http://www.ncbi.nlm.nih.gov/pubmed/28513453.
177. Mammen MJ, Sethi S. COPD and the microbiome. Respirology. 2016;21:590–9. http://www.ncbi.nlm.nih.gov/pubmed/26852737.
178. Caramori G, Casolari P, Barczyk A, Durham AL, Di Stefano A, Adcock I. COPD immunopathology. Semin Immunopathol. 2016;38:497–515. http://www.ncbi.nlm.nih.gov/pubmed/27178410.
179. Adcock IM. Role of epigenetic modifications in pathology of COPD. Tanaffos. 2017;16:S2. http://www.ncbi.nlm.nih.gov/pubmed/29158743.
180. Freeman CM, Curtis JL. Lung dendritic cells: shaping immune responses throughout COPD progression. Am J Respir Cell Mol Biol. 2016;56:152–9. http://www.atsjournals.org/doi/10.1165/rcmb.2016-0272TR.
181. Yang X, Huo B, Zhong X, Su W, Liu W, Li Y, et al. Imbalance between subpopulations of regulatory T cells in patients with acute exacerbation of COPD. COPD J Chronic Obstr Pulm Dis. 2017;14:618–25. http://www.ncbi.nlm.nih.gov/pubmed/29166179.
182. Panda SK, Colonna M. Innate lymphoid cells in mucosal immunity. Front Immunol. 2019;10:861. http://www.ncbi.nlm.nih.gov/pubmed/31134050.
183. Poh TY, Mac Aogáin M, Chan AKW, Yii ACA, Yong VFL, Tiew PY, et al. Understanding COPD-overlap syndromes. Expert Rev Respir Med. 2017;11:285–98. http://www.ncbi.nlm.nih.gov/pubmed/28282995.
184. Faiz A, Heijink IH, Vermeulen CJ, Guryev V, van den Berge M, Nawijn MC, et al. Cigarette smoke exposure decreases CFLAR expression in the bronchial epithelium, augmenting susceptibility for lung epithelial cell death and DAMP release. Sci Rep. 2018;8:12426. http://www.ncbi.nlm.nih.gov/pubmed/30127367.
185. Mizumura K, Maruoka S, Shimizu T, Gon Y. Autophagy, selective autophagy, and necroptosis in COPD. Int J Chron Obstruct Pulmon Dis. 2018;13:3165–72. http://www.ncbi.nlm.nih.gov/pubmed/30349225.
186. Künzi L, Holt GE. Cigarette smoke activates the parthanatos pathway of cell death in human bronchial epithelial cells. Cell Death Dis. 2019;5:127. http://www.nature.com/articles/s41420-019-0205-3.
187. Sauler M, Bazan IS, Lee PJ. Cell death in the lung: the apoptosis–necroptosis axis. Annu Rev Physiol. 2019;81:375–402. http://www.ncbi.nlm.nih.gov/pubmed/30485762.
188. Yoshida M, Minagawa S, Araya J, Sakamoto T, Hara H, Tsubouchi K, et al. Involvement of cigarette smoke-induced epithelial cell ferroptosis in COPD pathogenesis. Nat Commun. 2019;10:3145. http://www.nature.com/articles/s41467-019-10991-7.
189. Pouwels SD, Heijink IH, ten Hacken NH, Vandenabeele P, Krysko DV, Nawijn MC, et al. DAMPs activating innate and adaptive immune responses in COPD. Mucosal Immunol. 2014;7:215–26. http://www.ncbi.nlm.nih.gov/pubmed/24150257.
190. Pouwels SD, Hesse L, Faiz A, Lubbers J, Bodha PK, ten Hacken NHT, et al. Susceptibility for cigarette smoke-induced DAMP release and DAMP-induced inflammation in COPD. Am J Physiol Cell Mol Physiol. 2016;311:L881–92. http://www.ncbi.nlm.nih.gov/pubmed/27612964.
191. Brajer-Luftmann B, Nowicka A, Kaczmarek M, Wyrzykiewicz M, Yasar S, Piorunek T, et al. Molecules of damage-associated patterns in bronchoalveolar lavage fluid and serum in chronic obstructive pulmonary disease. Adv Exp Med Biol. 2018;1113:27–35. http://www.ncbi.nlm.nih.gov/pubmed/29429028.
192. Uh S-T, Koo SM, Kim Y, Kim K, Park S, Jang AS, et al. The activation of NLRP3-inflammsome by stimulation of diesel exhaust particles in lung tissues from emphysema model and RAW 264.7 cell line. Korean J Intern Med. 2017;32:865–74. http://www.ncbi.nlm.nih.gov/pubmed/28814068.

193. Zheng R, Tao L, Jian H, Chang Y, Cheng Y, Feng Y, et al. NLRP3 inflammasome activation and lung fibrosis caused by airborne fine particulate matter. Ecotoxicol Environ Saf. 2018;163:612–9. http://www.ncbi.nlm.nih.gov/pubmed/30092543.
194. Wang H, Lv C, Wang S, Ying H, Weng Y, Yu W. NLRP3 Inflammasome involves in the acute exacerbation of patients with chronic obstructive pulmonary disease. Inflammation. 2018;41:1321–33. http://link.springer.com/10.1007/s10753-018-0780-0.
195. Duvall MG, Bruggemann TR, Levy BD. Bronchoprotective mechanisms for specialized pro-resolving mediators in the resolution of lung inflammation. Mol Aspects Med. 2017;58:44–56. http://www.ncbi.nlm.nih.gov/pubmed/28455109.
196. Chen H, Li Z, Dong L, Wu Y, Shen H, Chen Z. Lipid metabolism in chronic obstructive pulmonary disease. Int J Chron Obstruct Pulmon Dis. 2019;14:1009–18. http://www.ncbi.nlm.nih.gov/pubmed/31190786.
197. Thatcher TH, Woeller CF, McCarthy CE, Sime PJ. Quenching the fires: pro-resolving mediators, air pollution, and smoking. Pharmacol Ther. 2019;197:212–24. http://www.ncbi.nlm.nih.gov/pubmed/30759375.
198. Hsiao H-M, Sapinoro RE, Thatcher TH, Croasdell A, Levy EP, Fulton RA, et al. A novel anti-inflammatory and pro-resolving role for resolvin D1 in acute cigarette smoke-induced lung inflammation. Yildirim AÖ, editor. PLoS One. 2013;8:e58258. http://dx.plos.org/10.1371/journal.pone.0058258.
199. Fritscher LG, Post M, Rodrigues MT, Silverman F, Balter M, Chapman KR, et al. Profile of eicosanoids in breath condensate in asthma and COPD. J Breath Res. 2012;6:026001. http://stacks.iop.org/1752-7163/6/i=2/a=026001?key=crossref.27de5bd610a6465aab9a684512ec18ce.
200. Croasdell A, Thatcher TH, Kottmann RM, Colas RA, Dalli J, Serhan CN, et al. Resolvins attenuate inflammation and promote resolution in cigarette smoke-exposed human macrophages. Am J Physiol Lung Cell Mol Physiol. 2015;309:L888–901. http://ajplung.physiology.org/lookup/doi/10.1152/ajplung.00125.2015.
201. Ftouh S, Lewington A. Acute Kidney Injury Guideline Development Group convened by the National Clinical Guidelines Centre and commissioned by the National Institute for Health and Care Excellence in association with TRC of PC. Prevention, detection and management of acute kidney injury: concise guideline. Clin Med (Northfield IL). 2014;14:61–5. http://www.ncbi.nlm.nih.gov/pubmed/24532748.
202. Uchino S, Bellomo R, Goldsmith D, Bates S, Ronco C. An assessment of the RIFLE criteria for acute renal failure in hospitalized patients. Crit Care Med. 2006;34:1913–7. https://insights.ovid.com/crossref?an=00003246-200607000-00008.
203. Ratanarat R, Skulratanasak P, Tangkawattanakul N, Hantaweepant C. Clinical accuracy of RIFLE and Acute Kidney Injury Network (AKIN) criteria for predicting hospital mortality in critically ill patients with multi-organ dysfunction syndrome. J Med Assoc Thai. 2013;96(Suppl 2):S224–31. http://www.ncbi.nlm.nih.gov/pubmed/23590046.
204. Raup-Konsavage WM, Wang Y, Wang WW, Feliers D, Ruan H, Reeves WB. Neutrophil peptidyl arginine deiminase-4 has a pivotal role in ischemia/reperfusion-induced acute kidney injury. Kidney Int. 2018;93:365–74. http://www.ncbi.nlm.nih.gov/pubmed/29061334.
205. Dellepiane S, Marengo M, Cantaluppi V. Detrimental cross-talk between sepsis and acute kidney injury: new pathogenic mechanisms, early biomarkers and targeted therapies. Crit Care. 2016;20:61. http://ccforum.com/content/20/1/61.
206. Kellum JA, Prowle JR. Paradigms of acute kidney injury in the intensive care setting. Nat Rev Nephrol. 2018;14:217–30. http://www.ncbi.nlm.nih.gov/pubmed/29355173.
207. Raghavan R, Shawar S. Mechanisms of drug-induced interstitial nephritis. Adv Chronic Kidney Dis. 2017;24:64–71. http://www.ncbi.nlm.nih.gov/pubmed/28284381.
208. Markowitz GS, Bomback AS, Perazella MA. Drug-induced glomerular disease: direct cellular injury. Clin J Am Soc Nephrol. 2015;10:1291–9. http://www.ncbi.nlm.nih.gov/pubmed/25862776.
209. Khan S, Loi V, Rosner MH. Drug-induced kidney injury in the elderly. Drugs Aging. 2017;34:729–41. http://link.springer.com/10.1007/s40266-017-0484-4.

210. Wu H, Huang J. Drug-induced nephrotoxicity: pathogenic mechanisms, biomarkers and prevention strategies. Curr Drug Metab. 2018;19:559–67. http://www.ncbi.nlm.nih.gov/pubmed/29119923.
211. Linkermann A, Chen G, Dong G, Kunzendorf U, Krautwald S, Dong Z. Regulated cell death in AKI. J Am Soc Nephrol. 2014;25:2689–701. http://www.jasn.org/cgi/doi/10.1681/ASN.2014030262.
212. Linkermann A, Bräsen JH, Darding M, Jin MK, Sanz AB, Heller J-O, et al. Two independent pathways of regulated necrosis mediate ischemia-reperfusion injury. Proc Natl Acad Sci U S A. 2013;110:12024–9. http://www.pnas.org/cgi/doi/10.1073/pnas.1305538110.
213. von Mässenhausen A, Tonnus W, Linkermann A. Cell death pathways drive necroinflammation during acute kidney injury. Nephron. 2018;140(2):144–7. http://www.ncbi.nlm.nih.gov/pubmed/29961062.
214. Anders H-J. Necroptosis in acute kidney injury. Nephron. 2018;139:342–8. http://www.ncbi.nlm.nih.gov/pubmed/29852497.
215. Linkermann A, Stockwell BR, Krautwald S, Anders H-J. Regulated cell death and inflammation: an auto-amplification loop causes organ failure. Nat Rev Immunol. 2014;14:759–67. http://www.nature.com/articles/nri3743.
216. Mulay SR, Linkermann A, Anders H-J. Necroinflammation in kidney disease. J Am Soc Nephrol. 2016;27:27–39. http://www.ncbi.nlm.nih.gov/pubmed/26334031.
217. Letteri JM. Post traumatic acute renal failure. Adv Exp Med Biol. 1987;212:211–8. http://www.ncbi.nlm.nih.gov/pubmed/3303851.
218. Menashe PI, Ross SA, Gottlieb JE. Acquired renal insufficiency in critically ill patients. Crit Care Med. 1988;16:1106–9. http://www.ncbi.nlm.nih.gov/pubmed/3168503.
219. Stene JK. Renal failure in the trauma patient. Crit Care Clin. 1990;6:111–9. http://www.ncbi.nlm.nih.gov/pubmed/2404542.
220. de Abreu KLS, Silva Júnior GB, Barreto AGC, Melo FM, Oliveira BB, Mota RMS, et al. Acute kidney injury after trauma: prevalence, clinical characteristics and RIFLE classification. Indian J Crit Care Med. 2010;14:121–8. http://www.ijccm.org/text.asp?2010/14/3/121/74170.
221. Makris K, Spanou L. Acute kidney injury: definition, pathophysiology and clinical phenotypes. Clin Biochem Rev. 2016;37:85–98. http://www.ncbi.nlm.nih.gov/pubmed/28303073.
222. Sun Y, Johnson C, Zhou J, Wang L, Li Y-F, Lu Y, et al. Uremic toxins are conditional danger- or shomeostasis-associated molecular patterns. Front Biosci (Landmark Ed). 2018;23:348–87. http://www.ncbi.nlm.nih.gov/pubmed/28930551.
223. Mulay SR, Kumar SV, Lech M, Desai J, Anders H-J. How kidney cell death induces renal necroinflammation. Semin Nephrol. 2016;36:162–73. https://linkinghub.elsevier.com/retrieve/pii/S0270929516000243.
224. Sharfuddin AA, Molitoris BA. Pathophysiology of ischemic acute kidney injury. Nat Rev Nephrol. 2011;7:189–200. http://www.ncbi.nlm.nih.gov/pubmed/21364518.
225. Bonventre JV, Yang L. Cellular pathophysiology of ischemic acute kidney injury. J Clin Invest. 2011;121:4210–21. http://www.jci.org/articles/view/45161.
226. Kanagasundaram NS. Pathophysiology of ischaemic acute kidney injury. Ann Clin Biochem. 2015;52:193–205. http://www.ncbi.nlm.nih.gov/pubmed/25293591.
227. Akcay A, Nguyen Q, Edelstein CL. Mediators of inflammation in acute kidney injury. Mediators Inflamm. 2009;2009:1–12. http://www.ncbi.nlm.nih.gov/pubmed/20182538.
228. Lee DW, Faubel S, Edelstein CL. Cytokines in acute kidney injury (AKI). Clin Nephrol. 2011;76:165–73. http://www.ncbi.nlm.nih.gov/pubmed/21888852.
229. Han HI, Skvarca LB, Espiritu EB, Davidson AJ, Hukriede NA. The role of macrophages during acute kidney injury: destruction and repair. Pediatr Nephrol. 2019;34:561–9. http://link.springer.com/10.1007/s00467-017-3883-1.
230. Wang J, Djudjaj S, Gibbert L, Lennartz V, Breitkopf DM, Rauen T, et al. YB-1 orchestrates onset and resolution of renal inflammation via IL10 gene regulation. J Cell Mol Med. 2017;21:3494–505. http://doi.wiley.com/10.1111/jcmm.13260.
231. Bernhardt A, Fehr A, Brandt S, Jerchel S, Ballhause TM, Philipsen L, et al. Inflammatory cell infiltration and resolution of kidney inflammation is orchestrated by the cold-shock pro-

tein Y-box binding protein-1. Kidney Int. 2017;92:1157–77. https://linkinghub.elsevier.com/retrieve/pii/S0085253817302405.
232. Dessing MC, Pulskens WP, Teske GJ, Butter LM, van der Poll T, Yang H, et al. RAGE does not contribute to renal injury and damage upon ischemia/reperfusion-induced injury. J Innate Immun. 2012;4:80–5. http://www.ncbi.nlm.nih.gov/pubmed/22067944.
233. Li J, Gong Q, Zhong S, Wang L, Guo H, Xiang Y, et al. Neutralization of the extracellular HMGB1 released by ischaemic damaged renal cells protects against renal ischaemia-reperfusion injury. Nephrol Dial Transplant. 2011;26:469–78. https://academic.oup.com/ndt/article-lookup/doi/10.1093/ndt/gfq466.
234. Wu H, Steenstra R, de Boer ECS, Zhao CY, Ma J, van der Stelt JM, et al. Preconditioning with recombinant high-mobility group box 1 protein protects the kidney against ischemia–reperfusion injury in mice. Kidney Int. 2014;85:824–32. http://www.ncbi.nlm.nih.gov/pubmed/24352152.
235. González-Guerrero C, Cannata-Ortiz P, Guerri C, Egido J, Ortiz A, Ramos AM. TLR4-mediated inflammation is a key pathogenic event leading to kidney damage and fibrosis in cyclosporine nephrotoxicity. Arch Toxicol. 2017;91:1925–39. http://www.ncbi.nlm.nih.gov/pubmed/27585667.
236. Park HS, Kim EN, Kim MY, Lim JH, Kim HW, Park CW, et al. The protective effect of neutralizing high-mobility group box1 against chronic cyclosporine nephrotoxicity in mice. Transpl Immunol. 2016;34:42–9. http://www.ncbi.nlm.nih.gov/pubmed/26603313.
237. Kim J. Poly(ADP-ribose) polymerase activation induces high mobility group box 1 release from proximal tubular cells during cisplatin nephrotoxicity. Physiol Res. 2016;65:333–40. http://www.ncbi.nlm.nih.gov/pubmed/26447520.
238. Tan X, Zheng X, Huang Z, Lin J, Xie C, Lin Y. Involvement of S100A8/A9-TLR4-NLRP3 inflammasome pathway in contrast-induced acute kidney injury. Cell Physiol Biochem. 2017;43:209–22. https://www.karger.com/Article/FullText/480340.
239. Westhoff JH, Seibert FS, Waldherr S, Bauer F, Tönshoff B, Fichtner A, et al. Urinary calprotectin, kidney injury molecule-1, and neutrophil gelatinase-associated lipocalin for the prediction of adverse outcome in pediatric acute kidney injury. Eur J Pediatr. 2017;176:745–55. http://www.ncbi.nlm.nih.gov/pubmed/28409285.
240. Azimi A. Could "calprotectin" and "endocan" serve as "tsroponin of nephrologists"? Med Hypotheses. 2017;99:29–34. http://www.ncbi.nlm.nih.gov/pubmed/28110693.
241. Brooks C, Wei Q, Cho S-G, Dong Z. Regulation of mitochondrial dynamics in acute kidney injury in cell culture and rodent models. J Clin Invest. 2009;119:1275–85. http://www.jci.org/articles/view/37829.
242. Ho PW-L, Pang W-F, Luk CC-W, Ng JK-C, Chow K-M, Kwan BC-H, et al. Urinary mitochondrial DNA level as a biomarker of acute kidney injury severity. Kidney Dis. 2017;3:78–83. http://www.ncbi.nlm.nih.gov/pubmed/28868295.
243. Zhang Q, Raoof M, Chen Y, Sumi Y, Sursal T, Junger W, et al. Circulating mitochondrial DAMPs cause inflammatory responses to injury. Nature. 2010;464:104–7. http://www.nature.com/articles/nature08780.
244. Emma F, Montini G, Parikh SM, Salviati L. Mitochondrial dysfunction in inherited renal disease and acute kidney injury. Nat Rev Nephrol. 2016;12:267–80. http://www.nature.com/articles/nrneph.2015.214.
245. Allam R, Scherbaum CR, Darisipudi MN, Mulay SR, Hägele H, Lichtnekert J, et al. Histones from dying renal cells aggravate kidney injury via TLR2 and TLR4. J Am Soc Nephrol. 2012;23:1375–88. http://www.jasn.org/cgi/doi/10.1681/ASN.2011111077.
246. Nakazawa D, Kumar SV, Marschner J, Desai J, Holderied A, Rath L, et al. Histones and neutrophil extracellular traps enhance tubular necrosis and remote organ injury in ischemic AKI. J Am Soc Nephrol. 2017;28:1753–68. http://www.jasn.org/lookup/doi/10.1681/ASN.2016080925.
247. Silk E, Zhao H, Weng H, Ma D. The role of extracellular histone in organ injury. Cell Death Dis. 2017;8:e2812. http://www.ncbi.nlm.nih.gov/pubmed/28542146.

248. Rosin DL, Okusa MD. Dying cells and extracellular histones in AKI: beyond a NET effect? J Am Soc Nephrol. 2012;23:1275–7. http://www.jasn.org/cgi/doi/10.1681/ASN.2012060615.
249. Devuyst O, Olinger E, Rampoldi L. Uromodulin: from physiology to rare and complex kidney disorders. Nat Rev Nephrol. 2017;13:525–44. http://www.ncbi.nlm.nih.gov/pubmed/28781372.
250. Anders H-J, Schaefer L. Beyond tissue injury-damage-associated molecular patterns, Toll-like receptors, and inflammasomes also drive regeneration and fibrosis. J Am Soc Nephrol. 2014;25:1387–400. http://www.ncbi.nlm.nih.gov/pubmed/24762401.
251. Säemann MD, Weichhart T, Zeyda M, Staffler G, Schunn M, Stuhlmeier KM, et al. Tamm-Horsfall glycoprotein links innate immune cell activation with adaptive immunity via a Toll-like receptor-4-dependent mechanism. J Clin Invest. 2005;115:468–75. http://www.ncbi.nlm.nih.gov/pubmed/15650774.
252. Darisipudi MN, Thomasova D, Mulay SR, Brech D, Noessner E, Liapis H, et al. Uromodulin triggers IL-1β-dependent innate immunity via the NLRP3 inflammasome. J Am Soc Nephrol. 2012;23:1783–9. http://www.jasn.org/cgi/doi/10.1681/ASN.2012040338.
253. Wu T-H, Li K-J, Yu C-L, Tsai C-Y. Tamm–Horsfall protein is a potent immunomodulatory molecule and a disease biomarker in the urinary system. Molecules. 2018;23:200. http://www.ncbi.nlm.nih.gov/pubmed/29361765.
254. Mulay SR, Shi C, Ma X, Anders HJ. Novel Insights into crystal-induced kidney injury. Kidney Dis. 2018;4:49–57. http://www.ncbi.nlm.nih.gov/pubmed/29998119.
255. Mulay SR, Kulkarni OP, Rupanagudi KV, Migliorini A, Darisipudi MN, Vilaysane A, et al. Calcium oxalate crystals induce renal inflammation by NLRP3-mediated IL-1β secretion. J Clin Invest. 2013;123:236–46. http://www.jci.org/articles/view/63679.
256. Wu J, Ren J, Liu Q, Hu Q, Wu X, Wang G, et al. Effects of changes in the levels of damage-associated molecular patterns following continuous veno–venous hemofiltration therapy on outcomes in acute kidney injury patients with sepsis. Front Immunol. 2019;9:3052. http://www.ncbi.nlm.nih.gov/pubmed/30666251.
257. Araujo LP, Truzzi RR, Mendes GE, Luz MAM, Burdmann EA, Oliani SM. Interaction of the anti-inflammatory annexin A1 protein and tacrolimus immunosuppressant in the renal function of rats. Am J Nephrol. 2010;31:527–33. http://www.ncbi.nlm.nih.gov/pubmed/20484890.
258. Facio FN, Sena AA, Araújo LP, Mendes GE, Castro I, Luz MAM, et al. Annexin 1 mimetic peptide protects against renal ischemia/reperfusion injury in rats. J Mol Med. 2011;89:51–63. http://www.ncbi.nlm.nih.gov/pubmed/20953576.
259. Araujo LP, Truzzi RR, Mendes GEF, Luz MAM, Burdmann EA, Oliani SM. Annexin A1 protein attenuates cyclosporine-induced renal hemodynamics changes and macrophage infiltration in rats. Inflamm Res. 2012;61:189–96. http://www.ncbi.nlm.nih.gov/pubmed/22101490.
260. Luo R, Kakizoe Y, Wang F, Fan X, Hu S, Yang T, et al. Deficiency of mPGES-1 exacerbates renal fibrosis and inflammation in mice with unilateral ureteral obstruction. Am J Physiol Physiol. 2017;312:F121–33. http://www.ncbi.nlm.nih.gov/pubmed/27784694.
261. Bauerle JD, Grenz A, Kim J-H, Lee HT, Eltzschig HK. Adenosine generation and signaling during acute kidney injury. J Am Soc Nephrol. 2011;22:14–20. http://www.ncbi.nlm.nih.gov/pubmed/21209250.
262. Venkatachalam MA, Weinberg JM, Kriz W, Bidani AK. Failed tubule recovery, AKI-CKD transition, and kidney disease progression. J Am Soc Nephrol. 2015;26:1765–76. http://www.ncbi.nlm.nih.gov/pubmed/25810494.
263. Romagnani P, Remuzzi G, Glassock R, Levin A, Jager KJ, Tonelli M, et al. Chronic kidney disease. Nat Rev Dis Primers. 2017;3:17088. http://www.ncbi.nlm.nih.gov/pubmed/29168475.
264. Nogueira A, Pires MJ, Oliveira P. Pathophysiological mechanisms of renal fibrosis: a review of animal models and therapeutic strategies. In Vivo (Brooklyn). 2017;31:1–22. http://www.ncbi.nlm.nih.gov/pubmed/28064215.
265. Higashi AY, Aronow BJ, Dressler GR. Expression profiling of fibroblasts in chronic and acute disease models reveals novel pathways in kidney fibrosis. J Am Soc Nephrol. 2019;30:80–94. http://www.ncbi.nlm.nih.gov/pubmed/30545984.

266. Yuan Q, Tan RJ, Liu Y. Myofibroblast in kidney fibrosis: origin, activation, and regulation. Adv Exp Med Biol. 2019;1165:253–83. http://www.ncbi.nlm.nih.gov/pubmed/31399969.
267. Tang PM-K, Nikolic-Paterson DJ, Lan H-Y. Macrophages: versatile players in renal inflammation and fibrosis. Nat Rev Nephrol. 2019;15:144–58. http://www.nature.com/articles/s41581-019-0110-2.
268. Zhan J, Wang K, Zhang C, Zhang C, Li Y, Zhang Y, et al. GSPE inhibits HMGB1 release, attenuating renal IR-induced acute renal injury and chronic renal fibrosis. Int J Mol Sci. 2016;17:1647. http://www.ncbi.nlm.nih.gov/pubmed/27690015.
269. Lynch J, Nolan S, Slattery C, Feighery R, Ryan MP, McMorrow T. High-mobility group box protein 1: a novel mediator of inflammatory-induced renal epithelial-mesenchymal transition. Am J Nephrol. 2010;32:590–602. https://www.karger.com/Article/FullText/320485.
270. Zhang M, Guo Y, Fu H, Hu S, Pan J, Wang Y, et al. Chop deficiency prevents UUO-induced renal fibrosis by attenuating fibrotic signals originated from Hmgb1/TLR4/NFκB/IL-1β signaling. Cell Death Dis. 2015;6:e1847. http://www.ncbi.nlm.nih.gov/pubmed/26247732.
271. Tammaro A, Florquin S, Brok M, Claessen N, Butter LM, Teske GJD, et al. S100A8/A9 promotes parenchymal damage and renal fibrosis in obstructive nephropathy. Clin Exp Immunol. 2018;193:361–75. http://www.ncbi.nlm.nih.gov/pubmed/29746703.
272. Li L, Tang W, Yi F. Role of inflammasome in chronic kidney disease. Adv Exp Med Biol. 2019;1165:407–21. http://link.springer.com/10.1007/978-981-13-8871-2_19.
273. Mulay SR, Anders H-J. Crystal nephropathies: mechanisms of crystal-induced kidney injury. Nat Rev Nephrol. 2017;13:226–40. http://www.nature.com/articles/nrneph.2017.10.
274. Komada T, Usui F, Shirasuna K, Kawashima A, Kimura H, Karasawa T, et al. ASC in renal collecting duct epithelial cells contributes to inflammation and injury after unilateral ureteral obstruction. Am J Pathol. 2014;184:1287–98. https://linkinghub.elsevier.com/retrieve/pii/S000294401400087X.
275. Komada T, Chung H, Lau A, Platnich JM, Beck PL, Benediktsson H, et al. Macrophage uptake of necrotic cell DNA activates the AIM2 inflammasome to regulate a proinflammatory phenotype in CKD. J Am Soc Nephrol. 2018;29:1165–81. http://www.jasn.org/lookup/doi/10.1681/ASN.2017080863.
276. Neymeyer H, Labes R, Reverte V, Saez F, Stroh T, Dathe C, et al. Activation of annexin A1 signalling in renal fibroblasts exerts antifibrotic effects. Acta Physiol. 2015;215:144–58. http://www.ncbi.nlm.nih.gov/pubmed/26332853.
277. Zhao S, Shen Z, Gao B, Han P. microRNA-206 overexpression inhibits epithelial-mesenchymal transition and glomerulosclerosis in rats with chronic kidney disease by inhibiting JAK/STAT signaling pathway. J Cell Biochem. 2019;120:jcb.28722. http://www.ncbi.nlm.nih.gov/pubmed/31148248.
278. Fontecha-Barriuso M, Martin-Sanchez D, Ruiz-Andres O, Poveda J, Sanchez-Niño MD, Valiño-Rivas L, et al. Targeting epigenetic DNA and histone modifications to treat kidney disease. Nephrol Dial Transplant. 2018;33(11):1875–86. http://www.ncbi.nlm.nih.gov/pubmed/29534238.
279. Chakraborty A, Viswanathan P. Methylation-demethylation dynamics: implications of changes in acute kidney injury. Anal Cell Pathol. 2018;2018:1–16. http://www.ncbi.nlm.nih.gov/pubmed/30073137.
280. Tang J, Zhuang S. Histone acetylation and DNA methylation in ischemia/reperfusion injury. Clin Sci. 2019;133:597–609. http://www.ncbi.nlm.nih.gov/pubmed/30804072.
281. Morgado-Pascual JL, Marchant V, Rodrigues-Diez R, Dolade N, Suarez-Alvarez B, Kerr B, et al. Epigenetic modification mechanisms involved in inflammation and fibrosis in renal pathology. Mediators Inflamm. 2018;2018:1–14. http://www.ncbi.nlm.nih.gov/pubmed/30647531.
282. Bower WA, Johns M, Margolis HS, Williams IT, Bell BP. Population-based surveillance for acute liver failure. Am J Gastroenterol. 2007;102:2459–63. http://www.nature.com/doifinder/10.1111/j.1572-0241.2007.01388.x.
283. Bernal W, Wendon J. Acute liver failure. N Engl J Med. 2013;369:2525–34. http://www.ncbi.nlm.nih.gov/pubmed/24369077.

284. Fyfe B, Zaldana F, Liu C. The pathology of acute liver failure. Clin Liver Dis. 2018;22:257–68. https://linkinghub.elsevier.com/retrieve/pii/S1089326118300035.
285. Moreau R. Acute-on-chronic liver failure: a new syndrome in cirrhosis. Clin Mol Hepatol. 2016;22:1–6. http://www.ncbi.nlm.nih.gov/pubmed/27044760.
286. Arroyo V, Moreau R, Kamath PS, Jalan R, Ginès P, Nevens F, et al. Acute-on-chronic liver failure in cirrhosis. Nat Rev Dis Primers. 2016;2:16041. http://www.nature.com/articles/nrdp201641.
287. Nishikawa H, Osaki Y. Liver cirrhosis: evaluation, nutritional status, and prognosis. Mediators Inflamm. 2015;2015:1–9. http://www.ncbi.nlm.nih.gov/pubmed/26494949.
288. Tittarelli R, Pellegrini M, Scarpellini MG, Marinelli E, Bruti V, di Luca NM, et al. Hepatotoxicity of paracetamol and related fatalities. Eur Rev Med Pharmacol Sci. 2017;21:95–101. http://www.ncbi.nlm.nih.gov/pubmed/28379590.
289. Mowry JB, Spyker DA, Brooks DE, McMillan N, Schauben JL. 2014 annual report of the American Association of Poison Control Centers' National Poison Data System (NPDS): 32nd annual report. Clin Toxicol (Phila). 2015;53:962–1147. http://www.ncbi.nlm.nih.gov/pubmed/26624241.
290. Lee WM. Recent developments in acute liver failure. Best Pract Res Clin Gastroenterol. 2012;26:3–16. http://www.ncbi.nlm.nih.gov/pubmed/22482521.
291. Akamatsu N, Sugawara Y, Kokudo N. Acute liver failure and liver transplantation. Intractable Rare Dis Res. 2013;2:77–87. http://www.ncbi.nlm.nih.gov/pubmed/25343108.
292. Bernal W, Lee WM, Wendon J, Larsen FS, Williams R. Acute liver failure: a curable disease by 2024? J Hepatol. 2015;62:S112–20. http://linkinghub.elsevier.com/retrieve/pii/S0168827814009374.
293. Koch DG, Speiser JL, Durkalski V, Fontana RJ, Davern T, McGuire B, et al. The natural history of severe acute liver injury. Am J Gastroenterol. 2017;112:1389–96. http://www.ncbi.nlm.nih.gov/pubmed/28440304.
294. Papadopoulos D, Siempis T, Theodorakou E, Tsoulfas G. Hepatic ischemia and reperfusion injury and trauma: current concepts. Arch trauma Res. 2013;2:63–70. http://archtrauma.kaums.ac.ir/article_62138.html.
295. Schwabe RF, Luedde T. Apoptosis and necroptosis in the liver: a matter of life and death. Nat Rev Gastroenterol Hepatol. 2018;15:738–52. http://www.ncbi.nlm.nih.gov/pubmed/30250076.
296. Tsurusaki S, Tsuchiya Y, Koumura T, Nakasone M, Sakamoto T, Matsuoka M, et al. Hepatic ferroptosis plays an important role as the trigger for initiating inflammation in nonalcoholic steatohepatitis. Cell Death Dis. 2019;10:449. http://www.nature.com/articles/s41419-019-1678-y.
297. Li P, He K, Li J, Liu Z, Gong J. The role of Kupffer cells in hepatic diseases. Mol Immunol. 2017;85:222–9. http://www.ncbi.nlm.nih.gov/pubmed/28314211.
298. Li Z, Weinman S. Regulation of hepatic inflammation via macrophage cell death. Semin Liver Dis. 2018;38:340–50. http://www.ncbi.nlm.nih.gov/pubmed/30357771.
299. Guo H, Xie M, Zhou C, Zheng M. The relevance of pyroptosis in the pathogenesis of liver diseases. Life Sci. 2019;223:69–73. http://www.ncbi.nlm.nih.gov/pubmed/30831126.
300. Iorga A, Dara L, Kaplowitz N. Drug-induced liver injury: cascade of events leading to cell death, apoptosis or necrosis. Int J Mol Sci. 2017;18(5):1018. http://www.ncbi.nlm.nih.gov/pubmed/28486401.
301. Iorga A, Dara L. Cell death in drug-induced liver injury. Adv Pharmacol. 2019;85:31–74. http://www.ncbi.nlm.nih.gov/pubmed/31307591.
302. Jaeschke H, Williams CD, Ramachandran A, Bajt ML. Acetaminophen hepatotoxicity and repair: the role of sterile inflammation and innate immunity. Liver Int. 2012;32:8–20. http://doi.wiley.com/10.1111/j.1478-3231.2011.02501.x.
303. Lancaster EM, Hiatt JR, Zarrinpar A. Acetaminophen hepatotoxicity: an updated review. Arch Toxicol. 2015;89:193–9. http://www.ncbi.nlm.nih.gov/pubmed/25537186.
304. Ramachandran A, Jaeschke H. Acetaminophen hepatotoxicity. Semin Liver Dis. 2019;39:221–34. http://www.thieme-connect.de/DOI/DOI?10.1055/s-0039-1679919.

305. Lee B-W, Jeon B-S, Yoon B-I. Exogenous recombinant human thioredoxin-1 prevents acetaminophen-induced liver injury by scavenging oxidative stressors, restoring the thioredoxin-1 system and inhibiting receptor interacting protein-3 overexpression. J Appl Toxicol. 2018;38:1008–17. http://doi.wiley.com/10.1002/jat.3609.
306. Paridaens A, Raevens S, Colle I, Bogaerts E, Vandewynckel Y-P, Verhelst X, et al. Combination of tauroursodeoxycholic acid and N-acetylcysteine exceeds standard treatment for acetaminophen intoxication. Liver Int. 2017;37:748–56. http://doi.wiley.com/10.1111/liv.13261.
307. Jaeschke H, Duan L, Akakpo JY, Farhood A, Ramachandran A. The role of apoptosis in acetaminophen hepatotoxicity. Food Chem Toxicol. 2018;118:709–18. http://www.ncbi.nlm.nih.gov/pubmed/29920288.
308. Du K, Ramachandran A, Jaeschke H. Oxidative stress during acetaminophen hepatotoxicity: sources, pathophysiological role and therapeutic potential. Redox Biol. 2016;10:148–56. http://www.ncbi.nlm.nih.gov/pubmed/27744120.
309. Lőrincz T, Jemnitz K, Kardon T, Mandl J, Szarka A. Ferroptosis is involved in acetaminophen induced cell death. Pathol Oncol Res. 2015;21:1115–21. http://link.springer.com/10.1007/s12253-015-9946-3.
310. Abdullah Z, Knolle PA. Liver macrophages in healthy and diseased liver. Pflügers Arch - Eur J Physiol. 2017;469:553–60. http://www.ncbi.nlm.nih.gov/pubmed/28293730.
311. Lefkowitch JH. The pathology of acute liver failure. Adv Anat Pathol. 2016;23:144–58. http://www.ncbi.nlm.nih.gov/pubmed/27058243.
312. Li M, Sun X, Zhao J, Xia L, Li J, Xu M, et al. CCL5 deficiency promotes liver repair by improving inflammation resolution and liver regeneration through M2 macrophage polarization. Cell Mol Immunol. 2020;17:753–64. http://www.nature.com/articles/s41423-019-0279-0.
313. Liu J, Zhang S, Cao H, Wang H, Sun C, Liu S, et al. Deficiency of p38α in macrophage ameliorates d-galactosamine/TNF-α-induced acute liver injury in mice. FEBS J. 2017;284:4200–15. http://doi.wiley.com/10.1111/febs.14294.
314. Krawitz S, Lingiah V, Pyrsopoulos NT. Acute liver failure. Clin Liver Dis. 2018;22:243–56. http://www.ncbi.nlm.nih.gov/pubmed/29605064.
315. Rutherford A, Chung RT. Acute liver failure: mechanisms of hepatocyte injury and regeneration. Semin Liver Dis. 2008;28:167–74. http://www.thieme-connect.de/DOI/DOI?10.1055/s-2008-1073116.
316. Hong J-M, Kim S-J, Lee S-M. Role of necroptosis in autophagy signaling during hepatic ischemia and reperfusion. Toxicol Appl Pharmacol. 2016;308:1–10. http://www.ncbi.nlm.nih.gov/pubmed/27521978.
317. Sui M, Jiang X, Chen J, Yang H, Zhu Y. Magnesium isoglycyrrhizinate ameliorates liver fibrosis and hepatic stellate cell activation by regulating ferroptosis signaling pathway. Biomed Pharmacother. 2018;106:125–33. http://www.ncbi.nlm.nih.gov/pubmed/29957462.
318. Al-Khafaji AB, Tohme S, Yazdani HO, Miller D, Huang H, Tsung A. Superoxide induces neutrophil extracellular trap formation in a TLR-4 and NOX-dependent mechanism. Mol Med. 2016;22:1. http://www.ncbi.nlm.nih.gov/pubmed/27453505.
319. Li Z, Zhao F, Cao Y, Zhang J, Shi P, Sun X, et al. DHA attenuates hepatic ischemia reperfusion injury by inhibiting pyroptosis and activating PI3K/Akt pathway. Eur J Pharmacol. 2018;835:1–10. http://www.ncbi.nlm.nih.gov/pubmed/30075219.
320. Zhao H, Huang H, Alam A, Chen Q, Suen KC, Cui J, et al. VEGF mitigates histone-induced pyroptosis in the remote liver injury associated with renal allograft ischemia-reperfusion injury in rats. Am J Transplant. 2018;18:1890–903. http://www.ncbi.nlm.nih.gov/pubmed/29446207.
321. Zhou W-C, Zhang Q-B, Qiao L. Pathogenesis of liver cirrhosis. World J Gastroenterol. 2014;20:7312. http://www.ncbi.nlm.nih.gov/pubmed/24966602.
322. Koyama Y, Brenner DA. Liver inflammation and fibrosis. J Clin Invest. 2017;127:55–64. http://www.ncbi.nlm.nih.gov/pubmed/28045404.
323. Yang R, Tonnesseen TI. DAMPs and sterile inflammation in drug hepatotoxicity. Hepatol Int. 2019;13:42–50. http://www.ncbi.nlm.nih.gov/pubmed/30474802.

324. Yang R, Zou X, Tenhunen J, Tønnessen TI. HMGB1 and extracellular histones significantly contribute to systemic inflammation and multiple organ failure in acute liver failure. Mediators Inflamm. 2017;2017:5928078. https://www.hindawi.com/journals/mi/2017/5928078/.
325. Tsung A, Sahai R, Tanaka H, Nakao A, Fink MP, Lotze MT, et al. The nuclear factor HMGB1 mediates hepatic injury after murine liver ischemia-reperfusion. J Exp Med. 2005;201:1135–43. http://www.jem.org/lookup/doi/10.1084/jem.20042614.
326. Huang H, Tohme S, Al-Khafaji AB, Tai S, Loughran P, Chen L, et al. Damage-associated molecular pattern-activated neutrophil extracellular trap exacerbates sterile inflammatory liver injury. Hepatology. 2015;62:600–14. http://doi.wiley.com/10.1002/hep.27841.
327. Basta G, Del Turco S, Navarra T, Lee WM, Acute Liver Failure Study Group. Circulating levels of soluble receptor for advanced glycation end products and ligands of the receptor for advanced glycation end products in patients with acute liver failure. Liver Transplant. 2015;21:847–54. http://www.ncbi.nlm.nih.gov/pubmed/25825217.
328. Yang R, Zou X, Tenhunen J, Tønnessen TI. HMGB1 and extracellular histones significantly contribute to systemic inflammation and multiple organ failure in acute liver failure. Mediators Inflamm. 2017;2017:1–6. http://www.ncbi.nlm.nih.gov/pubmed/28694564.
329. Yang R, Zhang S, Cotoia A, Oksala N, Zhu S, Tenhunen J. High mobility group B1 impairs hepatocyte regeneration in acetaminophen hepatotoxicity. BMC Gastroenterol. 2012;12:45. http://bmcgastroenterol.biomedcentral.com/articles/10.1186/1471-230X-12-45.
330. Lundbäck P, Lea JD, Sowinska A, Ottosson L, Fürst CM, Steen J, et al. A novel high mobility group box 1 neutralizing chimeric antibody attenuates drug-induced liver injury and postinjury inflammation in mice. Hepatology. 2016;64:1699–710. http://doi.wiley.com/10.1002/hep.28736.
331. Martin-Murphy BV, Holt MP, Ju C. The role of damage associated molecular pattern molecules in acetaminophen-induced liver injury in mice. Toxicol Lett. 2010;192:387–94. http://www.ncbi.nlm.nih.gov/pubmed/19931603.
332. Lea JD, Clarke JI, McGuire N, Antoine DJ. Redox-dependent HMGB1 isoforms as pivotal co-ordinators of drug-induced liver injury: mechanistic biomarkers and therapeutic targets. Antioxid Redox Signal. 2016;24:652–65. http://www.liebertpub.com/doi/10.1089/ars.2015.6406.
333. Dear JW, Clarke JI, Francis B, Allen L, Wraight J, Shen J, et al. Risk stratification after paracetamol overdose using mechanistic biomarkers: results from two prospective cohort studies lancet. Gastroenterol Hepatol. 2018;3:104–13. https://linkinghub.elsevier.com/retrieve/pii/S2468125317302662.
334. Antoine DJ, Jenkins RE, Dear JW, Williams DP, McGill MR, Sharpe MR, et al. Molecular forms of HMGB1 and keratin-18 as mechanistic biomarkers for mode of cell death and prognosis during clinical acetaminophen hepatotoxicity. J Hepatol. 2012;56:1070–9. https://linkinghub.elsevier.com/retrieve/pii/S0168827812000591.
335. Yamamoto T, Tajima Y. HMGB1 is a promising therapeutic target for acute liver failure. Expert Rev Gastroenterol Hepatol. 2017;11:673–82. http://www.ncbi.nlm.nih.gov/pubmed/28657371.
336. Wen Z, Liu Y, Li F, Ren F, Chen D, Li X, et al. Circulating histones exacerbate inflammation in mice with acute liver failure. J Cell Biochem. 2013;114:2384–91. http://doi.wiley.com/10.1002/jcb.24588.
337. Xu J, Zhang X, Monestier M, Esmon NL, Esmon CT. Extracellular histones are mediators of death through TLR2 and TLR4 in mouse fatal liver injury. J Immunol. 2011;187:2626–31. http://www.jimmunol.org/cgi/doi/10.4049/jimmunol.1003930.
338. Huang H, Chen H-W, Evankovich J, Yan W, Rosborough BR, Nace GW, et al. Histones activate the NLRP3 inflammasome in Kupffer cells during sterile inflammatory liver injury. J Immunol. 2013;191:2665–79. http://www.jimmunol.org/cgi/doi/10.4049/jimmunol.1202733.
339. Wen Z, Lei Z, Yao L, Jiang P, Gu T, Ren F, et al. Circulating histones are major mediators of systemic inflammation and cellular injury in patients with acute liver failure. Cell Death Dis. 2016;7:e2391. http://www.ncbi.nlm.nih.gov/pubmed/27685635.

340. Hayase N, Doi K, Hiruma T, Inokuchi R, Hamasaki Y, Noiri E, et al. Damage-associated molecular patterns in intensive care unit patients with acute liver injuries. Medicine (Baltimore). 2018;97:e12780. http://www.ncbi.nlm.nih.gov/pubmed/30313098.
341. McGill MR, Sharpe MR, Williams CD, Taha M, Curry SC, Jaeschke H. The mechanism underlying acetaminophen-induced hepatotoxicity in humans and mice involves mitochondrial damage and nuclear DNA fragmentation. J Clin Invest. 2012;122:1574–83. http://www.jci.org/articles/view/59755.
342. Marques PE, Oliveira AG, Pereira RV, David BA, Gomides LF, Saraiva AM, et al. Hepatic DNA deposition drives drug-induced liver injury and inflammation in mice. Hepatology. 2015;61:348–60. http://doi.wiley.com/10.1002/hep.27216.
343. Kono H, Chen C-J, Ontiveros F, Rock KL. Uric acid promotes an acute inflammatory response to sterile cell death in mice. J Clin Invest. 2010;120:1939–49. http://www.jci.org/articles/view/40124.
344. Hoque R, Sohail MA, Salhanick S, Malik AF, Ghani A, Robson SC, et al. P2X7 receptor-mediated purinergic signaling promotes liver injury in acetaminophen hepatotoxicity in mice. Am J Physiol Gastrointest Liver Physiol. 2012;302:G1171–9. http://www.physiology.org/doi/10.1152/ajpgi.00352.2011.
345. Amaral SS, Oliveira AG, Marques PE, Quintão JLD, Pires DA, Resende RR, et al. Altered responsiveness to extracellular ATP enhances acetaminophen hepatotoxicity. Cell Commun Signal. 2013;11:10. http://biosignaling.biomedcentral.com/articles/10.1186/1478-811X-11-10.
346. Xie Y, Woolbright BL, Kos M, McGill MR, Dorko K, Kumer SC, et al. Lack of direct cytotoxicity of extracellular ATP against hepatocytes: role in the mechanism of acetaminophen hepatotoxicity. J Clin Transl Res. 2015;1:100–6. http://www.ncbi.nlm.nih.gov/pubmed/26722668.
347. Locatelli I, Sutti S, Jindal A, Vacchiano M, Bozzola C, Reutelingsperger C, et al. Endogenous annexin A1 is a novel protective determinant in nonalcoholic steatohepatitis in mice. Hepatology. 2014;60:531–44. http://www.ncbi.nlm.nih.gov/pubmed/24668763.
348. Quiroga J, Prieto J. Liver cytoprotection by prostaglandins. Pharmacol Ther. 1993;58:67–91. http://www.ncbi.nlm.nih.gov/pubmed/8415874.
349. O'Brien A, China L, Massey KA, Nicolaou A, Winstanley A, Newson J, et al. Bile duct-ligated mice exhibit multiple phenotypic similarities to acute decompensation patients despite histological differences. Liver Int. 2016;36:837–46. http://www.ncbi.nlm.nih.gov/pubmed/26012885.
350. Yao L, Chen W, Song K, Han C, Gandhi CR, Lim K, et al. 15-hydroxyprostaglandin dehydrogenase (15-PGDH) prevents lipopolysaccharide (LPS)-induced acute liver injury. Mohanraj R, editor. PLoS One. 2017;12:e0176106. http://www.ncbi.nlm.nih.gov/pubmed/28423012.
351. Erceg D, Kelava T, Cavar I, Pasalić M, Culo F. The effect of cyclic adenosine monophosphate (cAMP) on acute liver toxicity in mice induced by D-galactosamine and lipopolysaccharide. Coll Antropol. 2010;34(Suppl 1):273–7. http://www.ncbi.nlm.nih.gov/pubmed/20402332.
352. Kang J-W, Lee S-M. Resolvin D1 protects the liver from ischemia/reperfusion injury by enhancing M2 macrophage polarization and efferocytosis. Biochim Biophys Acta - Mol Cell Biol Lipids. 1861;2016:1025–35. http://www.ncbi.nlm.nih.gov/pubmed/27317426.
353. Hangai S, Ao T, Kimura Y, Matsuki K, Kawamura T, Negishi H, et al. PGE2 induced in and released by dying cells functions as an inhibitory DAMP. Proc Natl Acad Sci. 2016;113:3844–9. http://www.ncbi.nlm.nih.gov/pubmed/27001836.
354. Dadhania VP, Muskhelishvili L, Latendresse JR, Mehendale HM. Hepatic overexpression of annexin A1 and A2 in thioacetamide-primed mice protects them against acetaminophen-induced liver failure and death. Int J Toxicol. 2016;35:654–65. http://journals.sagepub.com/doi/10.1177/1091581816659067.
355. Yang X, Zhan Y, Sun Q, Xu X, Kong Y, Zhang J. Adenosine 5′-monophosphate blocks acetaminophen toxicity by increasing ubiquitination-mediated ASK1 degradation. Oncotarget. 2017;8:6273–82. http://www.ncbi.nlm.nih.gov/pubmed/28031524.
356. Wiegand J, Berg T. The etiology, diagnosis and prevention of liver cirrhosis: part 1 of a series on liver cirrhosis. Dtsch Arztebl Int. 2013;110:85–91. https://www.aerzteblatt.de/10.3238/arztebl.2013.0085.

357. Moreau R, Jalan R, Gines P, Pavesi M, Angeli P, Cordoba J, et al. Acute-on-chronic liver failure is a distinct syndrome that develops in patients with acute decompensation of cirrhosis. Gastroenterology. 2013;144:1426–37, 1437.e1-9. https://linkinghub.elsevier.com/retrieve/pii/S0016508513002916.
358. Moreau R. The pathogenesis of ACLF: the inflammatory response and immune function. Semin Liver Dis. 2016;36:133–40. http://www.ncbi.nlm.nih.gov/pubmed/27172355.
359. Gustot T, Fernandez J, Garcia E, Morando F, Caraceni P, Alessandria C, et al. Clinical course of acute-on-chronic liver failure syndrome and effects on prognosis. Hepatology. 2015;62:243–52. http://doi.wiley.com/10.1002/hep.27849.
360. Clària J, Arroyo V, Moreau R. The acute-on-chronic liver failure syndrome, or when the innate immune system goes astray. J Immunol. 2016;197:3755–61. http://www.jimmunol.org/lookup/doi/10.4049/jimmunol.1600818.
361. Cai C, Zhu X, Li P, Li J, Gong J, Shen W, et al. NLRP3 deletion inhibits the non-alcoholic steatohepatitis development and inflammation in Kupffer cells induced by palmitic acid. Inflammation. 2017;40:1875–83. http://www.ncbi.nlm.nih.gov/pubmed/28730512.
362. Zhang W-J, Fang Z-M, Liu W-Q. NLRP3 inflammasome activation from Kupffer cells is involved in liver fibrosis of Schistosoma japonicum-infected mice via NF-κB. Parasit Vectors. 2019;12:29. http://www.ncbi.nlm.nih.gov/pubmed/30635040.
363. Ma X, Zheng X, Pan L, Zhang X. NLRP3 inflammasome activation in liver cirrhotic patients. Biochem Biophys Res Commun. 2018;505:40–4. http://www.ncbi.nlm.nih.gov/pubmed/30236988.
364. Tsuchida T, Friedman SL. Mechanisms of hepatic stellate cell activation. Nat Rev Gastroenterol Hepatol. 2017;14:397–411. http://www.nature.com/articles/nrgastro.2017.38.
365. Ebrahimi H, Naderian M, Sohrabpour AA. New concepts on reversibility and targeting of liver fibrosis; a review article. Middle East J Dig Dis. 2018;10:133–48. http://www.ncbi.nlm.nih.gov/pubmed/30186577.
366. Parola M, Pinzani M. Liver fibrosis: pathophysiology, pathogenetic targets and clinical issues. Mol Aspects Med. 2019;65:37–55. http://www.ncbi.nlm.nih.gov/pubmed/30213667.
367. Kao Y-H, Jawan B, Goto S, Hung C-T, Lin Y-C, Nakano T, et al. High-mobility group box 1 protein activates hepatic stellate cells in vitro. Transplant Proc. 2008;40:2704–5. http://www.ncbi.nlm.nih.gov/pubmed/18929840.
368. Gaskell H, Ge X, Nieto N. High-mobility group box-1 and liver disease. Hepatol Commun. 2018;2:1005–20. http://www.ncbi.nlm.nih.gov/pubmed/30202816.
369. Ge X, Arriazu E, Magdaleno F, Antoine DJ, dela Cruz R, Theise N, et al. High mobility group box-1 drives fibrosis progression signaling via the receptor for advanced glycation end products in mice. Hepatology. 2018;68:2380–404. http://www.ncbi.nlm.nih.gov/pubmed/29774570.
370. Chen L, Li J, Zhang J, Dai C, Liu X, Wang J, et al. S100A4 promotes liver fibrosis via activation of hepatic stellate cells. J Hepatol. 2015;62:156–64. http://www.ncbi.nlm.nih.gov/pubmed/25111176.
371. Jiang S, Zhang Y, Zheng J-H, Li X, Yao Y-L, Wu Y-L, et al. Potentiation of hepatic stellate cell activation by extracellular ATP is dependent on P2X7R-mediated NLRP3 inflammasome activation. Pharmacol Res. 2017;117:82–93. http://www.ncbi.nlm.nih.gov/pubmed/27940204.
372. Yaping Z, Ying W, Luqin D, Ning T, Xuemei A, Xixian Y. Mechanism of interleukin-1β-induced proliferation in rat hepatic stellate cells from different levels of signal transduction. APMIS. 2014;122:392–8. http://www.ncbi.nlm.nih.gov/pubmed/23992404.
373. Xu F, Liu C, Zhou D, Zhang L. TGF-β/SMAD pathway and its regulation in hepatic fibrosis. J Histochem Cytochem. 2016;64:157–67. http://www.ncbi.nlm.nih.gov/pubmed/26747705.
374. Musso G, Gambino R, Cassader M, Paschetta E, Sircana A. Specialized proresolving mediators: enhancing nonalcoholic steatohepatitis and fibrosis resolution. Trends Pharmacol Sci. 2018;39:387–401. https://linkinghub.elsevier.com/retrieve/pii/S0165614718300269.
375. Jung YK, Yim HJ. Reversal of liver cirrhosis: current evidence and expectations. Korean J Intern Med. 2017;32:213–28. http://kjim.org/journal/view.php?doi=10.3904/kjim.2016.268.

376. Poznyak V, Rekve DE. WHO | Global status report on alcohol and health 2018. WHO World Health Organization. 2018. https://www.who.int/substance_abuse/publications/global_alcohol_report/en/.
377. Lieber C. Alcoholic liver disease: new insights in pathogenesis lead to new treatments. J Hepatol. 2000;32:113–28. http://www.ncbi.nlm.nih.gov/pubmed/10728799.
378. Osna NA, Donohue TM, Kharbanda KK. Alcoholic liver disease: pathogenesis and current management. Alcohol Res. 2017;38:147–61. http://www.ncbi.nlm.nih.gov/pubmed/28988570.
379. Miniño AM, Heron MP, Smith BL. Deaths: preliminary data for 2004. Natl Vital Stat Rep. 2006;54:1–49. http://www.ncbi.nlm.nih.gov/pubmed/16850709.
380. Stickel F, Datz C, Hampe J, Bataller R. Pathophysiology and management of alcoholic liver disease: update 2016. Gut Liver. 2017;11:173–88. http://www.ncbi.nlm.nih.gov/pubmed/28274107.
381. Parlesak A, Schäfer C, Schütz T, Bode JC, Bode C. Increased intestinal permeability to macromolecules and endotoxemia in patients with chronic alcohol abuse in different stages of alcohol-induced liver disease. J Hepatol. 2000;32:742–7. http://www.ncbi.nlm.nih.gov/pubmed/10845660.
382. Rao R. Endotoxemia and gut barrier dysfunction in alcoholic liver disease. Hepatology. 2009;50:638–44. http://doi.wiley.com/10.1002/hep.23009.
383. Hartmann P, Seebauer CT, Schnabl B. Alcoholic liver disease: the gut microbiome and liver cross talk. Alcohol Clin Exp Res. 2015;39:763–75. http://doi.wiley.com/10.1111/acer.12704.
384. Tripathi A, Debelius J, Brenner DA, Karin M, Loomba R, Schnabl B, et al. The gut–liver axis and the intersection with the microbiome. Nat Rev Gastroenterol Hepatol. 2018;15:397–411. http://www.ncbi.nlm.nih.gov/pubmed/29748586.
385. Wang S, Pacher P, De Lisle RC, Huang H, Ding W-X. A mechanistic review of cell death in alcohol-induced liver injury. Alcohol Clin Exp Res. 2016;40:1215–23. http://www.ncbi.nlm.nih.gov/pubmed/27130888.
386. Gao B, Ahmad MF, Nagy LE, Tsukamoto H. Inflammatory pathways in alcoholic steatohepatitis. J Hepatol. 2019;70:249–59. http://www.ncbi.nlm.nih.gov/pubmed/30658726.
387. Mihm S. Danger-associated molecular patterns (DAMPs): molecular triggers for sterile inflammation in the liver. Int J Mol Sci. 2018;19:3104. http://www.mdpi.com/1422-0067/19/10/3104.
388. Zhou Z, Ye TJ, Bonavita G, Daniels M, Kainrad N, Jogasuria A, et al. Adipose-specific lipin-1 overexpression renders hepatic ferroptosis and exacerbates alcoholic steatohepatitis in mice. Hepatol Commun. 2019;3:656–69. http://www.ncbi.nlm.nih.gov/pubmed/31061954.
389. Ge X, Antoine DJ, Lu Y, Arriazu E, Leung T-M, Klepper AL, et al. High mobility group box-1 (HMGB1) participates in the pathogenesis of alcoholic liver disease (ALD). J Biol Chem. 2014;289:22672–91. http://www.ncbi.nlm.nih.gov/pubmed/24928512.
390. Saha B, Tornai D, Kodys K, Adejumo A, Lowe P, McClain C, et al. Biomarkers of macrophage activation and immune danger signals predict clinical outcomes in alcoholic hepatitis. Hepatology. 2019;70(4):1134–49. . http://www.ncbi.nlm.nih.gov/pubmed/30891779.
391. Sacleux S-C, Samuel D. A critical review of MELD as a reliable tool for transplant prioritization. Semin Liver Dis. 2019;39(4):403–13. http://www.ncbi.nlm.nih.gov/pubmed/31242526.
392. Szabo G, Csak T. Inflammasomes in liver diseases. J Hepatol. 2012;57:642–54. https://linkinghub.elsevier.com/retrieve/pii/S0168827812003340.
393. Petrasek J, Iracheta-Vellve A, Saha B, Satishchandran A, Kodys K, Fitzgerald KA, et al. Metabolic danger signals, uric acid and ATP, mediate inflammatory cross-talk between hepatocytes and immune cells in alcoholic liver disease. J Leukoc Biol. 2015;98:249–56. http://doi.wiley.com/10.1189/jlb.3AB1214-590R.
394. Heo MJ, Kim TH, You JS, Blaya D, Sancho-Bru P, Kim SG. Alcohol dysregulates miR-148a in hepatocytes through FoxO1, facilitating pyroptosis via TXNIP overexpression. Gut. 2019;68:708–20. http://www.ncbi.nlm.nih.gov/pubmed/29475852.
395. Bataller R, Gao B. Liver fibrosis in alcoholic liver disease. Semin Liver Dis. 2015;35:146–56. http://www.ncbi.nlm.nih.gov/pubmed/25974900.

396. Karvellas CJ, Tillman H, Leung AA, Lee WM, Schilsky ML, Hameed B, et al. Acute liver injury and acute liver failure from mushroom poisoning in North America. Liver Int. 2016;36:1043–50. http://www.ncbi.nlm.nih.gov/pubmed/26837055.
397. Debi U, Kaur R, Prasad KK, Sinha SK, Sinha A, Singh K. Pancreatic trauma: a concise review. World J Gastroenterol. 2013;19:9003. http://www.ncbi.nlm.nih.gov/pubmed/24379625.
398. Klochkov A, Sun Y. Alcoholic Pancreatitis. In: StatPearls [Internet]. Treasure Island: StatPearls Publishing; 2020. http://www.ncbi.nlm.nih.gov/pubmed/30725876.
399. Lankisch PG, Apte M, Banks PA. Acute pancreatitis. Lancet (London, England). 2015;386:85–96. https://linkinghub.elsevier.com/retrieve/pii/S0140673614606498.
400. Clemens DL, Schneider KJ, Arkfeld CK, Grode JR, Wells MA, Singh S. Alcoholic pancreatitis: new insights into the pathogenesis and treatment. World J Gastrointest Pathophysiol. 2016;7:48–58. http://www.wjgnet.com/2150-5330/full/v7/i1/48.htm.
401. Majumder S, Chari ST. Chronic pancreatitis. Lancet. 2016;387:1957–66. http://www.ncbi.nlm.nih.gov/pubmed/26948434.
402. Pham A, Forsmark C. Chronic pancreatitis: review and update of etiology, risk factors, and management. F1000Research. 2018;7:607. http://www.ncbi.nlm.nih.gov/pubmed/29946424.
403. Fortunato F, Kroemer G. Impaired autophagosome-lysosome fusion in the pathogenesis of pancreatitis. Autophagy. 2009;5:850–3. http://www.ncbi.nlm.nih.gov/pubmed/19458481.
404. Gu H, Werner J, Bergmann F, Whitcomb DC, Büchler MW, Fortunato F. Necro-inflammatory response of pancreatic acinar cells in the pathogenesis of acute alcoholic pancreatitis. Cell Death Dis. 2013;4:e816. http://www.ncbi.nlm.nih.gov/pubmed/24091659.
405. Ren Z, Wang X, Xu M, Yang F, Frank JA, Ke Z, et al. Binge ethanol exposure causes endoplasmic reticulum stress, oxidative stress and tissue injury in the pancreas. Oncotarget. 2016;7:54303–16. http://www.ncbi.nlm.nih.gov/pubmed/27527870.
406. Kang R, Lotze MT, Zeh HJ, Billiar TR, Tang D. Cell death and DAMPs in acute pancreatitis. Mol Med. 2014;20:466–77. http://www.ncbi.nlm.nih.gov/pubmed/25105302.
407. Merrick MA. Secondary injury after musculoskeletal trauma: a review and update. J Athl Train. 2002;37:209–17. http://www.ncbi.nlm.nih.gov/pubmed/16558673.
408. Kobbe P, Vodovotz Y, Kaczorowski DJ, Billiar TR, Pape H-C. The role of fracture-associated soft tissue injury in the induction of systemic inflammation and remote organ dysfunction after bilateral femur fracture. J Orthop Trauma. 2008;22:385–90. https://insights.ovid.com/crossref?an=00005131-200807000-00003.
409. Einhorn TA, Gerstenfeld LC. Fracture healing: mechanisms and interventions. Nat Rev Rheumatol. 2015;11:45–54. http://www.ncbi.nlm.nih.gov/pubmed/25266456.
410. Hauser CJ, Zhou X, Joshi P, Cuchens MA, Kregor P, Devidas M, et al. The immune microenvironment of human fracture/soft-tissue hematomas and its relationship to systemic immunity. J Trauma. 1997;42:895–903; discussion 903-4. http://www.ncbi.nlm.nih.gov/pubmed/9191672.
411. Bastian O, Pillay J, Alblas J, Leenen L, Koenderman L, Blokhuis T. Systemic inflammation and fracture healing. J Leukoc Biol. 2011;89:669–73. http://www.ncbi.nlm.nih.gov/pubmed/21208896.
412. Kobbe P, Vodovotz Y, Kaczorowski DJ, Mollen KP, Billiar TR, Pape H-C. Patterns of cytokine release and evolution of remote organ dysfunction after bilateral femur fracture. Shock. 2008;30:43–7. https://insights.ovid.com/crossref?an=00024382-200807000-00008.
413. Levy RM, Prince JM, Yang R, Mollen KP, Liao H, Watson GA, et al. Systemic inflammation and remote organ damage following bilateral femur fracture requires Toll-like receptor 4. Am J Physiol Regul Integr Comp Physiol. 2006;291:R970–6. http://www.physiology.org/doi/10.1152/ajpregu.00793.2005.
414. Pfeifer R, Darwiche S, Kohut L, Billiar TR, Pape H-C. Cumulative effects of bone and soft tissue injury on systemic inflammation: a pilot study. Clin Orthop Relat Res. 2013;471:2815–21. http://www.ncbi.nlm.nih.gov/pubmed/23479238.
415. Levy RM, Mollen KP, Prince JM, Kaczorowski DJ, Vallabhaneni R, Liu S, et al. Systemic inflammation and remote organ injury following trauma require HMGB1. Am J Physiol

Regul Integr Comp Physiol. 2007;293:R1538–44. http://www.physiology.org/doi/10.1152/ajpregu.00272.2007.
416. Sirait R, Hatta M, Ramli M, Islam A, Arief S. Systemic lidocaine inhibits high-mobility group box 1 messenger ribonucleic acid expression and protein in BALB/c mice after closed fracture musculoskeletal injury. Saudi J Anaesth. 2018;12:395. http://www.ncbi.nlm.nih.gov/pubmed/30100837.
417. Degos V, Maze M, Vacas S, Hirsch J, Guo Y, Shen F, et al. Bone fracture exacerbates murine ischemic cerebral injury. Anesthesiology. 2013;118:1362–72. http://anesthesiology.pubs.asahq.org/Article.aspx?doi=10.1097/ALN.0b013e31828c23f8.
418. Tsai W-H, Huang S-T, Liu W-C, Chen L-W, Yang K-C, Hsu K-C, et al. High risk of rhabdomyolysis and acute kidney injury after traumatic limb compartment syndrome. Ann Plast Surg. 2015;74:S158–61. http://www.ncbi.nlm.nih.gov/pubmed/25785380.
419. Torres PA, Helmstetter JA, Kaye AM, Kaye AD. Rhabdomyolysis: pathogenesis, diagnosis, and treatment. Ochsner J. 2015;15:58–69. http://www.ncbi.nlm.nih.gov/pubmed/25829882.
420. Huang R-S, Zhou J-J, Feng Y-Y, Shi M, Guo F, Gou S-J, et al. Pharmacological inhibition of macrophage Toll-like receptor 4/nuclear factor-kappa B alleviates rhabdomyolysis-induced acute kidney injury. Chin Med J (Engl). 2017;130:2163. http://www.ncbi.nlm.nih.gov/pubmed/28836571.
421. Chen L, Zhao H, Alam A, Mi E, Eguchi S, Yao S, et al. Postoperative remote lung injury and its impact on surgical outcome. BMC Anesthesiol. 2019;19:30. http://www.ncbi.nlm.nih.gov/pubmed/30832647.
422. Sanchez-Adams J, Leddy HA, McNulty AL, O'Conor CJ, Guilak F. The mechanobiology of articular cartilage: bearing the burden of osteoarthritis. Curr Rheumatol Rep. 2014;16(10):451.
423. Anderson DE, Johnstone B. Dynamic mechanical compression of chondrocytes for tissue engineering: a critical review. Front Bioeng Biotechnol. 2017;5:76. http://www.ncbi.nlm.nih.gov/pubmed/29322043.
424. Blagojevic M, Jinks C, Jeffery A, Jordan KP. Risk factors for onset of osteoarthritis of the knee in older adults: a systematic review and meta-analysis. Osteoarthr Cartil. 2010;18:24–33. https://doi.org/10.1016/j.joca.2009.08.010.
425. Robinson WH, Lepus CM, Wang Q, Raghu H, Mao R, Lindstrom TM, et al. Low-grade inflammation as a key mediator of the pathogenesis of osteoarthritis. Nat Rev Rheumatol. 2016;12:580–92. http://www.ncbi.nlm.nih.gov/pubmed/27539668.
426. Jonsson H, Olafsdottir S, Sigurdardottir S, Aspelund T, Eiriksdottir G, Sigurdsson S, et al. Incidence and prevalence of total joint replacements due to osteoarthritis in the elderly: risk factors and factors associated with late life prevalence in the AGES-Reykjavik Study. BMC Musculoskelet Disord. 2016;17:14. http://www.ncbi.nlm.nih.gov/pubmed/26759053.
427. Hwang HS, Kim HA. Chondrocyte apoptosis in the pathogenesis of osteoarthritis. Int J Mol Sci. 2015;16(11):26035–54. https://doi.org/10.3390/ijms161125943.
428. Riegger J, Brenner RE. Evidence of necroptosis in osteoarthritic disease: investigation of blunt mechanical impact as possible trigger in regulated necrosis. Cell Death Dis. 2019;10:683. https://doi.org/10.1038/s41419-019-1930-5.
429. Zhao L-R, Xing R-L, Wang P-M, Zhang N-S, Yin S-J, Li X-C, et al. NLRP1 and NLRP3 inflammasomes mediate LPS/ATP-induced pyroptosis in knee osteoarthritis. Mol Med Rep. 2018;17:5463–9. http://www.ncbi.nlm.nih.gov/pubmed/29393464.
430. Zhang L, Xing R, Huang Z, Zhang N, Zhang L, Li X, et al. Inhibition of synovial macrophage pyroptosis alleviates synovitis and fibrosis in knee osteoarthritis. Mediators Inflamm. 2019;2019:2165918. https://doi.org/10.1155/2019/2165918.
431. Lepetsos P, Papavassiliou AG. ROS/oxidative stress signaling in osteoarthritis. Biochim Biophys Acta. 2016;1862:576–91. https://doi.org/10.1016/j.bbadis.2016.01.003.
432. Abusarah J, Bentz M, Benabdoune H, Rondon PE, Shi Q, Fernandes JC, et al. An overview of the role of lipid peroxidation-derived 4-hydroxynonenal in osteoarthritis. Inflamm Res. 2017;66(8):637–51.

433. Hügle T, Geurts J. What drives osteoarthritis?-synovial versus subchondral bone pathology. Rheumatology (Oxford). 2017;56:1461–71. http://www.ncbi.nlm.nih.gov/pubmed/28003493.
434. Griffin TM, Scanzello CR. Innate inflammation and synovial macrophages in osteoarthritis pathophysiology. Clin Exp Rheumatol. 2019;37(Suppl 1):57–63. http://www.ncbi.nlm.nih.gov/pubmed/31621560.
435. Sokolove J, Lepus CM. Role of inflammation in the pathogenesis of osteoarthritis: latest findings and interpretations. Ther Adv Musculoskelet Dis. 2013;5:77–94. http://www.ncbi.nlm.nih.gov/pubmed/23641259.
436. Rosenberg JH, Rai V, Dilisio MF, Agrawal DK. Damage-associated molecular patterns in the pathogenesis of osteoarthritis: potentially novel therapeutic targets. Mol Cell Biochem. 2017;434:171–9. https://doi.org/10.1007/s11010-017-3047-4.
437. Mahon OR, Kelly DJ, McCarthy GM, Dunne A. Osteoarthritis-associated basic calcium phosphate crystals alter immune cell metabolism and promote M1 macrophage polarization. Osteoarthr Cartil. 2019;28(5):603–12. http://www.ncbi.nlm.nih.gov/pubmed/31730805.
438. Dadas A, Washington J, Diaz-Arrastia R, Janigro D. Biomarkers in traumatic brain injury (TBI): a review. Neuropsychiatr Dis Treat. 2018;14:2989–3000. http://www.ncbi.nlm.nih.gov/pubmed/30510421.
439. Wang KK, Yang Z, Zhu T, Shi Y, Rubenstein R, Tyndall JA, et al. An update on diagnostic and prognostic biomarkers for traumatic brain injury. Expert Rev Mol Diagn. 2018;18:165–80. http://www.ncbi.nlm.nih.gov/pubmed/29338452.
440. Posti JP, Takala RSK, Lagerstedt L, Dickens AM, Hossain I, Mohammadian M, et al. Correlation of blood biomarkers and biomarker panels with traumatic findings on computed tomography after traumatic brain injury. J Neurotrauma. 2019;36:2178–89. https://www.liebertpub.com/doi/10.1089/neu.2018.6254.
441. Paudel YN, Shaikh MF, Chakraborti A, Kumari Y, Aledo-Serrano Á, Aleksovska K, et al. HMGB1: a common biomarker and potential target for TBI, neuroinflammation, epilepsy, and cognitive dysfunction. Front Neurosci. 2018;12:628. http://www.ncbi.nlm.nih.gov/pubmed/30271319.
442. Hu Q, Ren J, Wu J, Li G, Wu X, Liu S, et al. Urinary mitochondrial DNA levels identify acute kidney injury in surgical critical illness patients. Shock. 2017;48:11–7. http://www.ncbi.nlm.nih.gov/pubmed/28060212.
443. Whitaker RM, Stallons LJ, Kneff JE, Alge JL, Harmon JL, Rahn JJ, et al. Urinary mitochondrial DNA is a biomarker of mitochondrial disruption and renal dysfunction in acute kidney injury. Kidney Int. 2015;88:1336–44. http://www.ncbi.nlm.nih.gov/pubmed/26287315.
444. Clarke JI, Dear JW, Antoine DJ. Recent advances in biomarkers and therapeutic interventions for hepatic drug safety – false dawn or new horizon? Expert Opin Drug Saf. 2016;15:1–10. http://www.ncbi.nlm.nih.gov/pubmed/26923482.
445. Yang L, Wang F, Yang L, Yuan Y, Chen Y, Zhang G, et al. HMGB1 a-box reverses brain edema and deterioration of neurological function in a traumatic brain injury mouse model. Cell Physiol Biochem. 2018;46:2532–42. https://www.karger.com/Article/FullText/489659.
446. Kobayashi M, Tamari K, Al Salihi MO, Nishida K, Takeuchi K. Anti-high mobility group box 1 antibody suppresses local inflammatory reaction and facilitates olfactory nerve recovery following injury. J Neuroinflammation. 2018;15:124. https://jneuroinflammation.biomedcentral.com/articles/10.1186/s12974-018-1168-7.
447. Okuma Y, Wake H, Teshigawara K, Takahashi Y, Hishikawa T, Yasuhara T, et al. Anti–high mobility group box 1 antibody therapy may prevent cognitive dysfunction after traumatic brain injury. World Neurosurg. 2019;122:e864–71. http://www.ncbi.nlm.nih.gov/pubmed/30391757.
448. Gao T, Chen Z, Chen H, Yuan H, Wang Y, Peng X, et al. Inhibition of HMGB1 mediates neuroprotection of traumatic brain injury by modulating the microglia/macrophage polarization. Biochem Biophys Res Commun. 2018;497:430–6. https://linkinghub.elsevier.com/retrieve/pii/S0006291X18303310.

449. Yan B, Chen F, Xu L, Xing J, Wang X. HMGB1-TLR4-IL23-IL17A axis promotes paraquat-induced acute lung injury by mediating neutrophil infiltration in mice. Sci Rep. 2017;7:597. http://www.ncbi.nlm.nih.gov/pubmed/28377603.
450. Shimazaki J, Matsumoto N, Ogura H, Muroya T, Kuwagata Y, Nakagawa J, et al. Systemic involvement of high-mobility group box 1 protein and therapeutic effect of anti–high-mobility group box 1 protein antibody in a rat model of crush injury. Shock. 2012;37:634–8. http://www.ncbi.nlm.nih.gov/pubmed/22392147.
451. Lau A, Wang S, Liu W, Haig A, Zhang Z-X, Jevnikar AM. Glycyrrhizic acid ameliorates HMGB1-mediated cell death and inflammation after renal ischemia reperfusion injury. Am J Nephrol. 2014;40:84–95. http://www.ncbi.nlm.nih.gov/pubmed/25059568.
452. Zhu F, Chong Lee Shin OL, Xu H, Zhao Z, Pei G, Hu Z, et al. Melatonin promoted renal regeneration in folic acid-induced acute kidney injury via inhibiting nucleocytoplasmic translocation of HMGB1 in tubular epithelial cells. Am J Transl Res. 2017;9:1694–707. http://www.ncbi.nlm.nih.gov/pubmed/28469775.
453. Bisicchia E, Sasso V, Catanzaro G, Leuti A, Besharat ZM, Chiacchiarini M, et al. Resolvin D1 halts remote neuroinflammation and improves functional recovery after focal brain damage via ALX/FPR2 receptor-regulated microRNAs. Mol Neurobiol. 2018;55:6894–905. http://www.ncbi.nlm.nih.gov/pubmed/29357041.
454. Liao W-I, Wu S-Y, Wu G-C, Pao H-P, Tang S-E, Huang K-L, et al. Ac2-26, an annexin A1 peptide, attenuates ischemia-reperfusion-induced acute lung injury. Int J Mol Sci. 2017;18:1771. http://www.ncbi.nlm.nih.gov/pubmed/28809781.
455. Serhan CN, Levy BD. Resolvins in inflammation: emergence of the pro-resolving superfamily of mediators. J Clin Invest. 2018;128:2657–69. http://www.ncbi.nlm.nih.gov/pubmed/29757195.

Atherosclerosis 10

10.1 Introduction

Atherosclerosis is an ancient disease, first signs of which have been found in mummies from four different geographical regions or populations spanning more than 4000 years: from ancient Egypt, ancient Peru, the Ancestral Puebloans of southwest America, and the Unangan of the Aleutian Islands [1]. As reminded by Wick et al. [2], the inflammatory hallmarks of the atherosclerotic disease were first described >150 years ago [3, 4], but interest in this topic has increased over the past 30–50 years [5–7]. During this period, innovative fields of basic scientific and clinical research have progressively developed [8], whereby the possible role of DAMPs in atherosclerosis was first described in 2003 [9].

Atherosclerosis is a multifactorial, large- and medium-sized arteries-affecting disease, in which genetic/epigenetic and lifestyle-dominated environmental risk factors interact. Pathogenetically, this vessel disease has experienced an extraordinary paradigm change. For many years, atherosclerosis was simply regarded as a consequence of the accumulation of lipids in the vessel walls and called a lipid (cholesterol) storage disease. Today, the picture has completely changed. Current notions in vascular biology hold that acute repetitive/chronic persistent, infectious/sterile injury-induced DAMPs elicit chronic nonresolving low-grade inflammatory, profibrotic, and adaptive autoimmune responses to promote atherogenesis as the underlying disorder of CVD [10–12].

Indeed, the atherosclerosis story is impressive and began during the mid-late 1990s, when various theories were proposed for the genesis of the arterial disease, most concentrating on the role of EC injury, in particular [13, 14].

Interestingly, these theories were based upon early hypotheses on the impact of arterial injuries raised by the German pathologist Rudolf Virchow. In 1856, Virchow proposed that the lesions of atherosclerosis result from injury to the artery wall. He believed that atherogenesis reflects a combination of inflammatory and proliferative responses within the artery wall preceding the degenerative changes that have been long recognized in the advanced lesions of atherosclerosis [15]. In fact, in the late

W. G. Land, *Damage-Associated Molecular Patterns in Human Diseases*,
https://doi.org/10.1007/978-3-030-53868-2_10

1990s, it was discussed in depth by many researchers that atherosclerotic lesions result from an excessive inflammatory–fibroproliferative response to various forms of injuries to ECs and VSMCs. It was particularly Russel Ross who first formulated the "response-to-injury" hypothesis, continuously modifying it until the end of the past millennium. The theory held that "the lesions of atherosclerosis arise as a result of some form of injury to arterial endothelium. This injury somehow results in alteration in endothelial cell-cell attachment or endothelial cell-connective tissue attachment, so that forces such as those derived from the shear in the flow of blood result in focal desquamation of endothelium. This is followed by adherence, aggregation, and release of platelets at the sites of focal injury. During the process of release, a mitogenic factor is secreted from the platelets which, together with plasma constituents, gains entry into the artery wall resulting in focal intimal proliferation of smooth muscle cells" [5, 16, 17]. In one of his reviews in 1993, he sketched the perspective of the pathogenesis of atherosclerosis for the 1990s [16]. The history from Ross's work onward was sketched by Tabas in his "2016 Russell Ross Memorial Lecture in Vascular Biology"; Tabas wrote [7]: "The evolution of Dr Ross's concepts on this topic is highly instructive, moving from an initial theory that imagined a role for overt endothelial injury and smooth muscle cell proliferation to one that considered the role of more subtle changes in endothelial function, including inflammatory changes. … Through the work of many researchers from this time forward, including leaders such as Peter Libby, Göran Hansson, and many past Ross Lectureship awardees, the concept that atherosclerosis is driven by inflammation—in essence, the most important response to lipoprotein retention—has been supported by thousands of papers using causation models in mice and observational studies in humans."

In 2003, it was Land [9] who—when coining the term DAMPs for HSPs regarding atherosclerosis as a characteristic feature of chronic allograft rejection (= alloatherosclerosis)—proposed: "ROS-induced HSPs may interact with and signal through TLRs of vascular cells. Local secretion of inflammatory cytokines, chemokines, adhesion molecules, and growth factors by activated vascular cells of the donor's innate immune system may initiate the process of graft atherogenesis."

In 2011, in his book on *Innate Alloimmunity*, Part 2, Land [18]—in describing the development of atherosclerosis in allografts—comprehensively reviewed the pathogenetic role of acute and chronic pathogen-mediated and sterile vascular injuries (e.g., IRI, hypertension, and hyperlipidemia) in the emission of various DAMPs to promoting atherogenesis.

Today, the concept that inflammation and (auto)immunity participate in the pathogenesis of vascular diseases has gained widespread recognition and stimulated work around the globe [19–21]. Nevertheless, although the last several decades have seen significant medical advances in the diagnosis and treatment of CVD given new insights into pathogenesis, atherosclerosis remains the major cause of morbidity and mortality worldwide [22]. In the following, the pathogenic role of vascular injury → DAMP-promoted innate immune inflammatory, adaptive autoimmune, and fibrotic responses is a bit further elucidated by designing a model of four waves of DAMPs that drive these processes.

10.2 Vascular Oxidative Stress: The Early Injurious Key Event in Atherogenesis

10.2.1 Introductory Remarks

The initial event in the development of atherosclerosis is the injury to the endothelium that—following the danger/injury model in Immunology—elicits innate inflammatory/adaptive (auto)immune responses at the vessel wall. Predominantly, it is the acute repetitive/persistent injurious insults to the arterial wall which possess atherogenic capacities. Among all potential vascular damages, oxidative stress—less strongly ER stress—plays a prominent role, in particular, in the initiating stage of atherogenesis, and this via promotion of the oxidative modification of retained low-density lipoprotein (LDL). Low-density lipoprotein is a spherical particle with a diameter of 220 nm and a mass of ~3000 kDa. Each particle contains ~1500 molecules of cholesteryl ester in an oily core that is shielded from the aqueous plasma by a hydrophilic coat composed of ~800 molecules of phospholipid, ~500 molecules of unesterified cholesterol, and 1 molecule of a 500-kDa protein, apolipoprotein B (ApoB).

Accordingly, oxidative stress can be considered a hallmark of atherosclerosis. In fact, since the 1950s, oxidative modifications of lipids and proteins have been detected in atherosclerotic lesions, and the degree of oxidation was recognized to be correlated with the severity of atherosclerosis [23]. Indeed, it was this observation that strongly indicated a role of oxidative stress in atherogenesis. From the perspective of this book, oxidative stress/injury to vascular cells is a critical source of DAMPs that promote arterial inflammation and shape autoimmune responses, the pathogenetic key features of atherosclerosis. Production of ROS in the vessel wall reflecting vascular oxidative stress is increased in most injurious conditions which are widely considered risk factors for atherosclerotic CVD, including oscillatory shear stress at sites of blood flow disturbance, hypertension, diabetes/hyperglycemia, smoking, dyslipidemia, drugs, chemical toxins, and aging.

At this point, however, for the reader's understanding, it seems worth noting a few remarks on oxidative "eustress," oxidative stress, and the oxidative stress response, as described in more detail in Sect. 4.2.3, as well as in Vol. 1 [24], Part V, Sect. 18.3.

10.2.2 Oxidative Eustress, Oxidative Stress, and the Oxidative Stress Response

Under homeostatic conditions, generation of ROS in physiological low/moderate concentrations—operating as second messenger molecules and causing so-called oxidative "eustress" (in contrast to stress in terms of distress) [25]—assists in intracellular signaling pathways and, thus, is essential for optimal cell functions and homeostasis of the vascular system. In other words, the biological effects of ROS at the vessel wall—beneficial or deleterious—considerably depend on the amounts of

ROS present. In action, this phenomenon is in agreement with the idea that cellular ROS generation has characteristics of hormesis, implying a dose-response phenomenon that is characterized by beneficial effects at low doses and deleterious effectivity at high toxic doses [26]. To guarantee this homeostatic function of vascular ROS, to keep these molecules within physiological limits, and to prevent their deleterious effects on the arterial walls, that is, to maintain hormesis, a smooth running of the oxidative stress (defense) response is of utmost importance (see also Sect. 4.2.3). This stress response of the innate immune system was originally divided into the three tiers of an antioxidative defense response: (1) antioxidant enzymes including SOD, catalase, and GPX; (2) detoxifying enzymes such as GPX, glutathione S-transferase, aldo-keto reductase, and aldehyde dehydrogenase; and (3) energy-dependent efflux pumps. More recently, however, the oxidant-promoted, Keap1 ↔ Nrf2-triggered antioxidant response element pathway has gained increasing attention. This Nrf2-triggered antioxidant response is initiated by activation of Keap1 that functions as a substrate adaptor protein for the degradation of Nrf2 and serves as an intracellular sensor for redox changes [27–29] reflecting the presence of Subclass IIC-4 DAMPs (for Keap1 ↔ Nrf2 pathway, see Sect. 4.2.3.2 and Vol. 1 [24], Part V, Sect. 18.3.3.3 and Fig. 18.4). Of note, Nrf2 activation was shown to protect ECs from oxidative damage and inflammatory reaction, suggesting Nrf2 as a novel therapeutic target for atherosclerosis (for further reading, see Refs. [30–33]).

If, however, these oxidative stress responses fail, for example, in case of excessive and/or persistent ROS production overriding the antioxidative capacities of the vessel wall, oxidative stress emerges that contributes to endothelial dysfunction, damage, and even death of vascular cells, thereby promoting atherogenesis. The detrimental effects of ROS to vascular cells are of multiple natures and related to alterations in cell signaling and/or direct irreversible oxidative damage of NAs, proteins, carbohydrates, and lipids.

The demonstration of oxidative stress at the vessel wall is by no means a surprising finding. Thus, a variety of critical enzyme systems are present in cells of the vascular wall (e.g., macrophages, ECs, and VSMCs) providing generation of excessive and/or persistent production of ROS including superoxide anion radicals ($O_2^{\bullet-}$) and peroxynitrite ($ONOO^-$) under pathological conditions [34–36]. They include NADPH oxidases (NOXes), xanthine oxidoreductase (XOR), and enzymes of the mitochondrial electron transport chain (ETC) (Fig. 10.1). More specifically in mitochondria, $O_2{\cdot}^-$ can be generated as a result of the premature univalent reduction of O_2 during OXPHOS in the ETC and as by-products of several enzyme reactions in the tricarboxylic acid (TCA) cycle (for ETC, OXPHOS, and the TCA cycle, also compare Vol. 1, Ref. [24], Part V, Sect. 18.3.2.2. and Fig. 18.3 as well as Part VI, Sect. 24.4.2). Also, ROS production under pathological conditions originates from a dysfunctional, uncoupled endothelial nitric oxide synthase (eNOS). Notably, various isoforms of NOXes have been investigated for their function in atherosclerosis, and importantly, there exists a crosstalk between these prooxidant systems, whereby NADPH oxidase can trigger XOR activity, mitochondrial ROS production, and eNOS uncoupling. Further sources of ROS with relevance in the cardiovascular system include COX and LOX but also members of the cytochrome P450 family

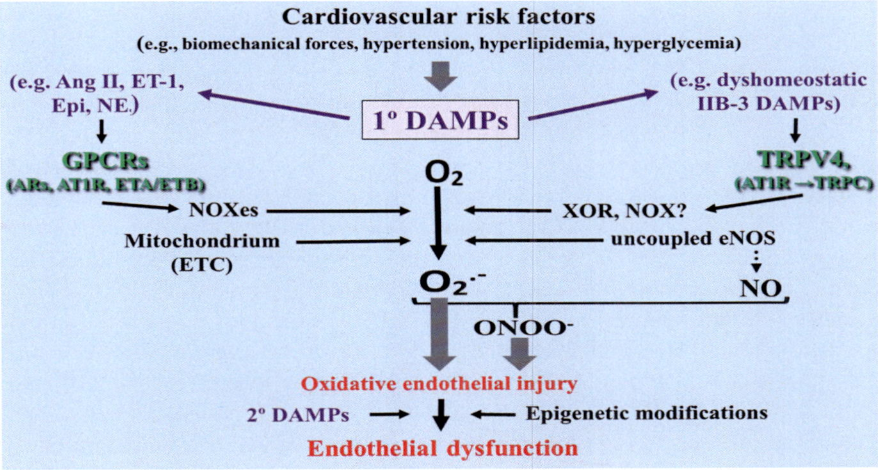

Fig. 10.1 A simplified diagrammatic model approach to the scenario of cardiovascular risk factors provoking emission of a first wave of "proatherosclerotic" DAMPs at the arterial wall, which trigger pathways contributing to ROS-mediated endothelial dysfunction. Inducible DAMPs (Ang II, ET-1, Epi, NE) are sensed by specific GPCRs to activate NOXes leading to production to ROS (superoxide anion radicals, $O2^{\cdot-}$). Cell-extrinsic dyshomeostatic DAMPs are sensed by mechanosensors (TRPV4, AT1R → TRPC) to activate XOR, contributing to generation of superoxide anion radicals. Superoxide anions can react with NO to form peroxynitrite $ONOO^-$. Together with mitochondria-derived ROS and uncoupled eNOS, the ROS-producing enzyme systems induce oxidative endothelial injury that—together with the second wave of DAMPs (e.g., OSEs) and under the influence of ROS-mediated epigenetic modifications—result in endothelial dysfunction. *Ang II* angiotensin II, *AT1R* angiotensin II AT1 receptor, *1°* DAMPs first wave of DAMPs, *eNOS* endothelial nitric oxide synthase, *Epi* epinephrine, *ETC* electron transport chain, *ET-1* endothelin-1, *GPCRs* G protein-coupled receptors, *NE* norepinephrine, *NO* nitric oxide, *NOXes* NADPH oxidases, *ONOO* $^-$ peroxynitrite, *ROS* reactive oxygen species, *TRPC* channels transient receptor potential canonical channels, *TRPV* channels transient receptor potential vanilloid channels, *XOR* xanthine oxidoreductase. (Sources: [43, 45, 46, 50, 54, 56, 63, 131, 134])

and some peroxisomal oxidases (for reviews, see Refs. [37–44]; compare also again Vol. 1, Ref. [24], Part V, Sect. 18.3.2 and Fig. 18.2). The pathogenetic role of these ROS-producing enzyme systems in atherosclerosis is convincingly proven, has been comprehensively reviewed by Konior et al. [42], Förstermann et al. [43], and Daiber et al. [45], and is briefly discussed in the following.

10.2.3 Reactive Oxygen Species-Producing Systems in Atherosclerosis: NADPH Oxidases

10.2.3.1 General Remarks

As the major players in oxidative stress involved in atherosclerosis, NOXes are expressed in resident innate immune cells, that is, ECs and VSMCs, but also infiltrating mobile innate immune cells such as neutrophils and macrophages. Notably,

NOXes are the only known class of enzymes whose sole purpose is to generate $O_2^{\cdot-}$. Interaction between $O_2^{\cdot-}$ and NO can form $ONOO^-$ that also causes cellular damages. So far, seven NOX isoforms have been identified in humans, denoted as NOX1 → NOX5, dual oxidase 1 (DUOX1), and DUOX2 [46] (for additional information also compare Vol. 1, Ref. [24], Part V, Sect. 18.3.2.2, p. 389, and Fig. 18.2, p. 389). Four of them are found in the vasculature (NOX1, NOX2, NOX4, and, most recently, NOX5), all with different distributions and control mechanisms and, thus, with distinct pathophysiological functions (reviewed in Refs. [47–49]). NOX1 is expressed primarily in VSMCs and at very low levels in ECs, whereas NOX2 can be found in ECs, adventitial fibroblasts, and invading innate immune cells of developing atherosclerotic lesions. Both NOX1 and NOX2—expressed at low levels in the vasculature under homeostatic conditions—become upregulated in cardiovascular risk settings including hypertension, diabetes, and hyperlipidemia. By contrast to NOX1 and NOX2, NOX4 is present at high levels under physiological conditions in all of the constitutive cell types of the vascular walls, while NOX5—just recently identified in humans—has been demonstrated to be upregulated in atherosclerotic vasculature and is reportedly implicated in both EC and VSMC proliferation.

Of three NOX isoforms found in the vascular wall of mice (NOX 1 and NOX4 in VSMCs and NOX2 and NOX4 predominantly in ECs), the superoxide-generating NOX1 and NOX2 were shown to have a pivotal proatherosclerotic role, whereas NOX4 possess a more protective role against atherosclerosis. Nevertheless, in other sets of studies, NOX4 was shown to regulate VSMC migration and differentiation, which is critical for neointima formation. In human atherosclerosis, NOX4 expression was found to be increased in intimal lesions of coronary arteries. Similarly, NOX1 overexpression in the media was demonstrated to result in increased neointima formation on vascular injury.

10.2.3.2 Regulation of NADPH Oxidases by Mechanosensitive G Protein-Coupled Receptors

Of note, the family of NADPH oxidases generates ROS in response to activated cell surface receptors, in particular, GPCRs, which were shown to activate NOXes through various signaling pathways (reviewed by Petry and Görlach [50]). The mechanosensitive GPCR angiotensin II receptor (abbreviated AT_1R), following recognition of Ang II, has been shown to activate these ROS-producing enzymes, that is, NADPH subunits [51, 52] (for AT_1R, see Sect. 2.4.3.2). As outlined in Sect. 2.4.3.2 and partially described in Vol. 1 [24] (Part II, Sect. 5.3.5 and Fig. 5.11), a central feature of GPCRs is their capability to interact with a large variety of ligands, that is, DAMPs, including lipid-based inflammatory mediators such as eicosanoids (prostaglandins, LTs; i.e., denoted as inducible IIIA-7 DAMPs), and platelet-activating factor, as well as vasoactive amines such as catecholamines, Ang II, and ETs, denoted as inducible vasoactive IIIA-8 DAMPs in this book (also compare Table 3.1 and Sects. 3.5.3.3–3.5.3.6).

Thus, one may argue that cardiovascular risk factors mediate stress and injury to the arterial wall in a process that is associated with the induction of "proatherosclerotic"

DAMPs, which are sensed by certain GPCRs to activate NOXes, thereby inducing oxidative stress/injury at this wall (Fig. 10.1). In other words, it may be this first wave of DAMPs sensed by GPCRs, which trigger signaling pathways leading to the development of vascular oxidative stress resulting in endothelial injury → endothelial dysfunction. Mechanistically, it is currently unclear how exactly GPCRs contribute to the activation of NADPH oxidase; also, other PRMs than GPCRs may be involved in the activation of NOXes. Together, despite the increasing number of data from innate immune research programs, the DAMP-promoted, PRM-triggered pathways responsible for NOX upregulation under vascular pathophysiological circumstances are not entirely understood. This burning topic—at least from the perspective of this book—will be resumed in Sect. 10.3.

10.2.3.3 Concluding Remarks

Together, given accumulating data from recent research, one may discuss the scenario that cardiovascular risk factors provoke emission of DAMPs at the arterial wall, which are sensed by specific GPCRs to activate NOXes leading to production to ROS. However, caution is appropriate in the broad acceptance of this scenario. Indeed, as warned by Petry and Görlach [50] in this context, "there is more precision needed to discriminate between increased ROS generation due to NADPH oxidase activation by subunit translocation, posttranslational modifications of subunits or recruitment of additional regulatory proteins, and enhanced ROS generation due to upregulation of NADPH oxidase subunit expression. … As NADPH oxidases have been associated with various pathophysiological conditions, and GPCRs are major drug targets for various diseases, a more detailed picture of the complex interactions between these signaling hubs is warranted."

10.2.4 Reactive Oxygen Species-Producing Systems in Atherosclerosis: Xanthine Oxidase and the Mitochondrial Electron Transport Chain

In addition to NOX-promoted ROS production, the activity of endothelial XOR was found to be increased in studies on experimental atherosclerosis models as well as in human atherosclerotic plaques, suggesting a contribution of XOR-derived superoxide to atherosclerosis. Of note, the expression and activity of endothelial XOR are reportedly enhanced by Ang II (denoted as an inducible DAMP) [53] sensed by the GPCR AT_1R [54] and oscillatory shear stress (OSS, reflecting the presence of dyshomeostatic IIB-3 DAMPs) [55] sensed by nonselective ion channel TRPV4 [56, 57]. Interestingly, other lines of studies provided evidence indicating that blockade of AT_1R inhibits ROS production [58]. These findings—when put together—lent support to the notion that Ang II may operate as a DAMP that, via interaction with AT_1R, triggers signaling pathways resulting in the activation of XOR (compare Fig. 10.1). The function of OSS sensed by TRPV4 as a mechanosensitive ion channel is poorly understood. A cautious explanation could be offered by referring to the concept of putative cell-extrinsic dyshomeostatic DAMPs described in Sect. 3.4.3.3: such shear stress-provoked DAMPs may induce conformational changes of the mechanosensor TRPV4 that get activated to convert shear stress-mediated mechanical stimuli into intracellular (bio)chemical signaling pathways (for mechanosensitive ion channels, compare Sect. 2.4.2).

Apart from this, however, the definitive proof of the role of XOR in atherosclerosis remains to be established.

Finally, mitochondrial oxidative stress induced by uncontrolled production of ROS and mediated by the ETC was observed to be associated with atherosclerosis in humans and found to be correlated with human plaque development [42, 43, 59]. By contrast to ligand ↔ PRM-triggered and NOX- and XOR-mediated oxidative stress, proatherosclerotic levels of mitochondrial ROS can be regarded as an excessively produced by-product of otherwise (i.e., under homeostatic conditions) normal mitochondrial metabolism. This may happen in the course of any damage to mitochondria, for example, under oxidative damage to mitochondria, then called "ROS-induced ROS release" [60, 61].

10.2.5 Reactive Oxygen Species-Producing Systems in Atherosclerosis: The Different Role of Nitric Oxide

By contrast to ROS, the role of NO in atherosclerosis is different [62]. Under homeostatic conditions, NO is produced in the vascular wall mainly by eNOS. Endothelial NO—as a vasoprotective factor for the endothelium—has atheroprotective properties mediated by various effects, including relaxation of blood vessels and inhibition of platelet activity, as well as inhibition of LDL oxidation, prevention of leukocyte migration into the vascular wall, and inhibition of VSMC proliferation (discussed in Ref. [43]). However, under pathological conditions associated with oxidative stress such as hypertension and hypercholesterolemia, eNOS may become uncoupled. Uncoupled eNOS generates superoxide at the expense of NO and contributes substantially to oxidative stress and endothelial dysfunction (Fig. 10.1). Mechanistically, deficiency of eNOS cofactor tetrahydrobiopterin (BH4), deficiency of eNOS substrate l-arginine, and eNOS S-glutathionylation have been supposed to be the major causes for eNOS uncoupling. Notably, ROS production from uncoupled eNOS has not only been shown experimentally in mouse models of atherosclerosis but also in patients with cardiovascular risk factor-associated atherosclerosis (reviewed in Refs. [43, 63, 64]).

Different from eNOS, expression of the proatherogenic iNOS in blood vessels is only upregulated in pathological situations such as oxidative stress and inflammation [65, 66]. The enzyme may generate large amounts of NO over long periods of time and has been shown to contribute to atherosclerosis, for example, via promotion of the generation of $ONOO^-$ as a key proatherosclerotic oxidant (see also Ref. [43]).

10.2.6 Regulation of ROS-Producing Systems Under the Influence of Epigenetic Mechanisms

Besides the model of regulation of ROS-producing systems via DAMP → PRM-triggered signaling pathways, including activation of transcription factors, epigenetic mechanisms reportedly play a critical role in contributing to cardiovascular pathophysiology (reviewed in Refs. [67, 68]). Indeed, there is increasing evidence suggesting vascular ROS to modulating the epigenetic landscape via DNA and histone modifications, the expression of ncRNAs, and ATP-dependent chromatin remodeling (for these modifications, see Sect. 5.6). Besides others, these modifications are increasingly discussed as contributing to endothelial dysfunction [69–71] (for endothelial dysfunction as a pre-lesion in atherogenesis, see Sect. 10.4.2).

10.2.7 Oxidative Stress ↔ Endoplasmic Reticulum Stress: The Two Integrated Stress Responses Involved in Atherogenesis

10.2.7.1 General Remarks

As outlined in Vol. 1 [24], Part V, Subchapter 18.5, the ER—as a subcellular organelle in the control of proteostasis—is responsible for calcium storage and lipid biosynthesis, as well as the synthesis, correct folding, processing, PTMs, and final maturation of proteins. Perturbation of any of those ER-associated functions such as accumulation of unfolded/misfolded proteins, hypoxia, calcium and glucose depletion, viral and bacterial infections, and, last but not least, excessive ROS production reflects stress of the organelle and results in activation of an ER stress-coping response, the evolutionary conserved UPR [72–75] (also compare Sect. 4.2.5).

10.2.7.2 Interrelationship Between Oxidative Stress and Endoplasmic Reticulum Stress

To remember, ROS-associated ER stress reflects the presence of cell-intrinsic dyshomeostatic DAMPs, that is, a subclass of IIC-4 DAMPs (see Sect. 4.2.5.2; for additional information see Vol. 1 [24], Part IV, Sect 13.4.5.2, p. 289, and Fig. 13.1, p. 279). Indeed, as highlighted by Ochoa et al. [76], a unique characteristic of the ER is its luminal redox tension. As pointed out by these authors, "the ER interior mimics the relatively oxidized extracellular environment and promotes crosslinking of sulfhydryl groups to form disulfides that would not survive the reduced cytosol. Accurate titration and strict compartmentalization of the oxidized intraluminal environment renders the ER sensitive to perturbations in overall cellular redox status, so the ER responds rapidly to both energetic and redox stresses. Perhaps related to this, the production of ROS has become an essential part of the ER stress response." Intriguingly and apparently, the ER is even able to distinguish between ROS production under homeostatic conditions when the free radicals act as second messenger molecules in commission of optimal cellular functions and, on the other hand, its excessive generation reflecting oxidative stress. Importantly, as accurately described by the authors [76], oxidative stress—in terms of an integrated stress response—can also induce a UPR via activation of eIF2α, for example, through NOX4-induced ROS (for eIF2α, also compare Vol. 1 [24], Part V, Fig. 18.6). On the other side, that is, in response to ER stress, ROS are reportedly also produced downstream as a consequence of the UPR, leading to cell death, pointing to a dual role of ROS in ER stress signaling.

10.2.7.3 Endoplasmic Reticulum Stress and the Unfolded Protein Response in Atherosclerosis

To cope with ER stress, cells—apparently also including vascular wall cells, in particular ECs—have the unique possibility to activate the UPR, a dynamic signaling network that orchestrates the recovery of homeostasis or triggers RCD modalities, depending on the level of damage (compare Sect. 4.2.5; for additional information see Vol. 1, Ref. [24], Part V, Sect. 18.5.2, p. 401, and Fig. 18.6, p. 402). Of note, ER stress has emerged as an essential component that influences the course of atherosclerosis, mainly in the advanced stages of the disease, and accumulating supportive data has been reported linking different pathways of the UPR with atherosclerosis (reviewed in Refs. [76, 77]). Besides others, this may be due to the ability of the ER to control many key lipogenic pathways. For example, the active transcription factor XBP1s (XBP1s, for X-box binding protein-1 whereby the "s" stands for the spliced form of XBP1; for additional information see also Vol. 1 [24], Part V, Fig. 18.6, p. 402) has a role in phosphatidylcholine synthesis and membrane expansion. A crucial target cell for ER stress in this regard is the macrophage that is recruited to the arterial subendothelial intima wall and promotes the removal of excessive low-density lipoprotein cholesterol (LDL-C) from vessel walls (see Sect. 10.4.3.2). The occurrence of ER stress in atherosclerosis is sufficiently documented by detection of molecules involved in the UPR. For example, the ER chaperone *binding immunoglobulin protein* (BiP)—keeping the three sensors of the ER homeostasis in an inactive state—is induced in atheroprone regions in human ECs exposed to disturbed shear stress before lesion development, suggesting a potential atheroprotective compensatory effect in response to ER stress within atherosclerotic lesions [78]. Moreover, in studies on a model of ER stress and activation of UPR in human aortic ECs, ATF4 and XBP1 branches of the UPR were observed to be strongly induced in the endothelium over inflammatory areas, in regional foam cell macrophages, and in areas rich with oxidized lipids [79].

What about the role of the H_2O_2-forming NOX4-induced ROS in ER stress? As mentioned above, NOX4, by contrast to NOX1, exerts primarily atheroprotective effects. Thus, both in humans and in mice, NOX4 has been shown to act as a negative modulator of inflammation and remodeling, thereby conveying atheroprotection [80]. Of note, as discussed by Ochoa et al. [76], NOX4 exerts its protective effect by presumably promoting homeostatic UPR responses. Thus, the appearance of ROS in atherosclerosis—eventually in combination with an ER stress—is apparently not always non-desirable oxidative stress but can also have protective effects.

In this context, a word to ER stress in relation to the role of autophagy in atherosclerosis should be allowed, a topic that seems to be complicated and complex in that both protective and detrimental effects at the site of vascular injury have been reportedly observed (for autophagy, see Sect. 4.2.2 and Vol. 1, Ref. [24], Part V, Sect. 18.2, and Fig. 18.1). Regarding the primary goal and task of adaptive stress responses to maintain and restore cellular homeostasis, autophagy appears to play a predominantly protective role during the development of atherosclerosis, at least in situations when there are mild homeostatic perturbations. In fact, as outlined by Perrotta and Aquila [81], the protective role of autophagy in atherosclerosis has been demonstrated in several in vitro systems. The authors also discuss that autophagy—as a special type called lipophagy—has also been shown to be directly involved in lipid homeostasis. As a matter of fact, as discussed by Ochoa et al. [76], autophagy/lipophagy in many if not most instances may originate from degradation of ER-derived accumulated lipids and, thus, is commonly activated as a novel signaling pathway in response to ER stress striving for cell survival. Together, these facts have led to the general consensus that basal autophagy can protect plaque cells against oxidative stress by degrading damaged intracellular material and promoting cell survival [81].

10.2.7.4 Concluding Remarks

Given the role of ER stress and UPR in the progression of atherosclerosis, therapeutic strategies to combat prolonged ER stress have been proposed, and several agents have been tested. The topic is not further pursued here.

The use of appropriate novel small molecular chemical chaperones has been considered as modulators of ER stress. The initial studies with these chemical chaperones are promising, but detailed studies are required to define their efficacy and adverse effects during therapeutic use in humans (further details of this topic can be found in Ref. [82]).

10.2.8 Résumé

In this section, some evidence is presented suggesting that oxidative stress/injury to the arterial wall is the crucial initial event in arterial wall inflammation leading to endothelial dysfunction as one of the first events in atherogenesis. Notably, there is growing evidence suggesting that certain PRMs, in particular, GPCRs and TRPV4 on vascular cells, trigger the activation of ROS-producing enzyme systems, that is, NOXes and XOR at the arterial wall. Recognition of DAMPs by these PRMs can be regarded as a new research field. However, as concluded by Petry and Görlach [50], "with regard to GPCRs, there is still limited information regarding the type and precise action of the heterotrimeric G proteins involved in NADPH oxidase activation under different conditions, thus leaving a wide field full of open questions to be resolved." Also, the nature of putative DAMPs sensed by GPCRs to regulate NOXes or XOR is still under investigation. Independently from this discussion, the concept is also of interest proposing that ROS, in turn, may promote epigenetic modifications with important implications for the development of endothelial dysfunction.

Last but not least, the two integrated stress responses, oxidative stress and ER stress, are involved in both the initiation and progression of atherosclerosis. Indeed, there is growing evidence suggesting that oxidative stress, ER stress, and inflammatory pathways triggered by both stress responses are closely entwined phenomena. They are involved in the pathogenesis of atherosclerosis, in particular, with focus on human atherosclerotic plaques.

10.3 Cardiovascular Risk Factors: Contributors to the First Wave of DAMPs → Promoting Oxidative Stress and Endoplasmic Reticulum Stress

10.3.1 Introductory Remarks

The pivotal role of vascular oxidative stress as the initial key event of atherogenesis has been touched in the previous section. Accordingly, and compellingly, pathological conditions identified as cardiovascular risk factors should promote the generation of ROS. In fact, as mentioned, increased oxidative stress has been described to be associated with many atherosclerotic risk factors, including sites of blood flow disturbance, hypertension, dyslipidemia, metabolic syndrome, diabetes, and obesity. In addition, vascular oxidative stress reportedly promotes endothelial dysfunction that is consequently defined as a well-established response to those cardiovascular risk factors and regarded as a predictor of atherosclerosis (for endothelial dysfunction, see Sect. 10.4.2). On the other hand, as briefly described above, there is increasing evidence suggesting that vascular oxidative stress is predominantly mediated by ROS-producing enzyme systems, which are activated by DAMPs. This line of argumentation lent support to the notion that cardiovascular risk factors trigger oxidative stress via induction of DAMPs, which activate ROS-producing enzyme systems. This concept is elaborated in the following by quoting recent findings in support of this model.

10.3.2 Biomechanical Forces (Oscillatory Shear Stress–Luminal Shear Stress)

10.3.2.1 General Remarks

Atherosclerosis is known to develop at curvatures, arterial bifurcations, and side branches preferentially, that is, regions that are exposed to non-uniform, disturbed patterns of blood flow mostly associated with OSS, multi-directional shear stress, and sometimes turbulence ("chaotic flow"). On the other hand, straight regions of the arterial tree are considered "protected" from atherogenesis by high levels of unidirectional laminar shear stress (LSS) (reviewed in Refs. [83–85]). The proatherosclerotic effect of shear stress is supposed to be mediated by both oxidative stress and stress of the ER, an exciting approach that deserves a few more words.

10.3.2.2 Oscillatory Shear Stress-Induced ROS Production

As reviewed and discussed already by Hsieh et al. [86], a regular flow pattern is supposed to produce lower levels of ROS and higher NO bioavailability, creating an antiatherogenic environment, whereas, on the other hand, an irregular flow pattern such as OSS results in higher levels of ROS and yet lower NO bioavailability, thus triggering proatherogenic effects. Based on available evidence, the authors further argue that this differential ROS production may modulate endothelial gene expression through complex mechanotransduction processes, to induce atheroprotective (laminar flow) or proatherogenic (disturbed flow) endothelial phenotype and formation of an early atherosclerotic plaque. In this context of importance is that OSS has been shown to stimulate the release of ROS from NOX1 [87]. Moreover, as demonstrated in other lines of studies [88], LSS and OSS differentially regulate NOX and eNOS pathways to affect the redox status of ECs. Thus, under OSS, NOX1 complexes with its regulator *NADPH oxidase organizer 1* (NOXO1), resulting in uncoupling of eNOS. This leads to increased production of superoxide and a decrease in NO bioavailability. By contrast, under LSS, however, NOX2 complexes with its regulatory subunit p47phox, causing a modest increase in H_2O_2, which results in activation of eNOS, a consequent increase in NO production, and a decline in superoxide levels.

Apart from NOX proteins, mitochondria represent another source of ROS production with altered shear as experimentally shown by release of ROS during cyclic strain in umbilical vein endothelium.

10.3.2.3 Mechanisms of ROS Production by Shear Stress: The Role of Mechanosensors and Transducers

There is increasing evidence suggesting that biomechanical shear stress promotes ROS production via mechanosensor-triggered signaling pathways (compare Fig. 10.1) (for mechanosensors and innate defense responses, see Sect. 2.4). The recognition of mechanosensing properties of the arterial wall is not a surprise. In fact, ECs and VSMCs are constantly exposed to mechanical forces such as shear stress generated by blood flow, as well as hydrostatic blood pressure and pulsatile stretch due to systolic–diastolic fluctuations. All these mechanical stimuli are sensed by a variety of mechanosensors and signaling molecules, locating, for example, on the EC surface, intra- and trans-EC membrane, and within the EC cytoskeleton. Following activation, these mechanosensors trigger signaling pathways leading to gene and protein expressions via transcriptional and translational processes. As a result, morphology and function of ECs and VSMCs are modulated to guarantee homeostasis of the circulatory system, for example, by secreting vasoactive substances to maintain vessel tonus (for reviews, see Refs. [89–91]). Plausibly, disruption of and failure in mechanosensing and transduction may contribute to various diseases such as atherosclerosis.

The mechanosensors and transducers so far discovered include cell adhesion proteins (e.g., vascular endothelial {VE}-cadherin, *platelet endothelial cell adhesion molecule 1* {PECAM-1}), ion channels (e.g., TRP channels), GPCRs (e.g.,

AT_1R), Piezo 1/2, primary cilia, actin filaments, integrins, and endothelial surface glycocalyx (ESG), which is a matrix-like thin layer covering the luminal surface of the EC (reviewed in Refs. [90–93]).

Here, mechanosensors and mechano-signaling molecules are of interest, which were proposed to contribute to ROS production. Concerning mechanosensors of ECs, only a few studies devoted to this topic are available. The GPCR AT_1R was shown to act as a mechanosensor [94]. Interestingly, in in vitro studies on a rat kidney proximal tubular EpC line [95], an AT_1R inhibitor was found able to inhibit NADPH oxidase and oxidative stress, suggesting indirectly a role of AT_1R in the production of ROS in ECs exposed to mechanical forces. In indirect support of this finding are more recent studies on the murine aorta, showing that inhibition of AT_1R results in reduction of human endothelial inflammation induced by low shear stress [96].

Also, intracellular mechano-signaling molecules in ECs promoting ROS production have been reported. For example, as reviewed by Naruse [91], stretching stimulation of ECs was demonstrated to increasing intracellular levels of cAMP and causing the production of superoxide and NO, as well as activating NF–κB. So far, however, studies on the role of mechanosensor-triggered pathways leading to activation of ROS-producing enzyme systems have not been published.

Plausibly, in light of the danger/injury model in Immunology, the crucial question here is: What are the mechanical shear stress-mediated ligands/agonists interacting with the various mechanosensors? To date, that is, as long as such ligands are not precisely identified, the answer could be the cell-extrinsic IIB-3 DAMPs introduced in Sect. 3.4.3.3. As outlined there, such cell-extrinsic dyshomeostasis-associated molecular patterns, reflecting cell stress/injury-induced molecular perturbations, promote conformational changes of mechanosensors, which get activated to convert extracellularly applied mechanical stimuli into intracellular (bio)chemical signaling pathways. For example, mechanical forces at the arterial wall may be associated with a change of ionic currents, activated by stretching of the plasma membrane reflecting ion perturbation; or mechanical forces may change the tension on the cytoskeleton, again leading to ion perturbations; or the forces act on ECs by altering cell membrane fluidity.

Together, the discovery of the mechanosensors, which sense stressful mechanical stimuli such as fluid shear stress and translate them into biochemical signals, may allow the conclusion to define these stimuli as DAMPs. Though not precisely defined yet—but like other well-defined DAMPs—their role is to regulate physiological cellular functions, thereby maintaining homeostasis, here, of the circulatory system. However, as with other classes of DAMPs, when emitted in excess, they may promote pathological responses, an example being shear stress-induced oxidative stress at the arterial wall promoting atherogenesis.

10.3.2.4 Atherosusceptible Shear Stress Promoting Stress of the Endoplasmic Reticulum

Of note, however, shear stress does not only provoke oxidative stress. Thus, several reports have been published addressing a role of "atherosusceptible" shear stress in activating ER stress to promote endothelial inflammation [97–100] (for ER stress → UPR-promoted inflammatory responses, also compare Vol. 1 [24], Part V, Sect. 18.5.2.2). Several mechanisms have been described which are not discussed here further. However, one may argue that the integrated crosstalk of both stress responses may contribute to atherogenesis via vascular wall inflammation.

10.3.2.5 Concluding Remarks

Clearly, this section should be regarded as a preliminary conceptual model approach to explain the ability of biomechanical forces such as OSS to trigger mechanosensor-mediated innate immune functions. Future studies in this exciting research field might reveal that biomechanical forces can induce distinct molecules that can really bind to mechanosensors physically.

10.3.3 Hypertension

10.3.3.1 General Remarks

The etiopathogenesis of hypertension is multifactorial and highly complex and involves an interplay between peripheral cardiovascular organs and the CNS. However, among the various etiopathogenetic factors, oxidative stress seems to play a vital role. A large variety of experimental and clinical studies has shown that excessive production of ROS contributes to hypertension and that scavenging of ROS decreases blood pressure. Additionally, hypertension increases oxidative stress in the kidney that, in turn, can augment blood pressure elevations, again associated with oxidative stress. Of note, hypertension was one of the first pathologies in which NOX-mediated oxidative stress was suspected to play a crucial atherogenetic role. Subsequent experimental studies in a variety of animal models let suggest NADPH oxidase to be the primary ROS source (reviewed in [101–104]). Prohypertensive inducible DAMPs sensed by GPCRs such as Ang II, ETs, and catecholamines [105]—or even in the form of biomechanically induced IIB-3 DAMPs—may be theoretically discussed to lead to generation of NADPH oxidases via GPCR signaling, thereby contributing to hypertension-mediated ROS production at the arterial wall (compare Fig. 10.1).

10.3.3.2 Activation by Stress-Induced Catecholamines and Angiotensin II of GPCRs: A Model of Hypertension-Induced Oxidative Stress

Physical or mental/emotional stress can lead to the "fight-or-flight" response in terms of an adaptive defense response mediated primarily via the catecholamines Epi and NE, operating as inducible DAMPs sensed by ARs that represent GPCRs (see also Fig. 1.1 and Sects. 1.2 and 3.5.3.4). The two circulating catecholamines derive from two major sources in the whole organism: The sympathetic nerve endings release NE on effector organs; and the chromaffin cells of the adrenal medulla are cells that synthesize, store, and release Epi (predominantly) and NE. All of the Epi in the body and a significant amount of circulating NE derive from the adrenal medulla. Here, it should not be forgotten to note that the other stress-induced neurohormonal system, the HPA axis, also maintains high levels of catecholamines in the adrenal medulla via glucocorticoid-mediated stimulation of the genes encoding catecholamine biosynthetic enzymes. In other words, there is crosstalk between these two stress-provoked outflow systems in promoting catecholamine release into the bloodstream (reviewed in Refs. [106, 107]).

In permanently stressed individuals, this stress response is associated with long-term elevated levels of circulating catecholamines, which can result in pathological conditions such as hypertension. For instance, chronic mental/psychological stress can lead to permanent activation of the sympathetic nervous system (SNS) [108]. In turn, the activation of the SNS in human hypertension has been convincingly demonstrated [109–111]. Moreover, the SNS is directly related to the RAAS that functions as an unusual endocrine axis in which the active hormone Ang II is formed in the extracellular space by sequential proteolytic cleavage of its precursors [112]. Indeed, among the various mechanisms contributing to the development of hypertension, the dysregulation of RAAS plays a critical role in the generation and maintenance of the disease. In the end, both the SNS and RAAS can promote the synthesis and release of Ang II and NE, the major functional "transmitters" of the two systems [113].

On the other hand, as described in Sects. 2.3.4.4 and 2.4.3.2, Epi, NE, and Ang II have been shown to be sensed by various GPCRs (ARs, AT_1R, AT_2R) that, in turn, as mentioned above, were found to activate NOXes to induce generation of ROS (Fig. 10.1). Moreover, activation of ARs causes multiple physiological reactions. Regarding vascular effects, vasoconstriction by catecholamines is mediated by α-ARs, whereas vasodilation is mediated by β-2 ARs. As reviewed by Tank and Lee Wong [106], α-1a ARs are present postsynaptically at synapses of the sympathetic nervous system and, hence, are stimulated by NE released from these nerve terminals. By contrast, α-2b ARs are present in VSMC nonsynaptic sites and, to a lesser degree, at sympathetic synapses. Together, both α-1 and α-2 ARs are stimulated by circulating catecholamines, and agonist occupation of these ARs produces vasoconstriction.

Importantly, there is first evidence suggesting a role of β1-ARs in promoting oxidative stress. Thus, signaling through β1-ARs in cardiac myocytes was shown to result in increased mitochondrial ROS generation via upregulation of NOX4 [114]. Other lines of studies in rat primary mesencephalic neuron–glia cultures showed that a β2-adrenoreceptor agonist selectively increases the production of ROS by NADPH oxidase [115]. However, further experiments are still required to prove whether or not catecholamine-activated ARs contribute to hypertension-associated vascular oxidative stress.

More data are available for Ang II and its cognate receptors AT_1R, which were shown to have multiple systemic and local actions in different tissues, including the blood vessels, kidneys, adrenal glands, heart, and CNS.

There is convincing ample evidence indicating that Ang II—via activation of RAS in terms of the angiotensin-converting enzyme/Ang II/AT_1R axis—is produced in response to stress, qualifying it as an important stress hormone [116].

In fact, many groups have shown that central AT_1R signaling plays a pivotal role in both the development and maintenance of hypertension via promotion of oxidative stress (reviewed in Refs. [117, 118]). Interestingly, already earlier experiments provided evidence indicating that the NADPH oxidase and its cytosolic subunit p47phox play a pivotal role in mediating hypertension caused by Ang II [52]. Subsequent studies have revealed that NOX-generated ROS, following activation of AT_1R by Ang II as the main peptide of RAAS, is the central mechanism involved in Ang II-derived hypertension (reviewed by de Queiroz et al. [118]).

10.3.3.3 Activation by Vasoactive Endothelin-1 of GPCRs: Another Model of Hypertension-Induced Oxidative Stress

Another vasoactive stress hormone known to be involved in hypertension is ET-1 that coordinates stress responses in close association with catecholamine metabolism (reviewed in Refs. [119–121]). This molecule has already been classified as a DAMP elsewhere [122, 123] and is denoted in this book as an inducible IIIA-8 DAMP (see Sect. 3.5.3.6 and Table 3.1). Endothelin-1 signals via ET receptor subtypes ET_A and ET_B, which are Gαq-coupled and belong to GPCRs of the β-group of rhodopsin receptors, which are 21 amino acid long peptides derived from longer prepro-endothelin precursors (see Ref. [124] and also compare Sect. 2.3.4.3). Endothelin-1 has been found in ECs in all types of vessels, from large conduit arteries, resistance arteries (contributing to the maintenance of blood pressure), large veins, and venules. Notably, ET-1 is constitutively released by ECs at a basal level, but this secretion can be stimulated through multiple pathways. The molecule is also stored in ECs' WBPs, allowing for rapid ET-1 export after stimulation (for additional information also compare Vol. 1, Ref. [24], Part IV, Sect. 14.2.5.3 and Fig. 14.2). The hormone is secondarily induced by Ang II but also expressed under the influence of numerous other factors, including shear stress, TGF-β, thrombin, bradykinin, hypoxia, and LDL either oxidized or acetylated (for comprehensive reviews, see Refs. [125, 126]).

Of note, ET-1, via ET_A-receptor-triggered signaling, has reportedly been demonstrated to activate NADPH oxidases [102, 127–129], suggesting another stress hormone-mediated mechanism of hypertension-associated oxidative stress at the arterial wall (compare Fig. 10.1).

10.3.3.4 Activation of GPCRs via Mechanotransduction in the Absence of Catecholamines, Angiotensin II, and Endothelin-1

Remarkably, there is some emerging evidence in support of the notion that the increased blood pressure per se—independently from the effect of catecholamines, Ang II, and ET-1—may lead to oxidative stress, and this via AT_1R. This is a mechanism that, for instance, might operate in case of arterial stiffness. Thus, the GPCR AT_1R (the AT_1B receptor isoform being more sensitive than the AT_1A receptor) have been proposed to act as a mechanosensors in a ligand-independent manner [130–133] (also compare Sect. 2.4.3). For example, in studies on small cerebral and renal arteries conducted by Mederos et al. [131], evidence was provided showing that Gq/11-coupled receptors are essential mechanosensing components in VSMCs and function as sensors of membrane stretch, leading to TRPC channel activation in a G protein- and phospholipase C-dependent manner (for TRPC channel, see Sect. 2.4.2.2). The study further provided evidence that spontaneously and mechanically activated receptors adopt an active conformation, allowing for productive G protein coupling and recruitment of β-arrestin (note: the issue of spontaneous activation of GPCRs is also discussed in Ref. [134]). The authors suggested that "$G_{q/11}$-coupled receptors, for example AT1R, serve as mechanosensors mediating pressure-dependent, TRPC-mediated membrane depolarization in cerebral and renal arteries, which is at least in part responsible for myogenic vasoconstriction" [131].

Notably, the concept of mechanotransduction-promoted oxidative stress is supported by earlier studies on rat VSMCs [135]. In this study, the investigators could show that mechanical stretch and Ang II synergistically increase NADPH oxidase expression in VSMCs, suggesting that part of this mechanism is mediated through upregulation of the AT_1R, induced by mechanical stretch. The authors concluded that the combined effects of mechanical stress and Ang II might promote vascular damage through the production of superoxide in a hypertensive state.

10.3.3.5 Role of Endoplasmic Reticulum Stress in Hypertension-Induced Oxidative Stress

Notably, first experimental evidence suggests that the ER stress (= reflecting cell-intrinsic dyshomeostatic IIC-4 DAMPs) induces a UPR that mediates changes in the vasculature which promote hypertension and also—in terms of a positive feedback loop—is involved in hypertension-promoted atherogenesis (discussed in Refs. [76, 136]). Indeed, chronic activation of ER stress and UPR pathways in ECs was demonstrated to result in increased oxidative stress and inflammation and often results in cell death [137]. For example, infusion of Ang II in mice leading to increase in blood pressure was shown to induce the UPR proteins BiP and CHOP in aortas, mesenteric arteries, and myocardium in response to hypertension [138]. Extended studies of the group using blood pressure normalization agents confirmed a vital role of ER stress in hypertension-dependent development of endothelial dysfunction. Indeed, these experimental observations are of high interest; however, further studies are needed to clarify the pathogenic role of hypertensive ER stress in atherogenesis settings.

10.3.3.6 Concluding Remarks

Together, there is growing evidence in support of a conceptual model proposing that hypertension-associated oxidative stress is caused, or at least promoted, by a first line of various prohypertensive DAMPs such as Epi, NE, Ang II, and ET-1, as well as by biomechanically induced dyshomeostatic DAMPs. The concept suggests that these DAMPs are sensed by PRMs, preferentially GPCRs, which trigger signaling pathways to generate NADPH oxidases, thereby contributing to hypertension-mediated ROS production at the arterial wall (compare Fig. 10.1).

Finally, and at this point, it should be mentioned that the development and maintenance of hypertension as a characteristic manifestation of vascular dysfunction have been proposed per se to be regulated and driven by DAMP ↔ PRM-triggered innate and adaptive immune responses of the vascular wall. The topic is not alluded to further here. Instead, the reader is referred to excellent articles for an in-depth discussion of this topic as published by the Webb group [123, 139, 140].

10.3.4 Hyperlipidemia/Hypercholesterolemia

Hyperlipidemia/hypercholesterolemia has also been shown to mediate oxidative stress to the arterial wall. For example, in hypercholesterolemic patients suffering from coronary artery disease (CAD), NADPH oxidases and XOR were proposed to be the major sources of superoxide in the coronary artery [141]. Importantly, both native LDL and OxLDL have been shown to stimulate superoxide/peroxynitrite production and to uncouple eNOS. Moreover, ROS production from uncoupled eNOS has been shown in hypercholesterolemic apolipoprotein E (ApoE) KO mice and in hypercholesterolemic patients (reviewed in [43]).

10.3.5 Diabetes Mellitus: Hyperglycemia

Of considerable clinical importance is the contribution of hyperglycemia to oxidative stress-mediated atherosclerosis in diabetes patients. Notably, hyperglycemia promotes excessive ROS production from different cellular sources. Among these, the mitochondrial ETC is supposed to represent the initial superoxide producer, but other systems of ROS production are also involved, including XOR, LOX, COX, NOS, and peroxidases (compare Fig. 10.1). Mechanistically, hyperglycemia was shown to activate a particular metabolic route that consists of the diacylglycerol (DAG) → protein kinase C (PKC) → advanced glycation end products (AGEs) → NADPH oxidase axis, culminating in ROS production (for competent articles and reviews, see Refs. [43, 142–146]). Notably, this sequelae of events have previously been proposed as the “dangerous metabolic route in diabetes” [147].

Interestingly, there is already first evidence suggesting a role of hyperglycemia-associated ER stress in atherogenesis. As recently reported [148], glycation of paraoxonase-1 by hyperglycemia can induce endothelial dysfunction through ER stress. High-density lipoprotein (HDL) associated paraoxonase-1 is an enzyme that is primarily responsible for the antioxidative properties of HDL in retarding the oxidation of LDL and cell membranes (see below). In this perspective, the authors considered paraoxonase-1 glycation a novel risk factor of hyperglycemia-induced endothelial dysfunction.

10.3.6 Cigarette Smoking

Cigarette smoking is one of the most severe health concerns worldwide and represents an established risk factor for the development of atherosclerosis and CVD. The critical underlying mechanism of smoking-induced CVD is certainly oxidative stress that leads to endothelial cell dysfunction. Typical pathological features associated with smoking—besides endothelial dysfunction—include a prothrombotic state, inflammation, altered lipid metabolism, and hypoxia. Mechanistically, multiple molecular events have been described to contribute to smoking-induced CVD. However, the excessive production of ROS is considered the most crucial process in promoting the development of diverse CVDs.

As highlighted by Golbidi et al. [149], cigarette smoke cannot only be regarded as a source of ROS per se but is also known to induce endogenous production of it by causing uncoupling of eNOS, altering the mitochondrial ETC, and interfering with NADPH oxidase and XOR function. Notably, it is the NADPH oxidase that has been established as a critical source of ROS responsible for the pathogenesis of CVD. As reviewed by Kim et al. [150], activation of NOX and subsequent ROS production by cigarette smoke administration have been widely observed in in vitro studies on isolated blood vessels and cultured vascular cells as well as in animal studies. Of the many cigarette smoke-containing compounds, nicotine, methyl vinyl ketone, and α,β-unsaturated aldehydes appear to be primarily responsible for the activation of endothelial NADPH oxidase and subsequent NOX-mediated cytotoxicity. According to the authors' conclusion [150], "a growing body of evidence suggests NOX contributes to smoking-related CVD. However, the clinical relevance of NOX activation by smoking requires further validation, because human studies conducted to date do not sufficiently support its contribution to the development of CVD."

Together, as pointedly concluded by Golbidi et al. [149], "smoking harms the CV system in many different ways; however, endothelial dysfunction can be considered a convergence point for the majority of these chain reactions. Cigarette smoke, as a source of oxidative materials and inducer of pro-oxidative radicals, destroys the protective homeostatic function of endothelial cells. This not only leads to tissue oedema and extravasation of blood components but also accelerates atherosclerosis. As e-cigarettes do not deliver toxins from tobacco combustion, they may be helpful in easing cigarette smoking cessation, but they can by no means be considered as being free of harm to the CV system."

10.3.7 Infectious Agents Contributing to Vascular Oxidative Stress and Endoplasmic Reticulum Stress in Atherosclerosis

10.3.7.1 General Remarks

According to the danger/injury model in Immunology, besides sterile damage, infectious injuries to the arterial wall may also contribute to atherogenesis, though they do not usually represent chronic persistent injurious insults. Accordingly, vascular injury, particularly oxidative stress, mediated directly or indirectly by several infectious agents, has been considered as risk co-factors for the development of CVD. As already described in Ref. [18] (Sect. 6.3.5.2, page 545) and recently reviewed by

Hemmat et al. [151] and di Pietro et al. [152], both bacteria and viruses have been identified as such proatherosclerotic infectious agents, which may contribute to the early and late stages of atherosclerotic processes.

10.3.7.2 Bacterial Infections

Among the numerous periodontal pathogens involved in the onset and/or development of CVDs, *P. gingivalis* and *A. actinomycetemcomitans* have been detected in atherosclerotic lesions (discussed in [152]). Considerable evidence was provided indicating that *P. gingivalis* and *A. actinomycetemcomitans* can disseminate in the bloodstream causing bacteremia and localize in the vascular wall contributing to the atherosclerotic process by inducing ROS-mediated LDL oxidation (reviewed in Ref. [153]). These interesting observations were supported by other lines of experiments. For example, in studies on ApoE KO mice, chronic intravenous infection with *P. gingivalis* was found to accelerate the development of atherosclerosis, possibly associated with mediating oxidative stress as well as inflammatory responses and disturbing the lipid profile [154].

As further highlighted by di Pietro et al. [152], *Chlamydia pneumoniae* reportedly disseminate via the bloodstream to the vascular wall as manifested by the presence of chlamydial DNA in peripheral blood mononuclear cells as well as in atherosclerotic lesions. As demonstrated by other lines of studies, this pathogen is also able to induce oxidative stress, thereby contributing to the early and late stages of the atherosclerotic process. Regarding the pathological effect of *C. pneumonia* on endothelial dysfunction, the pathogen was demonstrated to significantly facilitate the superoxide anion production in ECs through the upregulation of NOX and COX-2, as well as through the downregulation of antioxidant enzyme systems such as catalase, SOD-1, and TRX-1 [155].

10.3.7.3 Viral Infections

In principle, viruses may instigate atherosclerosis by two different pathways. They can exert their direct effects on atherogenesis by infecting vascular cells and then inducing inflammation in ECs and VSMCs. Alternatively, they can also apply indirect effects by infecting non-vascular cells and inducing systemic inflammation. Here, the capacity to promote oxidative stress in vascular cells is of significant interest (compare Ref. [156]).

Lifelong persistent infection with cytomegalovirus (CMV) has reportedly been associated with CVD. Recent data from a meta-analysis of prospective studies confirm this observation by reporting that CMV infection is associated with a significantly increased relative risk of CVD (ischemic heart disease, stroke, and cardiovascular death) [157]. As a causative factor, infection-promoted oxidative stress has been discussed. Thus, as reviewed [158], there is some evidence from primary infection of isolated cells that CMV can activate NADPH oxidase in VSMCs from coronary arteries and dysregulate eNOS in ECs. The authors contributed to this evidence by conducting studies in mice showing different functional roles for these enzymes during persistent CMV infection in the intact microvasculature. Thus, a gp91phox-containing NADPH oxidase was found to contribute to endothelium-dependent arteriolar vasodilation during persistent CMV infection and, in the presence of hypercholesterolemia, platelet adhesion. Also, eNOS was observed to mediate venular inflammatory and thrombogenic responses induced by CMV in mice under high cholesterol diet [158]. These early findings were subsequently supported by studies in in human heart transplant recipients with CMV infection, showing that CMV DNA in circulating leukocytes may serve as a marker of CMV-related oxidative stress in ECs associated with transplant arteriosclerosis (see Ref. [159] as also discussed in [152]). Moreover, as also observed in these clinical studies, PCR evidence of CMV DNA in leukocytes was associated with higher oxidative stress and subclinical atherosclerosis in healthy subjects. The increased oxidative stress was found to also result in mitochondrial DNA damage and dysfunction.

Human immunodeficiency virus infection is a well-known risk factor for premature CVD resulting from atherosclerosis, whereby this risk is even accentuated by particular antiretroviral combination therapies, independent of their effects on lipid metabolism and insulin sensitivity. Indeed, several vascular complications, including coronary heart disease, pulmonary hypertension, and atherosclerosis, have been described in HIV-1-infected patients (see Refs. [160–162]). Again, there is growing evidence suggesting that this proatherosclerotic effect of HIV is mainly due to its ability to induce oxidative stress [163, 164].

Interestingly, as highlighted by Marincowitz et al. [164], accumulating evidence indicates that HIV proteins such as Tat, glycoprotein 120, and HIV Nef, proinflammatory cytokines, and antiretroviral drugs all result in increased ROS production. The resulting oxidative stress, in turn, induces eNOS uncoupling and decreased NO bioavailability. Together, these mechanisms culminate in endothelial dysfunction. For example, in studies on cultured human ECs, transfer of intracellular HIV protein Nef was demonstrated to induce endothelial activation, dysfunction, and apoptosis [165]. These studies showed further that this Nef-mediated event occurred through an NADPH oxidase and ROS-dependent mechanism. As concluded by Marincowitz et al. [164], "Increased ROS production and oxidative stress, linked to decreased NO bioavailability and ensuing endothelial dysfunction, have emerged as the common underlying mechanisms afflicting the vascular endothelium in the wake of HIV and ART."

In addition, and of interest, in studies on exposure of human brain microvascular ECs exposed to HIV transactivator protein Tat, early induction of several major ER stress regulators could be demonstrated including BiP and ER stress sensors ATF6, PERK, and downstream mediators eIF2α and ATF4 [166] (again, compare Vol. 1 [24], Part V, Fig. 18.6). This is another intriguing example of an integratively operating pathogenetic role of oxidative stress and ER stress in contributing to atherogenesis.

Another viral infection discussed to promote vascular/proatherosclerotic oxidative stress refers to *hepatitis C virus* (HCV) infection that has been reported as a risk factor for subclinical and clinical atherosclerosis-driven CVD [167, 168]. Several factors are discussed to possibly contribute to oxidative stress in HCV-infected patients (reviewed in Ref. [152]). For example, hepatocellular mitochondrial alterations and iron accumulation—as typically observed in patients with chronic hepatitis C—have been proposed to be closely related to oxidative stress, since the mitochondria are the main site of ROS generation, and iron produces hydroxyl radicals via the Fenton reaction [169].

10.3.7.4 Concluding Remarks

Together, as concluded by di Pietro et al. [152], oxidative mechanisms activated by infectious agents during atherogenesis underlying CVDs are very complex and only poorly understood. "In future perspectives, a better awareness of infectious agents as cardiovascular risk factors may be helpful to comprehensively evaluate atherosclerosis progression in clinical practice."

10.3.8 Genetic Background of Risk Factor-Promoted Oxidative Stress (Polymorphisms)

It is a general observation that exposure to a given atherosclerotic factor provokes different clinical manifestations due to a genetically different susceptibility of individuals. In fact, atherosclerosis is a complex multifocal arterial disease involving interactions of multiple genetic and cardiovascular risk factors. Advances in techniques of molecular genetics have revealed that the genetic background significantly influences susceptibility to atherosclerotic vascular diseases. Besides further investigations of monogenetic diseases, candidate genes, genetic polymorphisms, and susceptibility loci associated with atherosclerotic diseases have been identified in recent years, and their number is rapidly increasing. A detailed discussion of this topic is beyond the scope of this book. For profound information, the reader is referred to comprehensive reviews in this field listed under Refs. [170–172].

10.3.9 Résumé

This section on cardiovascular risk factors is just a selection of stresses and injuries, which may potentially hit the arterial wall. Not all oxidative injuries have been listed (let alone potential non-oxidative damage that has not been mentioned at all). For example, the impact of persistent mental/psychological stress on atherogenesis may also use a pathway leading to oxidative stress at the arterial wall via bypassing the pathological event of hypertension. Such an unproven scenario is tentatively sketched in Fig. 10.2.

Nevertheless, the various oxidative injuries to the arterial wall touched here are generally regarded as the classical cardiovascular risk factors. The point tried to make here is that—according to the danger/injury model in Immunology—all potential arterial injuries are associated with the emission of DAMPs, which promote proinflammatory and adaptive immune responses at the vessel wall to initiate and maintain atherogenesis. Most important for this scenario is the accumulating

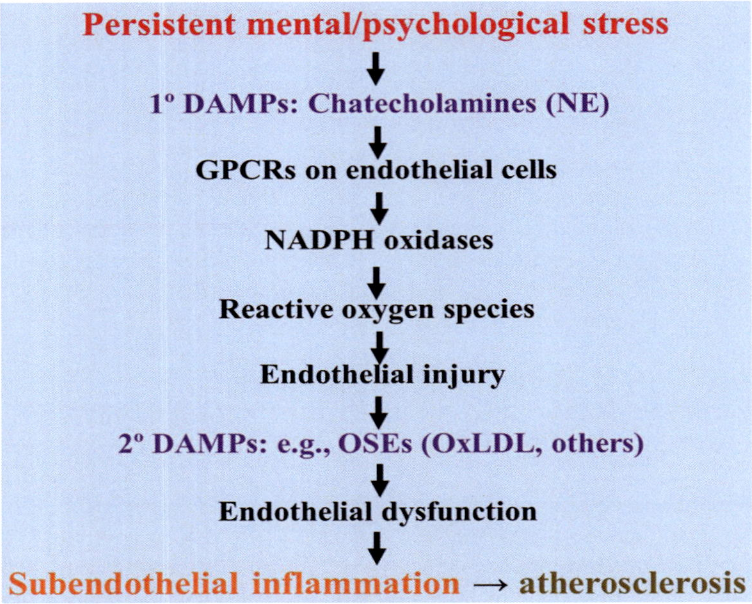

Fig. 10.2 A diagrammatic model approach to a theoretical, still unproven scenario illustrating that persistent psychological stress may contribute to atherosclerosis via bypassing hypertension as a known cardiovascular risk factor. *GPCRs* G protein-coupled receptors, *NADPH* oxidases nicotinamide adenine dinucleotide phosphate oxidases, *NE* norepinephrine, *OSEs* oxidation-specific epitopes, *OxLDL* oxidized low-density lipoproteins, *1°* and *2° DAMPs* first and second wave of DAMPs

evidence suggesting that oxidative stress-induced emission of DAMPs at the arterial wall is implicated in the development of endothelial dysfunction as an early sign of atherogenesis [173, 174]—an emerging topic that is highlighted in the following section.

10.4 DAMPs and SAMPs in the Pathogenesis of Atherosclerosis

10.4.1 Introductory Remarks

The pathogenesis of atherosclerosis is driven by the activities of cells of both the innate and adaptive immune system, which get activated in response to various infective/sterile injurious stimuli arising from all three layers of arteries. Many sessile and mobile PRM-bearing innate immune cells residing in or entering the arterial subendothelial intima such as ECs, VSMCs, neutrophils, monocytes and monocyte-derived macrophages, and DCs, as well as T-cell receptor (TCR)/B-cell receptor (BCR)-expressing adaptive immune T and B lymphocytes, are involved and interact with each other. The result of their interaction is mirrored by a complex interplay of subendothelial retention and deposition of lipids and lipoproteins, endothelial dysfunction, chronic low-grade inflammation, VSMC proliferation, and ECM remodeling (→ "vascular sclerosing"). The ultimate outcome of these pathological events is the formation of a typical atherosclerotic intimal plaque.

Instigation and propagation of all these processes are promoted by infectious/sterile injury-induced DAMPs, which activate those various PRM-expressing innate immune cells, including APCs such as autoreactive DCs, which, after engulfment of injury-induced vascular neoantigens, stimulate T cells to elicit an autoimmune response.

In fact, a large variety of stressful stimuli and inciting events to the arterial wall, including—as partially mentioned above—blood flow disturbances, hypertension, diabetes/hyperglycemia, hyperlipidemia, drugs, and chemical toxins, can lead to vascular injury associated with the creation of various DAMPs. As stressed above, most of these injuries are mediated by the generation of ROS and, thus, reflect oxidative damage.

Here, guided by competent review articles (see Refs. [19, 20, 102, 175–180]), some more details of the cellular and molecular pathobiology of atherosclerosis are added by focusing on the pivotal role of DAMPs.

10.4.2 The "Pre-lesions" in Atherogenesis: Retention and Modification of Lipoproteins Promoting Endothelial Dysfunction

10.4.2.1 General Remarks: Endothelial Dysfunction

Atherosclerosis is a spatially nonrandom and temporally non-linear process that initially affects so-called lesion-prone areas of the arterial tree which display a unique endothelial dysfunctional phenotype. As outlined above, the phenomenon of endothelial dysfunction is usually elicited by oxidative stress at the vessel wall mediated through atherosclerotic risk factors. Current notions hold that endothelial dysfunction, that is, alterations of the endothelial phenotype into a dysfunctional state, constitutes a vital risk factor in the pathobiology of atherosclerosis (reviewed in Refs. [181, 182]). The endothelial alterations observed are usually ubiquitous throughout the body, as patients with known atherosclerosis also have endothelial dysfunction in peripheral vascular beds that may not be affected by frank atherosclerosis. The progression of endothelial dysfunction is related to the intensity and duration of proven risk factors and the total risk of the individual subjects. Finally, however, the impact of endothelial dysfunction typically manifests in frank atherosclerosis (reviewed in Refs. [183, 184]).

Of note, the published characteristic features associated with endothelial dysfunction include two crucial events: increase in permeability of the endothelium for macromolecules and enhanced adhesion and transendothelial migration of leukocytes and monocytes/ macrophages, further, impaired bioavailability of NO, imbalance in the production of the vasodilator and vasoconstrictor factors, and changes in the expression of genes in ECs (reviewed in Refs. [185, 186]).

10.4.2.2 Increased Vascular Permeability and Subendothelial Retention/Accumulation of Atherosclerotic Lipoproteins

Increased vascular permeability as a typical sign of endothelial dysfunction may be regarded as the very first event in the initiation of atherosclerotic processes, all the more as there is evidence for oxidative stress at the vessel wall to lead to increased vascular permeability. For example, it could be shown that oxidative stress through the production of oxygen metabolites such as hydrogen peroxide (H_2O_2) increases vascular endothelial permeability, whereby, mechanistically, H_2O_2 was found to stimulate ADP-ribose formation, which in turn opens TRPM2 channels [187]. The increased vascular permeability allows transport of macromolecules across the endothelium that can reportedly occur through three potential pathways [188]: (1) transcytosis in vesicles, (2) paracellular transport through the regular breaks in the tight junction strand, and (3) through the leaky junction associated with cells undergoing apoptosis known to be induced by excessive oxidative stress.

This maneuver must be considered a critical atherosclerotic risk factor: increased vascular permeability allows LDL, more precisely LDL-C (or cholesterol-rich ApoB-containing lipoproteins), to cross the endothelium and to accumulate in the subendothelial space, preferentially in these pre-lesional but susceptible areas which then further exacerbates the endothelial dysfunctional phenotype. Here, one has to realize what has been impressively outlined by Taleb et al. [189]: "One LDL particle is composed of approximately 600 molecules of free cholesterol, 1600 molecules of cholesteryl esters, 700 molecules of phospholipids and 185 molecules of triglycerides… The polyunsaturated acyl chains of cholesteryl esters, polyunsaturated acyl and triglycerides are vulnerable to oxidation, as is the sterol of free cholesterol and cholesteryl esters. LDL contains one molecule of apoB-100, made up of 4536 amino acid residues with many exposed lysines, which can be directly oxidized or modified by lipid oxidation products …. Owing to its molecular composition, LDL is particularly susceptible to oxidation and OxLDL is considered among the strongest proinflammatory components of vulnerable plaques."

Typically, this retention/accumulation process of cholesterol/LDL-C takes place in the intimal space of medium-sized and large arteries, particularly, in regions in which the laminar blood flow is disturbed (i.e., injurious shear stress) by bends or branch points in the arteries [177, 190, 191]. Importantly, this process of entry and the amount of retention of cholesterol/LDL-C can be influenced and promoted not only by various injury-dependent degrees of endothelial permeability but also by genetic factors, the (increased) plasma level of LDL, the age, and metabolic state of the individual.

10.4.2.3 Oxidative Endothelial Injury-Induced Generation of Oxidation-Specific Epitopes: The Second Wave of DAMPs Promoting Endothelial Dysfunction

The process of retention and accumulation of cholesterol/LDL-C is even more critical from an atherogenic point of view as, during this maneuver, under the influence of risk factor-induced oxidative stress (see above), the lipoproteins undergo extracellular oxidative modifications to generate OSEs such as OxLDL. Indeed, there is a growing body of evidence suggesting that this second wave of IIB-1 DAMPs promotes the progressive process of endothelial dysfunction [192–194]. As argued in this context elsewhere [195], it is unlikely that a regular junction break would permit the passage of lipoproteins such as LDL, because the widest part of the junction is expected to be smaller than LDL. Thus, the leaky junction is mostly favored to provide the primary transport pathway for LDL, although cytokine-induced transcytosis across ECs has also been reported [196]. In fact, as one of the earliest events in both murine and human atherogenesis, the subendothelial retained lipoproteins undergo proteolytic, lipolytic, and oxidative PTMs that induce LDL aggregation (for PTMs, compare Vol. 1 [24], Part VI, Sect. 24.3 and Fig. 24.2). Oxidatively modified LDL generates OxLDL, minimally oxidized LDL (mmLDL), and OxPL which provide OSEs and, thus, act as immunogenic IIB-1 DAMPs (see Sect. 3.4.3.2 and Vol. 1 [24], Part IV, Sect. 13.3.2.2 and Refs. [197–199]). Of note, oxidation of LDL refers to a complex process during which both the protein and the lipids undergo oxidative changes and form complex products = adducts. Thus, the term OxLDL defines a variety of oxidative modifications of the PUFAs present in phospholipids, cholesteryl esters, and triglycerides of LDL. Such OSEs in OxLDL are present in both the lipid phase and covalently bound to ApoB-100 via the ε-amino group of lysines. Besides its function as a DAMP, OxLDL has been identified as a key disease-specific antigen in atherosclerosis, and earlier studies had documented its presence in animal and human arterial lesions (reviewed in Ref. [198]). From the perspective of the danger/injury model in Immunology, emission of OSEs may be regarded as the second wave of DAMPs operating in atherosclerosis (also see Fig. 10.3).

Oxidized LDL—containing, as mentioned, numerous cholesterol, cholesteryl ester, and other lipid products—is directly linked with atherogenesis due to uncontrolled uptake by cells in the vascular wall [23]. As outlined by Girotti and Korytowski in this context [200], "among the many intermediates/products of cholesterol oxidation, hydroperoxide species (ChOOHs) have multiple different damaging abilities. They include (1) damage-enhancement via iron-catalyzed one-electron reduction, (2) damage containment via two-electron reduction, and (3) inter-membrane, inter-lipoprotein, and membrane-lipoprotein translocation, which allows dissemination of one-electron damage or off-site suppression thereof depending on antioxidant location and capacity. In addition, ChOOHs can serve as reliable and conveniently detected mechanistic reporters of free radical-mediated reactions vs. non-radical (e.g., singlet oxygen)-mediated reactions."

All these sterile and infectious injurious processes in relation to the induction of endothelial dysfunction—preferentially mediated by oxidative stress as outlined

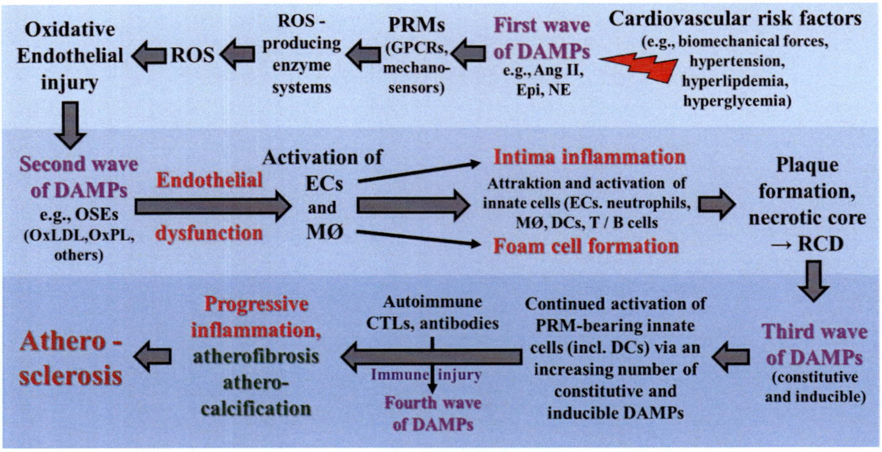

Fig. 10.3 A schematic diagram of a tentative narrative model illustrating four waves of DAMPs implicated in atherogenesis. The figure should be read in a meandering fashion, from top right to bottom left. Sources of the DAMPs are cardiovascular risk factors (first wave); endothelial oxidative stress/injury (second wave); RCD in the necrotic core (third wave); and adaptive autoimmune injuries (fourth wave). *Ang II* angiotensin II, *CTLs* cytotoxic T lymphocytes, *DCs* dendritic cells, *ECs* endothelial cells, *Epi* epinephrine, *GPCRs* G protein-coupled receptors, *MØ* macrophages, *NE* norepinephrine, *OSEs* oxidation-specific epitopes, *OxLDL* oxidized low-density lipoproteins, *OxPL* oxidized phospholipids, *PRMs* pattern recognition molecules, *RCD* regulated cell death, *ROS* reactive oxygen species

above—may affect arterial wall biology, including, besides oxidation of lipids and lipoproteins, variations in subendothelial PGs (e.g., biglycan and versican) that retain ApoB LPs [201]. It is proposed that structural changes in the GAG chains on PGs are the initial proatherogenic step that results in facilitated binding properties of PGs for those subendothelially retained atherogenic lipoproteins [202]. In other words, PGs and GAGs might operate as second-line DAMPs in atherogenesis as well (for PGs acting as IIA-1 DAMPs and GAGs working as IIA-2 DAMPs, see Table 3.1 and Vol. 1 [24], Part IV, Sects. 13.2.2 and 13.2.3).

It is also worth to note that OxLDL is capable of stimulating biglycan expression by VSMCs and enhancing the interaction of this PG with lipoproteins [203]. Mechanistically, oxidative stress-induced MMPs might contribute to the generation of those lipid-retaining properties of PGs (discussed in Ref. [204]). Here, it should also already be noted that, at this stage of atherogenesis, ROS is preferentially produced by vascular NADPH oxidases derived from ECs and VSMCs.

10.4.2.4 Enhanced Adhesion and Transendothelial Migration of Leukocytes and Monocytes/Macrophages: The Result of Second Wave DAMP-Induced Activation of Endothelial Cells

The other typical sign of endothelial dysfunction, that is, enhanced adhesion and transendothelial migration of innate immune cells such as leukocytes, monocytes/

macrophage, and mast cells, is proposed to be mediated by adhesion molecules and chemokines as secreted by ECs. Such atherogenic adhesion molecules expressed on the surface of ECs include PECAM-1, vascular cell adhesion molecule-1 (VCAM-1), intercellular adhesion molecule-1 (ICAM-1), and selectins (E-selectin and P-selectin) [205, 206]. Their work is accompanied by atherogenic chemokines described in relation to the initial stage of atherosclerosis, which include CXCL1 and CCL2 [207] (for leukocyte ↔ endothelial interaction, see Vol. 1, Ref. [24], Part VI, Sect. 22.2.2.2 and Fig. 22.2; for chemokines, see Part VIII, Sect. 22.5.11 and Tables 22.1 and 22.2).

Here, it should be insinuated that there is preliminary evidence in support of the notion that endothelial dysfunction may be the result of an activation of ECs ("type II activation") in response to MAMPs and DAMPs or DAMPs, that is, danger signals which induce proinflammatory, proliferative, and procoagulatory conditions favoring atherogenesis (also discussed in Refs. [182, 208–210]). The nature of the various potential DAMPs involved—except for OxLDL—has not clearly been defined yet; however, one can assume that their emission is caused by endothelial stress/injury, preferentially by vascular oxidative stress/injury (see Sect. 10.3).

Intriguingly, there is growing evidence suggesting that activation of ECs can be induced by OxLDL that signal mainly through their receptors TLR4 and LOX-1. Whereas LOX-1 supports the specific binding, internalization, and degradation of OxLDL in macrophages—that proceed to their formation into foam cells [211]—(see below), TLR4 was shown to trigger signaling pathways leading to secretion of adhesion molecules, chemokines, and other proinflammatory mediator substances [212]. Indeed, there is convincing experimental evidence confirming that the atherogenic effects of OxLDL can be mediated, at least in part, via the TLR4 → NF-κB pathway [213]. For example, OxLDL was shown to induce secretion by ECs of adhesion molecules such as VCAM-1, ICAM-1, and E-selectin [214], while other lines of studies could demonstrate that lysophosphatidic acid derived from the OSEs OxPL and OxLDL, respectively, can trigger release of chemokines such as CXCL1 [215] and CCL2 [216].

Together, these findings suggest that endothelial dysfunction as the initial event of atherosclerosis is promoted by the second wave of DAMPs, predominantly OxLDL. Further studies are needed to elucidate whether other DAMPs are involved in this initiating stage of atherosclerosis development. Of interest in this context is a discussion on the potential role of circulating bacterial and mitochondrial N-formyl peptides in SIRS-associated endothelial barrier dysfunction [217].

10.4.2.5 Concluding Remarks

In sum, endothelial dysfunction has been considered a critical pre-lesion of atherosclerosis that is caused by various factors, predominantly, however, by oxidative stress at the arterial wall. There is growing evidence in support of the notion that oxidative injury promotes emission of DAMPs and oxidative epigenetic modifications that are involved in the progression of endothelial dysfunction and may subsequently lead to CVD.

10.4.3 Post-Initiation Progression of Inflammation Within the Arterial Subendothelial Intima

10.4.3.1 General Remarks

Modern notions on atherogenesis and atherosclerotic plaque progression have been reviewed comprehensively by Hansson et al. [218] and Tabas and Lichtman [190]. Following the process of vascular (oxidative) injury → DAMP-favored entry, retention, accumulation, and oxidation of LDL in the pre-lesional but susceptible arterial intima areas in the course of endothelial dysfunction, the DAMP-driven inflammatory processes go on and expand and ultimately result in the formation of foam cells (Figs. 10.3 and 10.4; for global DAMP-induced inflammatory responses, also compare Vol. 1 [24], Part VI, Sects. 22.2.4 and 22.2.5).

However, the OSE on OxLDLs (and OxPLs) not only mediate uptake by PRM-bearing macrophages to generate foam cells but also—via activation of other PRM-bearing innate immune cells including ECs [182]—mediate many of the ongoing highly inflammatory events that ultimately lead to the development of plaques characteristic for later phases of atherogenesis (reviewed in Refs. [218–220]). Moreover, OxLDL-generated initial inflammatory stimuli (cytokines, chemokines, adhesion molecules, others) drive further recruitment of leukocytes, monocyte-derived macrophages, and other inflammatory cells to the vessel wall, which sustain chronic vascular inflammation (compare Figs. 10.3 and 10.4). This inflammatory process is particularly fired by OxLDL that, following receptor-mediated phagocytosis, activates—in terms of a priming and second activating stimulus—the NLRP3 inflammasome, resulting in release of the potent atherogenic cytokine IL-1β that operates as an inducible DAMP (see Sect. 10.6.2.5). It is this event of monocyte → macrophage extravasation into the vessel wall that is considered a critical step in the advancing development of atherosclerosis. And at this point, it should not be forgotten to note that the oxidation processes go on. Indeed, at this stage, the phagocytic oxidases derived from macrophages and neutrophils take over and may play a crucial role in the production of ROS, while monocytes and lymphocytes infiltrate vascular tissues and promote functional and structural alterations to form the plaques. As a characteristic sign within these lesions, the activated monocytes are reportedly the only cells capable of oxidizing LDL in the absence of added free metal ions through a reaction that is entirely dependent on the production of superoxide anion by the NADPH oxidase [221, 222]. In this scenario—as discussed by Perrotta and Aquila [81]—the NADPH oxidase activity may directly participate in lipid and lipoprotein oxidation, leading to foam cell formation and, one may add, in their function as OSE–DAMPs, continue to activate PRM-bearing innate immune cells to sustain vessel wall inflammation. As the formation of foam cells is discussed to be driven by DAMPs, the process deserves some more words.

10.4.3.2 OxLDL ↔ Scavenger Receptor-Triggered Foam Cell Formation

As mentioned, macrophages serve as the primary source of foam cells after they cross the endothelial barrier, accumulate in the subendothelial space, and engulf

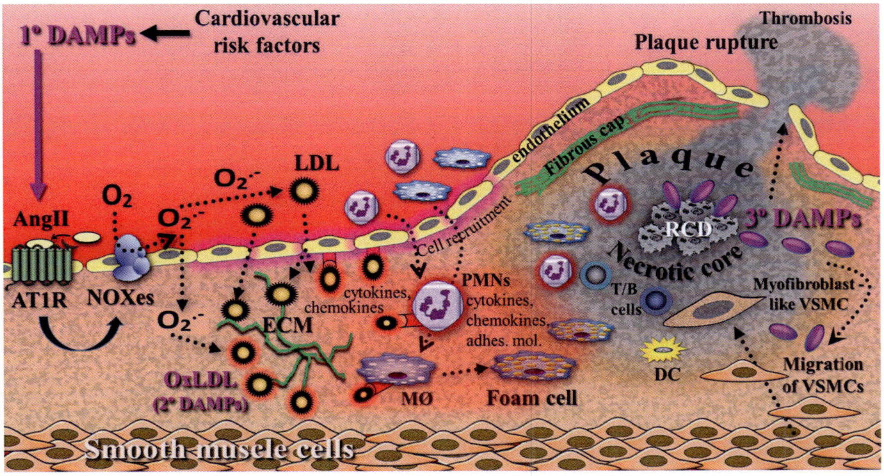

Fig. 10.4 A schematically depicted narrative model of cardiovascular risk factor-induced DAMPs (first wave of DAMPs) leading to sequelae of atherosclerosis-associated events in the arterial wall that culminate in the formation of atheromatous plaques. The scenario begins with crossing of serum LDL through the endothelium and retention in the subendothelial ECM that is considered the first step in atherosclerosis pathogenesis. Risk factor-induced first wave of DAMPs, here exemplified by Ang II, is sensed by PRMs, here exemplified by the G protein-coupled receptor AT1R to activate vascular NOXes, which, in turn, contribute the generation of superoxide anions. These ROS oxidate LDL into OxLDL (a member of OSEs acting as second wave DAMPs), which—via activation of endothelial cells and recruitment of PMNs—trigger a progressive inflammatory response in the subendothelial intimal space. In parallel, OxLDLs activate macrophages into foam cells. This scenario results in the formation of an atheromatous plaque that consists of many cells (foam cells, leukocytes, DCs, T and B cells, others) and is characterized by a central necrotic core. This necrotic area encompasses predominantly cells (such as foam cells and PMNs), which died from subroutines of regulated cell death associated with the release of large amounts of DAMPs. The third wave of DAMPs triggers further proinflammatory pathways that sustain the chronic intimal inflammatory milieu and, most important, can contribute to rupture of plaques (associated with thrombosis) as well as transition of VSMCs to myofibroblast-like cells. *adhes.mol.* adhesion molecules, *Ang II* angiotensin II, *DC* dendritic cell, *ECM* extracellular matrix, *LDL* low-density lipoproteins, *NOXes* NADPH oxidases, *OxLDL* oxidized low-density lipoproteins, O_2^- superoxide anions, *PMNs* polymorphonuclear neutrophils, *RCD* regulated cell death, *VSMCs* vascular smooth muscle cells, *1°, 2°, 3° DAMPs* first, second, third wave of DAMPs. (Sources: [50–52, 81, 197, 198, 224, 238, 239, 255, 258, 262])

excessive modified LDL and cholesterol esters. Also, however, a small part of foam cells reportedly originates from ECs and VSMCs [223]. Mechanisms underlying this foam cell formation process involve OxLDL in two ways: serving as the lipoprotein to be engulfed by the phagocytosing cells and function as DAMPs to trigger pathways that promote foam cell formation. Both events are driven by SRs such as LOX-1, SR-B2 (CD36), and SR-A1(for SRs see Vol. 1, Ref. [24], Part II, Sects. 5.2.7.3 and 5.3.3.2).

At the beginning of the atherosclerotic dynamics, expression of LOX-1 on macrophages is significantly upregulated due to increased generation of OxLDL; in turn, the upregulated LOX-1 receptor results in increased lipid uptake. Mechanistic details of further handling of excessively engulfed lipids in macrophages are reviewed by Chistiakov et al. [224]: For facilitation of uptake, macrophages sense and bind OxLDL with LOX-1 but also with several other SRs such as SR-A1 and SR-B2 (= SR-dependent endocytosis). Engulfed OxLDL is then shuttled to late endosomes/lysosomes, where lysosomal acid lipase degrades cholesteryl esters to free cholesterol and free fatty acids. Under homeostatic conditions, free cholesterol—via the ER—is transported outside the cells via ATP-binding cassette (ABC) transporters ABCA1 and ABCG1. However, in atherosclerosis, expression of ABCA1 and ABCG1 is suppressed, which diminishes cholesterol efflux and promotes cholesterol deposition in macrophages. This leads to accumulation of cholesteryl esters in the cell. Together, these mechanisms lead to excessive lipid deposits and transformation of macrophages to foam cells.

Of note, DAMPs such as the inducible IIIB-5 DAMP LPA (i.e., an LPL) and secreted HMGB1—as well as still unidentified NLRP3-inflammasome activating DAMPs—were reportedly found to promote indirectly or directly the formation of foam cells in both macrophages and VSMCs [225–228].

10.4.3.3 Concluding Remarks

Together, progression of inflammation within the arterial subendothelial intima up to the final formation of the atherosclerotic plaque is a complex scenario. The process is dominated by DAMP-promoted inflammatory responses that attract further innate immune inflammatory cells to the vessel wall, which sustain chronic vascular inflammation. Within this scenario, the DAMP-promoted foam cell formation can be considered a key event that is tightly associated with further progression of atherosclerosis.

10.4.4 The Atherosclerotic Plaque as a Prototypical Inflammatory Lesion in Arteries

10.4.4.1 General Remarks

As macrophages progressively take up oxidatively modified LDL, they give rise to steadily growing generation of those foam cells, which, however, as shown in other lines of studies, appear to respond weaker to the M1-polarizing factors, as indicated by reduced upregulation of the proinflammatory genes, reduced secretion of TNF, and a trend toward lower NF–κB activity [229]. Nevertheless, this scenario results in the formation of a cushion called atheroma or atheromatous or fibrofatty plaque, composed of a mixture of macrophages (recruited from circulating monocytes but also originated from macrophage proliferation within the plaque), DCs, NK cells, T lymphocytes, VSMCs, cholesterol crystals, OxLDL, lipid-laden foam cells, and debris from dead cells. The macrophages are undoubtedly the leading players in atherogenesis, whereas other innate immune cells, such as neutrophils, mast cells, NK cells, and NKT cells, are considered minor populations in the plaques.

DAMPs in Atherosclerotic Plaques

The atherosclerotic plaques can be regarded as "breeding places" for the production of proinflammatory mediator substances contributing to progression of vascular inflammation. Besides OSEs such as OxPL that are present in the plaques and found to be implicated in the generation of unstable and ruptured plaques [230], other DAMPs have been detected to contribute. For example, emerging evidence has uncovered a critical role of the NLRP3 inflammasome in sustaining vascular wall inflammation via production of the proatherosclerotic cytokines IL-1β and IL-18, thereby aggravating the progression of atherosclerosis (for NLRP3 inflammasome, see Vol. 1 [24], Part VI, Sect. 22.4.2). Already in 2010, Duewell et al. [231] could demonstrate the critical role of the NLRP3 inflammasomes in the progression of atherosclerosis. In the meantime, various DAMPs, including cholesterol crystals, calcium phosphate crystals, OxLDL, and HMGB1 have been shown to activate this inflammasome in macrophages to trigger inflammatory responses in the atherosclerotic plaque lesions (reviewed in Refs. [232, 233]). Interestingly, a recent study revealed that HMGB1 acts as a critical downstream signal molecule of NLRP 3 inflammasome activation and plays an essential role in VSMCs' foam cell formation and atherogenesis [227] (for the NLRP3 inflammasome, also see Sect. 10.6.2.5).

Here, it is also worth to mention that there is evidence for the action of inducible DAMPs, which—besides IL-1β—may also contribute to expansion of the inflammatory milieu. For example, in experiments on ApoE-deficient mice, GAL-3 (a IIIA-5 DAMP) was demonstrated to promote plaque progression and necrotic core formation [234].

Role of Myofibroblast in the Creation of the "Fibrous Cap"

As key drivers of intimal hyperplasia in the initiation and early progression of atherosclerosis, myofibroblasts (also called myofibroblast-like cells) derived and transformed from medial DAMP-activated VSMCs and possibly other sources enter the intima and lead to the formation of ECM compounds including collagen fibers that create a collagenous "fibrous cap" that overlies the lipid-rich plaque core [235, 236]. These typical lesions—in parallel accompanied by varying degrees of matrix remodeling and calcification—generally remain covered by an intact endothelium until the late stages of the disease. The eventual breakdown of endothelial continuity at a later stage can promote lesion progression and complications (see below).

10.4.4.2 The "Necrotic Core" of Atherosclerotic Plaques

Notably, the vast majority of dying cells in those advanced atherosclerotic plaques undergo necrosis. Various stressing and damaging stimuli within the plaques may cause necrotic cell death in their centers. Such cell-lethal stimuli include hypoxia, high levels of oxidative stress (see also below), ER stress, and DNA stress/damage, which ultimately result in a failure of the cognate adaptive stress responses (oxidative stress response, UPR, DDR) associated with the development of RCD (apoptosis and various forms of RN; for stress responses and subroutines of RCD, see Ref. [237], and Chap. 4). This "cell-dying scenario" leads to the typical picture of a highly inflammatory "necrotic core" (also known as lipid core) overlying by the "fibrous cap" in more stable lesions. Indeed, large necrotic cores can be seen as a hallmark of advanced atherosclerotic disease [238–240]. In other words, the large necrotic cores of atherosclerotic plaques must be regarded as critical sources for DAMPs emission in terms of a third wave (see below) (Figs. 10.3 and 10.4). Of note, however, as will be outlined in more detail in Sect. 10.4.8, besides DAMPs and proinflammatory cytokines, SAMPs and antiinflammatory cytokines are also produced by activated innate immune cells, and this delicate balance between DAMPs and SAMPs as well as pro- and antiinflammatory signals promotes a slowly progressive, nonresolving, chronic inflammation.

10.4.4.3 DAMP-Promoted Transition from Stable into Unstable Vulnerable Plaques → Plaque Rupture

The involved innate immune cells—activated by DAMPs derived from the necrotic core—further modulate the endothelial proinflammatory phenotype (via production of ROS, RNS, cytokines, chemokines, eicosanoids, others) and, thus, contribute to structural instability of the plaques that may lead to superficial erosion of plaques or plaque rupture (see Figs. 10.4 and 10.7). Moreover, along with the thickening of the plaque, its deeper layers may become hypoxic, triggering angiogenesis and microvascular proliferation from the adventitial vasa vasorum. These neovessels are prone to bleeding that may yield rapid changes in plaque size and composition and, thus, may promote the transition from a stable into an unstable vulnerable lesion that is characterized by a thin fibrous cap. As comprehensively described by Rai and Agrawal [241], this process of a growing plaque vulnerability is thought to be caused by MAMP/DAMP- or DAMP-induced increased secretion of the inflammatory cytokines and MMPs which mediate the proteolytic modification/degradation of the collagen content of ECM. For example, the OSE lysophosphatidic acid was shown to promote MMP9 expression and activation in THP-1 cells, partly through the TLR4 → NF–kB signaling pathway, whereby the finding of upregulated MMP9 expression was discussed by the authors to be one of the mechanisms contributing to the formation of unstable plaques [242] (THP-1 is a human leukemia monocytic cell line, which has been extensively used to study monocyte/macrophage functions). (For further reviews on plaque vulnerability mediated by MMPs, the reader is referred to articles listed under Refs. [6, 243–248].)

Other lines of studies supporting this concept provided evidence indicating that crosstalk between macrophages and VSMCs impairs collagen synthesis and promotes angiogenesis, that is, decreased synthesis of ECM components by VSMC, increased production of MMPs by both cells, and facilitated production of angiogenic factors [249].

Highly pathologically, these unstable, fragile "vulnerable plaques" (also called "thin-cap fibroatheroma") may result in a catastrophe, the plaque rupture that occurs very often at the weakest areas of the plaque, the "shoulders," where the plaque meets the normal arterial wall. Plaque rupture or endothelial cell erosion is associated with luminal release of the highly thrombogenic contents of the necrotic core, triggering an atherothrombotic occlusion, as seen in heart attack and stroke [218, 219, 250–252].

10.4.4.4 Concluding Remarks

Plaque development and rupture are hallmarks of atherosclerotic vascular disease and may be considered the work of three subsequently generated lines of DAMPs (compare Figs. 10.3 and 10.4). The increasing knowledge about the role of DAMPs in the promotion of plaque rupture may stimulate new diagnostic approaches to using them as prognostic imaging biomarkers for plaque vulnerability. Development of such new diagnostic means would be even more justified, given the fact that many diagnostic techniques have failed in providing satisfactory findings to detect or predict vulnerable plaques.

10.4.5 Source of the Third Wave of DAMPs: Plaque-Caused Regulated Cell Death in the Necrotic Core

Of note, as already touched above, the late atherosclerotic plaque-forming phase, associated with the formation of the necrotic core, is characterized by the development of subroutines of RCD of lesional cells, preferentially macrophages and VSMCs [253, 254], thereby providing the third wave of DAMPs emission (Fig. 10.4) (for subroutines of RCD, see Sect. 4.3 and Vol. 1 [24], Part V, Chapter 19 and Figs. 19.1 and 19.2). In fact, in experimental models, different types of RCD have been described in atherosclerosis such as apoptosis → secondary necrosis, autophagic cell death [255], necroptosis [255–257]), pyroptosis [258–261], and NETosis [262, 263]. Another subroutine of RCD, ferroptosis can be assumed to occur as well and has already been discussed elsewhere [200, 264]. Usually, RCD is the result of unsuccessful stress responses, and, indeed, this scenario—serving as robust sources of passively released DAMPs—has also been observed in atherosclerosis and, because of its pivotal pathological effect in the progression of this disease, will be separately detailed in Sect. 10.6.

Interestingly, much attention has been paid to autophagy-dependent cell death as observed in atherosclerosis. For example, as argued by Perrotta and Aquila [81], excessive stimulation of autophagy in VSMCs and/or ECs—for instance, via activation by excessive DAMPs emission—may cause autophagic cell death, leading to reduced synthesis of collagen, thinning of the fibrous cap, plaque destabilization, lesional thrombosis, and acute clinical events. Regarding autophagy-depending cell death as a type of RCD, one should pay regard to the recommendations of the *Nomenclature Committee on Cell Death 2018* [237]: "Proficient autophagic responses (which are under tight transcriptional and post-translational regulation) most often operate at the hub of adaptation to stress, hence mediating cytoprotective (rather than cytotoxic) effects. .... However, in a number of developmental and pathophysiological settings, the molecular machinery for autophagy etiologically contributes to cellular demise ...". It is conceivable that such a scenario may take place in the center of an atherosclerotic plaque, where excessive stimulation of autophagy in plaque macrophages, VSMCs, and ECs within the necrotic core may lead to RCD of these cells. In the context of macrophages, VSMC, and EC autophagy, another approach is of interest as discussed by Grootaert et al. [254,

265], who highlighted the recent insights into the causes and consequences of defective autophagy in atherosclerosis, with a particular focus on the role of autophagy and mitophagy in plaque macrophages, VSMCs, and ECs. In their review, the authors came to the conclusion that genetic disruption of the autophagic process can elicit opposing effects in plaque macrophages, VSMCs, and ECs. They argue that macrophages respond to autophagy impairment by undergoing apoptosis, while VSMCs engage the senescence program, though both phenomena have been shown to promote plaque progression. Here, one has to note that—according to the recommendations of the *Nomenclature Committee on Cell Death 2018* [237]—cellular senescence is defined as irreversible loss of proliferative potential associated with specific morphological and biochemical features, including the senescence-associated secretory phenotype (also compare Box 4.1). However, cellular senescence does not constitute a form of RCD. Grootaert et al. continue [265]: "In this regard, autophagy can be defined as a sensitive control switch between senescence and apoptosis. When autophagy is impaired, the cell has two main choices: either die (via apoptosis) or adapt (via senescence). However, autophagy-defective ECs do not favor one particular cell fate but can undergo both apoptosis and senescence. The reason for these cell type-specific differences remains poorly understood …".

10.4.6 Secondary Autoimmune Processes Sustaining Chronic Inflammation: An Interplay Between Innate and Adaptive Immunity

Adaptive immunity is not a prerequisite for atherogenesis, but its presence profoundly affects lesion formation and, on balance, is proatherogenic. Such adaptive immune responses involve Th1 cells primarily but also Th17 and Th2 cells and B cells, developing in conjunction with a progressive decrease in Tregs. In fact, the DAMP-promoted adaptive immune response is regulated primarily by mechanisms that affect the balance between regulatory and effector T cells. According to the autoimmune concept of atherosclerosis, the specific disease-associated adaptive immune response is not restricted to subendothelial plaques and draining lymph nodes. Microvessels, lymphatics, and small conduits are created to communicate between the plaque and the adventitia, leaving the media layer usually blank (for reviews, see Refs. [10–12, 20, 21, 218, 266, 267]).

Indeed, extensive data now support the notion that T cells, mainly Th1 cells in conjunction with IFN-γ, mediate proinflammatory and proatherogenic immune responses. The strong stimulatory effect of IFN-γ on autoantigen presentation is mediated via upregulation of MHC-II as well as the ability of this cytokine to inhibit VSMC proliferation and expression of α-SMA.

As reviewed by Wick et al. [2], autoantigens are presented by resident intimal vascular-associated DCs, which accumulate within the proinflammatory milieu or by DCs, which are believed to invade into the atherosclerotic lesions. The vascular-associated DCs are already present within the tertiary lymphoid structures in the adventitia of atherosclerotic vessels. On the other hand, newly invading DCs enter the atherosclerotic lesions from the circulation and the adventitia via the vasa vasorum. In these lesions, DCs often form clusters with T cells, which suggests that direct activation of DCs occurs within the arterial wall and that their accumulation in arterial lesions is associated with plaque growth and inflammation. Nota bene, for principles of uptake and processing of endogenous and exogenous antigens by DAMP-activated immunostimulatory DCs and their subsequent direct presentation and cross-presentation to naïve $CD4^+$ and $CD8^+$ naïve T cells, the reader is referred to Vol. 1 [24], Part VIII, Chaps. 31 and 32. The DAMP-promoted sequelae leading to autoimmune processes in atherosclerosis are briefly sketched as a model scenario in the following (being guided by excellent review articles cited in Refs. [10, 12, 20, 21, 190, 218, 266, 267]).

Initially, autostimulatory DCs—accumulated subendothelially in the arterial wall and activated after recognition of DAMPs through PRMs—engulf and process stress/injury-induced plaque-derived neoantigens in terms of native or modified self-proteins generated in early atherosclerotic lesions (or systemically), such as HSP60/65, the oxidatively modified ApoB-100 component of LDL, and others such as OSEs (Fig. 10.5). In other words, these molecules play a double role in atherogenesis in that they operate not only as DAMPs but also as neoantigens. A crucial question here is as to whether LDL in terms of oxidized LDL represents an altered-self antigen that is recognized by altered self-reactive T cells or whether LDL acts as an unmodified self, that is, bona fide self-antigen. While the first notion cannot be regarded—strictly speaking—as a breakdown of self-tolerance, only the last assumption would allow discussing a breakdown of self-tolerance in atherosclerotic plaques leading to autoimmune responses in atherosclerosis.

Regardless of this unsolved question, the vascular autostimulatory DCs, then, migrate from the atherosclerotic lesions—even from advanced plaques—to the secondary lymphoid tissues and present these self-proteins as peptide/major histocompatibility complex (pMHC) complexes to naïve altered self-reactive $CD4^+$ T cells leading to T-cell clonal expansion and differentiation into effector Th1 cells but also Th17 cells that can promote plaque fibrosis. Also, local presentation of antigens by DCs in atherosclerotic plaques can reactivate T cells in atherosclerotic plaques, leading to further differentiation and proliferation. By contrast to Th1 cells, Th2 cells can be found much less frequent in atherosclerotic plaques, and Th2-type cytokines have complex (and in part, opposite) effects on atherosclerosis. However, their exact role in atherogenesis is not yet clear. Similarly, conflicting effects of Th17 cells in atherosclerosis development have been reported. In sum, the findings so far published suggest that Th17 cells can differentiate in response to the development of atherosclerotic disease, promote plaque stability, and have a role in preventing cardiovascular events [268]. The effector T cells (i.e., CTLs) migrate into arterial lesions where they cause further vascular injury leading to induction of DAMPs (in terms of a fourth wave) that again initiate proinflammatory and/or profibrotic innate immune pathways (i.e., a vicious circle) (compare Figs. 10.4 and 10.5) (for details of DAMP-shaped adaptive immune responses, also see Vol. 1 [24], Part VIII, Chap. 32).

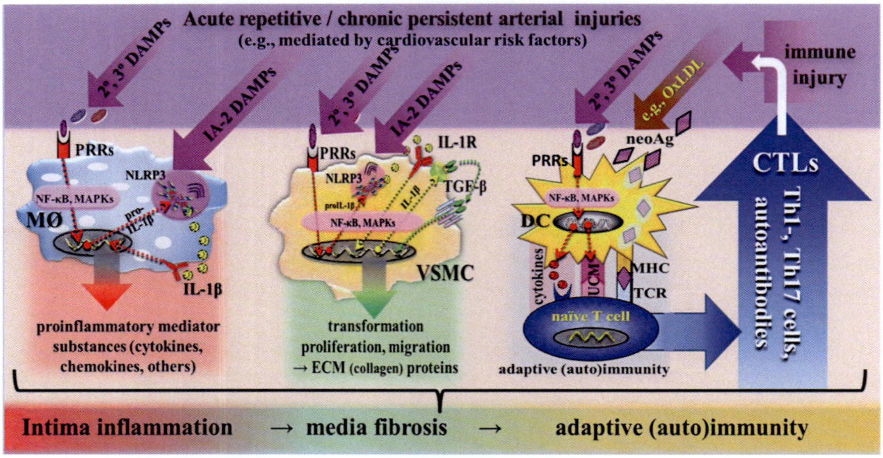

Fig. 10.5 Schematic scenario model of endothelial injury-induced, innate, and adaptive immune responses involved in atherogenesis. Vascular innate immune cells—here illustrated by PRR-bearing, NLRP3 inflammasome-expressing macrophages, vascular smooth muscle cells, and dendritic cells—are activated by the second and third wave of DAMPs induced by various vascular injuries. All three cell types exert different innate immune functions which orchestrate a network of processes leading to the characteristic features of atherosclerosis, that is, (1) macrophages, via function of the NLRP3 inflammasome (compare Fig. 2.1), contribute to creation of vessel wall inflammation; (2) activated smooth muscle cells (again via function of the NLRP3 inflammasome) contribute to development of vascular fibrosis via transition to myofibroblast-like cells (compare Fig. 10.4); and (3) vascular dendritic cells engulf and process neoantigens such as oxidation-specific epitopes (e.g., OxLDL), migrate to secondary lymphoid tissue, and present the peptide/MHC complex to naïve T cells. This leads to the initiation and induction of a specific adaptive Th17- and/or Th1 autoimmune response that, via CTLs and cytotoxic antibodies, may further aggravate the vascular injury. *CTLs* cytotoxic T lymphocytes, *DCs* dendritic cells, *ECM* extracellular matrix, *IL-1R* interleukin-1 receptor, *MØ* macrophage, *MAPKs* mitogen-activated protein kinases, *MHC* major histocompatibility complex, *neoAg* neoantigens, *NF-κB* nuclear factor-kappaB; *NLRP3* nucleotide binding and oligomerization domain-like receptor family, pyrin domain-containing 3, *OxLDL* oxidized low-density lipoproteins, *PRRs* pattern recognition receptors, *TCR* T cell receptor, *TGF-β* transforming growth factor-beta, *UCM* upregulation of costimulatory molecules, *VSMC* vascular smooth muscle cell, *2°, 3° DAMPs* second, third wave of DAMPs. (Source: [2, 11, 12, 20, 285, 286])

Of note, the cellular adaptive autoimmune response, in particular, during the early phases of atherogenesis, can also be atheroprotective as reflected by the generation of Tregs (for Tregs, see Vol. 1 [24], Part VIII, Sects. 33.2.3 and 33.4). Thus, experimental studies revealed that Tregs inhibit the activity of autoreactive Th1 effector T cells by release of antiinflammatory cytokines such as IL-10 and TGF-β. As the disease progresses, this control is gradually lost, and the immune responses toward plaque-associated neoantigens switch toward activation of Th1 or Th17 effector T cells and release of proinflammatory cytokines such as IFN-γ and TNF as well as profibrotic IL-17 (reviewed in [20, 21, 269]).

B cells are only occasionally found in atherosclerotic plaques, and their role in atherosclerosis remains controversial. Although most of the literature has indicated that B cells are protective in atherosclerosis, some studies have recently questioned this hypothesis. Nonetheless, some data suggest that B2 cells are proatherogenic, while B1a cells are atheroprotective. Both pro- and antiatherosclerotic mechanisms of B cells were shown to be driven by antibodies against OSEs on LDL that are found in the circulation and in plaques of animals and humans (reviewed in [20, 270]).

10.4.7 Atherofibrosis and Atherocalcification

10.4.7.1 General Remarks

Atherosclerosis is generally acknowledged to be associated with fibrogenic/fibrotic processes that promote the development of the disease. Specifically, one has to distinguish between the formation of a fibrous cap in intimal plaques and the real vascular fibrosis developing in the media.

10.4.7.2 Fibrous Cap Formation

According to traditional notions, fibrous cap formation is the product of resident medial VSMCs that undergo phenotypic modulation and migrate into the intima where they proliferate, produce ECM (e.g., collagen), and participate in fibrous cap formation/stabilization. The phenotypic plasticity of VSMCs is characterized by their unique ability to switch, upon environmental stress and injury, from a quiescent "contractile" state into an active "synthetic" phenotype, in which VSMCs display enhanced migration, proliferation, and secretory capacity (e.g., outlined and discussed in Refs. [271–274]). That this scenario of phenotypic transition of VSMCs is much more complicated and represents a future therapeutic challenge has been discussed elsewhere [272].

Nevertheless, this momentum of stress-promoted transformation of VSMCs is generally understood to play a significant role in the development of the phenomenon of intimal hyperplasia (= neointimal formation). Interestingly, first evidence has been reported in support of the notion that atherosclerotic risk factor-mediated stress/injury may provoke emission of DAMPs (OxLDL, HMGB1, NLRP3-activating DAMPs, GAL-3) which, in turn, promote VSMCs to toggle to the "synthetic" phenotype (compare Refs. [275–278]). It is tempting to speculate that DAMPs may even contribute to VSMCs transformation via promotion of epigenetic modifications, which have been discussed to regulate VSMCs plasticity [271] (also compare Sect. 6.6.3).

10.4.7.3 Vascular Fibrosis

Vascular fibrosis, also called atherosclerosis takes place in the vascular media and involves accumulation of ECM proteins, mainly collagen and fibronectin, associated with inhibition of matrix degradation. The ECM components contribute to structural remodeling and scar formation that is associated with arterial stiffening, which has been demonstrated to promote the development of atherosclerosis and be a typical natural consequence of advancing age (also compare Sect. 6.2). This fibroproliferative response is the result of an intercellular networking that occurs among macrophages (M2-like macrophages), VSMCs, ECs, and T cells, whereby ECM plays a dominant role (for reviews, see Refs. [279–284]). In particular, DAMP-driven phenotypic transformation of VSMCs from contraction to synthesis is widely accepted as the pivotal process in vascular remodeling [285, 286]. Mechanistically, the biomechanical properties of arteries are discussed to be largely dependent on the absolute and relative quantities of collagen and elastin, whereby both excessive collagen and a lack of elastin in the vascular wall lead to vascular fibrosis [287–289]. Among the various factors reported to promote vascular fibrosis, TGF-β plays a critical role in ECM accumulation and vascular remodeling via upregulating the production of several agents, including connective tissue growth factor and fibroblast growth factor (compare Sect. 6.5). An imbalance between MMPs and TIMPs results in collagen accumulation and adverse matrix remodeling (reviewed in Ref. [283]).

As with chronic intimal inflammation, atherofibrosis is initiated and sustained by injury, brought about by the typical risk factors such as those described above. Again, according to current notions, DAMPs are also implicated in vascular fibrogenesis in terms of a DAMP-induced maladaptive overshooting innate repairing response upon acute repetitive or chronic persistent vascular injury. In particular, as discussed in detail in Sect. 10.6.2.5, DAMPs that are known to activate the NLRP3 inflammasome appear to be the most critical danger signals in promoting vascular fibrosis. These observations are in line with current knowledge about the power of DAMPs to promote interstitial fibrosis in general (see Sects. 6.4 and 6.5, as well as Vol. 1 [24], Part VIII, Sect. 36.4). In other words, the growing evidence for a role of DAMPs in the formation of fibrous caps may also count for their fibrogenic function in the development of medial atherofibrosis (compare again Refs. [275–278]).

10.4.7.4 Vascular Calcification

In the context of atherofibrosis, it is worth touching the topic of ectopic arterial calcification as another typical late feature of atherosclerosis (for a recent review, see Hortell et al. Ref. [290]) Vascular calcification was once considered a passive and degenerative process evolving during aging in terms of "wear and tear," but it is now considered an active, possibly DAMP-induced biological process that shares many features of physiological bone formation and remodeling. The process is complex and is driven by atherosclerotic risk factors in the frame of a genetic background, although the precise mechanisms have not fully elucidated. As outlined [290], factors such as high levels of extracellular phosphate and calcium, ROS, oxidized lipoproteins, and proinflammatory cytokines contribute to driving VSMCs toward a calcifying phenotype, located preferentially in the media.

Excitingly, there is first evidence suggesting that certain DAMPs such as OSEs (e.g., modified LDL) and S100A12 proteins are implicated in the promotion of arterial calcification. Thus, the experiments so far designed and conducted in this research field let suggest a phenotypic switch of contractile VSMCs to osteoblast-like VSMCs by uptake of enzyme-modified LDL in the medial layer and neointima (reviewed by Chellan et al. [291]). Certainly, further studies are needed to clarify the underlying mechanisms, in particular, to explore the role of DAMPs in the transition of VSMCs into osteoblast-like cells.

10.4.7.5 Concluding Remarks

Atherofibrosis and atherocalcification are typical features of aging characterized by arterial remodeling, vascular fibrosis, and arterial stiffening, resembling interstitial ECM stiffness. Of note, as described for the DAMP-driven self-perpetuating process of interstitial fibrosis, the fibrogenic process in vascular fibrosis is also progressive, leading to further worsening of arterial stiffness and fibrosis that gradually extends into the neighboring interstitial space, causing tissue and organ damage [284]. However, whether similar mechanisms are involved in both scenarios is not known and has to be explored.

10.4.8 Pathogenetic Role of Nonresolving Inflammatory Responses in Atherogenesis

10.4.8.1 General Remarks on Resolution of Inflammation and Its Defects

The causative background of chronic inflammation of the arterial subendothelial space was and still is a major topic of research in atherosclerosis. Today, most researchers agree on the notion that chronic progressive inflammation of the arterial wall reflects an event of nonresolving inflammation. It is this event that drives the development of clinically dangerous atherosclerotic lesions by promoting sustained atheromatous plaque inflammation, large necrotic cores, thin fibrous caps prone to plaque rupture, and thrombosis. This process of defective resolution involves activation of both the innate and adaptive branches of the host immune system (for competent articles, see Refs. [292–299]).

Resolution of Inflammation

At this point, it seems worthwhile to briefly remember the nature of the process of inflammation resolution as already partially alluded to above in Sect. 5.3 (for additional information also compare Vol. 1 [24], Part VI, Sect. 22.2.3, p. 480, plus Fig. 22.1, p. 477). Indeed, the timely resolution of inflammation is essential to restore tissue homeostasis and to avoid chronic inflammatory diseases. This unique, highly coordinated program is governed by innate immune cells and specific mediators produced by them. Accordingly, cells of the innate immune system such as neutrophils and macrophages are not only innate immune cells to promote inflammation but also participate in its resolution. For example, resident macrophages, after clearance of injurious factors, replenish their populations by proliferation and a shift from proinflammatory M1-like phenotype to antiinflammatory/proresolving M2-like phenotype to promote the resolution of inflammation by clearing apoptotic cells/cell debris. In fact, there is recent evidence suggesting that M2-like macrophages enhance effective efferocytosis via upregulated MerTK receptor [300, 301] (for MerTK, see Sect. 2.3.2, and for the issue of M1 → "M1-like" and M2 → "M2-like"macrophages; for additional information compare also Vol. 1 [24], Part III, Sect. 8.2.2.2, p. 117, and Fig. 8.2, p. 119). Thus, promoting apoptosis of neutrophils and their phagocytic removal via efferocytosis by macrophages represent fundamental cellular mechanisms involved in the resolution of inflammation (reviewed in Refs. [302–304]) (for efferocytosis, see Sect. 5.3.2.2 and also compare Vol. 1 [24], Part VI, Sect. 22.6.3.3). As outlined in Vol. 1 [24], Part IV, Sect. 14.4 and in Sect. 5.3.3, it is the work of SAMPs that drives and sustains these resolution processes. Like DAMPs, SAMPs are emitted upon stress and injury, which—in parallel to proinflammatory responses—convey proresolving and antiinflammatory processes, as well as shape immunosuppressive responses aimed at maintaining tissue homeostasis. Accordingly, as reported by the Serhan group [305–309], several SPMs, particularly MaR1 and RvD2, have been demonstrated to limit further PMN infiltration in inflamed tissue and have an additional effect on macrophage phenotype by (1) favoring M2-like markers, (2) increasing efferocytic and phagocytic capacity, as well as (3) facilitating tissue regeneration.

In addition, and excitingly, recent hypothetical models hold that the resolving mechanisms of inflammation, at least in part, are influenced by epigenetic changes in innate immune cells that are involved in DAMP-promoted inflammatory processes [310] (for epigenetic modifications, see Sect. 5.6 and also Vol. 1 [24], Part VI, Sect. 24.2). For example, regarding posttranslational histone modifications, antiinflammatory macrophages reportedly express the histone JMJD3 (an H3K27 demethylase) in response to the "M2-like" polarization-promoting cytokine IL-4 [311]. Moreover, type I IFNs, especially IFN-β, have been shown to induce expression of the histone methyltransferase *SET domain bifurcated 2* (Setdb2) in macrophages, leading to epigenetic repression of proinflammatory genes through increased *histone H3 tri methyl K9* (H3K9me3) [312, 313]. In fact, as stressed elsewhere [314], histone methyltransferases are strongly associated with activation of antiinflammatory macrophages by repressing phenotype signature genes of inflammatory macrophages and promoting the transcription of genes of antiinflammatory macrophages, whereby repression may occur in the basal state or during inflammation.

Disturbance of the Process of Inflammation Resolution

However, the homeostatic process of inflammation resolution can be disturbed under pathological conditions. As also discussed in Vol. 1 [24], Part VI, Sects. 22.2.4.2 and 22.2.4.3, causes of inappropriate or inefficient resolving mechanisms can be found on a cellular or humoral level. Cellular roots mainly refer to (1) the failure of neutrophils to undergo timely apoptosis, or (2) failure of macrophages to clear those apoptotic neutrophilic cells by efferocytosis [315], or (3) an abnormal T cell response, for instance, as indicated by deficiency in Tregs. On the other hand, defective, that is, reduced or delayed expression of SAMPs such as SPMs or antiinflammatory cytokines may be the reason for ongoing inflammatory processes. For example, exudates from ongoing inflammation were shown to have a significant imbalance in the SPMs to proinflammatory leukotriene ratio compared with exudates from self-limited or resolving inflammation [316].

However, the most straightforward cause of nonresolving inflammation is the acute repetitive or chronic persistent emission of DAMPs in the course of acute repetitive/permanent sterile injury (e.g., ROS-mediated oxidative injury) as well as of autoimmune (e.g., autoantibodies)-mediated or pathogen-mediated injury. In these situations, large amounts of both constitutive and inducible DAMPs may be emitted/secreted and override the action of SAMPs and, thus, can operate as a molecular driver of chronic inflammatory responses.

Regarding the process of nonresolving inflammation in atherosclerosis, various causes may be discussed as briefly touched here.

10.4.8.2 Insufficient/Inferior Action of SAMPs in Nonresolving Arterial Wall Inflammation

First of all, SAMPs are definitely generated in atherosclerosis! For example, in studies on carotid endarterectomy specimens from patients with significant carotid stenosis, AnxA1 was found to be constitutively expressed in all plaques, but its gene expression was statistically higher in patients with asymptomatic disease compared with those with neurological symptoms [317]. Given these findings, the authors suggest that high AnxA1 expression may have a stabilizing effect in asymptomatic patients with less echolucent atherosclerotic plaques. They further postulated that this SAMP may play an essential role in preventing plaque complications or disease progression (for AnxA1, see Sect. 3.5.5.2 and Vol. 1 [24], Part IV, Sect. 14.4.3.2). Also, Ang-(1-7) was shown to protect endothelial cell function and prevent early atherosclerosis by inhibiting inflammatory responses [318]. Moreover, in studies on atherosclerosis models in mice, extracellular adenosine in mice resistant to atherosclerosis was found to exert antiinflammatory and antiatherosclerotic properties [319]. In turn, as also observed in these studies, mice with genetically induced hypercholesterolemia and atherosclerosis showed decreased production and increased degradation of extracellular adenosine. Lastly, the SPM RvD1 was found to enhance the clearance of necroptotic cells in advanced murine plaques [320].

However, defects in these or any other of the SAMP-governed proresolving pathways can impair resolution of arterial wall inflammation and, thus, may contribute to chronic inflammation observed in atherogenesis. Growing data from current research on SPMs underline this appraisal. In fact, as reviewed and emphasized by Kasikara et al. [297] and Bäck et al. [299], in human and murine advanced atherosclerosis, there is an imbalance between levels of SPMs and proinflammatory lipid mediators, resulting in the development of features of clinically significant plaques as reflected by sustained leukocyte influx into lesions and inflammatory macrophage polarization (compare Fig. 10.6; for imbalance of macrophage polarization, here M2-like macrophages → M1-like macrophages, also compare Vol. 1 [24], Part III, Sect. 8.2.2.2 and Fig. 8.2). For example, in studies on flash-frozen human plaques obtained from carotid endarterectomy, extended by appropriate experiments in a

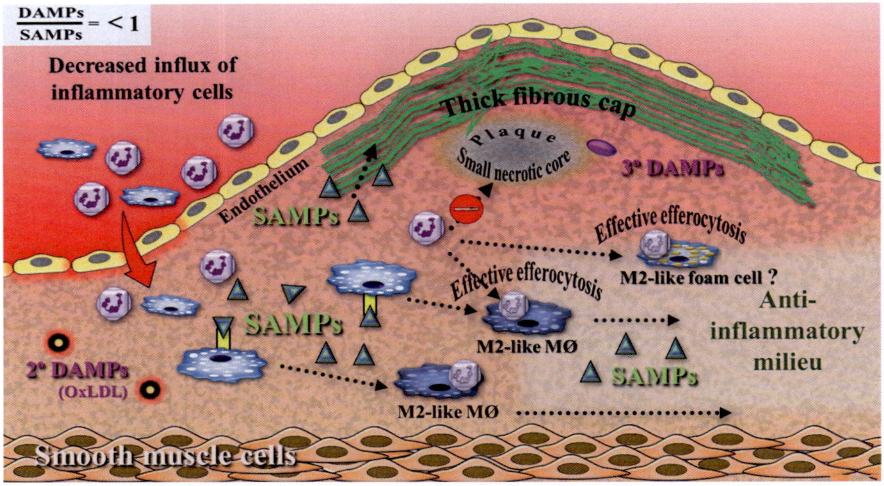

Fig. 10.6 Schematically designed narrative model of a scenario in atherosclerotic plaques, illustrating the role of antagonistically acting SAMPs overriding the agonistic function of DAMPs, that is, the DAMPs:SAMPs ratio, is less than 1 (based on evidence so far published; for references, see below). When non-defective SAMPs in efficient quantities dominate, they facilitate resolution of intimal inflammation via decreased influx of inflammatory cells; generation of M2-like macrophages (and M2-like foam cells) which in turn enhance effective efferocytosis; creation of a thick fibrous cap and small necrotic core; and promotion of an antiinflammatory milieu in the vessel wall. Conversely, an increase in the DAMPs:SAMPs ratio above 1 promotes instability of atherosclerotic plaques, see next Fig. 10.7. *MØ* macrophage, *OxLDL* oxidized low-density lipoproteins, *2°, 3° DAMPs* second, third wave of DAMPs. (Sources: [295, 297, 299–301, 317–320, 488–490])

murine atherosclerotic model [295], the authors could demonstrate that regions of atherosclerotic plaques, characterized by large necrotic cores and thin fibrous caps, have low levels of the proresolving mediator RvD1 but high levels of the proinflammatory mediator LTB4. The background of the discovery can explain this finding, as briefly sketched here.

Leukotriene B4 can be regarded as an inducible DAMP that is mainly produced by activated neutrophils and macrophages via enhancement of the nuclear localization of 5-LOX [321–323]; this inducible danger signal mediates its effects through two cognate GPCRs, BLT1, and BLT2 (also called LTB4R1 and LTB4R2) [323, 324] (for LTB4 acting as an inducible DAMPs, also see Sect. 3.5.3.3). Conversely, plaque regions containing less necrosis and thicker fibrous have high levels of RvD1 and relatively lower levels of LTB4 [295]. Indeed, these findings convincingly demonstrate that the ratio of RvD1 to LTB4 correlates with plaque severity and, thus, provide further support to the concept that defective resolution of inflammation contributes to atherosclerosis progression (for the role of the DAMPs:SAMPs ratio in inflammation and its switch from the proinflammatory to the proresolving phase, see Sect. 7.3.3.2 and Fig. 7.1).

In line with these observations are other studies showing that the plasma levels of the SPM LXA4 are decreased in patients with peripheral artery disease compared with healthy controls. Given that both SPMs signal through the GPCR ALX/FPR2, their decreased levels in these patients—according to Bäck et al. [299]—suggest "that the proresolving signaling through this receptor might be perturbed in advanced atherosclerosis, consistent with a failure in the resolution of inflammation" (for ALX/FPR2, see Sect. 2.3.4.6).

In another set of studies in atherosclerosis-prone mice (i.e., ApoE KO mice), Viola et al. [296] presented evidence for the imbalance between inflammatory and resolving lipid mediators during atheroprogression. Indeed, their studies revealed an expansion of inflammatory lipid mediator LTB4, associated in parallel with a decrease of the resolving lipid mediators RvD2 and MaR1, during advanced atherosclerosis. Notably, the increased level of LTB4 was observed to correlate directly with plaque vulnerability whereas RvD2 and MaR1 to be associated with plaque stability. In extended therapy-related experiments of this study, repetitive RvD2 and MaR1 delivery was observed to prevent atheroprogression as characterized by halted expansion of the necrotic core and accumulation of macrophages along with increased fibrous cap thickness and VSMC numbers. Mechanistically, RvD2 and MaR1 reportedly induced a shift in macrophage profile toward a reparative phenotype, which secondarily stimulated collagen synthesis in VSMCs. The authors argued [296] that delivery of resolving lipid mediators halts inflammation, possibly by instructing a positive feedback loop focused on the induction of reparative macrophages giving rise to a homeostasis-restoring environment that promotes plaque stability.

In support of these observations are experimental studies on ApoE KO mice reported by Laguna-Fernandez et al. [325]. They showed that deficiency of the E-resolvin receptor (ERV)/chemerin receptor 23 (ChemR23) (i.e., ERV1/ChemR23, the receptor for RvE1) increases atherosclerotic lesion size and macrophage content. Similar findings along with an increased necrotic core size were also observed in chimeric animals receiving ChemR23-deficient bone marrow grafts. This data, together with observations that ChemR23 localizes to a subset of lesional macrophages near the necrotic core in human atherosclerotic plaques, point to a specific role for RvE1 → ERV1/ChemR23 signaling in macrophages to limit necrotic core formation. Another highlight of these studies was the observation that RvE1 directly decreases the uptake of OxLDL by macrophages in vitro.

Interestingly, the imbalance between high levels of proinflammatory lipid mediators and low levels of SPMs in advanced atherosclerosis, as clinically manifested by significant plaques, was found to contribute to impaired efferocytosis (reviewed in Refs. [297, 299])—a topic that should be alluded to a bit more in detail in the next section.

10.4.8.3 Defective Efferocytosis in Atherosclerosis

As described in Sect. 5.3.2.2 and Vol. 1 [24], Part VI, Sect. 22.6.3.3, efferocytosis is a carefully orchestrated process by which phagocytes are recruited to sites of cell death, recognize and engulf apoptotically dying cells, and clear them in an "immunologically silent" manner, often associated with secretion of SAMPs before they become necrotic. Indeed, this process is essential for maintenance of normal tissue homeostasis and represents a vital step in successful resolution of

DAMP-induced lesional inflammation (reviewed in Refs. [326–328]; also compare Fig. 5.1). However, defects in any of the four steps of efferocytosis (mentioned in Sect. 5.3.2.2) can lead to secondary post-apoptotic necrosis associated with the release of large amounts of DAMPs which continue to activating innate immune cells. Pathogenetically, these DAMP-activated cells promote further inflammatory responses, which often become chronic and nonresolving (compare Sect. 5.5.2).

This pathogenetic principle is now agreed upon to apply to atherosclerosis, too (compare Fig. 10.7). Failure to clear apoptotic cells from atherosclerotic plaques in a timely fashion leads to secondary necrosis, which promotes persistent inflammation owing to the release of DAMPs from the necrotic cells, probably predominantly derived from the necrotic core of plaques (see Refs. [220, 294, 297, 299, 329]) (for apoptosis proceeding to secondary necrosis, see Vol. 1 [24], Part V, Sect. 19.2.3 and Fig. 19.2). Although the mechanisms of defective efferocytosis during atherosclerosis are still not precisely defined, distinct molecular and cellular dysfunctions in the process of engulfment of apoptotic cells have been uncovered. Thus, as reviewed by Bäck et al. [299], experimental studies have already provided evidence for a considerable dysfunction of apoptosis-facilitating receptors such as MerKT (a member of the TAM family) and TIM1/4 in progressive atherosclerosis (for apoptotic cell-recognizing receptors, compare Sect. 2.3.2). Also, apoptotic cells in mouse and human atherosclerotic lesions were shown to have variations in "eat-me" signal that renders them resistant to efferocytosis. For example, atherosclerotic plaques from patients carrying a genetic variation at the *9p21* locus (known to be associated with atherosclerosis) have reportedly reduced levels of the "eat-me" signal CALR compared with atherosclerotic plaques from non-carriers [330]. The studies further revealed that, as a result of decreased CALR, apoptotic bodies were resistant to efferocytosis and not efficiently cleared by neighboring macrophages (for CALR as an "eat-me" signal in terms of an exposed IB-1 DAMP, see Vol. 1 [24], Part IV, Sect. 12.3.2.2 and Fig. 12.5).

Taken together, defective efferocytosis has emerged as a critical pathogenetic momentum in atherosclerosis. In this context, Bäck et al. [299] concluded: "These studies demonstrate that defective efferocytosis transforms benign lesions into clinically relevant atheromas in both mice and humans. These atheromas are particularly sensitive to the accumulation of necrotic cells and to the loss of anti-inflammatory and pro-resolving responses that, as mentioned above, are inherent to the efferocytosis programme. These findings raise the possibility that therapeutic strategies that increase efferocytosis in the atherosclerotic lesion might reduce the risk of plaque rupture."

10.4.8.4 Impairment of the Action of T Regulatory Cells

Defective generation of SAMPs, here, SPMs also contribute to atherosclerosis since, under homeostatic conditions, SPMs were shown to promote Tregs and prevent activation of Th1 and Th17 cells (for a role of Tregs in atherosclerosis, see Sect. 10.4.6). As reviewed by Chiurchiu et al. [331], SPMs are able to prevent naïve $CD4^+$ T-cell differentiation into Th1 and Th17 by downregulating their signature transcription factors, T-bet and RORγt, in a mechanism mediated by the GPR32 and ALX/FPR2 receptors. Additionally, they concomitantly enhanced de novo generation and function of Foxp3$^+$ Tregs via the GPR32 receptor (for Th1,Th17 cells, Tregs, T-bet, and RORγt, see Vol. 1 [24], Part VIII, Sects. 32.4, and 33.4 and Fig. 32.4). This result is in line with a report of MaR1 in engaging Tregs in mice to promote resolution of lung inflammation [332]. Although further studies are needed to demonstrate the existence of an indirect modulation of Th1 and Th17 cells by an SPM-mediated sustained induction of Treg cells, these findings suggest that SPMs might modulate inflammatory responses via several selective mechanisms on specific adaptive immune cells. Chiurchiu et al. concluded [331]: "Although further studies are needed to demonstrate the existence of an indirect modulation of Th1 and Th17 cells by a SPM-mediated sustained induction of Treg cells, these findings suggest that SPMs might modulate inflammatory responses via several selective mechanisms on specific adaptive immune cells. This hypothesis is conceivable, also in the light of the recent discovery that Th17 cells transdifferentiate into Treg cells during resolution of inflammation… , where SPMs might be possible key players of such Th17 instability and plasticity."

10.4.8.5 Concluding Remarks

It has become evident that atherogenesis mirrors chronic inflammation of the arterial wall, today recognized and identified as the result of chronic nonresolving inflammatory responses. According to the homeostatic principle of DAMP-regulated proinflammatory and SAMP-governed counterbalancing proresolving pathways leading to *restitutio ad integrum*, the pathogenetic momentum in atherosclerosis may be sought in an imbalance of the DAMP:SAMP ratio in that DAMPs outweigh SAMPs (see Fig. 10.7 and compare Fig. 5.3). Indeed, there is already growing experimental and clinical evidence for impaired generation and dysregulated function of SAMPs, mutually interacting with impaired efferocytotic activities. Both findings underline the current view on atherosclerosis as an expression of ongoing chronic DAMP-promoted nonresolving inflammatory processes.

10.4.9 Résumé

Taken together, the pathogenetic role of DAMPs and SAMPs in terms of an imbalance in the homeostatic DAMP:SAMP ratio in atherosclerosis progression appears to be well established. In particular, increasing evidence has been reported indicating impaired generation and dysregulated function of SAMPs that results in a functional overbalance of atherogenic DAMPs. In other words, infectious/sterile stress/injury to the arterial wall—acute repetitively or persistently induced—leads to acute repetitive or permanent emission of DAMPs, which override the parallel emission of dysfunctional SAMPs. Consequently, DAMP-induced promotion of infectious/sterile inflammation of the arterial wall overrides SAMP-induced resolution of inflammation, the end result being chronic nonresolving inflammation that transitions into vascular fibrosis.

However, the role of poorly expressed and dysfunctional SAMPs (in association with impaired efferocytosis) as the sole reason for the imbalance of the DAMP:SAMPs ratio in atherogenesis may be questioned. Given the work of four subsequently occurring waves of DAMPs generation/emission, culminating in the release of large amounts of DAMPs from subroutines of RCD within the necrotic core of plaques, it can be suggested that these overwhelmingly emitted DAMPs override the work of SAMPs in their regular quantity and function.

This scenario may be even more detrimental in view of the phenomenon of trained immunity: this mechanism leads to MAMP and DAMP- or DAMP-induced activation of already epigenetically reprogrammed, that is, "overactivated" myeloid cells which contribute to progression of atherosclerotic lesions, a topic that deserves a few more words in the following.

10.5 The Role of Trained Immunity and Immunometabolism in Chronic Proatherosclerotic Inflammation

10.5.1 Introductory Remarks

Epigenetic modifications of the genome, such as DNA methylation and histone modifications, have been reported to play a critical role in atherosclerosis (reviewed in [333]). Here, some remarks are made to this hot topic in CVD, using the example of trained immunity. The defining feature of trained immunity as an innate immune memory is based on the innate immune cell's ability to retain and recall information about previous exposures to infectious or sterile insults. This cellular memory is fostered by crucial shifts in transcriptional and metabolic pathways. Current notions in this research branch of innate immunity hold that such alterations are inseparably and bi-directionally linked through epigenetic mechanisms at the level of histone methylation and acetylation (briefly discussed in Vol. 1 [24], Part VI, Sect. 24.2.4, and updated in Sects. 5.6.2.3, 5.6.3.3, and 5.6.3.4 and Fig. 5.4). There is good and bad news of trained immunity. While the beneficial effects of trained immunity may be numerous and multilocal and worthwhile, potential deleterious effects such as enhancing chronic infectious/sterile inflammatory processes must also be considered.

10.5.2 Trained Immunity of Innate Immune Cells in Chronic Proatherosclerotic Inflammation

Excitingly, headed by the Radboud University group, this mechanism has been proposed to contribute to the well-known association between acute and chronic infectious/sterile inflammation and atherosclerotic CVD [334–339]. The proposal was deduced from the typical persistent state of heightened innate immune cell activation in trained immunity that may also contribute to progression of atherosclerosis development and acute destabilization of existing atherosclerotic plaques [340].

In fact, trained immunity—as another explanation of chronically ongoing vascular inflammation—is not only induced by microbial products, that is, MAMPs, but also by endogenous sterile atherogenic stimuli, that is, DAMPs, such as OxLDL or lipoprotein(a) (Lp[a]) (reviewed in Refs. [334, 341, 342]).

First data from in vitro studies in support of this concept showed that brief OxLDL exposure of human monocytes induces epigenetic histone modifications (histone methylation—H3K4me3) that result in a long-lasting proinflammatory phenotype with increased production of proinflammatory cytokines (such as IL-6, TNF) and chemokines (such as MCP-1), augmented foam cell formation, and increased production of MMPs [343].

Remarkably, in vivo studies were conducted in support of this concept (reviewed in [334]. Thus, in studies on circulating monocytes from patients with risk factors for atherosclerosis or established atherosclerosis, Lp(a) was demonstrated to induce trained immunity, an effect related to the OSE OxPLs—that is, Subclass IIB-1 DAMPs—carried by this lipoprotein [344]. In this study, evidence was provided in support of the concept that the proinflammatory IIB-1DAMPs OxPLs are major contributors to the atherogenicity of Lp(a) by showing that (1) patients with elevated Lp(a) have pronounced arterial inflammation in vivo; (2) monocytes isolated from patients with elevated Lp(a) remain in a long-lasting ex vivo activated state; and (3) Lp(a) mounts the proinflammatory response in healthy monocytes in vitro. Similarly, cytokine production capacity was increased in patients with severe established coronary atherosclerosis [345]. The data of this study provided additional evidence in favor of the concept that trained innate immunity contributes to atherogenesis. In particular, this study revealed that circulating monocytes of patients with established atherosclerosis display a proinflammatory phenotype, associated with epigenetic remodeling at the level of histone methylation and increased expression of rate-limiting enzymes of the glycolysis pathway and the pentose phosphate pathway (PPP).

10.5.3 Immunometabolism of Innate Immune Cells in Chronic Proatherosclerotic Inflammation

As impressively highlighted by van der Heijden et al. [342], epigenetic reprogramming and reprogramming of intracellular metabolic pathways are two fundamental processes in trained immunity that are closely intertwined. This is also true for atherogenesis where a proatherosclerotic environment—reflected by the presence of DAMPs and their triggered inflammatory responses—reprograms the immunometabolism of monocytes and macrophages in the various developmental phases of atherosclerosis (reviewed by Riksen and Stienstra and Groh et al. [336, 346]). Accordingly, the epigenetic reprogramming of trained monocytes → macrophages is driven by a profound rewiring of, at least, three intracellular metabolic pathways (reviewed in Ref. [347]).

First, a characteristic feature of activated innate immune cells (monocytes → macrophages) is the shift from mitochondrial OXPHOS fueled by the β-oxidation of lipids to upregulation of anabolic pathways such as aerobic glycolysis (the "Warburg effect," also see Sect. 5.6.2.3 and Vol. 1 [24], Part VI, Sect. 24.4, Box 4.1); the PPP; glutaminolysis; and fatty acid synthesis. By contrast, catabolic pathways, such as fatty acid oxidation, are downregulated (for additional information also compare Vol. 1 [24], Part VI, Sect. 24.4, p. 649, and Part VIII, Chap. 35, p. 837). Importantly, these processes, in particular, activation of the glycolytic rate, also appear to play critical roles in the development of trained immunity. Furthermore, increased glutaminolysis and subsequent accumulation of fumarate occur and integrate immune and metabolic circuits to induce monocyte epigenetic reprogramming by inhibiting KDM5 histone demethylases (for histone demethylation, see Sect. 5.6.3.5).

Finally, the cholesterol synthesis pathway has also been reported to modulate trained immunity and epigenetic reprogramming, combining transcriptomic and epigenomic studies in OxLDL-trained monocytes [348]. The experiments concerned revealed that the cholesterol synthesis pathway is essential for activation and/or amplification of trained immunity and its inhibition by statins downregulated the increased cytokine production and epigenetic reprogramming induced by OxLDL. In their study, the authors could show that not the synthesis of cholesterol itself is essential but the accumulation of the metabolite mevalonate, an intermediate of the cholesterol biosynthetic pathway. According to the investigators' interpretation, this indicates that, next to fumarate, mevalonate is an essential metabolite in the metabolo-epigenetic pathways mediating trained immunity.

Of note, there is a growing body of evidence in support of the notion that the activation of the glycolytic rate in plaque macrophages is the work of MAMPs or DAMPs. As outlined in Sect. 10.4.5, within the microenvironment of a nascent atherosclerotic plaque associated with necrotic cores, multiple atherogenic DAMPs, including IIB-4 DAMPs (= OxLDL), passively released IA-1 and IA-2 DAMPs (uric acid and cholesterol crystals), as well as cell-intrinsic dyshomeostatic IIC-4 DAMPs (reflected by hypoxia), are emitted which affect the metabolism and drive glycolytic activation of plaque macrophages in the context of atherosclerosis (reviewed by Riksen and Stiensdra [336]). Interestingly, metabolic changes have also reportedly been observed in circulating monocytes and their bone marrow progenitors, driven by systemic DAMPs derived from hypercholesterolemia or hyperglycemia. Also, OSE such as OxPLs were shown to impact macrophage metabolism: thus, by activation of glycolysis and the PPP, OxPLs were found to drive the increased expression of antioxidant genes and increased glutathione production [349].

A critical and burning question is as to how the metabolic alterations, briefly touched here, ultimately interlink to gene expression and inflammatory phenotype of the cells (= "overactivated cells"). One explanation of this momentum refers to epigenetic reprogramming as the underlying key mechanism (for reviews, see [335, 336, 339, 346, 350]). Thus, various intermediate metabolites from the abovementioned pathways—serving as essential substrates or cofactors—coregulate the activity of epigenetic enzymes. This culminates in long-term activation of proinflammatory gene transcription by enrichment of activating histone marks and increase of chromatin accessibility (for histone marks and chromatin accessibility, see Sect. 5.6.2.2 and Fig. 5.4). For example, as outlined by Groh et al. [346], histone acetyltransferase applies acetyl-CoA as the acetyl donor during the acetylation of histone lysine residues. Additionally, acetylated histone marks such as H3K9ac and H3K27ac are associated with active promoters and enhancers. On the other hand, histone deacetylases reduce chromatin accessibility and inhibit gene transcription by removing acetyl groups from lysines. Importantly, these adaptations not only occur in circulating mature monocytes but have also been observed in hematopoietic stem and progenitor cells in the bone marrow niche, that is, a phenomenon which explains the finding that trained monocytes remain present in the circulation after initial stimulation for more than three months (reviewed in [346, 350]).

10.5.4 Résumé

Together, a main piece of evidence supports the concept that MAMP/DAMP- or DAMP-promoted training of monocytes and macrophages displays a profound pro-atherogenic phenotype, with increased production of proatherogenic cytokines/chemokines and enhanced foam cell formation. In this context, Riksen and Stienstra conclude [336]: "Evidence is rapidly accumulating that central metabolic pathways in bone marrow myeloid precursors, circulating monocytes, and in plaque macrophages, are profoundly reprogrammed in the context of atherosclerosis development. Activation of glycolysis, the PPP and FAS, and a reduction of FAO, and complex changes in the lysosomal handling of lipids all appear to facilitate atherogenesis. These processes also appear to play major roles in the development of trained immunity."

Also, in this context, Leentjens et al. conclude [334]: "Multiple levels of experimental evidence have now supported the concept that exposure of the innate immune system to a variety of microorganisms triggers a prolonged state of hyperactivation, which has been termed trained immunity."

Finally, given these new exciting insights into the role of trained immunity in atherosclerosis-mediated CVD, Norota concludes [338]): "We now have a clearer picture of molecular mechanisms controlling trained immunity. The next years of research will have to focus on a successful translation in the clinical setting of approaches aimed at controlling trained immunity with the purpose of improving cardiovascular outcomes; and at the same time, should carefully monitor any increase in the risk of infections."

10.6 DAMP-Promoted Inflammatory, Adaptive Immune, and Fibrotic Processes in Atherosclerosis

10.6.1 Introductory Remarks

Up to this point in the chapter, the sources of proatherogenic DAMPs, generated and emitted in terms of four sequentially emerging waves, as well as the various DAMP-promoted proatherogenic responses, have been neatly sketched. Here, this conceptual model is extended by describing some more details of the DAMPs and the innate/adaptive/fibrotic pathways triggered by them in atherosclerosis, as so far reported in the literature.

10.6.2 DAMP-Driven Vessel Wall Inflammation Resulting in Atherosclerosis

10.6.2.1 General Remarks

The DAMP-driven vessel wall inflammation can be regarded as the key momentum in atherogenesis and, thus, is resumed in more detail in the following by focusing on some typical molecules generated or emitted along various stress and injuries, impacting on the arterial wall (for a comprehensive review on DAMPs in atherosclerosis, see also publication of Goulopoulou et al. [139]). Notably, sterile insult-triggered danger signals such as cholesterol crystals, OxLDL, and modified phospholipids can trigger sterile arterial inflammation, whereas, in systemic or local vascular infection, MAMPs plus DAMPs mount infectious inflammatory responses. As with other innate immune diseases, PRMs on/in innate immune cells are fundamental for activating signaling pathways resulting in innate immune proinflammatory responses in atherosclerosis.

10.6.2.2 Oxidation-Specific Epitopes: The Second Wave of Prototypical DAMPs in Atherogenesis

Oxidation-specific epitopes denoted as Subclass IIB-1 DAMPs have been described in detail in Vol. 1 [24] (Part IV, Sect. 13.3.2) and briefly resumed in Sect. 3.4.3.2. Typically, the OSEs possess a dual role by not only functioning as DAMPs but also as altered-self antigens. For example, antibodies against OxLDL have been found in patients with atherosclerosis [351]. The role of this subclass of DAMPs in atherosclerosis has comprehensively reviewed by the Binder group [199, 352, 353]. Here, these reviews are briefly summarized.

As outlined above, the early stages of atherosclerosis are characterized by the subendothelial accumulation and retention of LDL from the circulation through interactions with the ECM components PGs [201]. Once retained, LDL is becoming modified oxidatively via enzymatic or nonenzymatic mechanisms (i.e., lipid peroxidation, also compare Sect. 4.3.4.2) to generate OSEs. Such modified structures (e.g., OxLDL and mmLDL) can be generated by extensive oxidative stress as promoted by the proatherosclerotic risk factors mentioned above. Importantly, OSEs are not only present on OxLDL but also on other autologous lipids and/or proteins, that is, in the membrane of dying cells, apoptotic blebs, and cellular debris. As already mentioned in Sect. 3.4.3.2, the most prominent examples of OSEs include PC of OxPLs, MDA-lysine epitopes, 4-HNE, oxidized PtdSer, CEP, and OxCL. Notably, OxPLs on ApoB-100 particles are strongly associated with Lp(a), qualifying this OSE as the leading carrier of PC-containing OxPL in human lipoproteins [354].

Various cellular and humoral PRMs have been identified to interact specifically with those OSEs: they include LOX-1, TLRs (such as TLR2 and TLR4), SRs (such as SR-B2 [CD36] and SR-A1, see Vol. 1 [24], Part II, Sect. 5.3.3.2), as well as natural IgM antibodies (nIgM receptor, see Vol. 1 [24], Part II, Sect. 5.4.2) and soluble proteins, such as C-reactive protein (CRP) and complement factor H (CFH) (for CFH, see Vol. 1 [24], Part VI, Sect. 23.2.3.4). It is the different sets of SRs and TLRs expressed by ECs and macrophages, which are major cellular sensors of OSEs to triggering atherosclerotic proinflammatory responses. For example, OxPLs promote the expression of chemoattractants, such as CC-chemokine ligand 2, fibronectin containing connecting segment 1, CXCL8, and P-selectin, and also trigger monocyte binding to ECs that is partly mediated by TLR4. Moreover, the SRs are typically located on the surface of atherosclerotic plaque macrophages and mediate the engulfment of OxLDL to generate foam cell formation. Also, OxLDL was found to promote sterile inflammation through assembly of TLR4 and TLR6 heterodimer under regulation by signals from the SR-B2 receptor. Of note, this signaling pathway—in terms of the priming step—paves the way for subsequent activation of the NLRP3 inflammasome by cholesterol crystals that are generated during foam cell formation (for NLRP3 inflammasome, see Sect. 10.6.2.5). In addition to cellular inflammatory processes, OSE-triggered proatherosclerotic humoral innate immune responses have been detected as well. For example, the humoral receptor CRP (a short pentraxin, see Vol. 1 [24], Part II, Sect. 5.4.6) specifically binds phosphocholine of OxPLs, and the key regulator of the alternative complement pathway CFH (see Vol. 1 [24], Part VI, Sect. 23.2.3.4) has been shown to bind MDA epitopes. Notably, the latter may have a critical role in the development of atherosclerotic lesions as CFH was demonstrated to neutralize the ability of MDA epitopes to stimulate the production of IL-8, known to promote lesion formation [355].

However, OSEs on OxLDL not only mediate uptake by macrophages to generate foam cells and trigger many of the chronic inflammatory events resulting in the development of plaques, but—when plaques rupture—they can also trigger thrombus formation, resulting in severe clinical manifestations such as MI and cerebral stroke. In fact, OSE-triggered prothrombotic responses characterized by modulation of activation state of ECs are remarkable. Mechanistically, exposure of ECs to OxLDL reportedly promotes a decreased endothelial barrier function and upregulates adhesion molecules such as VCAM-1, as well as modulates components of the coagulation cascade. This includes enhanced prothrombinase and protein C inhibitor activity, upregulation of TF expression and activity, downregulation of thrombomodulin, and inactivation of TF pathway inhibitor. These events then lead to an overall increased thrombogenic state of ECs (reviewed in [352]).

Together, OSEs operate as strong atherosclerotic DAMPs and are implicated not only in the initial stage of atherogenesis but also contribute to its progression and even may provoke acute thrombotic catastrophes. In their function as modified altered-self antigens, they promote elicitation of adaptive immune antibody responses that, by contrast, however, appear to serve protective functions [267, 356].

10.6.2.3 Extracellular Matrix Degradation Products: Often Underestimated DAMPs Involved in Atherogenesis

Extracellular matrix degradation products have been described as constitutively expressed, injury-modified molecules and denoted as Class IIA DAMPs in Vol. 1 [24] (Part IV, Sect. 13.2). More information about ECM fragment-triggered, MyD88-dependent signaling pathways through TLR2, TLR4, and TLR6 can be found in Vol. 1. [24], Part VI, Sect. 22.3.3.2 and Fig. 22.3.

Some ECM degradation products out of the families of PGs, GAGs, and glycoproteins have been proposed to act as DAMPs in atherosclerotic inflammatory responses (reviewed in Refs. [357, 358]). Evidence from reports so far available suggests that these DAMPs participate in triggering inflammatory responses during all stages of developing atherosclerosis, whereby their activation seems to be mainly the result of oxidative injury/DAMP-induced activation of MMPs. In line with this consideration are studies showing that elevated HMGB1 is associated with induction of MMPs and matrix degradation resulting in collagen, whereby loss and blockade of HMGB1 were found to lead to decreased inflammation and MMP activity [359] (for matrix degradation, see Sect. 6.2.2).

Proteoglycans

The major types of vascular PGs identified in blood vessels include versican, decorin, and biglycan [358]. In studies outside of atherosclerosis research, PGs were shown to trigger inflammatory responses through interaction with TLR2, TLR4, TLR6, and NLRP3 (compare Vol. 1 [24], Part IV, Sect. 13.2.2 and Table 13.1). However, the proatherosclerotic role of PGs has mainly been seen in their lipid-retaining properties [201]. Whether these DAMPs also trigger proatherosclerotic inflammatory responses is still not firmly elucidated. Nevertheless, an indirect clue for this unproven possibility are findings showing that oxidative stress can activate macrophages to secrete MMPs, reported to be involved in intimal thickening and plaque rupture, on the one hand [246]), and engaged in proteoglycans turnover, on the other side (discussed in [204, 360, 361]).

Glycosaminoglycans

Glycosaminoglycans, in particular, fHA, are also recognized as proatherosclerotic DAMPs (IIA-2 DAMPs), which promote inflammation via activation of TLR2, TLR4, and NLRP3, (see Vol. 1. [24], Part IV, Sect. 13.2.3.2 and Table 13.1). Under homeostatic conditions, HA is present predominantly in the tunica adventitia, produced by VSMCs, while during the atherosclerotic process, it is highly synthesized and deposited in the neointima contributing to the thickening of the arterial wall. Furthermore, HA reportedly modulates the immune response by increasing macrophage retention and by promoting the polarization of Th1 cells that enhance macrophage-driven inflammation as well (reviewed in [362, 363]). Notably, HA accumulates in human atherosclerotic plaques and plays a crucial role in their erosion and rupture [364].

Glycoproteins

Glycoproteins such as TNC and FNIII EDA were also demonstrated to be involved in atherosclerosis. Denoted as IIA-3 DAMPs, these molecules activate macrophages and fibroblasts and upregulate inflammatory cytokine expression through TLR4. In particular, TNC (see Vol. 1 [24], Part IV, Sect. 13.2.4.3, and Table 13.1) has been implicated in atherosclerosis progression. For example, TNC is reportedly expressed in advanced atherosclerotic plaque to induce platelet activation that is relevant to atherothrombosis [365]. Interestingly, the level of TNC in atherosclerotic plaque was found to be correlated with the infiltration of macrophages [366]. Similar functions have been described for FNIII EDA (see Vol. 1 [24], Part IV, Sect. 13.2.4.2 and Table 13.1). Thus, in experimental studies, mice lacking FNIII EDA were observed to develop significantly smaller atherosclerotic lesions when compared with controls [367]. Other ECM degradation products such as fibrinogen and heparan sulfate were also demonstrated to be involved in atherogenesis but are not quoted here.

Together, doubtlessly, various DAMPs released from the ECM are highly implicated in the onset and progression of atherosclerosis. Often, however, they are not appropriately addressed but neglected in the international literature. Indeed, more targeted experimental and clinical studies are needed to assess the full spectrum of their action in chronic atherosclerotic inflammatory processes.

10.6.2.4 Cell-Intrinsic Modified DAMPs Contributing to the Third Wave of DAMPs in Atherogenesis: A Closer Look

Cell-intrinsic modified DAMPs (IIC-DAMPs) are molecules that can induce adaptive cell-autonomous (cell-intrinsic) stress responses by using genetically encoded molecular machinery (see Sect. 4.2 as well as Vol. 1 [24], Part V, Chap. 18). For this book, they have been detailed and denoted as Subclass IIC-1 DAMPs (nuclear DNA breaks) and Subclass IIC-4 DAMPs (cell-intrinsic dyshomeostatic DAMPs), respectively (see Table 3.1 and Sect. 3.4.4; additionally, for dyshomeostatic DAMPs and their receptors, compare Vol. 1 [24], Part II, Sect. 5.3.2, Part IV, Sect. 13.4.5, and Part V, Sects. 18.3 and 18.5; and for DNA breaks and their receptors, see Part II, Sect. 5.2.6.4, Part IV, Sect. 13.4.2, and Part V, Sect. 18.6, respectively). As also outlined in Sect. 4.1 and in Vol. 1 [24], Part V, Chap. 17, unsuccessful stress responses as a result of excessive stress such as the oxidative stress response, the ER stress-induced UPR, and the DDR lose their protective effect. Instead, these defense responses result in a controlled destruction of the stressed cell, that is, RCD, whereby the event of RN is of utmost importance with respect to the emission of both constitutive and inducible DAMPs.

Of note, there is a growing body of evidence indicating that, in atherosclerotic plaques, the unsuccessful responses to oxidative stress [40, 368–370], ER stress [329, 370–373], and DNA stress/damage [374–376] promote apoptosis that may lead to secondary necrosis of lesional cells within the necrotic core. In all these situations, dyshomeostatic DAMPs and DNA breaks are initially operating to induce those (later unsuccessful) stress responses, which, at this point, deserve closer attention.

Oxidative Stress in Atherosclerotic Plaques

Independent from its role in promoting initial endothelial dysfunction, oxidative stress within formed atherosclerotic plaques is recognized as contributing to the expansion of the necrotic core, mainly driven by macrophage and VSMC apoptosis. Additionally, the oxidized derivatives of PUFA reportedly promote defective efferocytosis, with the final result of necrotic core expansion [370, 377, 378]. Moreover, trained macrophages are characterized by activation of the PPP that is important for NADPH generation, and, revealingly, ROS production was found to be upregulated in monocytes trained with OxLDL [379]. Together, though not published yet, the unproven possibility is imaginable that the protective oxidative stress response mediated by the Keap1 ↔ Nrf2 system fails in such situations of ROS production in atheromatous plaques (for the oxidative stress-induced Keap1 ↔ Nrf2 pathway, see Sect. 4.2.3.2 and Vol. 1 [24], Part V, Sect. 18.3.3.3 and Fig. 18.4). Plausibly, the expansion of the necrotic core by these excessive oxidative events is automatically associated with expansion of release of DAMPs. One mechanism leading to such a release of DAMPs from necrotic cells refers to ferroptosis. As oxidative stress-induced lipid peroxidation has been described to occur in atherosclerotic plaques [43, 380] and, on the other hand, as lipid peroxidation is considered the primary driver of ferroptosis [381], it is plausibly imaginable that this type of RN may well serve as an important source of passively released DAMPs from necrotic cells in atherosclerotic plaques (as also discussed in [264]).

Endoplasmic Reticulum Stress and the Unfolded Protein Response in Atherosclerotic Plaques

As already mentioned above (Sect. 4.2.5), ER stress—reflecting IIC-4 DAMPs—has emerged as an essential component that influences the course of atherosclerosis, notably, in the advanced stages of the disease. Indeed, accumulating supportive data have been reported linking different pathways of the UPR with atherosclerosis (reviewed in [76, 77]). In particular, ER stress in ECs, VSMCs, and vascular macrophages in combination with oxidative stress is considered mainly responsible for advanced lesional apoptotic cell death in atherosclerotic plaques. This kind of cellular stress can be evoked by those cardiovascular risk factors outlined above. Also, proapoptotic oxidative stress and ER stress inducers were shown to give rise to autophagy as another stress response in the macrophages [382] (for autophagy, compare Sect. 4.2.2).

Indeed, typically, the activation of the various UPR signaling pathways displays a temporal pattern of activation at different stages of atherogenesis [383] (for additional information also compare Vol. 1 [24], Part V, Fig. 18.6, p. 402). Thus, the ATF6 and IRE1α pathways are activated in ECs in atherosusceptible regions of pre-lesional arteries, whereas the PERK pathway is activated in VSMCs and macrophages in early lesions. With the progression of atherosclerosis, the extended duration and increased intensity of ER stress in advanced lesions lead to prolonged and enhanced UPR signaling. Under this circumstance, the PERK pathway induces the expression of death effectors, and, possibly, IRE1α activates apoptosis signaling pathways. This leads to apoptosis of macrophages, ECs, and VSMCs, thereby contributing to the expansion of necrotic cores. Again, the subsequent unavoidable elicitation of other classes of DAMPs released from necrotic cells, then, may promote what is now UPR-independent vascular inflammation. It is likely that this occurs in terms of a crosstalk with the NLRP3 inflammasomes located in macrophages, thereby contributing to the clinical progression of atherosclerosis [384].

Of note, mechanisms of ER stress-mediated apoptosis and inflammation in atherosclerosis have recently been reviewed by Hong et al. [385]. The authors discussed that, in atherosclerosis, the UPR fails to control misfolded proteins in the ER and upregulates the expression of CHOP with a progression of atherosclerosis (for CHOP, again compare Fig. 18.6 in Vol. 1. [24], Part V). Activation of CHOP-mediated (and JNK/p38 MAPK-mediated) apoptosis-signaling pathways regulates the Bcl-2 family, which controls the balance of pro-/antiapoptotic signaling; and ER stress-induced apoptosis signaling dampens eNOS expression with the increased oxidative stress. Furthermore, the authors discussed [385] that excessive ER stress and subsequent activation of the IRE1α-triggered pathway increase activation of TXNIP (a metabolic IIC-5 DAMP) that, in turn, contributes to NLRP3 inflammasome activation in atherosclerotic plaques (for TXNIP, see also Vol. 1 [24], Part IV, Sect. 13.4.6.3). As activation of the NLRP3 inflammasome results in pyroptosis, another source of released constitutive and inducible DAMPs is created, instigated by the action of dyshomeostatic DAMPs (for details of the ER stress → UPR, see also Sect. 4.2.5).

The DNA Damage Response in Atherosclerotic Plaques

There is growing evidence for a role of the DDR and its subsequent effects in the initiation and progression of atherosclerosis up to formation of atherosclerotic plaques (for reviews, see Refs. [374–376, 386, 387]; for details of the DDR, see Sect. 4.2.6 and also compare Vol. 1. [24], Part V, Sect. 18.6 and Fig. 18.7). As the canonical injury, oxidative stress is generally believed to mediate accumulation of DNA damage in atherosclerotic plaques. Indeed, advanced atherosclerotic plaques are characterized by accumulation of oxidatively modified DNA in macrophages, VSMCs, and ECs. Among the oxidative injury-induced DAMPs which trigger the activation of the DDR, SSBs and DSBs (= IIC-1 DAMPs), as well as cytosolic oxidized DNA (8-oxoguanine, i.e., IIC-2 DAMPs), have been detected in plaques (for SSBs and DSBs acting as DAMPs, see Sect. 3.4.4.2 and Vol. 1 [24], Part IV, Sect. 13.4.2 and Part V, Fig. 18.7). Outstanding in the perspective of this chapter are studies demonstrating that the consequences of DNA damage including cell senescence and apoptosis are all increased in atherosclerotic plaques. There is the unproven possibility that apoptotic cell death—in the hypoxic milieu of plaques and due to insufficient efferocytosis—may progress to a lytic phase, that is, secondary necrosis/pyroptosis, thereby counting as sources of DAMPs to promote vascular inflammation [388] (for secondary necrosis, see also Vol. 1. [24], Part V, Sect. 19.2.3 and Fig. 19.2).

10.6.2.5 DAMPs Activating Indirectly the NLRP3 Inflammasome in Atherosclerosis

DAMPs activating the NLRP3 inflammasome indirectly have been denoted as Subclass IA-2 DAMPs and addressed in Vol. 1, [24], Part IV, Sect. 12.2.5. Mechanisms of this indirect activation of the NLRP3 inflammasome (e.g., priming signal and second activating stimulus) were also highlighted in Sects. 2.2.5.2 and 2.2.5.3 and in Vol. 1 [24], Part VI, Sect. 22.4.2 and Fig. 22.11.

Modern experimental research in atherosclerosis has provided convincing evidence for a critical role of the NLRP3 inflammasome—located in vascular macrophages and VSMCs—in both the proinflammatory nonresolving and the fibrosclerotic phase of atherogenesis. Whereas activation of the inflammasome in macrophages mainly contributes to vascular inflammation, in VSMCs, it promotes their proliferation and transformation from a contractile phenotype to a synthetic phenotype associated with vascular remodeling ("phenotype switching" of VSMCs) [227, 276, 389, 390] (compare Fig. 10.5).

Of note, in 2010, Duewell et al. [231] were the first to demonstrate the critical role of NLRP3 inflammasomes in the progression of atherosclerosis. Knowing that cholesterol crystal formation is present in the early stages and can be detected in all stages of atherosclerosis, the investigators focused on cholesterol crystals as the candidate of DAMPs and revealed that these crystals strongly activated NLRP3 inflammasomes in macrophages. Subsequent studies on murine and human phagocytes and on in vivo settings then confirmed that crystals of cholesterol, operating as DAMPs, indirectly activate the NLRP3 inflammasome required for atherogenesis (Fig. 10.5) (for reviews, see [232, 233, 391–394]). The activation of this inflammasome is of peculiar importance for the chronic nature of proatherosclerotic inflammation: As outlined in Sect. 4.3.5, the assembly of the NLRP3 inflammasome results in pyroptotic cell death that is associated with the release of constitutive DAMPs as well as the inducible DAMP IL-1β, all able to expand the inflammatory process, thereby contributing to the progression of atherosclerosis (compare Vol. 1, [24], Part IV, Sect. 14.3.2.3, and Part V, Sect. 19.3.4 and Fig. 19.7). Concurrent activating mechanisms include the notion that phagocytosed cholesterol crystals or OxLDL, taken up via receptor-mediated phagocytosis, results in cholesterol crystal formation within phagolysosomes. Then, the crystals provoke phagolysosomal rupture that results in activation of the NLRP3 protein followed by assembly of the inflammasome (for details, including the process of "frustrated phagocytosis," see Vol. 1 [24], Part IV, Sect. 12.2.5.4, and Part VI, Sect. 22.4.2.2). However, one may add here that OxLDL may also contribute to NLRP3 inflammasome activation as the priming stimulus when interacting with TLR4 (Fig. 10.5). Interestingly, recent studies revealed that OxLDL immune complexes—through FcγR, TLR4, and CD36 signaling—trigger IL-1β production more potently than OxLDL alone resulting in increased Th17 polarization and cytokine secretion [395].

Besides OxLDL and cholesterol crystals, other proatherosclerotic DAMPs (operating at the level of the priming and the second activating step) have been identified to activate the NLRP3 inflammasome (for DAMPs indirectly activating the NLRP3 inflammasome, denoted as IA-2 DAMPs, see Vol. 1 [24], Part IV, Sect. 12.2.5).

These DAMPs include calcium phosphate crystals (hydroxylapatite and tricalcium phosphate) and lipotoxic species (ceramides and palmitate). Also, HMGB1 belongs to such DAMPs as it was found to activate the NLRP3 inflammasome in VSMCs associated with increased IL-1β production and promotion of foam cell formation [227, 390].

On the other hand, several mechanisms that negatively regulate NLRP3 inflammasome activation have been reported, such as autophagic processes, which, for example, were shown to capture and degrade the assembled complex of NLRP3 inflammasomes via its ubiquitination, thereby modulating its activity (reviewed in Ref. [233]).

Of note, recent results suggested the possible role of NLRP3 and its variants in human accelerating atherosclerosis [232]. This study—performed on carotid artery plaque tissues, obtained during endarterectomy surgery from 106 patients with ischemic cerebrovascular disease—showed that NLRP3 inflammasome-related genes are highly expressed in atherosclerotic plaque and sensitive to activation when exposed to TLR4 activation (priming step) and ATP or cholesterol crystals (second activating step).

Together, the DAMP-activated NLRP3 inflammasome is an essential player in atherogenesis via three seminal executing effects: contribution to vascular inflammation via IL-1β release; positive regulation of VSMC phenotypic transformation and proliferation associated with vascular wall remodeling; and, finally, induction of pyroptotic cell death as a critical source of further DAMPs release. Consequently, this outstanding proatherogenic effect has encouraged researchers to harness the inducible DAMP IL-1β as a target for the treatment of atherosclerosis in a clinical trial: the CANTOS trial (*Canakinumab Antiinflammatory Thrombosis Outcomes Study*) [396]—a therapeutic topic that will be touched in Sect. 10.7.3.3.

10.6.2.6 The Third Wave of DAMPs in Atherosclerosis

The various subroutines of RN observed in the necrotic core of plaques—including progression of apoptosis to secondary necrosis/pyroptosis—serve as pivotal sources of passively released DAMPs (compare Vol. 1 [24], Part IV, Sect. 12.2). Some of them have already been described to be involved in atherogenesis. For example, HMGB1 and HSPs, which are known to bind to TLR2, TLR4, and RAGE on vascular cells, in particular on vascular macrophages, were found to be implicated in establishing a vascular proinflammatory/profibrotic cascade contributing to atherogenesis. Also, other types of DAMPs released from severely damaged cells, such as S100A8/A9, sensed by TLR4 and RAGE have increasingly been recognized to contribute to vascular innate immunity-mediated inflammatory pathways involved in atherogenesis (see [10–12, 18, 397–399]). These Class IA-1 DAMPs—which may also be released from cells succumbing RN when induced by bacteria or viruses—are briefly addressed in the following.

High Mobility Group Box 1

In Vol. 1 [24], both forms of HMGB1, released as a constitutive IA-1 DAMP from necrotic cells and secreted as an inducible IIIB-2 DAMP by activated immune cells, are described in Part IV, Sects. 12.2.2 and 14.3.3, respectively. For detailed knowledge about HMGB1-triggered signaling pathways through TLR4 and RAGE, the reader is referred to Vol. 1 [24], Part VI, Sect. 22.3.2 and Fig. 22.3, as well as Sect. 22.3.9 and Fig. 22.10.

In recent years, this prominent DAMP has been studied experimentally and clinically for its roles in atherosclerosis, as comprehensively reviewed in several competent articles (see Refs. [241, 400–402]).

For example, in experiments on diabetic ApoE KO mice, increased expression of HMGB1 (also S100A8/A9, see below) was exhibited in atherosclerotic plaques [403]. In similar experiments on ApoE KO mice, HMGB1 was found to augment atherosclerotic lesion development by stimulating macrophage migration, modulating proinflammatory mediators (TNF and IL-1β), and encouraging the accumulation of VSMCs, DCs, and $CD4^+$ T cells [404]. The detection of VSMCs and IL-1β in this study is not surprising in light of other sets of studies demonstrating that HMGB1in terms of the primary signal increases IL-1β production [390] and promotes foam cell formation in VSMCs via activation of the NLRP3 inflammasome [227]. Indeed, the effect of this DAMP produced by or acting on VSMCs is obviously pronounced. Thus, an earlier study on human advanced atherosclerotic lesions provided evidence that HMGB1, produced by activated VSMCs in these lesions, directly stimulates the production of both CRP and MMP through RAGE [405]. The authors discussed that their findings provide evidence that HMGB1 produced by activated VSMCs may contribute to the progression and vulnerability of human atherosclerotic lesions toward rupture, a concept that is indirectly supported by studies on a potential role of *oleacein* in attenuation of carotid plaque destabilization ex vivo [406] (compare Sect. 10.4.4.3). In subsequent studies in mice, HMGB1, in turn, was observed to induce migration of VSMCs through a TLR4-dependent PI3K/Akt signaling pathway, which—as concluded by the authors—suggests a possible molecular mechanism for HMGB1 in the contribution to neointima formation in restenosis after vascular damage [407] (for PI3K/Akt pathway, see Vol. 1 [24], Part VI, Sect. 22.3.4.2).

Of note, an emerging link between HMGB1 and atherosclerosis has also been uncovered via clinical observations in patients suffering from CVD. For example, several investigations showed that serum HMGB1 levels are higher in patients with acute CAD (reviewed by Wu et al. in Ref. [402]). In line with these studies, upregulated HMGB1 levels and thrombosis were observed in patients with atherosclerotic plaque rupture compared with healthy subject volunteers [408]. Also, immunofluorescence microscopy studies revealed high HMGB1 expression levels in human coronary artery thrombi. Further, in these studies, HMGB1 was found to be highly expressed in platelet-rich human coronary artery thrombi pointing toward a central role for HMGB1 in atherothrombosis [409, 410].

As a logical consequence, these stimulating clinical data gave a reason for considerations to harness HMGB1 as a DAMP for diagnostic and prognostic assessment and an innovative therapeutic target in atherosclerotic patients as will be described below.

S100A Proteins

In Vol. 1 [24], both forms of S100A proteins, released as constitutive IA-1 DAMPs from necrotic cells and secreted as inducible IIIA-1 DAMPs by activated immune cells, are described in Part IV, Sects. 12.2.4.2 and 14.2.2.4, respectively. Some information about S100 protein-triggered signaling pathways through their two crucial receptors TLR4 and RAGE can be found in Vol. 1 [24], Part VI, Sect. 22.3.2 and Fig. 22.3, as well as Sect. 22.3.9 and Fig. 22.10.

Like HMGB1, S100A proteins (most intensely S100A8, S100A9, and S100A12 but also S100B and S100A4) have been investigated in both atherosclerotic animal models and clinical studies on atherosclerosis. The investigators in this research field consider these DAMPs important proinflammatory mediators of atherosclerosis but also proposed them, under certain circumstances and at different stages of atherogenesis, to have protective functions (reviewed in [400, 401, 411–414]; for molecules operating context-dependently as DAMPs or SAMPs, also compare Sect. 3.5.6).

Findings from early experiments on ApoE KO mice already showed infiltration of mainly S100A9-expressing cells in the atherosclerotic plaques of 6 months old mice, whereas S100A8-positive cells very rarely occurred in these lesions [415]. Subsequent studies then demonstrated that S100A12 in VSMCs accelerates atherosclerotic processes in ApoE KO mice as indicated by a significant increase in atherosclerotic plaque size and a substantial rise in necrotic core, calcified plaque area, and reduced ECM [416]. Notably, these signs of pathological vascular remodeling are characteristic histological features of vulnerable plaques and observed to be often associated with plaque rupture and MI in patients with coronary artery disease [417].

Similarly, as outlined by Rai and Agrawal [241], other lines of studies in non-atherosclerosis models have been reported that are suggestive for a critical role of S100A proteins in the promotion of MMP-mediated plaque rupture [418, 419]. As mentioned, such a significant pathological effect has also been described for HMGB1 [405]. At this point, the unproven possibility is imaginable that MMP-mediated ECM components acting as Class IIA DAMPs may even aggravate this plaque rupture-promoting effect of HMGB1 and S100A proteins (for Class IIA DAMPs, see Vol. 1 [24], Part IV, Sect. 13.2). Nevertheless, further experiments are needed to confirm and solidify this exciting model of a role of DAMPs in promoting atherosclerotic plaque rupture.

During the past decade, a growing number of publications have provided ample clinical evidence for the role of S100A proteins in human atherosclerosis (reviewed in [412, 413]). Already in 2004, an autopsy study of victims of sudden cardiac death revealed enhanced expression of S100A12 and RAGE in macrophages and VSMCs in the ruptured coronary artery plaque [420], suggesting a potential role of this locally expressed DAMP within the atherosclerotic lesion for a dangerous plaque instability. In another early study in 2005, S100A8 and S100A9 protein and mRNA were clinically demonstrated in macrophages, foam cells, and neovessels in human atheroma; additionally, S100A9 was found to be strongly expressed in calcifying areas and the surrounding ECM [421]. Subsequent investigations of human carotid plaques supported these early findings by revealing an increased expression of S100A8 and S100A9 on monocytes and macrophages, whereby S100A9 was shown to be strongly associated with the inflammatory status of rupture-prone atherosclerotic lesions [422].

In the following years, stimulated by these findings, the interest in conducting clinical studies on S100A DAMPs in CVD steadily grew [423]. For example, in a survey on patients with carotid atherosclerosis [424], all three S100A DAMPs were found to be elevated, with the highest levels of S100A12 in patients with the most recent symptoms. Moreover, mRNA levels of S100A8, S100A9, and S100A12 were found to be TLR2- and TLR4-dependently upregulated in atherosclerotic carotid plaques from patients with the most recent symptoms. The authors concluded from their data that, in particular, S100A12 may be related to plaque instability. Further, in another clinical analysis of data from patients with T2DM undergoing coronary angiography for the evaluation of CAD, plasma S100A12 levels were shown to be correlated with the presence and severity of the disease [425]. Again in another clinical study on patients suffering from systemic lupus erythematosus and simultaneous CVD, increased levels of S100A8 and S100A9 in the area of atherosclerotic plaque and thrombus could be demonstrated, believed by the authors to be derived from the activated platelets [426]. Last but not least, there is first evidence suggesting that S100A12 proteins are implicated in the promotion of arterial calcification (reviewed in [427]).

Clearly, these encouraging clinical observations gave rise to use this class of DAMPs as diagnostic and predictive criteria as well as harness them as therapeutic targets in atherosclerotic patients, a topic that will be resumed below.

Heat Shock Proteins

In Vol. 1 [24], both forms of HSPs, released as constitutive IA-1 DAMPs from necrotic cells and secreted as inducible IIIB-2 DAMPs by activated (stressed) cells, are described in Part IV, Sects. 12.2.3 and 14.2.2.2, respectively. For some knowledge about HSP-triggered signaling pathways through various cognate receptors, the reader is referred to Vol. 1 [24], Part IV, Sect. 12.2.3.3.

The property of HSPs to act as DAMPs is well accepted [428]. In several comprehensive reviews, experimental and clinical studies were described demonstrating the role of HSPs in atherosclerosis (see [2, 401, 429, 430]). Here, special attention is paid to HSP60 only. Indeed, awareness of a pathological role of HSPs in atherosclerosis is mainly focused on the function of HSP60 for which direct atherogenic potential has been proven in experimental and clinical studies. In particular, the atherogenic function of HSP60 is generally ascribed to its property to act as an autoantigen, whereby very few data on its role as an innate immune response-triggering DAMP in the context of atherosclerosis is available. A very early study on human peripheral blood mononuclear cells (PBMCs) and monocyte-derived macrophages provided first evidence for a role of HSP60 to activate the innate immune system through CD14 signaling and p38 MAPK [431], an observation that let the authors suggest molecular mechanisms by which extracellular HSPs may participate in atherosclerosis (for the CD14 molecule, see Vol. 1 [24], Part II, Sect. 5.2.2.3). A recent report has been published showing that HSP60 can stimulate the migration of VSMCs via TLR4 and MAPK activation [432]. Further support for HSP60 to act as a DAMP derives from observations showing that levels of its soluble form directly correlate with the presence of both classic risk factors for atherosclerosis and proinflammatory markers [433, 434].

Together, the whole HSP60-based autoimmune concept of atherosclerosis is preferentially based on its role as an autoantigen than on a DAMP. In fact, as discussed by Wick et al. [2], detailed investigations of atherosclerosis in animal models and studies of early atherosclerotic lesions in humans have shown that the disease starts as an HSP60-specific T cell-mediated immune response and that antibodies to HSP60 act as autoantibodies and accelerate and perpetuate atherogenesis.

10.6.2.7 Inducible DAMPs: Interleukin-1 Family Members, Tumor Necrosis Factor, and Interferon-Alpha

Without going into detail, a few remarks should be allowed on the role of those cytokines in atherosclerosis, denoted as inducible DAMPs in this book. The pro-atherogenic property of IL-1β has already been touched concerning its role as a product of pyroptotic cell death. Thus, in experiments in atherosclerosis models, this inducible DAMP was shown, besides others, to be involved in the upregulation of M1-like macrophage activation and adhesion molecules expression by ECs. Also, TNF has been found to play a key role in the development of atherosclerosis. Indeed, atherosclerosis progression was demonstrated to be always directly correlated with a local increase in TNF production in the atherosclerotic plaque and with TNF level in blood. Indeed, TNF, like IL-1β, was found to induce macrophage and foam cell apoptosis, causing them to release their lipid content into the intima of the artery and contribute toward the size of the necrotic core in the plaque. Moreover, experiments in mice with double knockout of *TNF* and *ApoE* genes revealed a significant reduction of plaque size in the aortic sinus due to decreased expression of ICAM-1, VCAM-1, and MCP-1 (for reviews, see [435, 436]).

In this context of interest are elegant in vitro experiments on the exploration of functional activities of the antiviral cytokine IFN-α in the atherosclerotic plaque as reported by Niessner et al. [437]. These studies provided evidence of synergistic proinflammatory effects of the plasmacytoid dendritic cell (pDC)-produced IFN-α (a type I IFN)—operating as an inducible IIIA-2 DAMP—and TLR4 ligands (MAMPs and DAMPs) within atherosclerotic plaques (for type I IFN in their role as inducible DAMPs, compare Vol. 1 [24], Part IV, Sect. 14.2.3.3). In these experiments, conventional TLR-bearing DCs—when clustered with plaque pDCs—were found to respond to IFN-α produced by pDCs with a marked change in their activation threshold, that is, with increased secretion of the other inducible IIIA-2 DAMP TNF and the cytokines IL-12 and IL-23, as well as the production of MMPs (!), all mediators implicated in rendering plaque susceptible to rupture. Given these findings, the authors argued that "this immune amplification loop assigns a critical function to IFN-α in adjusting the responsiveness of plaque-residing cells to stimulatory signals and identifies this innate immune marker as a key regulator in plaque inflammation and destabilization. IFN-α is typically induced during viral infections, raising the possibility that such infectious episodes expose patients to an immediate risk for acute complications of atherosclerosis." Furthermore, these data let the investigators suggest [437] "that viral infections trigger pDCs through TLR9 to secrete IFN-α in the atherosclerotic plaque. Furthermore, IFN-α enhances the expression of TLR4 on APCs with both pDC and cDC populations localized in close vicinity in the rupture-prone shoulder region. As a result, responses of these cell types to exogenous and endogenous TLR4 ligands are amplified." And further [437]: "This model predicts that host infections, particularly those being sensed by pDCs and even when colonizing distant tissues, represent an immediate risk for the inflamed atherosclerotic plaque."

10.6.2.8 Concluding Remarks

This brief overview of selected danger signals released in terms of a third wave of DAMPs from cells within the necrotic core succumbing RN should help to accept the concept of nonresolving vascular inflammation that is characterized—besides the action of dysfunctional SAMPs—by a dominance of DAMPs over SAMPs as generated in average amounts. The critical impact of these DAMPs (HMGB1, S100A proteins, inducible DAMPs such as IL-1β, TNF, and type I IFN) on a deleterious course of either sterile or infectious injury-induced atherosclerotic disease can be seen in their potency to promote the catastrophic atherosclerotic plaque rupture as thought to be caused via DAMP-induced MMP-mediated degradation of ECM components (Fig. 10.7).

10.6.3 DAMP-Activated Vascular Dendritic Cells Resulting in Autoimmunity

The role of DCs in atherosclerosis has recently been reviewed by Gil-Pulido and Zernecke [438]. As briefly mentioned in Sect. 10.4.6, APCs in atherosclerosis execute their tasks in a similar and analogous way as documented in other experimental models of autoimmunity and human autoimmune diseases: vascular autostimulatory DCs present vascular non-self neoantigens (or bona fide self-antigens?) as pMHC complexes to naïve autoreactive T cells leading to an adaptive anti-arterial T-cell autoimmune response. Both subsets of these key cells translating innate immune events into adaptive immune processes, that is, conventional DCs (cDCs) and pDCs have been found in mice and humans, located in the intima at regions prone to the development of atherosclerosis; and both subsets were shown to promote proatherogenic T-cell responses.

There is only limited data available in support of a direct role of DAMPs in inducing these auto-immunostimulatory DCs residing in or entering atherosclerotic lesions. Nonetheless, some immune responses with specificity for OxLDL have been reportedly documented in mice and humans plaques and reveal the potency of this DAMP to activate DCs in atherosclerosis settings. For example, in

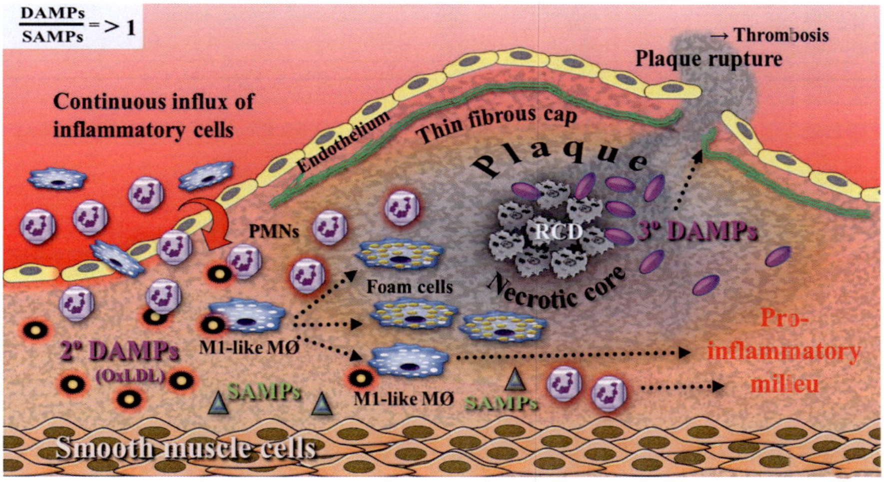

Fig. 10.7 Schematically designed narrative model of a scenario in atherosclerotic plaques, illustrating the role of agonistically acting DAMPs overriding the antagonistic function of SAMPs, that is, the DAMPs:SAMPs ratio, is higher than 1 (based on evidence so far published; for references, see below). When the DAMPs dominate the scene, resolution of inflammation is impaired, leading to a continuous influx of inflammatory cells such as PMNs and macrophages; polarization of M1-like macrophages; impaired efferocytosis; formation of only a thin fibrous cap; large necrotic cores in plaques; altogether the creation of a chronic nonresolving inflammatory milieu in the vessel wall. *MØ* macrophage, *OxLDL* oxidized low-density lipoproteins, *PMNs* polymorphonuclear neutrophils, *RCD* regulated cell death. (Sources: [229, 295, 297, 299–301, 488–490])

earlier experiments, T cells that were isolated from human carotid atherosclerotic lesions were found to proliferate specifically in response to OxLDL in an MHC-II-restricted manner. The response of the OxLDL-specific $CD4^+$ T cells was dependent on the presence of autologous, antigen-presenting monocytes and was blocked by antibodies to HLA–DR [439]. The authors discussed conclusively that the T-cell response is mounted against an HLA–DR-restricted, processed antigen derived from OxLDL. Parallel activation of DCs in this test model can at least be assumed. In other lines of studies, OxLDL through SR signaling was documented to promote a proinflammatory cytokine profile in human DCs leading to DC maturation and differentiation [440].

Notably, this concept could be confirmed by recent in vitro experiments showing that T cells, isolated from human carotid atherosclerotic plaques and exposed to OxLDL-treated autologous DCs, proliferated and produced IFN-γ and IL-17, thus with polarization to Th1 and/or Th17 subsets [441]. Similarly, in an analogous in vitro test model of human T cells derived from such plaques, HSP60 was shown to induce maturation of DCs and T-cell activation mainly of proinflammatory Th1/17 type. However, the DAMP could not clearly be shown to promote DC activation via HSP60 → cognate receptor-triggered signaling [442]. Of interest, however, from this study was the observation that AnxA5 could inhibit the HSP60-induced immune response effect, thereby qualifying this molecule —like AnxA1— as a putative SAMP, at least in this in vitro atherosclerosis test model (for the SAMP AnxA1, see Sect. 3.5.5.2 and Vol. 1 [24], Part IV, Sect. 14.4.3.2).

Regardless of a role of OxLDL as a "DAMP of the first hour" in the activation of DCs in atherosclerosis, the third wave of DAMPs emitted from the necrotic core of plaques such as HMGB1 or NAs can be supposed to activate lesional immature dendritic cells (iDCs) into immunostimulatory DCs which may contribute to chronic inflammation-sustaining autoimmune processes as observed in atherosclerosis.

In conclusion, the role of DAMPs in the contribution of DC-triggered autoimmune processes in atherosclerosis is well documented; however, this topic has still to be secured by further studies showing more clear-cut results. Since other lines of studies clearly demonstrated that adaptive immune processes can sustain chronic inflammatory processes, such an interplay between DAMP-promoted innate and adaptive autoimmune pathways in atherogenesis can be assumed (compare Fig. 10.5).

10.6.4 DAMP-Promoted Fibrogenic Processes in Atherosclerosis

As mentioned above, modern experimental research in atherosclerosis has provided convincing evidence for a critical role of the NLRP3 inflammasome—located in vascular macrophages and VSMCs—in the fibrosclerotic phase of atherogenesis. Hence, DAMPs identified to activate the inflammasome can be supposed to contribute to fibroproliferative responses in vascular fibrosis. Nevertheless, this is probably not the whole story. For example, in experiments on a mouse oxidative stress model, increased mitochondrial oxidative stress was found to increase intrinsic VSMC stiffness and induce aortic ECM remodeling and fibrosis [443], suggesting that other oxidative injury-induced DAMPs are involved. However, further targeted studies are needed to increase insights into the role of DAMPs in promoting fibroproliferative responses in vascular fibrosis

10.6.5 Résumé

The presentation of some selected studies on the role of DAMPs in atherosclerosis clearly shows that this research topic is in full swing. Indeed, there is a growing body of evidence in support of the notion that all waves of DAMPs generation and emission, as discussed above, contribute to the various proatherosclerotic innate/adaptive immune pathways. Consequently, their use as biomarkers and therapeutic targets in atherosclerosis is currently receiving much attention.

10.7 DAMPs and SAMPs as Diagnostics, Prognostics, Therapeutics, and Therapeutic Targets in Atherosclerosis

10.7.1 Introductory Remarks

The historical key biomarker in atherosclerosis—very well known to the public as the "bad" cholesterol—is the LDL-C. It is generally recognized as an important prognostic marker for the risk of developing CVD. In fact, the multifaceted path by which cholesterol became linked to coronary heart disease (CHD) is one of the great biomedical stories of the twentieth century [444]. Thus, in the famous Framingham study [445], a milestone in research on epidemiology and etiology of CVD, a total of 383 men and 227 women was observed to develop CHD during the 12 years of follow-up, which was significantly associated with LDL-C (besides other risk factors such as blood pressure). Today, pharmacies all over the world offer the service to their customers to measure LDL-C levels using a simple blood test. In the meantime, further molecules were added as biomarkers in this field, such as ApoB that turned out to improve risk assessment of future CHD events over and beyond LDL-C [446]. Today, this traditional tool to monitor the risk of atherosclerosis has been developed by leading expert groups to a highly scientific and sophisticated methodology. Plausibly, in light of all the various DAMP-triggered causal pathways implicated in atherogenesis as described above, these molecules may serve as ideal biomarkers by allowing proper decision-making in clinical management when their levels are measured. However, in the current era of DAMPs, the rationale to measure them in the plasma or in the vessel wall (in terms of molecule imaging) is not only limited to their use as a crutch to understanding the transition of occult atherosclerosis to clinically relevant CVD but also to target them to develop clinical tools to treat atherosclerosis-associated CVD in humans. In particular, the possibility to harness SAMPs in therapeutic efforts to tackle nonresolving inflammation of the arterial wall has gained increasing attention. In the following, some selected DAMPs and SAMPs will be discussed which have already raised great hope in their exploitation as diagnostics, prognostics, and therapeutics/therapeutic targets

10.7.2 DAMPs as Biomarkers in Atherosclerosis

10.7.2.1 General Remarks

Most work on proatherosclerotic DAMPs serving as biomarkers in atherosclerosis has been done in the field of OSEs. By contrast, and compared to these studies, reports on HMGB1and S100 proteins as biomarkers in atherosclerosis are not that straightforwardly designed and conducted. Nevertheless, they are also briefly touched here.

10.7.2.2 Oxidation-Specific Epitopes as Diagnostic and Prognostic Biomarkers in Atherosclerosis

As the "DAMPs of the first hour," OSEs, in particular, OxPL and MDA epitopes, have been developed as essential biomarkers in atherosclerosis. It is the group around Witztum and Tsimikas in San Diego, USA, who published first pathbreaking papers on this topic [447–449]. The investigators recognized OSEs as viable targets for developing in vitro diagnostics (biomarkers), therapeutic agents, and diagnostic molecular imaging probes (called by the group as "biotheranostics"). The group developed human and murine OSE-targeting antibodies that are being used as biomarkers in human studies and experimentally in translational applications of non-invasive molecular imaging of oxidation-rich plaques and immunotherapeutics. In other words, in these studies, the targets are the OSEs, present either in the circulation or in the vessel wall. Targeting agents directed to OSEs can be used for in vitro ELISA to detect circulating antigens, or coupled with imaging probes in detecting the presence and quantity of OSEs present in the artery wall, or used directly as therapeutic agents in neutralizing proinflammatory and proatherogenic effects of OSEs.

As a first result of the group's work [448], Lp(a)—the preferential lipoprotein carrier of the DAMP OxPL— has been generally recognized as a causal, independent, genetic risk factor for CVDs such as MI and has become a target of therapy for reducing cardiovascular risk. Since small Apo(a) isoforms are associated with high Lp(a) plasma levels, and because these lipoproteins contain the most OxPL content, the OxPL/ApoB measurement primarily reflects the most atherogenic Lp(a) particles. Hence, elevated levels of OxPL/ApoB were found to predict the presence and progression of coronary, femoral, and carotid artery disease, to be increased following acute coronary syndromes (ACS) and percutaneous coronary intervention, as well as predict the development of death, MI, stroke, and need for revascularization in unselected populations [189].

Also, for molecular OSEs imaging, oxidation-specific antibodies have been used intensely for immunostaining of atherosclerotic lesions in human artery specimens [448]. For example, in postmortem investigations on hearts with CAD, it could be demonstrated that human atherosclerotic lesions show differential expression of different OSEs and ApoAI as they progress, rupture, and become clinically symptomatic [230]. For example, MDA epitopes were observed to be more prominent in early lesions, such as in pathologic intimal thickening and early fibroatheromas, whereas OxPL and ApoAI were found to be more prevalent in advanced lesions, that is, in the necrotic core and ruptured plaques. As plausibly stressed by the authors [230], the presence of OSEs in clinically relevant human lesions provides a strong rationale to target such epitopes in plasma and in atherosclerotic plaques for clinical applications.

This concept was supported by subsequent ELISA studies on OxPL on human ApoB (OxPL/ApoB) in plasma, confirming that oxidation-specific biomarkers predict cardiovascular events in humans (described in detail in [449]). In these studies, OxPL/ApoB levels were demonstrated (1) to be elevated in patients with

ACSs and following percutaneous coronary intervention; (2) to predict the progression of femoral/carotid and coronary artery disease; (3) to predict death, MI, and stroke in unselected populations followed prospectively; and (4) to reclassify ~ 30% of patients to lower- or higher-risk categories based on clinical criteria and Framingham risk score.

Finally, on the basis of promising pre-clinical molecular imaging studies in mice, rabbits, and monkeys using murine and human OSE-specific antibodies as targeting agents, the group around Witztum and Tsimikas [449] developed radionuclide and magnetic resonance-based nanoparticles, containing gadolinium, manganese, or lipid-coated ultrasmall superparamagnetic iron oxide, to non-invasively image OSE within experimental atherosclerotic lesions. Excitingly, this methodology was shown to quantitate plaque burden and allow detection of lesion progression and regression, plaque stabilization, and accumulation of OSE within macrophage-rich areas of the artery wall. Under sophisticated experimental extension of such studies, these approaches—as concluded by the authors [449]—should enhance the clinical translation of this technique to image, monitor, evaluate efficacy of novel therapeutic agents, and guide optimal therapy of high-risk atherosclerotic lesions.

10.7.2.3 High Mobility Group Box 1, S100 Proteins, Heat Shock Proteins, and Cytosolic DNA as Biomarkers in Atherosclerosis

The function of DAMPs as biomarkers in atherosclerosis has already been briefly touched in Sect. 10.6.2.6.

Indeed, most of the DAMPs in this role have been addressed in relation to CADs and, thus, are mentioned in Sect. 11.4.2.3. Here, just a few remarks are made.

High Mobility Group Box 1

Current knowledge in this field has been thoroughly reviewed by de Souza et al. [398]. As could be expected, HMGB1was shown to be markedly increased in human atherosclerotic lesions from the aorta, carotid, and coronary arteries, whereby the DAMP was typically localized in the nuclei and in the cytoplasm of macrophages and VSMCs near the intima. Moreover, intense upregulated HMGB1expression has also been observed in areas adjacent to the necrotic core of atherosclerotic lesions [405, 450]. The prognostic power of this DAMP in atherosclerosis and CVD has already been demonstrated in some studies, mainly on patients who have CAD (described in more detail in Sect. 11.4.2.3).

S100A Proteins

Current knowledge of S100A proteins in their function as biomarkers has been reviewed by Oesterle and Bowman [412]. Early evidence for S100A proteins to act as a prognostic factor in CVD derived from a nested case study among patients with ACS enrolled in the *Pravastatin or Atorvastatin Evaluation and Infection Therapy: Thrombolysis in Myocardial Infarction 22* trial [451]. The topic is resumed with the description of further details in Sect. 11.4.2.3.

Cytosolic DNA and Heat Shock Proteins

There are a few reports on cytosol DNA and HSPs acting as biomarkers. For example, nDNA and mtDNA [452, 453] and HSP have been found in patients with acute MI [452, 453]. Moreover, HSP has been detected in the plasma of patients with ACS and MI, respectively. Thus, plasma HSPB7 concentration was found to be significantly higher in patients with ACS than in control patients with non-cardiac chest pain [454]. Furthermore, in patients presenting to the emergency department with acute chest pain, the HSPB7 level was observed to be an independent risk factor of ACS. The authors concluded that HSPB7 may serve as a potential early biomarker after MI, indicating an independent risk factor of ACS in patients with acute chest pain.

10.7.2.4 Concluding Remarks

In conclusion, the literature so far available provides a growing body of evidence for a critical role of DAMPs as diagnostic and prognostic biomarkers in atherosclerosis. Most of them have been examined in relation to CVDs. One does not need to be a prophet to predict that the great time of DAMPs in this role is still ahead and may change the diagnostic, prognostic, and predictive capabilities of clinicians and physicians at the bedside of patients suffering from CVDs drastically. Moreover, and probably, the SAMPs may join the DAMPs in this field of modern medicine very soon (see also Sect. 11.4.2).

10.7.3 DAMPs as Therapeutic Targets in Atherosclerosis

10.7.3.1 General Remarks

In principle, therapeutic options in atherosclerosis can be seen in different levels: inhibiting proinflammatory/proatherosclerotic responses may be critical at the onset of the disease. On the contrary, enhancing proresolving/atheroprotective processes by administration of SAMPs may be the best future therapeutic strategy in prevention of atherosclerosis progression. Vaccination approaches have also been successfully applied in experimental models; however, translation of these findings in clinical practice has only just started [455–458].

Interestingly, proposals of harnessing proatherosclerotic DAMPs as therapeutic targets in atherosclerosis can be increasingly noted in the international literature. Adequate trials appear to be "just around the corner." According to the concept of sequentially emitted waves of DAMPs as formulated above, blockade of the second wave, the OSEs, appears to be most efficient, because—at least theoretically—this therapeutic approach could prevent or mitigate the release of large amounts of constitutive and inducible DAMPs from RN dying cells (third wave) within the necrotic core (compare Fig. 10.7). Simultaneously, a source of neoantigens could be prevented. On the other hand, strategies to target the first wave of DAMPs (e.g., catecholamines, dyshomeostatic DAMPs) would imply to interfering with the various arteriosclerotic risk factors.

10.7.3.2 Blockade of Constitutive DAMPs in Atherogenesis

The background of therapeutic strategies to block DAMPs in atherogenesis is quite transparent and plausible: their capability to promote inflammatory and fibrogenic processes at the arterial wall. Except for the work on OSEs, however, the topic is still in its infancy—as outlined in the following.

Oxidation-Specific Epitopes

The topic of blocking OSEs is of high interest and has recently been reviewed by Hartley et al. [459]. Early reports on the possibility of using oxidation-specific antibodies as a therapeutic potential in atherosclerosis were published by the Tsimikas group [447, 449, 460]. The researchers utilized a special human anti-OSE (present on LDL)-specific antibody that inhibits uptake of OxLDL by macrophages. In a murine atherosclerosis model, intraperitoneal infusion of this mAb was shown to lead to a 29% decrease in atherosclerosis progression, in another model, even to 46% reduction. Also, these studies provided first evidence for this modified antibody to prevent foam cell formation by binding to OSE.

Regarding larger animals, in vivo administration of an antibody against OxLDL, here, a human recombinant IgG anti-MDA-LDL antibody, was examined in hypercholesterolemic minipigs, i.e., a porcine model of atherosclerosis [461]. The antibody was found to have no effect on the burden of atherosclerosis as assessed on histopathological analysis or fluorodeoxyglucose PET imaging. However, immunostaining of coronary lesions revealed reduced cathepsin S positivity in the treated group compared with placebo.

Of note, this human recombinant IgG anti-MDA-LDL antibody was also tested in a clinical study: the GLACIER (*Goal of Oxidized LDL and Activated Macrophage Inhibition by Exposure to a Recombinant Antibody*) trial that is the first multicenter, randomized, double-blind study evaluating an anti-OxLDL targeted mAb in patients with stable inflammatory vascular lesions (in carotid artery or aortic disease) [462]. As assessed with either imaging or circulating markers of inflammation at 3 months, treatment did not significantly reduce arterial inflammation. Given this disappointing result, the authors discussed—besides others—that the antibody binding may be restricted to OxLDL-rich inflamed plaques, which may have been less common in this population with stable CVD on background statins.

Another approach to interfere with OSEs should also be briefly touched here, namely, the use of inhibitors of secreted phospholipase A2, an enzyme that promoted hydrolysis of LDL to generate proatherogenic LDL [463]. Such an effect could be seen, for example, in a murine atherosclerosis model showing that group 1B phospholipase A2 inactivation suppresses atherosclerosis in LDL receptor-deficient mice [464].

Finally, aside from direct therapeutic utility, such oxidation-specific antibodies could also be used indirectly as therapeutic agents. In this context, Hartley et al. [459] argued that "targeting OxLDL may be used for delivery of nanoparticles with therapeutic cargo to the plaque, allowing the directed treatment of atherosclerotic lesions at risk. This could allow smaller doses for therapeutic efficacy and reduce systemic side."

High Mobility Group Box 1 and S100 Proteins

Regarding their essential pathogenetic role in atherosclerosis, HMGB1 and S100 proteins—representing mainly the third wave of DAMPs (Fig. 10.7)—have already been proposed as therapeutic targets in atherosclerosis [412, 465, 466]. Thus, reports of pre-clinical studies dedicated to this topic are expected with the highest interest.

10.7.3.3 Blockade of Inducible DAMPs in Atherogenesis

Besides interfering with constitutive DAMPs, therapeutic targeting IL-1β, denoted as an inducible DAMP in this book, has been considered as a complementary strategy for lowering the risk of atherosclerotic vascular disease. This idea recently made a quantum leap in plausibility with the publication of the CANTOS trial, which examined approximately 10,000 post-myocardial infarction patients to determine whether inhibition of the IL-1β with canakinumab could prevent recurrent vascular events in men and women who have a persistent proinflammatory response, defined as a high-sensitivity CRP levels [396, 467]. As known to cardiologists, the results showed that treatment with canakinumab reduces inflammation, indicated by decrease in both CRP and IL-6, as well as recurrent cardiovascular event rates with no effect on lipid concentrations. On the other side, patients treated with canakinumab showed a significantly higher incidence of fatal infection and sepsis. Given this data, Anay and Ridker concluded [467]: "With the publication of the CANTOS results, clinicians have definitive evidence that directly targeting inflammation is beneficial for the secondary prevention of CVD, and this benefit is independent of cholesterol. This serves as a reminder that there are emerging therapeutic options for individuals with residual inflammatory risk, as defined by persistently elevated levels of CRP despite adequate LDL-C Lowering."

10.7.3.4 Concluding Remarks

The findings briefly addressed in this section make obvious that therapeutic efforts to mitigate the function of DAMPs in atherosclerosis result in a beneficial effect, but, on the other hand, they are not entirely satisfactory.

The therapeutic failure of oxidation-specific antibodies in clinical atherosclerosis may be due to the fact that other DAMPs are still doing their work. Also, regarding the CANTOS trial, one has to realize that inhibition of an inducible DAMP such as IL-1β reflects antiinflammatory treatment that may also suppress critical host defense mechanisms as, for example, manifested by fatal infections in the CANTOS study patients.

10.7.4 Use of DAMPs as Vaccines in Atherosclerosis Models

10.7.4.1 General Remarks

There is considerable interest in boosting protective immunity related to atherosclerosis not only via administration of inhibitors such as antibodies but also by active immunization with oxidized or native LDL or derivatives, that is, vaccination procedures. The aim is clear: to induce adaptive immune CTLs and cytotoxic/neutralizing antibodies, which can interfere with molecules acting as both antigens and DAMPs, such as OSEs, thereby inhibiting their detrimental function at the arterial wall. The topic, comprehensively reviewed by Chyu et al. [468], will be briefly addressed in the following by focusing on preclinical experiments in atherosclerosis models.

10.7.4.2 Vaccination with Defined Epitopes of Low-Density Lipoproteins

A selected well-defined potential atheroprotective antigenic epitope in LDL is the peptide p210 (a 20 amino acid ApoB-100-related peptide) that has been used as a prototype antigen in vaccine formulations. In a murine model of atherosclerosis, immunization with the p210 vaccine resulted in a significant reduction of aortic atherosclerosis, shown to be mediated by robust $CD4^+$ and $CD8^+$ T-cell responses [469]. Similar results were obtained with the use of other peptide fragments such as MHC-II-restricted ApoB peptides [470]. Moreover, other lines of studies on a humanized mouse model of atherosclerosis revealed that two specific epitopes from human native ApoB100 can trigger T-cell activation and protect the transgenic mice against atherosclerosis when used in a vaccine [471]. Given these findings, the authors suggested that vaccination-induced protective mechanisms may be mediated at least in part through specific antibody responses to LDL that inhibit macrophage activation.

10.7.4.3 Vaccines Targeting Proatherogenic Heat Shock Proteins and Extracellular Matrix Molecules

The use of other proatherogenic DAMPs such as HSPs and ECM molecules as vaccines against atherosclerosis has also been tested experimentally in rodents. For example, intranasal vaccinations using either plasmid DNA encoding HSP65 or whole protein HSP65 in rabbits were demonstrated to reduce atherosclerosis accompanied by decreased cholesterol levels [472]. Similar observations were made using glycoproteins (IIA-3 DAMPs) as vaccines. For example, immunization with fibronectin formulated with alum as the adjuvant was found to reduce atherosclerosis in ApoE KO mice significantly [473]; and immunization with β2-glycoprotein I was shown to attenuate the development of early atherosclerosis, presumably by inducing tolerance against this molecule [474].

10.7.4.4 Concluding Remarks

The idea of developing vaccination strategies to interfere with proatherogenic molecules implicated in CVD is attractive. The experimental evidence for a beneficial effect of vaccination on mitigating atherosclerosis (as shown in rodent models) is promising (a few examples presented here). However, the concept is still in its infancy. As concluded in this context by Chyu et al. [468]: "We have the vision of moving this idea of vaccination to reduce atherosclerosis into clinical testing, but this goal cannot be achieved without academic investigators, professional societies, government agencies, funding organizations, and the pharmaceutical industries working together to initiate this long journey. With all of these challenges in mind, we are cautiously optimistic about the potential for future clinical application." A similar conclusion has been drawn by Amirfakhryan [458]: "However, there is a long distance to reach the ideal vaccination strategy, which could be utilized from early years of life to protect humans against atherosclerosis. It will not be achieved unless the investigators make inexhaustible attempts and funding organizations, governments, and universities provide financial support to research."

10.7.5 Administration of SAMPs as Therapeutics in Atherosclerosis

10.7.5.1 General Remarks

In the two previous sections, the emerging concept of inhibiting the proinflammatory/proatherosclerotic function of DAMPs in atherogenesis was briefly presented by focusing on some progress but also obstacles in DAMP-targeting antibodies (passive immunization) and vaccine procedures (active immunization). Given some still unsolved questions associated with these two options, another therapeutic strategy moves to the fore: the promotion of efforts aimed at facilitating inflammation resolving processes at the vessel wall without compromising host defense, that is, administering SAMPs.

Remarkably, but not being a big surprise, an increasing number of researchers can be noted working on the concept to administer SAMPs, here SPMs, in atherosclerosis [298, 475–482]. Indeed, regarding the multifactorial functions of SPMs in resolving inflammatory responses as formulated in Sect. 5.3.3.2 (including antioxidative efficacy, promotion of efferocytosis, mitigation of proinflammatory factors), their protective properties as observed in atherosclerosis models could be expected. In addition, as reviewed by Fredman [482], there is evidence from various studies suggesting that SPMs act on ECs to potentially inhibit superficial erosion associated with plaque rupture and play essential roles in regulating platelet activation, which could have important therapeutic implications for CVD.

10.7.5.2 Protective Role of SAMPs in Atherosclerosis Models

There are already reports of a protective role of SPMs and AnxA1 in models of atherosclerosis, which are briefly touched in the following.

Specialized Proresolving Mediators

One of the first insights into the role of SPMs in atherosclerosis was the clinical observation that atherosclerotic plaque rupture by balloon angioplasty releases detectable levels of LXs within the lumen of the vessel [483]. However, the first experimental study that demonstrated definitely a therapeutic role for SPMs in atherosclerosis was published by Hasturk et al. [484], showing that RvE1, when treated orally and topically, thwarted atherogenesis in a rabbit model of atherosclerosis. In subsequent studies in mice reviewed by Fredman [482], RvE1, RvD1, RvD2, and MaR1 were observed to be protective during atheroprogression as well. Among the most striking and consistent observations in those mice treated with SPMs was an increase in fibrous cap thickness and/or collagen synthesis in plaques

Annexin A1

The function of AnxA1 in these experimental settings is similar to the actions of SPMs. For example, AnxA1 was shown to limit atherogenesis and plaque necrosis. As reported in this context, administration of this SAMP moderates/reduces leukocyte recruitment to the vascular wall, stabilizes advanced atherosclerotic lesions, and reduces total plaque inflammation/necrosis (for more details, see [485–487]).

10.7.5.3 Concluding Remarks

The findings so far obtained from studies on SAMPs on atherosclerosis models let expect that they will become a constituent part of future treatment in patients with progressive atherosclerosis. However, there will be much work to do to prove that SAMPs can really reach this level of expectations. As Fredman [482] concluded in this context: "Nevertheless, inflammation-resolution is an emerging field and a deeper understanding of how SPMs signal will provide insight into which SPMs or combination of SPMs may be ideal to treat diseases, like atherosclerosis."

10.7.6 Résumé

The idea to use DAMPs and SAMPs as diagnostics, prognostics, therapeutics, and therapeutic targets in atherosclerosis is a natural consequence of the new insights into their emerging pathogenetic role in atherogenesis. However, before translating all the promising preclinical observations into the clinical arena, many challenging questions have to be answered while designing and conducting proper clinical studies. Indeed, it is still a long way to go until these molecules enter clinical routine, even if we would exclude the caveats of their therapeutic application as outlined in Sect. 7.3.3. Nevertheless, "where there is a will, there is a way"!

10.8 Outlook and Future Perspectives

In this chapter, based on an increasing number of reports from the international literature, a tentative model of the complex actions of DAMPs and SAMPs in atherosclerosis has been designed and sketched, parts of which are still theoretical. Although there is growing experimental and clinical evidence for a definite pathogenetic role of these molecules in this vessel disease, many questions remain unclear and have to be thoroughly explored in further targeted experimental and clinical studies. In particular, clinical trials, including cross-sectional, retrospective, and prospective studies, must be designed and conducted to prove whether or not the model of DAMP-driven proatherosclerotic inflammation and SAMP-promoted atheroprotective inflammation resolution outlined here will evolve from reasonable ideas to clinical reality. Also, although experimental data are promising, implementation of experimental therapies in the clinical setting presents challenges. Again, large-scale randomized clinical trials—by complying with the caveats addressed in Sect. 7.3—will be necessary to evaluate therapies that target DAMPs and SAMPs and ensure their effectiveness and possible unwanted actions.

References

1. Thompson RC, Allam AH, Lombardi GP, Wann LS, Sutherland ML, Sutherland JD, et al. Atherosclerosis across 4000 years of human history: the Horus study of four ancient populations. Lancet (London, England). 2013;381:1211–22. https://linkinghub.elsevier.com/retrieve/pii/S014067361360598X.
2. Wick G, Jakic B, Buszko M, Wick MC, Grundtman C. The role of heat shock proteins in atherosclerosis. Nat Rev Cardiol. 2014;11:516–29. http://www.ncbi.nlm.nih.gov/pubmed/25027488.
3. Rokitansky CA. A manual of pathological anatomy. Philadelphia: Blanchard and Lea; 1855. https://catalog.hathitrust.org/Record/006219914.
4. Mayerl C, Lukasser M, Sedivy R, Niederegger H, Seiler R, Wick G. Atherosclerosis research from past to present—on the track of two pathologists with opposing views, Carl von Rokitansky and Rudolf Virchow. Virchows Arch. 2006;449:96–103. http://link.springer.com/10.1007/s00428-006-0176-7.
5. Ross R. Atherosclerosis—an inflammatory disease. N Engl J Med. 1999;340:115–26. http://www.ncbi.nlm.nih.gov/pubmed/9887164.
6. Hansson GK, Libby P. The immune response in atherosclerosis: a double-edged sword. Nat Rev Immunol. 2006;6:508–19. http://www.nature.com/articles/nri1882.
7. Tabas I. 2016 Russell Ross memorial lecture in vascular biology: molecular-cellular mechanisms in the progression of atherosclerosis. Arterioscler Thromb Vasc Biol. 2017;37:183–9. http://atvb.ahajournals.org/lookup/doi/10.1161/ATVBAHA.116.308036.
8. Wick G, Grundtman C. Inflammation and atherosclerosis. 1st ed. Wien: Springer-Verlag; 2012. https://www.springer.com/us/book/9783709103371.
9. Land W. Allograft injury mediated by reactive oxygen species: from conserved proteins of drosophila to acute and chronic rejection of human transplants. Part III: Interaction of (oxidative) stress-induced heat shock proteins with Toll-like receptor-bearing cells. Transplant Rev. 2003;17:67–86. http://linkinghub.elsevier.com/retrieve/pii/S0955470X0380006X.
10. Hansson GK, Hermansson A. The immune system in atherosclerosis. Nat Immunol. 2011;12:204–12. http://www.ncbi.nlm.nih.gov/pubmed/21321594.
11. Land WG. Chronic allograft dysfunction: a model disorder of innate immunity. Biom J. 2013;36:209–28. http://biomedj.cgu.edu.tw/pdfs/2013/36/5/images/BiomedJ_2013_36_5_209_117622.pdf.
12. Witztum JL, Lichtman AH. The influence of innate and adaptive immune responses on atherosclerosis. Annu Rev Pathol. 2014;9:73–102. http://www.annualreviews.org/doi/10.1146/annurev-pathol-020712-163936.
13. French JE. Atherosclerosis in relation to the structure and function of the arterial intima, with special reference to the endothelium. Int Rev Exp Pathol. 1966;5:253–353. http://www.ncbi.nlm.nih.gov/pubmed/4877347.
14. Ross R, Glomset JA. Atherosclerosis and the arterial smooth muscle cell: proliferation of smooth muscle is a key event in the genesis of the lesions of atherosclerosis. Science. 1973;180:1332–9. http://www.ncbi.nlm.nih.gov/pubmed/4350926.
15. Virchow R. Thrombose und Embolie. Gefässentzündung und septische Infektion. In: Gesammelte Abhandlungen zur wissenschaftlichen Medicin. Frankfurt: Meidinger Sohn & Comp; 1856. https://www.medicusbooks.com/2-Medizin/Innere-Medizin/Kardiologie/Virchow-Rudolf-Thrombose-und-Embolie-Gefaessentzuendung-und-septische-Infektion-pp-219-752-In-Gesammelte-Abhandlungen-zur-wissenschaftlichen-Medicin::26800.html.
16. Ross R. The pathogenesis of atherosclerosis: a perspective for the 1990s. Nature. 1993;362:801–9. http://www.nature.com/doifinder/10.1038/362801a0.
17. Ross R. Cellular and molecular studies of atherogenesis. Atherosclerosis. 1997;131(Suppl):S3–4. http://www.ncbi.nlm.nih.gov/pubmed/9253466.
18. Land WG. Innate alloimmunity. Part 2. Innate immunity and allograft rejection. Ankara/Lengerich: Baskent University/Pabst Science Publishers; 2011. https://www.amazon.de/Innate-Alloimmunity-Immunity-Allograft-Rejection-ebook/.

19. Libby P, Hansson GK. Inflammation and immunity in diseases of the arterial tree: players and layers. Circ Res. 2015;116:307–11. http://www.ncbi.nlm.nih.gov/pubmed/25593275.
20. Ketelhuth DFJ, Hansson GK. Adaptive response of T and B cells in atherosclerosis. Circ Res. 2016;118:668–78. http://www.ncbi.nlm.nih.gov/pubmed/26892965.
21. Gisterå A, Hansson GK. The immunology of atherosclerosis. Nat Rev Nephrol. 2017;13: 368–80. http://www.ncbi.nlm.nih.gov/pubmed/28392564.
22. Mozaffarian D, Benjamin EJ, Go AS, Arnett DK, Blaha MJ, Cushman M, et al. Heart disease and stroke statistics—2016 update. Circulation. 2016;133:e38–360. http://www.ncbi.nlm.nih.gov/pubmed/26673558.
23. Stocker R, Keaney JF. Role of oxidative modifications in atherosclerosis. Physiol Rev. 2004;84:1381–478. http://www.physiology.org/doi/10.1152/physrev.00047.2003.
24. Land WG. Damage-associated molecular patterns in human diseases: Vol. 1. Injury-induced innate immune responses. New York: Springer International Publishing AG; 2018. https://www.springer.com/de/book/9783319786544.
25. Sies H, Berndt C, Jones DP. Oxidative stress. Annu Rev Biochem. 2017;86:715–48. http://www.annualreviews.org/doi/10.1146/annurev-biochem-061516-045037.
26. Schieber M, Chandel NS. ROS function in redox signaling and oxidative stress. Curr Biol. 2014;24:R453–62. http://www.ncbi.nlm.nih.gov/pubmed/24845678.
27. Saito R, Suzuki T, Hiramoto K, Asami S, Naganuma E, Suda H, et al. Characterizations of three major cysteine sensors of Keap1 in stress response. Mol Cell Biol. 2015;36:MCB.00868-15. http://www.ncbi.nlm.nih.gov/pubmed/26527616.
28. Dinkova-Kostova AT, Kostov RV, Canning P. Keap1, the cysteine-based mammalian intracellular sensor for electrophiles and oxidants. Arch Biochem Biophys. 2017;617:84–93. http://www.ncbi.nlm.nih.gov/pubmed/27497696.
29. Sihvola V, Levonen A-L. Keap1 as the redox sensor of the antioxidant response. Arch Biochem Biophys. 2017;617:94–100. http://www.ncbi.nlm.nih.gov/pubmed/27769838.
30. Chen X-L, Dodd G, Thomas S, Zhang X, Wasserman MA, Rovin BH, et al. Activation of Nrf2/ARE pathway protects endothelial cells from oxidant injury and inhibits inflammatory gene expression. Am J Physiol Heart Circ Physiol. 2006;290:H1862–70. http://www.physiology.org/doi/10.1152/ajpheart.00651.2005.
31. Ding Y, Zhang B, Zhou K, Chen M, Wang M, Jia Y, et al. Dietary ellagic acid improves oxidant-induced endothelial dysfunction and atherosclerosis: role of Nrf2 activation. Int J Cardiol. 2014;175:508–14. https://linkinghub.elsevier.com/retrieve/pii/S0167527314011127.
32. Jiang S, Yang Y, Li T, Ma Z, Hu W, Deng C, et al. An overview of the mechanisms and novel roles of Nrf2 in cardiovascular diseases. Expert Opin Ther Targets. 2016;20:1413–24. https://www.tandfonline.com/doi/full/10.1080/14728222.2016.1250887.
33. Lu M-C, Ji J-A, Jiang Z-Y, You Q-D. The Keap1-Nrf2-ARE pathway as a potential preventive and therapeutic target: an update. Med Res Rev. 2016;36:924–63. http://doi.wiley.com/10.1002/med.21396.
34. Zhang M, Shah AM. ROS signalling between endothelial cells and cardiac cells. Cardiovasc Res. 2014;102:249–57. https://academic.oup.com/cardiovascres/article-lookup/doi/10.1093/cvr/cvu050.
35. Brown DI, Griendling KK. Regulation of signal transduction by reactive oxygen species in the cardiovascular system. Circ Res. 2015;116:531–49. http://www.ncbi.nlm.nih.gov/pubmed/25634975.
36. Görlach A, Dimova EY, Petry A, Martínez-Ruiz A, Hernansanz-Agustín P, Rolo AP, et al. Reactive oxygen species, nutrition, hypoxia and diseases: problems solved? Redox Biol. 2015;6:372–85. https://linkinghub.elsevier.com/retrieve/pii/S2213231715001068.
37. Rosenblat M, Aviram M. Oxysterol-induced activation of macrophage NADPH-oxidase enhances cell-mediated oxidation of LDL in the atherosclerotic apolipoprotein E deficient mouse: inhibitory role for vitamin E. Atherosclerosis. 2002;160:69–80. http://www.ncbi.nlm.nih.gov/pubmed/11755924.

38. Rueckschloss U, Duerrschmidt N, Morawietz H. NADPH oxidase in endothelial cells: impact on atherosclerosis. Antioxid Redox Signal. 2003;5:171–80. http://www.ncbi.nlm.nih.gov/pubmed/12716477.
39. Cathcart MK. Regulation of superoxide anion production by NADPH oxidase in monocytes/macrophages: contributions to atherosclerosis. Arterioscler Thromb Vasc Biol. 2004;24:23–8. http://atvb.ahajournals.org/cgi/doi/10.1161/01.ATV.0000097769.47306.12.
40. Peluso I, Morabito G, Urban L, Ioannone F, Serafini M. Oxidative stress in atherosclerosis development: the central role of LDL and oxidative burst. Endocr Metab Immune Disord Drug Targets. 2012;12:351–60. http://www.ncbi.nlm.nih.gov/pubmed/23061409.
41. Kattoor AJ, Pothineni NVK, Palagiri D, Mehta JL. Oxidative stress in atherosclerosis. Curr Atheroscler Rep. 2017;19:42. http://www.ncbi.nlm.nih.gov/pubmed/28921056.
42. Konior A, Schramm A, Czesnikiewicz-Guzik M, Guzik TJ. NADPH oxidases in vascular pathology. Antioxid Redox Signal. 2014;20:2794–814. http://www.ncbi.nlm.nih.gov/pubmed/24180474.
43. Förstermann U, Xia N, Li H. Roles of vascular oxidative stress and nitric oxide in the pathogenesis of atherosclerosis. Circ Res. 2017;120:713–35. http://www.ncbi.nlm.nih.gov/pubmed/28209797.
44. Pignatelli P, Menichelli D, Pastori D, Violi F. Oxidative stress and cardiovascular disease: new insights. Kardiol Pol. 2018;76:713–22. http://www.ncbi.nlm.nih.gov/pubmed/29537483.
45. Daiber A, Di Lisa F, Oelze M, Kröller-Schön S, Steven S, Schulz E, et al. Crosstalk of mitochondria with NADPH oxidase via reactive oxygen and nitrogen species signalling and its role for vascular function. Br J Pharmacol. 2017;174:1670–89. http://www.ncbi.nlm.nih.gov/pubmed/26660451.
46. Bedard K, Krause K-H. The NOX family of ROS-generating NADPH oxidases: physiology and pathophysiology. Physiol Rev. 2007;87:245–313. http://www.ncbi.nlm.nih.gov/pubmed/17237347.
47. Madamanchi NR, Runge MS. NADPH oxidases and atherosclerosis: unraveling the details. Am J Physiol Heart Circ Physiol. 2010;298:H1–2. http://www.physiology.org/doi/10.1152/ajpheart.01020.2009.
48. Yin W, Voit EO. Function and design of the Nox1 system in vascular smooth muscle cells. BMC Syst Biol. 2013;7:20. http://bmcsystbiol.biomedcentral.com/articles/10.1186/1752-0509-7-20.
49. Breitenbach M, Rinnerthaler M, Weber M, Breitenbach-Koller H, Karl T, Cullen P, et al. The defense and signaling role of NADPH oxidases in eukaryotic cells. Wien Med Wochenschr. 2018;168:286–99. http://www.ncbi.nlm.nih.gov/pubmed/30084091.
50. Petry A, Görlach A. Regulation of NADPH oxidases by G protein-coupled receptors. Antioxid Redox Signal. 2018;30(1):74–94. http://www.ncbi.nlm.nih.gov/pubmed/29466865.
51. Griendling KK, Minieri CA, Ollerenshaw JD, Alexander RW. Angiotensin II stimulates NADH and NADPH oxidase activity in cultured vascular smooth muscle cells. Circ Res. 1994;74:1141–8. http://www.ncbi.nlm.nih.gov/pubmed/8187280.
52. Landmesser U, Cai H, Dikalov S, McCann L, Hwang J, Jo H, et al. Role of p47(phox) in vascular oxidative stress and hypertension caused by angiotensin II. Hypertension. 2002;40:511–5. http://www.ncbi.nlm.nih.gov/pubmed/12364355.
53. Landmesser U, Spiekermann S, Preuss C, Sorrentino S, Fischer D, Manes C, et al. Angiotensin II induces endothelial xanthine oxidase activation: role for endothelial dysfunction in patients with coronary disease. Arterioscler Thromb Vasc Biol. 2007;27:943–8. https://www.ahajournals.org/doi/10.1161/01.ATV.0000258415.32883.bf.
54. Forrester SJ, Booz GW, Sigmund CD, Coffman TM, Kawai T, Rizzo V, et al. Angiotensin II signal transduction: an update on mechanisms of physiology and pathophysiology. Physiol Rev. 2018;98:1627–738. http://www.ncbi.nlm.nih.gov/pubmed/29873596.
55. McNally JS, Davis ME, Giddens DP, Saha A, Hwang J, Dikalov S, et al. Role of xanthine oxidoreductase and NAD(P)H oxidase in endothelial superoxide production in response to oscillatory shear stress. Am J Physiol Heart Circ Physiol. 2003;285:H2290–7. http://www.physiology.org/doi/10.1152/ajpheart.00515.2003.

56. Köhler R, Hoyer J. Role of TRPV4 in the mechanotransduction of shear stress in endothelial cells. In: TRP ion channel function in sensory transduction and cellular signaling cascades. Boca Raton, FL: CRC Press/Taylor & Francis; 2007. http://www.ncbi.nlm.nih.gov/pubmed/21204499.
57. Mendoza SA, Fang J, Gutterman DD, Wilcox DA, Bubolz AH, Li R, et al. TRPV4-mediated endothelial Ca^{2+} influx and vasodilation in response to shear stress. Am J Physiol Heart Circ Physiol. 2010;298:H466–76. http://www.physiology.org/doi/10.1152/ajpheart.00854.2009.
58. Kim D, Pattamatta U, Kelly E, Healey PR, Carnt N, Zoellner H, et al. Inhibitory effects of angiotensin II receptor blockade on human Tenon fibroblast migration and reactive oxygen species production in cell culture. Transl Vis Sci Technol. 2018;7:20. http://www.ncbi.nlm.nih.gov/pubmed/29657902.
59. Martínez-Reyes I, Diebold LP, Kong H, Schieber M, Huang H, Hensley CT, et al. TCA cycle and mitochondrial membrane potential are necessary for diverse biological functions. Mol Cell. 2016;61:199–209. https://linkinghub.elsevier.com/retrieve/pii/S1097276515009363.
60. Zorov DB, Filburn CR, Klotz LO, Zweier JL, Sollott SJ. Reactive oxygen species (ROS)-induced ROS release: a new phenomenon accompanying induction of the mitochondrial permeability transition in cardiac myocytes. J Exp Med. 2000;192:1001–14. http://www.ncbi.nlm.nih.gov/pubmed/11015441.
61. Zandalinas SI, Mittler R. ROS-induced ROS release in plant and animal cells. Free Radic Biol Med. 2018;122:21–7. http://www.ncbi.nlm.nih.gov/pubmed/29203327.
62. Liu VWT, Huang PL. Cardiovascular roles of nitric oxide: a review of insights from nitric oxide synthase gene disrupted mice. Cardiovasc Res. 2008;77:19–29. https://academic.oup.com/cardiovascres/article-lookup/doi/10.1016/j.cardiores.2007.06.024.
63. Li H, Förstermann U. Uncoupling of endothelial NO synthase in atherosclerosis and vascular disease. Curr Opin Pharmacol. 2013;13:161–7. http://www.ncbi.nlm.nih.gov/pubmed/23395155.
64. Karbach S, Wenzel P, Waisman A, Munzel T, Daiber A. eNOS uncoupling in cardiovascular diseases—the role of oxidative stress and inflammation. Curr Pharm Des. 2014;20:3579–94. http://www.ncbi.nlm.nih.gov/pubmed/24180381.
65. Pautz A, Art J, Hahn S, Nowag S, Voss C, Kleinert H. Regulation of the expression of inducible nitric oxide synthase. Nitric Oxide Biol Chem. 2010;23:75–93. http://linkinghub.elsevier.com/retrieve/pii/S1089860310000583.
66. Lind M, Hayes A, Caprnda M, Petrovic D, Rodrigo L, Kruzliak P, et al. Inducible nitric oxide synthase: good or bad? Biomed Pharmacother. 2017;93:370–5. http://www.ncbi.nlm.nih.gov/pubmed/28651238.
67. Manea S-A, Constantin A, Manda G, Sasson S, Manea A. Regulation of Nox enzymes expression in vascular pathophysiology: focusing on transcription factors and epigenetic mechanisms. Redox Biol. 2015;5:358–66. https://linkinghub.elsevier.com/retrieve/pii/S2213231715000634.
68. Kietzmann T, Petry A, Shvetsova A, Gerhold JM, Görlach A. The epigenetic landscape related to reactive oxygen species formation in the cardiovascular system. Br J Pharmacol. 2017;174:1533–54. http://doi.wiley.com/10.1111/bph.13792.
69. Coco C, Sgarra L, Potenza MA, Nacci C, Pasculli B, Barbano R, et al. Can epigenetics of endothelial dysfunction represent the key to precision medicine in type 2 diabetes mellitus? Int J Mol Sci. 2019;20:2949. http://www.ncbi.nlm.nih.gov/pubmed/31212911.
70. Costantino S, Mohammed SA, Ambrosini S, Paneni F. Epigenetic processing in cardiometabolic disease. Atherosclerosis. 2019;281:150–8. http://www.ncbi.nlm.nih.gov/pubmed/30290963.
71. Cross D, Drury R, Hill J, Pollard AJ. Epigenetics in sepsis: understanding its role in endothelial dysfunction, immunosuppression, and potential therapeutics. Front Immunol. 2019;10:1363. http://www.ncbi.nlm.nih.gov/pubmed/31275313.
72. Schröder M, Kaufman RJ. The mammalian unfolded protein response. Annu Rev Biochem. 2005;74:739–89. http://www.ncbi.nlm.nih.gov/pubmed/15952902.

73. Ron D, Walter P. Signal integration in the endoplasmic reticulum unfolded protein response. Nat Rev Mol Cell Biol. 2007;8:519–29. http://www.ncbi.nlm.nih.gov/pubmed/17565364.
74. Wang Q, Groenendyk J, Michalak M. Glycoprotein quality control and endoplasmic reticulum stress. Molecules. 2015;20:13689–704. http://www.ncbi.nlm.nih.gov/pubmed/26225950.
75. Díaz-Villanueva JF, Díaz-Molina R, García-González V. Protein folding and mechanisms of proteostasis. Int J Mol Sci. 2015;16:17193–230. http://www.ncbi.nlm.nih.gov/pubmed/26225966.
76. Ochoa CD, Wu RF, Terada LS. ROS signaling and ER stress in cardiovascular disease. Mol Asp Med. 2018;63:18–29. https://linkinghub.elsevier.com/retrieve/pii/S009829971730136X.
77. Sano R, Reed JC. ER stress-induced cell death mechanisms. Biochim Biophys Acta. 1833;2013:3460–70. http://www.ncbi.nlm.nih.gov/pubmed/23850759.
78. Feaver RE, Hastings NE, Pryor A, Blackman BR. GRP78 upregulation by atheroprone shear stress via p38-, α2β1-dependent mechanism in endothelial cells. Arterioscler Thromb Vasc Biol. 2008;28:1534–41. http://www.ncbi.nlm.nih.gov/pubmed/18556570.
79. Gargalovic PS, Gharavi NM, Clark MJ, Pagnon J, Yang W-P, He A, et al. The unfolded protein response is an important regulator of inflammatory genes in endothelial cells. Arterioscler Thromb Vasc Biol. 2006;26:2490–6. http://www.ncbi.nlm.nih.gov/pubmed/16931790.
80. Gray SP, Di Marco E, Kennedy K, Chew P, Okabe J, El-Osta A, et al. Reactive oxygen species can provide atheroprotection via NOX4-dependent inhibition of inflammation and vascular remodeling. Arterioscler Thromb Vasc Biol. 2016;36:295–307. http://www.ncbi.nlm.nih.gov/pubmed/26715682.
81. Perrotta I, Aquila S. The role of oxidative stress and autophagy in atherosclerosis. Oxidative Med Cell Longev. 2015;2015:1–10. http://www.ncbi.nlm.nih.gov/pubmed/25866599.
82. Mohan S, Preetha Rani MR, Brown L, Ayyappan P, Raghu KG. Endoplasmic reticulum stress: a master regulator of metabolic syndrome. Eur J Pharmacol. 2019;860:172553. https://linkinghub.elsevier.com/retrieve/pii/S0014299919305059.
83. Mowbray AL, Kang D-H, Rhee SG, Kang SW, Jo H. Laminar shear stress up-regulates peroxiredoxins (PRX) in endothelial cells: PRX 1 as a mechanosensitive antioxidant. J Biol Chem. 2008;283:1622–7. http://www.jbc.org/lookup/doi/10.1074/jbc.M707985200.
84. Kwak BR, Bäck M, Bochaton-Piallat M-L, Caligiuri G, Daemen MJAP, Davies PF, et al. Biomechanical factors in atherosclerosis: mechanisms and clinical implications. Eur Heart J. 2014;35:3013–20, 3020a–d. https://academic.oup.com/eurheartj/article-lookup/doi/10.1093/eurheartj/ehu353.
85. Dabagh M, Jalali P, Butler PJ, Randles A, Tarbell JM. Mechanotransmission in endothelial cells subjected to oscillatory and multi-directional shear flow. J R Soc Interface. 2017;14:20170185. http://rsif.royalsocietypublishing.org/lookup/doi/10.1098/rsif.2017.0185.
86. Hsieh H-J, Liu C-A, Huang B, Tseng AH, Wang D. Shear-induced endothelial mechanotransduction: the interplay between reactive oxygen species (ROS) and nitric oxide (NO) and the pathophysiological implications. J Biomed Sci. 2014;21:3. http://www.ncbi.nlm.nih.gov/pubmed/24410814.
87. Sorescu GP, Song H, Tressel SL, Hwang J, Dikalov S, Smith DA, et al. Bone morphogenic protein 4 produced in endothelial cells by oscillatory shear stress induces monocyte adhesion by stimulating reactive oxygen species production from a nox1-based NADPH oxidase. Circ Res. 2004;95:773–9. https://www.ahajournals.org/doi/10.1161/01.RES.0000145728.22878.45.
88. Siu KL, Gao L, Cai H. Differential roles of protein complexes NOX1-NOXO1 and NOX2-p47phox in mediating endothelial redox responses to oscillatory and unidirectional laminar shear stress. J Biol Chem. 2016;291:8653–62. http://www.ncbi.nlm.nih.gov/pubmed/26826128.
89. Mammoto A, Mammoto T, Ingber DE. Mechanosensitive mechanisms in transcriptional regulation. J Cell Sci. 2012;125:3061–73. http://jcs.biologists.org/lookup/doi/10.1242/jcs.093005.
90. Zeng Y, Zhang XF, Fu BM, Tarbell JM. The role of endothelial surface glycocalyx in mechanosensing and transduction. Adv Exp Med Biol. 2018;1097:1–27. http://www.ncbi.nlm.nih.gov/pubmed/30315537.
91. Naruse K. Mechanomedicine. Biophys Rev. 2018;10:1257–62. http://www.ncbi.nlm.nih.gov/pubmed/30269290.

92. Chatterjee S, Fisher AB. Mechanotransduction in the endothelium: role of membrane proteins and reactive oxygen species in sensing, transduction, and transmission of the signal with altered blood flow. Antioxid Redox Signal. 2014;20:899–913. http://www.liebertpub.com/doi/10.1089/ars.2013.5624.
93. Lim C-G, Jang J, Kim C. Cellular machinery for sensing mechanical force. BMB Rep. 2018;51:623–9. http://www.ncbi.nlm.nih.gov/pubmed/30293551.
94. Storch U, Mederos y Schnitzler M, Gudermann T. G protein-mediated stretch reception. Am J Physiol Heart Circ Physiol. 2012;302:H1241–9. http://www.physiology.org/doi/10.1152/ajpheart.00818.2011.
95. Qin B, Wang Q, Lu Y, Li C, Hu H, Zhang J, et al. Losartan ameliorates calcium oxalate-induced elevation of stone-related proteins in renal tubular cells by inhibiting NADPH oxidase and oxidative stress. Oxidative Med Cell Longev. 2018;2018:1–12. http://www.ncbi.nlm.nih.gov/pubmed/29849862.
96. Chao Y, Zhu L, Qu X, Zhang J, Zhang J, Kong X, et al. Inhibition of angiotension II type 1 receptor reduced human endothelial inflammation induced by low shear stress. Exp Cell Res. 2017;360:94–104. http://www.ncbi.nlm.nih.gov/pubmed/28843962.
97. Davies PF, Civelek M. Endoplasmic reticulum stress, redox, and a proinflammatory environment in athero-susceptible endothelium in vivo at sites of complex hemodynamic shear stress. Antioxid Redox Signal. 2011;15:1427–32. http://www.ncbi.nlm.nih.gov/pubmed/21126204.
98. Tabas I. The role of endoplasmic reticulum stress in the progression of atherosclerosis. Circ Res. 2010;107:839–50. http://www.ncbi.nlm.nih.gov/pubmed/20884885.
99. Bailey KA, Haj FG, Simon SI, Passerini AG. Atherosusceptible shear stress activates endoplasmic reticulum stress to promote endothelial inflammation. Sci Rep. 2017;7:8196. http://www.ncbi.nlm.nih.gov/pubmed/28811527.
100. Pan L, Hong Z, Yu L, Gao Y, Zhang R, Feng H, et al. Shear stress induces human aortic endothelial cell apoptosis via interleukin-1 receptor-associated kinase 2-induced endoplasmic reticulum stress. Mol Med Rep. 2017;16:7205–12. http://www.ncbi.nlm.nih.gov/pubmed/28944871.
101. Harrison DG, Gongora MC. Oxidative stress and hypertension. Med Clin North Am. 2009;93:621–35. http://www.ncbi.nlm.nih.gov/pubmed/19427495.
102. Montezano AC, Dulak-Lis M, Tsiropoulou S, Harvey A, Briones AM, Touyz RM. Oxidative stress and human hypertension: vascular mechanisms, biomarkers, and novel therapies. Can J Cardiol. 2015;31:631–41. http://www.ncbi.nlm.nih.gov/pubmed/25936489.
103. Sinha N, Dabla PK. Oxidative stress and antioxidants in hypertension—a current review. Curr Hypertens Rev. 2015;11:132–42. http://www.ncbi.nlm.nih.gov/pubmed/26022210.
104. Peng J-J, Liu B, Xu J-Y, Peng J, Luo X-J. NADPH oxidase: its potential role in promotion of pulmonary arterial hypertension. Naunyn Schmiedebergs Arch Pharmacol. 2017;390:331–8. http://www.ncbi.nlm.nih.gov/pubmed/28190244.
105. Wang X, Bosonea A-M, Odenbach J, Fernandez-Patron C. Molecular signals elicited by GPCR agonists in hypertension, cardiovascular remodeling: are MMPs and ADAMs elusive therapeutic targets? Curr Hypertens Rev. 2012;8:159–80. http://www.ncbi.nlm.nih.gov/pubmed/24976815.
106. Tank AW, Lee WD. Peripheral and central effects of circulating catecholamines. Compr Physiol. 2015;5:1–15. http://doi.wiley.com/10.1002/cphy.c140007.
107. Lymperopoulos A, Brill A, McCrink KA. GPCRs of adrenal chromaffin cells & catecholamines: the plot thickens. Int J Biochem Cell Biol. 2016;77:213–9. https://linkinghub.elsevier.com/retrieve/pii/S1357272516300218.
108. Esler M. Mental stress and human cardiovascular disease. Neurosci Biobehav Rev. 2017;74:269–76. http://www.ncbi.nlm.nih.gov/pubmed/27751732.
109. Oparil S, Zaman MA, Calhoun DA. Pathogenesis of hypertension. Ann Intern Med. 2003;139:761–76. http://www.ncbi.nlm.nih.gov/pubmed/14597461.
110. Ziegler MG, Milic M. Sympathetic nerves and hypertension in stress, sleep apnea, and caregiving. Curr Opin Nephrol Hypertens. 2017;26:26–30. http://www.ncbi.nlm.nih.gov/pubmed/27755119.

111. Hering D, Trzebski A, Narkiewicz K. Recent advances in the pathophysiology of arterial hypertension—potential implications for clinical practice. Pol Arch Intern Med. 2017;127:195–204. http://www.ncbi.nlm.nih.gov/pubmed/28377560.
112. Atlas SA. The renin-angiotensin aldosterone system: pathophysiological role and pharmacologic inhibition. J Manag Care Pharm. 2007;13:9–20. http://www.ncbi.nlm.nih.gov/pubmed/17970613.
113. Mancia G, Dell'Oro R, Quarti-Trevano F, Scopelliti F, Grassi G. Angiotensin–sympathetic system interactions in cardiovascular and metabolic disease. J Hypertens. 2006;24:S51–6. http://www.ncbi.nlm.nih.gov/pubmed/16601574.
114. Theccanat T, Philip JL, Razzaque AM, Ludmer N, Li J, Xu X, et al. Regulation of cellular oxidative stress and apoptosis by G protein-coupled receptor kinase-2; the role of NADPH oxidase 4. Cell Signal. 2016;28:190–203. http://www.ncbi.nlm.nih.gov/pubmed/26631573.
115. Qian L, Hu X, Zhang D, Snyder A, Wu H-M, Li Y, et al. β2 adrenergic receptor activation induces microglial NADPH oxidase activation and dopaminergic neurotoxicity through an ERK-dependent/protein kinase A-independent pathway. Glia. 2009;57:1600–9. http://www.ncbi.nlm.nih.gov/pubmed/19330844.
116. Saavedra JM, Benicky J. Brain and peripheral angiotensin II play a major role in stress. Stress. 2007;10:185–93. http://www.ncbi.nlm.nih.gov/pubmed/17514587.
117. Leenen FHH, Blaustein MP, Hamlyn JM. Update on angiotensin II: new endocrine connections between the brain, adrenal glands and the cardiovascular system. Endocr Connect. 2017;6:R131–45. http://www.ncbi.nlm.nih.gov/pubmed/28855243.
118. de Queiroz TM, Monteiro MMO, Braga VA. Angiotensin-II-derived reactive oxygen species on baroreflex sensitivity during hypertension: new perspectives. Front Physiol. 2013;4:105. http://www.ncbi.nlm.nih.gov/pubmed/23717285.
119. Kurihara Y, Kurihara H, Morita H, Cao W-H, Ling G-Y, Kumada M, et al. Role of endothelin-1 in stress response in the central nervous system. Am J Physiol Integr Comp Physiol. 2000;279:R515–21. http://www.ncbi.nlm.nih.gov/pubmed/10938240.
120. Yammine L, Kang D-H, Baun MM, Meininger JC. Endothelin-1 and psychosocial risk factors for cardiovascular disease. Psychosom Med. 2014;76:109–21. http://www.ncbi.nlm.nih.gov/pubmed/24434952.
121. Sandoval Y-HG, Atef ME, Levesque L-O, Li Y, Anand-Srivastava MB. Endothelin-1 signaling in vascular physiology and pathophysiology. Curr Vasc Pharmacol. 2014;12:202–14. http://www.ncbi.nlm.nih.gov/pubmed/24568156.
122. Erridge C. Endogenous ligands of TLR2 and TLR4: agonists or assistants? J Leukoc Biol. 2010;87:989–99. http://www.ncbi.nlm.nih.gov/pubmed/20179153.
123. McCarthy CG, Goulopoulou S, Wenceslau CF, Spitler K, Matsumoto T, Webb RC. Toll-like receptors and damage-associated molecular patterns: novel links between inflammation and hypertension. Am J Physiol Heart Circ Physiol. 2014;306:H184–96. http://www.physiology.org/doi/10.1152/ajpheart.00328.2013.
124. Braasch I, Schartl M. Evolution of endothelin receptors in vertebrates. Gen Comp Endocrinol. 2014;209:21–34. http://www.ncbi.nlm.nih.gov/pubmed/25010382.
125. Davenport AP, Hyndman KA, Dhaun N, Southan C, Kohan DE, Pollock JS, et al. Endothelin. Pharmacol Rev. 2016;68:357–418. http://pharmrev.aspetjournals.org/cgi/doi/10.1124/pr.115.011833.
126. Houde M, Desbiens L, D'Orléans-Juste P. Endothelin-1: biosynthesis, signaling and vasoreactivity. Adv Pharmacol. 2016;77:143–75. https://linkinghub.elsevier.com/retrieve/pii/S1054358916300333.
127. Dammanahalli KJ, Sun Z. ENDOTHELINS and NADPH oxidases in the cardiovascular system. Clin Exp Pharmacol Physiol. 2008;35:2–6. http://www.ncbi.nlm.nih.gov/pubmed/18047620.
128. Chen D-D, Dong Y-G, Yuan H, Chen AF. Endothelin 1 activation of ENDOTHELIN A receptor/NADPH oxidase pathway and diminished antioxidants critically contribute to endothelial progenitor cell reduction and dysfunction in salt-sensitive hypertension. Hypertension. 2012;59:1037–43. http://www.ncbi.nlm.nih.gov/pubmed/22431579.

129. Sánchez A, Martínez P, Muñoz M, Benedito S, García-Sacristán A, Hernández M, et al. Endothelin-1 contributes to endothelial dysfunction and enhanced vasoconstriction through augmented superoxide production in penile arteries from insulin-resistant obese rats: role of ET A and ET B receptors. Br J Pharmacol. 2014;171:5682–95. http://www.ncbi.nlm.nih.gov/pubmed/25091502.
130. Zou Y, Akazawa H, Qin Y, Sano M, Takano H, Minamino T, et al. Mechanical stress activates angiotensin II type 1 receptor without the involvement of angiotensin II. Nat Cell Biol. 2004;6:499–506. http://www.nature.com/articles/ncb1137.
131. Mederos y Schnitzler M, Storch U, Meibers S, Nurwakagari P, Breit A, Essin K, et al. Gq-coupled receptors as mechanosensors mediating myogenic vasoconstriction. EMBO J. 2008;27:3092–103. http://emboj.embopress.org/cgi/doi/10.1038/emboj.2008.233.
132. Mederos y Schnitzler M, Storch U, Gudermann T. Mechanosensitive G q/11 protein-coupled receptors mediate myogenic vasoconstriction. Microcirculation. 2016;23:621–5. http://www.ncbi.nlm.nih.gov/pubmed/27344060.
133. Hong K, Li M, Nourian Z, Meininger GA, Hill MA. Angiotensin II type 1 receptor mechanoactivation involves RGS5 (regulator of G protein signaling 5) in skeletal muscle arteries: impaired trafficking of RGS5 in hypertension. Hypertension. 2017;70:1264–72. https://www.ahajournals.org/doi/10.1161/HYPERTENSIONAHA.117.09757.
134. Sato J, Makita N, Iiri T. Inverse agonism: the classic concept of GPCRs revisited [Review]. Endocr J. 2016;63:507–14. https://www.jstage.jst.go.jp/article/endocrj/63/6/63_EJ16-0084/_article.
135. Hitomi H, Fukui T, Moriwaki K, Matsubara K, Sun G-P, Rahman M, et al. Synergistic effect of mechanical stretch and angiotensin II on superoxide production via NADPH oxidase in vascular smooth muscle cells. J Hypertens. 2006;24:1089–95. https://insights.ovid.com/crossref?an=00004872-200606000-00018.
136. Shanahan CM, Furmanik M. Endoplasmic reticulum stress in arterial smooth muscle cells: a novel regulator of vascular disease. Curr Cardiol Rev. 2017;13:94–105. http://www.ncbi.nlm.nih.gov/pubmed/27758694.
137. Lenna S, Han R, Trojanowska M. Endoplasmic reticulum stress and endothelial dysfunction. IUBMB Life. 2014;66:530–7. http://www.ncbi.nlm.nih.gov/pubmed/25130181.
138. Kassan M, Galán M, Partyka M, Saifudeen Z, Henrion D, Trebak M, et al. Endoplasmic reticulum stress is involved in cardiac damage and vascular endothelial dysfunction in hypertensive mice. Arterioscler Thromb Vasc Biol. 2012;32:1652–61. https://www.ahajournals.org/doi/10.1161/ATVBAHA.112.249318.
139. Goulopoulou S, McCarthy CG, Webb RC. Toll-like receptors in the vascular system: sensing the dangers within. Pharmacol Rev. 2015;68:142–67. http://www.ncbi.nlm.nih.gov/pubmed/26721702.
140. McCarthy CG, Goulopoulou S, Webb RC. Paying the toll for inflammation. Hypertension. 2019;73:514–21. http://www.ncbi.nlm.nih.gov/pubmed/30661480.
141. Guzik TJ, Sadowski J, Guzik B, Jopek A, Kapelak B, Przybylowski P, et al. Coronary artery superoxide production and nox isoform expression in human coronary artery disease. Arterioscler Thromb Vasc Biol. 2006;26:333–9. http://atvb.ahajournals.org/cgi/doi/10.1161/01.ATV.0000196651.64776.51.
142. Giacco F, Brownlee M. Oxidative stress and diabetic complications. Circ Res. 2010;107:1058–70. http://www.ncbi.nlm.nih.gov/pubmed/21030723.
143. Shah MS, Brownlee M. Molecular and cellular mechanisms of cardiovascular disorders in diabetes. Circ Res. 2016;118:1808–29. http://www.ncbi.nlm.nih.gov/pubmed/27230643.
144. Wilson AJ, Gill EK, Abudalo RA, Edgar KS, Watson CJ, Grieve DJ. Reactive oxygen species signalling in the diabetic heart: emerging prospect for therapeutic targeting. Heart. 2017;104:heartjnl-2017-311448. http://www.ncbi.nlm.nih.gov/pubmed/28954833.
145. Jha JC, Ho F, Dan C, Jandeleit-Dahm K. A causal link between oxidative stress and inflammation in cardiovascular and renal complications of diabetes. Clin Sci. 2018;132:1811–36. http://www.ncbi.nlm.nih.gov/pubmed/30166499.

146. Volpe CMO, Villar-Delfino PH, dos Anjos PMF, Nogueira-Machado JA. Cellular death, reactive oxygen species (ROS) and diabetic complications. Cell Death Dis. 2018;9:119. http://www.ncbi.nlm.nih.gov/pubmed/29371661.
147. Nogueira-Machado JA, Chaves MM. From hyperglycemia to AGE-RAGE interaction on the cell surface: a dangerous metabolic route for diabetic patients. Expert Opin Ther Targets. 2008;12:871–82. http://www.tandfonline.com/doi/full/10.1517/14728222.12.7.871.
148. Yu W, Liu X, Feng L, Yang H, Yu W, Feng T, et al. Glycation of paraoxonase 1 by high glucose instigates endoplasmic reticulum stress to induce endothelial dysfunction in vivo. Sci Rep. 2017;7:45827. http://www.ncbi.nlm.nih.gov/pubmed/28374834.
149. Golbidi S, Edvinsson L, Laher I. Smoking and endothelial dysfunction. Curr Vasc Pharmacol. 2020;18:1–11. http://www.ncbi.nlm.nih.gov/pubmed/30210003.
150. Kim M, Han C-H, Lee M-Y. NADPH oxidase and the cardiovascular toxicity associated with smoking. Toxicol Res. 2014;30:149–57. http://www.ncbi.nlm.nih.gov/pubmed/25343008.
151. Hemmat N, Ebadi A, Badalzadeh R, Memar MY, Baghi HB. Viral infection and atherosclerosis. Eur J Clin Microbiol Infect Dis. 2018;37:2225–33. http://link.springer.com/10.1007/s10096-018-3370-z.
152. Di Pietro M, Filardo S, Falasca F, Turriziani O, Sessa R. Infectious agents in atherosclerotic cardiovascular diseases through oxidative stress. Int J Mol Sci. 2017;18:2459. http://www.ncbi.nlm.nih.gov/pubmed/29156574.
153. Kurita-Ochiai T, Yamamoto M. Periodontal pathogens and atherosclerosis: implications of inflammation and oxidative modification of LDL. Biomed Res Int. 2014;2014:595981. http://www.hindawi.com/journals/bmri/2014/595981/.
154. Xuan Y, Shi Q, Liu G-J, Luan Q-X, Cai Y. Porphyromonas gingivalis infection accelerates atherosclerosis mediated by oxidative stress and inflammatory responses in ApoE−/− mice. Clin Lab. 2017;63:1627–37. http://www.ncbi.nlm.nih.gov/pubmed/29035447.
155. Kreutmayer S, Csordas A, Kern J, Maass V, Almanzar G, Offterdinger M, et al. Chlamydia pneumoniae infection acts as an endothelial stressor with the potential to initiate the earliest heat shock protein 60-dependent inflammatory stage of atherosclerosis. Cell Stress Chaperones. 2013;18:259–68. http://link.springer.com/10.1007/s12192-012-0378-7.
156. Schwarz KB. Oxidative stress during viral infection: a review. Free Radic Biol Med. 1996;21:641–9. http://www.ncbi.nlm.nih.gov/pubmed/8891667.
157. Wang H, Peng G, Bai J, He B, Huang K, Hu X, et al. Cytomegalovirus infection and relative risk of cardiovascular disease (ischemic heart disease, stroke, and cardiovascular death): a meta-analysis of prospective studies up to 2016. J Am Heart Assoc. 2017;6:e005025. http://www.ncbi.nlm.nih.gov/pubmed/28684641.
158. Leskov IL, Whitsett J, Vasquez-Vivar J, Stokes KY. NAD(P)H oxidase and eNOS play differential roles in cytomegalovirus infection-induced microvascular dysfunction. Free Radic Biol Med. 2011;51:2300–8. http://www.ncbi.nlm.nih.gov/pubmed/22033010.
159. Weis M, Kledal TN, Lin KY, Panchal SN, Gao SZ, Valantine HA, et al. Cytomegalovirus infection impairs the nitric oxide synthase pathway: role of asymmetric dimethylarginine in transplant arteriosclerosis. Circulation. 2004;109:500–5. http://www.ncbi.nlm.nih.gov/pubmed/14732750.
160. Laurence J, Elhadad S, Ahamed J. HIV-associated cardiovascular disease: importance of platelet activation and cardiac fibrosis in the setting of specific antiretroviral therapies. Open Heart. 2018;5:e000823. http://www.ncbi.nlm.nih.gov/pubmed/30018781.
161. Aurpibul L, Sugandhavesa P, Srithanaviboonchai K, Sitthi W, Tangmunkongvorakul A, Chariyalertsak C, et al. Peripheral artery disease in HIV-infected older adults on antiretroviral treatment in Thailand. HIV Med. 2019;20:54–9. http://doi.wiley.com/10.1111/hiv.12671.
162. Kirichenko TV, Myasoedova VA, Shimonova TE, Melnichenko AA, Sviridov D, Sobenin IA, et al. Atherosclerosis in subjects newly diagnosed with human immunodeficiency virus infection. Biosci Rep. 2018;38:BSR20180597. http://www.ncbi.nlm.nih.gov/pubmed/29961673.
163. Lambert CT, Sandesara PB, Hirsh B, Shaw LJ, Lewis W, Quyyumi AA, et al. HIV, highly active antiretroviral therapy and the heart: a cellular to epidemiological review. HIV Med. 2016;17:411–24. http://doi.wiley.com/10.1111/hiv.12346.

164. Marincowitz C, Genis A, Goswami N, De Boever P, Nawrot TS, Strijdom H. Vascular endothelial dysfunction in the wake of HIV and ART. FEBS J. 2019;286:1256–70. https://onlinelibrary.wiley.com/doi/abs/10.1111/febs.14657.
165. Wang T, Green LA, Gupta SK, Kim C, Wang L, Almodovar S, et al. Transfer of intracellular HIV Nef to endothelium causes endothelial dysfunction. PLoS One. 2014;9:e91063. http://dx.plos.org/10.1371/journal.pone.0091063.
166. Ma R, Yang L, Niu F, Buch S. HIV tat-mediated induction of human brain microvascular endothelial cell apoptosis involves endoplasmic reticulum stress and mitochondrial dysfunction. Mol Neurobiol. 2016;53:132–42. http://www.ncbi.nlm.nih.gov/pubmed/25409632.
167. Adinolfi LE, Restivo L, Zampino R, Guerrera B, Lonardo A, Ruggiero L, et al. Chronic HCV infection is a risk of atherosclerosis. Role of HCV and HCV-related steatosis. Atherosclerosis. 2012;221:496–502. http://linkinghub.elsevier.com/retrieve/pii/S0021915012001141.
168. Voulgaris T, Sevastianos VA. Atherosclerosis as extrahepatic manifestation of chronic infection with hepatitis C virus. Hepat Res Treat. 2016;2016:1–8. http://www.ncbi.nlm.nih.gov/pubmed/26885388.
169. Hino K, Nishina S, Sasaki K, Hara Y. Mitochondrial damage and iron metabolic dysregulation in hepatitis C virus infection. Free Radic Biol Med. 2019;133:193–9. https://linkinghub.elsevier.com/retrieve/pii/S0891584918317295.
170. Kovacic S, Bakran M. Genetic susceptibility to atherosclerosis. Stroke Res Treat. 2012;2012:1–5. http://www.ncbi.nlm.nih.gov/pubmed/22550613.
171. Forgo B, Medda E, Hernyes A, Szalontai L, Tarnoki DL, Tarnoki AD. Carotid artery atherosclerosis: a review on heritability and genetics. Twin Res Hum Genet. 2018;21:333–46. http://www.ncbi.nlm.nih.gov/pubmed/29976271.
172. Labos C, Thanassoulis G. Genetic risk prediction for primary and secondary prevention of atherosclerotic cardiovascular disease: an update. Curr Cardiol Rep. 2018;20:36. http://www.ncbi.nlm.nih.gov/pubmed/29574623.
173. Bhayadia R, Schmidt BMW, Melk A, Hömme M. Senescence-induced oxidative stress causes endothelial dysfunction. J Gerontol Ser A Biol Sci Med Sci. 2016;71:161–9. http://www.ncbi.nlm.nih.gov/pubmed/25735595.
174. Cai X, She M, Xu M, Chen H, Li J, Chen X, et al. GLP-1 treatment protects endothelial cells from oxidative stress-induced autophagy and endothelial dysfunction. Int J Biol Sci. 2018;14:1696–708. http://www.ncbi.nlm.nih.gov/pubmed/30416384.
175. Simon DI. Inflammation and vascular injury: basic discovery to drug development. Circ J. 2012;76:1811–8. http://www.ncbi.nlm.nih.gov/pubmed/22785436.
176. Hopkins PN. Molecular biology of atherosclerosis. Physiol Rev. 2013;93:1317–542. http://www.ncbi.nlm.nih.gov/pubmed/23899566.
177. Tabas I, García-Cardeña G, Owens GK. Recent insights into the cellular biology of atherosclerosis. J Cell Biol. 2015;209:13–22. http://www.jcb.org/lookup/doi/10.1083/jcb.201412052.
178. Ketelhuth DFJ, Hansson GK. Modulation of autoimmunity and atherosclerosis—common targets and promising translational approaches against disease. Circ J. 2015;79:924–33. https://www.jstage.jst.go.jp/article/circj/79/5/79_CJ-15-0167/_article.
179. Geovanini GR, Libby P. Atherosclerosis and inflammation: overview and updates. Clin Sci. 2018;132:1243–52. http://www.ncbi.nlm.nih.gov/pubmed/29930142.
180. Wu M-Y, Li C-J, Hou M-F, Chu P-Y. New insights into the role of inflammation in the pathogenesis of atherosclerosis. Int J Mol Sci. 2017;18:2034. http://www.ncbi.nlm.nih.gov/pubmed/28937652.
181. Sitia S, Tomasoni L, Atzeni F, Ambrosio G, Cordiano C, Catapano A, et al. From endothelial dysfunction to atherosclerosis. Autoimmun Rev. 2010;9:830–4. http://linkinghub.elsevier.com/retrieve/pii/S1568997210001540.
182. Gimbrone MA, García-Cardeña G. Endothelial cell dysfunction and the pathobiology of atherosclerosis. Circ Res. 2016;118:620–36. http://www.ncbi.nlm.nih.gov/pubmed/26892962.
183. Lerman A, Burnett JC. Intact and altered endothelium in regulation of vasomotion. Circulation. 1992;86:III12–9. http://www.ncbi.nlm.nih.gov/pubmed/1424046.

184. Widmer RJ, Lerman A. Endothelial dysfunction and cardiovascular disease. Glob Cardiol Sci Pract. 2014;2014:291–308. http://www.ncbi.nlm.nih.gov/pubmed/25780786.
185. Hadi HAR, Carr CS, Al Suwaidi J. Endothelial dysfunction: cardiovascular risk factors, therapy, and outcome. Vasc Health Risk Manag. 2005;1:183–98. http://www.ncbi.nlm.nih.gov/pubmed/17319104.
186. Incalza MA, D'Oria R, Natalicchio A, Perrini S, Laviola L, Giorgino F. Oxidative stress and reactive oxygen species in endothelial dysfunction associated with cardiovascular and metabolic diseases. Vasc Pharmacol. 2018;100:1–19. http://www.ncbi.nlm.nih.gov/pubmed/28579545.
187. Hecquet CM, Ahmmed GU, Vogel SM, Malik AB. Role of TRPM2 channel in mediating H_2O_2-induced Ca^{2+} entry and endothelial hyperpermeability. Circ Res. 2008;102:347–55. http://www.ncbi.nlm.nih.gov/pubmed/18048770.
188. Tarbell JM. Mass transport in arteries and the localization of atherosclerosis. Annu Rev Biomed Eng. 2003;5:79–118. http://www.annualreviews.org/doi/10.1146/annurev.bioeng.5.040202.121529.
189. Taleb A, Witztum JL, Tsimikas S. Oxidized phospholipids on apoB-100-containing lipoproteins: a biomarker predicting cardiovascular disease and cardiovascular events. Biomark Med. 2011;5:673–94. https://www.futuremedicine.com/doi/10.2217/bmm.11.60.
190. Tabas I, Lichtman AH. Monocyte-macrophages and T cells in atherosclerosis. Immunity. 2017;47:621–34. http://www.ncbi.nlm.nih.gov/pubmed/29045897.
191. Williams KJ, Tabas I. The response-to-retention hypothesis of early atherogenesis. Arterioscler Thromb Vasc Biol. 1995;15:551–61. http://www.ncbi.nlm.nih.gov/pubmed/7749869.
192. Hu J, Liu T, Zhang Z, Xu Y, Zhu F. Oxidized low-density lipoprotein promotes vascular endothelial cell dysfunction by stimulating miR-496 expression and inhibiting the Hippo pathway effector YAP. Cell Biol Int. 2019;43:528–38. https://onlinelibrary.wiley.com/doi/abs/10.1002/cbin.11120.
193. Patel R, Varghese JF, Singh RP, Yadav UCS. Induction of endothelial dysfunction by oxidized low-density lipoproteins via downregulation of Erk-5/Mef2c/KLF2 signaling: amelioration by fisetin. Biochimie. 2019;163:152–62. https://linkinghub.elsevier.com/retrieve/pii/S0300908419301725.
194. Singh S, Gautam AS. Upregulated LOX-1 receptor: key player of the pathogenesis of atherosclerosis. Curr Atheroscler Rep. 2019;21:38. http://link.springer.com/10.1007/s11883-019-0801-y.
195. Cancel LM, Ebong EE, Mensah S, Hirschberg C, Tarbell JM. Endothelial glycocalyx, apoptosis and inflammation in an atherosclerotic mouse model. Atherosclerosis. 2016;252:136–46. https://linkinghub.elsevier.com/retrieve/pii/S002191501631231X.
196. Zhang Y, Yang X, Bian F, Wu P, Xing S, Xu G, et al. TNF-α promotes early atherosclerosis by increasing transcytosis of LDL across endothelial cells: crosstalk between NF-κB and PPAR-γ. J Mol Cell Cardiol. 2014;72:85–94. http://www.ncbi.nlm.nih.gov/pubmed/24594319.
197. Harkewicz R, Hartvigsen K, Almazan F, Dennis EA, Witztum JL, Miller YI. Cholesteryl ester hydroperoxides are biologically active components of minimally oxidized low density lipoprotein. J Biol Chem. 2008;283:10241–51. http://www.jbc.org/lookup/doi/10.1074/jbc.M709006200.
198. Steinberg D, Witztum JL. Oxidized low-density lipoprotein and atherosclerosis. Arterioscler Thromb Vasc Biol. 2010;30:2311–6. http://www.ncbi.nlm.nih.gov/pubmed/21084697.
199. Binder CJ, Papac-Milicevic N, Witztum JL. Innate sensing of oxidation-specific epitopes in health and disease. Nat Rev Immunol. 2016;16:485–97. http://www.ncbi.nlm.nih.gov/pubmed/27346802.
200. Girotti AW, Korytowski W. Cholesterol hydroperoxide generation, translocation, and reductive turnover in biological systems. Cell Biochem Biophys. 2017;75:413–9. http://link.springer.com/10.1007/s12013-017-0799-0.
201. Nakashima Y, Fujii H, Sumiyoshi S, Wight TN, Sueishi K. Early human atherosclerosis: accumulation of lipid and proteoglycans in intimal thickenings followed by macrophage infiltration. Arterioscler Thromb Vasc Biol. 2007;27:1159–65. https://www.ahajournals.org/doi/10.1161/ATVBAHA.106.134080.

202. Ballinger ML, Nigro J, Frontanilla KV, Dart AM, Little PJ. Regulation of glycosaminoglycan structure and atherogenesis. Cell Mol Life Sci. 2004;61:1296–306. http://link.springer.com/10.1007/s00018-004-3389-4.
203. Chang MY, Potter-Perigo S, Tsoi C, Chait A, Wight TN. Oxidized low density lipoproteins regulate synthesis of monkey aortic smooth muscle cell proteoglycans that have enhanced native low density lipoprotein binding properties. J Biol Chem. 2000;275:4766–73. http://www.ncbi.nlm.nih.gov/pubmed/10671509.
204. Chen Q, Wang Q, Zhu J, Xiao Q, Zhang L. Reactive oxygen species: key regulators in vascular health and diseases. Br J Pharmacol. 2018;175:1279–92. http://www.ncbi.nlm.nih.gov/pubmed/28430357.
205. Galkina E, Ley K. Vascular adhesion molecules in atherosclerosis. Arterioscler Thromb Vasc Biol. 2007;27:2292–301. http://www.ncbi.nlm.nih.gov/pubmed/17673705.
206. Golia E, Limongelli G, Natale F, Fimiani F, Maddaloni V, Pariggiano I, et al. Inflammation and cardiovascular disease: from pathogenesis to therapeutic target. Curr Atheroscler Rep. 2014;16:435. http://www.ncbi.nlm.nih.gov/pubmed/25037581.
207. Zernecke A, Weber C. Chemokines in atherosclerosis: proceedings resumed. Arterioscler Thromb Vasc Biol. 2014;34:742–50. https://www.ahajournals.org/doi/10.1161/ATVBAHA.113.301655.
208. Pober JS, Sessa WC. Evolving functions of endothelial cells in inflammation. Nat Rev Immunol. 2007;7:803–15. http://www.nature.com/articles/nri2171.
209. Sun X, Jiao X, Ma Y, Liu Y, Zhang L, He Y, et al. Trimethylamine N-oxide induces inflammation and endothelial dysfunction in human umbilical vein endothelial cells via activating ROS-TXNIP-NLRP3 inflammasome. Biochem Biophys Res Commun. 2016;481:63–70. http://www.ncbi.nlm.nih.gov/pubmed/27833015.
210. He Y-E, Qiu H-X, Wu R-Z, Rong X, Xu H-T, Xiang R-L, et al. Oxidised low-density lipoprotein and its receptor-mediated endothelial dysfunction are associated with coronary artery lesions in Kawasaki disease. J Cardiovasc Transl Res. 2019. http://www.ncbi.nlm.nih.gov/pubmed/31428922.
211. Varghese JF, Patel R, Yadav UCS. Sterol regulatory element binding protein (SREBP)-1 mediates oxidized low-density lipoprotein (oxLDL) induced macrophage foam cell formation through NLRP3 inflammasome activation. Cell Signal. 2019;53:316–26. http://www.ncbi.nlm.nih.gov/pubmed/30389501.
212. Feng Y, Cai ZR, Tang Y, Hu G, Lu J, He D, et al. TLR4/NF-κB signaling pathway-mediated and oxLDL-induced up-regulation of LOX-1, MCP-1, and VCAM-1 expressions in human umbilical vein endothelial cells. Genet Mol Res. 2014;13:680–95. http://www.ncbi.nlm.nih.gov/pubmed/24615033.
213. Geng H, Wang A, Rong G, Zhu B, Deng Y, Chen J, et al. The effects of ox-LDL in human atherosclerosis may be mediated in part via the toll-like receptor 4 pathway. Mol Cell Biochem. 2010;342:201–6. http://link.springer.com/10.1007/s11010-010-0484-8.
214. Su Q, Sun Y, Ye Z, Yang H, Kong B, Li L. Pinocembrin protects endothelial cells from oxidized LDL-induced injury. Cytokine. 2018;111:475–80. http://www.ncbi.nlm.nih.gov/pubmed/29914794.
215. Zhou Z, Subramanian P, Sevilmis G, Globke B, Soehnlein O, Karshovska E, et al. Lipoprotein-derived lysophosphatidic acid promotes atherosclerosis by releasing CXCL1 from the endothelium. Cell Metab. 2011;13:592–600. http://www.ncbi.nlm.nih.gov/pubmed/21531341.
216. Su J, Zhou H, Liu X, Nilsson J, Fredrikson GN, Zhao M. oxLDL antibody inhibits MCP-1 release in monocytes/macrophages by regulating Ca^{2+}/K^{+} channel flow. J Cell Mol Med. 2017;21:929–40. http://www.ncbi.nlm.nih.gov/pubmed/27995732.
217. Martinez-Quinones P, Komic A, McCarthy CG, Webb RC, Wenceslau CF. Targeting endothelial barrier dysfunction caused by circulating bacterial and mitochondrial N-formyl peptides with deformylase. Front Immunol. 2019;10:1270. http://www.ncbi.nlm.nih.gov/pubmed/31244835.
218. Hansson GK, Libby P, Tabas I. Inflammation and plaque vulnerability. J Intern Med. 2015;278:483–93. http://doi.wiley.com/10.1111/joim.12406.

219. Libby P. Mechanisms of acute coronary syndromes and their implications for therapy. N Engl J Med. 2013;368:2004–13. http://www.ncbi.nlm.nih.gov/pubmed/23697515.
220. Yurdagul A, Doran AC, Cai B, Fredman G, Tabas IA. Mechanisms and consequences of defective efferocytosis in atherosclerosis. Front Cardiovasc Med. 2018;4:86. http://www.ncbi.nlm.nih.gov/pubmed/29379788.
221. Xing X, Baffic J, Sparrow CP. LDL oxidation by activated monocytes: characterization of the oxidized LDL and requirement for transition metal ions. J Lipid Res. 1998;39:2201–8. http://www.ncbi.nlm.nih.gov/pubmed/9799806.
222. Bey EA, Cathcart MK. In vitro knockout of human p47phox blocks superoxide anion production and LDL oxidation by activated human monocytes. J Lipid Res. 2000;41:489–95. http://www.ncbi.nlm.nih.gov/pubmed/10706597.
223. Lao KH, Zeng L, Xu Q. Endothelial and smooth muscle cell transformation in atherosclerosis. Curr Opin Lipidol. 2015;26:449–56. http://content.wkhealth.com/linkback/openurl?sid=WKPTLP:landingpage&an=00041433-201510000-00015.
224. Chistiakov DA, Melnichenko AA, Myasoedova VA, Grechko AV, Orekhov AN. Mechanisms of foam cell formation in atherosclerosis. J Mol Med. 2017;95:1153–65. http://www.ncbi.nlm.nih.gov/pubmed/28785870.
225. An D, Hao F, Zhang F, Kong W, Chun J, Xu X, et al. CD14 is a key mediator of both lysophosphatidic acid and lipopolysaccharide induction of foam cell formation. J Biol Chem. 2017;292:14391–400. http://www.jbc.org/lookup/doi/10.1074/jbc.M117.781807.
226. Dai Y, Cao Y, Zhang Z, Vallurupalli S, Mehta JL. Xanthine oxidase induces foam cell formation through LOX-1 and NLRP3 activation. Cardiovasc Drugs Ther. 2017;31:19–27. http://link.springer.com/10.1007/s10557-016-6706-x.
227. Wang R, Wu W, Li W, Huang S, Li Z, Liu R, et al. Activation of NLRP3 inflammasome promotes foam cell formation in vascular smooth muscle cells and atherogenesis via HMGB1. J Am Heart Assoc. 2018;7:e008596. http://www.ncbi.nlm.nih.gov/pubmed/30371306.
228. Wu H, Chen Z, Chen J-Z, Pei L-G, Xie J, Wei Z-H, et al. High mobility group B-1 (HMGB-1) promotes apoptosis of macrophage-derived foam cells by inducing endoplasmic reticulum stress. Cell Physiol Biochem. 2018;48:1019–29. https://www.karger.com/Article/FullText/491970.
229. da Silva RF, Lappalainen J, Lee-Rueckert M, Kovanen PT. Conversion of human M-CSF macrophages into foam cells reduces their proinflammatory responses to classical M1-polarizing activation. Atherosclerosis. 2016;248:170–8. http://www.ncbi.nlm.nih.gov/pubmed/27038418.
230. van Dijk RA, Kolodgie F, Ravandi A, Leibundgut G, Hu PP, Prasad A, et al. Differential expression of oxidation-specific epitopes and apolipoprotein(a) in progressing and ruptured human coronary and carotid atherosclerotic lesions. J Lipid Res. 2012;53:2773–90. http://www.ncbi.nlm.nih.gov/pubmed/22969153.
231. Duewell P, Kono H, Rayner KJ, Sirois CM, Vladimer G, Bauernfeind FG, et al. NLRP3 inflammasomes are required for atherogenesis and activated by cholesterol crystals. Nature. 2010;464:1357–61. http://www.nature.com/articles/nature08938.
232. Paramel Varghese G, Folkersen L, Strawbridge RJ, Halvorsen B, Yndestad A, Ranheim T, et al. NLRP3 inflammasome expression and activation in human atherosclerosis. J Am Heart Assoc. 2016;5. https://www.ahajournals.org/doi/10.1161/JAHA.115.003031.
233. Karasawa T, Takahashi M. Role of NLRP3 inflammasomes in atherosclerosis. J Atheroscler Thromb. 2017;24:443–51. http://www.ncbi.nlm.nih.gov/pubmed/28260724.
234. MacKinnon AC, Liu X, Hadoke PW, Miller MR, Newby DE, Sethi T. Inhibition of galectin-3 reduces atherosclerosis in apolipoprotein E-deficient mice. Glycobiology. 2013;23:654–63. https://academic.oup.com/glycob/article-lookup/doi/10.1093/glycob/cwt006.
235. Jonasson L, Holm J, Skalli O, Bondjers G, Hansson GK. Regional accumulations of T cells, macrophages, and smooth muscle cells in the human atherosclerotic plaque. Arteriosclerosis. 1986;6:131–8. http://www.ncbi.nlm.nih.gov/pubmed/2937395.
236. Lusis AJ. Atherosclerosis. Nature. 2000;407:233–41. http://www.ncbi.nlm.nih.gov/pubmed/11001066.

237. Galluzzi L, Vitale I, Aaronson SA, Abrams JM, Adam D, Agostinis P, et al. Molecular mechanisms of cell death: recommendations of the Nomenclature Committee on Cell Death 2018. Cell Death Differ. 2018;25:486–541. http://www.nature.com/articles/s41418-017-0012-4.
238. Martinet W, Schrijvers DM, De Meyer GRY. Necrotic cell death in atherosclerosis. Basic Res Cardiol. 2011;106:749–60. http://www.ncbi.nlm.nih.gov/pubmed/21611880.
239. Fok P-W. Growth of necrotic cores in atherosclerotic plaque. Math Med Biol. 2012;29:301–27. http://www.ncbi.nlm.nih.gov/pubmed/21908792.
240. Gonzalez L, Trigatti BL. Macrophage apoptosis and necrotic Core development in atherosclerosis: a rapidly advancing field with clinical relevance to imaging and therapy. Can J Cardiol. 2017;33:303–12. http://www.ncbi.nlm.nih.gov/pubmed/28232016.
241. Rai V, Agrawal DK. The role of damage- and pathogen-associated molecular patterns in inflammation-mediated vulnerability of atherosclerotic plaques. Can J Physiol Pharmacol. 2017;95:1245–53. http://www.ncbi.nlm.nih.gov/pubmed/28746820.
242. Zhou Z-B, Yang B, Li X, Liu H, Lei G. Lysophosphatidic acid promotes expression and activation of matrix metalloproteinase 9 (MMP9) in THP-1 cells via toll-like receptor 4/nuclear factor-κB (TLR4/NF-κB) signaling pathway. Med Sci Monit. 2018;24:4861–8. https://www.medscimonit.com/abstract/index/idArt/906450.
243. Libby P. Inflammation in atherosclerosis. Nature. 2002;420:868–74. http://www.ncbi.nlm.nih.gov/pubmed/12490960.
244. Moreno PR, Purushothaman KR, Fuster V, Echeverri D, Truszczynska H, Sharma SK, et al. Plaque neovascularization is increased in ruptured atherosclerotic lesions of human aorta: implications for plaque vulnerability. Circulation. 2004;110:2032–8. https://www.ahajournals.org/doi/10.1161/01.CIR.0000143233.87854.23.
245. Hansson GK. Inflammation, atherosclerosis, and coronary artery disease. N Engl J Med. 2005;352:1685–95. http://www.ncbi.nlm.nih.gov/pubmed/15843671.
246. Newby AC. Metalloproteinases promote plaque rupture and myocardial infarction: a persuasive concept waiting for clinical translation. Matrix Biol. 2015;44–46:157–66. https://linkinghub.elsevier.com/retrieve/pii/S0945053X15000293.
247. Spacek M, Zemanek D, Hutyra M, Sluka M, Taborsky M. Vulnerable atherosclerotic plaque—a review of current concepts and advanced imaging. Biomed Pap Med Fac Univ Palacky Olomouc Czech Repub. 2018;162:10–7. http://www.ncbi.nlm.nih.gov/pubmed/29467545.
248. Johnson JL. Metalloproteinases in atherosclerosis. Eur J Pharmacol. 2017;816:93–106. http://www.ncbi.nlm.nih.gov/pubmed/28893577.
249. Butoi E, Gan AM, Tucureanu MM, Stan D, Macarie RD, Constantinescu C, et al. Cross-talk between macrophages and smooth muscle cells impairs collagen and metalloprotease synthesis and promotes angiogenesis. Biochim Biophys Acta. 1863;2016:1568–78. https://linkinghub.elsevier.com/retrieve/pii/S0167488916300829.
250. Fuster V, Moreno PR, Fayad ZA, Corti R, Badimon JJ. Atherothrombosis and high-risk plaque: Part I. Evolving concepts. J Am Coll Cardiol. 2005;46:937–54. http://linkinghub.elsevier.com/retrieve/pii/S0735109705013963.
251. Schwartz SM, Galis ZS, Rosenfeld ME, Falk E. Plaque rupture in humans and mice. Arterioscler Thromb Vasc Biol. 2007;27:705–13. http://www.ncbi.nlm.nih.gov/pubmed/17332493.
252. Yahagi K, Kolodgie FD, Otsuka F, Finn AV, Davis HR, Joner M, et al. Pathophysiology of native coronary, vein graft, and in-stent atherosclerosis. Nat Rev Cardiol. 2016;13:79–98. http://www.nature.com/articles/nrcardio.2015.164.
253. Chistiakov DA, Myasoedova VA, Melnichenko AA, Grechko AV, Orekhov AN. Calcifying matrix vesicles and atherosclerosis. Biomed Res Int. 2017;2017:1–7. http://www.ncbi.nlm.nih.gov/pubmed/29238720.
254. Grootaert MOJ, Moulis M, Roth L, Martinet W, Vindis C, Bennett MR, et al. Vascular smooth muscle cell death, autophagy and senescence in atherosclerosis. Cardiovasc Res. 2018;114:622–34. http://www.ncbi.nlm.nih.gov/pubmed/29360955.
255. Kavurma MM, Rayner KJ, Karunakaran D. The walking dead: macrophage inflammation and death in atherosclerosis. Curr Opin Lipidol. 2017;28:91–8. http://insights.ovid.com/crossref?an=00041433-201704000-00002.

256. Lin J, Li H, Yang M, Ren J, Huang Z, Han F, et al. A role of RIP3-mediated macrophage necrosis in atherosclerosis development. Cell Rep. 2013;3:200–10. http://linkinghub.elsevier.com/retrieve/pii/S2211124712004573.
257. Zhe-Wei S, Li-Sha G, Yue-Chun L. The role of necroptosis in cardiovascular disease. Front Pharmacol. 2018;9:721. http://www.ncbi.nlm.nih.gov/pubmed/30034339.
258. Pan J, Han L, Guo J, Wang X, Liu D, Tian J, et al. AIM2 accelerates the atherosclerotic plaque progressions in ApoE−/− mice. Biochem Biophys Res Commun. 2018;498:487–94. http://www.ncbi.nlm.nih.gov/pubmed/29510138.
259. Wu X, Zhang H, Qi W, Zhang Y, Li J, Li Z, et al. Nicotine promotes atherosclerosis via ROS-NLRP3-mediated endothelial cell pyroptosis. Cell Death Dis. 2018;9:171. http://www.ncbi.nlm.nih.gov/pubmed/29416034.
260. Zhaolin Z, Jiaojiao C, Peng W, Yami L, Tingting Z, Jun T, et al. OxLDL induces vascular endothelial cell pyroptosis through miR-125a-5p/TET2 pathway. J Cell Physiol. 2019;234:7475–91. https://onlinelibrary.wiley.com/doi/abs/10.1002/jcp.27509.
261. Jia C, Chen H, Zhang J, Zhou K, Zhuge Y, Niu C, et al. Role of pyroptosis in cardiovascular diseases. Int Immunopharmacol. 2019;67:311–8. http://www.ncbi.nlm.nih.gov/pubmed/30572256.
262. Warnatsch A, Ioannou M, Wang Q, Papayannopoulos V. Neutrophil extracellular traps license macrophages for cytokine production in atherosclerosis. Science. 2015;349:316–20. http://www.ncbi.nlm.nih.gov/pubmed/26185250.
263. Qi H, Yang S, Zhang L. Neutrophil extracellular traps and endothelial dysfunction in atherosclerosis and thrombosis. Front Immunol. 2017;8:928. http://www.ncbi.nlm.nih.gov/pubmed/28824648.
264. Martinet W, Coornaert I, Puylaert P, De Meyer GRY. Macrophage death as a pharmacological target in atherosclerosis. Front Pharmacol. 2019;10:306. http://www.ncbi.nlm.nih.gov/pubmed/31019462.
265. Grootaert MOJ, Roth L, Schrijvers DM, De Meyer GRY, Martinet W. Defective autophagy in atherosclerosis: to die or to senesce? Oxidative Med Cell Longev. 2018;2018:1–12. http://www.ncbi.nlm.nih.gov/pubmed/29682164.
266. Björkbacka H, Fredrikson GN, Nilsson J. Emerging biomarkers and intervention targets for immune-modulation of atherosclerosis—a review of the experimental evidence. Atherosclerosis. 2013;227:9–17. https://linkinghub.elsevier.com/retrieve/pii/S0021915012007873.
267. Lichtman AH, Binder CJ, Tsimikas S, Witztum JL. Adaptive immunity in atherogenesis: new insights and therapeutic approaches. J Clin Invest. 2013;123:27–36. http://www.jci.org/articles/view/63108.
268. Taleb S, Tedgui A, Mallat Z. IL-17 and Th17 cells in atherosclerosis. Arterioscler Thromb Vasc Biol. 2015;35:258–64. http://www.ncbi.nlm.nih.gov/pubmed/25234818.
269. Meng X, Yang J, Dong M, Zhang K, Tu E, Gao Q, et al. Regulatory T cells in cardiovascular diseases. Nat Rev Cardiol. 2016;13:167–79. http://www.ncbi.nlm.nih.gov/pubmed/26525543.
270. Tsiantoulas D, Diehl CJ, Witztum JL, Binder CJ. B cells and humoral immunity in atherosclerosis. Circ Res. 2014;114:1743–56. http://www.ncbi.nlm.nih.gov/pubmed/24855199.
271. Liu R, Leslie KL, Martin KA. Epigenetic regulation of smooth muscle cell plasticity. Biochim Biophys Acta. 1849;2015:448–53. http://www.ncbi.nlm.nih.gov/pubmed/24937434.
272. Bennett MR, Sinha S, Owens GK. Vascular smooth muscle cells in atherosclerosis. Circ Res. 2016;118:692–702. http://www.ncbi.nlm.nih.gov/pubmed/26892967.
273. Baumer Y, McCurdy S, Alcala M, Mehta N, Lee B-H, Ginsberg MH, et al. CD98 regulates vascular smooth muscle cell proliferation in atherosclerosis. Atherosclerosis. 2017;256:105–14. http://www.ncbi.nlm.nih.gov/pubmed/28012647.
274. Low EL, Baker AH, Bradshaw AC. TGFβ, smooth muscle cells and coronary artery disease: a review. Cell Signal. 2019;53:90–101. http://www.ncbi.nlm.nih.gov/pubmed/30227237.
275. Tian L, Chen K, Cao J, Han Z, Gao L, Wang Y, et al. Galectin-3-induced oxidized low-density lipoprotein promotes the phenotypic transformation of vascular smooth muscle cells. Mol Med Rep. 2015;12:4995–5002. https://www.spandidos-publications.com/10.3892/mmr.2015.4075.

276. Sun H-J, Ren X-S, Xiong X-Q, Chen Y-Z, Zhao M-X, Wang J-J, et al. NLRP3 inflammasome activation contributes to VSMC phenotypic transformation and proliferation in hypertension. Cell Death Dis. 2017;8:e3074. http://www.ncbi.nlm.nih.gov/pubmed/28981106.
277. Wang K, Li W, Yu Q, Guo B, Yang B, Zhang C, et al. High mobility group box 1 mediates interferon-γ-induced phenotypic modulation of vascular smooth muscle cells. J Cell Biochem. 2017;118:518–29. http://doi.wiley.com/10.1002/jcb.25682.
278. Lee G-L, Wu J-Y, Tsai C-S, Lin C-Y, Tsai Y-T, Lin C-S, et al. TLR4-activated MAPK-IL-6 axis regulates vascular smooth muscle cell function. Int J Mol Sci. 2016;17:1394. http://www.ncbi.nlm.nih.gov/pubmed/27563891.
279. Touyz RM. Intracellular mechanisms involved in vascular remodelling of resistance arteries in hypertension: role of angiotensin II. Exp Physiol. 2005;90:449–55. http://doi.wiley.com/10.1113/expphysiol.2005.030080.
280. Shirwany NA, Zou M. Arterial stiffness: a brief review. Acta Pharmacol Sin. 2010;31:1267–76. http://www.nature.com/articles/aps2010123.
281. Katsuda S, Kaji T. Atherosclerosis and extracellular matrix. J Atheroscler Thromb. 2003;10:267–74. http://www.ncbi.nlm.nih.gov/pubmed/14718743.
282. Vassiliadis E, Barascuk N, Karsdal MA. Atherofibrosis—a unique and common process of the disease pathogenesis of atherosclerosis and fibrosis—lessons for biomarker development. Am J Transl Res. 2013;5:1–14. http://www.ncbi.nlm.nih.gov/pubmed/23390561.
283. Lan T-H, Huang X-Q, Tan H-M. Vascular fibrosis in atherosclerosis. Cardiovasc Pathol. 2013;22:401–7. https://linkinghub.elsevier.com/retrieve/pii/S1054880713000069.
284. Harvey A, Montezano AC, Lopes RA, Rios F, Touyz RM. Vascular fibrosis in aging and hypertension: molecular mechanisms and clinical implications. Can J Cardiol. 2016;32:659–68. http://www.ncbi.nlm.nih.gov/pubmed/27118293.
285. Shi N, Chen S-Y. Mechanisms simultaneously regulate smooth muscle proliferation and differentiation. J Biomed Res. 2014;28:40–6. http://www.ncbi.nlm.nih.gov/pubmed/24474962.
286. Li F-J, Zhang C-L, Luo X-J, Peng J, Yang T-L. Involvement of the MiR-181b-5p/HMGB1 pathway in Ang II-induced phenotypic transformation of smooth muscle cells in hypertension. Aging Dis. 2019;10:231. http://www.ncbi.nlm.nih.gov/pubmed/31011475.
287. Arteaga-Solis E, Gayraud B, Ramirez F. Elastic and collagenous networks in vascular diseases. Cell Struct Funct. 2000;25:69–72. http://www.ncbi.nlm.nih.gov/pubmed/10885576.
288. Jacob MP. Extracellular matrix remodeling and matrix metalloproteinases in the vascular wall during aging and in pathological conditions. Biomed Pharmacother. 2003;57:195–202. http://www.ncbi.nlm.nih.gov/pubmed/12888254.
289. Arribas SM, Hinek A, González MC. Elastic fibres and vascular structure in hypertension. Pharmacol Ther. 2006;111:771–91. http://www.ncbi.nlm.nih.gov/pubmed/16488477.
290. Hortells L, Sur S, St. Hilaire C. Cell phenotype transitions in cardiovascular calcification. Front Cardiovasc Med. 2018;5:27. http://www.ncbi.nlm.nih.gov/pubmed/29632866.
291. Chellan B, Sutton NR, Hofmann Bowman MA. S100/RAGE-Mediated Inflammation and Modified Cholesterol Lipoproteins as Mediators of Osteoblastic Differentiation of Vascular Smooth Muscle Cells. Frontiers in Cardiovascular Medicine 5. 2018
292. Merched AJ, Ko K, Gotlinger KH, Serhan CN, Chan L. Atherosclerosis: evidence for impairment of resolution of vascular inflammation governed by specific lipid mediators. FASEB J. 2008;22:3595–606. http://www.fasebj.org/doi/10.1096/fj.08-112201.
293. Tabas I. Macrophage death and defective inflammation resolution in atherosclerosis. Nat Rev Immunol. 2010;10:36–46. http://www.ncbi.nlm.nih.gov/pubmed/19960040.
294. Viola J, Soehnlein O. Atherosclerosis—a matter of unresolved inflammation. Semin Immunol. 2015;27:184–93. https://linkinghub.elsevier.com/retrieve/pii/S1044532315000214.
295. Fredman G, Hellmann J, Proto JD, Kuriakose G, Colas RA, Dorweiler B, et al. An imbalance between specialized pro-resolving lipid mediators and pro-inflammatory leukotrienes promotes instability of atherosclerotic plaques. Nat Commun. 2016;7:12859. http://www.nature.com/doifinder/10.1038/ncomms12859.

296. Viola JR, Lemnitzer P, Jansen Y, Csaba G, Winter C, Neideck C, et al. Resolving lipid mediators Maresin 1 and Resolvin D2 prevent Atheroprogression in mice. Circ Res. 2016;119:1030–8. http://circres.ahajournals.org/lookup/doi/10.1161/CIRCRESAHA.116.309492.
297. Kasikara C, Doran AC, Cai B, Tabas I. The role of non-resolving inflammation in atherosclerosis. J Clin Invest. 2018;128:2713–23. http://www.ncbi.nlm.nih.gov/pubmed/30108191.
298. Conte MS, Desai TA, Wu B, Schaller M, Werlin E. Pro-resolving lipid mediators in vascular disease. J Clin Invest. 2018;128:3727–35. http://www.ncbi.nlm.nih.gov/pubmed/30168805.
299. Bäck M, Yurdagul A, Tabas I, Öörni K, Kovanen PT. Inflammation and its resolution in atherosclerosis: mediators and therapeutic opportunities. Nat Rev Cardiol. 2019;16:389–406. http://www.ncbi.nlm.nih.gov/pubmed/30846875.
300. Lai Y-S, Putra RBDS, Aui S-P, Chang K-T. M2 C polarization by Baicalin enhances efferocytosis via upregulation of MERTK receptor. Am J Chin Med. 2018;46:1899–914. http://www.ncbi.nlm.nih.gov/pubmed/30518232.
301. Bi Y, Chen J, Hu F, Liu J, Li M, Zhao L. M2 macrophages as a potential target for anti-atherosclerosis treatment. Neural Plast. 2019;2019:1–21. http://www.ncbi.nlm.nih.gov/pubmed/30923552.
302. Wynn TA, Vannella KM. Macrophages in tissue repair, regeneration, and fibrosis. Immunity. 2016;44:450–62. http://www.ncbi.nlm.nih.gov/pubmed/26982353.
303. Martin K, Ohayon D, Witko-Sarsat V. Promoting apoptosis of neutrophils and phagocytosis by macrophages: novel strategies in the resolution of inflammation. Swiss Med Wkly. 2015;145:w14056. http://www.ncbi.nlm.nih.gov/pubmed/25701669.
304. Robb CT, Regan KH, Dorward DA, Rossi AG. Key mechanisms governing resolution of lung inflammation. Semin Immunopathol. 2016;38:425–48. http://www.ncbi.nlm.nih.gov/pubmed/27116944.
305. Serhan CN, Dalli J, Karamnov S, Choi A, Park C-K, Xu Z-Z, et al. Macrophage proresolving mediator maresin 1 stimulates tissue regeneration and controls pain. FASEB J. 2012;26:1755–65. http://www.fasebj.org/doi/10.1096/fj.11-201442.
306. Serhan CN, Yang R, Martinod K, Kasuga K, Pillai PS, Porter TF, et al. Maresins: novel macrophage mediators with potent antiinflammatory and proresolving actions. J Exp Med. 2009;206:15–23. http://www.jem.org/lookup/doi/10.1084/jem.20081880.
307. Dalli J, Zhu M, Vlasenko NA, Deng B, Haeggström JZ, Petasis NA, et al. The novel 13S,14S-epoxy-maresin is converted by human macrophages to maresin 1 (MaR1), inhibits leukotriene A4 hydrolase (LTA4H), and shifts macrophage phenotype. FASEB J. 2013;27:2573–83. http://www.fasebj.org/doi/10.1096/fj.13-227728.
308. Chiang N, Dalli J, Colas RA, Serhan CN. Identification of resolvin D2 receptor mediating resolution of infections and organ protection. J Exp Med. 2015;212:1203–17. http://www.jem.org/lookup/doi/10.1084/jem.20150225.
309. Serhan CN, Dalli J, Colas RA, Winkler JW, Chiang N. Protectins and maresins: new proresolving families of mediators in acute inflammation and resolution bioactive metabolome. Biochim Biophys Acta. 1851;2015:397–413. http://linkinghub.elsevier.com/retrieve/pii/S1388198114001619.
310. Carson WF, Kunkel SL. Regulation of cellular immune responses in sepsis by histone modifications. Adv Protein Chem Struct Biol. 2017;106:191–225. http://www.ncbi.nlm.nih.gov/pubmed/28057212.
311. Kittan NA, Allen RM, Dhaliwal A, Cavassani KA, Schaller M, Gallagher KA, et al. Cytokine induced phenotypic and epigenetic signatures are key to establishing specific macrophage phenotypes. PLoS One. 2013;8:e78045. http://dx.plos.org/10.1371/journal.pone.0078045.
312. Kroetz DN, Allen RM, Schaller MA, Cavallaro C, Ito T, Kunkel SL. Type I interferon induced epigenetic regulation of macrophages suppresses innate and adaptive immunity in acute respiratory viral infection. PLoS Pathog. 2015;11:e1005338. http://dx.plos.org/10.1371/journal.ppat.1005338.
313. Schliehe C, Flynn EK, Vilagos B, Richson U, Swaminathan S, Bosnjak B, et al. The methyltransferase Setdb2 mediates virus-induced susceptibility to bacterial superinfection. Nat Immunol. 2015;16:67–74. http://www.nature.com/doifinder/10.1038/ni.3046.

314. Kapellos TS, Iqbal AJ. Epigenetic control of macrophage polarisation and soluble mediator gene expression during inflammation. Mediat Inflamm. 2016;2016:1–15. http://www.ncbi.nlm.nih.gov/pubmed/27143818.
315. Novak ML, Thorp EB. Shedding light on impaired efferocytosis and nonresolving inflammation. Circ Res. 2013;113:9–12. http://www.ncbi.nlm.nih.gov/pubmed/23788501.
316. Fredman G, Li Y, Dalli J, Chiang N, Serhan CN. Self-limited versus delayed resolution of acute inflammation: temporal regulation of pro-resolving mediators and microRNA. Sci Rep. 2012;2:639. http://www.nature.com/articles/srep00639.
317. Cheuk BLY, Cheng SWK. Annexin A1 expression in atherosclerotic carotid plaques and its relationship with plaque characteristics. Eur J Vasc Endovasc Surg. 2011;41:364–71. http://linkinghub.elsevier.com/retrieve/pii/S1078588410007094.
318. Zhang Y-H, Zhang Y, Dong X-F, Hao Q-Q, Zhou X-M, Yu Q-T, et al. ACE2 and Ang-(1–7) protect endothelial cell function and prevent early atherosclerosis by inhibiting inflammatory response. Inflamm Res. Birkhauser Verlag AG; 2015;64:253–60. http://link.springer.com/10.1007/s00011-015-0805-1
319. Kutryb-Zajac B, Bulinska A, Zabielska MA, Mierzejewska P, Slominska EM, Smolenski RT. Vascular extracellular adenosine metabolism in mice correlates with susceptibility to atherosclerosis. Nucleosides Nucleotides Nucleic Acids. 2018;37:653–62. http://www.ncbi.nlm.nih.gov/pubmed/30587087.
320. Gerlach BD, Marinello M, Heinz J, Rymut N, Sansbury BE, Riley CO, et al. Resolvin D1 promotes the targeting and clearance of necroptotic cells. Cell Death Differ. 2019. http://www.nature.com/articles/s41418-019-0370-1.
321. Tavares N, Afonso L, Suarez M, Ampuero M, Prates DB, Araújo-Santos T, et al. Degranulating neutrophils promote leukotriene B 4 production by infected macrophages to kill Leishmania amazonensis parasites. J Immunol. 2016;196:1865–73. http://www.ncbi.nlm.nih.gov/pubmed/26800873.
322. Lai X-F, Qin H-D, Guo L-L, Luo Z-G, Chang J, Qin C-C. Hypercholesterolemia increases the production of leukotriene B4 in neutrophils by enhancing the nuclear localization of 5-lipoxygenase. Cell Physiol Biochem. 2014;34:1723–32. http://www.ncbi.nlm.nih.gov/pubmed/25428728.
323. Brandt SL, Klopfenstein N, Wang S, Winfree S, McCarthy BP, Territo PR, et al. Macrophage-derived LTB4 promotes abscess formation and clearance of *Staphylococcus aureus* skin infection in mice. PLoS Pathog. 2018;14:e1007244. http://www.ncbi.nlm.nih.gov/pubmed/30102746.
324. Yokomizo T, Kato K, Terawaki K, Izumi T, Shimizu T. A second leukotriene B(4) receptor, BLT2. A new therapeutic target in inflammation and immunological disorders. J Exp Med. 2000;192:421–32. http://www.ncbi.nlm.nih.gov/pubmed/10934230.
325. Laguna-Fernandez A, Checa A, Carracedo M, Artiach G, Petri MH, Baumgartner R, et al. ERV1/ChemR23 signaling protects against atherosclerosis by modifying oxidized low-density lipoprotein uptake and phagocytosis in macrophages. Circulation. 2018;138:1693–705. https://www.ahajournals.org/doi/10.1161/CIRCULATIONAHA.117.032801.
326. Green DR, Oguin TH, Martinez J. The clearance of dying cells: table for two. Cell Death Differ. 2016;23:915–26. http://www.nature.com/articles/cdd2015172.
327. Elliott MR, Koster KM, Murphy PS. Efferocytosis signaling in the regulation of macrophage inflammatory responses. J Immunol. 2017;198:1387–94. http://www.ncbi.nlm.nih.gov/pubmed/28167649.
328. Greenlee-Wacker MC. Clearance of apoptotic neutrophils and resolution of inflammation. Immunol Rev. 2016;273:357–70. http://www.ncbi.nlm.nih.gov/pubmed/27558346.
329. Linton MF, Babaev VR, Huang J, Linton EF, Tao H, Yancey PG. Macrophage apoptosis and efferocytosis in the pathogenesis of atherosclerosis. Circ J. 2016;80:2259–68. http://www.ncbi.nlm.nih.gov/pubmed/27725526.
330. Kojima Y, Downing K, Kundu R, Miller C, Dewey F, Lancero H, et al. Cyclin-dependent kinase inhibitor 2B regulates efferocytosis and atherosclerosis. J Clin Invest. 2014;124:1083–97. http://www.ncbi.nlm.nih.gov/pubmed/24531546.

331. Chiurchiù V, Leuti A, Dalli J, Jacobsson A, Battistini L, Maccarrone M, et al. Proresolving lipid mediators resolvin D1, resolvin D2, and maresin 1 are critical in modulating T cell responses. Sci Transl Med. 2016;8:353ra111. http://stm.sciencemag.org/lookup/doi/10.1126/scitranslmed.aaf7483.
332. Krishnamoorthy N, Burkett PR, Dalli J, Abdulnour R-EE, Colas R, Ramon S, et al. Cutting edge: maresin-1 engages regulatory T cells to limit type 2 innate lymphoid cell activation and promote resolution of lung inflammation. J Immunol. 2015;194:863–7. http://www.jimmunol.org/lookup/doi/10.4049/jimmunol.1402534.
333. Muka T, Koromani F, Portilla E, O'Connor A, Bramer WM, Troup J, et al. The role of epigenetic modifications in cardiovascular disease: a systematic review. Int J Cardiol. 2016;212:174–83. http://www.ncbi.nlm.nih.gov/pubmed/27038728.
334. Leentjens J, Bekkering S, Joosten LAB, Netea MG, Burgner DP, Riksen NP. Trained innate immunity as a novel mechanism linking infection and the development of atherosclerosis. Circ Res. 2018;122:664–9. http://www.ncbi.nlm.nih.gov/pubmed/29367213.
335. Lacy M, Atzler D, Liu R, de Winther M, Weber C, Lutgens E. Interactions between dyslipidemia and the immune system and their relevance as putative therapeutic targets in atherosclerosis. Pharmacol Ther. 2019;193:50–62. http://www.ncbi.nlm.nih.gov/pubmed/30149100.
336. Riksen NP, Stienstra R. Metabolism of innate immune cells. Curr Opin Lipidol. 2018;29:1. http://www.ncbi.nlm.nih.gov/pubmed/30020200.
337. Dominguez-Andres J, Netea MG. Long-term reprogramming of the innate immune system. J Leukoc Biol. 2019;105:329–38. http://www.ncbi.nlm.nih.gov/pubmed/29999546.
338. Norata GD. Trained immunity and cardiovascular disease: is it time for translation to humans? Cardiovasc Res. 2018;114:e41–2. http://www.ncbi.nlm.nih.gov/pubmed/29897493.
339. Pirillo A, Bonacina F, Norata GD, Catapano AL. The interplay of lipids, lipoproteins, and immunity in atherosclerosis. Curr Atheroscler Rep. 2018;20:12. http://www.ncbi.nlm.nih.gov/pubmed/29445885.
340. Christ A, Bekkering S, Latz E, Riksen NP. Long-term activation of the innate immune system in atherosclerosis. Semin Immunol. 2016;28:384–93. https://linkinghub.elsevier.com/retrieve/pii/S1044532316300185.
341. Riksen NP, Netea MG. Be aware, innate immune cells remember. Aging (Albany NY). 2018;10:2218–9. http://www.ncbi.nlm.nih.gov/pubmed/30215600.
342. van der Heijden CDCC, Noz MP, Joosten LAB, Netea MG, Riksen NP, Keating ST. Epigenetics and trained immunity. Antioxid Redox Signal. 2018;29:1023–40. http://www.ncbi.nlm.nih.gov/pubmed/28978221.
343. Bekkering S, Quintin J, Joosten LAB, van der Meer JWM, Netea MG, Riksen NP. Oxidized low-density lipoprotein induces long-term proinflammatory cytokine production and foam cell formation via epigenetic reprogramming of monocytes. Arterioscler Thromb Vasc Biol. 2014;34:1731–8. http://atvb.ahajournals.org/cgi/doi/10.1161/ATVBAHA.114.303887.
344. van der Valk FM, Bekkering S, Kroon J, Yeang C, Van den Bossche J, van Buul JD, et al. Oxidized phospholipids on lipoprotein(a) elicit arterial wall inflammation and an inflammatory monocyte response in humans. Circulation. 2016;134:611–24. https://www.ahajournals.org/doi/10.1161/CIRCULATIONAHA.116.020838.
345. Bekkering S, van den Munckhof I, Nielen T, Lamfers E, Dinarello C, Rutten J, et al. Innate immune cell activation and epigenetic remodeling in symptomatic and asymptomatic atherosclerosis in humans in vivo. Atherosclerosis. 2016;254:228–36. https://linkinghub.elsevier.com/retrieve/pii/S0021915016314228.
346. Groh L, Keating ST, Joosten LAB, Netea MG, Riksen NP. Monocyte and macrophage immunometabolism in atherosclerosis. Semin Immunopathol. 2018;40:203–14. http://www.ncbi.nlm.nih.gov/pubmed/28971272.
347. Stienstra R, Netea-Maier RT, Riksen NP, Joosten LAB, Netea MG. Specific and complex reprogramming of cellular metabolism in myeloid cells during innate immune responses. Cell Metab. 2017;26:142–56. http://www.ncbi.nlm.nih.gov/pubmed/28683282.

348. Bekkering S, Arts RJW, Novakovic B, Kourtzelis I, van der Heijden CDCC, Li Y, et al. Metabolic induction of trained immunity through the mevalonate pathway. Cell. 2018;172:135–146.e9. https://linkinghub.elsevier.com/retrieve/pii/S0092867417313727.
349. Serbulea V, Upchurch CM, Ahern KW, Bories G, Voigt P, DeWeese DE, et al. Macrophages sensing oxidized DAMPs reprogram their metabolism to support redox homeostasis and inflammation through a TLR2-Syk-ceramide dependent mechanism. Mol Metab. 2018;7:23–34. https://linkinghub.elsevier.com/retrieve/pii/S2212877817307846.
350. Mitroulis I, Ruppova K, Wang B, Chen L-S, Grzybek M, Grinenko T, et al. Modulation of myelopoiesis progenitors is an integral component of trained immunity. Cell. 2018;172:147–161.e12. http://www.ncbi.nlm.nih.gov/pubmed/29328910.
351. Samson S, Mundkur L, Kakkar VV. Immune response to lipoproteins in atherosclerosis. Cholesterol. 2012;2012:1–12. http://www.ncbi.nlm.nih.gov/pubmed/22957222.
352. Bartolini Gritti B, Binder C. Oxidation-specific epitopes are major targets of innate immunity in atherothrombosis. Hamostaseologie. 2016;36:89–96. http://www.ncbi.nlm.nih.gov/pubmed/25682990.
353. Papac-Milicevic N, Busch CJ-L, Binder CJ. Malondialdehyde epitopes as targets of immunity and the implications for atherosclerosis. Adv Immunol. 2016;131:1–59. http://www.ncbi.nlm.nih.gov/pubmed/27235680.
354. Bergmark C, Dewan A, Orsoni A, Merki E, Miller ER, Shin M-J, et al. A novel function of lipoprotein [a] as a preferential carrier of oxidized phospholipids in human plasma. J Lipid Res. 2008;49:2230–9. http://www.jlr.org/lookup/doi/10.1194/jlr.M800174-JLR200.
355. Boisvert WA, Santiago R, Curtiss LK, Terkeltaub RA. A leukocyte homologue of the IL-8 receptor CXCR-2 mediates the accumulation of macrophages in atherosclerotic lesions of LDL receptor-deficient mice. J Clin Invest. 1998;101:353–63. http://www.jci.org/articles/view/1195.
356. Miller YI, Choi S-H, Wiesner P, Fang L, Harkewicz R, Hartvigsen K, et al. Oxidation-specific epitopes are danger-associated molecular patterns recognized by pattern recognition receptors of innate immunity. Circ Res. 2011;108:235–48. http://www.ncbi.nlm.nih.gov/pubmed/21252151.
357. Zimmer S, Grebe A, Latz E. Danger signaling in atherosclerosis. Circ Res. 2015;116:323–40. https://www.ahajournals.org/doi/10.1161/CIRCRESAHA.116.301135.
358. Viola M, Karousou E, D'Angelo ML, Moretto P, Caon I, De Luca G, et al. Extracellular matrix in atherosclerosis: hyaluronan and proteoglycans insights. Curr Med Chem. 2016;23:2958–71. http://www.ncbi.nlm.nih.gov/pubmed/27281127.
359. Kohno T, Anzai T, Kaneko H, Sugano Y, Shimizu H, Shimoda M, et al. High-mobility group box 1 protein blockade suppresses development of abdominal aortic aneurysm. J Cardiol. 2012;59:299–306. http://www.ncbi.nlm.nih.gov/pubmed/22365948.
360. Kar S, Subbaram S, Carrico PM, Melendez JA. Redox-control of matrix metalloproteinase-1: a critical link between free radicals, matrix remodeling and degenerative disease. Respir Physiol Neurobiol. 2010;174:299–306. http://linkinghub.elsevier.com/retrieve/pii/S156990481000323X.
361. Apte SS, Parks WC. Metalloproteinases: a parade of functions in matrix biology and an outlook for the future. Matrix Biol. 2015;44–46:1–6. http://www.ncbi.nlm.nih.gov/pubmed/25916966.
362. Viola M, Bartolini B, Vigetti D, Karousou E, Moretto P, Deleonibus S, et al. Oxidized low density lipoprotein (LDL) affects hyaluronan synthesis in human aortic smooth muscle cells. J Biol Chem. 2013;288:29595–603. http://www.jbc.org/lookup/doi/10.1074/jbc.M113.508341.
363. Fischer JW. Role of hyaluronan in atherosclerosis: current knowledge and open questions. Matrix Biol. 2019;78–79:324–36. https://linkinghub.elsevier.com/retrieve/pii/S0945053X17304675.
364. Wight TN. A role for extracellular matrix in atherosclerotic plaque erosion. J Am Coll Cardiol. 2018;72:1504–5. http://www.ncbi.nlm.nih.gov/pubmed/30236313.

365. Schaff M, Receveur N, Bourdon C, Wurtz V, Denis CV, Orend G, et al. Novel function of tenascin-C, a matrix protein relevant to atherosclerosis, in platelet recruitment and activation under flow. Arterioscler Thromb Vasc Biol. 2011;31:117–24. https://www.ahajournals.org/doi/10.1161/ATVBAHA.110.206375.
366. Wallner K, Li C, Shah PK, Fishbein MC, Forrester JS, Kaul S, et al. Tenascin-C is expressed in macrophage-rich human coronary atherosclerotic plaque. Circulation. 1999;99:1284–9. http://www.ncbi.nlm.nih.gov/pubmed/10077510.
367. Tan MH, Sun Z, Opitz SL, Schmidt TE, Peters JH, George EL. Deletion of the alternatively spliced fibronectin EIIIA domain in mice reduces atherosclerosis. Blood. 2004;104:11–8. http://www.bloodjournal.org/cgi/doi/10.1182/blood-2003-09-3363.
368. Sorescu D, Weiss D, Lassègue B, Clempus RE, Szöcs K, Sorescu GP, et al. Superoxide production and expression of nox family proteins in human atherosclerosis. Circulation. 2002;105:1429–35. http://www.ncbi.nlm.nih.gov/pubmed/11914250.
369. Manea A, Simionescu M. Nox enzymes and oxidative stress in atherosclerosis. Front Biosci (Schol Ed). 2012;4:651–70. http://www.ncbi.nlm.nih.gov/pubmed/22202083.
370. Cominacini L, Garbin U, Mozzini C, Stranieri C, Pasini A, Solani E, et al. The atherosclerotic plaque vulnerability: focus on the oxidative and endoplasmic reticulum stress in orchestrating the macrophage apoptosis in the formation of the necrotic core. Curr Med Chem. 2015;22:1565–72. http://www.ncbi.nlm.nih.gov/pubmed/25760090.
371. Myoishi M, Hao H, Minamino T, Watanabe K, Nishihira K, Hatakeyama K, et al. Increased endoplasmic reticulum stress in atherosclerotic plaques associated with acute coronary syndrome. Circulation. 2007;116:1226–33. http://circ.ahajournals.org/cgi/doi/10.1161/CIRCULATIONAHA.106.682054.
372. Ying R, Li S-W, Chen J-Y, Zhang H-F, Yang Y, Gu Z-J, et al. Endoplasmic reticulum stress in perivascular adipose tissue promotes destabilization of atherosclerotic plaque by regulating GM-CSF paracrine. J Transl Med. 2018;16:105. http://www.ncbi.nlm.nih.gov/pubmed/29669585.
373. Sun Y, Zhang D, Liu X, Li X, Liu F, Yu Y, et al. Endoplasmic reticulum stress affects lipid metabolism in atherosclerosis via CHOP activation and over-expression of miR-33. Cell Physiol Biochem. 2018;48:1995–2010. http://www.ncbi.nlm.nih.gov/pubmed/30092598.
374. Cervelli T, Borghini A, Galli A, Andreassi MG. DNA damage and repair in atherosclerosis: current insights and future perspectives. Int J Mol Sci. 2012;13:16929–44. http://www.mdpi.com/1422-0067/13/12/16929.
375. Shah NR, Mahmoudi M. The role of DNA damage and repair in atherosclerosis: a review. J Mol Cell Cardiol. 2015;86:147–57. http://www.ncbi.nlm.nih.gov/pubmed/26211712.
376. Gray K, Kumar S, Figg N, Harrison J, Baker L, Mercer J, et al. Effects of DNA damage in smooth muscle cells in atherosclerosis. Circ Res. 2015;116:816–26. http://www.ncbi.nlm.nih.gov/pubmed/25524056.
377. Lilledahl MB, Gustafsson H, Ellingsen PG, Zachrisson H, Hallbeck M, Hagen VS, et al. Combined imaging of oxidative stress and microscopic structure reveals new features in human atherosclerotic plaques. J Biomed Opt. 2015;20:020503. http://www.ncbi.nlm.nih.gov/pubmed/25714991.
378. Yang X, Li Y, Li Y, Ren X, Zhang X, Hu D, et al. Oxidative stress-mediated atherosclerosis: mechanisms and therapies. Front Physiol. 2017;8:600. http://www.ncbi.nlm.nih.gov/pubmed/28878685.
379. Bekkering S, Blok BA, Joosten LAB, Riksen NP, van Crevel R, Netea MG. In vitro experimental model of trained innate immunity in human primary monocytes. Clin Vaccine Immunol. 2016;23:926–33. http://cvi.asm.org/lookup/doi/10.1128/CVI.00349-16.
380. Ellulu MS, Patimah I, Khaza'ai H, Rahmat A, Abed Y, Ali F. Atherosclerotic cardiovascular disease: a review of initiators and protective factors. Inflammopharmacology. 2016;24:1–10. http://www.ncbi.nlm.nih.gov/pubmed/26750181.
381. Yang WS, Stockwell BR. Ferroptosis: death by lipid peroxidation. Trends Cell Biol. 2016;26:165–76. http://www.ncbi.nlm.nih.gov/pubmed/26653790.

382. Liao X, Sluimer JC, Wang Y, Subramanian M, Brown K, Pattison JS, et al. Macrophage autophagy plays a protective role in advanced atherosclerosis. Cell Metab. 2012;15:545–53. http://linkinghub.elsevier.com/retrieve/pii/S1550413112000629.
383. Zhou AX, Tabas I. The UPR in atherosclerosis. Semin Immunopathol. 2013;35:321–32. http://link.springer.com/10.1007/s00281-013-0372-x.
384. Menu P, Mayor A, Zhou R, Tardivel A, Ichijo H, Mori K, et al. ER stress activates the NLRP3 inflammasome via an UPR-independent pathway. Cell Death Dis. 2012;3:e261. http://www.nature.com/articles/cddis2011132.
385. Hong J, Kim K, Kim J-H, Park Y. The role of endoplasmic reticulum stress in cardiovascular disease and exercise. Int J Vasc Med. 2017;2017:1–9. http://www.ncbi.nlm.nih.gov/pubmed/28875043.
386. Ishida T, Ishida M, Tashiro S, Yoshizumi M, Kihara Y. Role of DNA damage in cardiovascular disease. Circ J. 2014;78:42–50. http://www.ncbi.nlm.nih.gov/pubmed/24334614.
387. Shah A, Gray K, Figg N, Finigan A, Starks L, Bennett M. Defective base excision repair of oxidative DNA damage in vascular smooth muscle cells promotes atherosclerosis. Circulation. 2018;138:1446–62. http://www.ncbi.nlm.nih.gov/pubmed/29643057.
388. Sachet M, Liang YY, Oehler R. The immune response to secondary necrotic cells. Apoptosis. 2017;22:1189–204. http://www.ncbi.nlm.nih.gov/pubmed/28861714.
389. Ren X-S, Tong Y, Ling L, Chen D, Sun H-J, Zhou H, et al. NLRP3 gene deletion attenuates angiotensin II-induced phenotypic transformation of vascular smooth muscle cells and vascular remodeling. Cell Physiol Biochem. 2017;44:2269–80. http://www.ncbi.nlm.nih.gov/pubmed/29262411.
390. Kim EJ, Park SY, Baek SE, Jang MA, Lee WS, Bae SS, et al. HMGB1 increases IL-1β production in vascular smooth muscle cells via NLRP3 inflammasome. Front Physiol. 2018;9:313. http://www.ncbi.nlm.nih.gov/pubmed/29643819.
391. Ding Z, Liu S, Wang X, Dai Y, Khaidakov M, Deng X, et al. LOX-1, mtDNA damage, and NLRP3 inflammasome activation in macrophages: implications in atherogenesis. Cardiovasc Res. 2014;103:619–28. https://academic.oup.com/cardiovascres/article-lookup/doi/10.1093/cvr/cvu114.
392. Zhou W, Chen C, Chen Z, Liu L, Jiang J, Wu Z, et al. NLRP3: a novel mediator in cardiovascular disease. J Immunol Res. 2018;2018:1–8. http://www.ncbi.nlm.nih.gov/pubmed/29850631.
393. Grebe A, Hoss F, Latz E. NLRP3 inflammasome and the IL-1 pathway in atherosclerosis. Circ Res. 2018;122:1722–40. http://www.ncbi.nlm.nih.gov/pubmed/29880500.
394. Hoseini Z, Sepahvand F, Rashidi B, Sahebkar A, Masoudifar A, Mirzaei H. NLRP3 inflammasome: its regulation and involvement in atherosclerosis. J Cell Physiol. 2018;233:2116–32. http://doi.wiley.com/10.1002/jcp.25930.
395. Rhoads JP, Lukens JR, Wilhelm AJ, Moore JL, Mendez-Fernandez Y, Kanneganti T-D, et al. Oxidized low-density lipoprotein immune complex priming of the Nlrp3 inflammasome involves TLR and FcγR cooperation and is dependent on CARD9. J Immunol. 2017;198:2105–14. http://www.jimmunol.org/lookup/doi/10.4049/jimmunol.1601563.
396. Ridker PM, Everett BM, Thuren T, MacFadyen JG, Chang WH, Ballantyne C, et al. Antiinflammatory therapy with canakinumab for atherosclerotic disease. N Engl J Med. 2017;377:1119–31. http://www.nejm.org/doi/10.1056/NEJMoa1707914.
397. Weismann D, Binder CJ. The innate immune response to products of phospholipid peroxidation. Biochim Biophys Acta. 1818;2012:2465–75. http://www.ncbi.nlm.nih.gov/pubmed/22305963.
398. de Souza AWS, Westra J, Limburg PC, Bijl M, Kallenberg CGM. HMGB1 in vascular diseases: its role in vascular inflammation and atherosclerosis. Autoimmun Rev. 2012;11:909–17. http://linkinghub.elsevier.com/retrieve/pii/S1568997212000766.
399. Schiopu A, Cotoi OS. S100A8 and S100A9: DAMPs at the crossroads between innate immunity, traditional risk factors, and cardiovascular disease. Mediat Inflamm. 2013;2013:828354. http://www.hindawi.com/journals/mi/2013/828354/.

400. Fan Z, Yang J, Yang J, Yang C, Guo X. HMGB1: a promising therapeutic approach for atherosclerosis. Int J Cardiol. 2016;202:507–8. http://www.ncbi.nlm.nih.gov/pubmed/26440462.
401. Boteanu RM, Suica VI, Uyy E, Ivan L, Dima SO, Popescu I, et al. Alarmins in chronic non-communicable diseases: atherosclerosis, diabetes and cancer. J Proteome. 2017;153:21–9. https://linkinghub.elsevier.com/retrieve/pii/S1874391916304730.
402. Wu H, Li R, Pei L-G, Wei Z-H, Kang L-N, Wang L, et al. Emerging role of high mobility group box-1 in thrombosis-related diseases. Cell Physiol Biochem. 2018;47:1319–37. http://www.ncbi.nlm.nih.gov/pubmed/29940562.
403. Soro-Paavonen A, Watson AMD, Li J, Paavonen K, Koitka A, Calkin AC, et al. Receptor for advanced glycation end products (RAGE) deficiency attenuates the development of atherosclerosis in diabetes. Diabetes. 2008;57:2461–9. http://diabetes.diabetesjournals.org/cgi/doi/10.2337/db07-1808.
404. Kanellakis P, Agrotis A, Kyaw TS, Koulis C, Ahrens I, Mori S, et al. High-mobility group box protein 1 neutralization reduces development of diet-induced atherosclerosis in apolipoprotein e-deficient mice. Arterioscler Thromb Vasc Biol. 2011;31:313–9. https://www.ahajournals.org/doi/10.1161/ATVBAHA.110.218669.
405. Inoue K, Kawahara K, Biswas KK, Ando K, Mitsudo K, Nobuyoshi M, et al. HMGB1 expression by activated vascular smooth muscle cells in advanced human atherosclerosis plaques. Cardiovasc Pathol. 2007;16:136–43. http://linkinghub.elsevier.com/retrieve/pii/S1054880706001931.
406. Filipek A, Czerwińska ME, Kiss AK, Polański JA, Naruszewicz M. Oleacein may inhibit destabilization of carotid plaques from hypertensive patients. Impact on high mobility group protein-1. Phytomedicine. 2017;32:68–73. http://www.ncbi.nlm.nih.gov/pubmed/28732809.
407. Yang J, Chen L, Yang J, Ding J, Rong H, Dong W, et al. High mobility group box-1 induces migration of vascular smooth muscle cells via TLR4-dependent PI3K/Akt pathway activation. Mol Biol Rep. 2012;39:3361–7. http://link.springer.com/10.1007/s11033-011-1106-6.
408. Su Z, Lu H, Jiang H, Zhu H, Li Z, Zhang P, et al. IFN-γ-producing Th17 cells bias by HMGB1-T-bet/RUNX3 axis might contribute to progression of coronary artery atherosclerosis. Atherosclerosis. 2015;243:421–8. https://linkinghub.elsevier.com/retrieve/pii/S0021915015301441.
409. Ahrens I, Chen Y-C, Topcic D, Bode M, Haenel D, Hagemeyer CE, et al. HMGB1 binds to activated platelets via the receptor for advanced glycation end products and is present in platelet rich human coronary artery thrombi. Thromb Haemost. 2015;114:994–1003. http://www.thieme-connect.de/DOI/DOI?10.1160/TH14-12-1073.
410. Yamashita A, Nishihira K, Matsuura Y, Ito T, Kawahara K, Hatakeyama K, et al. Paucity of CD34-positive cells and increased expression of high-mobility group box 1 in coronary thrombus with type 2 diabetes mellitus. Atherosclerosis. 2012;224:511–4. https://linkinghub.elsevier.com/retrieve/pii/S0021915012004996.
411. Geczy CL, Chung YM, Hiroshima Y. Calgranulins may contribute vascular protection in atherogenesis. Circ J. 2014;78:271–80. http://www.ncbi.nlm.nih.gov/pubmed/24389598.
412. Oesterle A, Bowman MAH. S100A12 and the S100/calgranulins: emerging biomarkers for atherosclerosis and possibly therapeutic targets. Arterioscler Thromb Vasc Biol. 2015;35:2496–507. http://atvb.ahajournals.org/lookup/doi/10.1161/ATVBAHA.115.302072.
413. Nazari A, Khorramdelazad H, Hassanshahi G, Day AS, Sardoo AM, Fard ET, et al. S100A12 in renal and cardiovascular diseases. Life Sci. 2017;191:253–8. http://www.ncbi.nlm.nih.gov/pubmed/29080693.
414. Farokhzadian J, Mangolian Shahrbabaki P, Bagheri V. S100A12-CD36 axis: a novel player in the pathogenesis of atherosclerosis? Cytokine. 2019;122:154104. https://linkinghub.elsevier.com/retrieve/pii/S1043466617302119.
415. Eue I, Langer C, Eckardstein A, Sorg C. Myeloid related protein (MRP) 14 expressing monocytes infiltrate atherosclerotic lesions of ApoE null mice. Atherosclerosis. 2000;151:593–7. http://www.ncbi.nlm.nih.gov/pubmed/10944082.
416. Hofmann Bowman MA, Gawdzik J, Bukhari U, Husain AN, Toth PT, Kim G, et al. S100A12 in vascular smooth muscle accelerates vascular calcification in apolipoprotein

E-null mice by activating an osteogenic gene regulatory program. Arterioscler Thromb Vasc Biol. 2011;31:337–44. https://www.ahajournals.org/doi/10.1161/ATVBAHA.110.217745.
417. Virmani R, Kolodgie FD, Burke AP, Farb A, Schwartz SM. Lessons from sudden coronary death: a comprehensive morphological classification scheme for atherosclerotic lesions. Arterioscler Thromb Vasc Biol. 2000;20:1262–75. http://www.ncbi.nlm.nih.gov/pubmed/10807742.
418. Schelbergen RFP, Blom AB, van den Bosch MHJ, Slöetjes A, Abdollahi-Roodsaz S, Schreurs BW, et al. Alarmins S100A8 and S100A9 elicit a catabolic effect in human osteoarthritic chondrocytes that is dependent on Toll-like receptor 4. Arthritis Rheum. 2012;64:1477–87. http://doi.wiley.com/10.1002/art.33495.
419. Moz S, Basso D, Padoan A, Bozzato D, Fogar P, Zambon C-F, et al. Blood expression of matrix metalloproteinases 8 and 9 and of their inducers S100A8 and S100A9 supports diagnosis and prognosis of PDAC-associated diabetes mellitus. Clin Chim Acta. 2016;456:24–30. https://linkinghub.elsevier.com/retrieve/pii/S0009898116300638.
420. Burke AP, Kolodgie FD, Zieske A, Fowler DR, Weber DK, Varghese PJ, et al. Morphologic findings of coronary atherosclerotic plaques in diabetics: a postmortem study. Arterioscler Thromb Vasc Biol. 2004;24:1266–71. https://www.ahajournals.org/doi/10.1161/01.ATV.0000131783.74034.97.
421. McCormick MM, Rahimi F, Bobryshev YV, Gaus K, Zreiqat H, Cai H, et al. S100A8 and S100A9 in human arterial wall. Implications for atherogenesis. J Biol Chem. 2005;280:41521–9. http://www.jbc.org/lookup/doi/10.1074/jbc.M509442200.
422. Ionita MG, Vink A, Dijke IE, Laman JD, Peeters W, van der Kraak PH, et al. High levels of myeloid-related protein 14 in human atherosclerotic plaques correlate with the characteristics of rupture-prone lesions. Arterioscler Thromb Vasc Biol. 2009;29:1220–7. https://www.ahajournals.org/doi/10.1161/ATVBAHA.109.190314.
423. Averill MM, Kerkhoff C, Bornfeldt KE. S100A8 and S100A9 in cardiovascular biology and disease. Arterioscler Thromb Vasc Biol. 2012;32:223–9. https://www.ahajournals.org/doi/10.1161/ATVBAHA.111.236927.
424. Abbas A, Aukrust P, Dahl TB, Bjerkeli V, Sagen EBL, Michelsen A, et al. High levels of S100A12 are associated with recent plaque symptomatology in patients with carotid atherosclerosis. Stroke. 2012;43:1347–53. http://www.ncbi.nlm.nih.gov/pubmed/22382154.
425. Zhao P, Wu M, Yu H, Huang Y, Wang Y, Wang W, et al. Serum S100A12 levels are correlated with the presence and severity of coronary artery disease in patients with type 2 diabetes mellitus. J Investig Med. 2013;61:861–6. http://www.ncbi.nlm.nih.gov/pubmed/23609464.
426. Lood C, Tydén H, Gullstrand B, Jönsen A, Källberg E, Mörgelin M, et al. Platelet-derived S100A8/A9 and cardiovascular disease in systemic lupus erythematosus. Arthritis Rheumatol. 2016;68:1970–80. http://doi.wiley.com/10.1002/art.39656.
427. Chellan B, Sutton NR, Hofmann Bowman MA. S100/RAGE-mediated inflammation and modified cholesterol lipoproteins as mediators of osteoblastic differentiation of vascular smooth muscle cells. Front Cardiovasc Med. 2018;5:163. https://www.frontiersin.org/article/10.3389/fcvm.2018.00163/full.
428. Giuliano JS, Lahni PM, Wong HR, Wheeler DS. Pediatric sepsis—Part V: Extracellular heat shock proteins: alarmins for the host immune system. Open Inflamm J. 2011;4:49–60. http://benthamopen.com/ABSTRACT/TOINFJ-4-49.
429. Deniset JF, Pierce GN. Heat shock proteins: mediators of atherosclerotic development. Curr Drug Targets. 2015;16:816–26. http://www.ncbi.nlm.nih.gov/pubmed/25882217.
430. Khandia R, Munjal AK, Iqbal HMN, Dhama K. Heat shock proteins: therapeutic perspectives in inflammatory disorders. Recent Patents Inflamm Allergy Drug Discov. 2017;10:94–104. http://www.eurekaselect.com/openurl/content.php?genre=article&issn=1872-213X&volume=10&issue=2&spage=94.
431. Kol A, Lichtman AH, Finberg RW, Libby P, Kurt-Jones EA. Cutting edge: heat shock protein (HSP) 60 activates the innate immune response: CD14 is an essential receptor for HSP60 activation of mononuclear cells. J Immunol. 2000;164:13–7. http://www.ncbi.nlm.nih.gov/pubmed/10604986.

432. Zhao Y, Zhang C, Wei X, Li P, Cui Y, Qin Y, et al. Heat shock protein 60 stimulates the migration of vascular smooth muscle cells via Toll-like receptor 4 and ERK MAPK activation. Sci Rep. 2015;5:15352. http://www.ncbi.nlm.nih.gov/pubmed/26477505.
433. Shamaei-Tousi A, Halcox JP, Henderson B. Stressing the obvious? Cell stress and cell stress proteins in cardiovascular disease. Cardiovasc Res. 2007;74:19–28. https://academic.oup.com/cardiovascres/article-lookup/doi/10.1016/j.cardiores.2006.10.025.
434. Lewthwaite J, Owen N, Coates A, Henderson B, Steptoe A. Circulating human heat shock protein 60 in the plasma of British civil servants: relationship to physiological and psychosocial stress. Circulation. 2002;106:196–201. http://www.ncbi.nlm.nih.gov/pubmed/12105158.
435. Fatkhullina AR, Peshkova IO, Koltsova EK. The role of cytokines in the development of atherosclerosis. Biochemist. 2016;81:1358–70. http://www.ncbi.nlm.nih.gov/pubmed/27914461.
436. Moss JW, Ramji DP. Cytokines: roles in atherosclerosis disease progression and potential therapeutic targets. Future Med Chem. 2016;8:1317–30. http://www.ncbi.nlm.nih.gov/pubmed/27357616.
437. Niessner A, Shin MS, Pryshchep O, Goronzy JJ, Chaikof EL, Weyand CM. Synergistic proinflammatory effects of the antiviral cytokine interferon-alpha and Toll-like receptor 4 ligands in the atherosclerotic plaque. Circulation. 2007;116:2043–52. https://www.ahajournals.org/doi/10.1161/CIRCULATIONAHA.107.697789.
438. Gil-Pulido J, Zernecke A. Antigen-presenting dendritic cells in atherosclerosis. Eur J Pharmacol. 2017;816:25–31. http://www.ncbi.nlm.nih.gov/pubmed/28822856.
439. Stemme S, Faber B, Holm J, Wiklund O, Witztum JL, Hansson GK. T lymphocytes from human atherosclerotic plaques recognize oxidized low density lipoprotein. Proc Natl Acad Sci U S A. 1995;92:3893–7. http://www.ncbi.nlm.nih.gov/pubmed/7732003.
440. Nickel T, Schmauss D, Hanssen H, Sicic Z, Krebs B, Jankl S, et al. oxLDL uptake by dendritic cells induces upregulation of scavenger-receptors, maturation and differentiation. Atherosclerosis. 2009;205:442–50. http://www.ncbi.nlm.nih.gov/pubmed/19203752.
441. Liu A, Frostegård J. PCSK9 plays a novel immunological role in oxidized LDL-induced dendritic cell maturation and activation of T cells from human blood and atherosclerotic plaque. J Intern Med. 2018;284:193–210. http://www.ncbi.nlm.nih.gov/pubmed/29617044.
442. Rahman M, Steuer J, Gillgren P, Hayderi A, Liu A, Frostegård J. Induction of dendritic cell-mediated activation of T cells from atherosclerotic plaques by human heat shock protein 60. J Am Heart Assoc. 2017;6. http://www.ncbi.nlm.nih.gov/pubmed/29151033.
443. Canugovi C, Stevenson MD, Vendrov AE, Hayami T, Robidoux J, Xiao H, et al. Increased mitochondrial NADPH oxidase 4 (NOX4) expression in aging is a causative factor in aortic stiffening. Redox Biol. 2019;26:101288. https://linkinghub.elsevier.com/retrieve/pii/S2213231719306573.
444. Goldstein JL, Brown MS. A century of cholesterol and coronaries: from plaques to genes to statins. Cell. 2015;161:161–72. https://linkinghub.elsevier.com/retrieve/pii/S0092867415000793.
445. Andersson C, Johnson AD, Benjamin EJ, Levy D, Vasan RS. 70-year legacy of the Framingham Heart Study. Nat Rev Cardiol. 2019. http://www.nature.com/articles/s41569-019-0202-5.
446. Pencina MJ, D'Agostino RB, Zdrojewski T, Williams K, Thanassoulis G, Furberg CD, et al. Apolipoprotein B improves risk assessment of future coronary heart disease in the Framingham Heart Study beyond LDL-C and non-HDL-C. Eur J Prev Cardiol. 2015;22:1321–7. http://www.ncbi.nlm.nih.gov/pubmed/25633587.
447. Miller YI, Tsimikas S. Oxidation-specific epitopes as targets for biotheranostic applications in humans. Curr Opin Lipidol. 2013;24:426–37. http://www.ncbi.nlm.nih.gov/pubmed/23995232.
448. Leibundgut G, Witztum JL, Tsimikas S. Oxidation-specific epitopes and immunological responses: translational biotheranostic implications for atherosclerosis. Curr Opin Pharmacol. 2013;13:168–79. http://www.ncbi.nlm.nih.gov/pubmed/23541680.
449. Briley-Saebo K, Yeang C, Witztum JL, Tsimikas S. Imaging of oxidation-specific epitopes with targeted nanoparticles to detect high-risk atherosclerotic lesions: progress and

future directions. J Cardiovasc Transl Res. 2014;7:719–36. http://www.ncbi.nlm.nih.gov/pubmed/25297940.
450. Kalinina N, Agrotis A, Antropova Y, DiVitto G, Kanellakis P, Kostolias G, et al. Increased expression of the DNA-binding cytokine HMGB1 in human atherosclerotic lesions: role of activated macrophages and cytokines. Arterioscler Thromb Vasc Biol. 2004;24:2320–5. https://www.ahajournals.org/doi/10.1161/01.ATV.0000145573.36113.8a.
451. Morrow DA, Wang Y, Croce K, Sakuma M, Sabatine MS, Gao H, et al. Myeloid-related protein 8/14 and the risk of cardiovascular death or myocardial infarction after an acute coronary syndrome in the Pravastatin or Atorvastatin Evaluation and Infection Theraphy: Thrombolysis in Myocardial Infarction (PROVE IT-TIMI 22) trial. Am Heart J. 2008;155:49–55. http://linkinghub.elsevier.com/retrieve/pii/S0002870307007041.
452. Wang L, Xie L, Zhang Q, Cai X, Tang Y, Wang L, et al. Plasma nuclear and mitochondrial DNA levels in acute myocardial infarction patients. Coron Artery Dis. 2015;26:296–300. http://www.ncbi.nlm.nih.gov/pubmed/25714070.
453. Simmons JD, Gillespie MN. Plasma nuclear and mitochondrial DNA levels in acute myocardial infarction patients. Coron Artery Dis. 2015;26:286–8. http://www.ncbi.nlm.nih.gov/pubmed/25909176.
454. Chiu T-F, Li C-H, Chen C-C, Chen C-H, Cheng C-J, Yan Y-T, et al. Association of plasma concentration of small heat shock protein B7 with acute coronary syndrome. Circ J. 2012;76:2226–33. http://www.ncbi.nlm.nih.gov/pubmed/22785082.
455. Shah PK, Chyu K-Y, Dimayuga PC, Nilsson J. Vaccine for atherosclerosis. J Am Coll Cardiol. 2014;64:2779–91. http://www.ncbi.nlm.nih.gov/pubmed/25541132.
456. Kimura T, Tse K, Sette A, Ley K. Vaccination to modulate atherosclerosis. Autoimmunity. 2015;48:152–60. http://www.ncbi.nlm.nih.gov/pubmed/25683179.
457. Welsh P, Grassia G, Botha S, Sattar N, Maffia P. Targeting inflammation to reduce cardiovascular disease risk: a realistic clinical prospect? Br J Pharmacol. 2017;174:3898–913. http://doi.wiley.com/10.1111/bph.13818.
458. Amirfakhryan H. Vaccination against atherosclerosis: an overview. Hell J Cardiol. 2019. pii: S1109-9666(19)30125-3.
459. Hartley A, Haskard D, Khamis R. Oxidized LDL and anti-oxidized LDL antibodies in atherosclerosis—novel insights and future directions in diagnosis and therapy. Trends Cardiovasc Med. 2019;29:22–6. http://www.ncbi.nlm.nih.gov/pubmed/29934015.
460. Tsimikas S, Miyanohara A, Hartvigsen K, Merki E, Shaw PX, Chou M-Y, et al. Human oxidation-specific antibodies reduce foam cell formation and atherosclerosis progression. J Am Coll Cardiol. 2011;58:1715–27. http://www.ncbi.nlm.nih.gov/pubmed/21982317.
461. Poulsen CB, Al-Mashhadi AL, von Wachenfeldt K, Bentzon JF, Nielsen LB, Al-Mashhadi RH, et al. Treatment with a human recombinant monoclonal IgG antibody against oxidized LDL in atherosclerosis-prone pigs reduces cathepsin S in coronary lesions. Int J Cardiol. 2016;215:506–15. https://linkinghub.elsevier.com/retrieve/pii/S0167527316306234.
462. Lehrer-Graiwer J, Singh P, Abdelbaky A, Vucic E, Korsgren M, Baruch A, et al. FDG-PET imaging for oxidized LDL in stable atherosclerotic disease: a phase II study of safety, tolerability, and anti-inflammatory activity. JACC Cardiovasc Imaging. 2015;8:493–4. https://linkinghub.elsevier.com/retrieve/pii/S1936878X14007803.
463. Webb NR. Secretory phospholipase A2 enzymes in atherogenesis. Curr Opin Lipidol. 2005;16:341–4. http://www.ncbi.nlm.nih.gov/pubmed/15891396.
464. Hollie NI, Konaniah ES, Goodin C, Hui DY. Group 1B phospholipase A2 inactivation suppresses atherosclerosis and metabolic diseases in LDL receptor-deficient mice. Atherosclerosis. 2014;234:377–80. http://www.ncbi.nlm.nih.gov/pubmed/24747111.
465. Buyukterzi Z, Can U, Alpaydin S, Guzelant A, Karaarslan S, Kocyigit D, et al. Enhanced S100A9 and S100A12 expression in acute coronary syndrome. Biomark Med. 2017;11:229–37. http://www.ncbi.nlm.nih.gov/pubmed/28157385.
466. Vijayakumar EC, Bhatt LK, Prabhavalkar KS. High Mobility Group Box-1 (HMGB1): a potential target in therapeutics. Curr Drug Targets. 2019;20:1474–85. http://www.ncbi.nlm.nih.gov/pubmed/31215389.

467. Aday AW, Ridker PM. Antiinflammatory therapy in clinical care: the CANTOS trial and beyond. Front Cardiovasc Med. 2018;5:62. http://www.ncbi.nlm.nih.gov/pubmed/29922680.
468. Chyu K-Y, Dimayuga PC, Shah PK. Vaccine against arteriosclerosis: an update. Ther Adv Vaccines. 2017;5:39–47. http://journals.sagepub.com/doi/10.1177/2051013617693753.
469. Chyu K-Y, Zhao X, Dimayuga PC, Zhou J, Li X, Yano J, et al. CD8+ T cells mediate the atheroprotective effect of immunization with an ApoB-100 peptide. PLoS One. 2012;7:e30780. http://dx.plos.org/10.1371/journal.pone.0030780.
470. Kimura T, Tse K, McArdle S, Gerhardt T, Miller J, Mikulski Z, et al. Atheroprotective vaccination with MHC-II-restricted ApoB peptides induces peritoneal IL-10-producing CD4 T cells. Am J Physiol Circ Physiol. 2017;312:H781–90. http://www.ncbi.nlm.nih.gov/pubmed/28087520.
471. Gisterå A, Hermansson A, Strodthoff D, Klement ML, Hedin U, Fredrikson GN, et al. Vaccination against T-cell epitopes of native ApoB100 reduces vascular inflammation and disease in a humanized mouse model of atherosclerosis. J Intern Med. 2017;281:383–97. http://www.ncbi.nlm.nih.gov/pubmed/28194913.
472. Long J, Lin J, Yang X, Yuan D, Wu J, Li T, et al. Nasal immunization with different forms of heat shock protein-65 reduced high-cholesterol-diet-driven rabbit atherosclerosis. Int Immunopharmacol. 2012;13:82–7. http://www.ncbi.nlm.nih.gov/pubmed/22465386.
473. Dunér P, To F, Beckmann K, Björkbacka H, Fredrikson GN, Nilsson J, et al. Immunization of apoE−/− mice with aldehyde-modified fibronectin inhibits the development of atherosclerosis. Cardiovasc Res. 2011;91:528–36. https://academic.oup.com/cardiovascres/article-lookup/doi/10.1093/cvr/cvr101.
474. De Haro J, Esparza L, Bleda S, Varela C, Sanchez C, Acin F. Attenuation of early atherosclerotic lesions by immunotolerance with β2 glycoprotein I and the immunomodulatory effectors interleukin 2 and 10 in a murine model. J Vasc Surg. 2015;62:1625–31. https://linkinghub.elsevier.com/retrieve/pii/S0741521414011227.
475. Heinz J, Marinello M, Fredman G. Pro-resolution therapeutics for cardiovascular diseases. Prostaglandins Other Lipid Mediat. 2017;132:12–6. https://linkinghub.elsevier.com/retrieve/pii/S1098882317300539.
476. Fredman G, Tabas I. Boosting inflammation resolution in atherosclerosis: the next frontier for therapy. Am J Pathol. 2017;187:1211–21. https://linkinghub.elsevier.com/retrieve/pii/S0002944017301359.
477. Fredman G, Spite M. Specialized pro-resolving mediators in cardiovascular diseases. Mol Asp Med. 2017;58:65–71. https://linkinghub.elsevier.com/retrieve/pii/S0098299717300171.
478. de Gaetano M, McEvoy C, Andrews D, Cacace A, Hunter J, Brennan E, et al. Specialized pro-resolving lipid mediators: modulation of diabetes-associated cardio-, reno-, and retino-vascular complications. Front Pharmacol. 2018;9:1488. https://www.frontiersin.org/article/10.3389/fphar.2018.01488/full.
479. Doyle R, Sadlier DM, Godson C. Pro-resolving lipid mediators: agents of anti-ageing? Semin Immunol. 2018;40:36–48. https://linkinghub.elsevier.com/retrieve/pii/S1044532318300204.
480. Abdolmaleki F, Kovanen PT, Mardani R, Gheibi-Hayat SM, Bo S, Sahebkar A. Resolvins: emerging players in autoimmune and inflammatory diseases. Clin Rev Allergy Immunol. 2019. http://link.springer.com/10.1007/s12016-019-08754-9.
481. Satish M, Agrawal DK. Pro-resolving lipid mediators in the resolution of neointimal hyperplasia pathogenesis in atherosclerotic diseases. Expert Rev Cardiovasc Ther. 2019;17:177–84. https://www.tandfonline.com/doi/full/10.1080/14779072.2019.1563483.
482. Fredman G. Can inflammation-resolution provide clues to treat patients according to their plaque phenotype? Front Pharmacol. 2019;10:205. https://www.frontiersin.org/article/10.3389/fphar.2019.00205/full.
483. Brezinski DA, Nesto RW, Serhan CN. Angioplasty triggers intracoronary leukotrienes and lipoxin A4. Impact of aspirin therapy. Circulation. 1992;86:56–63. https://www.ahajournals.org/doi/10.1161/01.CIR.86.1.56.
484. Hasturk H, Abdallah R, Kantarci A, Nguyen D, Giordano N, Hamilton J, et al. Resolvin E1 (RvE1) attenuates atherosclerotic plaque formation in diet and inflammation-induced ath-

erogenesis. Arterioscler Thromb Vasc Biol. 2015;35:1123–33. https://www.ahajournals.org/doi/10.1161/ATVBAHA.115.305324.

485. Fredman G, Kamaly N, Spolitu S, Milton J, Ghorpade D, Chiasson R, et al. Targeted nanoparticles containing the proresolving peptide Ac2-26 protect against advanced atherosclerosis in hypercholesterolemic mice. Sci Transl Med. 2015;7:275ra20. http://www.ncbi.nlm.nih.gov/pubmed/25695999.
486. Kusters DHM, Chatrou ML, Willems BAG, De Saint-Hubert M, Bauwens M, van der Vorst E, et al. Pharmacological treatment with Annexin A1 reduces atherosclerotic plaque burden in LDLR−/− mice on Western type diet. PLoS One. 2015;10:e0130484. https://dx.plos.org/10.1371/journal.pone.0130484.
487. de Jong R, Leoni G, Drechsler M, Soehnlein O. The advantageous role of Annexin A1 in cardiovascular disease. Cell Adhes Migr. 2017;11:261–74. http://www.ncbi.nlm.nih.gov/pubmed/27860536.
488. Li Y, Cai L, Wang H, Wu P, Gu W, Chen Y, et al. Pleiotropic regulation of macrophage polarization and tumorigenesis by formyl peptide receptor-2. Oncogene. 2011;30:3887–99. http://www.nature.com/articles/onc2011112.
489. Titos E, Rius B, González-Périz A, López-Vicario C, Morán-Salvador E, Martínez-Clemente M, et al. Resolvin D1 and its precursor docosahexaenoic acid promote resolution of adipose tissue inflammation by eliciting macrophage polarization toward an M2-like phenotype. J Immunol. 2011;187:5408–18. http://www.jimmunol.org/lookup/doi/10.4049/jimmunol.1100225.
490. Herová M, Schmid M, Gemperle C, Hersberger M. ChemR23, the receptor for chemerin and resolvin E1, is expressed and functional on M1 but not on M2 macrophages. J Immunol. 2015;194:2330–7. http://www.jimmunol.org/lookup/doi/10.4049/jimmunol.1402166.

Cerebro-Cardiovascular Diseases

11

11.1 Introduction

According to the WHO definition, CVDs are a group of disorders of the heart and blood vessels. In general, CVDs can be divided into two major subgroups: disorders that arise due to atherosclerosis such as CHD (e.g., heart attack, MI), cerebrovascular disease (stroke, cerebral hemorrhage), and peripheral vascular disease or disorders that are independent of atherosclerotic processes, including congenital and rheumatic heart diseases, cardiomyopathies, arrhythmias, and venous thromboembolism [1]. According to the WHO, CVDs with atherogenic origin are responsible for 80% of CVD deaths. As reported by the *European Cardiovascular Disease Statistics* [2], CVD accounts for 45% of all deaths in Europe and 37% of all deaths in the EU, thus remaining the leading cause of mortality in Europe. Interestingly, death rates from both ischemic heart disease (IHD) and cerebral stroke are generally higher in Central and Eastern Europe than in Northern, Southern, and Western Europe. However, CVD mortality is currently falling in most European countries, including Central and Eastern European countries. Encouragingly, downward trends in several key CVD risk factors can be noticed, including smoking, alcohol consumption, and levels of mean blood cholesterol, with the observed increases in rates of CVD treatment. Nevertheless, levels of other CVD risk factors, particularly the prevalence of overweight/obesity and diabetes, have increased considerably in recent decades, raising concerns about the sustainability of the observed reduction in CVD mortality.

Here, rather than a comprehensive review of all facets of CVD, the most common manifestations of vascular injury-promoted atherogenesis, that is, cerebrovascular disorders and CAD, are briefly described and emphasized in light of the danger/injury model in Immunology.

W. G. Land, *Damage-Associated Molecular Patterns in Human Diseases*,
https://doi.org/10.1007/978-3-030-53868-2_11

11.2 Cerebrovascular Diseases

11.2.1 Introductory Remarks

A neurologic symptom or symptomatic complex caused by cerebral ischemia or bleeding is commonly denoted as a cerebrovascular accident or stroke, clinically featured by sudden or subacute onset. Cerebrovascular diseases are subdivided into ischemic events and cerebral hemorrhages, with many etiologies for each. Typically, ischemic events—besides others—are further classified by the duration of symptoms, whereby transient ischemic attacks (TIAs) seldom last more than a few minutes and never more than 24 h, and ischemic stroke has been present more than 24 h and may be progressive, stable, or resolving. Cerebrovascular diseases, including ischemic and hemorrhagic conditions, are leading causes of death and disability worldwide (for reviews, see [3–5]). Pathogenetically, these disorders can be categorized as caused by occlusive injury intrinsic to blood vessels, occlusive injury extrinsic to blood vessels, cerebral hypoperfusion, and cerebral bleeding (reviewed in [6]).

11.2.2 Experimental Models of Stroke (in Brief)

Although there is a considerable gap between ischemic or hemorrhagic stroke in experimental models and the reality of stroke in human patients, many aspects of the pathophysiology of focal brain ischemia or hemorrhage have been primarily identified in experimental models and could be confirmed later also in the setting of human stroke.

The most frequently used experimental model of ischemic stroke in rodents is the middle cerebral artery occlusion (MCAO) model, which does not require craniectomy. By contrast, the intraluminal monofilament model of MCAO involves the insertion of a surgical filament into the external carotid artery and threading it forward into the internal carotid artery until the tip occludes the origin of the middle cerebral artery, resulting in a cessation of blood flow and subsequent brain infarction in the middle cerebral artery territory. This technique can be used to model permanent or transient occlusion. If the suture is removed after a certain interval (e.g., 30 min, 1 h, or 2 h) and reperfusion is achieved, researchers talk about transient MCAO. If the filament is left in place (e.g., 24 h), the methodology is suitable as a model of permanent MCAO (reviewed in [7]).

The two most commonly used models of intracerebral hemorrhage (ICH) are (1) the collagenase model, where injection of a bacterial enzyme digests the collagen present in the basal lamina of the blood vessels to produce spontaneous brain hemorrhage, and (2) the blood infusion model, where a fixed amount of blood (autologous or donor-derived) is injected into the brain parenchyma to mimic a primary accumulation as observed in human ICH (reviewed in [8]). Moreover, regarding subarachnoid hemorrhage (SAH), the anterior circulation mouse model, where blood is injected into the prechiasmatic cistern, is often used. The model allows for the recreation of clinically relevant findings such as large vessel vasospasm, oxidative stress, microcirculatory spasm, microthrombosis, and delayed neuronal injury—all of which appear in human cases of SAH (reviewed in [9]).

As briefly reviewed in this subchapter, ischemic and hemorrhagic stroke are pathogenetically complex processes, and besides DAMPs, a multitude of other modifying factors matter, such as the duration and severity of ischemia or hemorrhage, etiology, and localization of the infarct or hemorrhage, but also the genetic background. Concerning this scenario, experimental models of stroke are valuable tools to analyze specific facets of stroke, here DAMPs, more or less close to human stroke. Therefore, a word of caution, being aware of the limitations of the individual experimental models used and ideally having support from studies using human tissues are of utmost importance before drawing any final conclusions concerning the role of DAMPs in patients with strokes.

11.2.3 Ischemic Stroke (Cerebral Infarction)

11.2.3.1 General Remarks

The major type of stroke is the ischemic stroke that is caused by thrombosis, embolism, or focal hypoperfusion, all of which can lead to a reduction in or cessation of cerebral blood flow. The consequence of arterial occlusion is an infarction of a circumscribed focus or area of brain tissue. According to the *Global Burden of Diseases, Injuries, and Risk Factors Study* (GBD), stroke (including ischemic and hemorrhagic stroke), as a consequence of high mortality and disability, the economic costs of treatment, and poststroke care are substantial worldwide. Thus, the study revealed that in 2016, there were 5.5 million deaths and 116.4 million disability-adjusted life-years due to stroke (for review, see [10]). Risk factors of stroke can be divided into nonmodifiable factors, including age, gender, ethnicity, and genetic predisposition, and modifiable factors, such as hypertension, dyslipidemia, diabetes mellitus, and smoking (reviewed in [11]).

11.2.3.2 Regulated Cell Death in the Penumbra Around Cerebral Infarction

Ischemic neuronal injury that occurs following loss of oxygen and glucose, failure of energetic metabolism, and accumulation of acidic by-products in brain tissue leads initially to immediate ACD in the affected region ("core zone") that may serve as a source of a first wave of DAMPs to induce initial neuroinflammation. The core surrounding tissues, containing still metabolically active cells, are denoted the "ischemic penumbra zone." The penumbra reflects less severely affected tissue that is considerably hypoperfused and hypoxic due to moderately reduced blood flow, which makes this area a functionally and electrically silent, at-risk, but not yet infarcted tissue zone. However, after reperfusion, neurons within the penumbra may restore their membrane potentials (reviewed in [12, 13]). It is this region in which cells may die from various subroutines of RCD to release further DAMPs able to potentiate neuroinflammatory responses [14] (compare Fig. 11.1).

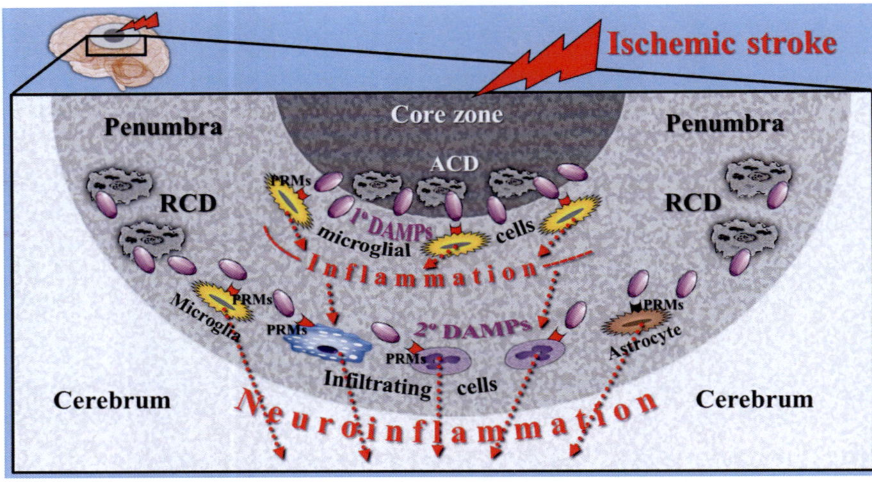

Fig. 11.1 Schematic diagram of a conceptual narrative model illustrating the ischemic stroke-induced emission of DAMPs leading to poststroke neuroinflammatory responses. The first wave of DAMPs (1° DAMPs) derives from necrotic cells located in the core zone (infarction area); the second wave (2° DAMPs) is released/secreted by cells in the penumbra succumbing from various subroutines of regulated cell death. Following ischemic brain injury, the initial inflammatory response is mediated by 1° DAMP-activated PRM-bearing microglial cells; subsequent progression and propagation of neuroinflammation are the results of 2° DAMP-activated recruited and infiltrated PRM-bearing macrophages and neutrophils, as well as further PRM-expressing microglial cell and astrocytes. *ACD* accidental cell death, *RCD* regulated cell death. (Sources: [15, 17, 41, 42])

As experimentally shown, various subroutines of RCD occur in ischemic stroke as promoted by typical pathogenetic prooxidative processes such as overproduction of ROS, Ca^{2+} overload, and excitotoxicity (defined below); they include apoptosis, necroptosis, ferroptosis, and pyroptosis (reviewed in [15]; for RCD, see also Sect. 4.3; for additional information, see Vol. 1 [16], Part V, Chpt. 19, p. 427).

Apoptosis

Intrinsic and extrinsic pathways of caspase-mediated RCD, as well as activation of the caspase-independent signaling pathway of apoptosis, have been proposed to be involved in the pathogenesis of ischemic stroke (reviewed in [13, 17]; for intrinsic and extrinsic apoptotic pathways, see Vol. 1 [16], Part V, Sect. 19.2.2). Evidence has been provided for apoptosis to contribute to a significant proportion of neuron death following acute brain ischemia. For example, it has been reported from studies in rats that intrinsic caspase proteins are activated in the penumbra zone and their inhibition could protect against their detrimental role in focal ischemia injuries [18]. Other lines of studies have revealed that expressions of caspase-1, caspase-3, caspase-8, and caspase-9 and cleaved caspase-8 are enhanced in the ischemic penumbra zone [19]. It is imaginable that cells dying from apoptosis at an early stage or conversion from apoptosis to secondary necrosis may be associated with secretion or release of DAMPs (for additional information, compare Vol. 1 [16], Part V, Sect. 19.2.3, p. 434, and Fig. 19.2, p. 429).

Autophagy-Dependent Cell Death

Accumulating evidence shows that autophagy is activated in various cell types in the brain, such as neurons, glia cells, and brain microvascular cells upon ischemic stroke. As reviewed [15, 20], acute or severe autophagic processes may contribute to cell death of ischemic astrocytes. Although the exact mechanism of autophagy in stroke is unclear, yet it was found that inhibition of autophagy causes lysosomal membrane stabilization that retains the signaling of lysosomal proteases such as cathepsins, which subsequently inhibit the mitochondria-mediated apoptotic pathway in ischemic astrocytes. Other authors have proposed a crosstalk between autophagy, necroptosis, and apoptosis that contribute to ischemic stroke [20] (for the nature of the autophagic process, see Sect. 4.2.2; also compare Vol. 1 [16], Part V, Sect. 18.2 and Fig. 18.1).

Necroptosis

The necroptotic pathways have been addressed in Sect. 4.3.3 and Vol. 1 [16], Part V, Sect. 19.3.2 and Figs. 19.4 and 19.5). Given the broad area of damaged cells in ischemic stroke, it is amazing that, at least so far, most studies have been published showing only indirect biochemical and morphological evidence for the role of the necroptotic pathway in stroke-associated pathological processes.

In earlier experiments, intracerebroventricular injection of necrostatin-1, an RIPK1 inhibitor, that is, a necroptosis inhibitor, was already shown to reduce the infarction area in the MCAO model significantly [21] (for necrostatins, also see [22]). In more recent experimental studies on a transient MCAO model in rats (i.e., transient internal carotid artery occlusion with subsequent postischemic reperfusion) confirming these data [23], cerebral ischemia was found to stimulate phosphorylation of RIPK1 and increase RIPK3 and MLKL expression levels in the brain. Moreover, necrostatin-1 was shown to effectively inhibit ischemia-induced changes while it protected the brain against ischemic injury and functional deficits. Based on their findings, the authors suggested that RIPK1 participates in RIPK3/MLKL-dependent neuronal necroptosis after cerebral ischemia.

In other studies on models of transient MCAO followed by postischemic reperfusion after 1 h occlusion and oxygen–glucose deprivation in mice, GSK'872, a specific RIP3 inhibitor, was also shown to mitigate ischemic brain injury-related necroptosis [24]. Notably, these models are used to mimic the pathogenesis of ischemic stroke and provide the experimental basis for the mechanism study of ischemic stroke. The investigators could demonstrate that the inhibitor GSK'872 (but also a RIP3 siRNA) blocks RIP1–RIP3–MLKL-dependent necroptosis and promote neuroprotective effect following application of the two models, mimicking the pathogenesis of ischemic stroke (for RIP1–RIP3–MLKL-signaling pathways, see Vol. 1 [16], Part V, Fig. 19.4).

Excitingly, a recent study provided already direct evidence for the involvement of necroptosis in ischemic stroke [25]. These studies on a transient MCAO model in rats provided convincing evidence suggesting that endothelial necroptosis is activated in ischemic penumbra after IRI and can increase BBB permeability and ischemic brain injury. Additional findings from their experiments let the authors suggest that M1-like microglia-derived TNF induces endothelial necroptosis and that NF-κB nuclear translocation increased the expression of TNF in M1-like microglia after IRI (for activation of necroptosis by TNF, again compare Fig. 19.4 in Vol. 1 [16], Part V).

Ferroptosis

Emerging evidence implicates ferroptosis as a bona fide mechanism of acute brain cell death in ischemic stroke (reviewed in [26]; see also Sect. 4.3.4 and Fig. 4.2a, b and Vol. 1 [16], Part V, Sect. 19.3.3). For example, in studies on the model of unilateral transient MCAO followed by postischemic reperfusion 1 h after occlusion (again mimicking the pathogenesis of ischemic stroke) [27], elevated iron levels were found in the lesioned hemisphere that correlated with a reduction in iron export. The authors hypothesized that this proferroptotic iron accumulation could sensitize to, or perhaps even induce, ferroptosis. Consistent with such a model, intranasal treatment with liproxstatin-1 and ferrostatin-1 (both potent and specific ferroptosis inhibitors) limited the infarct size and reduced the neurological deficits induced by this stroke model, even when administered 6 h after IRI (for ferrostatins, also see [22]).

Parthanatos

Interestingly, another subroutine of RN, namely, parthanatos, has also been described to be implicated in ischemic stroke [28]. Parthanatos is a unique and highly choreographed form of cell death, which occurs through injury-induced overactivation of the nuclear enzyme, poly (ADP-ribose) synthetase-1 (PARP-1), also known as poly (ADP-ribose) glycohydrolase or poly (ADP-ribose) transferase-1. Such cellular injuries include stimuli which can induce DNA damage directly, such as ROS, alkylating agents, UV radiation, and ionizing radiation (reviewed in [29–32]; also see Vol. 1 [16], Part V, Sect. 19.3.5.3, and Box 4.1). Thus, in studies on male mice subjected to 2 h of transient focal cerebral ischemia [33], first evidence was provided suggesting implication of parthanatos in ischemic stroke.

NETosis

As mentioned in Vol. 1 [16], Part V, Sect. 19.3.6, and in Box 4.1, the subroutine of RN performed by activated neutrophils, that is, NETosis, is a form of neutrophil-specific cell death characterized by the release of chromatin-derived, weblike structures released into the extracellular space, referred to as NETs (reviewed in [34–36]). Thus, it should not go unmentioned here that in studies on the permanent stroke model of MCAO-induced focal cerebral ischemia in rats, HMGB1was observed not only to induce NETosis but to be included as a part of the extruded NETs, thereby contributing to NETosis-mediated neuronal death.

In Sum

These first observations give rise to suggest that subroutines of RCD act as critical sources of a second wave of DAMPs, which trigger necro-neuroinflammatory responses involved in the pathogenesis of ischemic stroke. Moreover, but not detailed here, further RCD may occur in the case of subsequent reperfusion therapy, that is, intravenous thrombolysis and endovascular thrombectomy, which is known to improve the clinical outcome in patients with acute ischemic stroke remarkably [37]. For example, in studies on experimental brain IRI models, some evidence was obtained indicating cerebral IRI to induce necroptosis, ferroptosis, and pyroptosis [38–40]. Indeed, these experimental observations may strongly suggest the emission of another wave of DAMPs in the context of therapeutic reperfusion/recanalization strategies considered after the patient's hospital admission.

Again, as discussed already in the context of TBI (Sect. 9.2.3), the molecular mechanisms responsible for the development of the stroke-associated conditions—as briefly touched in the next section—are still not fully understood, but there is growing evidence in support of the notion that the DAMPs play a vital role in these pathologies.

11.2.3.3 Pathogenesis of Ischemic Stroke: Neuroinflammation (in Brief)

The pathogenesis of stroke—similar to that described for TBI (see Sect. 9.2.4)—is extremely complex and involves numerous processes, including initial energy failure, excitotoxicity, excess of Ca^{2+} influx, and oxidative and nitrous stress, all known to contribute to the generation of RCD, associated with emission of DAMPs. These DAMPs then promote proinflammatory pathways to establish neuroinflammation. Guided by comprehensive review articles [17, 41, 42], some points are briefly and selectively highlighted in the following.

Prooxidative Processes

Excitotoxicity refers to sequelae of events induced by excessive accumulation of excitatory amino acids (i.e., neurotransmitters that can transmit a nerve message across a synapse), leading to toxic increases in intracellular calcium. As a second messenger, calcium ions activate various signaling pathways, which eventually lead to cell death. Other mechanisms contributing to excitotoxicity refer to activation of NMDA and AMPA type of glutamate receptors that leads to membrane depolarization. As already set out in Sect. 9.2.4.2 [43], excessive glutamate at the synaptic junction that in turn activates its NMDA and AMPA receptors facilitates excessive calcium influx into the neuronal cells and promotes oxidative stress that further leads to mitochondrial dysfunction and oxidation of lipids, proteins, and DNA.

Further neuronal cell damage is mediated by nitrative and oxidative stresses that override the antioxidative stress response (compare Sect. 4.2.3). Thus, during ischemic stroke, several mechanisms contribute to the generation of ROS, including NMDA receptor-mediated excitotoxicity, excess of Ca^{2+} influx, activation of mitochondrial ETC, and activation of ROS-producing enzyme systems such as NOXes and XOR. Notably, these systems become activated and may aggravate the oxidative injury by postischemic reperfusion in case the blood flow is restored after only a short period of ischemia or in case the revascularization procedures via recombinant tissue plasminogen activator or mechanical thrombectomy are too late performed [44].

DAMP-Driven Promotion of Neuroinflammatory Processes in the Penumbra

As plausibly imaginable, these various injuries, particularly oxidative damage, may induce the emission of both primary DAMPs such as OSEs and secondary DAMPs derived from subroutines of RCD (described above). Following, these DAMPs induce activation of several types of PRM-bearing cells, which in turn mount postischemic neuroinflammation in the area of the penumbra that is associated with edema formation and increase in intracranial pressure (reviewed in [45]). Characteristically, these cells, including the dominating proliferating microglial cells (i.e., resident macrophages) and infiltrating macrophages and neutrophils, but also ECs, astrocytes, and swelling neurons, produce proinflammatory mediator substances such as cytokines, chemokines, and adhesion molecules (compare Fig. 11.1). These molecules, including TNF and IL-1β in their function as inducible IIIA-2 and IIIB-1 DAMPs, potentiate neuroinflammation via disruption of the BBB, thereby promoting—besides creation of cerebral edema and hemorrhagic transformation—recruitment and infiltration of neutrophils, macrophages, NK cells, DCs, T cells (i.e., $CD4^+$ Th cells and $CD8^+$ CTLs) and B cells (for global DAMP-induced inflammatory responses, also compare Vol. 1 [16], Part VI, Sects. 22.2.4 and 22.2.5).

Of note, key mediators of the disruption of the BBB are MMPs that are responsible for protein digestion and ECM (see Sect. 6.2.2). Microglia are major sources of MMPs which appear within a few hours in the ischemic core and stay increased above basal levels for up to 1 week. Although different types of MMPs act differently, there is accumulating evidence that MMP2, MMP9, and MMP12 are involved in the pathogenesis of BBB disruption and cerebral edema formation during ischemic stroke (for review, see [46]).

Several months after a stroke, astrocytes form a dense network of glial fibers mixed with capillaries and connective tissue (astrogliosis). Of note, the dominant role of microglial cells and macrophages in provoking innate immune responses has also been observed in human ischemic infarcts. Remarkably, the detection of T and B cells has given rise to the assumption that stroke may induce adaptive autoreactive immune responses. Indeed, experimental and clinical evidence has been reported that such poststroke adaptive immune responses really occur (for further reading, see [47, 48]; for DAMP-shaped adaptive immune responses, also compare Vol. 1, [16], Part VIII, Chpt. 32).

Thromboinflammation in Ischemic Stroke

Importantly, in ischemic stroke, downstream microvascular thrombosis in cortical venules as an early response to proximal cerebral arterial occlusion, as well as IRI after recanalization procedures, promotes another inflammatory event referred to as thromboinflammation, that is, a complex process that may facilitate further cerebral infarction development. In particular, cerebral postischemic reperfusion is known to trigger interactions among the vessel wall, platelets, leukocytes, and coagulation that can impair reperfusion and destabilize the BBB [49–51].

Downstream thromboinflammation is characterized by leukocyte margination in cortical microvessels where blood flow is markedly reduced despite collateral circulation from pial anastomoses. As reviewed by Desilles et al. [49], leukocyte margination facilitates fibrinogen deposition and secondary venous thrombosis, as well as rupture of the BBB in both cortical venules and arterioles. Moreover, the thrombi can persist, and leukocyte extravasation can continue progressing in venules after recanalization that only partially corrects blood flow in cortical microvessels. Given these observations, the authors suggested that hemorrhagic transformation might be a consequence of persisting occlusion rather than postischemic reperfusion.

Thromboinflammation as a consequence of recanalization develops mechanistically differently. Thus, as reviewed by Stoll and Nieswandt [51] regarding acute experimental stroke, T cells contribute to IRI after recanalization in an antigen-independent manner. The detrimental T-cell effects were shown to be platelet-dependent. Glycoprotein Ib- and glycoprotein VI-mediated platelet activation were demonstrated to be a crucial checkpoint that orchestrates thrombotic and proinflammatory pathways and downstream activation of coagulation factor XII to be a driving force of IRI in acute stroke.

SAMP-Promoted Resolution of Neuroinflammatory Processes

As typical for inflammatory responses in general (as outlined in Sect. 5.3), the neuroinflammatory response persists into the subacute/late inflammation-resolving and repair phase of stroke and participates in all brain repair elements, including neurogenesis, angiogenesis, synaptogenesis, remyelination, and axonal sprouting, a scenario that sheds new light on poststroke brain recovery. This restoring phase following ischemic stroke is critical for improving poststroke neurological recovery and cognitive functions. Accumulating evidence suggests that the myeloid cells, including both the resident microglia and infiltrating monocytes/macrophages and neutrophils, are highly plastic in response to the environmental cues (for reviews, see Wang et al. [52] and Zhu et al. [53]). As characteristic for the resolving phase—but as also demonstrated in studies on a murine model of ischemic stroke [54]— 3 days after stroke onset, infiltrating macrophages and neutrophils were detected to shift from their initial inflammatory roles to a proresolving function.

Proresolving macrophages were shown to express high levels of SRs such as the *macrophage scavenger receptor 1* (MSR1) and *macrophage receptor with collagenous structure* (MARCO), also known as SR-A6, responsible for clearing work in the ischemic brain. The receptor MSR1 was found to recognize DAMPs such as HMGB1, PRDXs, S100A8, and S100A9 and engulf them into the cell for degradation in the lysosome [54]. Also, as reviewed in [52, 53], there is growing evidence indicating that there are different phenotypes of microglia, denoted as "alternatively activated" M2-microglia that may promote brain recovery. Moreover, after ischemic stroke, the expression MerTK (a receptor known to be expressed on M2-like macrophages) was shown to be transiently upregulated. Inhibition of MerTK may prevent delayed neuronal loss after stroke (for MerTK, see Sect. 2.3.2, and for the issue of M1 → "M1-like" and M2 → "M2-like" macrophages, also compare Vol. 1 [16], Part III, Sect. 8.2.2.2 and Fig. 8.2). Moreover, invading Tregs have been shown to contribute to neuroprotection in later recovering phase after stroke by secreting cerebral IL-10 [55, 56]. To stress here is that—like M2-like macrophages— N2 neutrophils have also been observed to mediate neuroprotection after stroke [57] (compare Sect. 5.3.2.3).

Of note, in this subacute late phase after stroke, in human patients and experimental stroke models, a stroke-induced immunosuppression syndrome has been described that contributes to increased susceptibility of stroke patients to bacterial infections, a critical cause of mortality and secondary morbidity [58]. Remarkably, this observation is reminiscent of increased susceptibility of patients to infection during the hyperresolution phase in CARS following SIRS (see Fig. 8.1 and Sect. 8.3.2). As discussed in terms of a conceptual model, an uncontrolled overshooting generation of SAMPs was proposed to be implicated in this immunosuppressive phase (see Sect. 8.3.4.2). So indeed, there has been already some evidence reported indicating a role of SAMPs such as AnxA1 and SPMs in promoting resolution of neuroinflammation, as shown in various models of ischemic stroke [59–61] (see below).

Epigenetic Regulation of Inflammation in Ischemic Stroke

Stroke is one example of tissue injury for which the impact of epigenetic regulation has already been reviewed (for key articles, see [62–64]; for epigenetic modifications, also compare Sect. 5.6 and Figs. 5.4, 5.5, and 5.6). As outlined and discussed by Ng et al. [64], epigenetics, such as DNA methylation, histone modification, and microRNAs, involves the differential regulation of gene expression, including those involved in brain inflammation and remodeling after stroke.

For example, as also reviewed in [64], it has been suggested that DNA hypomethylation may promote stroke-induced inflammation and thereby exacerbate stroke injury. Other lines of studies reportedly showed that acetylation at histone 3 lysine 9 is upregulated in the ischemic territory and is associated with microglial activation. On the other hand, HDAC inhibitors were found to lead to decreased cytokines indicating a neuroprotective action of HDAC inhibitors, a finding that was confirmed by many other studies showing that inhibition of histone deacetylation was favorable for stroke outcome. Together, while HDAC may be an essential mediator of inflammatory responses during stroke, targeting HDAC may attenuate inflammatory damage and promote functional outcome.

Moreover, there is clinical and convincing experimental evidence for a regulatory role of miRNA in stroke (also reviewed in [64]). Such clinical evidence derives, for example, from ischemic stroke patients showing reduced blood levels of miR-30a and miR-126 for 24 weeks. Experimentally, miR-155 has been identified as a proinflammatory miRNA that is involved in the inflammatory process during stroke and was also shown to induce proinflammatory signaling in microglia. Of interest is also the observation that inflammasome activity, known to play a role in ischemic stroke, may be regulated via the action of miRNAs.

Finally, Ng et al. [64] argue: "Careful consideration and further studies are needed to gain a deeper understanding of the roles of DNA methylation in different stroke subtypes. Nonetheless, it has been recently proposed that the level of DNA methylation correlates with the chronological age of patients and serves as a good prognostic marker to assess stroke risk."

11.2.3.4 DAMPs in Ischemic Stroke

As briefly mentioned above, DAMPs in ischemic stroke may be emitted in terms of three waves: (1) released by cells dying from ACD in the "core zone," (2) released or secreted by cells dying from RCD in the ischemic penumbra zone, and (3) released or secreted by dying cells from RCD induced by therapeutic recanalization/reperfusion strategies. Indeed, there are an increasing number of experimental and clinical reports on the pathogenetic role of DAMPs in inducing neuroinflammation after ischemic stroke [45, 65, 66]; they are briefly and selectively summarized here.

High Mobility Group Box 1

High mobility group box 1 has been addressed in Vol. 1 [16], Part IV, Sect. 12.2.2, as a constitutive IA-1 DAMP passively released from necrotic cells and as an inducible IIIB-2 DAMP actively secreted as acetylated HMGB1 in Vol. 1[16], Part IV, Sect. 14.3.3 and Fig. 14.4. In ischemic stroke models and patients with ischemic stroke, emission of HMGB1 has been convincingly documented as pivotal proinflammatory DAMP. For example, in studies at autopsy, the immunolocalization of HMGB1 was investigated in brains of patients with acute and chronic cerebral infarction [67]. In 3 out of 10 acute cerebral infarction cases, the cytoplasm of neurons located in the penumbra was found positive for HMGB1. On the other hand, in the chronic stage of cerebral infarction, macrophages located in some ischemic regions were positive for HMGB1.

In fact, HMGB1 that is passively released from damaged nerve cells already 2–4 h after the onset of ischemic stroke to enter the blood circulation through the damaged BBB has been identified as a key DAMP in promoting pathogenetic innate immune mechanisms in ischemic stroke (for reviews, see [68–70]). For example, in the acute phase, this proinflammatory IA-1 DAMP was shown to cause excitotoxic injury, promote the disruption of the BBB, and activate microglia and macrophages to amplify inflammatory responses by recognizing TLRs or RAGE receptors. During the advanced/late stages of ischemic stroke, HMGB1is thought to promote the regeneration of nerve cells, remodeling of blood vessels, and recovery of neurological function. Notably, in this later phase, microglia and astrocytes are activated, and intracellular HMGB1 is modified by a series of acetylation and phosphorylation reaction, leading to active secretion of HMGB1 into extracellular space.

Importantly, when an ischemic stroke occurs, HMGB1 is not only locally released and secreted in the brain but also released into peripheral blood from the CNS, a phenomenon that could be observed in experimental stroke models and patients with stroke. Thus, a systematic review and meta-analysis revealed that—compared with controls—patients with ischemic stroke had significantly higher circulating blood HMGB1 levels and the HMGB1 level was positively correlated with severity and infarct volume (reviewed in [69]). Given this data, the authors concluded that HMGB1 can serve as a new prognostic biomarker and therapeutic target in the diagnosis and management of ischemic stroke.

Peroxiredoxins

As briefly touched in Sect. 3.5.4.4, PRXs or PRDXs, in their role as inducible IIIB-6 DAMPs, are a family of antioxidant proteins that are sensed by TLR2 and TLR4 on infiltrating myeloid cells. Studies on a murine ischemic stroke model showed that extracellular release of PRXs such as PRX-1, PRX-2, PRX-5, and PRX-6 increases in the cerebral infarct lesion 12–24 h after stroke onset. This PRX release coincides with the beginning of myeloid infiltration in the ischemic brain, suggesting its critical role in triggering the postischemic inflammation by neutrophils and macrophages. Remarkably, the neutralization of extracellular PRXs with antibodies was found to suppress inflammatory cytokine expression and infarct volume growth and, further, to be neuroprotective, even if administered 12 h after stroke onset [71]. Interestingly, these DAMPs were discovered to be present in a mass spectrometry analysis of extracellular fluids collected from the infarct lesions of ischemic stroke patients [72]. Other studies in humans revealed high levels of PRX-1 during the first hours after stroke onset [73]. Based on their data, the authors recommended this inducible DAMP to use as biomarkers for determining cerebral infarction onset.

Heat Shock Proteins

Heat shock proteins have been addressed in Vol. 1 [16], Part IV, Sect. 12.2.3, as constitutive IA-1 DAMPs passively released from necrotic cells and in Sect. 14.2.2.2 as actively secreted inducible IIIA-1 DAMPs. Here, instead of reviewing all HSPs, only some aspects of the prototypical HSP70 are briefly highlighted. Thus, in ischemic stroke models, studies over the past two decades have shown that HSP70 mainly protects against multiple types of RCD, whereas its role in modulating inflammatory pathways has also been reported (reviewed in [74]). Interestingly, the neuroprotective properties of HSP70 have been proposed to harness therapeutically, for example, in using this molecule to improve neurological outcome synergistically or to extend the time window of existing interventions, thereby increasing the numbers of stroke victims eligible for treatment (reviewed in [74]).

S100 Proteins

S100 proteins have been addressed in Vol. 1 [16], Part IV, Sect. 12.2.4.2, as constitutive IA-1 DAMPs passively released from necrotic cells and in Sect. 14.2.2.4 as actively secreted inducible IIIA-1 DAMPs. Regarding their prominent role in inflammatory processes (for additional information, compare Sect. 12.2.4.2, p. 229, in Vol. 1 [16], Part IV), evidence for their participation in the pathogenesis of ischemic stroke was expectably reported. Thus, in earlier clinical trials, S100 proteins were already measured in patients with acute ischemic stroke aimed at assessing them as biomarkers [75]. The study revealed that S100 is significantly increased after stroke onset and correlates with infarct volume, stroke severity, and functional outcome, that is, all of which are features that qualify this DAMP as a possible marker of ongoing ischemia. In continuation of this study, an integrative review including 48 studies until March 2017 provided convincing data for S100B protein to be considered as a potent neurobiochemical marker that can play a pathognomonic role in the diagnosis of stroke [76].

Some more in-depth information about the mechanistic function of S100 proteins in cerebral ischemia has been provided by studies on the MCAO model in mice showing that S100B promotes microglia M1 polarization with enhanced migration ability and inhibits M2 polarization, thereby aggravating cerebral ischemia [77].

Extracellular ATP

Extracellular ATP has been denoted as a IA-2 DAMP to contribute indirectly to NLRP3 inflammasome activation (for additional information, compare Vol. 1 [16], Part IV, Sect. 12.2.5.2, p. 238, and Part VI, Sect. 22.4.2.2, p. 516, and Fig. 22.11, p. 517). Extracellular ATP is, like glutamate, a major excitatory neurotransmitter in the CNS via activation of ionotropic P2X receptors. Thus, it is not a surprise that evidence for its involvement in ischemic stroke has also been reported. As discussed by An et al. [78], microglial P2X7 receptors are upregulated in response to cerebral ischemia, and P2X7 receptor antagonists have been shown to protect against transient global cerebral IRI by reducing inflammatory responses (for indirect activation of the NLRP3 inflammasome via eATP ↔ P2X7R, see Fig. 2.1). Further evidence in support of a role of eATP in contributing to ischemic stroke-associated neuroinflammation has been discussed elsewhere [79].

Together, eATP appears to operate as a DAMP in ischemic stroke; however, more targeted studies are obviously needed to get a clearer picture of their function in promoting neuroinflammatory processes. In particular, its role in the activation of the NLRP3 inflammasome warrants further investigations. Such studies may also be applied to other DAMPs that are known to activate the NLRP3 inflammasome indirectly.

Histones and Extracellular Nucleosomes

Histones and nucleosomes are critical nuclear proteins that contribute to the structural organization and stability of chromatin. When released from dying cells (succumbing to ACD or RCD such as NETosis) into the extracellular space, histones, that is, free histones and DNA-bound histones (nucleosomes), have been recognized as candidates of the DAMP family (for additional information, see Vol. 1 [16], Part IV, Sect. 12.2.4.4, p. 233). As reviewed by Silk et al. [80], evidence for a pathogenetic role of extracellular histones—nucleosomes in ischemic stroke—is growing. For example, models of ischemic stroke could demonstrate a sevenfold serum nucleosome increase. Moreover, in human observational trials, measuring serum nucleosome after stroke confirmed this evidence, suggesting that poor oxygen perfusion stimulates the release of nucleosomes from cells into the systemic circulation. In other lines of studies on the formation of NETs (containing histones) [81], NETs were found to be significantly elevated in the plasma of patients with acute ischemic stroke and even increased in patients with a history of atrial fibrillation. Further, as revealed by multivariate analysis, elevated levels of the citrullinated histone 3 (the most specific marker of NETs) at onset of stroke were independently associated with atrial fibrillation and all-cause mortality at 1-year follow-up. The authors concluded that citrullinated histone 3 may constitute a useful prognostic marker and therapeutic target in patients with acute stroke.

Inducible DAMPs in Ischemic Stroke: Members of the Interleukin-1 Family and Tumor Necrosis Factor

Infiltrating neutrophils and macrophages in the ischemic brain, activated by DAMPs via PRMs, produce various inflammatory cytokines, including members of the IL-1 family and TNF, which play a dominant role in ischemic stroke.

Members of the IL-1 family, such as processed IL-1α and IL-1β, have been described in Vol. 1 [16], Part IV, Sect. 14.3.2, and Part VI, Sect. 22.5.6. Acting as inducible IIIB-1 DAMPs, they play a prominent role in ischemic stroke (reviewed in [68, 82]). Such evidence, for example, derived from studies on the murine transient MCAO model, showed that mice deficient in both IL-1α and IL-1β have marked reductions in lesion volume. Clinically, several studies have demonstrated elevated concentrations of the proinflammatory cytokine IL-1 in blood and the CSF of patients with acute ischemic stroke that correlated with neurological deficits suggesting a localized CNS IL-1-mediated inflammatory response to ischemic injury. Moreover, levels of IL-1β in ischemic stroke have been consistently shown to be lower in serum compared with CSF suggesting intrathecal production of these proinflammatory mediators by DAMP-activated cells.

The other most extensively studied cytokine in experimental stroke is the proinflammatory and immune regulatory cytokine TNF. Like IL-1β, it can operate as an inducible IIIA-2 DAMP, as described in Vol. 1 [16], Part IV, Sect. 14.2.3.2, and Part VI, Sect. 22.5.7. The considerable impact of TNF on the progression of neuroinflammation lies in the fact that it can induce a subroutine of RN, that is, necroptosis, as another source of DAMPs release (for additional information, also compare Vol. 1 [16], Part V, Sect. 19.3.2.2 and Fig. 19.4, p. 437). As reviewed [83], TNF is primarily produced by microglia in the early phase after experimental stroke and sustained by macrophages at later time points, although other cell types such as astrocytes and neuronal cells have also been reported to produce TNF during ischemic damage. In the model of permanent MCAO, TNF was found to be acutely and significantly upregulated, remaining elevated for days to make this inducible DAMP a key player both in acute and chronic ischemia and in postischemic neuronal plasticity.

Inducible DAMPs: ASC Specks in NLRP3 Inflammasome Activation

In Sects. 2.2.5.4 and 3.5.4.2, the scenario of ASC specks was briefly outlined. Excitingly, in studies on a mouse model of recurrent stroke, increased activation of the NLRP3 inflammasome was observed that exacerbate the brain damage and the proinflammatory response [84]. Additionally, in these studies, the investigators found that ASC protein level surrounding the infarct area was increased and the number of ASC specks surrounding the second infarct area was positively correlated to the damage scores. Given their findings (including some others not quoted here), the authors concluded that the NLRP3 inflammasome is activated by two attacks of stroke, which act together with ASC to exacerbate recurrent strokes.

11.2.3.5 SAMPs in Ischemic Stroke

The detection of inflammation-resolving processes in ischemic stroke under involvement of M2-like macrophages and M2-microglia cells was briefly touched above. Notably, there is already first evidence suggesting a role of SAMPs in these processes.

For example, AnxA1 has been shown to act in various ways to mitigate cerebral IRI (for AnxA1, see Vol. 1 [16], Part IV, Sect.14.4.3). Thus, in studies on murine models of ischemic stroke, AnxA1 and its peptide mimetics were observed to diminishing leukocyte adhesion and trafficking, inhibiting the release of proinflammatory and prothrombotic cytokines, and regulating neutrophil ↔ platelet interactions. Moreover, human recombinant AnxA1 and its peptide mimetics were shown to markedly reduce the lesion size, clinical score, and markers of leukocyte infiltration in the murine MCAO model (reviewed b Ansari et al. [59]). Also, in other lines of studies, AnxA1 was found to afford protection by altering the platelet phenotype in cerebral IRI from propathogenic to regulatory and reducing the propensity for platelets to aggregate and cause thrombosis [61].

In addition, extracellular adenosine that increases in the brain dramatically during ischemia has been identified as another SAMP implicated in ischemic stroke (for extracellular adenosine, see Sect. 3.5.5.4; for further reading, see [85–87]). Extracellular adenosine is known to operate as a neuroprotective endogenous agent mainly by activating A1 adenosine receptors (A1ARs), which control calcium influx, glutamate release, membrane potential, and metabolism (for purinergic receptors, see Sect. 2.3.3 and Vol. 1 [16], Part II, Sect. 5.3.4 and Figs. 5.9 and 5.10). Findings in support of this inflammation-resolving function derive, for example, from studies on an ischemic mouse model showing that the neuroprotective effect of *mitochondrial division inhibitor 1* (Mdivi-1) is mediated through increasing the concentration of extracellular adenosine [86]. (Notably, in this study, Mdivi-1 was observed to protect against excitotoxic Ca^{2+} overload and necrotic cell death, associated with significantly reduced infarct volume and neurological scores.)

Also, as reviewed by Yin et al. [60], there is accumulating evidence from studies on various in vitro and in vivo models of ischemic stroke suggesting that SPMs decrease leukocyte infiltration, enhance efferocytosis, reduce local neuronal injury, and decrease both oxidative stress and the production of inflammatory cytokines. In fact, in first human cell in vitro and murine in vivo models of ischemic stroke, neuroprotectively acting SPMs and their aspirin-triggered forms were shown to be endogenously produced [88–90] (for SMPs, see Sect. 3.5.5.5 and Vol. 1 [16], Part IV, Sect. 14.4.4).

Concluding, the detection of a neuroprotective effect of SAMPs on ischemic stroke-associated neuroinflammation opens the door for applying new therapeutic options in patients with cerebral stroke. In this context, Yin et al. [60] concluded: "Stable synthetic mimetics to endogenous SPMs and synthetic SPM receptor agonists are under development for various chronic inflammatory disease models ... ; however, the side effects accompanying these need to be investigated further .... It is our hope that the results from these studies will provide new stroke treatments by controlling resolution."

11.2.3.6 Concluding Remarks

Together, the dominating role of DAMP-driven neuroinflammatory responses in ischemic stroke is well documented. Plausibly, this property licenses DAMPs to be used as promising diagnostic and prognostic biomarkers as well as therapeutic targets. On the other hand, there is a growing body of evidence suggesting administration of SAMPs as a new promising therapeutic approach in patients with ischemic stroke. For the future, it appears to be the order of the day, to harness DAMPs as therapeutic targets and apply SAMPs as therapeutics in all situations of recanalization procedures: it is these recanalization attempts that lead to the release of large quantities of DAMPs in the course of postischemic reperfusion (also compare Sect. 11.4.3.2).

11.2.4 Hemorrhagic Stroke

11.2.4.1 General Remarks

Hemorrhagic stroke refers to SAH, ICH, and intraventricular hemorrhage, also known as hemorrhagic cerebrovascular accidents. Intracerebral hemorrhage accounts for about 10–20% of all strokes and is associated with higher morbidity, more severe disability, and mortality than ischemic strokes. Subarachnoid hemorrhage, in about 85% as a consequence of the rupture of an intracranial aneurysm, accounts for only 5% of all the stroke events but is associated with the mortality by about 50% (for reviews, see [91–95]).

11.2.4.2 Regulated Cell Death in Hemorrhagic Stroke

Intracerebral hemorrhage and SAH due to rupture of a blood vessel cause physical disruption to the cellular architecture of the brain surrounding the hemorrhagic site due to shearing force and the mass effect of the hemorrhage. This process is associated with increased intracranial hydrostatic pressure that can compress brain regions and potentially impact blood flow, causing direct destruction of adjacent tissue and cells via mechanical and ischemic damage. This primary mechanical/ischemic injury may result in ACD, but rather RCD in the immediate vicinity of the bleeding, releasing a first wave of DAMPs. Indeed, apoptosis, necroptosis, ferroptosis, and pyroptosis have already been identified in animal models of intracerebral hemorrhage as well as in the perihematomal region after surgical evacuation in humans. They are briefly touched here.

Apoptosis

In earlier studies on an ICH model in rabbits, a high burden of apoptotic cells was already observed, located in the matrix of the hematoma [96]. Interestingly, in a more recent study on a rat ICH model investigating the role of PERK signaling in the pathophysiology of secondary brain injury, the PERK pathway was found to be activated, as evidenced by increased protein levels of eIF2α and ATF4. The resultant ER stress induced neuronal apoptosis [97]. Based on their findings, the authors proposed that PERK signaling pathway plays an essential role in ICH-induced apoptosis and could be a critical endogenous physiological regulatory signal pathway in neurons (for PERK-triggered proapoptotic signaling, see Sect. 4.2.5.3 and Fig. 4.1, and compare Fig. 18.6 in Vol. 1 [16], Part V, Sect. 18.5.2).

Autophagy-Dependent Cell Death

Several studies have provided evidence for a role of autophagy in hemorrhagic stroke. For example, experiments on a collagenase-induced ICH model in mice showed that autophagy activation may regulate ICH-induced brain injury and neural damage may be related to regulating of NF-κB pathway, thereby promoting inflammation and apoptosis [98]. Another line of studies could demonstrate that autophagy promotes microglia activation through Beclin-1-ATG5 pathway in ICH (for the nature of the autophagic process, also compare Sect. 4.2.2 and Vol. 1 [16], Part V, Sect. 18.2 and Fig. 18.1). Altogether, however, the role of autophagy in ICH remains elusive.

Necroptosis

Earlier studies have already confirmed that the microglia is rapidly activated in brain tissues after ICH to secrete proinflammatory mediators, including TNF, which can induce necroptosis [99] (for activation of necroptosis by TNF, again compare Fig. 19.4 in Vol. 1 [16], Part V). More recently reported studies on an ICH model in rats showed that TNF secreted from activated microglia can induce necroptosis of neurons after ICH [100]. Indeed, the investigators found that necroptosis exists in brain tissues after ICH and plays a critical role in neuronal dysfunction, brain edema, and BBB permeability. Moreover, the RIP1 inhibitor necrostatin-1 was found to attenuate neurological dysfunction, brain edema, and BBB injury. Based on their data, the authors discussed that their findings contribute to modern views on the relationship between RCD and neuroinflammation in brain injury after ICH, thereby providing a potential therapeutic target for secondary brain injury after ICH.

Ferroptosis

Given the knowledge that hemorrhagic stroke is associated with release of iron from red blood cells, the growing interest in research on an iron-dependent form of RCD in ICH, that is, ferroptosis, is not a surprise (for further reading, see [101–106]; also compare Sect. 4.3.4 and Fig. 4.2a, b, and Vol. 1 [16], Part V, Sect. 19.3.3). Indeed, first studies on hemorrhagic stroke models in vitro or in vivo indicated that ferroptosis contributes to neuronal death after ICH and that administration of ferrostatin-1 protects hemorrhagic brain [107] (for ferrostatins, also see [22]). Remarkably, in more recent studies on a collagenase-induced mouse model of ICH, it could be shown that pharmacological *selenium* supplementation effectively inhibits GPX4-dependent ferroptotic death as well as cell death induced by excitotoxicity or ER stress, which are GPX4-independent events [105]. Moreover, systemic administration of a brain-penetrant selenopeptide was found to activate homeostatic transcription to inhibit cell death and improve function when delivered after hemorrhagic stroke [105]. In fact, these studies suggest a critical role of ferroptosis in ICH, but further targeted experiments are needed to confirm these observations.

Pyroptosis

Interestingly, there is already first evidence suggesting an involvement of pyroptosis in hemorrhagic stroke. For instance, as reviewed in [108], in experiments on a SAH and ICH model, respectively, in rats [109, 110], findings were observed suggesting that P2X7R suppression significantly reduces NLRP3 inflammasome-associated caspase-1 activation, indicating that P2X7R-mediated pyroptosis is obviously involved in the pathological process of brain injury after hemorrhagic stroke. Again, further studies are required to confirm the assumption that this subroutine of RN is also implicated in hemorrhagic stroke.

In Sum

Together, these observations point to subroutines of RCD, which can be considered a hallmark of secondary brain injury after hemorrhagic stroke. The RCDs may induce a second wave of DAMPs that drive necro-neuroinflammatory responses involved in the pathogenesis of hemorrhagic stroke. Again, as discussed already in the context of ischemic stroke, the molecular mechanisms responsible for the development of the hemorrhagic stroke-associated neuroinflammation are still not fully understood, but there is growing evidence in support of the notion that the DAMPs play a dominant role in these pathologies.

11.2.4.3 Pathogenesis of Hemorrhagic Stroke: Neuroinflammation (in Brief)

Compared to ischemic stroke, hemorrhagic strokes lead to a similar type of cellular and molecular dysfunction and orchestrated events of repair with the addition of blood extravasation and resorption. As mentioned, the primary injury in intracerebral hemorrhage is characterized by physical disruption of parenchymal architecture associated with increased intracranial pressure and subsequent global ischemia, which, altogether, can induce RCD of various cerebral cells. Following, these DAMPs induce activation of several types of PRM-bearing cells to initiate post-bleeding neuroinflammatory processes (reviewed in [111]) that, in turn, promote secondary brain injury (for SAH, a first phase, early brain injury, and a delayed phase, neurological deterioration, is described; compare Fig. 11.2).

Increasing evidence suggests that after ICH, the DAMP-activated, PRM-expressing M1-polarized microglial cells are the major cell type responsible for secondary neuroinflammation owing to their release of cytokines, chemokines, prostaglandins, proteases, ferrous iron, and other immunoactive molecules. Similar

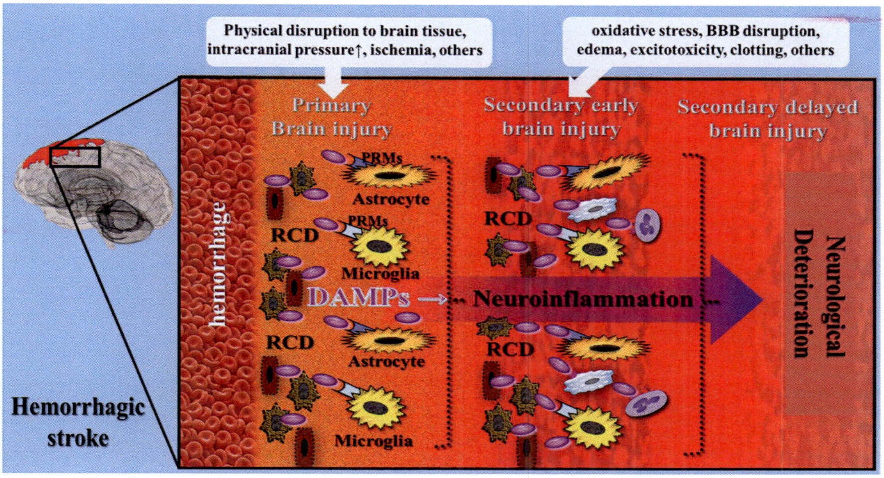

Fig. 11.2 Schematic diagram of a conceptual narrative model illustrating the hemorrhagic stroke-induced emission of DAMPs leading to posthemorrhage neuroinflammatory responses, characterized by involvement of PRM-bearing microglial cells and astrocytes, as well as infiltrating PRM-expressing neutrophils and macrophages. The first wave of DAMPs derives from various cells dying from RCD, occurring during hemorrhage-provoked primary brain injury. The second wave of DAMPs is emitted by various cells dying from RCD, occurring during secondary brain injury and induced by multiple neuroinflammation-promoted pro-death pathways. In subarachnoid hemorrhage, the secondary brain injury occurs in two phases, an early phase and a delayed phase, where posthemorrhage complications can develop and cause neurological deterioration. *BBB* blood-brain barrier, *PRMs* pattern recognition molecules, *RCD* regulated cell death. (Sources: [95, 111–117])

to observations in ischemic stroke, the microglia can switch to an M2-polarized neuroprotective phenotype by promoting hematoma and cell debris absorption and inducing neurogenesis and angiogenesis (reviewed in [112, 113].

Notably, the neuroinflammation-provoked secondary brain injury occurring within the first days of the primary hemorrhagic insult is characterized by complex and complicated processes, including oxidative stress, delayed BBB disruption, excitatory amino acid toxicity, perihematomal edema formation, infiltration of leukocytes, release of hemoglobin, heme, and iron from lysed red blood cells [114, 115]. In addition, by contrast to ischemic stroke and as reviewed by An et al. [95], in ICH, the secondary mechanism of brain injury is related to a clotting cascade, in particular thrombin, after endothelial damage and hemoglobin breakdown. Thrombin causes inflammatory cells to infiltrate the brain, proliferation of mesenchymal cells, and creation of brain edema. Heme influx in the neuron after endothelial damage leads to iron release and neuronal insult [92, 114]. Altogether, one may discuss that this complex secondary brain injury may lead to multiple pro-death pathways, which further contribute to various subroutines of RCD, serving as the source of a secondary wave of DAMP emission (Fig. 11.2).

To add here is that in SAH, this early neuroinflammation-provoked early brain injury may be followed by a secondary delayed phase of brain damage over a period of 3–14 days, reflecting the time frame where, for example, post-SAH complications can develop and cause neurological deterioration (reviewed in [116]).

11.2.4.4 DAMPs in Hemorrhagic Stroke

As could be expected, based on convincing data from experimental and clinical research, DAMPs are pathogenetically involved not only in ischemic but also in hemorrhagic stroke. The molecules are briefly and selectively touched in the following (also see the review of Chaudhry et al. [117]).

Experimental Evidence for a Role of DAMPs in Hemorrhagic Stroke

Studies on experimental ICH or SAH models have revealed the emission of both constitutive and inducible DAMPs which trigger posthemorrhage neuroinflammatory responses; they include HMGB1 [118–120], HSPs [121], S100 proteins [122], peroxiredoxin-1 [123], TNC [124], IL-1β [108], and TNF [125]. Since these molecules (without TNC) have been briefly described above with ischemic stroke, they are not resumed and discussed here further. Instead, some molecules typical for the emission of DAMPs in hemorrhage, that is, heme and fibrinogen, are listed here, which are known to arise from hemorrhage.

Thus, a critical DAMP emitted from lysed erythrocytes in hemorrhagic processes is heme, denoted as a IA-1 DAMP (for additional information, see Vol. 1 [16], Part IV, Sect. 12.2.4.8, p. 237, and also [126]). Plausibly, heme represents a DAMP that may contribute to posthemorrhagic stroke neuroinflammation. So indeed, findings from a study on a mouse ICH model showed that heme potentiates microglial activation via TLR4, in turn inducing NF-κB activation and ultimately increasing cytokine expression and neuroinflammatory responses [127]. Also, fibrinogen, a IIA-3 DAMP (for more details, see Vol. 1 [16], Part IV, Sect. 13.2.4.4, p. 276) was demonstrated to contribute to microglial activation and neuronal damage after stroke [128]. In line with these experimental findings are clinical observations showing that poor-grade aneurysmal SAH patients with reduced admission fibrinogen levels have a higher risk of delayed cerebral ischemia and 6-month mortality compared to those without [129].

Together, these findings highlight the role of red blood cell-derived DAMPs in contributing to the ongoing neuroinflammation in hemorrhagic stroke.

Detection of DAMPs in Patients with Hemorrhagic Stroke

Excitingly, clinical studies in patients with hemorrhagic stroke have also provided ample evidence for the emission of both constitutive and inducible DAMPs that are believed to trigger deleterious posthemorrhage neuroinflammatory responses.

For example, elevated HMGB1 levels were found to be higher in the CSF of patients with an unfavorable clinical outcome after aneurysmal SAH and HMGB1 levels correlated with proinflammatory cytokines suggesting an indispensable role of HMGB1 in ongoing inflammation [130]. Other investigators [131] measured HMGB1 levels in the systemic circulation of patients with aneurysmal SAH and, based on multivariate analysis, showed that the plasma HMGB1 level was an independent predictor of poor functional outcome and mortality after 1 year, in-hospital mortality, and cerebrovasospasm. Indeed, a receiver operating characteristic curve showed that plasma HMGB1 level on admission statistically significantly predicted these outcomes. Given these data, the authors [131] concluded that "HMGB1 level is a useful, complementary tool to predict functional outcome and mortality after aneurysmal subarachnoid hemorrhage. However, HMGB1 determination does not add to the accuracy of prediction of the clinical outcomes." Further clinical data obtained from patients with hemorrhagic stroke, not quoted here, have confirmed these crucial observations.

Other DAMPs already detected in patients with hemorrhagic stroke are S100 proteins. For example, elevated S100B levels were measured in patients with aneurysmal SAH [132]. However, obviously, their clinical usefulness in the diagnosis and prognosis of stroke has a limitation due to its low discriminating ability in stroke diagnosis and prognosis [133]. On the other hand, elevated S100A proteins (S100A12) measured in patients with ICH [134] were found to be positively associated with inflammation, hemorrhagic severity, and short-term mortality, indicating this DAMP to be a biomarker for predicting poor outcome after hemorrhagic stroke.

Mitochondrial DNA has joint the group of DAMPs involved in hemorrhagic stroke. Thus, as reported by Chaudhry et al. [135], systemic levels of mtDNA are elevated in aneurysmal SAH patients and display differential correlations with different aneurysmal SAH-associated characters, complications, and clinical outcome.

11.2.4.5 SAMPs in Hemorrhagic Stroke

Remarkably, there is already some experimental evidence for a role of SAMPs in hemorrhagic stroke. For example, as investigated in the mouse collagenase-induced ICH model, administration of AnxA1 was demonstrated to attenuate brain edema effectively, improve short-term neurological function, and ameliorate microglial activation after ICH [136]. Also, the investigators observed AnxA1 enhancing memory function at 28 days after ICH. In another line of studies on a two-hemorrhage SAH model in rats [137], a beneficial effect of 17beta-estradiol, an adenosine receptor agonist, in the attenuating SAH-induced vasospasm and apoptosis was found and suggested to be due to an increased expression of the adenosine receptor A2AAR, indicating a neuroprotective function of extracellular adenosine in ICH. Again other lines of studies on mouse ICH models provided evidence suggesting that PGE2 may promote neuroprotective responses in hemorrhagic stroke [138, 139].

11.2.4.6 Concluding Remarks

Amazingly, the concluding remarks on the topic of hemorrhagic stroke will be similar to those on ischemic stroke. So, the paramount role of DAMPs in promoting neuroinflammatory responses in ICH or SAH is experimentally well established and has clinically been observed in first orienting studies. Plausibly, this property licenses DAMPs to be used as promising diagnostic and prognostic biomarkers as well as therapeutic targets. Though evidence for a counterbalancing function of

SAMPs is just beginning to be examined, their future use as therapeutics in hemorrhagic stroke can, at least, already be discussed.

11.2.5 Résumé

As stated already in the concluding remarks, the pivotal role of DAMPs in cerebrovascular diseases is well established. This understanding opens the door to new innovative diagnostic and prognostic options. In this context and addressing the role of DAMPs in aneurysmal SAH, Chaudhry et al. [117] stated: "Finally, investigation of the time course of various DAMPs may have a diagnostic and prognostic potential and will be helpful for early identification of the patients at increased risk of developing different complications and achieving poor clinical outcome. Therefore, it will aid in addressing early and aggressive treatment and management in these patients. Further, DAMPs may be used as treatment response markers. Systemic S100B and HMGB1 represent interesting DAMP molecules that have been investigated in aSAH associated complications and may serve as potential biomarkers. Our knowledge, regarding DAMPs and their implication in complex pathophysiological events triggered after brain injury, is still in infancy and further investigations aimed at combined multifaceted role of DAMPs in brain injury after aSAH are warranted."

More difficult to assess is the future use of DAMPs and SAMPs as therapeutic targets and therapeutics, respectively. Choosing DAMPs as therapeutic targets may be considered, in particular, when the whole spectrum of DAMPs in a given situation has been measured. Harnessing SAMPs as therapeutics—should they ever been developed for clinical use—may be indicated, as mentioned above, in case of any recanalization therapies in acute ischemic stroke. However, such treatment strategies should only be considered in compliance with the caveats described in Sect. 7.3.3. Indeed, the observation of a poststroke immunosuppressive syndrome—probably influenced by the generation of SAMPs—should be regarded as a warning sign. The burning issue will be resumed in Sect. 11.4.

11.3 Cardiovascular Diseases: Myocardial Infarction

11.3.1 Introductory Remarks

As cited by the WHO, CHD, together with stroke, are the world's biggest killers, accounting for a combined 15.2 million deaths in 2016 [140]. According to a report from the American Heart Association, referring to data from the *National Health and Nutrition Examination Survey* from 2011 to 2014 [141], an estimated 16.5 million Americans $\geq$20 years of age have a CHD. In 2018, ~720,000 Americans were supposed to have a new coronary event (defined as first hospitalized MI or coronary heart death), and ~335,000 were supposed to have a recurrent event. Certainly, the routine use of early reperfusion strategies has significantly reduced acute mortality in patients with MI. Nonetheless—as will be outlined in this chapter in more details— this achievement in modern MI therapy resulted in the extension of the pool of patients who, although surviving the acute disease, develop detrimental cardiac remodeling and are prone to develop chronic heart failure. In other words, following MI, the two sides, beneficial and detrimental, of DAMP-promoted innate immune events become evident again. The infarct-associated sudden death of up to a billion cardiomyocytes triggers an acute inflammatory → fibrogenic response that, when controlled and regulated, leads to complete scarring repair of the infarcted heart. On the other hand, when uncontrolled and dysregulated, infarction-elicited innate immune responses may result in further pathologies such as infarct expansion, increased cardiac fibrosis → chronic heart failure, and/or systemic inflammation under involvement of other organs (for the two sites of the coin of innate immune responses, also compare Vol. 1 [16], Part II, Sect. 4.4, and Fig. 4.1).

11.3.1.1 Classification of Myocardial Infarction

Acute MI is a classic example of an atherosclerosis-associated acute disease that, with or without ST-segment elevation in the electrocardiogram (ECG) (= STEMI or NSTEMI), has the potential for considerable morbidity and mortality. As an event of myocardial necrosis caused by an unstable ischemic syndrome, STEMI or NSTEMI are further classified into six types: spontaneous infarction due to coronary atherothrombosis, e.g., due to atherosclerotic plaque rupture (type 1); infarction secondary to an ischemic imbalance, e.g., due to a supply–demand mismatch that is not the result of acute atherothrombosis (type 2); infarction causing sudden death without the opportunity for biomarker or ECG confirmation (type 3); infarction related to a percutaneous coronary intervention (PCI) (type 4a); infarction related to thrombosis of a coronary stent (type 4b); and infarction related to coronary artery bypass grafting (type 5) (reviewed in [142, 143]).

11.3.1.2 Clinical Management: A Brief Overview

Following urgent prehospital care of MI-suspected patients and initial inpatient management and treatment (antithrombotic therapy) of ACS, further therapeutic strategies depend on the diagnosis of either STEMI or NSTEMI. Emergency reperfusion of ischemic myocardium that is in the process of becoming infarcted is the most important advance in the treatment of STEMI over the past three decades and is the primary therapeutic goal. Coronary reperfusion is accomplished by means of primary PCI (angioplasty and stenting) or intravenous fibrinolytic therapy. However, given residual perfusion in the ischemic zone in ACS without ST-segment elevation, the urgency of and approach to revascularization differ from that in STEMI. Once a definite or likely diagnosis of an NSTEMI has been made, the patient is triaged to either an invasive strategy or an ischemia-guided strategy (i.e., an initial medical strategy with angiography reserved for evidence of spontaneous or provoked ischemia) (for details, see [143, 144]).

11.3.2 Experimental Models of Myocardial Ischemia and Infarction

11.3.2.1 General Remarks

Animal models of myocardial ischemia and infarction are necessary to understand the complex mechanistic scenario of this cardiovascular event that includes the process of myocardial reperfusion. In particular, such (in vitro or in vivo) models of myocardial ischemia and infarction are valuable tools to analyze and assess—besides the other specific facets of MI—the role of DAMPs in MI. In the following, the models are briefly and selectively addressed; for more in-depth information, the reader is referred to the excellent review article published by Lindsey et al. [145].

11.3.2.2 In Vitro Models

As a useful in vitro model of ischemia → reperfusion, isolated fresh or cultured cardiomyocytes can be used, whereby ischemia is simulated with hypoxia and reperfusion with reoxygenation. This system allows precise control of the specific impact of hypoxia and subsequent reoxygenation on cardiomyocytes without confounding influences of other cell types or circulating factors (reviewed in [145]). The most common use of this model system is for in vitro testing of specific factors proposed to be involved in IRI or cardioprotection, here, for DAMPs and SAMPs. The most common in vitro conditions used to simulate in vivo ischemia are anoxia and complete substrate depletion (serum-free, glucose-free medium). There are many variations to the protocol with additional conditions that more closely mimic the ischemic heart, such as partial hypoxia, partial or no substrate depletion, hyperkalemia, acidosis, and use of electrical stimulation [146]. Nevertheless, even with the most carefully designed experimental protocol, in vitro conditions can never fully recapitulate the full spectrum of IRI in vivo [145].

11.3.2.3 The Isolated Perfused Heart Model

A powerful in vivo model refers to the isolated perfused heart that is a reproducible model to test mechanisms of myocardial injury and cardioprotection [147]. Perfused hearts can be studied in a working heart mode or a nonworking Langendorff mode. In the Langendorff mode, the perfusate enters the coronary arteries to perfuse and oxygenate the heart, which continues to beat for several hours [148], whereas in the working heart mode, the perfusate enters the atrium at a filling pressure set by the operator, and the heart pumps perfusate against a hydrostatic pressure set to different levels [149]. The model has been used with considerable success. For example, much of the information about the molecular signaling pathways responsible for cardioprotection was established in perfused heart models [150].

11.3.2.4 In Vivo Model

As reviewed [145], in vivo models of myocardial ischemia and infarction include models to examine (1) coronary stenosis and stress-induced myocardial ischemia; (2) coronary microembolization; (3) stunning, short-term and chronic hibernation; (4) ischemic cardiomyopathy; and (5) noninvasive imaging. Of special interest here are MI models, that is, permanent coronary artery occlusion with nonreperfused and reperfused MI, which can also be performed in larger animals such as pigs and dogs. Of particular interest is the reperfused MI model that allows estimation of additional myocardial damage by reperfusion, associated with emission of DAMPs.

11.3.2.5 Concluding Remarks

As apparent, there are various in vitro and in vivo models of myocardial ischemia and infarction available, which have been touched only cursorily here but have been extensively reviewed by Lindsey et al. [145]. The authors concluded: " .... all of the approaches described above may be considered good and a gold standard if appropriate to address the target hypothesis. In vitro studies using isolated cardiomyocytes or even isolated organelles ... are well suited to identify single molecular targets of injury and protection ... . isolated, buffer-perfused heart models can be used to study the acute biochemical and functional mechanisms of myocardial I/R injury and cardioprotection. ... Permanent coronary occlusion MI and reperfused MI models are both well suited to study repair and remodeling. I/R models are mandatory to study cardioprotection, and the ischemia must be of sufficient severity and duration to cause some infarction."

11.3.3 Pathogenesis of Myocardial Infarction (in Brief): Inflammation and Fibrosis

The sequelae of pathogenetic events after MI can be divided into three phases. The initial stage encompasses the first minutes to hours or a few days of the acute proinflammatory phase. The inflammation–resolution phase lasts a few days to weeks and consists of the reparative or proresolving phase. Finally, the progression phases persist weeks to months or years depending on the strength of the resolution phase, which, if defective, may lead to left ventricular dysfunction, chronic heart failure, morbidity, and mortality.

In the following sections and guided by review articles of Frangogiannis [151–154], the most important experimental and clinical pathophysiological events are presented which characterize the nature and course of this acute disease: post-infarction inflammation and fibrosis.

In fact, following infarction, sudden death of up to a billion cardiomyocytes triggers a necroinflammatory response that plays a crucial healing role in repair of the infarcted heart but is also implicated in the pathogenesis of adverse ventricular remodeling processes. As typical for various types of aberrant inflammatory responses leading to severe pathologies (here, also compare Vol. 1 [16], Part VI, Sects. 22.2.4 and 22.2.5), excessive, sustained, or dysregulated inflammatory processes following MI were shown to be associated with accentuated dilation and infarct expansion and observed to progress to overshooting fibrosis that may worsen ventricular dysfunction.

Indeed, although improved medical treatment and revascularization/reperfusion strategies have increased the survival rates after acute MI significantly over the last decades [141, 155], patients surviving MI often develop a chronically deteriorating cardiac function as a consequence of left ventricular fibrotic remodeling. This post-MI complication can be defined as the change in shape, size, and function of the left ventricle, characterized by the alteration in the structure of the heart in response to the cardiac injury in association with neurohormonal activation. This serious chronic disease is clinically known to have a poor prognosis that is comparable to or worse than most cancers, a decreased quality of life, and considerable healthcare costs [156].

In the following, the pathogenetic role of DAMPs in these scenarios will be examined and, under the perspective of the book, particularly highlighted.

11.3.4 Post-infarct-Induced Promotion and Resolution of Myocardial Inflammation

11.3.4.1 General Remarks

The pathophysiology of MI is mirrored by distinctly orchestrated and complex series of events, instigated by intense cell death → DAMP-promoted sterile necro-inflammation that transitions into a reparative phase with resolution of inflammation, (myo)fibroblast proliferation, scar formation, and neovascularization.

In this section, the early DAMP-promoted inflammation phase is briefly sketched, which can be regarded as the initial necessary step for the transition to subsequent reparative and proliferative processes.

11.3.4.2 Initiating Mechanisms of Acute Myocardial Infarction

As mentioned in Sect. 10.4.4, the usual initiating mechanism for acute MI is rupture or erosion of a vulnerable, lipid-laden, atherosclerotic coronary plaque, resulting in exposure of circulating blood to highly thrombogenic core and matrix materials in the plaque. More recently—on the basis of postmortem studies and in vivo studies using intravascular imaging— this scenario has been redefined and extended by proposing four pathologic pathways to ACS: (1) plaque rupture with systemic inflammation, (2) plaque rupture without systemic inflammation, (3) plaque erosion, or (4) plaque without thrombus (reviewed in [157–159]). Importantly, this modern view includes the notion that ACS can occur without apparent epicardial coronary artery thrombus or stenosis. Such events may arise from spasm, microvascular disease, or other pathways. Indeed, epicardial coronary vasospasm (also called "functional CAD") may reportedly occur in patients in whom coronary angiography does not demonstrate an obstructive atherosclerotic plaque [160].

11.3.4.3 Myocardial Infarction-Induced Cell Death

In MI, various infarct regions have been defined with different pathophysiology: the central zone and the peri-infarct border zone that are reportedly still perfused [161, 162]. Accordingly, the affected areas of the myocardium are obviously gradually damaged at different degrees resulting in either myocardial ACD or RCD, involving both cardiomyocytes and non-myocytes (Fig. 11.3). However, the occurrence of RCD is not clearly documented, neither in the central nor the border zone.

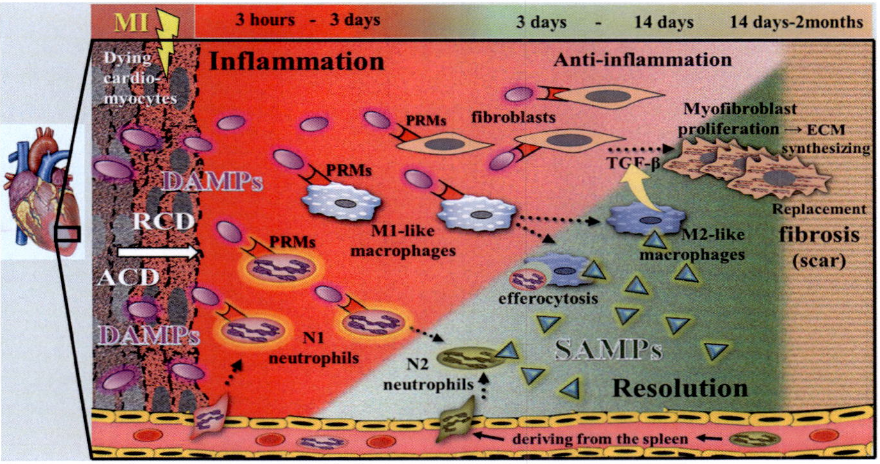

Fig. 11.3 Simplified diagram of a conceptual narrative model of the action of DAMPs and SAMPs in myocardial infarction. Constitutive and inducible DAMPs, emitted by cardiomyocytes dying from ACD or RCD, activate PRM-bearing M1 macrophages, infiltrating N1 neutrophils, and resident fibroblasts (and other cells such as ECs and mast cells not shown) to promote a sterile inflammatory response within the first 3 days following infarction. Following, DAMP-(epigenetically?) driven macrophage polarization and neutrophil phenotype switch lead to generation of M2-like macrophages and N2 neutrophils. These cells, together with neutrophils originating from the spleen, produce SAMPs (i.e., SPMs) that drive resolution of inflammation. This stage (lasting ~3–14 days) is characterized, for example, by promotion of antiinflammatory pathways and phagocytic clearance of the infarct lesion from dead cells, cell debris, and apoptotic neutrophils (efferocytosis). The resolving processes then set the stage for the proliferative phase of cardiac repair (during the next 14 days to ~2 months). In this phase, DAMPs (e.g., TGF-β) promote transdifferentiation of fibroblasts to myofibroblasts that proliferate. In orchestration with other cells such as ECs, mast cells, and M2-like macrophages, myofibroblasts drive fibrotic processes by secreting fibrogenic mediators and ECM proteins (for details of fibrotic processes, see Sects. 6.4 and 6.5, and compare Figs. 6.1 and 6.2). The reparative healing program then ends up with replacement fibrosis forming a scar. *ACD* accidental cell death, *ECM* extracellular matrix, *MI* myocardial infarction, *PRMs* pattern recognition molecules, *RCD* regulated cell death. (Sources: [153, 154, 163, 164, 183, 191, 192, 197, 215, 223, 226])

Coronary Artery Occlusion-Induced Accidental Cell Death

Acute occlusion of the coronary artery in the STEMI patients leads to acute myocardial anoxia and ischemia that, if prolonged more than 20 min, promotes an abrupt reduction in oxygen supply and, thus, cellular energy associated with impairment of the sodium–potassium pump and loss in membrane integrity, the result being subsequent irreversible cardiomyocyte death (reviewed in [163]). It can be assumed, or at least discussed, that such markedly prolonged occlusion of the coronary artery may lead to immediate, irreversible cell death in terms of ACD in an increasing number of parenchymal cells and cardiomyocytes. Subendocardial cardiomyocytes are more susceptible to ischemic injury; thus, a "wave front" of necrosis is noted that extends from the subendocardial area to the subepicardium—as documented by early experiments on dogs which showed that, after 40 min of ischemia, myocyte necrosis was subendocardial but, with increasing duration of coronary occlusion, extends transmurally over time toward the subepicardium [164].

Postischemic Reperfusion-Induced Regulated Cell Death

However, in almost all of the scenarios listed above, the pathophysiology of MI is continued as a typical consequence of IRI creating additional damage, here, to the myocardium, mediated by a burst of ROS—in particular, mitochondria-derived ROS [165, 166]. Thus, the event of reperfusion of the myocardium is either a consequence of successful PCI (angioplasty and stenting) or intravenous fibrinolytic therapy or, in case of "functional CAD," resolution of an epicardial coronary vasospasm (for myocardial IRI, see [167–170]). Along with reperfusion, a maladaptive remodeling phase might occur that is associated with inflammation as well as a reduced ability to recover metabolism homeostasis [171].

As outlined in detail by Hausenloy and Yellon [168], the reperfusion of acutely ischemic myocardium can independently induce cardiomyocyte death, whereby the so-called lethal myocardial reperfusion injury is of particular interest that refers to reperfusion-induced death of cardiomyocytes that were viable at the end of the index ischemic event [172]. This phenomenon is deduced from observations in both experimental MI models and in patients with STEMI, suggesting that lethal myocardial reperfusion injury may account for up to 50% of the final MI size. In the words of Hausenloy and Yellon [168]: "Lethal myocardial reperfusion injury attenuates the full benefits of myocardial reperfusion in terms of MI size reduction and thus represents an important target for cardioprotection in PPCI patients" (PPCI stands for primary percutaneous coronary intervention). Quite expectedly, the process of *lethal myocardial reperfusion injury* is accompanied by induction of various subroutines of RCD (reviewed in [170, 173]; for RCD, see Sect. 4.3 and also Vol. 1 [16], Part V, Chpt. 19). In fact, an early report already suggested that myocardial IRI includes two pivotal mechanisms, including apoptosis and necrosis [174]. Moreover, recent reports have provided accumulating evidence for MI → myocardial IRI-induced subroutines of RN contributing to MI-related inflammation and subsequent remodeling (for recent reviews, see [173, 175]).

Necroptosis

The classic pathway of necroptosis plays an essential role in IRI. Accordingly, this subroutine of RN is reportedly implicated in post-infarct myocardial IRI after MI [176, 177]. For example, as reviewed by Del Re et al. [175], inhibition of necroptosis by necrostatin-1 or global deletion of RIPK3, applied at the time of or before reperfusion in mouse and pig IRI models, was found to reduce infarct size and ameliorate cardiac dysfunction. Interestingly, as recently reported, in addition to the well-established formation of complexes involving RIP3, RIP1, and MLKL (compare Sect. 4.3.3 and [22] Fig. 4.2; for additional information, see Vol. 1, Part V [16], Sect. 19.3.2, p. 436 , and Fig. 19.4, p. 437), RIP3 can also trigger myocardial necroptosis through activation of *Ca^{2+}/calmodulin-dependent protein kinase II* (CaMKII). CaMKII is a newly identified RIP3 substrate that helps delineate a RIP3 → CaMKII → MPT pore myocardial necroptosis pathway (for details, see [176]).

Ferroptosis

Perhaps more intense than necroptosis, ferroptosis is considered a key factor in the pathogenesis of IRI-evoked disorders (compare Sect. 4.3.4 and Fig. 4.2a, b and [22] and Fig. 4.3; for additional information, see Vol. 1 [16], Part V, Sect. 19.3.3, p. 442, and Fig. 19.6, p. 445). Accordingly, this iron-dependent RN has also been discussed to be involved in MI-associated myocardial IRI [178]. Indeed, five studies involving ferroptosis are directly relevant to the heart (reviewed in [175]). For example, in first in vitro experiment on cultured adult mouse cardiomyocytes, it could be demonstrated that the mechanistic target of rapamycin plays an important role in protecting cardiomyocytes against excess iron and ferroptosis [179]. Another recent study could show that the ferroptosis inhibitor ferrostatin-1 reduces cardiomyocyte death both in heart transplantation and the traditional coronary artery ligation IRI models in vivo [180]. So, further studies on in vivo MI models are required in order to confirm these first observations and establish therapies that could target this iron-dependent RN more efficiently in MI.

Pyroptosis

A growing body of evidence has been reported indicating a pivotal role of NLRP3 inflammasome-mediated cardiomyocyte pyroptosis in post-MI-occurring inflammatory and fibrogenic responses (see [181–185]; for more information about the pyroptotic death pathway, also compare Sects. 2.2.5 and Sect. 4.3.5 and Fig. 2.1 and Fig. 4 in [22] and; for additional information, see Vol. 1, Part V [16], Sect. 19.3.4, p. 447, and Fig. 19.7, p. 448). For example, Lei et al. [182], as a synopsis of in vitro and in vivo studies on MI models in rats, could demonstrate that NLRP3 inflammasome-mediated pyroptosis is critical in the process of cardiomyocyte loss induced by MI and further that the NF-κB → GSDMD axis functions as a bridge between oxidative stress (as inducer) and NLRP3 inflammasome- mediated cardiomyocyte pyroptosis. Nevertheless, the cell types in which inflammasome assembly and the resulting release of DAMPs occur remain elusive. Indeed, it appears that inflammasome assembly is significantly more robust in non-cardiomyocytes such as macrophages and fibroblasts that infiltrate into the heart during infarction, as compared to cardiomyocytes themselves [186, 187].

NETosis

Ultimately, it should not go unmentioned that a role of NETosis in MI has also been reported [188, 189]. For example, in studies on coronary plaque segments of acute MI patients, NETs were found to be present in all types of complicated, but not in intact, plaques [188]. They were found in thrombus, hemorrhages, and at the thrombus–plaque interface, with no significant differences in extent between ruptures, erosions, and intraplaque hemorrhages. Interestingly, the investigators also observed adjacent perivascular tissue of complicated, but not of intact, plaques to contain high numbers of NETs.

In Sum

These impressive experimental observations indicate that the different forms of RCD serve as sources of emission of constitutive and inducible DAMPs, which can trigger necroinflammatory and (necro)fibrotic responses involved in the pathogenesis of MI. Again, as discussed previously in the context of other diseases, the molecular mechanisms responsible for the development of the inflammatory and fibrogenic processes are still not fully understood, but there is growing evidence in support of the notion that the DAMPs play a vital role in these pathologies.

11.3.4.4 DAMP-Induced Lesional Inflammation

In MI, as already mentioned above, emission of constitutive DAMPs, released by cardiac cells dying from ACD and RCD, as well as inducible DAMPs secreted by activated cells, triggers proinflammatory responses which—under involvement of PRM-expressing phagocytosing cells and fibroblasts—serve to clear the wound and initiate wound healing that proceeds to fibrogenesis resulting in final fibrosis (Fig. 11.3). In fact, sterile myocardial inflammation is a typical pathological event following MI in successfully treated surviving patients (for reviews, see [154, 190–192]).

Many of the cellular and molecular pathways implicated in the post-infarct sterile inflammatory response comply substantially with the DAMP-induced, PRM-bearing cell-mediated efferent innate immune responses as comprehensively outlined in Vol. 1 [16], Part III and Part VI. For example, in MI, constitutive and inducible DAMPs interacting with PRMs on/in myocardial sessile and mobile innate immune cells (such as surviving parenchymal cells, ECs, fibroblasts, M1-like macrophages, mast cells, and infiltrating leukocytes) have been described to promote (1) recruitment of inflammatory cells (e.g., via leukocyte-endothelial interaction); (2) secretion of proinflammatory mediators, including cytokines, chemokines, and cell adhesion molecules; and (3) leukocyte/macrophage –performed phagocytic clearance of the infarct lesion from dead cells and cell debris. In addition, these DAMPs were shown to activate the complement cascade (see [152, 153, 193–196]).

Interestingly, in recent studies on the various phenotypes of neutrophils harvested and isolated from the infarcted left ventricle of mice, cardiac neutrophils could be demonstrated showing a predominantly proinflammatory N1 phenotype [197]. Of note, further findings observed in these studies revealed that DAMPs released from necrotic myocytes promote polarization of neutrophils to this proinflammatory N1 phenotype, which can be regarded as functionally cooperating partner cells of M1-like macrophages (Fig. 11.3).

As a key player in mounting post-MI sterile inflammation, again, the DAMP-activated NLRP3 inflammasome was identified whose formation typically requires the two independent steps: priming and triggering. In the heart, NLRP3 and the other inflammasome components are located in cardiomyocytes, leukocytes, and other non-cardiomyocyte resident cells such as fibroblasts and ECs (reviewed in [198]; for NLRP3 inflammasome, compare Sect. 2.2.5 and Fig. 2.1 and also Vol. 1, [16], Part VI, Sect. 22.4.2 and Fig. 22.11). Although most data for a role of the

NLRP3 inflammasome in MI derive from preclinical studies, some information about its activation in patients in the context of MI was provided by measurement of plasma levels of NLRP3 and caspase 1 [199] (for further details, see below).

11.3.4.5 DAMP-Induced Systemic Inflammation

A typical complication of acute MI is the induction of AKI that occurs in 16% of patients and is associated with altered synchrony between the heart and kidney (for AKI, see Sect. 9.4). Indeed, the MI-induced bi-directional interaction between progressive left ventricle remodeling and kidney dysfunction is considered a cardiorenal network as a unique momentum of comprehensive systems biology that integrates with renal dysfunction and increases inflammatory markers in heart failure [200, 201]. Of note, the background of this complication may refer to profound post-infarct systemic inflammatory responses as revealed by determination in the plasma of MI patients of (1) cytokines including the inducible DAMPs TNF [202] and IL-1β [203]; (2) chemokines such as MCP-1, fractalkine/CX3CR1, and CCL4, CXCL16, and CXCL10 [204]; and (3) adhesion molecules such as ICAM-1 and VCAM-1 [205] (also reviewed by Fang et al. in [206]; for chemokines, for additional information, compare Vol. 1, [16], Part VI, Sect. 22.5.11, p. 552, and Tables 22.1/22.2, p. 553). The detection of these inflammatory mediators in plasma is generally believed to be due to their release from the infarction lesion. However, one may also discuss that they are produced by extramyocardial innate immune cells that are activated by DAMPs released from the MI lesion into the circulation. For example, plasma levels of key DAMPs such as HMGB1 [207], S100A8/9 and S100A12 [208, 209], nDNA and mtDNA [210, 211], and HSPB7 [212] have documented in patients with ACS and acute MI, respectively (for DAMPs as biomarkers in CVD, see also Sect. 11.4.2.3).

Also and of high interest is a report showing that post-MI systemic inflammation can accelerate and aggravate atherosclerosis [213]: in experiments on ApoE KO mice, the investigators could show that after MI (or stroke !), the animals developed larger atherosclerotic plaque lesions with a more advanced morphology. This disease acceleration was observed to persist over many weeks and to be associated with markedly increased monocyte recruitment. On their search for a plausible explanation of this observation, the authors found that MI may liberate hematopoietic stem and progenitor cells from bone marrow niches via SNS signaling. The progenitors then seeded the spleen yielding a sustained boost in monocyte production.

It should not be forgotten to note here that—besides systemic inflammatory responses—systemic DC-triggered autoimmune pathways have been suggested to be involved in the pathophysiology of MI. Indeed, cardiac-specific autoreactive T cells were shown to get activated by mature DCs following MI [214]. As concluded by the authors, this finding could be used as a future therapeutic strategy to limit the onset of pathological cardiac autoimmunity following MI. Of course, further studies are needed to prove that the potential involvement of autoimmune processes does really extend or exacerbate the primary infarction-mediated injury.

11.3.4.6 SAMP-Controlled and SAMP-Uncontrolled Resolution of Post-infarct Inflammation

Following the rules as established in modern inflammation research, post-infarct promotion of inflammation is reportedly also counterbalanced with resolution of inflammation. This process is mainly regulated by cardioprotectively operating resident cardiac M2-like macrophages and N2 neutrophils that were polarized from M1-like macrophages and N1 neutrophils, respectively, to produce SAMPs (i.e., SPMs) (compare Fig. 11.3) [197, 215–219]. In other words, the initial DAMP-promoted proinflammatory response is immediately followed by SAMP-driven inflammation-resolving processes which can be regarded as transition processes leading to final healing tissue repair and homeostasis (for SAMPs, see Sect. 5.3.3 and Fig. 5.1; for additional information, see Vol. 1, [16], Part IV, Sect. 14.4, p. 330, and Part VI, Sect. 22.2.3, p. 480, and Fig. 22.1, p. 477). This SAMP-driven and SAMP-regulated resolution of inflammation is believed to also occur in cases of normal post-MI healing without any further complications (discussed in [151, 220, 221]). Support for this concept comes from studies on a murine model of experimental coronary occlusion, demonstrating that efferocytosis is implicated in resolution by bridging clearance of dying cardiac cells to subsequent repair and, in turn, mitigating progression to heart failure (reviewed in [222]). Moreover, in another set of supportive studies on a murine model of MI, the investigators showed that post-MI, SPMs (LXs, RVs, MaRs, and Pds) are produced by leukocytes that were mobilized from the spleen to the infarcted heart (compare Fig. 11.3). Macrophages were observed to be necessary for SPM generation because specific depletion of macrophages was associated with the lack of SPM biosynthesis [223]. Of note, the authors further demonstrated that the plethora of SPMs in the spleen before MI and the increase of SPMs in the infarcted left ventricle within 24 h after MI are temporally correlated with the resolution of inflammation (also see Sect. 11.3.6.4).

However, under certain circumstances, similar to disturbed resolution of inflammation in atherosclerosis (compare Sect. 10.4.8), nonresolving chronic inflammation—reflecting a preponderance of DAMPs possibly due to inferior production of SAMPs—may develop that is considered a significant trigger of post-MI pathologies such as adverse remodeling leading to advanced heart failure. In other words, in these cases, the myocardium is unable to restore homeostasis. This nonresolving inflammatory scenario is mirrored by pronounced leukocytosis as a cardinal sign of post-MI inflammation and sustained leukocytosis, which has emerged as a powerful predictor of morbidity and mortality in patients with advanced heart failure [224]. Moreover, and importantly, the SAMP *15-epi-LXA4* levels were observed to be lower than normal values in patients experiencing the progressive development of chronic heart failure due to the defective resolution of inflammation [225]. There is growing experimental evidence in support of these clinical observations, confirming that adequate resolution of inflammation can be pathologically disturbed in MI, thereby promoting persistent post-MI inflammation [221, 224]. For example, recent in vitro experiments and studies on an MI model in mice provided convincing evidence for a role of the SAMP *15-epi-lipoxin A4* in early activation of the resolving phase in post-MI healing [226] (see below).

11.3.4.7 Epigenetic Modifications in Post-infarct Inflammation

Of note, recent studies have provided accumulating evidence indicating that epigenetic regulation is critically involved in the pathogenesis of ischemic reperfusion-induced tissue injury, including IHD (reviewed by Tang and Zhang in [227]; see also Sect. 5.6).

For example, in several studies, aberrant DNA methylation was identified in ACS and CHD [228–230]. In one of such studies [228], a novel and reproducible relationship between ACS and blood methylation levels at 47 CpG sites was uncovered (for DNA methylation at CpG islands, compare Fig. 5.4). Given this data, the authors suggested that immune signaling and cellular functions might be regulated at an epigenetic level in ACS. Also, growing studies have revealed a crucial role of reversible protein acetylation involving in pathological cardiac remodeling in the settings of IRI. For example, acetylation induced by HDACs was found to be implicated in IHD, as shown by blunting pathological cardiac remodeling in the settings of pressure overload and IRI (reviewed in [231]). Mechanistically, the authors of this article discussed that HDAC inhibitors reduce stress-induced cardiomyocyte death, hypertrophy, and ventricular fibrosis (for HDACs, compare Fig. 5.4).

11.3.4.8 Concluding Remarks

Together, as briefly overviewed in this section, the classical sequelae of events involved in the scenario of injury-induced inflammation are also operating in MI-triggered inflammation, as there are initial mechanisms of arterial occlusion/IRI-conveying tissue injury → occurrence of ACD and subroutines of RCD → emission of DAMPs to trigger promotion of inflammation and generation of SAMPs to drive controlled repairing or uncontrolled pathological resolution of inflammation. Uncontrolled resolution of inflammation following MI can transition to fibrosis as reflected by adverse left ventricular remodeling that constitutes the structural basis for ischemic heart failure. In the following section, these pathological processes are briefly described by highlighting the potential role of DAMPs.

11.3.5 Myocardial Infarction-Induced Cardiac Fibrosis

11.3.5.1 General Remarks: The Sequelae of Cardiac Remodeling

Not surprisingly, cardiac fibrosis has been identified as an autonomous risk factor in heart failure: it predisposes heart failure patients to sudden cardiac death, for example, caused by fibrosis-induced arrhythmia, and increases overall mortality independently of the ejection fraction [232]. Thus, a closer look at this chronic disease is mandatory.

In response to MI, the injury-induced, DAMP-orchestrated wound healing response of the left ventricle is characterized by four overlapping phases, whereby the (1) initial inflammatory response (during the initial minutes to hours or few days) is followed by an (2) inflammation-resolving process (lasting a few days to weeks) that proceeds to a (3) proliferative phase marked by fibroblast proliferation and migration to the site of injury and ends up with a (4) maturation phase (lasting weeks to months or years depending on the resolution phase). This final maturation phase is characterized by cardiac ECM remodeling, fibroblast-to-myofibroblast phenotype conversion, and de novo ECM synthesis (Fig. 11.3; also compare Sects. 6.3 and 6.4). In fact, cardiac fibrosis—like sterile myocardial inflammation—is generally considered a typical event following MI.

Of note, however, the post-infarct fibrogenic response can be classified into two types of fibrosis, namely, reparative (replacement) and reactive fibrosis, both of which are mediated by fibroblast → myofibroblast transdifferentiation (discussed and reviewed in [154, 190–192, 233, 234]). Replacement fibrosis refers to a controlled repairing response that leads to wound healing without further complications and is observed in successfully treated surviving patients (compare Fig. 11.3). By contrast, reactive fibrosis is an uncontrolled and dysregulated progredient fibrogenic response that may result in late heart failure (compare Fig. 11.4; and for reviews, see [151, 154, 190–192]). This deleterious version of fibrosis after MI is further discussed in Sect. 11.3.5.4.

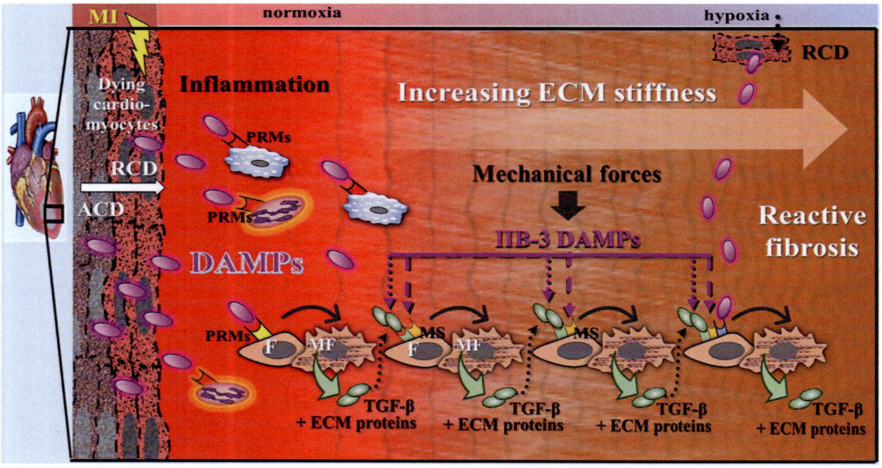

Fig. 11.4 Simplified diagram of a conceptual narrative model of DAMP-driven self-perpetuating processes in post-MI reactive fibrosis. DAMPs, emitted by cardiomyocytes dying from ACD or RCD, activate PRM-bearing innate immune cells such as proinflammatory macrophages, neutrophils, and fibroblasts, which transdifferentiate to myofibroblasts. The sterile inflammatory response—via chronic nonresolving inflammatory and fibrogenic responses—proceeds to progressive ECM formation. Increasing ECM stiffness is associated with enhanced mechanical/tensile forces reflecting the presence of dyshomeostatic IIB-3 DAMPs. These DAMPs activate mechanosensitive sensors (such as integrins and transient receptor potential channels, not shown) that trigger mechanotransduction-mediated positive feed-forward loops that contribute to further activation of myofibroblasts which, in turn, promote profibrotic ECM stiffness (also compare Fig. 6.1). Also, IIB-3DAMPs promote integrin-mediated release of TGF-β from the ECM that contributes to transdifferentiation of fibroblasts into contractile myofibroblasts to secrete further ECM components and TGF-β (also compare Fig. 6.2). Finally, severe fibrosis-associated hypoxia may result in RCD serving as a continuous source of DAMPs emission in very late post-infarct phases. *ACD* accidental cell death, *ECM* extracellular matrix, *MI* myocardial infarction, *MS* mechanosensors, *PRMs* pattern recognition molecules, *RCD* regulated cell death, *TGF-β* transforming growth factor-beta. (Sources: [154, 253–262])

11.3.5.2 The Role of DAMPs in Cardiac Fibrosis

As with all forms of injury-induced fibrotic tissue remodeling, cardiac fibrosis is considered the result of a classical fibrogenic response upon global cardiomyocyte injury, whereby DAMPs, during the proliferative phase of infarct healing, were shown to promote stimulation of fibroblast proliferation and migration, transdifferentiation into myofibroblasts, as well as activation of macrophages (M1-like → M2-like macrophages [154, 235, 236] (for the role of DAMPs in tissue repair and fibrosis, see Sects. 6.4 and 6.5, and also compare Vol. 1 [16], Part VIII, Chpt. 36 and Figs. 36.1 and 36.2). Indeed, there is a considerable body of evidence suggesting a pivotal role of DAMPs in the development of post-infarct cardiac fibrosis. For example, in experiments on necrotic myocardial cells containing multiple DAMPs, including HMGB1, S100A8, S100A9, GAL-3, and IL-1α, the necrotic cells were found to provoke a significant increase in fibroblast proliferation, α-SMA activation, and *COL1A1* and *COL3A1* mRNA expression [237].

Also, it should be noted here that there is some, though rather weak, evidence provided by experimental MI models suggesting a role of several fibrogenic growth factors and neurohumoral mediators—denoted as inducible DAMPs in this book—in the contribution to cardiac fibrosis via stimulating fibroblast proliferation, migration, and activation, as well as triggering their conversion into myofibroblast. They include inducible DAMPs such as TNF, members of the IL-1 family, ET-1, NE, and Ang II (reviewed in [154, 191, 236, 238, 239]) (for ET-1, NE, and Ang II, see also Sects. 3.5.3.5 and 3.5.3.6; for more details on DAMPs, see Sect. 11.3.6).

The favorable role of DAMPs in MI is impressively documented by their ability to promote replacement fibrosis. As mentioned above, this type of post-infarct fibrosis reflects the end result of a lesional reparative response to primary necrotic injury of cardiomyocytes. In terms of a collagen-based scar formation, this type of fibrosis is a beneficial process: after a transmural infarction, the fibrous scar is critical to protect the heart from rupture, by preserving the structural integrity of the ventricle and by protecting from dilative remodeling [240, 241]. Indeed, this is a vital step: as adult mammalian hearts have poor regenerative capacity, the loss of a significant number of cardiomyocytes must necessarily trigger a reparative program, leading to a life-saving formation of fibrous tissue (compare Fig. 11.3).

11.3.5.3 The Cellular Effectors of Cardiac Fibrosis and Their Activation by DAMPs

As already frequently mentioned and here stressed again, there is accumulating evidence for DAMPs to promote the transdifferentiation of fibroblasts into secretory and contractile cells termed myofibroblasts (believed mostly derived from resident populations), a process that is considered a major cellular event in fibrogenesis. As touched in Sects. 6.1 and 6.4.2, this process is characterized by the expression and incorporation of contractile proteins such as α-SMA into the cytoskeleton and the synthesis and deposition of structural and matricellular ECM proteins (also compare Fig. 6.1). Following activation by DAMPs, myofibroblasts promote the fibrotic response in MI (but also many other conditions associated with cardiac inflammation and heart failure) (see [154, 242, 243]; and for PRM-bearing fibroblasts/myofibroblasts and their different origins, see Vol. 1 [16], Part III, Sect. 9.3, and compare

Fig. 9.1). Additionally, several other cell types such as macrophages, mast cells, ECs, and cardiomyocytes are reportedly also implicated in fibrotic remodeling of the heart, either by secreting fibrogenic mediators and matricellular proteins or, in some cases, by undergoing conversion to activated myofibroblasts (reviewed in [154]) (for additional information, compare also Vol. 1 [16], Part VIII, Sect. 36.2, p. 845, and Fig. 36.1, p. 846).

Doubtlessly, however, it is the activated myofibroblasts that can be regarded as one of the main sources of collagen and other structural ECM protein production in cardiac fibrosis. These PRM-bearing cells of the innate immune system have been identified as vital cellular components of replacement fibrosis, in particular, of post-MI left ventricular remodeling, due to their location, numbers, and ECM scar-generating capabilities (compare Fig. 11.3). These cells regulate matrix remodeling by producing preferentially cytokines, chemokines, and proteases, such as MMPs and their inhibitors (reviewed in [233, 244, 245]).

The exact role of DAMPs in the MI-dependent transdifferentiation of PRM-bearing fibroblasts into myofibroblasts, particularly what subclasses of DAMPs are involved, is not entirely clear. Nevertheless, there is first experimental evidence suggesting a role of constitutive DAMPs such as HMGB1 [246, 247], NLRP3-activating DAMPs [248–250], and ED-A fibronectin [251] in the activation of cardiac fibroblasts (for more details, see below). Interestingly, in in vitro and in vivo studies, the function of the inducible DAMPs TNF and IL-1β on fibroblasts has also been documented but shown to vary.

Another crucial population of PRM-bearing innate immune cells involved in cardiac fibrosis is DAMP-activated macrophages known to produce large amounts of profibrotic growth factors, such as TGF-β, but also proteases and modified ECM proteins [154]. Especially, polarized M2-like macrophages in the myocardium have been argued to be associated with cardiac fibrogenesis [252]. Besides myofibroblasts and macrophages, other innate immune cells such as mast cells, granulocytes, and ECs were found to contribute to cardiac fibrosis and are supposed to be activated by DAMPs (reviewed in [154]); they are not further alluded to here (for further details of the role of DAMPs in activating fibroblasts and macrophages, see Sect. 11.3.6).

11.3.5.4 Evidence for a Detrimental Role of DAMPs in Post-infarct Reactive Fibrosis

As mentioned above, MI-associated cardiomyocyte injury not only always results in a controlled beneficial fibrotic replacement response but can also lead to a dysregulated detrimental process known as reactive fibrosis. This type of fibrosis, also called interstitial/perivascular fibrosis, develops in areas remote to infarction spared from initial cell death-induced necroinflammation. Reactive fibrosis is generally thought to be the result of prolonged or uncontrolled chronic inflammation in terms of nonresolving inflammation or other post-infarct injurious stimuli such as mechanical stress due to pressure overload, myocardial inflammation, or metabolic dysregulation (for chronic inflammation in terms of nonresolving inflammation, compare again Sect. 5.5).

The Concept of a DAMP-Driven Self-Perpetuating Process in Progressive Fibrosis

Here, however, one should discuss another mechanistic approach to this severe complication of MI that has already been presented in Chap. 6: the phenomenon of a DAMP-driven self-perpetuating process in fibrosis. According to this model approach, DAMPs, initially released during MI from infarction-associated ACD and IRI-induced RCD of cardiomyocytes, promote fibrogenic responses, which may subsequently transition to progressive fibrosis in terms of a self-perpetuating process. As summarized in Sect. 6.5.5 and illustrated in Figs. 6.1 and 6.2 and resumed here, three mechanisms occurring in parallel may be involved in such a process (Fig. 11.4): First, there is growing evidence suggesting that increasing ECM stiffness, associated with enhanced tension force generated by interaction with contractile myofibroblasts, generates mechanical stimuli in terms of putative cell-extrinsic dyshomeostatic IIB-3 DAMPs which activate mechanosensitive sensors such as integrins and TRPs (reviewed in [253]). These sensors trigger then mechanotransduction-mediated positive feed-forward loops that may contribute to activation of myofibroblasts, which in turn can promote profibrotic ECM stiffness. Second, via similar mechanisms, IIB-3DAMP-promoted, integrin-mediated release of TGF-β from the ECM (and consequent availability of soluble TGF-β) triggers signaling pathways that contribute to transdifferentiation of fibroblasts into contractile myofibroblasts to secrete further ECM components and TGF-β (also compare Fig. 6.2). In this way, integrin-mediated cell tensile force causes a steady release of the active TGF-β that drives Smad-dependent and Smad-independent signaling pathways in other fibroblasts (compare Fig. 6.3). Third, fibrotic tissues, in general, are associated with microvascular rarefication and diminished perfusion. This leads to decreased microvasculature that is often associated with chronic hypoxia, which may result in RCD serving as a continuous source of DAMP emission.

Evidence in Support of the Concept of a DAMP-Driven Self-Perpetuating Process in Reactive Fibrosis

Indeed, evidence in support of this concept has been reported or is at least discussed (compare [154, 254–257]). Of great interest is the observation that cardiac fibroblasts can respond to mechanical cues and physical forces deriving from the cardiac ECM [258]. In fact, in response to increased stiffness of the fibrosing myocardium and the resulting increased transmission of forces between fibroblasts and the ECM, cardiac fibroblasts were shown to convert to the myofibroblast phenotype. Various mechanotransduction pathways appear to be engaged in this process, whereby integrins, TRPs, and Piezo 1 have already been described as possible triggering sensors. Indeed, these mechanosensors were shown to play a role in cardiac fibrosis and a heart failing process induced by MI (for a comprehensive review, see Saucerman et al. [253] and also further Refs. [259, 260]; for mechanosensors such as TRPs, Piezo 1, and integrins, see Sects. 2.4.2 and 2.4.4). As comprehensively reviewed by Frangogiannis [154], cardiac fibroblasts can sense changes in ECM composition and stiffness by activating promiscuous integrin or PG receptors that initiate or modulate signaling cascades. Moreover, as further discussed by Frangogiannis

[154], a substantial body of evidence suggests a critical role of focal adhesion complexes (i.e., FAK) and the RhoA/ROCK pathway in the pathogenesis of cardiac fibrosis. Also, the SRF/MRTF axis has been suggested to play a dominant role in the regulation of α-SMA transcription and subsequent myofibroblast conversion, through interactions that may involve Smad3 and the Rho/ROCK system (for FAK, Rho/ROCK, and SRF/MRTF pathways, compare Sects. 6.3.3 and 6.3.4 and Fig. 6.1). Other lines of evidence also presented in [154] suggest that both the canonical and noncanonical TGF-β-triggered signaling pathways mediate cardiac fibrosis (see Sect. 6.5.3 and Figs. 6.2 and 6.3). These interesting observations are in support of the unproven possibility that post-MI reactive fibrosis, once established, is sustained by the action of cell-extrinsic dyshomeostatic DAMPs, which are continuously generated by increasing tensile forces and provoked by ECM ↔ myofibroblast interaction. It would be these IIB-3 DAMPs that contribute to a permanent activation of cardiac fibroblasts as well as their transdifferentiated myofibroblasts (for IIB-3 DAMPs, compare Sect. 3.4.3.3).

Besides the possible contribution of mechanotransduction-mediated pathways to progredient reactive fibrosis, another mechanism may also play a role: the known phenomenon that fibrotic tissue is often associated with a hypoxic milieu that may lead to various subroutines of hypoxia-induced RCD as a source of further DAMP release. Indeed, evidence has been reported indicating that chronic hypoxia may drive the process of fibrosis leading to scarring and compromised organ function (reviewed in [261, 262]).

Finally, it should be noted here that in MI, activation of interstitial cells and cardiomyocytes can produce and activate proteolytic enzymes, which together with an intense inflammatory reaction trigger degradation of the native cardiac ECM, resulting in the generation of matrix fragments acting as ECM-derived DAMPs (see below).

Clinical Consequences of Reactive Fibrosis

The concept of the DAMP-driven self-perpetuating process in reactive fibrosis deserves special attention because it is an urgent topic clinically. So, reactive interstitial fibrotic changes in the infarct border zone and in the remote uninjured myocardium are typically associated with diastolic dysfunction, altered chamber compliance, and increased ventricular stiffness, thereby compromising cardiac output. Of note, this type of fibrosis is also characterized by parallel expansion of connective tissue associated with deposition of ECM components in areas remote to the infarction site, indicating an active fibrogenic/fibrotic process (outlined in [154, 192]).

Notably, it is the ECM composition of the fibrotic heart that determines the mechanical properties of the ventricle and may regulate detrimental cellular function. As outlined in [154, 245], increased deposition of ECM proteins as the hallmark of fibrotic changes facilitates the progression of arrhythmia and cardiac dysfunction.

11.3.5.5 Epigenetic Regulation of Cardiac Fibrosis

The emerging impact of epigenetic regulation on fibrotic processes has briefly been outlined in Sect. 6.6. Here, a few remarks are briefly and selectively added on the implication of epigenetic modifications in cardiac fibrosis, by focusing on epigenetic regulation of stress-induced inflammation and fibroblast activation (for reviews, see [263–266]). From the perspective of the book, this is a burning topic in so far as DAMPs are currently discussed to promote a critical feature of the innate immune system, namely, trained immunity (see Sect. 5.6.2.3, and compare Vol. 1 [16], Part VI, Sect. 24.2.4).

Indeed, DNA methylation, histone acetylation, histone methylation, and activity of miRNAs and specific ncRNAs are currently appreciated as epigenetic events that may contribute to the pathogenesis of cardiac fibrosis and heart failure. Of critical importance are studies focusing on epigenetic modulation of myofibroblast differentiation that have mostly concentrated on the regulation of α-SMA gene expression.

DNA Methylation

Evidence for a role of DNA methylation in cardiac fibrosis has already been provided by studies on models of hypoxia-induced epigenetic modifications associated with cardiac tissue (reviewed in [264]). In recent studies on in vitro and in vivo MI models [267], α-SMA could be demonstrated to be overexpressed and DNMT1 expression downregulated in the infarct area after MI (for DNA methylation, compare Sect. 5.6.3.2 and Fig. 5.4). Also, treatment of cardiac fibroblast with TGF-β1 in vitro was found to upregulate α-SMA expression via epigenetic modifications. The investigators further observed that TGF-β1 can inhibit DNMT1 expression and activity during cardiac fibroblast differentiation and α-SMA expression is regulated by DNMT1. Conversely, increasing DNMT1 expression levels were shown to rescue the TGF-β1-induced upregulation of α-SMA expression. Given these findings, the authors concluded that inhibition of the DNMT1-mediated DNA methylation of the α-SMA promoter plays an essential role in differentiation of cardiac fibroblasts.

Histone Acetylation and Deacetylation

Accumulating evidence has demonstrated that HDACs are dysregulated in cardiac fibrosis (histone acetylation and deacetylation; compare Sect. 5.6.3.3 and Fig. 5.4). Whereas studies examining the role of HATs in fibrogenesis of the heart are missing, an accumulating body of in vivo evidence using small molecule HDAC inhibitors has been demonstrated to potently block cardiac fibroblast proliferation in association with enhanced histone acetylation and expression of antiproliferative genes and mitigate fibrotic remodeling in response to cardiac injury [263, 268–270]. Other lines of studies (reviewed in [271]) showed that downregulation of HDAC1 and HDAC2 could attenuate cardiac fibrosis in rat primary cardiac fibroblasts and in hypertensive mice and that suppression of HDAC3 limits ventricular fibrosis.

MicroRNAs and Long Noncoding RNAs

A growing body of evidence has also indicated that the expression of miRNAs and specific ncRNAs is strongly correlated with the onset and progression of cardiac fibrosis (reviewed in [264, 272, 273]; also compare Sects. 5.6.4 and 5.6.5, as well as Fig. 5.5 and 5.6). For example, in studies on a mouse model for coronary artery occlusion and reperfusion, evidence was presented documenting changes in miR expression following myocardial IRI in vivo [274]. The investigators conducted comprehensive expression profiling to identify clusters of miRs that significantly changed in expression on days 2 and 7 post-IRI and noted that IRI rapidly induces miR-21 in the heart and elevated miR-21 levels on day 7 post-IRI as well.

In other sets of studies, including experiments on an MI model [275], expression of the noncoding RNA *lncR-30245* was demonstrated to be significantly increased in MI hearts and TGF-β1-treated cardiac fibroblasts. The lncRNA tested was found to be mainly located in the cytoplasm and, when overexpressed, to promote collagen production and cardiac fibroblast proliferation. Moreover, the researchers observed that knockdown of *lncR-30245* significantly inhibits TGF-β1-induced collagen production and cardiac fibroblast proliferation.

In Sum

The impressive findings from experimental research in epigenetics involved in cardiac fibrosis have raised considerable interest in treating cardiac fibrosis in patients. However, proposals to treat cardiac fibrosis and heart failure with small-molecule inhibitors of epigenetic regulators are often met with skepticism because the regulators to be targeted are ubiquitously expressed and vital and govern fundamental physiological transcriptional mechanisms in a multitude of cell types. Confronted with this problem, Felisbino et al. [266] concluded: "Advances in the basic science of epigenetics, nonhistone epigenetic marks, and cardiac fibrosis promise to be rapidly forthcoming and to facilitate the clinical translation of innovative "epigenetic therapies" for patients who have heart disease."

11.3.5.6 Concluding Remarks

Together, heart failure associated with cardiac fibrosis, most often caused by MI, is a significant public health issue that affects more than 23 million people globally [276]. The problem here is that the adult mammalian heart has a minimal capacity to regenerate after injury and the lost cardiomyocytes are replaced by epigenetically regulated fibrotic tissue of the surrounding myocardium that may eventually lead to heart failure. Although the molecular signals and environmental cues that drive the dramatic phenotypic changes of cardiac fibroblasts in remodeling hearts following MI are not precisely identified yet, there is increasing evidence suggesting a role of DAMPs in activating those effector cells in cardiac fibrosis. To confirm this concept, more targeted studies have to be done on the role of DAMPs as main players in the development of post-infarct reactive fibrosis.

11.3.6 DAMPs and SAMPs in Myocardial Infarction

11.3.6.1 General Remarks

Current conceptual notions hold that emission of proinflammatory and profibrotic DAMPs occurs at the time of the catastrophic occlusion of a coronary artery (the first wave released from ACD, a second wave in the border zone released during RCD, not well studied) and after reperfusion therapy (the third wave released/ secreted during RCD). According to this model, DAMP-activated innate immune cells such as macrophages and neutrophils then produce SAMPs, which are generated immediately after the onset of MI. In line with this message—as often emphasized in this book— the primary function of DAMPs and SAMPs is to initiate homeostatic repairing responses, which can lead to full recovery of the patient. However, when these responses occur uncontrolled and dysregulated—for example, in case of excessive emission of DAMPs or impaired generation of SAMPs—reactive fibrosis may develop. By contrast, impaired emission of DAMPs may have fatal consequences in promoting cardiac rupture and aggravating dilative remodeling due to a marked reduction in the tensile strength of the scar.

Of particular importance in this context is interventional reperfusion because—as stressed by Heusch and Gersh [170]—despite widespread access to this therapy, mortality from STEMI is still substantial, as is the development of heart failure, particularly among an expanding older population. This knowledge has led to experimental and clinical proof-of-concept trials to develop additional cardioprotective strategies beyond timely interventional reperfusion. Disappointingly, however, translation of these trials into clinical practice often failed. Given this problem, Heusch and Gersh [170] discussed potential reasons for such failures in the application of additional cardiac protection beyond timely reperfusion.

It is at this point to discuss whether or not the use of DAMPs as therapeutic targets during intervention reperfusion might perhaps be a better therapeutic option. The role of DAMPs and SAMPs in post-MI inflammation and fibrosis has already been partially mentioned in the previous sections. Here, some more information is briefly and selectively added, whereby the role of DAMP-induced signaling pathways in cardiac fibrosis is discussed in both MI-dependent and MI-independent fibrosis (for review, see also [193–195, 277, 278]).

11.3.6.2 Promotion of Myocardial Inflammation and Fibrosis by Constitutive DAMPs

In the previous sections, sources and functions of DAMPs in ACS have been context-related outlined in brief. Here, a few more details of some of them should be briefly added.

High Mobility Group Box 1

Earlier studies have already documented HMGB1 to play a major role in the early event of IRI of the heart by binding to RAGE, resulting in the activation of proinflammatory pathways and enhanced myocardial injury [279].

In subsequent experimental studies on MI/IRI models, the pivotal role of HMGB1 in promoting proinflammatory responses has been convincingly confirmed and documented (see, for example, [280–282]). Moreover, as already touched above, other lines of studies revealed that HMGB1—if inflammation is not appropriately resolved—can also contribute to detrimental cardiac fibrosis [230, 246]. In support of these investigations is a recent study in rats showing that long-term oral atazanavir—an agent supposed to block the HMGB1↔TLR9 pathway—attenuates MI-induced cardiac fibrosis [283].

Notably, as a typical evolution-determined function of DAMPs in their primary role to restore homeostasis upon injury, HMGB1 has been shown to possess regenerative/repairing properties after MI (already described in Vol. 1 [16], Part VIII, Sect. 36.3.2). Thus, it should be noted here that there are also other lines of studies demonstrating such a favorable effects of HMGB1 in terms of preserving cardiac function after MI, for instance, via processes of stimulating cardiac fibroblast activities, promotion of cardiac stem cell proliferation and differentiation, and neoangiogenesis ([284, 285], see also reviews in [195, 277, 286]). These contradictory results may partly be explained by the different models used, in which the well-known tissue repairing capacity of HBMB1 (particularly when overexpressed) was dominating. Further, in some studies, SAMPs were not simultaneously measured, a circumstance that may blur these findings.

Of note, HMGB1 has qualified as an important biomarker in MI patients but has also been detected in ACS patients (reviewed by Wu et al. [287]). For instance, immunofluorescence microscopy studies on human coronary artery thrombi revealed high HMGB1 expression. Further, in these studies, HMGB1 was found to be highly expressed in platelet-rich coronary artery thrombi pointing toward a central role for HMGB1 in atherothrombosis [288]. Such findings could also be demonstrated in examinations of acute coronary thrombi from T2DM patients [289]. Of outstanding importance, however, are several investigations showing that HMGB1 serum levels are higher in ACS patients compared with normal values in healthy persons (reported in [290–294]). In one of such studies on STEMI patients successfully treated with PCI [292], elevated plasma HMGB1 levels were shown to be independently associated with increased mortality in those patients. Given these observations, the authors suggested plasma HMGB1 to be used as a new prognostic biomarker in STEMI patients. Similar investigations in patients with first-time STEMI or NSTEMI revealed HMGB1 to be related to infarct size and residual ejection fraction in patients with STEMI and NSTEMI, respectively [293]. Again, the investigators concluded that HMGB1 serum levels represent a highly valuable surrogate marker for infarct transmurality and the prediction of residual left ventricular function after MI. The role of HMGB1 as predictive DAMP in ACS patients could be confirmed in a subsequent study on patients with unstable angina and NSTEMI [294]. The obtained trial data motivated the investigators to conclude that circulating concentration of HMGB1 on admission may be a potential and independent predictor of cardiovascular mortality in patients hospitalized for unstable angina and NSTEMI within 24 h of onset. Similar results were obtained in other lines of trials in patients with acute MI, demonstrating that all patients have higher levels of

HMGB1, whereby those patients complicated with cerebral infarction, HMGB1 was found to be positively associated with acute MI [295].

Heat Shock Proteins

The function of HSPs in the presence of ischemic cardiac injury has also been investigated. In fact, as reviewed by van Hout et al. [277], HSP27, HSP60, and HSP72 are reportedly upregulated in studies on a rat model of MI. However, whereas HSP60 was found to be strongly associated with the development of heart failure after MI, HSP72 seems to protect the rodent heart against ischemic cardiac injury. Indeed, in line with reports on the role of HSP70 as a DAMP or a SAMP (compare Sect. 3.5.6), this heat shock molecule was experimentally found not only to stimulate proinflammatory responses but also to promote cardiomyocyte survival and attenuate cardiac damage.

S100 Proteins

As reflected by a growing number of reports [209, 296–304], S100 proteins have been accepted to playing an essential pathogenetic role in post-infarct inflammation and fibrosis. Earlier studies in rats already revealed that cardiac levels of a member of S100A proteins, S100A4, are significantly upregulated in injured myocardium and promote growth and survival of cardiac myocytes [296]. Besides experimental demonstration of S100A4 emission, expression of S100A8/9 proteins has been documented and more precisely quantified in various tissues in mouse models of MI [304].

Also, clinically, S100A proteins, here S100A8/A9, could be demonstrated in patients with acute MI as well as in patients with unstable angina pectoris. In earlier studies reported by Katashima et al. [297], increasing serum S100A8/A9 levels were measured in the MI patients and patients suffering from acute angina. On days 3–5 during monitoring, serum S100A8/A9 levels in acute MI patients reached a peak value and were significantly higher than the values in angina pectoris patients (1690 ± 144 ng/mL vs. 844 ± 100 ng/mL; $P < 0.0001$). In patients with acute infarction, peak S100A8/A9 levels were found to be positively correlated with peak white blood cell and neutrophil counts, peak creatine kinase muscle–brain (CK-MB), and peak CRP levels. Interestingly, examination of immunohistochemically proven expression of S100A8/A9 in the infarcted myocardium of autopsied patients, also performed in this study, revealed S100A8/A9 to be specifically expressed in neutrophils and macrophages infiltrating the infarcted myocardium. A short time after this report, another similar study on ACS patients and patients with stable angina was published [298] by presenting findings indicating that serum levels of S100B, S100A6, and S100P are associated with ACS. Subsequently, again similar studies in patients with ACS confirmed these early clinical observations by providing clinical data indicating that S100A8/A9 concentration increases in coronary artery blood in association with thrombus formation in ACS, co-localizes with leukocytes, and is associated with leukocyte activation [209]. Another examination of the S100 protein S100A4, emitted in patients with acute MI showed that, in accordance with S100A8/9, its serum levels are significantly higher in MI patients compared to healthy controls [302].

Together these clinical data qualify S100 proteins as pivotal DAMPs to be harnessed as biomarkers in both MI patients and patients experiencing acute angina pectoris (further details are added in Sect.11.4.2.3).

Nucleic Acids

Nucleic acids have been addressed in Vol. 1 [16], Part IV, Sect. 12.2.4.3 and Fig. 12.3 as constitutive IA-1 DAMPs passively released from necrotic cells. There is accumulating experimental and clinical evidence for a critical role of NAs in promoting proinflammatory pathways after MI. For example, in studies on a myocardial coronary artery occlusion/reperfusion model in genetically modified mice, RNA released from injured macrophages and cardiomyocytes was found to induce a cytokine response supposed by the investigators to contribute to myocardial inflammation and infarction [305]. In other sets of in vitro and in vivo studies, extracellular mtDNA was shown to activate NF-κB via TLR9 to induce cell death in cardiomyocytes [306].

Excitingly, extracellular nDNA and mtDNA have already been detected in the circulation of patients with acute MI [210, 211, 307, 308] (details are described in Sect. 11.4.2.3).

DAMP-Activated NLRP3 Inflammasome

Of note, activation of the NLRP3 inflammasome in various cardiac cells (e.g., macrophages, fibroblasts, ECs) by DAMPs (e.g., IA-1, IA-2 DAMPs)—particularly IRI-included activation—plays an eminent role in the creation of a myocardial inflammatory and fibrogenic responses. Indeed, the outstanding impact of NLRP3 inflammasome activation on MI-elicited proinflammatory and fibrogenic processes results from regulated pyroptotic cell death as a typical consequence of inflammasome activation. This subroutine of RCD may serve as an additional source for emission of both constitutive and inducible DAMPs (i.e., IL-1β), which in turn can aggravate proinflammatory and fibrogenic responses. Impressively, this subject has been abundantly discussed in the literature (for reviews, see [184, 198, 248–250, 309–313]).

Here again, it is worthwhile to briefly stress the primarily homeostatic role of the DAMP-induced NLRP3 inflammasome activation in MI. Hence, as pointed out above, the inflammasome-triggered pyroptotic cell death contributes to a robust inflammatory response, aimed at promoting a healing repairing response (thereby preventing cardiac muscle rupture)—even at the expense of further detrimental myocardial damage associated with increased infarct size (compare Fig. 2.1). On the other hand, however, when uncontrolled and dysregulated, the NLRP3 inflammasome, for example, expressed in M1-like macrophages, has been shown to also play a role in adverse remodeling that may contribute to reactive fibrosis [314, 315].

Interestingly, whereas evidence supporting the pathogenetic role of the NLRP3 inflammasome and the GSDMD-driven release of inducible DAMPs (IL-1β, IL-18) in MI is convincingly presented, the action of well-defined constitutive IA-1/IA-2 DAMPs contributing to the initial inflammasome activation is not explicit and remains to be elucidated.

Interleukin-1alpha

The pro-form of IL-1α is bioactive and, thus, when released from necrotic cells, operates as a DAMP, as described in Vol. 1 [16], Part IV, Sect. 12.2.4.5. In studies on necrotic cardiomyocytes and an IRI-MI model in mice [316], necrotic cardiomyocytes were found to release IL-1α, and the immune activation of cardiac fibroblasts shown to be abrogated by an IL-1R antagonist and an IL-1α-blocking antibody. In vivo, mice exposed to MI were observed to release IL-1α in the plasma, and postischemic inflammation was attenuated in *IL1a* KO mice. The authors concluded that their findings identify IL-1α as a crucial early danger signal triggering post-MI inflammation.

Extracellular Matrix Components

As mentioned above, ECM-derived DAMPs are implicated in cardiac fibrosis (for these IIA DAMPs, see Vol. 1, [16], Part IV, Sect. 13.2). As reviewed [154], these DAMPs include type I and type III collagen, fibrin, and FNIII EDA, TNC, and small leucine-rich proteoglycans (SLRPs). Some of these DAMPs have been shown to interact with PRM-bearing cells and induce post-MI inflammatory and fibrotic responses.

Here, as an example, SLRPs are briefly addressed which, following cardiac injury, are reportedly implicated in the regulation of the fibrotic response (reviewed in [317, 318]; for SLRPs, also compare Vol. 1 [16], Part IV, Sect. 13.2.2.2). Indeed, SLRPs but also syndecans are believed to play crucial roles in cardiac remodeling. These DAMPs reportedly regulate the hypertrophic growth of cardiomyocytes; inflammation, activation, and profibrotic activity of cardiac fibroblasts; and organization of the ECM. For example, as reviewed in [318], the levels of biglycan and decorin were shown to increase in experimental models of heart failure, that is, after MI and pressure overload. Clinically, elevated levels of both DAMPs were found in explanted hearts from patients with terminal heart failure, and biglycan has been detected in the healed infarct scar, co-localizing with tightly packed collagen fibers. Moreover (as also reviewed in [318]), biglycan is reportedly upregulated in cardiac fibroblasts after pressure overload. Also, upon MI, biglycan KO mice were observed to undergo increased mortality due to cardiac rupture, increased dilatation, less tensile strength, and severely impaired collagen matrix organization. These studies impressively demonstrate biglycan to be critical for extracellular remodeling in the heart. Given these findings and others not quoted here, PGs are considered excellent biomarkers for post-MI matrix remodeling and fibrosis. In addition, other lines of studies have even indicated PGs as new therapeutic targets for cardiac disease [318].

Cell-Extrinsic Dyshomeostatic DAMPs in Post-infarct Fibrosis

The putative contribution of cell-extrinsic dyshomeostatic DAMPs to cardiac fibrogenesis has already been addressed above in the context of myofibroblast transdifferentiation, triggered by the mechanosensors integrins and Piezo 1. Further support for an implication of putative dyshomeostatic DAMPs in cardiac fibrosis derives from observations on mechanosensitive ion channels such as TRPs generally and TRPV4 specifically (reviewed in [253]). Already in earlier studies on rat cultured cardiac fibroblasts [319], TRPV4 was found to be required for TGF-β-induced differentiation of cardiac fibroblasts into myofibroblasts. These experiments further revealed that TGF-β1-induced myofibroblast differentiation depends on ECM stiffness, a response that was attenuated by TRPV4 blockade. Given these findings, the authors suggested [319] that TRPV4 can regulate cardiac fibroblast differentiation to myofibroblasts by integrating signals from TGF-β and mechanical factors. Indeed, these interesting observations are in excellent agreement with the view of IIB-3 DAMP-driven, mechanosensor-triggered cardiac fibrosis as a self-perpetuating process (see also Sect. 6.3). Further support of this concept is provided by other lines of studies showing that TRPV4 ion channel is also involved in the regulation of dermal myofibroblast differentiation [320] and that TRPC3 mediates pressure overload-induced cardiac fibrosis [321].

11.3.6.3 Role of Inducible DAMPs in Post-infarct Inflammation and Fibrosis

Several cytokines and vasoactive neurohumoral mediators, known to be induced by stress/injury and denoted as inducible DAMPs in this book, are reportedly implicated in cardiac fibrosis. The role of Il-1β has already been cursorily alluded to above in the context of pyroptosis; here, some other molecules are briefly touched.

Tumor Necrosis Factor

Ample evidence has been published indicating a critical pathogenetic role of TNF in MI. After MI, activated cardiomyocytes and resident macrophages were shown to cause the myocardium in the infarcted zone and infarction border zone to produce large amounts of TNF, together with upregulation of its receptors, TNFRI and TNFRII (reviewed in [322]; also compare Vol. 1 [16], Part VI, Sect. 22.5.7, and Fig. 22.12). Besides its proinflammatory properties, TNF was demonstrated to cause adaptive hypertrophy of cardiomyocytes, thereby contributing to left ventricular hypertrophy and dilation, and to increase the transcription of hypertrophic genes by activation of MAPK and NF-κB pathways (also presented in [322]). However, no clear-cut data have been reported so far, showing a role of TNF in the activation of post-infarct necroptosis (for additional information, compare Vol. 1 [16], Part V, Sect. 19.3.2.2, and Fig. 19.4, p. 437).

Vasoactive Inducible DAMPs

Interestingly, there are already reports on a role of some neurohumoral mediators denoted as inducible DAMPs in this book (also see Sects. 3.5.3.5 and 3.5.3.6). Given their obvious function in contributing to cardiac fibroblast activation, they are briefly sketched in the following.

Angiotensin II Some evidence has been presented, indicating Ang II to be critically involved in myofibroblast activation, proliferation, and migration in the healing infarct. In fact, the fibrogenic actions of this putative inducible DAMP are mainly mediated through AT_1R-triggered signaling pathways, whereas, by contrast, the AT_2R is supposed to exert inhibitory functions, suppressing fibroblast proliferation and ECM synthesis (reviewed in [236]). In support of this concept are genetic studies and pharmacologic intervention experiments with ACE inhibitor or AT_1R antagonist that have proven effective in attenuating scar tissue metabolic activity and minimizing adverse accumulation of fibrous tissue in noninfarcted myocardium, thereby demonstrating a crucial role for Ang II in activation of the matrix synthetic capacity in infarct myofibroblasts [119, 323]. In addition, other lines of studies on transgenic animal models and an MI model in rats [324, 325] suggest that myocardial generation of Ang II may contribute to local fibroblast activation and matrix deposition.

Endothelin-1 Endothelin-1, also denoted as an inducible DAMP in this book, is reportedly an essential participant in the pathophysiology of CAD and MI. In a study on an IRI-MI model in rats [326], the expression of both ET-1 and ET_B receptors was found to be upregulated in the distal postischemic part of the occluded artery wall and in adjacent myocardium. As outlined in [327], during acute MI, ET-1 can enhance myocardial necrosis and arrhythmogenesis but seems to exert a favorable effect on subsequent infarct healing and early ventricular remodeling. In lines with these observations are investigations showing that in the chronic post-infarct phase, ET-1 increases left ventricular afterload and participates in the myocardial fibrotic process. Further supportive studies on an ET-1-induced model of cardiomyopathy provided evidence suggesting that ET-1, secreted by stimulated ECs, may stimulate fibroblast proliferation, myofibroblast conversion, and ECM synthesis [328]. Notably, plasma ET-1 levels have already been widely studied as potential risk biomarkers for cardiovascular events (reviewed in [329]). For example, in one of those clinical studies, ET-1 was found to be an independent predictor for major adverse cardiovascular events in MI patients younger than 35 years old [330].

11.3.6.4 Inflammation-Resolving Properties of SAMPs in Myocardial Infarction

In the course of elucidating mechanisms implicated in post-infarct resolution of inflammation, increasing evidence for a role of SAMPs in this scenario has become available. A few exciting aspects will be addressed in the following.

Annexin A1

There is an accumulating body of evidence indicating a cardioprotective role of AnxA1 in MI [331–333]. For example, in recent studies on an MI model in AnxA1 KO mice, AnxA1 was shown to have a direct action on cardiac macrophage polarization toward a proangiogenic, reparative phenotype that controls myocardial neoangiogenesis [332]. The AnxA1-stimulated cardiac macrophages were found to release high amounts of VEGF-A, thereby inducing neovascularization and cardiac repair. In another set of studies on cultured cardiomyocytes and cardiac fibroblasts and an MI-IRI model in mice, the N-terminal-derived peptide of annexin A1, “Ac2-26,” could be demonstrated not only to preserve cardiomyocyte survival in vitro but also to offer cardioprotection beyond the first few hours after an ischemic insult in vivo [333].

Adenosine

Although endogenous adenosine is produced by the heart during postischemic reperfusion as a natural cardioprotectant, reports on a distinct role in inflammation resolution are scarce. As outlined in an earlier review [334], two independent sites of adenosine formation in the heart—the myocytes and the ECs—are discussed that are differentially regulated. Indeed, there is evidence implicating the vascular endothelium as a potentially important site of both adenosine formation and action that subserves the cardioprotective effects of the nucleoside. Interestingly, the known protective effect of adenosine has been harnessed in adenosine receptor preconditioning studies. For example, in investigations on an MI-IRI model in rats, in vivo adenosine receptor preconditioning was shown to reduce MI size via subcellular ERK signaling [335].

Of note, in large randomized, placebo-controlled clinical trials in patients with acute MI within the first hours of infarction onset, infusion of high-dose adenosine in adjunction with recanalization treatment, administered prior to reperfusion, was reported to result in a significant reduction in infarct size, though clinical outcomes were not significantly improved [336, 337]. An updated meta-analysis of randomized controlled trials reported by Bulluck et al. [338] demonstrated a positive effect of adenosine treatment on heart failure outcomes in STEMI patients after reperfusion therapy. The authors concluded: "We hope that the findings from our meta-analysis will add to the positive evidence supporting the benefits of adenosine as an adjunct to reperfusion in STEMI patients and pave the way for large-scale prospective RCTs to confirm this beneficial effect of adenosine on major clinical outcomes." (For a more recent review, see also [339].)

Prostaglandin E2

In earlier studies on the role of endogenous prostaglandin endoperoxides, using a rabbit MI-IRI model, the contribution of PGE2 to thromboxane A2 synthase inhibitor-mediated cardioprotection was already suspected [340]. Subsequent experiments on a rat MI-IRI model then revealed that the myocardial content of PGE2, increased by pretreatment with atorvastatin, can mediate the statin-induced cardioprotective effects [341]. These findings were supported by studies on a rat MI-IRI model showing that pharmacological activation of the PGE2 receptor EP4 improves cardiac function after myocardial IRI [342]. The researchers of this study observed that the administration of an EP4 selective agonist significantly reduces infarction area, improves left ventricular contraction and dilatation, and also attenuates the recruitment of inflammatory cells and interstitial fibrosis in hearts (also reviewed in [343]). In more recent studies on a porcine model of MI-IRI exploring underlying mechanisms, the cardioprotective properties of PGE2 that may shelter the heart from IRI were demonstrated to be mediated via enhancement of VEGF and eNOS expression levels [344].

Specialized Proresolving Mediators

There is a growing body of valid clues from experimental and clinical studies indicating a pivotal role of SPMs in the post-infarct inflammation-resolving phase (compare [215, 223, 226, 345–350]).

The story of the pathogenetic role of SMPs in MI began with the discovery of Kain et al. [345] made in experiments on murine MI models that RvD1 promotes the post-infarct resolution of acute inflammation, thereby delaying the onset of heart failure. In these experiments, RvD1 was observed to limit neutrophil recruitment in the left ventricular and the spleen, increased resolving lipid mediators, and altered the macrophages phenotype post-MI.

Extended studies of this group then demonstrated that the lipoxin 15-epi-LXA4 initiates early activation of the resolving phase, thereby improving the left ventricular function post-MI [226]. Additionally, 15-epi-LXA4 was observed to activate neutrophil clearance in the left ventricle during the resolving phase with an increase in its cognate receptor FPR2 during the acute inflammatory phase (for FPR2 and other SPM-sensing GPCRs, see Sects. 2.3.4.5 and 2.3.4.6). Halade et al. [215] then performed similar experiments on a murine model of acute heart failure to study the temporal acute and resolving responses after MI and could show that the SAMP RvD1 improves left ventricular function, strain, and cardiac performance by promoting marked leukocyte clearance without affecting the acute innate immune inflammatory response. Interestingly and in relation to the MI-induced, DAMP-promoted bi-directional interaction between progressive left ventricle remodeling and kidney dysfunction (discussed in Sect. 11.3.4.5), the investigators [215] found RvD1 to attenuate MI-induced renal inflammation by increasing resolving leukocytes, decreasing neutrophil gelatinase-associated lipocalin and proinflammatory cytokines and chemokines in the kidney, and thereby facilitating renoprotective mechanisms to limit cardiorenal syndrome in acute and chronic heart failure. Given these exciting findings, Halade et al. [215] concluded that their study had identified the mechanistic circuit and cardioprotective role of RvD1 in post-MI cardiorenal resolution physiology. Further extended studies by the group on their murine MI model then revealed that the spleen not only serves as a leukocyte reservoir but also is the site where SPMs are actively generated, whereby their biosynthesis is driven by macrophages [223]. In fact, the researchers observed an abundance of SPMs in the spleen before MI and increased SPM concentrations in the infarcted left ventricle within 24 h after MI that were temporally correlated with the resolution of inflammation.

Excitingly, a first report on the regulation of SPMs during acute MI in humans was recently published (see [348]). In a recent clinical prospective observational study on STEMI patients during the first week following MI, plasma SPM concentrations were measured at three time points and compared with stable CAD patients and healthy controls. The main clinical findings observed by the investigators were as follows: (1) immediately after onset of MI, the levels of SPMs increased markedly in STEMI patients as compared with those measured in healthy controls and stable CAD patients, with levels of these SAMPs declining during follow-up; (2) the increase in SPMs primarily reflected an increase in Pds; and (3) several individual Pds were correlated with elevation of neutrophil counts [348]. The authors concluded that "… that pro-resolving mechanisms are increased early during STEMI, indicating that the "inflammation breaks" are activated immediately after MI onset. These findings could contribute to the start of a new era in relation to targeting inflammation during MI, focusing not only on anti-inflammatory intervention, but also on enhancing the pro-resolving capacity."

11.3.6.5 Concluding Remarks

As mentioned at the beginning, current notions hold that emission of proinflammatory and profibrotic DAMPs occurs at the time of coronary artery occlusion and after reperfusion therapy, associated with generation of SAMPs, which are generated immediately after the onset of MI. As reflected by a growing number of reports quoted in this section, substantial evidence in support of this concept is steadily increasing. The experimental and clinical findings described here in the context of MI again generalize the idea of injury-induced DAMPs and SAMPs, which are determined by evolution to induce inflammation-promoting and inflammation-resolving pathways, aimed at restoring homeostasis. If uncontrolled and dysregulated, these responses may lead to pathologies, here, in particular, life-threatening cardiac fibrosis.

11.3.7 Résumé

The growing knowledge on the role of DAMP-triggered proinflammatory and SAMP-driven proresolving cascades in inflammation, repair, and remodeling of the infarcted heart has revealed new therapeutic targets for patients surviving acute MI. Unfortunately, the action of multiple DAMPs and the various pathogenetic pathways implicated in cardiac remodeling, including DAMP-driven self-perpetuating processes, in human patients pose major challenges for clinical implementation of strategies targeting the post-infarct inflammatory and fibrotic responses. The use of DAMPs and SAMPs as biomarkers as well as the development of strategies to harness DAMPs as therapeutic targets and SAMPs as therapeutics may not only hold promise as protective measures to prevent reactive fibrosis and heart failure but may also prove critical in realizing the unrealistic goal of myocardial regeneration. Indeed, exploring innovative methods to improve cardiac function through regeneration of damaged and nonfunctioning myocardium has become a new direction for research. However, the results so far obtained with transplantation of bone marrow-derived stem cells are not satisfactory, whereby the essential goal appears to be to improve the survival rate of bone marrow stem cells after infarction transplantation (for review, see [351]).

Nevertheless, to mention in this context is that in experiments on a rat model of transplant arteriosclerosis, HMGB1 was shown to stimulate MSCs to migrate and differentiate to ECs via RAGE signaling [352]. An attempt to explore DAMPs in their capacity to stimulate stem cells in the setting of MI could, therefore, also be worthwhile to envisage. This burning topic is briefly resumed in Sect. 10.4.4.

11.4 DAMPs and SAMPs as Diagnostics, Prognostics, Therapeutic Targets, and Therapeutics in Cerebro-cardiovascular Diseases

11.4.1 Introductory Remarks

Given the increasing attention to the new approach to precision medicine (also known as personalized medicine; compare Sect. 7.2.1), the introduction of DAMPs and SAMPs as future biomarkers in CVDs appears to be the order of the day. Indeed, in accordance with the requirements for precise biomarkers, they should reflect the molecular pathology of the disease, allowing to improve patient's stratification and guide selection of the most effective targeted therapy. As traditionally known, patients and treatment responses may vary because of variables like genetic predisposition, epigenetic factors, ethnicity, and pharmacogenomically/pharmacokinetically substantial slow or fast metabolizers. These parameters affect whether a given individual will be a good or poor responder to a specific treatment but will not enable clinicians to make ad hoc, efficiently and accurately appropriate, diagnostic, prognostic, and therapeutic decisions.

In CVDs such as cerebral stroke or MI, DAMPs and SAMPs appear to fulfill the criteria of precise biomarkers by reflecting the controlled dynamics of post-infarct promotion and resolution of inflammatory responses on an individual basis or—as the case may be—by revealing, at the earliest possible moment, their uncontrolled dysregulation in the form, for example, of acute cerebral edema or cardiac reactive fibrosis.

Although there is a long way to go from current theory to clinical practice, some issues are addressed in this section, which should be considered a first approach to proper clinical use of DAMPs and SAMPs in CVD, rather than a presentation of routine clinical guidelines.

11.4.2 DAMPs and SAMPs as Biomarkers in Cerebro-cardiovascular Diseases

11.4.2.1 General Remarks

As outlined above, DAMPs and SAMPs in CVDs may originate in two waves from the initial infarcted region (i.e., first from ACD in the central zone, second from RCD in the border zone) as well as in terms of a third wave, during subsequent therapeutic recanalization/reperfusion strategies. Following their release into the blood circulation, they can be harnessed as robust diagnostic and prognostic biomarkers. In fact, as quoted already in part in the previous sections, a growing number of investigators have already addressed this new diagnostic tool in the discussion part of their papers. Here, a few more aspects are added that have not been previously discussed.

11.4.2.2 DAMPs as Biomarkers in Cerebral Stroke

It is now well accepted that the inflammatory response immediately following ischemic stroke can be evaluated as central or peripheral, based on the brain or peripheral tissue origin [353]. Accordingly, therapeutic blocking of proinflammatory cytokines or supplement of antiinflammatory cytokines has been proposed to be applied in patients with acute ischemic stroke and other inflammatory neurological diseases [354]. Plausibly, DAMPs and SAMPs should now be included in such strategies, and, indeed, for DAMPs, some reports have already been published.

High Mobility Group Box 1

As already mentioned above, HMGB1 that is passively released from damaged nerve cells already 2–4 h after the onset of ischemic stroke was found to enter the blood circulation through the damaged BBB. As also mentioned, a systematic review and meta-analysis revealed that patients with ischemic stroke had elevated circulating blood HMGB1 levels that correlate with severity and infarct volume (reviewed in [69]). The authors concluded that "HMGB1 may serve as a new prognostic biomarker and therapeutic target in the diagnosis and management of ischemic stroke."

S100 Proteins in Cerebral Stroke

Remarkably, serum S100B levels have been extensively studied as a biomarker in acute ischemic stroke. For example, data from large clinical studies on patients with acute cerebral stroke could demonstrate good correlation of S100B levels with clinical and radiographic features [355, 356]. In a review on S100 proteins as a marker of acute brain ischemia, already briefly touched above [75], S100 protein was found to increase after stroke onset significantly and to correlate with infarct volume, stroke severity, and functional outcome and, moreover, was assessed as a possible marker for ongoing ischemia. The authors concluded that the serum concentration of S100 protein during acute stroke is a useful marker of infarct size and long-term clinical outcome. In continuation of this study, an integrative review including 48 studies until March 2017 provided convincing data for S100B protein to be considered as a potent neurobiochemical marker that can play a pathognomonic role in the diagnosis of stroke [76]. In another observational, prospective study on patients hospitalized for ischemic stroke [357], S100B protein levels in peripheral blood at 48 h poststroke were demonstrated to reflect acute stroke severity and predict functional outcome at 12 weeks with a cutoff value of 140.5 ng/dL. The investigators emphasized that further clinical research and clinical practice should focus on the value of S100B as a predictor of functional recovery after stroke.

Of note, S100 proteins have also been discovered as biomarkers in hemorrhagic stroke. For example, in a prospective, observational study of patients with nontraumatic ICH and SAH, serum S100B was found to correspond with the severity of neurological insult and predict poor outcome in patients with nontraumatic ICH [122]. Also, a prospective study on ICH patients revealed that higher S100A12 concentrations are positively associated with hemorrhagic severity and short-term mortality among those patients, indicating that also this DAMP may represent a biomarker for predicting poor outcome after hemorrhagic stroke[134].

Nuclear and Mitochondrial DNA

Already in earlier clinical studies, plasma nDNA and mtDNA levels were serially examined in 50 acute ischemic stroke patients and in 50 at-risk control subjects during the study period [358]. The investigators reported that both plasma nDNA and mtDNA levels in patients with stroke were significantly higher than those in the controls. Elevated circulating nDNA in plasma was observed to persist until 1 month after the acute stroke and correlated positively to the clinical severity of stroke, as reflected by the National Institutes of Health Stroke Scale. Consequently, the authors stressed that assay of plasma DNA levels can be considered a neuropathologic marker of patients with acute ischemic stroke. In support of these findings is a more recent study on patients with acute ischemic stroke suggesting a putative role of circulating mtDNA as a new biomarker of stroke-associated infections and thus a clinical target for preventing poststroke infection [359].

Oxidation-Specific Epitopes

In a study on patients with CVDs including ischemic stroke and TIAs but also other diseases such as MI, new-onset unstable angina, acute coronary interventions, and vascular death [360], OSE biomarkers were found to predict 15-year CVD and stroke outcomes and provide potential clinical utility by reclassifying a significant proportion of individuals into higher- or lower-risk categories after traditional risk assessment. The authors discussed that "These data support the unifying hypothesis that OSEs, such as OxPL and MDA epitopes, represent DAMPs that are detrimental to the host." .... and further, ... " In response to such DAMPs, evolutionary processes have preserved and amplified innate immune effector proteins to bind and neutralize their proinflammatory effects."

11.4.2.3 DAMPs as Biomarkers in Coronary Artery Disease

The use of DAMPs as biomarkers in CAD appears to be more advanced compared to their use in cerebral stroke. In fact, the number of reports in the literature is steadily increasing and comprises a considerable spectrum.

Oxidation-Specific Epitopes

As the "DAMPs of the first hour," OSEs, in particular OxPL and MDA epitopes, have been developed as essential biomarkers in atherosclerosis. It is the group around Witztum and Tsimikas in San Diego, USA, who published first pathbreaking papers on this topic [360–363] (see Sect. 10.7.2.2). As a first result of the group's work [362], Lp(a)—the preferential lipoprotein carrier of the DAMP OxPL—has been generally recognized as a causal, independent, genetic risk factor for MI and has become a target of therapy for reducing cardiovascular risk. Since small Apo(a) isoforms are associated with high Lp(a) plasma levels and because these lipoproteins contain the most OxPL content, the OxPL/ApoB measurement primarily reflects the most atherogenic Lp(a) particles. Hence, elevated levels of OxPL/ApoB were found to predict the presence and progression of coronary, femoral, and carotid artery disease, to be increased following ACSs and PCI, as well as predict the development of death, MI, stroke, and need for revascularization in unselected populations [364]. In a study on patients with CVDs including MI (already mentioned above) [360], OSE biomarkers were found to predict 15-year CVD outcomes and provide potential clinical utility by reclassifying a significant proportion of individuals into higher- or lower-risk categories after traditional risk assessment.

This concept was supported by subsequent ELISA studies on OxPL on human ApoB (OxPL/ApoB) in plasma, confirming that oxidation-specific biomarkers predict cardiovascular events in humans (described in detail in [363]). In these studies, OxPL/ApoB levels were demonstrated to be elevated in patients with ACSs and following PCI, to predict the progression of femoral/carotid and coronary artery disease, to predict death and MI in unselected populations followed prospectively, and to reclassify ~30% of patients to lower- or higher-risk categories based on clinical criteria and Framingham risk score (further details are addressed in Sect. 10.7.2.2).

High Mobility Group Box 1

The outstanding role of HMGB1 as a useful biomarker in MI and acute angina pectoris—already briefly touched in Sect. 11.3.6.2—has already been addressed in earlier articles [365–367]. As could be expected, HMGB1was shown to be markedly increased in human atherosclerotic lesions from the aorta, carotid, and coronary arteries, whereby the DAMP was typically localized in the nuclei and in the cytoplasm of macrophages and VSMCs near the intima. Moreover, intense upregulated HMGB1expression was also observed in areas adjacent to the necrotic core of atherosclerotic lesions. Indeed, as comprehensively reviewed by Marsh et al. [368] and recently updated by Raucci et al. [286], serum HMGB1 concentration early after the acute MI is predictive of the infarct size and risk of death and is considered a critical prognostic biomarker for risk stratification and cardiovascular mortality in patients with MI. A few more details are added here.

The prognostic power of this DAMP in atherosclerosis and CVD has been impressively demonstrated in patients suffering from CAD (also compare Sect. 10.7.2.3). In general, plasma HMGB1 concentrations in this disease were observed to be significantly higher in patients with chest pain than in those with no symptomatology [369–372]. In line with these clinical observations are studies in diabetic patients: in an analysis of data from T2DM and non-T2DM patients with or without CAD, regardless of symptoms of ACS, HMGB1 serum levels were found to be significantly higher in diabetic and nondiabetic patients with CAD compared to those without CAD [370]. Together, these findings point to an important impact of HMGB1 on an increased risk of coronary heart atherosclerosis [371–373]. In support of this assumption is a clinical study showing that circulating concentration of HMGB1 on admission may be a strong and independent predictor of cardiovascular mortality in patients hospitalized for unstable angina and non-ST-segment elevation myocardial infarction within 24 h of onset [294]. Given these clinical observations, the authors argued that measurements of HMGB1 on admission may substantially improve the early risk stratification of such patients. In other lines of studies on STEMI and NSTEMI patients, HMGB1 serum levels were shown to be significantly correlated with infarct size as measured by cardiac magnetic resonance imaging [293]. Moreover, as observed in this study, cardiac magnetic resonance imaging, repeated 6 months after MI to estimate residual ventricular function, showed an inverse correlation between HMGB1 levels during MI and the residual ejection fraction both in STEMI and NSTEMI, respectively. From their findings, the authors concluded that HMGB1 serum levels reflect a highly valuable surrogate marker for infarct transmurality and for the prediction of residual left ventricular function after MI. In similar clinical investigations of patients with STEMI reported elsewhere, a higher peak HMGB1 level was associated with marked adverse clinical outcomes such as pump failure, cardiac rupture, and in-hospital cardiac death [374].

The prognostic value of HMGB1 as a biomarker was also documented in another study demonstrating that highly elevated HMGB1 plasma levels are associated with increased mortality in patients with STEMI treated with primary PCI [207]. The investigators found that a doubling of plasma HMGB1 levels was associated with a 75% increased risk of mortality, even after adjustment for age, sex, troponin I, and CK-MB. Moreover, in another study on the evaluation of a predictive value of preoperative HMGB1 on myocardial injury post-PCI, the investigators found that the occurrence of post-procedural myocardial injury was higher in the patients with elevated HMGB1 levels, which were associated with the worst clinical outcomes during 1-year follow-up [375]. On the other hand, a clinical study on HMGB1 expression level in circulating platelets was found not to be significantly associated with outcomes in symptomatic CAD—a finding that may not serve as a prognostic biomarker for this disease state [376]. Last but not least, and of interest, in other lines of studies on post-infarct patients, HMGB1 levels were found to be lower in those patients who underwent a 6-month exercise-based cardiac rehabilitation program [377].

Together, these studies demonstrate that serum/plasma HMGB1 levels are higher in patients with subclinical CAD and in those with overt ACS as compared to healthy individuals. Also, this DAMP fulfills the criteria of a powerful prognostic factor in ACS since its blood levels correlate with larger infarct size, transmurality, residual cardiac function, and cardiovascular mortality.

Heat Shock Proteins

Amazingly, there are only a few reports on the use of HSPs as biomarkers in MI. In an earlier study on patients with acute MI [378], HSP70 was found to be rapidly released into circulation after infarction. The investigators suggested already that circulating HSP70 may be a useful marker of myocardial damage and may have a role in the inflammatory response after acute MI. A few years later, these findings were supported by another investigation of patients with ACS and stable angina [379] demonstrating that plasma levels of HSP70 are markedly higher in patients with ACS (i.e., within 12 h of the onset of symptoms) than in the controls and, also, HSP70 levels are higher in ACS than in stable angina. In more recent studies on patients with ACS, plasma concentration of HSPB7 was also shown to be significantly higher in those patients compared with control patients with non-cardiac chest pain. Moreover, plasma HSPB7 was detected as early as 1–3 h after MI and remained detectable up to 24 h. Furthermore, in patients presenting to the emergency department with acute chest pain, HSPB7 level was found to be an independent risk factor of ACS [212]. The authors concluded that HSPB7 is a potential early biomarker after MI and serves as an independent risk factor of ACS in patients with acute chest pain. In another clinical study on patients with ACS, similar results were obtained with the determination of HSP70.

S100A Proteins

The outstanding role of S100 proteins as useful biomarkers in MI and acute angina pectoris has already been highlighted in Sect. 11.3.6.2 (for Refs., see [209, 297, 298, 302]). Here, a few more remarks are added.

Current knowledge on S100A proteins in their function as biomarkers has been reviewed by Oesterle and Bowman [301]. Early evidence for S100A proteins to act as a prognostic factor in CVD derived from a nested case study among patients with ACSs enrolled in the *Pravastatin or Atorvastatin Evaluation and Infection Therapy: Thrombolysis in Myocardial Infarction 22* trial [380]: patients with cardiovascular death or MI after 30 days were found to have higher median serum concentration of S100A8/9 levels than patients who remained free of recurrent events. From these data, the authors concluded that S100A8/9 may be a useful biomarker of inflammatory disease activity in atherothrombosis. This property of predicting cardiovascular events could also be shown for S100A12, namely, in studies of patients with stable CAD undergoing PCI and successful revascularization [208]. A subsequent study on patients with CAD could specify these data by demonstrating that serum S100A12 concentrations were independently associated with the presence of complex lesion in patients with stable angina pectoris [381]. Additionally, among patients with ACS who had higher serum S100A12 concentrations than patients with stable angina pectoris, those with multi-complex lesions were found to have significantly higher serum S100A12 concentrations than those with no or one complex lesion, that is, findings indicating that S100A12 may be a marker for plaque vulnerability in humans. Notably, these clinical observations could be confirmed by a recent study of patients who underwent coronary angiography and/or PCI [382]: the investigations confirmed serum S100A8, S100A9, and S100A12 levels to be valid markers of ACS. Specifically, S100A12 was identified as an independent associate of ACS suggesting again that this DAMP may serve as a marker of coronary plaque instability.

In studies of uremic patients, a similar predictive power could be demonstrated for serum S100A12 concentration: in a study of chronic kidney disease stage 5 patients and in two cross-sectional studies of maintenance hemodialysis patients, elevated serum S100A12 levels were shown to be markedly associated with the prevalence of CVD and increased mortality [383–385]. Interestingly, in a similar cross-sectional study of peritoneal dialysis patients, elevated plasma S100A12 level was also observed to be closely associated with atherosclerosis [386].

Similar clinical data have also been raised in diabetic patients. For example, in studies on patients with T2DM undergoing coronary angiography for the evaluation of CAD, serum S100A12 levels were shown to be significantly higher in the subjects with T2DM with CAD than in those without CAD [387]. In addition, the researchers observed that serum S100A12 levels are associated with the presence and severity of CAD. In view of their findings, they suggested that S100A12 might represent a novel biomarker for predicting the development and progression of CAD in patients with T2DM.

A more recent study in ACS patients, the S100A8/9 level in coronary artery blood obtained at thrombus aspiration was found to be higher in patients, in whom aspirated thrombus was confirmed [209], letting the authors conclude that S100A8/9 level is positioned as a unique biomarker at the interface of inflammation and thrombosis in ACS.

Mitochondrial DNA

Measurement of plasma levels of nDNA and mtDNA has joined the list of biomarkers in ACS [210, 211]. For example, Wang et al. [210], in examinations of plasma nDNA and mtDNA levels in the patients with acute MI before and after PCI, found that the concentrations of nDNA and mtDNA are significantly higher in patients with acute MI on hospital day 1 as compared with those observed in non-MI and healthy control patients. In the following time, the investigators could notice that the values of both NAs return to normal levels immediately after PCI, prompting them to suggest that they are potentially novel biomarkers for acute MI.

In this context, it seems worthwhile mentioning a systematic review and meta-analysis aimed to assess the role of circulating mtDNA in evaluating CVDs [388]. According to this review, the overall performance test of mtDNA for evaluating CVD and sudden cardiac death revealed that the mtDNA copy number presents the potential to be a biomarker for CVD and sudden cardiac death prediction. Given this observation, the authors concluded that fewer copies of mtDNA reflect the higher risk of CVD.

SAMPs as Biomarkers in Cardiovascular Disease

The great time for SAMPs to be used as biomarkers in CVD has not been yet realized and is still ahead. The monitoring of their plasma levels in CVD will be probably of particular importance regarding establishing a valid DAMP/SAMP ratio for designing targeted therapeutic strategies (i.e., use of DAMPs as therapeutic targets or SAMPs as therapeutics; see next section).

11.4.2.4 Concluding Remarks

In conclusion, the literature so far available—as only quoted in a nutshell here—provides ample evidence for a critical role of constitutive DAMPs as diagnostic and prognostic/predictive biomarkers in CVDs. Probably, inducible DAMPs such as TNF and IL-1β may also be harnessed for this purpose. In the future, detection of DAMPs in the early hours of ACS may become standard procedures, particularly in a situation when the ECG does not provide a clear-cut diagnosis. Nevertheless, as already stressed in Sect. 8.4.2.4, one has to state again—and this applies to all previous sections on the use of DAMPs as biomarkers—that standardization of DAMP protocols and the completion of large, prospective, multicenter trials may be warranted to firmly establish the clinical usefulness of DAMPs as biomarkers in CVDs.

11.4.3 DAMPs and SAMPs as Future Therapeutic Targets and Therapeutics in Cerebro-cardiovascular Diseases

11.4.3.1 General Remarks

Logically, all the following statements and remarks about DAMPs as future therapeutic targets and SAMPs as therapeutics in CVD are made in full confidence that in the foreseeable future, DAMP inhibiting agents (small molecules, synthetic small molecular mimetics, biologicals) and therapeutically applicable SAMPs such as

SPMs will be developed for clinical use. Indeed, inhibitors of DAMPs or activators of SAMPs such as SPM biosynthesis may become part of the potential future within the "resolution pharmacology" pharmacopeia [389]. To be optimistic, a look back shows us that the vast majority of approved drugs have been speedily developed to inhibit, block, or antagonize specific biological pathways involved in inflammatory conditions.

The goals of using DAMPs as therapeutic targets and SAMPs as therapeutics in stroke and MI are different: in stroke, the main aim is to prevent secondary injury-induced complications such as severe brain edema; in MI, the main objective is to avoid chronic inflammation that may transition to development of detrimental reactive fibrosis.

In both situations, clinicians, who take action in using DAMPs and SAMPs therapeutically, should always be aware that DAMPs and SAMPs are primarily responsible for a controlled post-injury repairing response that should lead to wound healing without further complications. This homeostatic process is based on sequelae of proinflammatory → proresolving → profibrotic responses resulting in healing replacement fibrosis. The meticulous monitoring of the homeostatic DAMP/SAMP ratio might serve as a guide for the preservation of these healing processes, whenever the therapeutic use of DAMPs and SAMPs is considered (for details, see Sect. 7.3.3).

11.4.3.2 Inhibition of DAMPs and Administration of SAMPs in Cerebral Stroke

Both therapeutic interventions, using DAMPs as therapeutic targets and administering SAMPs as therapeutics, can be discussed as game-changing innovative therapeutic strategies in both ischemic and hemorrhagic stroke. Also, regarding the observation of a poststroke immunosuppressive phase, the use of SAMPs as therapeutic targets at a later stage may be envisaged, if indicated at all. However, as outlined in the previous sections on this issue, special caveats of these new therapeutic approaches should be adhered to carefully.

The Use of DAMPs as Therapeutic Targets in Cerebral Stroke

The reason to think of blocking DAMPs in patients with cerebral stroke is evident: to find an innovative treatment option for ameliorating the secondary complications, particularly for preventing malignant cerebral edema, a therapeutic modality that is indicated in particular for any recanalization/reperfusion procedure.

There are already a few studies on experimental models demonstrating a protective effect DAMP inhibitors in ischemic and hemorrhagic stroke. For example, as shown in earlier experiments on a rat focal cerebral ischemia model [390], intravenous administration of *arundic acid* (an agent able to suppress astrocytic S100B synthesis), initiated immediately after induction of cerebral ischemia, was shown to significantly reduce cerebral infarct volume at 168 h (but not at 72 h). To the surprise of the researchers, the agent did not inhibit acute infarct expansion during the first 24 h but almost completely inhibited delayed infarct expansion.

As already mentioned in Sect. 8.4.4.2, *Affibody* molecules targeting HMGB1 has been investigated in different preclinical ischemic stroke models (*Affibody* molecules are small (6.5-kDa) affinity proteins based on a three-helix bundle domain framework and act as mimics with a favorable tissue distribution). According to a final report summary on these experiments (https://cordis.europa.eu/project/rcn/110068/reporting/en), HMGB1 blockage by these *Affibody* molecules as a treatment for stroke was not successful. As outlined in this report: "The negative results above could have several explanations. The two most likely are either the inability of the selected Affibody molecules in the selected doses to neutralize HMGB1 released during stroke, and the second is the redundancy in the inflammatory mechanisms activated after a stroke. In that scenario, neutralization of HMGB1 alone is not sufficient to impact inflammation ensuing ischemic stroke."

In more recent studies on both ischemic and hemorrhagic stroke models, intravenous injection of neutralizing anti-HMGB1 mAb was shown to significantly protect against BBB disruption induced by ischemia and hemorrhage in rats (see articles by the Nishibori group under [391–394]). Indeed, the experiments on an ischemic stroke model [392] revealed that this antibody is able to inhibit the development of brain edema through the protection of the BBB and the efficient clearance of circulating HMGB1. In experiments on the hemorrhagic stroke model [393], administration of anti-HMGB1 mAb was found to inhibit the release of HMGB1 into the extracellular space in the peri-hematomal region, reduce serum HMGB1 levels, and decrease brain edema by protecting BBB integrity. The authors concluded that their findings "strongly indicate that HMGB1 plays a critical role in the development of ICH-induced secondary injury through the amplification of plural inflammatory responses."

Regarding future clinical application of this innovative therapeutic intervention in stroke patients, the action should begin with initial measurement of the pattern of DAMPs—emitted poststroke and/or eventually post-recanalization— whereby the key DAMPs as found in a given patient may be chosen as therapeutic targets.

The challenge to neurologists here is not to interfere prematurely and too aggressively with the DAMP-promoted essential inflammatory response followed by a SAMP-triggered inflammation-resolving process, aimed at leading to the healing process without further complications. To avoid this potential treatment error, meticulous monitoring of the DAMP/SAMP ratio is recommended to be carried out that would allow applying DAMP inhibitors at the right time and in the right dose (for details, see Sect. 7.3.3).

Administration of SAMPs as Therapeutics in Cerebral Stroke

Therapeutic attempts to administer SAMPs in ischemic or hemorrhagic stroke are based on similar reasonable grounds as outlined for using DAMPs as therapeutic targets: to support poststroke resolution of inflammation, thereby preventing secondary complications, in particular cerebral edema. Indeed, as mentioned above, SAMPs such as AnxA1 and SPMs have already been shown to promote resolution of neuroinflammation [59–61].

The challenge to neurologists here is similar to that posed in using DAMPs as therapeutic targets: not to interfere prematurely with the DAMP-promoted homeostatic inflammatory response that contributes to a healing process. Again, this inappropriate decision could be circumvented by meticulous monitoring of the DAMP/SAMP ratio that would allow applying SAMPs at the right time and in the right dose.

Excitingly, there are already several reports from animal experiments showing a protective role of SAMPs in cerebral stroke that are briefly reviewed.

Annexin A1 Already in earlier investigations on a permanent MCAO model in rats, intracerebroventricular administration of a lipocortin-1 fragment (annexin-1 fragment) was found to cause marked inhibition of infarct size and cerebral edema [395]. In later investigations on a transient MCAO model in rats, administration of a short AnxA1 peptidomimetic (Ac2-26), given during the reperfusion phase, was also shown to reduce infarct sizes, associated with marked attenuation of cell adhesion and markers of inflammation [396]. In more recent studies on an ICH model in mice (already mentioned above), AnxA1 was found to effectively attenuate brain edema, improve short-term neurological function, and ameliorate microglia activation after ICH [136]. Given their findings, the authors concluded that AnxA1 could be a potential therapeutic strategy for ICH patients.

Extracellular Adenosine As touched above, extracellular adenosine is known to operate as an endogenous neuroprotective agent mainly by activating A1ARs. Interestingly, the neuroprotective potential of two A1AR partial agonists, namely, 2′-dCCPA and 3′-dCCPA, was recently evaluated in in vitro and ex vivo experimental models of cerebral ischemia [87]. Within the experimental paradigm of oxygen–glucose deprivation in vitro in human neuroblastoma (SH-SY5Y) cells, both A1AR partial agonists were found to increase cell viability. The investigators concluded that their findings demonstrate A1AR and its partial agonists to be still of interest to cerebral ischemia therapy.

Specialized Proresolving Mediators in Cerebral Stroke The neuroprotective role of SPMs in experimental cerebral IRI models has been comprehensively reviewed by Yin et al. [60]. Already in earlier studies on a mouse stroke model, specific novel bioactive docosanoids, generated in vivo, were shown to counteract leukocyte-mediated injury as well as proinflammatory gene induction [88]. Subsequent studies on various stroke models could specify these observations. For example, in experiments on a permanent MCAO model in mice, LXA4, biosynthesized by 5-LOX, was shown to mediate neuroprotective effects [397]. Further, experiments on a permanent MCAO model in rats revealed aspirin-triggered NPD1 to attenuate cerebral ischemic injury [398]. In more recent studies on a transient MCAO model in mice, intracerebroventricular injection of MaR1 could be demonstrated to reduce significantly the infarct volume and neurological defects, protect the brain tissue and neurons from injury efficiently, and alleviate proinflammatory reactions [399]. Also of interest is a recent study on a permanent MCAO model in rats showing that the DHA-derived mediator NPD1 counteracts neurological deficits by increasing "Iduna" expression in neurons and astrocytes after stroke onset [400]. Indeed, "Iduna" (*ring finger protein 146*) is known to facilitate DNA repair and protects against cell death induced by cerebral ischemia. In ischemic stroke, "Iduna" expression is downregulated in the penumbra and is associated with neurological deficits. The authors [400] concluded that "further unraveling of the molecular details of DHA-NPD1-Iduna expression signaling may contribute to possible therapeutic interventions for retinal degenerations and ischemic stroke."

11.4.3.3 Blockade of DAMPs and Administration of SAMPs in Myocardial Infarction

Both therapeutic interventions, choosing DAMPs as therapeutic targets and applying SAMPs as therapeutics, can also be discussed as innovative therapeutic strategies in acute MI. Again, however, special caveats of these new therapeutic approaches should be adhered to carefully.

The Use of DAMPs as Therapeutic Targets in Myocardial Infarction

The reason to think of blocking DAMPs in patients with acute MI is plausible: to find a novel treatment for limiting myocardial infarct size, a therapeutic modality that is indicated in particular for any recanalization/reperfusion procedure. Indeed, this therapeutic approach seems to be justified regarding a statement made by Bolli in this context [401], … "the field of cardioprotection has not been translated into any clinical therapy despite 40 years of intense work and billions of taxpayer dollars spent by the NIH and other bodies to find a drug that limits myocardial infarct size."

The aim of inhibiting the emission of DAMPs post-infarct is to mitigate/prevent the progression of the inflammatory response that may be associated with further demise of cardiomyocytes, may lead to systemic inflammation, and can result in detrimental development of reactive fibrosis (also compare Fig. 11.4 and [402]). As said, this therapeutic maneuver would be of outstanding importance when applied during recanalization/reperfusion therapy.

At first, one has to note that targeting DAMPs is not a new therapeutic approach for patients with MI when accepting IL-1β as inducible DAMPs. Indeed, the *Canakinumab Antiinflammatory Thrombosis Outcomes Study* (CANTOS) has provided convincing evidence that an antiinflammatory intervention with the human anti-IL-1β mAb (canakinumab) in patients with previous MI reduces recurrent cardiovascular events in high-risk patients with atherosclerotic disease [403]. However, according to a recent report, there remains reportedly substantial residual inflammatory risk related to both IL-18 and IL-6 after IL-1β inhibition with canakinumab (for more details, see [404]). These recent clinical observations support the concept that constitutive DAMPs should also be considered as additional therapeutic targets.

More precisely, the pattern of DAMP-emitted post-infarct and/or post-recanalization should be identified, whereby the key DAMPs, as measured in a given patient, could be chosen as therapeutic targets.

The challenge to cardiologists here is not to interfere prematurely and too aggressively with the DAMP-promoted inflammatory response and SAMP-triggered resolving processes that lead to healing replacement fibrosis and, thus, prevent infarction rupture. In other words, too early inhibition of DAMP emission may lead to infarct rupture due to an insufficient DAMP-promoted repairing response. Therefore, it would be critical to delivering DAMP inhibitors after the infarct scar has formed and matured to prevent aneurysm. On the other hand, a too late inhibition of DAMP emission may lead to progressive initial profibrotic responses, which, when fibrosis is once established, may result in a self-perpetuating process (→ reactive fibrosis associated with eventual heart failure). Again, these adverse effects might be avoided by meticulous monitoring of the DAMP/SAMP ratio that would allow applying DAMP inhibitors at the right time and in the right dose (for details, see Sect. 7.3.3).

It does not take a prophet to foresee that experimental studies on the inhibition of DAMPs in MI will be published soon that will show us the way to appropriate clinical trials.

Administration of SAMPs in Myocardial Infarction

The reason to think of administering SAMPs to patients with acute MI is similar but slightly different from that discussed in the context of using DAMPs as therapeutic targets, namely, to support post-MI resolution of inflammation, thereby preventing the development of detrimental reactive fibrosis, often associated with heart failure pathology. Such a therapeutic strategy is all the more indicated as a panoply of pharmacologic modifiers as antiinflammatory treatment for patients with acute MI has failed (expressis verbis stressed by Tourki and Halade [224]). The challenge to cardiologists here is the same as posed in using DAMPs as therapeutic targets: not to interfere prematurely with the DAMP-promoted essential inflammatory and fibrogenic response that leads to healing replacement fibrosis and, thus, prevents infarction rupture. Again, this adverse effect might be prevented by meticulous monitoring of the DAMP/SAMP ratio that would allow applying SAMPs at the right time and in the right dose.

Of note, as already mentioned above [336–338], the application of SAMPs to MI patients is not that a novel idea but has already been realized with the use of adenosine. Two large multicenter trials, the *Acute Myocardial Infarction Study of Adenosine 1 and 2* studies, examined the effects of adenosine in STEMI patients. Although adenosine was shown to reduce the size of the infarct, no effects on clinical outcome were noted.

Also, a combined treatment of AnxA1 (together with LXA4) in MI patients undergoing recanalization procedure was already proposed by de Jong et al. [405] to be beneficial.

To improve this novel therapeutic approach in MI, SPMs appear currently to be the ideal candidates for starting a new exciting era in relation to targeting chronic nonresolving inflammation during MI (also compare [226, 348, 406])).

11.4.3.4 Concluding Remarks

DAMPs and SAMPs, as future therapeutic targets and therapeutics in cerebro-cardiovascular events, herald a new era in the treatment of patients with CVDs. It is hoped that increasing numbers of targeted experimental studies as well as growing clinical experience of clinicians in handling the DAMP/SAMP ratio may expand the arsenal of new safe therapeutic options needed in those life-threatening diseases.

11.4.4 Future Role of DAMPs in Regeneration Approaches After Myocardial Infarction

An ambitious aim of cardiologists is to reverse reparative replacement fibrosis at the infarct site to induce regeneration of the cardiac muscle. Indeed, the use of various types of stem cells has emerged as a promising therapeutic approach to MI and ischemic heart failure with high expectations for patients with limited treatment options. Thus, the use of cells from various sources has been reported, classified as either embryonic, induced pluripotent stem cells, or adult/tissue stem cells. The most studied cell types are skeletal myoblasts, hematopoietic stem cells, endothelial progenitor cells, MSCs, and cardiac stem/progenitor cells (for reviews, see [407, 408]). However, poor performance of transplanted cells was frequently observed due to obstacles such as rejection after transplantation; poor engraftment, retention, and survival of the transplanted cells; occurrence of ventricular arrhythmias; and risk for tumor formation (reviewed in [409]).

Given these challenges and based on the hypothesis that cell therapy mainly functions through paracrine mechanisms, cell-free approaches have emerged as potential new therapeutic strategies, mainly including the administration/regulation of growth factors, noncoding RNAs, and, in particular, application of exosomes (for exosomes, EVs, and exosome-transferred secreted inducible DAMPs, see Sect. 3.5.3.2). Indeed, exosomes derived from various cellular sources, including stem cells and bodily fluids, were found to exert MI-repairing and regenerative effects both in vitro and in vivo (reviewed in [410]).

These new findings have given rise to reasonable hope for new therapeutic approaches to substituting the limited regenerative capacity of the human heart following myocardial injury. In this context, Adamiak and Sahoo conclude [410]: "Such a novel form of a therapeutic intervention, whereby cells could be exclusively used in vitro for the production of EVs, which would then be the only medicinal product given to the patient, would probably aid in overcoming many hurdles associated with conventional cell transplantation."

However, this thread can be woven even further. As outlined in Sect. 3.5.3.2, exosomes contain various subclasses of IIIA-1DAMPs, that is, a fact giving rise to the assumption that these molecules exert regenerative properties. On the other hand, DAMPs were demonstrated to promote both proliferation and trafficking of MSCs, identifying HMGB1 as a key factor in the regulation of these processes [411–413]. Other DAMPs, namely, S100A4 proteins and uric acid, have dose dependently been shown to induce chemotaxis of MSCs with synergistic effects when combined [414]. Moreover, novel insights were already gained from the role of DAMP-promoted inflammatory response in myocardial injury, repair, and remodeling [415]. For example, studies on a model of acute MI in transgenic mice exhibiting the cardiac-specific overexpression of HMGB1 in cardiomyocytes or local administration of HMGB1 provided first in vivo evidence that this DAMP induces myocardial regeneration by enhancing angiogenesis, restoring cardiac function, and improving survival after myocardial infarction [416]. In other lines of studies, nucleotide release from dying cells after AKI was found to promote proliferation of neighboring tubular cells, thus promoting wound closure via the downstream activation of Akt [417]. In the liver, the DAMP eATP released after partial hepatectomy, both from hepatocytes and from Kupffer cells, was shown to contribute to liver regeneration by activating cell cycle progression in hepatocytes [418]. A more recent report provided evidence for an early release by degenerating neurons of eATP that contributes to the activation of a series of intracellular pathways within Schwann cells that are crucial for nerve regeneration (Ca^{2+}, cAMP, ERK1/2, and CREB) [419].

Together, there seems to be a promising future of DAMPs to be harnessed as therapeutic molecules with regenerative capacities in MI, eventually administered jointly with stem cells such as MSCs. In support of such a concept are recent studies showing that combinatorial delivery of exosomes and stem cells in a sequential manner effectively reduces scar size and restores heart function after acute MI [420]. As concluded by the authors, "this approach may represent as an alternative promising strategy for stem cell-based heart repair and therapy." Self-evidently, such future studies have to analyze and assess DAMPs such as HMGB1, ATP, or NAs for their situative regenerative capacity in the injured myocardium.

11.4.5 Résumé

The topic of DAMPs and SAMPs in their role as diagnostics, prognostics, therapeutics, and therapeutic targets in cerebro-cardiovascular diseases as briefly described here can be seen as the beginning of an exciting area in this group of disorders of the heart and blood vessels. The introduction into clinical practices of DAMPs and SAMPs as biomarkers may allow for improving clinical decision-making and therapeutic monitoring in acute stroke and acute MI management. Indeed, their use as biomarkers for precise diagnostic procedures and therapeutic monitoring may soon become a clinical reality. On the other hand, the clinical use of DAMPs and SAMPs as therapeutic targets or therapeutics has not reached clinical maturation, although, in an increasing number of publications, such a future therapeutic option is seriously discussed. Above all, certain caveats for this kind of therapy—as described in Sect. 7.3.4—are recommended to be worked out in the recognition that DAMPs and SAMPs serve primarily to maintain and restore life-sustaining homeostasis following any tissue injury.

11.5 Outlook and Future Perspectives

This chapter presents a brief review of new insights into the pathogenesis of cerebrovascular disorders (stroke, cerebral hemorrhage) and CAD (i.e., MI) by focusing on the pathogenetic role of various subclasses of constitutive and inducible DAMPs and inducible SAMPs. According to the title of the book, the role of DAMPs and SAMPs as diagnostics, prognostics, therapeutics, and therapeutic targets in cerebro-cardiovascular diseases is highlighted. Doubtlessly, one can state that this topic is at the beginning of dramatic development. Their use as biomarkers for diagnostics and therapeutic monitoring may soon become a clinical reality, whereby the speed of introduction will also depend on the input of the pharmaceutical industry in launching suitable and reliable laboratory tests for their determination in body fluids and tissues. Also, the expectations of academia, federal governments, health insurances, professional societies, and the public media for a future high-level standard of personalized medicine may play a role.

On the other hand, the use of DAMPs and SAMPs as therapeutic targets or therapeutics will require more time before entering the clinic as a supplement to routine therapy of patients with CVDs. The promise of new targeted therapies developed from an improved understanding of inflammatory disease as a DAMP-driven inflammation-promoting, and a SAMP-driven inflammation-resolving process has now been experimentally realized, with necessary and mandatory safety guidelines for clinical use still awaiting clarification. The challenge here is not to interfere with the vital and life-saving work of DAMPs and SAMPs to restore homeostasis following tissue injury. As with traditional cytotoxic drugs, learning how to effectively utilize biologically significant agents introduces an inevitable delay in how quickly they can be safely applied to patients. The elaboration of a homeostatic DAMP/SAMP ratio in a given situation aimed at defining a "homeostatic window" for DAMPs and SAMPs concentrations, which should not be violated, may be helpful and advantageous here (also compare Sect. 7.3.3). To comply with those caveats, many translational studies are still needed: the ultimate goal for translational research being to design the best agents and therapeutic strategies that will achieve high efficacy with minimal toxicity.

References

1. WHO Report. Cardiovascular diseases (CVDs) [Internet]. 2017. https://www.who.int/news-room/fact-sheets/detail/cardiovascular-diseases-(cvds).
2. Timmis A, Townsend N, Gale C, Grobbee R, Maniadakis N, Flather M, et al. European Society of Cardiology: cardiovascular disease statistics 2017. Eur Heart J. 2018;39:508–79. http://www.ncbi.nlm.nih.gov/pubmed/29190377.
3. Good DC. Cerebrovascular Disease [Internet]. Third Edition. In: Walker HK, Hall WD, Hurst J, editors. Clinical methods: the history, physical, and laboratory examinations. Boston: Butterworth; 1990. http://www.ncbi.nlm.nih.gov/pubmed/21250219.
4. Hasan TF, Rabinstein AA, Middlebrooks EH, Haranhalli N, Silliman SL, Meschia JF, et al. Diagnosis and management of acute ischemic stroke. Mayo Clin Proc. 2018;93:523–38. http://www.ncbi.nlm.nih.gov/pubmed/29622098.
5. Gross BA, Jankowitz BT, Friedlander RM. Cerebral intraparenchymal hemorrhage. JAMA. 2019;321:1295. http://www.ncbi.nlm.nih.gov/pubmed/30938800.
6. Chandra A, Stone CR, Li WA, Geng X, Ding Y. The cerebral circulation and cerebrovascular disease II: pathogenesis of cerebrovascular disease. Brain Circ. 2017;3:57–65. http://www.ncbi.nlm.nih.gov/pubmed/30276306.
7. Chiang T, Messing RO, Chou W-H. Mouse model of middle cerebral artery occlusion. J Vis Exp. 2011;(48):2761. http://www.ncbi.nlm.nih.gov/pubmed/21372780.
8. Kathirvelu B, Carmichael ST. Intracerebral hemorrhage in mouse models: therapeutic interventions and functional recovery. Metab Brain Dis. 2015;30:449–59. http://link.springer.com/10.1007/s11011-014-9559-7.

9. Attia MS, Macdonald RL. Anterior circulation model of subarachnoid hemorrhage in mice. Neurovascular events after subarachnoid hemorrhage. Cham: Springer International Publishing; 2015. p. 311–4. http://www.ncbi.nlm.nih.gov/pubmed/25366643.
10. Johnson CO, Nguyen M, Roth GA, Nichols E, Alam T, Abate D, et al. Global, regional, and national burden of stroke, 1990–2016: a systematic analysis for the Global Burden of Disease Study 2016. Lancet Neurol. 2019;18:439–58. http://www.ncbi.nlm.nih.gov/pubmed/30871944.
11. Chandra A, Stone CR, Du X, Li WA, Huber M, Bremer R, et al. The cerebral circulation and cerebrovascular disease III: stroke. Brain Circ. 2017;3:66–77. http://www.ncbi.nlm.nih.gov/pubmed/30276307.
12. Paciaroni M, Caso V, Agnelli G. The concept of ischemic penumbra in acute stroke and therapeutic opportunities. Eur Neurol. 2009;61:321–30. https://www.karger.com/Article/FullText/210544.
13. Radak D, Katsiki N, Resanovic I, Jovanovic A, Sudar-Milovanovic E, Zafirovic S, et al. Apoptosis and acute brain ischemia in ischemic stroke. Curr Vasc Pharmacol. 2017;15:115–22. http://www.ncbi.nlm.nih.gov/pubmed/27823556.
14. Baron J-C. Protecting the ischaemic penumbra as an adjunct to thrombectomy for acute stroke. Nat Rev Neurol. 2018;14:325–37. http://www.ncbi.nlm.nih.gov/pubmed/29674752.
15. Sekerdag E, Solaroglu I, Gursoy-Ozdemir Y. Cell death mechanisms in stroke and novel molecular and cellular treatment options. Curr Neuropharmacol. 2018;16:1396–415. http://www.ncbi.nlm.nih.gov/pubmed/29512465.
16. Land WG. Damage-associated molecular patterns in human diseases; Vol. 1: injury-induced innate immune responses. Cham: Springer International Publishing AG; 2018. https://www.springer.com/de/book/9783319786544.
17. Khoshnam SE, Winlow W, Farzaneh M, Farbood Y, Moghaddam HF. Pathogenic mechanisms following ischemic stroke. Neurol Sci. 2017;38:1167–86. http://www.ncbi.nlm.nih.gov/pubmed/28417216.
18. Li H, Colbourne F, Sun P, Zhao Z, Buchan AM. Caspase inhibitors reduce neuronal injury after focal but not global cerebral ischemia in rats. Stroke. 2000;31:176–82. https://www.ahajournals.org/doi/10.1161/01.STR.31.1.176.
19. Ferrer I, Planas AM. Signaling of cell death and cell survival following focal cerebral ischemia: life and death struggle in the penumbra. J Neuropathol Exp Neurol. 2003;62:329–39. http://www.ncbi.nlm.nih.gov/pubmed/12722825.
20. Wang P, Shao B-Z, Deng Z, Chen S, Yue Z, Miao C-Y. Autophagy in ischemic stroke. Prog Neurobiol. 2018;163–164:98–117. http://www.ncbi.nlm.nih.gov/pubmed/29331396.
21. Degterev A, Huang Z, Boyce M, Li Y, Jagtap P, Mizushima N, et al. Chemical inhibitor of nonapoptotic cell death with therapeutic potential for ischemic brain injury. Nat Chem Biol. 2005;1:112–9. http://www.nature.com/articles/nchembio711.
22. Sarhan M, Land WG, Tonnus W, Hugo CP, Linkermann A. Origin and consequences of necroinflammation. Physiol Rev. 2018;98:727–80. http://www.physiology.org/doi/10.1152/physrev.00041.2016.
23. Deng X-X, Li S-S, Sun F-Y. Necrostatin-1 prevents necroptosis in brains after ischemic stroke via inhibition of RIPK1-mediated RIPK3/MLKL signaling. Aging Dis. 2019;10:807. http://www.ncbi.nlm.nih.gov/pubmed/31440386.
24. Yang X-S, Yi T-L, Zhang S, Xu Z-W, Yu Z-Q, Sun H-T, et al. Hypoxia-inducible factor-1 alpha is involved in RIP-induced necroptosis caused by in vitro and in vivo ischemic brain injury. Sci Rep. 2017;7:5818. http://www.nature.com/articles/s41598-017-06088-0.
25. Chen A-Q, Fang Z, Chen X-L, Yang S, Zhou Y-F, Mao L, et al. Microglia-derived TNF-α mediates endothelial necroptosis aggravating blood brain–barrier disruption after ischemic stroke. Cell Death Dis. 2019;10:487. http://www.ncbi.nlm.nih.gov/pubmed/31221990.
26. Magtanong L, Dixon SJ. Ferroptosis and brain injury. Dev Neurosci. 2018;40:382–95. http://www.ncbi.nlm.nih.gov/pubmed/30820017.

27. Tuo Q-Z, Lei P, Jackman KA, Li X-L, Xiong H, Li X-L, et al. Tau-mediated iron export prevents ferroptotic damage after ischemic stroke. Mol Psychiatry. 2017;22:1520–30. http://www.nature.com/articles/mp2017171.
28. Dawson TM, Dawson VL. Mitochondrial mechanisms of neuronal cell death: potential therapeutics. Annu Rev Pharmacol Toxicol. 2017;57:437–54. http://www.annualreviews.org/doi/10.1146/annurev-pharmtox-010716-105001.
29. Andrabi SA, Dawson TM, Dawson VL. Mitochondrial and nuclear cross talk in cell death: parthanatos. Ann N Y Acad Sci. 2008;1147:233–41. http://doi.wiley.com/10.1196/annals.1427.014.
30. David KK, Andrabi SA, Dawson TM, Dawson VL. Parthanatos, a messenger of death. Front Biosci (Landmark Ed). 2009;14:1116–28. http://www.ncbi.nlm.nih.gov/pubmed/19273119.
31. Wang Y, Kim NS, Haince J-F, Kang HC, David KK, Andrabi SA, et al. Poly(ADP-ribose) (PAR) binding to apoptosis-inducing factor is critical for PAR polymerase-1-dependent cell death (parthanatos). Sci Signal. 2011;4:ra20. http://stke.sciencemag.org/cgi/doi/10.1126/scisignal.2000902.
32. Fatokun AA, Dawson VL, Dawson TM. Parthanatos: mitochondrial-linked mechanisms and therapeutic opportunities. Br J Pharmacol. 2014;171:2000–16. http://www.ncbi.nlm.nih.gov/pubmed/24684389.
33. Li X, Klaus JA, Zhang J, Xu Z, Kibler KK, Andrabi SA, et al. Contributions of poly(ADP-ribose) polymerase-1 and -2 to nuclear translocation of apoptosis-inducing factor and injury from focal cerebral ischemia. J Neurochem. 2010;113:1012–22. http://doi.wiley.com/10.1111/j.1471-4159.2010.06667.x.
34. Delgado-Rizo V, Martínez-Guzmán MA, Iñiguez-Gutierrez L, García-Orozco A, Alvarado-Navarro A, Fafutis-Morris M. Neutrophil extracellular traps and its implications in inflammation: an overview. Front Immunol. 2017;8:81. http://www.ncbi.nlm.nih.gov/pubmed/28220120.
35. Grayson PC, Kaplan MJ. At the bench: neutrophil extracellular traps (NETs) highlight novel aspects of innate immune system involvement in autoimmune diseases. J Leukoc Biol. 2016;99:253–64. http://www.ncbi.nlm.nih.gov/pubmed/26432901.
36. Yang H, Biermann MH, Brauner JM, Liu Y, Zhao Y, Herrmann M. New Insights into neutrophil extracellular traps: mechanisms of formation and role in inflammation. Front Immunol. 2016;7:302. http://www.ncbi.nlm.nih.gov/pubmed/27570525.
37. Goyal M, Menon BK, van Zwam WH, Dippel DWJ, Mitchell PJ, Demchuk AM, et al. Endovascular thrombectomy after large-vessel ischaemic stroke: a meta-analysis of individual patient data from five randomised trials. Lancet (London, England). 2016;387:1723–31. https://linkinghub.elsevier.com/retrieve/pii/S014067361600163X.
38. Nikseresht S, Khodagholi F, Ahmadiani A. Protective effects of ex-527 on cerebral ischemia-reperfusion injury through necroptosis signaling pathway attenuation. J Cell Physiol. 2019;234:1816–26. http://www.ncbi.nlm.nih.gov/pubmed/30067864.
39. Guan X, Li X, Yang X, Yan J, Shi P, Ba L, et al. The neuroprotective effects of carvacrol on ischemia/reperfusion-induced hippocampal neuronal impairment by ferroptosis mitigation. Life Sci. 2019;235:116795. http://www.ncbi.nlm.nih.gov/pubmed/31470002.
40. Zhou Y, Gu Y, Liu J. BRD4 suppression alleviates cerebral ischemia-induced brain injury by blocking glial activation via the inhibition of inflammatory response and pyroptosis. Biochem Biophys Res Commun. 2019;519:481–8. http://www.ncbi.nlm.nih.gov/pubmed/31530390.
41. Xing C, Arai K, Lo EH, Hommel M. Pathophysiologic cascades in ischemic stroke. Int J Stroke. 2012;7:378–85. http://www.ncbi.nlm.nih.gov/pubmed/22712739.
42. Guo Y, Li P, Guo Q, Shang K, Yan D, Du S, et al. Pathophysiology and biomarkers in acute ischemic stroke—a review. Trop J Pharm Res. 2014;12:1097. http://www.ajol.info/index.php/tjpr/article/view/99924.
43. Khatri N, Thakur M, Pareek V, Kumar S, Sharma S, Datusalia AK. Oxidative stress: major threat in traumatic brain injury. CNS Neurol Disord Drug Targets. 2018;17:689–95. http://www.eurekaselect.com/163257/article.

44. Mizuma A, Yenari MA. Anti-inflammatory targets for the treatment of reperfusion injury in stroke. Front Neurol. 2017;8:467. http://www.ncbi.nlm.nih.gov/pubmed/28936196.
45. Nakamura K, Shichita T. Cellular and molecular mechanisms of sterile inflammation in ischaemic stroke. J Biochem. 2019;165:459–64. http://www.ncbi.nlm.nih.gov/pubmed/30796426.
46. Yang C, Hawkins KE, Doré S, Candelario-Jalil E. Neuroinflammatory mechanisms of blood-brain barrier damage in ischemic stroke. Am J Physiol Physiol. 2019;316:C135–53. http://www.ncbi.nlm.nih.gov/pubmed/30379577.
47. Planas AM, Gómez-Choco M, Urra X, Gorina R, Caballero M, Chamorro Á. Brain-derived antigens in lymphoid tissue of patients with acute stroke. J Immunol. 2012;188:2156–63. http://www.jimmunol.org/lookup/doi/10.4049/jimmunol.1102289.
48. Ortega SB, Noorbhai I, Poinsatte K, Kong X, Anderson A, Monson NL, et al. Stroke induces a rapid adaptive autoimmune response to novel neuronal antigens. Discov Med. 2015;19:381–92. http://www.ncbi.nlm.nih.gov/pubmed/26105701.
49. Desilles J-P, Syvannarath V, Di Meglio L, Ducroux C, Boisseau W, Louedec L, et al. Downstream microvascular thrombosis in cortical venules is an early response to proximal cerebral arterial occlusion. J Am Heart Assoc. 2018;7(5):e007804. https://www.ahajournals.org/doi/10.1161/JAHA.117.007804.
50. De Meyer SF, Denorme F, Langhauser F, Geuss E, Fluri F, Kleinschnitz C. Thromboinflammation in stroke brain damage. Stroke. 2016;47:1165–72. https://www.ahajournals.org/doi/10.1161/STROKEAHA.115.011238.
51. Stoll G, Nieswandt B. Thrombo-inflammation in acute ischaemic stroke — implications for treatment. Nat Rev Neurol. 2019;15:473–81. http://www.nature.com/articles/s41582-019-0221-1.
52. Wang X, Xuan W, Zhu Z-Y, Li Y, Zhu H, Zhu L, et al. The evolving role of neuro-immune interaction in brain repair after cerebral ischemic stroke. CNS Neurosci Ther. 2018;24:1100–14. http://www.ncbi.nlm.nih.gov/pubmed/30350341.
53. Zhu Z, Zheng L, Li Y, Huang T, Chao Y-C, Pan L, et al. Potential immunotherapeutic targets on myeloid cells for neurovascular repair after ischemic stroke. Front Neurosci. 2019;13:758. https://www.frontiersin.org/article/10.3389/fnins.2019.00758/full.
54. Shichita T, Ito M, Morita R, Komai K, Noguchi Y, Ooboshi H, et al. MAFB prevents excess inflammation after ischemic stroke by accelerating clearance of damage signals through MSR1. Nat Med. 2017;23:723–32. http://www.nature.com/articles/nm.4312.
55. Liesz A, Zhou W, Na S-Y, Hämmerling GJ, Garbi N, Karcher S, et al. Boosting regulatory T cells limits neuroinflammation in permanent cortical stroke. J Neurosci. 2013;33:17350–62. http://www.jneurosci.org/cgi/doi/10.1523/JNEUROSCI.4901-12.2013.
56. Liesz A, Hu X, Kleinschnitz C, Offner H. Functional role of regulatory lymphocytes in stroke: facts and controversies. Stroke. 2015;46:1422–30. http://stroke.ahajournals.org/cgi/doi/10.1161/STROKEAHA.114.008608.
57. García-Culebras A, Durán-Laforet V, Peña-Martínez C, Moraga A, Ballesteros I, Cuartero MI, et al. Role of TLR4 (Toll-like receptor 4) in N1/N2 neutrophil programming after stroke. Stroke. 2019;50:2922–32. http://www.ncbi.nlm.nih.gov/pubmed/31451099.
58. Liesz A, Rüger H, Purrucker J, Zorn M, Dalpke A, Möhlenbruch M, et al. Stress mediators and immune dysfunction in patients with acute cerebrovascular diseases. Arumugam TV., editor. PLoS One. 2013;8:e74839. https://dx.plos.org/10.1371/journal.pone.0074839.
59. Ansari J, Kaur G, Gavins F. Therapeutic potential of annexin A1 in ischemia reperfusion injury. Int J Mol Sci. 2018;19:1211. http://www.mdpi.com/1422-0067/19/4/1211.
60. Yin P, Wei Y, Wang X, Zhu M, Feng J. Roles of specialized pro-resolving lipid mediators in cerebral ischemia reperfusion injury. Front Neurol. 2018;9:617. https://www.frontiersin.org/article/10.3389/fneur.2018.00617/full.
61. Senchenkova EY, Ansari J, Becker F, Vital SA, Al-Yafeai Z, Sparkenbaugh EM, et al. Novel role for the AnxA1-Fpr2/ALX signaling axis as a key regulator of platelet function to promote resolution of inflammation. Circulation. 2019;140:319–35. https://www.ahajournals.org/doi/10.1161/CIRCULATIONAHA.118.039345.

62. Zhao H, Han Z, Ji X, Luo Y. Epigenetic regulation of oxidative stress in ischemic stroke. Aging Dis. 2016;7:295. http://www.ncbi.nlm.nih.gov/pubmed/27330844.
63. Narne P, Pandey V, Phanithi PB. Interplay between mitochondrial metabolism and oxidative stress in ischemic stroke: an epigenetic connection. Mol Cell Neurosci. 2017;82:176–94. http://www.ncbi.nlm.nih.gov/pubmed/28552342.
64. Ng GY-Q, Lim Y-A, Sobey CG, Dheen T, Fann DY-W, Arumugam TV. Epigenetic regulation of inflammation in stroke. Ther Adv Neurol Disord. 2018;11:1756286418771815. http://journals.sagepub.com/doi/10.1177/1756286418771815.
65. Goulopoulou S, McCarthy CG, Webb RC. Toll-like receptors in the vascular system: sensing the dangers within. Pharmacol Rev. 2015;68:142–67. http://www.ncbi.nlm.nih.gov/pubmed/26721702.
66. Gülke E, Gelderblom M, Magnus T. Danger signals in stroke and their role on microglia activation after ischemia. Ther Adv Neurol Disord. 2018;11:175628641877425. http://www.ncbi.nlm.nih.gov/pubmed/29854002.
67. Umahara T, Uchihara T, Hirokawa K, Hirao K, Shimizu S, Hashimoto T, et al. Time-dependent and lesion-dependent HMGB1-selective localization in brains of patients with cerebrovascular diseases. Histol Histopathol. 2018;33:215–22. http://www.ncbi.nlm.nih.gov/pubmed/28671243.
68. Singh V, Roth S, Veltkamp R, Liesz A. HMGB1 as a key mediator of immune mechanisms in ischemic stroke. Antioxid Redox Signal. 2016;24:635–51. http://www.ncbi.nlm.nih.gov/pubmed/26493086.
69. Le K, Mo S, Lu X, Idriss Ali A, Yu D, Guo Y. Association of circulating blood HMGB1 levels with ischemic stroke: a systematic review and meta-analysis. Neurol Res. 2018;40:907–16. http://www.ncbi.nlm.nih.gov/pubmed/30015578.
70. Ye Y, Zeng Z, Jin T, Zhang H, Xiong X, Gu L. The role of high mobility group box 1 in ischemic stroke. Front Cell Neurosci. 2019;13:127. http://www.ncbi.nlm.nih.gov/pubmed/31001089.
71. Shichita T, Hasegawa E, Kimura A, Morita R, Sakaguchi R, Takada I, et al. Peroxiredoxin family proteins are key initiators of post-ischemic inflammation in the brain. Nat Med. 2012;18:911–7. http://www.nature.com/articles/nm.2749.
72. Dayon L, Turck N, Garcí-Berrocoso T, Walter N, Burkhard PR, Vilalta A, et al. Brain extracellular fluid protein changes in acute stroke patients. J Proteome Res. 2011;10:1043–51. https://pubs.acs.org/doi/abs/10.1021/pr101123t.
73. Richard S, Lapierre V, Girerd N, Bonnerot M, Burkhard PR, Lagerstedt L, et al. Diagnostic performance of peroxiredoxin 1 to determine time-of-onset of acute cerebral infarction. Sci Rep. 2016;6:38300. http://www.nature.com/articles/srep38300.
74. Kim JY, Han Y, Lee JE, Yenari MA. The 70-kDa heat shock protein (Hsp70) as a therapeutic target for stroke. Expert Opin Ther Targets. 2018;22:191–9. http://www.ncbi.nlm.nih.gov/pubmed/29421932.
75. Nash DL, Bellolio MF, Stead LG. S100 as a marker of acute brain ischemia: a systematic review. Neurocrit Care. 2008;8:301–7. http://www.ncbi.nlm.nih.gov/pubmed/17968519.
76. Rezaei O, Pakdaman H, Gharehgozli K, Simani L, Vahedian-Azimi A, Asaadi S, et al. S100 B: a new concept in neurocritical care. Iran J Neurol. 2017;16:83–9. http://www.ncbi.nlm.nih.gov/pubmed/28761630.
77. Zhou S, Zhu W, Zhang Y, Pan S, Bao J. S100B promotes microglia M1 polarization and migration to aggravate cerebral ischemia. Inflamm Res. 2018;67:937–49. http://www.ncbi.nlm.nih.gov/pubmed/30229393.
78. An C, Shi Y, Li P, Hu X, Gan Y, Stetler RA, et al. Molecular dialogs between the ischemic brain and the peripheral immune system: dualistic roles in injury and repair. Prog Neurobiol. 2014;115:6–24. https://linkinghub.elsevier.com/retrieve/pii/S0301008213001421.
79. Cisneros-Mejorado A, Pérez-Samartín A, Gottlieb M, Matute C. ATP signaling in brain: release, excitotoxicity and potential therapeutic targets. Cell Mol Neurobiol. 2015;35:1–6. http://link.springer.com/10.1007/s10571-014-0092-3.
80. Silk E, Zhao H, Weng H, Ma D. The role of extracellular histone in organ injury. Cell Death Dis. 2017;8:e2812. http://www.ncbi.nlm.nih.gov/pubmed/28542146.

81. Vallés J, Lago A, Santos MT, Latorre AM, Tembl J, Salom J, et al. Neutrophil extracellular traps are increased in patients with acute ischemic stroke: prognostic significance. Thromb Haemost. 2017;117:1919–29. http://www.ncbi.nlm.nih.gov/pubmed/28837206.
82. Sobowale OA, Parry-Jones AR, Smith CJ, Tyrrell PJ, Rothwell NJ, Allan SM. Interleukin-1 in stroke. Stroke. 2016;47:2160–7. http://www.ncbi.nlm.nih.gov/pubmed/26931154.
83. Lambertsen KL, Finsen B, Clausen BH. Post-stroke inflammation—target or tool for therapy? Acta Neuropathol. 2019;137:693–714. http://www.ncbi.nlm.nih.gov/pubmed/30483945.
84. He X-F, Zeng Y-X, Li G, Feng Y-K, Wu C, Liang F-Y, et al. Extracellular ASC exacerbated the recurrent ischemic stroke in an NLRP3-dependent manner. J Cereb Blood Flow Metab. 2019;40(5):1048–60. http://journals.sagepub.com/doi/10.1177/0271678X19856226.
85. Pedata F, Pugliese AM, Coppi E, Dettori I, Maraula G, Cellai L, et al. Adenosine A 2A receptors modulate acute injury and neuroinflammation in brain ischemia. Mediators Inflamm. 2014;2014:1–16. http://www.ncbi.nlm.nih.gov/pubmed/25165414.
86. Cui M, Ding H, Chen F, Zhao Y, Yang Q, Dong Q. Mdivi-1 protects against ischemic brain injury via elevating extracellular adenosine in a cAMP/CREB-CD39-dependent manner. Mol Neurobiol. 2016;53:240–53. http://www.ncbi.nlm.nih.gov/pubmed/25428621.
87. Martire A, Lambertucci C, Pepponi R, Ferrante A, Benati N, Buccioni M, et al. Neuroprotective potential of adenosine A 1 receptor partial agonists in experimental models of cerebral ischemia. J Neurochem. 2019;149:211–30. http://www.ncbi.nlm.nih.gov/pubmed/30614535.
88. Marcheselli VL, Hong S, Lukiw WJ, Tian XH, Gronert K, Musto A, et al. Novel docosanoids inhibit brain ischemia-reperfusion-mediated leukocyte infiltration and pro-inflammatory gene expression. J Biol Chem. 2003;278:43807–17. http://www.ncbi.nlm.nih.gov/pubmed/12923200.
89. Mukherjee PK, Marcheselli VL, Serhan CN, Bazan NG. From the cover: neuroprotectin D1: a docosahexaenoic acid-derived docosatriene protects human retinal pigment epithelial cells from oxidative stress. Proc Natl Acad Sci. 2004;101:8491–6. http://www.ncbi.nlm.nih.gov/pubmed/15152078.
90. Serhan CN, Gotlinger K, Hong S, Lu Y, Siegelman J, Baer T, et al. Anti-inflammatory actions of neuroprotectin D1/protectin D1 and its natural stereoisomers: assignments of dihydroxy-containing docosatrienes. J Immunol. 2006;176:1848–59. http://www.jimmunol.org/lookup/doi/10.4049/jimmunol.176.3.1848.
91. van Gijn J, Kerr RS, Rinkel GJ. Subarachnoid haemorrhage. Lancet. 2007;369:306–18. http://www.ncbi.nlm.nih.gov/pubmed/17258671.
92. Qureshi AI, Mendelow AD, Hanley DF. Intracerebral haemorrhage. Lancet (London, England). 2009;373:1632–44. https://linkinghub.elsevier.com/retrieve/pii/S0140673609603718.
93. van Asch CJ, Luitse MJ, Rinkel GJ, van der Tweel I, Algra A, Klijn CJ. Incidence, case fatality, and functional outcome of intracerebral haemorrhage over time, according to age, sex, and ethnic origin: a systematic review and meta-analysis. Lancet Neurol. 2010;9:167–76. https://linkinghub.elsevier.com/retrieve/pii/S1474442209703400.
94. Macdonald RL. Delayed neurological deterioration after subarachnoid haemorrhage. Nat Rev Neurol. 2014;10:44–58. http://www.ncbi.nlm.nih.gov/pubmed/24323051.
95. An SJ, Kim TJ, Yoon B-W. Epidemiology, risk factors, and clinical features of intracerebral hemorrhage: an update. J Stroke. 2017;19:3–10. http://j-stroke.org/journal/view.php?doi=10.5853/jos.2016.00864.
96. Qureshi AI, Ling GS, Khan J, Suri MF, Miskolczi L, Guterman LR, et al. Quantitative analysis of injured, necrotic, and apoptotic cells in a new experimental model of intracerebral hemorrhage. Crit Care Med. 2001;29:152–7. https://insights.ovid.com/crossref?an=00003246-200101000-00030.
97. Meng C, Zhang J, Dang B, Li H, Shen H, Li X, et al. PERK pathway activation promotes intracerebral hemorrhage induced secondary brain injury by inducing neuronal apoptosis both in vivo and in vitro. Front Neurosci. 2018;12:111. http://journal.frontiersin.org/article/10.3389/fnins.2018.00111/full.

98. Shen X, Ma L, Dong W, Wu Q, Gao Y, Luo C, et al. Autophagy regulates intracerebral hemorrhage induced neural damage via apoptosis and NF-κB pathway. Neurochem Int. 2016;96:100–12. http://www.ncbi.nlm.nih.gov/pubmed/26964766.
99. Nguyen HX, O'Barr TJ, Anderson AJ. Polymorphonuclear leukocytes promote neurotoxicity through release of matrix metalloproteinases, reactive oxygen species, and TNF-alpha. J Neurochem. 2007;102:900–12. http://doi.wiley.com/10.1111/j.1471-4159.2007.04643.x.
100. Shen H, Liu C, Zhang D, Yao X, Zhang K, Li H, et al. Role for RIP1 in mediating necroptosis in experimental intracerebral hemorrhage model both in vivo and in vitro. Cell Death Dis. 2017;8:e2641. http://www.nature.com/articles/cddis201758.
101. Zille M, Karuppagounder SS, Chen Y, Gough PJ, Bertin J, Finger J, et al. Neuronal death after hemorrhagic stroke in vitro and in vivo shares features of ferroptosis and necroptosis. Stroke. 2017;48:1033–43. http://stroke.ahajournals.org/lookup/doi/10.1161/STROKEAHA.116.015609.
102. Stockwell BR, Friedmann Angeli JP, Bayir H, Bush AI, Conrad M, Dixon SJ, et al. Ferroptosis: a regulated cell death nexus linking metabolism, redox biology, and disease. Cell. 2017;171:273–85. http://www.ncbi.nlm.nih.gov/pubmed/28985560.
103. Wu J, Tuo Q, Lei P. Ferroptosis, a recent defined form of critical cell death in neurological disorders. J Mol Neurosci. 2018;66:197–206. http://www.ncbi.nlm.nih.gov/pubmed/30145632.
104. Weiland A, Wang Y, Wu W, Lan X, Han X, Li Q, et al. Ferroptosis and its role in diverse brain diseases. Mol Neurobiol. 2019;56:4880–93. http://www.ncbi.nlm.nih.gov/pubmed/30406908.
105. Alim I, Caulfield JT, Chen Y, Swarup V, Geschwind DH, Ivanova E, et al. Selenium drives a transcriptional adaptive program to block ferroptosis and treat stroke. Cell. 2019;177:1262–1279.e25. http://www.ncbi.nlm.nih.gov/pubmed/31056284.
106. Wan J, Ren H, Wang J. Iron toxicity, lipid peroxidation and ferroptosis after intracerebral haemorrhage. Stroke Vasc Neurol. 2019;4:93–5. http://www.ncbi.nlm.nih.gov/pubmed/31338218.
107. Li Q, Han X, Lan X, Gao Y, Wan J, Durham F, et al. Inhibition of neuronal ferroptosis protects hemorrhagic brain. JCI Insight. 2017;2(7):e90777. https://insight.jci.org/articles/view/90777.
108. Zhao H, Chen Y, Feng H. P2X7 receptor-associated programmed cell death in the pathophysiology of hemorrhagic stroke. Curr Neuropharmacol. 2018;16:1282–95. http://www.ncbi.nlm.nih.gov/pubmed/29766811.
109. Chen S, Ma Q, Krafft PR, Hu Q, Rolland W, Sherchan P, et al. P2X7R/cryopyrin inflammasome axis inhibition reduces neuroinflammation after SAH. Neurobiol Dis. 2013;58:296–307. https://linkinghub.elsevier.com/retrieve/pii/S096999611300185X.
110. Feng L, Chen Y, Ding R, Fu Z, Yang S, Deng X, et al. P2X7R blockade prevents NLRP3 inflammasome activation and brain injury in a rat model of intracerebral hemorrhage: involvement of peroxynitrite. J Neuroinflammation. 2015;12:190. http://jneuroinflammation.biomedcentral.com/articles/10.1186/s12974-015-0409-2.
111. Zhou Y, Wang Y, Wang J, Anne Stetler R, Yang Q-W. Inflammation in intracerebral hemorrhage: from mechanisms to clinical translation. Prog Neurobiol. 2014;115:25–44. http://www.ncbi.nlm.nih.gov/pubmed/24291544.
112. Zhang Z, Zhang Z, Lu H, Yang Q, Wu H, Wang J. Microglial polarization and inflammatory mediators after intracerebral hemorrhage. Mol Neurobiol. 2017;54:1874–86. http://link.springer.com/10.1007/s12035-016-9785-6.
113. Shao Z, Tu S, Shao A. Pathophysiological mechanisms and potential therapeutic targets in intracerebral hemorrhage. Front Pharmacol. 2019;10:1079. http://www.ncbi.nlm.nih.gov/pubmed/31607923.
114. Keep RF, Hua Y, Xi G. Intracerebral haemorrhage: mechanisms of injury and therapeutic targets. Lancet Neurol. 2012;11:720–31. http://www.ncbi.nlm.nih.gov/pubmed/22698888.
115. Keep RF, Andjelkovic AV, Xiang J, Stamatovic SM, Antonetti DA, Hua Y, et al. Brain endothelial cell junctions after cerebral hemorrhage: changes, mechanisms and therapeutic targets. J Cereb Blood Flow Metab. 2018;38:1255–75. http://www.ncbi.nlm.nih.gov/pubmed/29737222.
116. Macdonald RL, Schweizer TA. Spontaneous subarachnoid haemorrhage. Lancet (London, England). 2017;389:655–66. http://www.ncbi.nlm.nih.gov/pubmed/27637674.

117. Chaudhry SR, Hafez A, Rezai Jahromi B, Kinfe TM, Lamprecht A, Niemelä M, et al. Role of damage associated molecular pattern molecules (DAMPs) in aneurysmal subarachnoid hemorrhage (aSAH). Int J Mol Sci. 2018;19:2035. http://www.mdpi.com/1422-0067/19/7/2035.
118. Murakami K, Koide M, Dumont TM, Russell SR, Tranmer BI, Wellman GC. Subarachnoid hemorrhage induces gliosis and increased expression of the pro-inflammatory cytokine high mobility group box 1 protein. Transl Stroke Res. 2011;2:72–9. http://link.springer.com/10.1007/s12975-010-0052-2.
119. Sun Q, Wu W, Hu Y-C, Li H, Zhang D, Li S, et al. Early release of high-mobility group box 1 (HMGB1) from neurons in experimental subarachnoid hemorrhage in vivo and in vitro. J Neuroinflammation. 2014;11:106. http://jneuroinflammation.biomedcentral.com/articles/10.1186/1742-2094-11-106.
120. Tian X, Sun L, Feng D, Sun Q, Dou Y, Liu C, et al. HMGB1 promotes neurovascular remodeling via rage in the late phase of subarachnoid hemorrhage. Brain Res. 2017;1670:135–45. https://linkinghub.elsevier.com/retrieve/pii/S0006899317302378.
121. Shao A, Zhou Y, Yao Y, Zhang W, Zhang J, Deng Y. The role and therapeutic potential of heat shock proteins in haemorrhagic stroke. J Cell Mol Med. 2019;23:5846–58. http://www.ncbi.nlm.nih.gov/pubmed/31273911.
122. Junttila EK, Koskenkari J, Ohtonen PP, Karttunen A, Ala-Kokko TI. Serum S100β as a prognostic marker in patients with non-traumatic intracranial hemorrhag. Minerva Anestesiol. 2016;82:1189–98. http://www.ncbi.nlm.nih.gov/pubmed/27629991.
123. Liu D-L, Zhao L-X, Zhang S, Du J-R. Peroxiredoxin 1-mediated activation of TLR4/NF-κB pathway contributes to neuroinflammatory injury in intracerebral hemorrhage. Int Immunopharmacol. 2016;41:82–9. https://linkinghub.elsevier.com/retrieve/pii/S1567576916304416.
124. Suzuki H, Fujimoto M, Kawakita F, Liu L, Nakano F, Nishikawa H, et al. Toll-like receptor 4 and tenascin-C signaling in cerebral vasospasm and brain injuries after subarachnoid hemorrhage. Acta Neurochir Suppl. 2020;127:91–6. http://link.springer.com/10.1007/978-3-030-04615-6_15.
125. Rendevski V, Aleksovski B, Stojanov D, Aleksovski V, Rendevska AM, Kolevska M, et al. Peripheral glutamate and TNF-α levels in patients with intracerebral hemorrhage: their prognostic values and interactions toward the formation of the edemal volume. Neurol Neurochir Pol. 2018;52:207–14. http://www.ncbi.nlm.nih.gov/pubmed/29096921.
126. Jeney V. Pro-inflammatory actions of red blood cell-derived DAMPs. Exp Suppl. 2018;108:211–33. http://link.springer.com/10.1007/978-3-319-89390-7_9.
127. Lin S, Yin Q, Zhong Q, Lv F-L, Zhou Y, Li J-Q, et al. Heme activates TLR4-mediated inflammatory injury via MyD88/TRIF signaling pathway in intracerebral hemorrhage. J Neuroinflammation. 2012;9:548. http://www.ncbi.nlm.nih.gov/pubmed/22394415.
128. Adhami F, Liao G, Morozov YM, Schloemer A, Schmithorst VJ, Lorenz JN, et al. Cerebral ischemia-hypoxia induces intravascular coagulation and autophagy. Am J Pathol. 2006;169:566–83. https://linkinghub.elsevier.com/retrieve/pii/S0002944010627381.
129. Xie B, Lin Y, Wu X, Yu L, Zheng S, Kang D. Reduced admission serum fibrinogen predict 6-month mortality of poor-grade aneurysmal subarachnoid hemorrhage. World Neurosurg. 2019;136:e24–32. http://www.ncbi.nlm.nih.gov/pubmed/31476464.
130. Nakahara T, Tsuruta R, Kaneko T, Yamashita S, Fujita M, Kasaoka S, et al. High-mobility group box 1 protein in CSF of patients with subarachnoid hemorrhage. Neurocrit Care. 2009;11:362–8. http://link.springer.com/10.1007/s12028-009-9276-y.
131. Zhu X-D, Chen J-S, Zhou F, Liu Q-C, Chen G, Zhang J-M. Relationship between plasma high mobility group box-1 protein levels and clinical outcomes of aneurysmal subarachnoid hemorrhage. J Neuroinflammation. 2012;9:194. http://jneuroinflammation.biomedcentral.com/articles/10.1186/1742-2094-9-194.
132. Kiiski H, Långsjö J, Tenhunen J, Ala-Peijari M, Huhtala H, Hämäläinen M, et al. S100B, NSE and MMP-9 fail to predict neurologic outcome while elevated S100B associates with milder initial clinical presentation after aneurysmal subarachnoid hemorrhage. J Neurol Sci. 2018;390:129–34. http://www.ncbi.nlm.nih.gov/pubmed/29801873.

133. He Y, Cai Z, Chen Y. Role of S-100β in stroke. Int J Neurosci. 2018;128:1180–7. http://www.ncbi.nlm.nih.gov/pubmed/29792379.
134. Qian S-Q, He S-R, Li B-B, Qian J, Zheng X-D. Serum S100A12 and 30-day mortality after acute intracerebral hemorrhage. Clin Chim Acta. 2018;477:1–6. https://linkinghub.elsevier.com/retrieve/pii/S0009898117304758.
135. Chaudhry SR, Frede S, Seifert G, Kinfe TM, Niemelä M, Lamprecht A, et al. Temporal profile of serum mitochondrial DNA (mtDNA) in patients with aneurysmal subarachnoid hemorrhage (aSAH). Mitochondrion. 2019;47:218–26. https://linkinghub.elsevier.com/retrieve/pii/S1567724918300175.
136. Ding Y, Flores J, Klebe D, Li P, McBride DW, Tang J, et al. Annexin A1 attenuates neuroinflammation through FPR2/p38/COX-2 pathway after intracerebral hemorrhage in male mice. J Neurosci Res. 2019;98(1):168–78. http://www.ncbi.nlm.nih.gov/pubmed/31157469.
137. Lin C-L, Dumont AS, Tsai Y-J, Huang J-H, Chang K-P, Kwan A-L, et al. 17β-estradiol activates adenosine A2a receptor after subarachnoid hemorrhage. J Surg Res. 2009;157:208–15. http://www.ncbi.nlm.nih.gov/pubmed/19181336.
138. Leclerc JL, Ahmad AS, Singh N, Soshnik-Schierling L, Greene E, Dang A, et al. Intracerebral hemorrhage outcomes following selective blockade or stimulation of the PGE2 EP1 receptor. BMC Neurosci. 2015;16:48. http://www.ncbi.nlm.nih.gov/pubmed/26232001.
139. Wu H, Wu T, Han X, Wan J, Jiang C, Chen W, et al. Cerebroprotection by the neuronal PGE 2 receptor EP2 after intracerebral hemorrhage in middle-aged mice. J Cereb Blood Flow Metab. 2017;37:39–51. http://www.ncbi.nlm.nih.gov/pubmed/26746866.
140. WHO. World Health Organization: the top 10 causes of death. https://www.who.int/news-room/fact-sheets/detail/the-top-10-causes-of-death.
141. Benjamin EJ, Virani SS, Callaway CW, Chamberlain AM, Chang AR, Cheng S, et al. Heart disease and stroke statistics—2018 update: a report from the American Heart Association. Circulation. 2018;137:e67–492. http://www.ncbi.nlm.nih.gov/pubmed/29386200.
142. Thygesen K, Alpert JS, Jaffe AS, Simoons ML, Chaitman BR, White HD, et al. Third universal definition of myocardial infarction. J Am Coll Cardiol. 2012;60:1581–98. http://www.ncbi.nlm.nih.gov/pubmed/22958960.
143. Anderson JL, Morrow DA. Acute myocardial infarction. Campion EW, editor. N Engl J Med. 2017;376:2053–64. http://www.ncbi.nlm.nih.gov/pubmed/28538121.
144. Amsterdam EA, Wenger NK, Brindis RG, Casey DE, Ganiats TG, Holmes DR, et al. AHA/ACC guideline for the management of patients with non–ST-elevation acute coronary syndromes. J Am Coll Cardiol. 2014;64:e139–228. http://www.ncbi.nlm.nih.gov/pubmed/25260718.
145. Lindsey ML, Bolli R, Canty JM, Du X-J, Frangogiannis NG, Frantz S, et al. Guidelines for experimental models of myocardial ischemia and infarction. Am J Physiol Circ Physiol. 2018;314:H812–38. http://www.ncbi.nlm.nih.gov/pubmed/29351451.
146. Maddaford TG, Hurtado C, Sobrattee S, Czubryt MP, Pierce GN. A model of low-flow ischemia and reperfusion in single, beating adult cardiomyocytes. Am J Physiol. 1999;277:H788–98. https://www.physiology.org/doi/10.1152/ajpheart.1999.277.2.H788.
147. Liao R, Podesser BK, Lim CC. The continuing evolution of the Langendorff and ejecting murine heart: new advances in cardiac phenotyping. Am J Physiol Heart Circ Physiol. 2012;303:H156–67. https://www.physiology.org/doi/10.1152/ajpheart.00333.2012.
148. Sutherland FJ, Hearse DJ. The isolated blood and perfusion fluid perfused heart. Pharmacol Res. 2000;41:613–27. https://linkinghub.elsevier.com/retrieve/pii/S1043661899906539.
149. Bux AS, Lindsey ML, Vasquez HG, Taegtmeyer H, Harmancey R. Glucose regulates the intrinsic inflammatory response of the heart to surgically induced hypothermic ischemic arrest and reperfusion. Physiol Genomics. 2017;49:37–52. https://www.physiology.org/doi/10.1152/physiolgenomics.00102.2016.
150. Heusch G. Molecular basis of cardioprotection: signal transduction in ischemic pre-, post-, and remote conditioning. Circ Res. 2015;116:674–99. https://www.ahajournals.org/doi/10.1161/CIRCRESAHA.116.305348.

151. Frangogiannis NG. Regulation of the inflammatory response in cardiac repair. Rosenzweig A, editor. Circ Res. 2012;110:159–73. http://www.ncbi.nlm.nih.gov/pubmed/22223212.
152. Frangogiannis NG. Pathophysiology of myocardial infarction. Compr Physiol. 2015;5(4):1841–75. http://www.ncbi.nlm.nih.gov/pubmed/26426469.
153. Frangogiannis NG. Cell biological mechanisms in regulation of the post-infarction inflammatory response. Curr Opin Physiol. 2018;1:7–13. http://www.ncbi.nlm.nih.gov/pubmed/29552674.
154. Frangogiannis NG. Cardiac fibrosis: cell biological mechanisms, molecular pathways and therapeutic opportunities. Mol Aspects Med. 2019;65:70–99. https://linkinghub.elsevier.com/retrieve/pii/S0098299718300670.
155. Mendis S, Abegunde D, Yusuf S, Ebrahim S, Shaper G, Ghannem H, et al. WHO study on Prevention of REcurrences of Myocardial Infarction and StrokE (WHO-PREMISE). Bull World Health Organ. 2005;83:820–9. http://www.ncbi.nlm.nih.gov/pubmed/16302038.
156. Bleumink GS, Knetsch AM, Sturkenboom MCJM, Straus SMJM, Hofman A, Deckers JW, et al. Quantifying the heart failure epidemic: prevalence, incidence rate, lifetime risk and prognosis of heart failure The Rotterdam Study. Eur Heart J. 2004;25:1614–9. https://academic.oup.com/eurheartj/article-lookup/doi/10.1016/j.ehj.2004.06.038.
157. Libby P. Mechanisms of acute coronary syndromes and their implications for therapy. N Engl J Med. 2013;368:2004–13. http://www.ncbi.nlm.nih.gov/pubmed/23697515.
158. Bairey Merz CN, Pepine CJ, Walsh MN, Fleg JL, Camici PG, Chilian WM, et al. Ischemia and No Obstructive Coronary Artery Disease (INOCA): developing evidence-based therapies and research agenda for the next decade. Circulation. 2017;135:1075–92. https://www.ahajournals.org/doi/10.1161/CIRCULATIONAHA.116.024534.
159. Crea F, Libby P. Acute coronary syndromes:the way forward from mechanisms to precision treatment. Circulation. 2017;136:1155–66. http://www.ncbi.nlm.nih.gov/pubmed/28923905.
160. Beltrame JF, Crea F, Kaski JC, Ogawa H, Ong P, Sechtem U, et al. The who, what, why, when, how and where of vasospastic angina. Circ J. 2016;80:289–98. https://www.jstage.jst.go.jp/article/circj/80/2/80_CJ-15-1202/_article.
161. Jackson BM, Gorman JH, Moainie SL, Guy TS, Narula N, Narula J, et al. Extension of borderzone myocardium in postinfarction dilated cardiomyopathy. J Am Coll Cardiol. 2002;40:1160–7. https://linkinghub.elsevier.com/retrieve/pii/S0735109702021216.
162. Jin P, Wang E, Wang Y-H, Huang W, Kuang W, Sun C, et al. Central zone of myocardial infarction: a neglected target area for heart cell therapy. J Cell Mol Med. 2012;16:637–48. http://doi.wiley.com/10.1111/j.1582-4934.2011.01408.x.
163. Frangogiannis NG. The immune system and the remodeling infarcted heart: cell biological insights and therapeutic opportunities. J Cardiovasc Pharmacol. 2014;63:185–95. https://insights.ovid.com/crossref?an=00005344-201403000-00001.
164. Reimer KA, Lowe JE, Rasmussen MM, Jennings RB. The wavefront phenomenon of ischemic cell death. 1. Myocardial infarct size vs duration of coronary occlusion in dogs. Circulation. 1977;56:786–94. http://www.ncbi.nlm.nih.gov/pubmed/912839.
165. Chen Y-R, Zweier JL. Cardiac mitochondria and reactive oxygen species generation. Circ Res. 2014;114:524–37. http://www.ncbi.nlm.nih.gov/pubmed/24481843.
166. Ouyang Y-B, Stary CM, White RE, Giffard RG. The use of microRNAs to modulate redox and immune response to stroke. Antioxid Redox Signal. 2015;22:187–202. http://www.liebertpub.com/doi/10.1089/ars.2013.5757.
167. Yellon DM, Hausenloy DJ. Myocardial reperfusion injury. N Engl J Med. 2007;357:1121–35. http://www.ncbi.nlm.nih.gov/pubmed/17855673.
168. Hausenloy DJ, Yellon DM. Myocardial ischemia-reperfusion injury: a neglected therapeutic target. J Clin Invest. 2013;123:92–100. http://www.ncbi.nlm.nih.gov/pubmed/23281415.
169. Neri M, Riezzo I, Pascale N, Pomara C, Turillazzi E. Ischemia/reperfusion injury following acute myocardial infarction: a critical issue for clinicians and forensic pathologists. Mediators Inflamm. 2017;2017:1–14. http://www.ncbi.nlm.nih.gov/pubmed/28286377.

170. Heusch G, Gersh BJ. The pathophysiology of acute myocardial infarction and strategies of protection beyond reperfusion: a continual challenge. Eur Heart J. 2017;38:774–84. http://eurheartj.oxfordjournals.org/lookup/doi/10.1093/eurheartj/ehw224.
171. Bonezzi F, Piccoli M, Dei Cas M, Paroni R, Mingione A, Monasky MM, et al. Sphingolipid synthesis inhibition by myriocin administration enhances lipid consumption and ameliorates lipid response to myocardial ischemia reperfusion injury. Front Physiol. 2019;10:986. https://www.frontiersin.org/article/10.3389/fphys.2019.00986/full.
172. Piper HM, García-Dorado D, Ovize M. A fresh look at reperfusion injury. Cardiovasc Res. 1998;38:291–300. http://www.ncbi.nlm.nih.gov/pubmed/9709390.
173. Zhu H, Sun A. Programmed necrosis in heart disease: molecular mechanisms and clinical implications. J Mol Cell Cardiol. 2018;116:125–34. http://www.ncbi.nlm.nih.gov/pubmed/29426003.
174. Škėmienė K, Jablonskienė G, Liobikas J, Borutaitė V. Protecting the heart against ischemia/reperfusion-induced necrosis and apoptosis: the effect of anthocyanins. Medicina (Kaunas). 2013;49:84–8. http://www.ncbi.nlm.nih.gov/pubmed/23888344.
175. Del Re DP, Amgalan D, Linkermann A, Liu Q, Kitsis RN. Fundamental mechanisms of regulated cell death and implications for heart disease. Physiol Rev. 2019;99:1765–817. http://www.ncbi.nlm.nih.gov/pubmed/31364924.
176. Zhe-Wei S, Li-Sha G, Yue-Chun L. The role of necroptosis in cardiovascular disease. Front Pharmacol. 2018;9:721. http://www.ncbi.nlm.nih.gov/pubmed/30034339.
177. Gupta K, Phan N, Wang Q, Liu B. Necroptosis in cardiovascular disease—a new therapeutic target. J Mol Cell Cardiol. 2018;118:26–35. http://www.ncbi.nlm.nih.gov/pubmed/29524460.
178. Kobayashi M, Suhara T, Baba Y, Kawasaki NK, Higa JK, Matsui T. Pathological roles of iron in cardiovascular disease. Curr Drug Targets. 2018;19:1068–76. http://www.ncbi.nlm.nih.gov/pubmed/29874997.
179. Baba Y, Higa JK, Shimada BK, Horiuchi KM, Suhara T, Kobayashi M, et al. Protective effects of the mechanistic target of rapamycin against excess iron and ferroptosis in cardiomyocytes. Am J Physiol Circ Physiol. 2018;314:H659–68. http://www.ncbi.nlm.nih.gov/pubmed/29127238.
180. Li W, Feng G, Gauthier JM, Lokshina I, Higashikubo R, Evans S, et al. Ferroptotic cell death and TLR4/Trif signaling initiate neutrophil recruitment after heart transplantation. J Clin Invest. 2019;129:2293–304. https://www.jci.org/articles/view/126428.
181. Audia JP, Yang X-M, Crockett ES, Housley N, Haq EU, O'Donnell K, et al. Caspase-1 inhibition by VX-765 administered at reperfusion in P2Y12 receptor antagonist-treated rats provides long-term reduction in myocardial infarct size and preservation of ventricular function. Basic Res Cardiol. 2018;113:32. http://www.ncbi.nlm.nih.gov/pubmed/29992382.
182. Lei Q, Yi T, Chen C. NF-κB-Gasdermin D (GSDMD) axis couples oxidative stress and NACHT, LRR and PYD domains-containing protein 3 (NLRP3) inflammasome-mediated cardiomyocyte pyroptosis following myocardial infarction. Med Sci Monit. 2018;24:6044–52. http://www.ncbi.nlm.nih.gov/pubmed/30161099.
183. Takahashi M. Cell-specific roles of NLRP3 inflammasome in myocardial infarction. J Cardiovasc Pharmacol. 2019;74:188–93. http://www.ncbi.nlm.nih.gov/pubmed/31356542.
184. Takahashi M. Role of NLRP3 inflammasome in cardiac inflammation and remodeling after myocardial infarction. Biol Pharm Bull. 2019;42:518–23. http://www.ncbi.nlm.nih.gov/pubmed/30930410.
185. Jia C, Chen H, Zhang J, Zhou K, Zhuge Y, Niu C, et al. Role of pyroptosis in cardiovascular diseases. Int Immunopharmacol. 2019;67:311–8. http://www.ncbi.nlm.nih.gov/pubmed/30572256.
186. Du Y, Gu X, Meng H, Aa N, Liu S, Peng C, et al. Muscone improves cardiac function in mice after myocardial infarction by alleviating cardiac macrophage-mediated chronic inflammation through inhibition of NF-κB and NLRP3 inflammasome. Am J Transl Res. 2018;10:4235–46. http://www.ncbi.nlm.nih.gov/pubmed/30662666.
187. Kawaguchi M, Takahashi M, Hata T, Kashima Y, Usui F, Morimoto H, et al. Inflammasome activation of cardiac fibroblasts is essential for myocardial ischemia/reperfusion

injury. Circulation. 2011;123:594–604. https://www.ahajournals.org/doi/10.1161/CIRCULATIONAHA.110.982777.
188. Pertiwi K, van der Wal A, Pabittei D, Mackaaij C, van Leeuwen M, Li X, et al. Neutrophil extracellular traps participate in all different types of thrombotic and haemorrhagic complications of coronary atherosclerosis. Thromb Haemost. 2018;118:1078–87. http://www.ncbi.nlm.nih.gov/pubmed/29672788.
189. Vajen T, Koenen RR, Werner I, Staudt M, Projahn D, Curaj A, et al. Blocking CCL5-CXCL4 heteromerization preserves heart function after myocardial infarction by attenuating leukocyte recruitment and NETosis. Sci Rep. 2018;8:10647. http://www.ncbi.nlm.nih.gov/pubmed/30006564.
190. Rischpler C. Acute myocardial infarction. Q J Nucl Med Mol Imaging. 2016;60:236–51. http://www.ncbi.nlm.nih.gov/pubmed/27225319.
191. Prabhu SD, Frangogiannis NG. The biological basis for cardiac repair after myocardial infarction. Circ Res. 2016;119:91–112. http://www.ncbi.nlm.nih.gov/pubmed/27340270.
192. Talman V, Ruskoaho H. Cardiac fibrosis in myocardial infarction—from repair and remodeling to regeneration. Cell Tissue Res. 2016;365:563–81. http://www.ncbi.nlm.nih.gov/pubmed/27324127.
193. Mann DL. The emerging role of innate immunity in the heart and vascular system: for whom the cell tolls. Kirschenbaum L, editor. Circ Res. 2011;108:1133–45. https://www.ahajournals.org/doi/10.1161/CIRCRESAHA.110.226936.
194. Timmers L, Pasterkamp G, de Hoog VC, Arslan F, Appelman Y, de Kleijn DPV. The innate immune response in reperfused myocardium. Cardiovasc Res. 2012;94:276–83. http://www.ncbi.nlm.nih.gov/pubmed/22266751.
195. de Haan JJ, Smeets MB, Pasterkamp G, Arslan F. Danger signals in the initiation of the inflammatory response after myocardial infarction. Mediators Inflamm. 2013;2013:206039. http://www.hindawi.com/journals/mi/2013/206039/.
196. Ghigo A, Franco I, Morello F, Hirsch E. Myocyte signalling in leucocyte recruitment to the heart. Cardiovasc Res. 2014;102:270–80. https://academic.oup.com/cardiovascres/article-lookup/doi/10.1093/cvr/cvu030.
197. Ma Y, Yabluchanskiy A, Iyer RP, Cannon PL, Flynn ER, Jung M, et al. Temporal neutrophil polarization following myocardial infarction. Cardiovasc Res. 2016;110:51–61. http://www.ncbi.nlm.nih.gov/pubmed/26825554.
198. Toldo S, Abbate A. The NLRP3 inflammasome in acute myocardial infarction. Nat Rev Cardiol. 2017;15:203–14. http://www.ncbi.nlm.nih.gov/pubmed/29143812.
199. Wang L, Qu P, Zhao J, Chang Y. NLRP3 and downstream cytokine expression elevated in the monocytes of patients with coronary artery disease. Arch Med Sci. 2014;10:791–800. http://www.termedia.pl/doi/10.5114/aoms.2014.44871.
200. Fox CS, Muntner P, Chen AY, Alexander KP, Roe MT, Wiviott SD. Short-term outcomes of acute myocardial infarction in patients with acute kidney injury. Circulation. 2012;125:497–504. http://www.ncbi.nlm.nih.gov/pubmed/22179533.
201. Damman K, Testani JM. The kidney in heart failure: an update. Eur Heart J. 2015;36:1437–44. http://www.ncbi.nlm.nih.gov/pubmed/25838436.
202. Valgimigli M, Ceconi C, Malagutti P, Merli E, Soukhomovskaia O, Francolini G, et al. Tumor necrosis factor-alpha receptor 1 is a major predictor of mortality and new-onset heart failure in patients with acute myocardial infarction: the Cytokine-Activation and Long-Term Prognosis in Myocardial Infarction (C-ALPHA) study. Circulation. 2005;111:863–70. https://www.ahajournals.org/doi/10.1161/01.CIR.0000155614.35441.69.
203. Ørn S, Ueland T, Manhenke C, Sandanger Ø, Godang K, Yndestad A, et al. Increased interleukin-1β levels are associated with left ventricular hypertrophy and remodelling following acute ST segment elevation myocardial infarction treated by primary percutaneous coronary intervention. J Intern Med. 2012;272:267–76. http://doi.wiley.com/10.1111/j.1365-2796.2012.02517.x.
204. Orn S, Breland UM, Mollnes TE, Manhenke C, Dickstein K, Aukrust P, et al. The chemokine network in relation to infarct size and left ventricular remodeling following acute myocar-

dial infarction. Am J Cardiol. 2009;104:1179–83. http://linkinghub.elsevier.com/retrieve/pii/S0002914909012545.
205. Luc G, Arveiler D, Evans A, Amouyel P, Ferrieres J, Bard J-M, et al. Circulating soluble adhesion molecules ICAM-1 and VCAM-1 and incident coronary heart disease: the PRIME study. Atherosclerosis. 2003;170:169–76. http://www.ncbi.nlm.nih.gov/pubmed/12957696.
206. Fang L, Moore X-L, Dart AM, Wang L-M. Systemic inflammatory response following acute myocardial infarction. J Geriatr Cardiol. 2015;12:305–12. http://www.ncbi.nlm.nih.gov/pubmed/26089856.
207. Sørensen MV, Pedersen S, Møgelvang R, Skov-Jensen J, Flyvbjerg A. Plasma high-mobility group box 1 levels predict mortality after ST-segment elevation myocardial infarction. JACC Cardiovasc Interv. 2011;4:281–6. http://linkinghub.elsevier.com/retrieve/pii/S193687981100015X.
208. Saito T, Hojo Y, Ogoyama Y, Hirose M, Ikemoto T, Katsuki T, et al. S100A12 as a marker to predict cardiovascular events in patients with chronic coronary artery disease. Circ J. 2012;76:2647–52. http://www.ncbi.nlm.nih.gov/pubmed/22786469.
209. Sakuma M, Tanaka A, Kotooka N, Hikichi Y, Toyoda S, Abe S, et al. Myeloid-related protein-8/14 in acute coronary syndrome. Int J Cardiol. 2017;249:25–31. http://www.ncbi.nlm.nih.gov/pubmed/28986057.
210. Wang L, Xie L, Zhang Q, Cai X, Tang Y, Wang L, et al. Plasma nuclear and mitochondrial DNA levels in acute myocardial infarction patients. Coron Artery Dis. 2015;26:296–300. http://www.ncbi.nlm.nih.gov/pubmed/25714070.
211. Simmons JD, Gillespie MN. Plasma nuclear and mitochondrial DNA levels in acute myocardial infarction patients. Coron Artery Dis. 2015;26:286–8. http://www.ncbi.nlm.nih.gov/pubmed/25909176.
212. Chiu T-F, Li C-H, Chen C-C, Chen C-H, Cheng C-J, Yan Y-T, et al. Association of plasma concentration of small heat shock protein B7 with acute coronary syndrome. Circ J. 2012;76:2226–33. http://www.ncbi.nlm.nih.gov/pubmed/22785082.
213. Dutta P, Courties G, Wei Y, Leuschner F, Gorbatov R, Robbins CS, et al. Myocardial infarction accelerates atherosclerosis. Nature. 2012;487:325–9. http://www.nature.com/articles/nature11260.
214. Van der Borght K, Scott CL, Nindl V, Bouché A, Martens L, Sichien D, et al. Myocardial infarction primes autoreactive T cells through activation of dendritic cells. Cell Rep. 2017;18:3005–17. http://www.ncbi.nlm.nih.gov/pubmed/28329691.
215. Halade GV, Kain V, Serhan CN. Immune responsive resolvin D1 programs myocardial infarction–induced cardiorenal syndrome in heart failure. FASEB J. 2018;32:3717–29. http://www.ncbi.nlm.nih.gov/pubmed/29455574.
216. Schmidt T, Carmeliet P. Bridges that guide and unite. Nature. 2010;465:697–9. http://www.ncbi.nlm.nih.gov/pubmed/20535192.
217. Dick SA, Macklin JA, Nejat S, Momen A, Clemente-Casares X, Althagafi MG, et al. Self-renewing resident cardiac macrophages limit adverse remodeling following myocardial infarction. Nat Immunol. 2019;20:29–39. http://www.ncbi.nlm.nih.gov/pubmed/30538339.
218. Cheng Y, Yang C, Luo D, Li X, Le XC, Rong J. N-propargyl caffeamide skews macrophages towards a resolving M2-like phenotype against myocardial ischemic injury via activating Nrf2/HO-1 pathway and inhibiting NF-κB pathway. Cell Physiol Biochem. 2018;47:2544–57. http://www.ncbi.nlm.nih.gov/pubmed/29996121.
219. Werz O, Gerstmeier J, Libreros S, De la Rosa X, Werner M, Norris PC, et al. Human macrophages differentially produce specific resolvin or leukotriene signals that depend on bacterial pathogenicity. Nat Commun. 2018;9:59. http://www.ncbi.nlm.nih.gov/pubmed/29302056.
220. Mann DL. Innate immunity and the failing heart: the cytokine hypothesis revisited. Circ Res. 2015;116:1254–68. https://www.ahajournals.org/doi/10.1161/CIRCRESAHA.116.302317.
221. Kain V, Prabhu SD, Halade GV. Inflammation revisited: inflammation versus resolution of inflammation following myocardial infarction. Basic Res Cardiol. 2014;109:444. http://link.springer.com/10.1007/s00395-014-0444-7.

222. Thorp EB. Contrasting inflammation resolution during atherosclerosis and post myocardial infarction at the level of monocyte/macrophage phagocytic clearance. Front Immunol. 2012;3:39. http://www.ncbi.nlm.nih.gov/pubmed/22566922.
223. Halade GV, Norris PC, Kain V, Serhan CN, Ingle KA. Splenic leukocytes define the resolution of inflammation in heart failure. Sci Signal. 2018;11:eaao1818. http://www.ncbi.nlm.nih.gov/pubmed/29511119.
224. Tourki B, Halade G. Leukocyte diversity in resolving and nonresolving mechanisms of cardiac remodeling. FASEB J. 2017;31:4226–39. http://www.fasebj.org/doi/10.1096/fj.201700109R.
225. Reina-Couto M, Carvalho J, Valente MJ, Vale L, Afonso J, Carvalho F, et al. Impaired resolution of inflammation in human chronic heart failure. Eur J Clin Invest. 2014;44:527–38. http://doi.wiley.com/10.1111/eci.12265.
226. Kain V, Liu F, Kozlovskaya V, Ingle KA, Bolisetty S, Agarwal A, et al. Resolution agonist 15-epi-lipoxin A4 programs early activation of resolving phase in post-myocardial infarction healing. Sci Rep. 2017;7:9999. http://www.ncbi.nlm.nih.gov/pubmed/28855632.
227. Tang J, Zhuang S. Histone acetylation and DNA methylation in ischemia/reperfusion injury. Clin Sci. 2019;133:597–609. http://www.ncbi.nlm.nih.gov/pubmed/30804072.
228. Li J, Zhu X, Yu K, Jiang H, Zhang Y, Deng S, et al. Genome-wide analysis of DNA methylation and acute coronary syndrome. Circ Res. 2017;120:1754–67. https://www.ahajournals.org/doi/10.1161/CIRCRESAHA.116.310324.
229. Wang X, Liu A-H, Jia Z-W, Pu K, Chen K-Y, Guo H. Genome-wide DNA methylation patterns in coronary heart disease. Herz. 2018;43:656–62. http://link.springer.com/10.1007/s00059-017-4616-8.
230. Li D, Yan J, Yuan Y, Wang C, Wu J, Chen Q, et al. Genome-wide DNA methylome alterations in acute coronary syndrome. Int J Mol Med. 2018;41:220–32. http://www.spandidos-publications.com/10.3892/ijmm.2017.3220.
231. Xie M, Hill JA. HDAC-dependent ventricular remodeling. Trends Cardiovasc Med. 2013;23:229–35. https://linkinghub.elsevier.com/retrieve/pii/S105017381200463X.
232. Gulati A, Jabbour A, Ismail TF, Guha K, Khwaja J, Raza S, et al. Association of fibrosis with mortality and sudden cardiac death in patients with nonischemic dilated cardiomyopathy. JAMA. 2013;309:896. http://www.ncbi.nlm.nih.gov/pubmed/23462786.
233. Krenning G, Zeisberg EM, Kalluri R. The origin of fibroblasts and mechanism of cardiac fibrosis. J Cell Physiol. 2010;225:631–7. http://doi.wiley.com/10.1002/jcp.22322.
234. Liaudet L, Rosenblatt-Velin N. Role of innate immunity in cardiac inflammation after myocardial infarction. Front Biosci (Schol Ed). 2013;5:86–104. http://www.ncbi.nlm.nih.gov/pubmed/23277038.
235. Shiraishi M, Shintani Y, Shintani Y, Ishida H, Saba R, Yamaguchi A, et al. Alternatively activated macrophages determine repair of the infarcted adult murine heart. J Clin Invest. 2016;126:2151–66. https://www.jci.org/articles/view/85782.
236. Humeres C, Frangogiannis NG. Fibroblasts in the infarcted, remodeling, and failing heart. JACC Basic to Transl Sci. 2019;4:449–67. http://www.ncbi.nlm.nih.gov/pubmed/31312768.
237. Zhang W, Lavine KJ, Epelman S, Evans SA, Weinheimer CJ, Barger PM, et al. Necrotic myocardial cells release damage-associated molecular patterns that provoke fibroblast activation in vitro and trigger myocardial inflammation and fibrosis in vivo. J Am Heart Assoc. 2015;4:e001993. http://www.ncbi.nlm.nih.gov/pubmed/26037082.
238. Leicht M. Comitogenic effect of catecholamines on rat cardiac fibroblasts in culture. Cardiovasc Res. 2000;48:274–84. https://academic.oup.com/cardiovascres/article-lookup/doi/10.1016/S0008-6363(00)00170-X.
239. Sun Y, Weber KT. Angiotensin converting enzyme and myofibroblasts during tissue repair in the rat heart. J Mol Cell Cardiol. 1996;28:851–8. http://www.ncbi.nlm.nih.gov/pubmed/8762025.
240. van den Borne SWM, Diez J, Blankesteijn WM, Verjans J, Hofstra L, Narula J. Myocardial remodeling after infarction: the role of myofibroblasts. Nat Rev Cardiol. 2010;7:30–7. http://www.nature.com/articles/nrcardio.2009.199.

241. Shinde AV, Frangogiannis NG. Fibroblasts in myocardial infarction: a role in inflammation and repair. J Mol Cell Cardiol. 2014;70:74–82. https://linkinghub.elsevier.com/retrieve/pii/S0022282813003477.
242. Boza P, Ayala P, Vivar R, Humeres C, Cáceres FT, Muñoz C, et al. Expression and function of toll-like receptor 4 and inflammasomes in cardiac fibroblasts and myofibroblasts: IL-1β synthesis, secretion, and degradation. Mol Immunol. 2016;74:96–105. http://www.ncbi.nlm.nih.gov/pubmed/27174187.
243. Moore-Morris T, Cattaneo P, Guimarães-Camboa N, Bogomolovas J, Cedenilla M, Banerjee I, et al. Infarct fibroblasts do not derive from bone marrow lineages. Circ Res. 2018;122:583–90. https://www.ahajournals.org/doi/10.1161/CIRCRESAHA.117.311490.
244. Ma Y, Iyer RP, Jung M, Czubryt MP, Lindsey ML. Cardiac fibroblast activation post-myocardial infarction: current knowledge gaps. Trends Pharmacol Sci. 2017;38:448–58. http://www.ncbi.nlm.nih.gov/pubmed/28365093.
245. Li L, Zhao Q, Kong W. Extracellular matrix remodeling and cardiac fibrosis. Matrix Biol. 2018;68–69:490–506. http://www.ncbi.nlm.nih.gov/pubmed/29371055.
246. Di Maggio S, Milano G, De Marchis F, D'Ambrosio A, Bertolotti M, Palacios BS, et al. Non-oxidizable HMGB1 induces cardiac fibroblasts migration via CXCR4 in a CXCL12-independent manner and worsens tissue remodeling after myocardial infarction. Biochim Biophys Acta - Mol Basis Dis. 2017;1863:2693–704. http://www.ncbi.nlm.nih.gov/pubmed/28716707.
247. Wang Y, Ouyang M, Wang Q, Jian Z. MicroRNA-142-3p inhibits hypoxia/reoxygenation-induced apoptosis and fibrosis of cardiomyocytes by targeting high mobility group box 1. Int J Mol Med. 2016;38:1377–86. http://www.ncbi.nlm.nih.gov/pubmed/28025989.
248. Takahashi M. NLRP3 in myocardial ischaemia-reperfusion injury: inflammasome-dependent or -independent role in different cell types. Cardiovasc Res. 2013;99:4–5. http://www.ncbi.nlm.nih.gov/pubmed/23737495.
249. Sandanger Ø, Ranheim T, Vinge LE, Bliksøen M, Alfsnes K, Finsen AV, et al. The NLRP3 inflammasome is up-regulated in cardiac fibroblasts and mediates myocardial ischaemia-reperfusion injury. Cardiovasc Res. 2013;99:164–74. https://academic.oup.com/cardiovascres/article-lookup/doi/10.1093/cvr/cvt091.
250. Takahashi M. NLRP3 inflammasome as a novel player in myocardial infarction. Int Heart J. 2014;55:101–5. http://www.ncbi.nlm.nih.gov/pubmed/24632952.
251. Dobaczewski M, de Haan JJ, Frangogiannis NG. The extracellular matrix modulates fibroblast phenotype and function in the infarcted myocardium. J Cardiovasc Transl Res. 2012;5:837–47. http://link.springer.com/10.1007/s12265-012-9406-3.
252. Falkenham A, de Antueno R, Rosin N, Betsch D, Lee TDG, Duncan R, et al. Nonclassical resident macrophages are important determinants in the development of myocardial fibrosis. Am J Pathol. 2015;185:927–42. https://linkinghub.elsevier.com/retrieve/pii/S0002944015000243.
253. Saucerman JJ, Tan PM, Buchholz KS, McCulloch AD, Omens JH. Mechanical regulation of gene expression in cardiac myocytes and fibroblasts. Nat Rev Cardiol. 2019;16:361–78. http://www.nature.com/articles/s41569-019-0155-8.
254. Santiago J-J, Dangerfield AL, Rattan SG, Bathe KL, Cunnington RH, Raizman JE, et al. Cardiac fibroblast to myofibroblast differentiation in vivo and in vitro: expression of focal adhesion components in neonatal and adult rat ventricular myofibroblasts. Dev Dyn. 2010;239:1573–84. http://doi.wiley.com/10.1002/dvdy.22280.
255. Herum KM, Lunde IG, McCulloch AD, Christensen G. The soft- and hard-heartedness of cardiac fibroblasts: mechanotransduction signaling pathways in fibrosis of the heart. J Clin Med. 2017;6:53. http://www.mdpi.com/2077-0383/6/5/53.
256. Kim P, Chu N, Davis J, Kim D-H. Mechanoregulation of myofibroblast fate and cardiac fibrosis. Adv Biosyst. 2018;2:1700172. http://doi.wiley.com/10.1002/adbi.201700172.
257. Czubryt MP. Cardiac fibroblast to myofibroblast phenotype conversion-an unexploited therapeutic target. J Cardiovasc Dev Dis. 2019;6:28. https://www.mdpi.com/2308-3425/6/3/28.

258. Herum KM, Choppe J, Kumar A, Engler AJ, McCulloch AD. Mechanical regulation of cardiac fibroblast profibrotic phenotypes. Mol Biol Cell. 2017;28:1871–82. http://www.ncbi.nlm.nih.gov/pubmed/28468977.
259. Chen C, Li R, Ross RS, Manso AM. Integrins and integrin-related proteins in cardiac fibrosis. J Mol Cell Cardiol. 2016;93:162–74. http://www.ncbi.nlm.nih.gov/pubmed/26562414.
260. Liang J, Huang B, Yuan G, Chen Y, Liang F, Zeng H, et al. Stretch-activated channel Piezo1 is up-regulated in failure heart and cardiomyocyte stimulated by AngII. Am J Transl Res. 2017;9:2945–55. http://www.ncbi.nlm.nih.gov/pubmed/28670382.
261. Ruthenborg RJ, Ban J-J, Wazir A, Takeda N, Kim J. Regulation of wound healing and fibrosis by hypoxia and hypoxia-inducible factor-1. Mol Cells. 2014;37:637–43. http://www.ncbi.nlm.nih.gov/pubmed/24957212.
262. Darby IA, Hewitson TD. Hypoxia in tissue repair and fibrosis. Cell Tissue Res. 2016;365:553–62. http://link.springer.com/10.1007/s00441-016-2461-3.
263. Stratton MS, McKinsey TA. Epigenetic regulation of cardiac fibrosis. J Mol Cell Cardiol. 2016;92:206–13. http://www.ncbi.nlm.nih.gov/pubmed/26876451.
264. Grimaldi V, De Pascale MR, Zullo A, Soricelli A, Infante T, Mancini FP, et al. Evidence of epigenetic tags in cardiac fibrosis. J Cardiol. 2017;69:401–8. https://linkinghub.elsevier.com/retrieve/pii/S091450871630243X.
265. Ghosh AK, Rai R, Flevaris P, Vaughan DE. Epigenetics in reactive and reparative cardiac fibrogenesis: the promise of epigenetic therapy. J Cell Physiol. 2017;232:1941–56. http://doi.wiley.com/10.1002/jcp.25699.
266. Felisbino MB, McKinsey TA. Epigenetics in cardiac fibrosis. JACC Basic to Transl Sci. 2018;3:704–15. http://www.ncbi.nlm.nih.gov/pubmed/30456341.
267. He Y, Ling S, Sun Y, Sheng Z, Chen Z, Pan X, et al. DNA methylation regulates α-smooth muscle actin expression during cardiac fibroblast differentiation. J Cell Physiol. 2019;234:7174–85. http://www.ncbi.nlm.nih.gov/pubmed/30362530.
268. Nural-Guvener HF, Zakharova L, Nimlos J, Popovic S, Mastroeni D, Gaballa MA. HDAC class I inhibitor, mocetinostat, reverses cardiac fibrosis in heart failure and diminishes CD90+ cardiac myofibroblast activation. Fibrogenesis Tissue Repair. 2014;7:10. http://fibrogenesis.biomedcentral.com/articles/10.1186/1755-1536-7-10.
269. Williams SM, Golden-Mason L, Ferguson BS, Schuetze KB, Cavasin MA, Demos-Davies K, et al. Class I HDACs regulate angiotensin II-dependent cardiac fibrosis via fibroblasts and circulating fibrocytes. J Mol Cell Cardiol. 2014;67:112–25. https://linkinghub.elsevier.com/retrieve/pii/S0022282813003623.
270. Schuetze KB, Stratton MS, Blakeslee WW, Wempe MF, Wagner FF, Holson EB, et al. Overlapping and divergent actions of structurally distinct histone deacetylase inhibitors in cardiac fibroblasts. J Pharmacol Exp Ther. 2017;361:140–50. http://jpet.aspetjournals.org/lookup/doi/10.1124/jpet.116.237701.
271. Lyu X, Hu M, Peng J, Zhang X, Sanders YY. HDAC inhibitors as antifibrotic drugs in cardiac and pulmonary fibrosis. Ther Adv Chronic Dis. 2019;10:204062231986269. http://www.ncbi.nlm.nih.gov/pubmed/31367296.
272. Piccoli M-T, Bär C, Thum T. Non-coding RNAs as modulators of the cardiac fibroblast phenotype. J Mol Cell Cardiol. 2016;92:75–81. https://linkinghub.elsevier.com/retrieve/pii/S0022282815301619.
273. Tao H, Yang J-J, Hu W, Shi K-H, Deng Z-Y, Li J. Noncoding RNA as regulators of cardiac fibrosis: current insight and the road ahead. Pflugers Arch. 2016;468:1103–11. http://link.springer.com/10.1007/s00424-016-1792-y.
274. Roy S, Khanna S, Hussain S-RA, Biswas S, Azad A, Rink C, et al. MicroRNA expression in response to murine myocardial infarction: miR-21 regulates fibroblast metalloprotease-2 via phosphatase and tensin homologue. Cardiovasc Res. 2009;82:21–9. https://academic.oup.com/cardiovascres/article-lookup/doi/10.1093/cvr/cvp015.
275. Zhuang Y, Li T, Zhuang Y, Li Z, Yang W, Huang Q, et al. Involvement of lncR-30245 in myocardial infarction–induced cardiac fibrosis through peroxisome proliferator-activated

receptor-γ–mediated connective tissue growth factor signalling pathway. Can J Cardiol. 2019;35:480–9. http://www.ncbi.nlm.nih.gov/pubmed/30935639.
276. Bui AL, Horwich TB, Fonarow GC. Epidemiology and risk profile of heart failure. Nat Rev Cardiol. 2011;8(1):30–41.
277. van Hout GP, Arslan F, Pasterkamp G, Hoefer IE. Targeting danger-associated molecular patterns after myocardial infarction. Expert Opin Ther Targets. 2016;20:223–39. http://www.ncbi.nlm.nih.gov/pubmed/26420647.
278. Roche PL, Filomeno KL, Bagchi RA, Czubryt MP. Intracellular signaling of cardiac fibroblasts. Compr Physiol. 2015;5:721–60. http://doi.wiley.com/10.1002/cphy.c140044.
279. Andrassy M, Volz HC, Igwe JC, Funke B, Eichberger SN, Kaya Z, et al. High-mobility group box-1 in ischemia-reperfusion injury of the heart. Circulation. 2008;117:3216–26. http://circ.ahajournals.org/cgi/doi/10.1161/CIRCULATIONAHA.108.769331.
280. Ding H-S, Yang J, Chen P, Yang J, Bo S-Q, Ding J-W, et al. The HMGB1-TLR4 axis contributes to myocardial ischemia/reperfusion injury via regulation of cardiomyocyte apoptosis. Gene. 2013;527:389–93. https://linkinghub.elsevier.com/retrieve/pii/S037811191300677X.
281. Hu G, Zhang Y, Jiang H, Hu X. Exendin-4 attenuates myocardial ischemia and reperfusion injury by inhibiting high mobility group box 1 protein expression. Cardiol J. 2013;20:600–4. http://www.ncbi.nlm.nih.gov/pubmed/24338536.
282. Lin Y, Chen L, Li W, Fang J. Role of high-mobility group box-1 in myocardial ischemia/reperfusion injury and the effect of ethyl pyruvate. Exp Ther Med. 2015;9:1537–41. http://www.ncbi.nlm.nih.gov/pubmed/25780465.
283. Zhang G, Zhang X, Li D, Tian J, Jiang W. Long-term oral atazanavir attenuates myocardial infarction-induced cardiac fibrosis. Eur J Pharmacol. 2018;828:97–102. http://www.ncbi.nlm.nih.gov/pubmed/29605419.
284. Bauzá M del R, Giménez CS, Locatelli P, De Lorenzi A, Hnatiuk A, Capogrossi MC, et al. High-dose intramyocardial HMGB1 induces long-term cardioprotection in sheep with myocardial infarction. Drug Deliv Transl Res. 2019;9:935–44. http://link.springer.com/10.1007/s13346-019-00628-z.
285. Liu F-Y, Fan D, Yang Z, Tang N, Guo Z, Ma S-Q, et al. TLR9 is essential for HMGB1-mediated post-myocardial infarction tissue repair through affecting apoptosis, cardiac healing, and angiogenesis. Cell Death Dis. 2019;10:480. http://www.ncbi.nlm.nih.gov/pubmed/31209243.
286. Raucci A, Di Maggio S, Scavello F, D'Ambrosio A, Bianchi ME, Capogrossi MC. The Janus face of HMGB1 in heart disease: a necessary update. Cell Mol Life Sci. 2019;76:211–29. http://www.ncbi.nlm.nih.gov/pubmed/30306212.
287. Wu H, Li R, Pei L-G, Wei Z-H, Kang L-N, Wang L, et al. Emerging role of high mobility group box-1 in thrombosis-related diseases. Cell Physiol Biochem. 2018;47:1319–37. http://www.ncbi.nlm.nih.gov/pubmed/29940562.
288. Ahrens I, Chen Y-C, Topcic D, Bode M, Haenel D, Hagemeyer CE, et al. HMGB1 binds to activated platelets via the receptor for advanced glycation end products and is present in platelet rich human coronary artery thrombi. Thromb Haemost. 2015;114:994–1003. http://www.thieme-connect.de/DOI/DOI?10.1160/TH14-12-1073.
289. Yamashita A, Nishihira K, Matsuura Y, Ito T, Kawahara K, Hatakeyama K, et al. Paucity of CD34-positive cells and increased expression of high-mobility group box 1 in coronary thrombus with type 2 diabetes mellitus. Atherosclerosis. 2012;224:511–4. https://linkinghub.elsevier.com/retrieve/pii/S0021915012004996.
290. Goldstein RS, Gallowitsch-Puerta M, Yang L, Rosas-Ballina M, Huston JM, Czura CJ, et al. Elevated high-mobility group box 1 levels in patients with cerebral and myocardial ischemia. Shock. 2006;25:571–4. https://insights.ovid.com/crossref?an=00024382-200606000-00003.
291. Cirillo P, Giallauria F, Pacileo M, Petrillo G, D'Agostino M, Vigorito C, et al. Increased high mobility group box-1 protein levels are associated with impaired cardiopulmonary and echocardiographic findings after acute myocardial infarction. J Card Fail. 2009;15:362–7. https://linkinghub.elsevier.com/retrieve/pii/S1071916408010890.

292. Sørensen MV, Pedersen S, Møgelvang R, Skov-Jensen J, Flyvbjerg A. Plasma high-mobility group box 1 levels predict mortality after ST-segment elevation myocardial infarction. JACC Cardiovasc Interv. 2011;4:281–6. http://www.ncbi.nlm.nih.gov/pubmed/21435605.
293. Andrassy M, Volz HC, Riedle N, Gitsioudis G, Seidel C, Laohachewin D, et al. HMGB1 as a predictor of infarct transmurality and functional recovery in patients with myocardial infarction. J Intern Med. 2011;270:245–53. http://doi.wiley.com/10.1111/j.1365-2796.2011.02369.x.
294. Hashimoto T, Ishii J, Kitagawa F, Yamada S, Hattori K, Okumura M, et al. Circulating high-mobility group box 1 and cardiovascular mortality in unstable angina and non-ST-segment elevation myocardial infarction. Atherosclerosis. 2012;221:490–5. https://linkinghub.elsevier.com/retrieve/pii/S0021915012000731.
295. Chen J, Zhang W, Wu Y-Q, Chen H, Zhao J-F. Correlations of acute myocardial infarction complicated by cerebral infarction with insulin resistance, adiponectin and HMGB1. Eur Rev Med Pharmacol Sci. 2019;23:4425–31. http://www.ncbi.nlm.nih.gov/pubmed/31173318.
296. Schneider M, Kostin S, Strøm CC, Aplin M, Lyngbaek S, Theilade J, et al. S100A4 is upregulated in injured myocardium and promotes growth and survival of cardiac myocytes. Cardiovasc Res. 2007;75:40–50. https://academic.oup.com/cardiovascres/article-lookup/doi/10.1016/j.cardiores.2007.03.027.
297. Katashima T, Naruko T, Terasaki F, Fujita M, Otsuka K, Murakami S, et al. Enhanced expression of the S100A8/A9 complex in acute myocardial infarction patients. Circ J. 2010;74:741–8. http://joi.jlc.jst.go.jp/JST.JSTAGE/circj/CJ-09-0564?from=CrossRef.
298. Cai XY, Lu L, Wang YN, Jin C, Zhang RY, Zhang Q, et al. Association of increased S100B, S100A6 and S100P in serum levels with acute coronary syndrome and also with the severity of myocardial infarction in cardiac tissue of rat models with ischemia–reperfusion injury. Atherosclerosis. 2011;217:536–42. http://www.ncbi.nlm.nih.gov/pubmed/21663912.
299. Schiopu A, Cotoi OS. S100A8 and S100A9: DAMPs at the crossroads between innate immunity, traditional risk factors, and cardiovascular disease. Mediators Inflamm. 2013;2013:828354. http://www.hindawi.com/journals/mi/2013/828354/.
300. Wang Y, Fang C, Gao H, Bilodeau ML, Zhang Z, Croce K, et al. Platelet-derived S100 family member myeloid-related protein-14 regulates thrombosis. J Clin Invest. 2014;124:2160–71. http://www.ncbi.nlm.nih.gov/pubmed/24691441.
301. Oesterle A, Bowman MAH. S100A12 and the S100/calgranulins: emerging biomarkers for atherosclerosis and possibly therapeutic targets. Arterioscler Thromb Vasc Biol. 2015;35:2496–507. http://atvb.ahajournals.org/lookup/doi/10.1161/ATVBAHA.115.302072.
302. Gong X-J, Song X-Y, Wei H, Wang J, Niu M. Serum S100A4 levels as a novel biomarker for detection of acute myocardial infarction. Eur Rev Med Pharmacol Sci. 2015;19:2221–5. http://www.ncbi.nlm.nih.gov/pubmed/26166646.
303. Qian L, Hong J, Zhang Y, Zhu M, Wang X, Zhang Y, et al. Downregulation of S100A4 alleviates cardiac fibrosis via Wnt/β-catenin pathway in mice. Cell Physiol Biochem. 2018;46:2551–60. http://www.ncbi.nlm.nih.gov/pubmed/29758552.
304. Sreejit G, Nooti SK, Athmanathan B, Nagareddy PR. S100A8/A9 in myocardial infarction. Methods Mol Biol. 2019;1929:739–54. http://www.ncbi.nlm.nih.gov/pubmed/30710308.
305. Chen C, Feng Y, Zou L, Wang L, Chen HH, Cai J-Y, et al. Role of extracellular RNA and TLR3-Trif signaling in myocardial ischemia-reperfusion injury. J Am Heart Assoc. 2014;3:e000683. https://www.ahajournals.org/doi/10.1161/JAHA.113.000683.
306. Bliksøen M, Mariero LH, Torp MK, Baysa A, Ytrehus K, Haugen F, et al. Extracellular mtDNA activates NF-κB via toll-like receptor 9 and induces cell death in cardiomyocytes. Basic Res Cardiol. 2016;111:42. http://link.springer.com/10.1007/s00395-016-0553-6.
307. Bliksøen M, Mariero LH, Ohm IK, Haugen F, Yndestad A, Solheim S, et al. Increased circulating mitochondrial DNA after myocardial infarction. Int J Cardiol. 2012;158:132–4. https://linkinghub.elsevier.com/retrieve/pii/S0167527312004688.
308. Qin C, Gu J, Liu R, Xu F, Qian H, He Q, et al. Release of mitochondrial DNA correlates with peak inflammatory cytokines in patients with acute myocardial infarction. Anatol J Cardiol. 2017;17:224–8. http://www.anakarder.com/jvi.aspx?pdir=anatoljcardiol&plng=eng&un=AJC-71602.

309. Mezzaroma E, Toldo S, Farkas D, Seropian IM, Van Tassell BW, Salloum FN, et al. The inflammasome promotes adverse cardiac remodeling following acute myocardial infarction in the mouse. Proc Natl Acad Sci U S A. 2011;108:19725–30. http://www.pnas.org/cgi/doi/10.1073/pnas.1108586108.
310. Mezzaroma E, Marchetti C, Toldo S. Letter by Mezzaroma, et al regarding article, "NLRP3 inflammasome as a therapeutic target in myocardial infarction". Int Heart J. 2014;55:379. http://www.ncbi.nlm.nih.gov/pubmed/24942779.
311. van Hout GPJ, Bosch L. The inflammasomes in cardiovascular disease. Exp Suppl. 2018;108:9–40. http://link.springer.com/10.1007/978-3-319-89390-7_2.
312. Zhou W, Chen C, Chen Z, Liu L, Jiang J, Wu Z, et al. NLRP3: a novel mediator in cardiovascular disease. J Immunol Res. 2018;2018:5702103. https://www.hindawi.com/journals/jir/2018/5702103/.
313. Mauro AG, Bonaventura A, Mezzaroma E, Quader M, Toldo S. NLRP3 inflammasome in acute myocardial infarction. J Cardiovasc Pharmacol. 2019;74:175–87. http://insights.ovid.com/crossref?an=00005344-201909000-00002.
314. Liu W, Zhang X, Zhao M, Zhang X, Chi J, Liu Y, et al. Activation in M1 but not M2 macrophages contributes to cardiac remodeling after myocardial infarction in rats: a critical role of the calcium sensing receptor/NRLP3 inflammasome. Cell Physiol Biochem. 2015;35:2483–500. http://www.ncbi.nlm.nih.gov/pubmed/25967877.
315. Gao R, Shi H, Chang S, Gao Y, Li X, Lv C, et al. The selective NLRP3-inflammasome inhibitor MCC950 reduces myocardial fibrosis and improves cardiac remodeling in a mouse model of myocardial infarction. Int Immunopharmacol. 2019;74:105575. http://www.ncbi.nlm.nih.gov/pubmed/31299609.
316. Lugrin J, Parapanov R, Rosenblatt-Velin N, Rignault-Clerc S, Feihl F, Waeber B, et al. Cutting edge: IL-1α is a crucial danger signal triggering acute myocardial inflammation during myocardial infarction. J Immunol. 2015;194:499–503. http://www.jimmunol.org/lookup/doi/10.4049/jimmunol.1401948.
317. Nastase MV, Janicova A, Roedig H, Hsieh LT-H, Wygrecka M, Schaefer L. Small leucine-rich proteoglycans in renal inflammation: two sides of the coin. J Histochem Cytochem. 2018;66:261–72. http://journals.sagepub.com/doi/10.1369/0022155417738752.
318. Christensen G, Herum KM, Lunde IG. Sweet, yet underappreciated: proteoglycans and extracellular matrix remodeling in heart disease. Matrix Biol. 2019;75–76:286–99. https://linkinghub.elsevier.com/retrieve/pii/S0945053X17302718.
319. Adapala RK, Thoppil RJ, Luther DJ, Paruchuri S, Meszaros JG, Chilian WM, et al. TRPV4 channels mediate cardiac fibroblast differentiation by integrating mechanical and soluble signals. J Mol Cell Cardiol. 2013;54:45–52. https://linkinghub.elsevier.com/retrieve/pii/S0022282812003987.
320. Sharma S, Goswami R, Merth M, Cohen J, Lei KY, Zhang DX, et al. TRPV4 ion channel is a novel regulator of dermal myofibroblast differentiation. Am J Physiol Cell Physiol. 2017;312:C562–72. https://www.physiology.org/doi/10.1152/ajpcell.00187.2016.
321. Numaga-Tomita T, Kitajima N, Kuroda T, Nishimura A, Miyano K, Yasuda S, et al. TRPC3-GEF-H1 axis mediates pressure overload-induced cardiac fibrosis. Sci Rep. 2016;6:39383. http://www.nature.com/articles/srep39383.
322. Tian M, Yuan Y-C, Li J-Y, Gionfriddo MR, Huang R-C. Tumor necrosis factor-α and its role as a mediator in myocardial infarction: a brief review. Chronic Dis Transl Med. 2015;1:18–26. https://linkinghub.elsevier.com/retrieve/pii/S2095882X15000031.
323. Sun Y, Weber KT. Infarct scar: a dynamic tissue. Cardiovasc Res. 2000;46:250–6. http://www.ncbi.nlm.nih.gov/pubmed/10773228.
324. Bader M. Role of the local renin-angiotensin system in cardiac damage: a minireview focussing on transgenic animal models. J Mol Cell Cardiol. 2002;34:1455–62. https://linkinghub.elsevier.com/retrieve/pii/S0022282802920778.
325. Leenen FH, Skarda V, Yuan B, White R. Changes in cardiac ANG II postmyocardial infarction in rats: effects of nephrectomy and ACE inhibitors. Am J Physiol. 1999;276:H317–25. https://www.physiology.org/doi/10.1152/ajpheart.1999.276.1.H317.

326. Skovsted GF, Kruse LS, Berchtold LA, Grell A-S, Warfvinge K, Edvinsson L. Myocardial ischemia-reperfusion enhances transcriptional expression of endothelin-1 and vasoconstrictor ETB receptors via the protein kinase MEK-ERK1/2 signaling pathway in rat. Wang M, editor. PLoS One. 2017;12:e0174119. https://dx.plos.org/10.1371/journal.pone.0174119.
327. Kolettis TM, Barton M, Langleben D, Matsumura Y. Endothelin in coronary artery disease and myocardial infarction. Cardiol Rev. 2013;21:249–56. http://content.wkhealth.com/linkback/openurl?sid=WKPTLP:landingpage&an=00045415-201309000-00005.
328. Mueller EE, Momen A, Massé S, Zhou Y-Q, Liu J, Backx PH, et al. Electrical remodelling precedes heart failure in an endothelin-1-induced model of cardiomyopathy. Cardiovasc Res. 2011;89:623–33. https://academic.oup.com/cardiovascres/article-lookup/doi/10.1093/cvr/cvq351.
329. Jankowich M, Choudhary G. Endothelin-1 levels and cardiovascular events. Trends Cardiovasc Med. 2019;30(1):1–8. https://linkinghub.elsevier.com/retrieve/pii/S1050173818302330.
330. Zhou B-Y, Gao X-Y, Zhao X, Qing P, Zhu C-G, Wu N-Q, et al. Predictive value of big endothelin-1 on outcomes in patients with myocardial infarction younger than 35 years old. Per Med. 2018;15:25–33. https://www.futuremedicine.com/doi/10.2217/pme-2017-0044.
331. Qin CX, Finlayson SB, Al-Sharea A, Tate M, De Blasio MJ, Deo M, et al. Endogenous annexin-A1 regulates haematopoietic stem cell mobilisation and inflammatory response post myocardial infarction in mice in vivo. Sci Rep. 2017;7:16615. http://www.ncbi.nlm.nih.gov/pubmed/29192208.
332. Ferraro B, Leoni G, Hinkel R, Ormanns S, Paulin N, Ortega-Gomez A, et al. Pro-angiogenic macrophage phenotype to promote myocardial repair. J Am Coll Cardiol. 2019;73:2990–3002. https://linkinghub.elsevier.com/retrieve/pii/S0735109719348600.
333. Qin CX, Rosli S, Deo M, Cao N, Walsh J, Tate M, et al. Cardioprotective actions of the annexin-A1 N-terminal peptide, Ac2-26, against myocardial infarction. Front Pharmacol. 2019;10:269. http://www.ncbi.nlm.nih.gov/pubmed/31001111.
334. Mullane K. Harnessing an endogenous cardioprotective mechanism: cellular sources and sites of action of adenosine. J Mol Cell Cardiol. 1995;27:1041–54. https://linkinghub.elsevier.com/retrieve/pii/002228289590073X.
335. Reid EA, Kristo G, Yoshimura Y, Ballard-Croft C, Keith BJ, Mentzer RM, et al. In vivo adenosine receptor preconditioning reduces myocardial infarct size via subcellular ERK signaling. Am J Physiol Heart Circ Physiol. 2005;288:H2253–9. https://www.physiology.org/doi/10.1152/ajpheart.01009.2004.
336. Mahaffey KW, Puma JA, Barbagelata NA, DiCarli MF, Leesar MA, Browne KF, et al. Adenosine as an adjunct to thrombolytic therapy for acute myocardial infarction: results of a multicenter, randomized, placebo-controlled trial: the Acute Myocardial Infarction STudy of ADenosine (AMISTAD) trial. J Am Coll Cardiol. 1999;34:1711–20. http://www.ncbi.nlm.nih.gov/pubmed/10577561.
337. Ross AM, Gibbons RJ, Stone GW, Kloner RA, Alexander RW, AMISTAD-II Investigators. A randomized, double-blinded, placebo-controlled multicenter trial of adenosine as an adjunct to reperfusion in the treatment of acute myocardial infarction (AMISTAD-II). J Am Coll Cardiol. 2005;45:1775–80. https://linkinghub.elsevier.com/retrieve/pii/S073510970500536X.
338. Bulluck H, Sirker A, Loke YK, Garcia-Dorado D, Hausenloy DJ. Clinical benefit of adenosine as an adjunct to reperfusion in ST-elevation myocardial infarction patients: an updated meta-analysis of randomized controlled trials. Int J Cardiol. 2016;202:228–37. https://linkinghub.elsevier.com/retrieve/pii/S0167527315304460.
339. Hausenloy DJ, Botker HE, Engstrom T, Erlinge D, Heusch G, Ibanez B, et al. Targeting reperfusion injury in patients with ST-segment elevation myocardial infarction: trials and tribulations. Eur Heart J. 2016;38:ehw145. http://www.ncbi.nlm.nih.gov/pubmed/27118196.
340. Golino P, Ambrosio G, Villari B, Ragni M, Focaccio A, Pace L, et al. Endogenous prostaglandin endoperoxides may alter infarct size in the presence of thromboxane synthase inhibition: studies in a rabbit model of coronary artery occlusion-reperfusion. J Am Coll Cardiol. 1993;21:493–501. https://linkinghub.elsevier.com/retrieve/pii/073510979390694V.

341. Birnbaum Y, Ye Y, Rosanio S, Tavackoli S, Hu Z-Y, Schwarz ER, et al. Prostaglandins mediate the cardioprotective effects of atorvastatin against ischemia-reperfusion injury. Cardiovasc Res. 2005;65:345–55. https://academic.oup.com/cardiovascres/article-lookup/doi/10.1016/j.cardiores.2004.10.018.
342. Hishikari K, Suzuki J, Ogawa M, Isobe K, Takahashi T, Onishi M, et al. Pharmacological activation of the prostaglandin E2 receptor EP4 improves cardiac function after myocardial ischaemia/reperfusion injury. Cardiovasc Res. 2009;81:123–32. https://academic.oup.com/cardiovascres/article-lookup/doi/10.1093/cvr/cvn254.
343. Pang L, Cai Y, Tang EHC, Irwin MG, Ma H, Xia Z. Prostaglandin E receptor subtype 4 signaling in the heart: role in ischemia/reperfusion injury and cardiac hypertrophy. J Diabetes Res. 2016;2016:1324347. http://www.hindawi.com/journals/jdr/2016/1324347/.
344. Zhou Y, Yang P, Li A, Ye X, Ren S, Li X. Prostaglandin E2 reduces swine myocardial ischemia reperfusion injury via increased endothelial nitric oxide synthase and vascular endothelial growth factor expression levels. Biomed Rep. 2017;6:188–94. https://www.spandidos-publications.com/10.3892/br.2016.834.
345. Kain V, Ingle KA, Colas RA, Dalli J, Prabhu SD, Serhan CN, et al. Resolvin D1 activates the inflammation resolving response at splenic and ventricular site following myocardial infarction leading to improved ventricular function. J Mol Cell Cardiol. 2015;84:24–35. https://linkinghub.elsevier.com/retrieve/pii/S0022282815001042.
346. Fredman G, Spite M. Specialized pro-resolving mediators in cardiovascular diseases. Mol Aspects Med. 2017;58:65–71. http://www.ncbi.nlm.nih.gov/pubmed/28257820.
347. Leoni G, Soehnlein O. (Re) solving repair after myocardial infarction. Front Pharmacol. 2018;9:1342. http://www.ncbi.nlm.nih.gov/pubmed/30534069.
348. Fosshaug LE, Colas RA, Anstensrud AK, Gregersen I, Nymo S, Sagen EL, et al. Early increase of specialized pro-resolving lipid mediators in patients with ST-elevation myocardial infarction. EBioMedicine. 2019;46:264–73. http://www.ncbi.nlm.nih.gov/pubmed/31345784.
349. Halade GV, Tourki B. Specialized pro-resolving mediators directs cardiac healing and repair with activation of inflammation and resolution program in heart failure. Adv Exp Med Biol. 2019;1161:45–64. http://www.ncbi.nlm.nih.gov/pubmed/31562621.
350. Liu R, Li Z, Wang Q. Resolvin D1 attenuates myocardial infarction in a rodent model with the participation of the HMGB1 pathway. Cardiovasc Drugs Ther. 2019;33:399–406. http://link.springer.com/10.1007/s10557-019-06884-y.
351. Miao C, Lei M, Hu W, Han S, Wang Q. A brief review: the therapeutic potential of bone marrow mesenchymal stem cells in myocardial infarction. Stem Cell Res Ther. 2017;8:242. http://www.ncbi.nlm.nih.gov/pubmed/29096705.
352. Meng X, Chen M, Su W, Tao X, Sun M, Zou X, et al. The differentiation of mesenchymal stem cells to vascular cells regulated by the HMGB1/RAGE axis: its application in cell therapy for transplant arteriosclerosis. Stem Cell Res Ther. 2018;9:85. http://www.ncbi.nlm.nih.gov/pubmed/29615103.
353. Bonaventura A, Liberale L, Vecchié A, Casula M, Carbone F, Dallegri F, et al. Update on inflammatory biomarkers and treatments in ischemic stroke. Int J Mol Sci. 2016;17:1967. http://www.mdpi.com/1422-0067/17/12/1967.
354. Azodi S, Jacobson S. Cytokine therapies in neurological disease. Neurotherapeutics. 2016;13:555–61. http://link.springer.com/10.1007/s13311-016-0455-1.
355. Jauch EC, Lindsell C, Broderick J, Fagan SC, Tilley BC, Levine SR, et al. Association of serial biochemical markers with acute ischemic stroke: the National Institute of Neurological Disorders and Stroke recombinant tissue plasminogen activator Stroke Study. Stroke. 2006;37:2508–13. https://www.ahajournals.org/doi/10.1161/01.STR.0000242290.01174.9e.
356. Missler U, Wiesmann M, Friedrich C, Kaps M. S-100 protein and neuron-specific enolase concentrations in blood as indicators of infarction volume and prognosis in acute ischemic stroke. Stroke. 1997;28:1956–60. https://www.ahajournals.org/doi/10.1161/01.STR.28.10.1956.

357. Branco JP, Oliveira S, Sargento-Freitas J, Santos Costa J, Cordeiro G, Cunha L, et al. S100β protein as a predictor of poststroke functional outcome: a prospective study. J Stroke Cerebrovasc Dis. 2018;27:1890–6. http://www.ncbi.nlm.nih.gov/pubmed/29571758.
358. Tsai N-W, Lin T-K, Chen S-D, Chang W-N, Wang H-C, Yang T-M, et al. The value of serial plasma nuclear and mitochondrial DNA levels in patients with acute ischemic stroke. Clin Chim Acta. 2011;412:476–9. http://www.ncbi.nlm.nih.gov/pubmed/21130757.
359. Hernández-Jiménez E, Gutierrez-Fernández M, Cubillos-Zapata C, Otero-Ortega L, Rodríguez-Frutos B, Toledano V, et al. Circulating monocytes exhibit an endotoxin tolerance status after acute ischemic stroke: mitochondrial DNA as a putative explanation for poststroke infections. J Immunol. 2017;198:2038–46. http://www.jimmunol.org/lookup/doi/10.4049/jimmunol.1601594.
360. Tsimikas S, Willeit P, Willeit J, Santer P, Mayr M, Xu Q, et al. Oxidation-specific biomarkers, prospective 15-year cardiovascular and stroke outcomes, and net reclassification of cardiovascular events. J Am Coll Cardiol. 2012;60:2218–29. http://www.ncbi.nlm.nih.gov/pubmed/23122790.
361. Miller YI, Tsimikas S. Oxidation-specific epitopes as targets for biotheranostic applications in humans. Curr Opin Lipidol. 2013;24:426–37. http://www.ncbi.nlm.nih.gov/pubmed/23995232.
362. Leibundgut G, Witztum JL, Tsimikas S. Oxidation-specific epitopes and immunological responses: translational biotheranostic implications for atherosclerosis. Curr Opin Pharmacol. 2013;13:168–79. http://www.ncbi.nlm.nih.gov/pubmed/23541680.
363. Briley-Saebo K, Yeang C, Witztum JL, Tsimikas S. Imaging of oxidation-specific epitopes with targeted nanoparticles to detect high-risk atherosclerotic lesions: progress and future directions. J Cardiovasc Transl Res. 2014;7:719–36. http://www.ncbi.nlm.nih.gov/pubmed/25297940.
364. Taleb A, Witztum JL, Tsimikas S. Oxidized phospholipids on apoB-100-containing lipoproteins: a biomarker predicting cardiovascular disease and cardiovascular events. Biomark Med. 2011;5:673–94. https://www.futuremedicine.com/doi/10.2217/bmm.11.60.
365. de Souza AWS, Westra J, Limburg PC, Bijl M, Kallenberg CGM. HMGB1 in vascular diseases: its role in vascular inflammation and atherosclerosis. Autoimmun Rev. 2012;11:909–17. http://linkinghub.elsevier.com/retrieve/pii/S1568997212000766.
366. Inoue K, Kawahara K, Biswas KK, Ando K, Mitsudo K, Nobuyoshi M, et al. HMGB1 expression by activated vascular smooth muscle cells in advanced human atherosclerosis plaques. Cardiovasc Pathol. 2007;16:136–43. http://linkinghub.elsevier.com/retrieve/pii/S1054880706001931.
367. Kalinina N, Agrotis A, Antropova Y, DiVitto G, Kanellakis P, Kostolias G, et al. Increased expression of the DNA-binding cytokine HMGB1 in human atherosclerotic lesions: role of activated macrophages and cytokines. Arterioscler Thromb Vasc Biol. 2004;24:2320–5. https://www.ahajournals.org/doi/10.1161/01.ATV.0000145573.36113.8a.
368. Marsh AM, Nguyen AH, Parker TM, Agrawal DK. Clinical use of high mobility group box 1 and the receptor for advanced glycation end products in the prognosis and risk stratification of heart failure: a literature review. Can J Physiol Pharmacol. 2017;95:253–9. http://www.ncbi.nlm.nih.gov/pubmed/28092162.
369. Su Z, Lu H, Jiang H, Zhu H, Li Z, Zhang P, et al. IFN-γ-producing Th17 cells bias by HMGB1-T-bet/RUNX3 axis might contribute to progression of coronary artery atherosclerosis. Atherosclerosis. 2015;243:421–8. https://linkinghub.elsevier.com/retrieve/pii/S0021915015301441.
370. Yan XX, Lu L, Peng WH, Wang LJ, Zhang Q, Zhang RY, et al. Increased serum HMGB1 level is associated with coronary artery disease in nondiabetic and type 2 diabetic patients. Atherosclerosis. 2009;205:544–8. http://linkinghub.elsevier.com/retrieve/pii/S0021915008008927.
371. Haghjooy-Javanmard S, Sadeghi M, Safavi S, Gheraati M, Dana N. Prognostic value of the high-mobility group box-1 in young patients with chest pain. ARYA Atheroscler. 2014;10:154–8. http://www.ncbi.nlm.nih.gov/pubmed/25161686.

372. Hu X, Jiang H, Bai Q, Zhou X, Xu C, Lu Z, et al. Increased serum HMGB1 is related to the severity of coronary artery stenosis. Clin Chim Acta. 2009;406:139–42. http://linkinghub.elsevier.com/retrieve/pii/S0009898109003283.
373. Andrassy M, Volz HC, Maack B, Schuessler A, Gitsioudis G, Hofmann N, et al. HMGB1 is associated with atherosclerotic plaque composition and burden in patients with stable coronary artery disease. Zirlik A, editor. PLoS One. 2012;7:e52081. https://dx.plos.org/10.1371/journal.pone.0052081.
374. Kohno T, Anzai T, Naito K, Miyasho T, Okamoto M, Yokota H, et al. Role of high-mobility group box 1 protein in post-infarction healing process and left ventricular remodelling. Cardiovasc Res. 2008;81:565–73. http://www.ncbi.nlm.nih.gov/pubmed/18984601.
375. Jin P, Zhou Q, Song S, Xu J, Zhang M, Zhu M, et al. Elevated preoperative HMGB1 as predictor of myocardial injury post-percutaneous coronary intervention. Medicine (Baltimore). 2016;95:e5149. http://content.wkhealth.com/linkback/openurl?sid=WKPTLP:landingpage&an=00005792-201611150-00010.
376. Rath D, Geisler T, Gawaz M, Vogel S. HMGB1 expression level in circulating platelets is not significantly associated with outcomes in symptomatic coronary artery disease. Cell Physiol Biochem. 2017;43:1627–33. https://www.karger.com/Article/FullText/482026.
377. Giallauria F, Cirillo P, D'agostino M, Petrillo G, Vitelli A, Pacileo M, et al. Effects of exercise training on high-mobility group box-1 levels after acute myocardial infarction. J Card Fail. 2011;17:108–14. https://linkinghub.elsevier.com/retrieve/pii/S1071916410011255.
378. Dybdahl B, Slørdahl SA, Waage A, Kierulf P, Espevik T, Sundan A. Myocardial ischaemia and the inflammatory response: release of heat shock protein 70 after myocardial infarction. Heart. 2005;91:299–304. http://www.ncbi.nlm.nih.gov/pubmed/15710705.
379. Zhang X, Xu Z, Zhou L, Chen Y, He M, Cheng L, et al. Plasma levels of Hsp70 and anti-Hsp70 antibody predict risk of acute coronary syndrome. Cell Stress Chaperones. 2010;15:675–86. http://www.ncbi.nlm.nih.gov/pubmed/20300983.
380. Morrow DA, Wang Y, Croce K, Sakuma M, Sabatine MS, Gao H, et al. Myeloid-related protein 8/14 and the risk of cardiovascular death or myocardial infarction after an acute coronary syndrome in the Pravastatin or Atorvastatin Evaluation and Infection Therapy: Thrombolysis in Myocardial Infarction (PROVE IT-TIMI 22) tria. Am Heart J. 2008;155:49–55. http://linkinghub.elsevier.com/retrieve/pii/S0002870307007041.
381. Liu J, Ren Y-G, Zhang L-H, Tong Y-W, Kang L. Serum S100A12 concentrations are correlated with angiographic coronary lesion complexity in patients with coronary artery disease. Scand J Clin Lab Invest. 2014;74:149–54. http://www.tandfonline.com/doi/full/10.3109/00365513.2013.864786.
382. Buyukterzi Z, Can U, Alpaydin S, Guzelant A, Karaarslan S, Kocyigit D, et al. Enhanced S100A9 and S100A12 expression in acute coronary syndrome. Biomark Med. 2017;11:229–37. http://www.ncbi.nlm.nih.gov/pubmed/28157385.
383. Nakashima A, Carrero JJ, Qureshi AR, Miyamoto T, Anderstam B, Bárány P, et al. Effect of circulating soluble receptor for advanced glycation end products (sRAGE) and the proinflammatory RAGE ligand (EN-RAGE, S100A12) on mortality in hemodialysis patients. Clin J Am Soc Nephrol. 2010;5:2213–9. http://cjasn.asnjournals.org/cgi/doi/10.2215/CJN.03360410.
384. Shiotsu Y, Mori Y, Nishimura M, Sakoda C, Tokoro T, Hatta T, et al. Plasma S100A12 level is associated with cardiovascular disease in hemodialysis patients. Clin J Am Soc Nephrol. 2011;6:718–23. http://www.ncbi.nlm.nih.gov/pubmed/21258041.
385. Isoyama N, Leurs P, Qureshi AR, Bruchfeld A, Anderstam B, Heimburger O, et al. Plasma S100A12 and soluble receptor of advanced glycation end product levels and mortality in chronic kidney disease Stage 5 patients. Nephrol Dial Transplant. 2015;30:84–91. http://www.ncbi.nlm.nih.gov/pubmed/25074436.
386. Yayar O, Eser B, Buyukbakkal M, Erdogan B, Ercan Z, Merhametsiz O, et al. Do elevated plasma S100A12 levels predict atherosclerosis in peritoneal dialysis patients? Ren Fail. 2015;37:845–50. http://www.ncbi.nlm.nih.gov/pubmed/26016405.

387. Zhao P, Wu M, Yu H, Huang Y, Wang Y, Wang W, et al. Serum S100A12 levels are correlated with the presence and severity of coronary artery disease in patients with type 2 diabetes mellitus. J Investig Med. 2013;61:861–6. http://www.ncbi.nlm.nih.gov/pubmed/23609464.
388. Yue P, Jing S, Liu L, Ma F, Zhang Y, Wang C, et al. Association between mitochondrial DNA copy number and cardiovascular disease: current evidence based on a systematic review and meta-analysis. Cheungpasitporn W, editor. PLoS One. 2018;13:e0206003. http://www.ncbi.nlm.nih.gov/pubmed/30403687.
389. Serhan CN. Treating inflammation and infection in the 21st century: new hints from decoding resolution mediators and mechanisms. FASEB J. 2017;31:1273–88. http://www.ncbi.nlm.nih.gov/pubmed/28087575.
390. Mori T, Asano T, Town T. Targeting S100B in cerebral ischemia and in Alzheimer's disease. Cardiovasc Psychiatry Neurol. 2010;2010:1–14. http://www.ncbi.nlm.nih.gov/pubmed/20862385.
391. Liu K, Mori S, Takahashi HK, Tomono Y, Wake H, Kanke T, et al. Anti-high mobility group box 1 monoclonal antibody ameliorates brain infarction induced by transient ischemia in rats. FASEB J. 2007;21:3904–16. http://www.fasebj.org/doi/10.1096/fj.07-8770com.
392. Zhang J, Takahashi HK, Liu K, Wake H, Liu R, Maruo T, et al. Anti-high mobility group box-1 monoclonal antibody protects the blood-brain barrier from ischemia-induced disruption in rats. Stroke. 2011;42:1420–8. https://www.ahajournals.org/doi/10.1161/STROKEAHA.110.598334.
393. Wang D, Liu K, Wake H, Teshigawara K, Mori S, Nishibori M. Anti-high mobility group box-1 (HMGB1) antibody inhibits hemorrhage-induced brain injury and improved neurological deficits in rats. Sci Rep. 2017;7:46243. http://www.nature.com/articles/srep46243.
394. Nishibori M, Mori S, Takahashi HK. Anti-HMGB1 monoclonal antibody therapy for a wide range of CNS and PNS diseases. J Pharmacol Sci. 2019;140:94–101. http://www.ncbi.nlm.nih.gov/pubmed/31105025.
395. Relton JK, Strijbos PJ, O'Shaughnessy CT, Carey F, Forder RA, Tilders FJ, et al. Lipocortin-1 is an endogenous inhibitor of ischemic damage in the rat brain. J Exp Med. 1991;174:305–10. http://www.jem.org/cgi/doi/10.1084/jem.174.2.305.
396. Gavins FNE, Dalli J, Flower RJ, Granger DN, Perretti M. Activation of the annexin 1 counter-regulatory circuit affords protection in the mouse brain microcirculation. FASEB J. 2007;21:1751–8. http://www.fasebj.org/doi/10.1096/fj.06-7842com.
397. Sobrado M, Pereira MP, Ballesteros I, Hurtado O, Fernández-López D, Pradillo JM, et al. Synthesis of lipoxin A4 by 5-lipoxygenase mediates PPARgamma-dependent, neuroprotective effects of rosiglitazone in experimental stroke. J Neurosci. 2009;29:3875–84. http://www.jneurosci.org/cgi/doi/10.1523/JNEUROSCI.5529-08.2009.
398. Bazan NG, Eady TN, Khoutorova L, Atkins KD, Hong S, Lu Y, et al. Novel aspirin-triggered neuroprotectin D1 attenuates cerebral ischemic injury after experimental stroke. Exp Neurol. 2012;236:122–30. https://linkinghub.elsevier.com/retrieve/pii/S0014488612001598.
399. Xian W, Wu Y, Xiong W, Li L, Li T, Pan S, et al. The pro-resolving lipid mediator Maresin 1 protects against cerebral ischemia/reperfusion injury by attenuating the pro-inflammatory response. Biochem Biophys Res Commun. 2016;472:175–81. https://linkinghub.elsevier.com/retrieve/pii/S0006291X16302790.
400. Belayev L, Mukherjee PK, Balaszczuk V, Calandria JM, Obenaus A, Khoutorova L, et al. Neuroprotectin D1 upregulates Iduna expression and provides protection in cellular uncompensated oxidative stress and in experimental ischemic stroke. Cell Death Differ. 2017;24:1091–9. http://www.nature.com/articles/cdd201755.
401. Bolli R. Reflections on the irreproducibility of scientific papers. Circ Res. 2015;117:665–6. https://www.ahajournals.org/doi/10.1161/CIRCRESAHA.115.307496.
402. Seropian IM, Toldo S, Van Tassell BW, Abbate A. Anti-inflammatory strategies for ventricular remodeling following ST-segment elevation acute myocardial infarction. J Am Coll Cardiol. 2014;63:1593–603. https://linkinghub.elsevier.com/retrieve/pii/S0735109714003258.
403. Ridker PM, Everett BM, Thuren T, MacFadyen JG, Chang WH, Ballantyne C, et al. Antiinflammatory therapy with canakinumab for atherosclerotic disease. N Engl J Med. 2017;377:1119–31. http://www.nejm.org/doi/10.1056/NEJMoa1707914.

404. Ridker PM, MacFadyen JG, Thuren T, Libby P. Residual inflammatory risk associated with interleukin-18 and interleukin-6 after successful interleukin-1β inhibition with canakinumab: further rationale for the development of targeted anti-cytokine therapies for the treatment of atherothrombosis. Eur Heart J. 2019;41(23):2153–63. http://www.ncbi.nlm.nih.gov/pubmed/31504417.
405. de Jong R, Leoni G, Drechsler M, Soehnlein O. The advantageous role of annexin A1 in cardiovascular disease. Cell Adh Migr. 2017;11:261–74. https://www.tandfonline.com/doi/full/10.1080/19336918.2016.1259059.
406. Leoni G, Soehnlein O. (Re) solving repair after myocardial infarction. Front Pharmacol. 2018;9:1342. https://www.frontiersin.org/article/10.3389/fphar.2018.01342/full.
407. Madigan M, Atoui R. Therapeutic use of stem cells for myocardial infarction. Bioeng (Basel, Switzerland). 2018;5:28. http://www.mdpi.com/2306-5354/5/2/28.
408. Lalu MM, Mazzarello S, Zlepnig J, Dong YYR, Montroy J, McIntyre L, et al. Safety and efficacy of adult stem cell therapy for acute myocardial infarction and ischemic heart failure (safecell heart): a systematic review and meta-analysis. Stem Cells Transl Med. 2018;7:857–66. http://doi.wiley.com/10.1002/sctm.18-0120.
409. Cambria E, Pasqualini FS, Wolint P, Günter J, Steiger J, Bopp A, et al. Translational cardiac stem cell therapy: advancing from first-generation to next-generation cell types. NPJ Regen Med. 2017;2:17. http://www.nature.com/articles/s41536-017-0024-1.
410. Adamiak M, Sahoo S. Exosomes in myocardial repair: advances and challenges in the development of next-generation therapeutics. Mol Ther. 2018;26:1635–43. https://linkinghub.elsevier.com/retrieve/pii/S1525001618302028.
411. Pistoia V, Raffaghello L. Damage-associated molecular patterns (DAMPs) and mesenchymal stem cells: a matter of attraction and excitement. Eur J Immunol. 2011;41:1828–31. http://www.ncbi.nlm.nih.gov/pubmed/21706488.
412. Lotfi R, Eisenbacher J, Solgi G, Fuchs K, Yildiz T, Nienhaus C, et al. Human mesenchymal stem cells respond to native but not oxidized damage associated molecular pattern molecules from necrotic (tumor) material. Eur J Immunol. 2011;41:2021–8. http://www.ncbi.nlm.nih.gov/pubmed/21538978.
413. Prockop DJ, Oh JY. Mesenchymal stem/stromal cells (MSCs): role as guardians of inflammation. Mol Ther. 2012;20:14–20. http://www.ncbi.nlm.nih.gov/pubmed/22008910.
414. Eisenbacher JL, Schrezenmeier H, Jahrsdörfer B, Kaltenmeier C, Rojewski MT, Yildiz T, et al. S100A4 and uric acid promote mesenchymal stromal cell induction of IL-10+/IDO+ lymphocytes. J Immunol. 2014;192:6102–10. http://www.ncbi.nlm.nih.gov/pubmed/24795458.
415. Frangogiannis NG. The inflammatory response in myocardial injury, repair, and remodelling. Nat Rev Cardiol. 2014;11:255–65. http://www.ncbi.nlm.nih.gov/pubmed/24663091.
416. Kitahara T, Takeishi Y, Harada M, Niizeki T, Suzuki S, Sasaki T, et al. High-mobility group box 1 restores cardiac function after myocardial infarction in transgenic mice. Cardiovasc Res. 2008;80:40–6. http://www.ncbi.nlm.nih.gov/pubmed/18558628.
417. Nakagawa S, Omura T, Yonezawa A, Yano I, Nakagawa T, Matsubara K. Extracellular nucleotides from dying cells act as molecular signals to promote wound repair in renal tubular injury. Am J Physiol Renal Physiol. 2014;307:F1404–11. http://www.ncbi.nlm.nih.gov/pubmed/25354940.
418. Gonzales E, Julien B, Serrière-Lanneau V, Nicou A, Doignon I, Lagoudakis L, et al. ATP release after partial hepatectomy regulates liver regeneration in the rat. J Hepatol. 2010;52:54–62. http://www.ncbi.nlm.nih.gov/pubmed/19914731.
419. Negro S, Bergamin E, Rodella U, Duregotti E, Scorzeto M, Jalink K, et al. ATP released by injured neurons activates Schwann cells. Front Cell Neurosci. 2016;10:134. http://www.ncbi.nlm.nih.gov/pubmed/27242443.
420. Huang P, Wang L, Li Q, Xu J, Xu J, Xiong Y, et al. Combinatorial treatment of acute myocardial infarction using stem cells and their derived exosomes resulted in improved heart performance. Stem Cell Res Ther. 2019;10:300. https://stemcellres.biomedcentral.com/articles/10.1186/s13287-019-1353-3.

Part IV

Epilogue

The "DAMPome" as a Key Player in the Pathogenesis of Human Diseases

12

As the field of Immunology continues to become broader beyond its original definition, its boundaries continue to grow blurred. Nevertheless, the essential core role played by the immune system across the tree of life appears to be to defend the life of all living creatures and organisms on our planet against any insult – a function that would fit in the term "defensology." Throughout life, an organism encounters multiple perturbations, stresses, and injuries that interrupt and destroy homeostasis. Indeed, infections, traumatic injuries, dangerous emotional disturbances, abnormal metabolic changes, extreme temperature fluctuations, and exposure to toxins may be encountered daily. The mammalian immune system – in a crosstalk with the nervous/psychoneural system and the hypothalamic → pituitary → adrenal axis – must sense and cope with all these permanently occurring insults and restore homeostasis to survive. According to the danger/injury model in Immunology, three crucial steps must happen before the mammalian organism returns to homeostasis: first, perturbation/stress/injury-induced DAMPs are sensed through PRMs; second, an appropriate tailor-made DAMP-promoted efferent inflammatory response is implemented; and third, a SAMP-driven inflammation-resolving, tissue-repairing response restores and reconstitutes homeostasis. Of note, there is increasing evidence suggesting that both inflammation-promoting and inflammation-resolving processes are mediated by DAMP-triggered epigenetic modifications in cells of the innate immune system. Together, it is the dynamic homeostatic DAMPs:SAMPs ratio that guarantees successful restoration of homeostasis and, thus, survival.

However, as described in this book, any imbalance of the homeostatic DAMPs:SAMPs ratio may initiate a disorder. In fact, a disturbed DAMP:SAMP ratio may even be the pathogenetic key event in instigating a disease. For example, in the case DAMPs override and outweigh SAMPs, a chronic inflammation-nonresolving disease may occur. Such models are presented in the previous chapters when discussing the pathogenesis of traumatic diseases and CVDs, where the nature of the injury that leads to DAMPs emission is reasonably evident. But there are other disorders where the quality and nature of the initial tissue stress/injury are less

W. G. Land, *Damage-Associated Molecular Patterns in Human Diseases*,
https://doi.org/10.1007/978-3-030-53868-2_12

clear, but the pathogenetic role of DAMPs has nevertheless been described. Such diseases include infectious, autoimmune, and neurodegenerative diseases. For example, emission of DAMPs and their systemic distribution in severe viral infections reportedly lead to the full symptomatology of life-threatening sepsis [1]; also, DAMPs have been pathogenetically linked to many autoimmune diseases, such as rheumatoid arthritis, systemic lupus erythematosus, psoriasis, and systemic sclerosis by promoting activation of different innate immune cells, including autoreactive DCs, and proinflammatory cytokine production associated with these diseases [2–4]; moreover, in Alzheimer's disease, DAMPs, including amyloid β, reportedly drive and sustain neuroinflammation [5].

On the other hand, and by the contrary, in cancer diseases, the generation and emission of DAMPs are even desirable and reflect a promising therapeutic option. Thus, there is emerging evidence indicating that induction of ICD of tumor cells, associated with the emission of DAMPs, eventually results in long-lasting protective antitumor immunity [6]. Together, as discussed in this book, the pathogenetic role of DAMPs and SAMPs qualifies these molecules as informative diagnostic and prognostic biomarkers in many diseases and, thus, may become part of network medicine [7].

Logically, if one defines a disturbed homeostatic DAMPs:SAMPs ratio upon cell stress/tissue injury as the pathogenetic principle in human diseases, therapeutic efforts should be directed to restore this dynamic imbalanced DAMPs: SAMPs ratio. For chronic inflammatory, inflammation-nonresolving disorders such as atherosclerosis, this would imply to use DAMPs as therapeutic targets or administer SAMPs as therapeutics, or even both, in a time-adjusted manner. In the book, several proposals, recommendations, and caveats have been discussed in the conceivable realization of such a therapeutic strategy.

Of note, in the future, such therapeutic maneuvers may be expanded by another emerging therapeutic option: the prevention of DAMPs emission by previous inhibition of the event of injury-induced RCD, using, for example, anti-necroptosis or antiferroptosis agents [8, 9]. In fact, the development of novel drugs for selectively intercepting the RCD pathway holds considerable promise for preventing and treating human diseases in which cell death-associated DAMPs emission must be avoided. Plausibly, in cancer diseases, the opposite therapeutic strategy has to be applied: first, as mentioned above, to develop potent ICD inducers for enhancing the emission of DAMPs [6] or, second, to design agents for selectively activating the RCD pathway as a prerequisite to release DAMPs [10], the aim always being to induce a robust antitumor immune response that may cure cancer.

Indeed, DAMPs and DAMPome seem to be moving to the forefront as novel therapeutic principles in medicine, and one can state that exciting time is ahead of us.

References

1. Denning N-L, Aziz M, Gurien SD, Wang P. DAMPs and NETs in sepsis. Front Immunol. 2019;10:2536. http://www.ncbi.nlm.nih.gov/pubmed/31736963.
2. Álvarez K, Vasquez G. Damage-associated molecular patterns and their role as initiators of inflammatory and auto-immune signals in systemic lupus erythematosus. Int Rev Immunol. 2017;36(5):259–70.
3. Di Ceglie I, Kruisbergen NNL, van den Bosch MHJ, van Lent PLEM. Fc-gamma receptors and S100A8/A9 cause bone erosion during rheumatoid arthritis. Do they act as partners in crime? Rheumatology (Oxford). 2019;58:1331–43.
4. Choudhary V, Uaratanawong R, Patel RR, Patel H, Bao W, Hartney B, et al. Phosphatidylglycerol inhibits Toll-like receptor–mediated inflammation by danger-associated molecular patterns. J Invest Dermatol. 2019;139:868–77.
5. Venegas C, Heneka MT. Danger-associated molecular patterns in Alzheimer's disease. J Leukoc Biol. 2017;101:87–98. http://www.ncbi.nlm.nih.gov/pubmed/28049142.
6. Zhou J, Wang G, Chen Y, Wang H, Hua Y, Cai Z. Immunogenic cell death in cancer therapy: present and emerging inducers. J Cell Mol Med. 2019;23(8):4854–65.
7. Sonawane AR, Weiss ST, Glass K, Sharma A. Network medicine in the age of biomedical big data. Front Genet. 2019;10:294.
8. Tonnus W, Meyer C, Paliege A, Belavgeni A, von Mässenhausen A, Bornstein SR, et al. The pathological features of regulated necrosis. J Pathol. 2019;247(5):697–707.
9. Mishima E, Sato E, Ito J, Yamada K, Suzuki C, Oikawa Y, et al. Drugs repurposed as antiferroptosis agents suppress organ damage, including AKI, by functioning as lipid peroxyl radical scavengers. J Am Soc Nephrol. 2020;31(2):280–96. http://www.jasn.org/lookup/doi/10.1681/ASN.2019060570.
10. Khing TM, Po WW, Sohn UD. Fluoxetine enhances anti-tumor activity of paclitaxel in gastric adenocarcinoma cells by triggering apoptosis and necroptosis. Anticancer Res. 2019;39:6155–63.

The manufacturer's authorised representative in the EU is Springer Nature Customer Service Centre GmbH, Europaplatz 3, 69115 Heidelberg, Germany. If you have any concerns regarding our products, please contact ProductSafety@springernature.com

Printed and bound by CPI Group (UK) Ltd, Croydon, CR0 4YY
30/09/2026
02224058-0002